D0710709

Blood Banking
and Transfusion Medicine

Blood Banking and Transfusion Medicine

Basic Principles & Practice

Christopher D. Hillyer, MD
Director, Transfusion Medicine Program
Professor, Department of Pathology and Laboratory Medicine
Emory University School of Medicine
Atlanta, Georgia

Leslie E. Silberstein, MD
Director, Joint Program in Transfusion Medicine
Children's Hospital Boston, Dana-Farber Cancer Institute
and Brigham and Women's Hospital
Professor of Pathology (Pediatrics)
Harvard Medical School
Boston, Massachusetts

Paul M. Ness, MD
Director, Transfusion Medicine Division
The Johns Hopkins Hospital
Professor, Departments of Pathology and Medicine
The Johns Hopkins University School of Medicine
Baltimore, Maryland

Kenneth C. Anderson, MD
Director, Jerome Lipper Multiple Myeloma Center
Dana-Farber Cancer Institute
Professor of Medicine
Joint Program in Transfusion Medicine
Harvard Medical School
Boston, Massachusetts

Associate Editor:
Karen S. Roush, MD
Director, Transfusion Medicine
Methodist Medical Center
Dallas, Texas

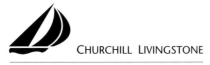

CHURCHILL LIVINGSTONE

An Imprint of Elsevier Science

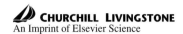
CHURCHILL LIVINGSTONE
An Imprint of Elsevier Science

The Curtis Center
Independence Square West
Philadelphia, Pennsylvania 19106

BLOOD BANKING AND TRANSFUSION MEDICINE
Copyright 2003, Elsevier Science (USA). All rights reserved.   ISBN 0-443-06542-X

No part of this publication may be reproduced, stored in a retrieval system, or transmitted in any form or by any means, electronic, mechanical, photocopying, recording, or otherwise, without prior permission of the publisher (Churchill Livingstone, The Curtis Center, Independence Square West, Philadelphia, PA 19106).

Distributed in the United Kingdom by Churchill Livingstone, Robert Stevenson House, 1-3 Baxter's Place, Leith Walk, Edinburgh EH1 3AF, and by associated companies, branches, and representatives throughout the world.

Churchill Livingstone and the sailboat design are registered trademarks.

Cover photograph copyright Dennis Kunkel Microscopy, Inc; with permission.

Notice

Medicine is an ever-changing field. Standard safety precautions must be followed, but as new research and clinical experience broaden our knowledge, changes in treatment and drug therapy may become necessary or appropriate. Readers are advised to check the most current product information provided by the manufacturer of each drug to be administered to verify the recommended dose, the method and duration of administration, and contraindications. It is the responsibility of the treating physician, relying on experience and knowledge of the patient, to determine dosages and the best treatment for each individual patient. Neither the Publisher nor the editor(s) assume any liability for any injury and/or damage to persons or property arising from this publication.

The Publisher

Library of Congress Cataloging-in-Publication Data

Blood banking and transfusion medicine: basic principles and practice / [edited by] Christopher D. Hillyer ... [et al.].– 1st ed.
  p. ; cm.
  ISBN 0-443-06542-X
  1. Blood–Transfusion. 2. Blood Banks. I. Hillyer, Christopher D.
  [DNLM: 1. Blood Transfusion–methods. 2. Blood Banks–organization & administration.
WB 356 P9565 2003]
RM171 .P745 2003
615'.39–dc21   2002073321

Acqusitions Editor: Dolores Meloni
Senior Project Manager: Natalie Ware

CE/MVY

Printed in the United States of America
Last digit is the print number: 9   8   7   6   5   4   3   2   1

*We wish to dedicate this text to our many mentors,
colleagues, trainees, and patients, who continue to teach
us new lessons and make transfusion medicine meaningful
to each of us.*

Contributors

Mary Beth Allen, MS, MT(ASCP)
Administrative Director, Emory Hospitals Laboratories, Emory University Hospital, Atlanta, Georgia
Component Preparation and Storage

Barbara M. Alving, MD
Professor of Medicine, Uniformed Services University of the Health Sciences; Deputy Director, National Heart, Lung, and Blood Institute, National Institutes of Health, Bethesda, Maryland
Transfusion of the Patient with Acquired Coagulation Defects

Daniel R. Ambruso, MD
Associate Medical Director for Bonfils Blood Center; Professor of Pediatrics; Associate Professor of Pathology, University of Colorado School of Medicine, Denver, Colorado
Acute Hemolytic Transfusion Reactions

Kenneth C. Anderson, MD
Director, Jerome Lipper Multiple Myeloma Center, Dana Farber Cancer Institute; Professor of Medicine, Harvard Medical School, Boston, Massachusetts

James P. AuBuchon, MD
E. Elizabeth French Professor and Chair of Pathology and Professor of Medicine, Dartmouth-Hitchcock Medical Center; Medical Director, Blood Bank and Transfusion Service, Lebanon, New Hampshire
Evolution to the 21st Century

Nicholas Bandarenko, MD
Associate Professor of Pathology and Laboratory Medicine, Transfusion Medicine Service, University of North Carolina Chapel Hill, Chapel Hill, North Carolina
Practical and Technical Issues and Adverse Reactions in Therapeutic Apheresis

Richard J. Benjamin, MBChB, PhD
Medical Director, Adult Transfusion Service, Brigham and Women's Hospital; Assistant Professor of Pathology, Harvard Medical School, Boston, Massachusetts
Quality Improvement and Control

Morris A. Blajchman, MD, FRCP(C)
Professor of Pathology and Molecular Medicine, Departments of Pathology and Medicine, McMaster University; Medical Director, Hamilton Centre, Canadian Blood Services, Hamilton, Ontario, Canada
Bacterial Infections

Mark E. Brecher, MD
Professor, Transfusion Medicine Service, University of North Carolina Hospitals, Chapel Hill, North Carolina
Practical and Technical Issues and Adverse Reactions in Therapeutic Apheresis

Silvana Z. Bucur, MD
Assistant Professor of Hematology/Oncology, Winship Cancer Institute, Emory University School of Medicine, Atlanta, Georgia
Fresh Frozen Plasma and Related Products; Cryoprecipitate and Related Products; Albumin, IVIG, and Derivatives

Michael P. Busch, MD, PhD
Professor, Laboratory Medicine, University of California, San Francisco; Vice President, Research and Scientific Affairs, Blood Centers of the Pacific and Blood Systems, Inc., San Francisco, California
Microchimerism and Graft-Versus-Host Disease; Human Immunodeficiency Virus, Human T-cell Lymphotrophic Viruses, and Other Retroviruses

Sally A. Campbell-Lee, MD
Fellow, Division of Transfusion Medicine, Johns Hopkins Medical Institutions, Baltimore, Maryland
Packed RBCs and Related Products

Richard Champlin, MD
Chairman, Department of Blood and Marrow Transplantation, M.D. Anderson Cancer Center, Houston, Texas
Bone Marrow and Peripheral Blood Stem Cell Transplantation

Raymond L. Comenzo, MD
Director, Cytotherapy Laboratory, Memorial Sloan-Kettering Cancer Center, New York, New York
Transfusion to Bone Marrow or Solid Organ Transplant Recipients and HIV-Positive Patients

Laurence Corash, MD
Professor, Laboratory Medicine, University of California, San Francisco; Attending Physician, Laboratory Medicine and Medicine-Hematology Division, The Medical Center at the University of California, San Francisco; Chief Medical Officer and Vice President, Research and Medical Affairs, Cerus Corporation, Concord, California
Virus "Safe" Products/Pathogen Reduction

Melody J. Cunningham, MD
Clinical Fellow in Transfusion Medicine, Pathology Department, Boston Children's Hospital, Boston, Massachusetts
Autoimmune Hemolytic Anemias

Roger Y. Dodd, PhD
Executive Director, Biomedical Safety, American Red Cross, Holland Laboratory, Rockville, Maryland
Infectious Disease Testing; Hepatitis A, Hepatitis B, and Non-A, Non-B, Non-C Viruses; Hepatitis C

Walter H. Dzik, MD
Associate Professor of Pathology, Harvard Medical School; Co-Director, Blood Transfusion Service, Department of Pathology and Laboratory Medicine, Massachusetts General Hospital, Boston, Massachusetts
Leukocyte Reduced Products

James R. Eckman, MD
Professor of Hematology, Oncology, and Medicine, Winship Cancer Institute; Adjunct Professor of Pediatrics, Emory University School of Medicine; Chief, Emory Hematology at Grady Memorial Hospital; Director, Georgia Comprehensive Sickle Cell Center, Atlanta, Georgia
Transfusion in the Hemoglobinopathies, Transfusion in the Hemolytic Anemias

Eberhard W. Fiebig, MD
Chief, Division of Hematology/Transfusion Medicine, Clinical Laboratories at San Francisco General Hospital, San Francisco, California
Microchimerism and Graft-Versus-Host Disease; Human Immunodeficiency Virus, Human T-cell Lymphotrophic Viruses, and Other Retroviruses

Mindy Goldman, MD
Premier Directeur Adjoint, Affaires Médicales, Hématologie, Héma-Québec, Saint-Laurent, Québec, Canada
Bacterial Infections

Ian S. Gourley, MD, MRCP
Clinical Research Pathologist, Eli Lilly & Company, Indianapolis, Indiana
Immunomodulation

Alfred J. Grindon, MD
Professor, Department of Pathology and Laboratory Medicine, Emory University School of Medicine, Atlanta, Georgia
Blood Donation; Lookback Investigations and Product Recall/Withdrawal

Christopher D. Hillyer, MD
Professor, Department of Pathology and Laboratory Medicine, Emory University School of Medicine; Director, Transfusion Medicine Program, Emory University, Atlanta, Georgia
Fresh Frozen Plasma and Related Products; Cryoprecipitate and Related Products

Krista Lankford Hillyer, MD
Assistant Professor, Department of Pathology and Laboratory Medicine, Emory University School of Medicine; Medical Director, American Red Cross Blood Services, Southern Region, Atlanta, Georgia
Transfusion in the Hemoglobinopathies

Edahn Isaak, MD
Assistant Professor of Pathology, Department of Pathology, Emory University School of Medicine, Grady Memorial Hospital Blood Bank, Atlanta, Georgia
Therapeutic Cytapheresis

Helen G. Jones, RN
Supervisor or Therapeutic Apheresis Unit, Transfusion Medicine Services, University of North Carolina Hospitals, Chapel Hill, North Carolina
Practical and Technical Issues and Adverse Reactions in Therapeutic Apheresis

Thomas S. Kickler, MD
Professor of Medicine and Pathology, The Johns Hopkins University School of Medicine, Baltimore, Maryland
Transfusion of the Platelet-Refractory Patient

Karen E. King, MD
Associate Medical Director, Transfusion Medicine Division, Johns Hopkins University School of Medicine, Baltimore, Maryland
Delayed Hemolytic Transfusion Reactions

Margot S. Kruskall, MD
Associate Professor of Pathology and Medicine, Harvard Medical School; Director, Division of Laboratory and Transfusion Medicine, Beth Israel Deaconess Medical Center, Boston, Massachusetts
Autologous Blood and Related Alternatives to Allogeneic Transfusion

Thomas J. Kunicki, PhD
Associate Professor, Molecular and Experimental Medicine, The Scripps Research Institute, LaJolla, California
Human Platelet Antigens

Joanne Kurtzberg, MD
Professor of Pediatrics and Director, Pediatric Bone Marrow and Stem Cell Transplant Program, and Associate Professor of Pathology, Duke University Medical Center; Director, Carolinas Cord Blood Bank at Duke University Medical Center, Durham, North Carolina
Umbilical Cord Blood Banking and Transplantation

Tzong-Hae Lee, MD, PhD
Director of Molecular Biology, Blood Centers of the Pacific, Irwin Center, San Francisco, California
Microchimerism and Graft-Versus-Host Disease

Naomi L.C. Luban, MD
Professor of Pediatrics and Pathology/Vice Chair of Academic Affairs, Department of Pediatrics, George Washington University School of Medicine; Chair, Laboratory Medicine and Pathology, Children's Hospital, National Medical Center, Washington, District of Columbia
Irradiated Products and Washed/Volume Reduced Products

Catherine S. Manno, MD
Associate Professor, Pediatrics, The University of Pennsylvania School of Medicine; Acting Chief, Division of Hematology, Department of Pediatrics, The Children's Hospital of Philadelphia, Philadelphia, Pennsylvania
Transfusion of the Patient with Congenital Coagulation Defects

Bruce C. McLeod, MD
Professor, Medicine and Pathology, Rush Medical College; Director, Blood Center, Rush-Presbyterian-St. Luke's Medical Center; Assistant Medical Director, Badger-Hawkeye Region, American Red Cross, Chicago, Illinois
Therapeutic Plasma Exchange

Jay E. Menitove, MD
Clinical Professor, Internal Medicine, University of Kansas School of
Medicine, Kansas City, Kansas; Executive Director and Medical Director,
Community Blood Center of Greater Kansas City, Kansas City, Missouri
Additional Infectious Complications

Edward L. Murphy, MD, MPH
Professor, Laboratory Medicine and Epidemiology/Biostatistics,
University of California San Francisco, San Francisco, California
*Human Immunodeficiency Virus, Human T-cell
Lymphotrophic Viruses, and Other Retroviruses*

Paul M. Ness, MD
Professor of Pathology, Medicine, and Oncology, and Director, Transfusion
Medicine Division, The Johns Hopkins Hospital, Baltimore, Maryland
Packed RBCs and Related Products; Delayed Hemolytic Transfusion Reactions

Bruce Newman, MD
Medical Director, American Red Cross, Southeastern Michigan Region,
Detroit, Michigan
Blood Donation

Diane J. Nugent, MD
Director of Hematology; Director of Hemostasis and Thrombosis; Director,
Blood Donor Service, Children's Hospital of Orange County, Orange,
California
Human Platelet Antigens

Keren Osman, MD
Clinical Scholar/Research Associate, Laboratory of Tumor Immunology
and Immunotherapy, Rockefeller University, New York, New York
*Transfusion to Bone Marrow or Solid Organ Transplant Recipients and
HIV-Positive Patients*

Peter L. Perrotta, MD
Assistant Professor, Pathology, University Hospital, State University of
New York at Stoney Brook, Stoney Brook, New York
Platelets and Related Products

Patricia T. Pisciotto, MD
Professor, Laboratory Medicine, University of Connecticut Health Sciences
Center; Director, Blood Bank, John Dempsey Hospital, Farmington,
Connecticut
Platelets and Related Products

Thomas H. Price, MD
Professor of Medicine, University of Washington; Medical Director,
Executive Vice President, Puget Sound Blood Center, Seattle, Washington
Granulocytes

M. Joleen Randels, RN
Director of Operations, Coral Blood Services, Durham, North Carolina
*Practical and Technical Issues and Adverse Reactions in
Therapeutic Apheresis*

William Reed, MD
Assistant Medical Director, Research, Blood Centers of the Pacific, San
Francisco, California; Medical Director, Sibling Donor Cord Blood Program,
Childrens Hospital Oakland Research Institute, Oakland, California
Microchimerism and Graft-Versus-Host Disease

Marion E. Reid, PhD
Director of Immunohematology, New York Blood Center, New York, New York
*Membrane Blood Group Antigens and Antibodies; ABO and Related
Antigens; Rh, Kell, Duffy, and Kidd Blood Group Systems; Other
Blood Group Systems and Antigens*

John D. Roback, MD, PhD
Assistant Professor, Transfusion Medicine Program, Department of Pathology
and Laboratory Medicine, Emory University School of Medicine,
Atlanta, Georgia
Human Herpesvirus Infections

Glenn E. Rodey, MD
Professor, Pathology, Baylor College of Medicine; Director, Histocompatibility
and Transplant Immunology Laboratory, The Methodist Hospitals,
Houston, Texas
HLA and Granulocyte Antigens

Nancy C. Rose, MD
Clinical Associate Professor of Obstetrics and Gynecology, Thomas
Jefferson School of Medicine, Philadelphia, Pennsylvania
Obstetric and Intrauterine Transfusion

Karen S. Roush, MD
Medical Director, Transfusion Medicine and Clinical Pathology,
Department of Pathology, Methodist Medical Center, Dallas, Texas
Febrile, Allergic, and Other Noninfectious Transfusion Reactions

Avichai Shimoni, MD
Senior BMT Physician, Department of Hematology and Bone Marrow
Transplantation, Chaim Sheba Medical Center, Isreal
Bone Marrow and Peripheral Blood Stem Cell Transplantation

R. Sue Shirey, MS, MT(ASCP) SBB
Technical Specialist, Transfusion Medicine Division, Johns Hopkins
Hospital, Baltimore, Maryland
Delayed Hemolytic Transfusion Reactions

Suzanne Shusterman, MD
Assistant in Pediatrics, Division of Oncology, The Children's Hospital of
Philadelphia, Philadelphia, Pennsylvania
Transfusion of the Patient with Congenital Coagulation Defects

Leslie E. Silberstein, MD
Professor of Pathology (Pediatrics), Joint Program in Transfusion Medicine,
Harvard Medical School, Boston, Massachusetts
Autoimmune Hemolytic Anemias, Immunomodulation

Edward L. Snyder, MD
Professor, Laboratory Medicine, Yale University School of Medicine;
Director, Blood Bank, Yale-New Haven Hospital, New Haven,
Connecticut
Platelets and Related Products

Ronald G. Strauss, MD
Professor of Pathology and Pediatrics, University of Iowa College of
Medicine; Medical Director, DeGowin Blood Center, University of Iowa
Hospitals and Clinics, Iowa City, Iowa
Transfusion of the Neonate and Pediatric Patient

Zbigniew M. Szczepiorkowski, MD, PhD
Associate Director, Blood Transfusion Service, Massachusetts General
Hospital; Instructor in Pathology, Harvard Medical School, Boston,
Massachusetts
Leukocyte Reduced Products

Gary E. Tegtmeier, PhD
Director, Viral Testing Laboratories, Community Blood Center of Greater
Kansas City; Clinical Associate Professor, University of Missouri—Kansas
City, Kanas City Missouri
Additional Infectious Complications

Pearl Toy, MD
Professor, University of California, San Francisco, San Francisco, California
*Red Blood Cell Transfusion and the Transfusion Trigger, Including the
Surgical Setting*

Iain J. Webb, MD
Currently, Associate Director, Clinical Research, Millennium
Pharmaceuticals, Inc., Cambridge, Massachusetts; formerly, Medical
Director, Cell Manipulation Core Facility, Dana Farber Cancer Institute,
Boston, Massachusetts
Mononuclear Cell Preparations

Constance M. Westhoff, SBB, PhD
Research Associate, Department of Pathology and Laboratory Medicine,
University of Pennsylvania, Philadelphia, Pennsylvania
*Membrane Blood Group Antigens and Antibodies; ABO and Related
Antigens; Rh, Kell, Duffy, and Kidd Blood Group Systems; Other Blood
Group Systems and Antigens*

Robert M. Winslow, MD
Adjunct Professor, Bioengineering, University of California San Diego,
San Diego, California
Blood Substitutes

Edward C.C. Wong, MD
Assistant Professor of Pediatrics and Pathology, Department of Laboratory
Medicine, George Washington School of Medicine; Director of Hematology/
Associate Director of Transfusion Medicine, Department of Laboratory
Medicine, Children's National Medical Center, Washington,
District of Columbia
Irradiated Products and Washed/Volume Reduced Products

David Wuest, MD
Director of Blood Bank and Transfusion Services, Blood Bank at Memorial
Sloan-Kettering Cancer Center, New York, New York
*Transfusion to Bone Marrow or Solid Organ Transplant Recipients and
HIV-Positive Patients*

Preface

Blood Banking and Transfusion Medicine was conceived to be a comprehensive textbook that would combine the traditional field of blood banking (with its focus on immunohematologic, manufacturing, laboratory, testing, and storage issues) with the practical field of transfusion medicine (with its focus on patient-based issues, including specialized components and patient needs, complications of transfusion, and the treatment of patients requiring therapeutic apheresis). The concept is always been that the scientific bases underlying both of these fields, blood banking and transfusion medicine, would be used as the foundation for this text, utilizing data from basic, translational, and clinical studies to provide a rationale for what we as blood bankers and transfusion medicine specialists actually do. In addition, blood banking and transfusion medicine have grown to be multi-disciplinary fields, encompassing specialists in hematology, pathology, anesthesiology, pediatrics, surgery, and other practitioners. Scientific contributions to these fields have come from an equally diverse group, ranging from virologists and molecular biologists to tissue and mechanical engineers. To these many specialists who have contributed to the wealth of knowledge accumulated in blood banking and transfusion medicine, we are grateful. We hope all of you will find *Blood Banking and Transfusion Medicine* a valuable reference and resource. As such, we would welcome any comments or input that could improve the content or layout of this text in future editions.

CD Hillyer
LE Silberstein
PM Ness
KC Anderson

Acknowledgments

We, the editors, would like to acknowledge the outstanding technical and professional support of Sue Rollins and Natalie Ware, and the expertise and guidance of Dolores Meloni, all of whom were instrumental in the creation of this textbook. We would also like to thank our friends and families for their unconditional love and support, without which this project could not have come to fruition, especially Krista, Whitney, Peter, and Margot Hillyer; the family and friends of Les Silberstein; Barbara, Jennie, Steven, and Molly Ness; and Cynthia, Emily, David, and Peter Anderson.

Contents

PART I

Introduction

Chapter 1

Evolution to the 21st Century

James P. AuBuchon

Much has transpired in the realm of transfusion medicine since the enabling work performed in a Viennese microbiology laboratory a century ago. Once the means were identified through which human transfusion could be accomplished without immunohematologic disaster, other researchers could sequentially address the problems of anticoagulation, storage sterility, blood groups, components, derivatives, infectious disease transmission, and pathogen inactivation. Each of these developments was built on the base of previous investigators' accomplishments, and each opened another opportunity for further improvements in transfusion practice. That process continues today, with the success in one endeavor allowing attention to be focused on the thread perceived to be the next most important. The challenges of safety and availability remain the same today (with a powerful economic overlay)—that is, to direct our efforts to providing the greatest benefits for the patients and the society we serve in the context of greatest safety.

Transfusion medicine today, as both a science and an art, consists of practices that could not be dreamed of a decade ago, let alone at the time of Landsteiner's insightful observations. Provision of well-preserved cellular or plasma components with predictable effects and uncommon severe side effects has become so commonplace that research and development efforts can head in other directions. Rapid advances, paralleled in other fields of medicine, have prompted us to dream of explorations in new fields that, at first blush, may appear to be only peripherally related to transfusion therapy but that, on investigation, represent the culmination of the craft. We can imagine replacement of human-derived biologic components with universally compatible pharmaceuticals derived through ex vivo expansion of progenitor cells. Already, we can apply hematopoietic stimulants to reduce the clinical need for blood components through increases in endogenous production, and we are well along in developing gene therapy as a means to replace the function of certain cells in patients who are unable to produce adequate numbers of cells with normal function. Admittedly, advancements such as these will pose new problems—of suitability, access, and appropriate application—and the field will continue to struggle with complex clinical issues, such as transfusion thresholds, as it has in the past. How will the "path forward" be illuminated?

■ Building on the Past

For the next decades, at least, it is likely that many of the same tenets and attributes that have made transfusion medicine so safe and successful will continue to be requisite qualities. The gravity and solemnity with which the field of transfusion medicine is addressed reflect the awesome, concomitant potentials for clinical benefit and patient harm implicit in transfusion; these considerations will continue to be paramount until transfusion is predictable and without significant side effects. The detection of alloantibodies and the provision of blood lacking corresponding antigens will continue to be the primary focus of transfusion services. Key problems that have plagued the field since its modern inception—such as giving a patient an incompatible unit of blood because of misidentification—will require continued diligence and new insights to be overcome. The specter of infectious disease risks that have terrorized patients and the public over the last 15 to 20 years will continue to demand extraordinary responses to a threat of even seemingly minute proportions (e.g., the risk of transmitting spongiform encephalopathy).

Both blood banking and transfusion medicine will continue to learn about and learn from efforts to ensure the quality of their services. Both have moved beyond rudimentary "quality control" concepts to include total quality management (TQM) and ongoing quality improvement initiatives in their efforts to ensure the quality of their services. To some, the jargon and conceptualizations of the practitioners of this field are still as uninterpretable as the discussion of red blood cell antigens and antibodies among experienced serologists is to a neophyte. The prominence of this subject in the *Technical Manual* of the American Association of Blood Banks (AABB)[1] and the use of these concepts as the basis of the AABB's assessment program[2] reflect not only the importance many believe these concepts have for the fields but also the imperative that they be adopted promptly.[3] Undoubtedly, these concepts will be refined over time, becoming more streamlined and simplified, allowing them to become more widely adopted. Continued appearance of success stories will also encourage further applications.[4-6] With mounting pressures for more efficient and more effective operations—that is, safer blood and lower health care costs—the adoption of these principles of operations will become necessary even beyond regulatory imperatives.

Several advantages of this new management approach have already become apparent. Focusing on the processes rather than on their individual steps or even on individual staff has allowed new insights to be brought to bear on old problems. Although "human error" remains the attributed immediate cause in most cases of mistranfusion, we have come to recognize that the process of sampling and testing patients and transfusing blood to them must have interlocking, coordinated steps with embedded process controls that ensure that all the critical steps have been performed correctly.[7-10] Humans will always err, but such a process should be robust enough to ensure detection of the errors at key points or to prevent them. As in other fields, machines (especially computers) are used with growing frequency to reduce the possibility of errors and take on the key control functions. Use of a mechanical barrier device to ensure that the recipient of the unit is the same person who gave the pretransfusion specimen has been demonstrated to interdict mistransfusion[11, 12]; hand-held computer devices have now been developed to provide similar process control steps.[13] These steps can help reduce the continuing occurrence of preventable disasters. It is to be hoped that we will employ this *systems* approach more broadly among transfusion services and blood center operations to reduce the frequency with which the end results of our efforts do not meet clinician or patient expectations.

The use of automation has also increased for the purpose of efficiency. Automated testing has long been a part of blood center operations, where large instruments with high throughput capacity are used for blood grouping and infectious disease testing. The capability of these instruments to generate data in a controlled manner that meets the requirements of good manufacturing practice (GMP) has added further impetus for their use, and their large capacities have supported the trend toward consolidation of testing operations. The transfusion service end of the field has been much slower to automate. Only recently have instruments been developed that are economically feasible for the smaller volumes encountered in a hospital laboratory. These instruments have the potential, however, to provide dependable output with direct interface with the laboratory information system, thus eliminating several possible avenues for imprecise capturing and reporting of the results. Computerization capabilities are still limited in smaller hospitals; although slowly expanding, this vital

capacity will need to become essentially universal for all laboratories to practice total quality management and good manufacturing practice to the fullest.

It is perhaps ironic that the same instrumentation that allows efficiency and process improvement in hospital laboratories also facilitates centralization of transfusion service functions to other locations. Several communities "grew up" in blood banking using a centralized crossmatching service, but only later have other communities begun to adapt this approach to their local system. Using dedicated staff and equipment, these facilities can provide more efficient laboratory support of a hospital's hemotherapy needs.[14] Logistics concerns regarding rapid response for emergencies remain extant, however, and making the best use of the educational and consultative capabilities of a service's transfusion medicine specialist requires new approaches to the practice of this field of medicine.[15] Although centralization is not likely to eliminate all the hospital transfusion services, many of those in urban areas may find the pressures to economize and, at the same time, perhaps to offer expanded technical and medical consultative services an irresistible combination.

■ Continuing Dilemmas

This society's optimistic dependence on the ability of rational thought and technology to solve all our problems provides encouragement to continue pressing ahead, but the interface between society and medicine is a complex one. In blood banking, the importance of health and longevity becomes entangled with power, economics, politics, and media forces to yield conflicting imperatives.[16]

Continued constraints on health care resources may be expected to have more visible effects on blood banking in the next few years. Financial resources have been lean for several years, and many blood centers are now operating on marginal financial reserves. Their ability to respond to new opportunities to expand the safety of the blood supply will be increasingly limited unless they can persuade their hospital customers of the medical or legal necessities of new interventions.

Hospital transfusion services are shielded from direct pressure from politicians and media to improve blood safety; individually, any one hospital is statistically unlikely to encounter an "unsafe" unit, and thus, hospitals are less focused on reducing infectious risks. In addition, they certainly have their own financial pressures, which can have detrimental effects on the overall safety of the transfusion experience for a patient. In a survey performed by the College of American Pathologists,[17] 8% of hospital transfusion services replied that fiscal restraints had forced operational changes that reduced the level of protection afforded transfusion recipients. As economic pressures mount, the willingness to pay for "improvements" in the blood supply that seem to offer insubstantial benefits will diminish.

The ambivalence of many transfusion specialists toward leukoreduction is an example of this dilemma. Reducing the leukocyte content for certain patients is clearly medically beneficial and may even save money.[18] The universal implementation of this practice may or may not provide substantial benefits in reducing the risk of bacterial infection. Without unequivocal data to justify the additional annual expenditure of $500 to $700 million to perform leukoreduction on all units in the United States, and without a clear demonstration that the leukocytes' presence is wreaking havoc, adoption of this approach has been slow. Resolution of this dilemma, so that the public's desire for "safer" blood is matched by a corresponding distribution of society's resources to achieve this end, will require political interaction of the kind to which blood banking specialists are not accustomed.

The media can be expected to "keep an eye on" blood banking because the general population has been sensitized to the risks of transfusion. Although the public's focus is sensitive to media direction and to (possibly disproportionate) fears of the "latest disease," the public voice is clear that it wants transfusion options without risks. Heretofore, steps toward this goal have focused on the addition of criteria to screen out donors or the units suspected of having a higher probability of disease transmission. The "costs" of these steps, up to now, have been primarily financial or logistic in nature. In the future, however, because of the current high level of safety in allogeneic transfusion, efforts to improve safety may generate new risks that dwarf the risks being avoided.

The case of solvent-detergent (SD) treatment of plasma is illustrative. A decade ago, the opportunity to make plasma free of the risk of human immunodeficiency virus (HIV) would have led quickly to universal application of this approach. With the risks of HIV and hepatitis C virus (HCV) now several orders of magnitude lower, however, the risk of transmitting nonenveloped viruses through the pooling process used in solvent-detergent plasma manufacture suddenly looms large in comparison with the risk of the viruses being inactivated.[19] Indeed, any viral inactivation protocol must take into account the small risk from the process or residual chemicals and must compare it with the risk of microbial transmission if the inactivation process is not performed.[20] Although both risks may be small in magnitude, they must be compared to ensure that such efforts do not create more morbidity than they avoid. The public's dread of certain kinds of disease may tip the scales in one direction or the other when the magnitude of these risks is small, but the comparative risks of a "safety" initiative must be understood.[16, 21, 22]

This issue of competing risks extends also to the adequacy of the blood supply. Exclusion of certain donors to reduce the risks of disease transmission is laudable and is appreciated by transfusion recipients, but continued winnowing of the blood supply through increasingly stringent donor qualification criteria and expanded unit testing (neither of which has 100% specificity) will ultimately result in the availability of too few units for a necessary transfusion. The subsequent catastrophe will emphasize the point that is beginning to be understood: Adequacy of the blood supply is also a *safety* issue. An era of chronic blood shortage is approaching at a pace accelerated by the "graying" of the population, a phenomenon that places more of us in the category likely to need a transfusion and fewer in the category able to give it. Data from the National Blood Data Resources Center suggests that the excess capacity in the current system has been utilized and that chronic, significant blood shortages are close to the horizon unless current collection and usage trends are reversed.

Implementation of more precise screening tests and the advent of viral inactivation technologies may allow the historical criteria for donors and the testing protocol for units to be relaxed slightly. However, it is more likely that increased resources will have to be directed toward donor recruitment and retention to ensure that the low risks of allogeneic transfusion will be matched by a high probability of its being available when needed. The automation of the collection process so as to direct donors toward donating one or more multiple components that can be separated, in their presence and during donation, according to blood type, platelet count, or hematocrit may improve the "yield" from each donor as well and can be expected to be explored extensively.[23, 24] Nevertheless, careful, informed choices need to be made so that lack of blood availability does not create a new safety hazard in transfusion.

Reliance on technology to solve the unsolvable problems continues to be a hope frequently fulfilled. Nucleic acid testing for key infectious diseases, for instance, was in its infancy a decade ago, was not practical for transfusible components just a few years ago, and yet has been fully implemented for all donations. The risks of bacterial contamination may finally yield to technological advances as well. The risk of bacterial contamination of platelets, which is approximately 1 per 3000 units, dwarfs the risk of viral contaminants, and the dire consequences of endotoxin infusion make the rare contamination of red blood cell units one that often leads to a disastrous outcome.[25] A variety of detection techniques have been investigated, but each offers less than sterling sensitivity and specificity (approaching only 70% at best).[26–30] However, most of the viral inactivation techniques under development for cellular components also inactivate contaminating bacteria.[31] For platelet units, at least, this advantage may be the primary driver in implementation of the techniques, because the risks of viral transmission have dropped so markedly. However, use of cultures to address the problem of bacterial contamination in platelets may provide a direct and successful means of reducing the danger of bacteria with less cost and fewer "competing risk" concerns.[32]

Against this backdrop of economic constraints and technologic advances stand the glowing and growing opportunities for the application of scientific wizardry to support or replace 20th century–style hemotherapy. The harvesting, processing, and even selection of hematopoietic progenitor cells for stem cell reconstitution are now common practice, and ex vivo expansion of stem cells is already feasible and may soon be practical. Hematopoietic stimulants have already greatly reduced the need for transfusion in one segment of the transfused population, patients with end-stage renal diseases, and may be helpful in reducing the risks of neutropenia and thrombocytopenia during chemotherapy. Gene therapy still has many hurdles to pass before becoming proficient in correcting genetic defects, but this endpoint now appears more a matter of "when" than "if" for a variety of inherited disorders.[33–35] Whether the "artificial" means of delivering oxygen via hemoglobin or perfluorocarbon solutions or via liposomes will provide clinically useful *substitutes* for red blood cells is uncertain, and the ability to achieve hemostasis with platelet microvesicles or artificial analogues requires additional investigation; however, the abilities of these creations to at least serve as augmentations of natural processes seem promising.[36, 37]

■ The Role of the Transfusion Specialist

With these limitations and opportunities facing the field, what is our future role as transfusion medicine specialists? Certain functions, such as therapeutic apheresis, medical decisions regarding donor acceptability, and planning a course of transfusion in light of unclear immunohematologic data, will continue to remain vital for the appropriate care of those entrusted to us. The importance of the traditional role of gatekeeper to minimize unnecessary transfusion[38, 39] because of infectious risks will decline concomitantly with these risks, and maintaining this focus for economic gain is anathema to a physician's credo. Selection of policies and methods that provide the best in patient care while minimizing costs requires insight and investigation, but the dividends will accrue in both recipient welfare and dollars.[40]

Some transfusion medicine practitioners have already moved beyond this point, emphasizing instead their educational role because most clinicians are inadequately trained in hemotherapy.[41–43] Consultations are then utilized to directly improve patient outcomes (as opposed to avoiding potential future difficulties). Synthesizing a cohesive picture of all laboratory data (which may be more readily available to the transfusion specialist) to present a plan of hemotherapeutic action can provide direction that is useful to the clinician and vital to the bleeding patient.[44, 45] This role may become even more central as the options in transfusion become more varied and interwoven. Few surgeons, for example, have the time to determine how best to provide hemotherapy support with hematopoietic agents, autologous transfusion options, and "blood substitutes." Consultation in the treatment of coagulopathies is another field in which a number of options other than the transfusion of routine components may be underutilized,[46] and sharing of expertise from the field of transfusion may positively affect the patients' as well as the facility's costs.

Expansion of these roles of the transfusion medicine specialist may require some new skills.[47, 48] The requisite knowledge base in serology and infectious disease will remain, and thorough comprehension of the molecular basis of what we have practiced successfully in the 20th century will be needed so that we may apply and extend these concepts into the practice of 21st-century medicine. The requirement for good communication skills will continue, because transfusion medicine is likely to become more complex before it becomes less so, and practicing clinicians will increasingly be at the disadvantage of having inadequate knowledge of the field to practice state-of-the-art hemotherapy. The transfusion medicine specialist will also need to learn the applications and implications of outcomes research and decision analysis. Increasingly, new therapies are expected to be able to demonstrate that they actually represent improvements in care before they garner support for implementation.

Furthermore, as transfusion safety improves, a keen eye will be needed even more to distinguish interventions that are "window dressing" and not likely to yield benefit from those that offer true assistance toward safer, more abundant units for transfusion. The public may, in the end, demand implementation of certain improvements despite low yields, high costs, or poor cost-effectiveness projections.[49, 50] The role of the transfusion medicine specialist in such deliberations should be to detail the risks, benefits, and alternatives so that the public can make an informed choice. The motivations for the decisions may not be "logical" from a specialist's viewpoint, but to the extent that society's resources are being expended in the effort, the public's will should be predominant. It is incumbent on all in the field, however, to continue diligent education efforts—ongoing in the background as well as on-demand for specific issues—so that the public can participate in the discussions as a knowledgeable partner and so that we "technocrats" can remain sensitive to their emotions and concerns.

Ultimately, however, the field of transfusion medicine will remain vibrant as long as it represents the practice of medicine dedicated to the good of the patient. The field has advanced far with seemingly small steps of important insight. Numerous "giants" of the field have taught us much about immunology, biochemistry, and physiology, and now it is our turn to harness these concepts and apply them through techniques that are based on molecular and genetic interactions.

The practical exigencies of budgets, reimbursements, and staffing levels, for example, cannot be ignored, but continued focus on the welfare of the patients under our care must remain our central precept as we expand our diagnostic and therapeutic capabilities. It is this fiduciary responsibility from which our professional position derives; it is the entrée to the respect accorded our professional opinions and advice. The complexity of this facet of our profession has grown just as the scientific side has. We can—and must—operate to the benefit of patients by seeking out those efficiencies that do not compromise patient care or safety and by highlighting the best means of applying a new approach to maximize benefit and minimize risks and costs.[40] This is a thin tightrope that does not need to be walked by every medical specialist, but it is intrinsic to the field of transfusion medicine, in which physicians take on greater responsibilities for administrative functions and societal interactions. As a profession, we are still learning how best to balance these claims, which at times appear to have arisen from diametrically opposed camps.

William Jennings Bryan once said, "It is a poor mind that cannot find plausible reason for what the heart wants to do." Our challenge for the future is to clarify the focus of our field of medicine and then practice our specialty so as to deliver the best possible care to all patients within the resource limitations we are given. The challenge can be both exasperating and exhilarating. It is to be hoped that we will continue to devise new strategies, uncover new facts, and develop new solutions to continue to move toward the universal goals of improved transfusion safety and supply while balancing economic pressure and patient and society needs. Each new intervention will likely provide a smaller incremental gain in health benefit (or another problem would have been targeted for attention at the outset).[16] By directing the field's attention to the greatest current risk or focusing attention on those interventions with which the greatest health yield can be obtained, we can satisfy our responsibilities to both individual patients and society.

REFERENCES

1. Brecher M (ed): Technical Manual, 13th ed. Bethesda, MD, American Association of Blood Banks, 1999.
2. Menitove J (ed): Standards for Blood Banks and Transfusion Services. Bethesda, MD, American Association of Blood Banks, 1999.
3. Berte LM, Nevalainen DE: The laboratory's role in assessing patient outcomes. Lab Med 1998;29:114–119.
4. Geurtsen M, Greene D, Floss A, Strauss R: Cost analysis of quality improvement initiatives. Transfusion 1996;36:84S.

5. Herman JH, Klumpp TR, Christman RA, et al: The effect of platelet dose on the outcome of prophylactic platelet transfusion. Transfusion 1995;18:46S.
6. Berte LM, Nevalainen DE: Quality pays—in every business. Transfus Sci 1997;18:586–596.
7. Sazama K: Reports of 355 transfusion-associated deaths: 1976 through 1985. Transfusion 1990;30:583–590.
8. Linden JV, Paul B, Dressler KP. A report of 104 transfusion errors in New York State. Transfusion 1992;32:601–606.
9. Wenz B, Mercuriali F, AuBuchon JP: Practical methods to improve transfusion safety by using novel blood unit and patient identification systems. Am J Clin Pathol 1997;107(Suppl 4);S12–S16.
10. Steane EA, Steane SM: Closing the loop: Standardization is the key. Transfusion 1996;Mar;36(3):200–202.
11. Wenz B, Burns ER: Improvements in transfusions safety using a new blood unit and patient identification system as part of safe transfusion practice. Transfusion 1991;31:401–403.
12. AuBuchon JP, Littenberg B: A cost-effectiveness analysis of the use of a barrier system to reduce the risk of mistransfusion. Transfusion 1996;36:222–226.
13. Jenson NJ, Cross JT: An automated system for bedside verification of the match between patient identification and blood unit identification. Transfusion 1996;36:216–221.
14. Triulzi DJ: Advantages of outsourcing the transfusion service. Transfus Sci 1997;18:559–563.
15. Domen RE: The transfusion service is an integral and important component of the hospital and should not be outsourced. Transfus Sci 1997;18:565–573.
16. AuBuchon JP, Birkmeyer JD, Busch MP: Blood safety: Challenges and opportunities. Ann Intern Med 1997;127:904–909.
17. College of American Pathologists: Comprehensive Transfusion Medicine Survey, Set 1997 J-B. Northfield, IL, College of American Pathologists, 1997.
18. Canadian Coordinating Office for Health Technology Assessment: Leukoreduction: The Technique Used, Their Effectiveness and Costs. Ottawa, Canadian Coordinating Office for Health Technology Assessment (CCOHTA), 1998.
19. AuBuchon JP, Birkmeyer JD: Safety and cost effectiveness of solvent-detergent treated plasma: In search of a zero-risk blood supply. JAMA 1994;272:1210–1214.
20. AuBuchon JP, Dodd RY: Inactivation of microbial contaminants of blood components. Clin Lab Med 1992;12:787–803.
21. Dinman BD: The reality and acceptance of risk. JAMA 1980;244:1226–1228.
22. Morgon MG: Risk analysis and management. Sci Am 1993;269:32–41.
23. Valbonesi M, De Luigi MC, Florio G, et al: The Cobe Trima system as a tool for optimizing component collection: A further step towards total apheresis. Int J Artif Organs 1999;22;58–59.
24. Knutson F, Roder J, Frank V, et al: A new apheresis procedure for the preparation of high-quality red cells and plasma. Transfusion 1999;39:565–571.
25. Blajchman MA: Bacterial contaminations of blood products and the value of pre-transfusion testing. Immunol Invest 1995;24:163–170.
26. Mitchell K-MT, Brecher ME: Approaches to the detection of bacterial contamination in cellular blood products. Transfus Med Rev 1999;13:132–144.
27. Kim DM, Brecher ME, Bland LA, et al: Visual identification of bacterially contaminated red cells. Transfusion 1992;32:221–225.
28. Leach MF, Pickard CA, Herschel LH, et al: Evaluation of glucose and pH test strips for detection of microbial contaminants in apheresis platelets. Transfusion 1998;38:89S.
29. Burstain JM, Brecher ME, Workman K, et al: Rapid identification of bacterially contaminated platelets using reagent strips: Glucose and pH analysis as markers of metabolism. Transfusion 1997;37:255–258.
30. Pickard C, Herschel LH, Seery P, AuBuchon JP: Visual identification of bacterially contaminated red cells. Transfusion 1998;38:12S.
31. Lin L, Cook DN, Wiesehahn GP, et al: Photochemical inactivation of viruses and bacteria in platelets concentrates by use of novel psoralen and long-wavelength ultraviolet light. Transfusion 1997;37:423–435.
32. Au Buchon JP, Cooper LK, Leach MF, et al: Bacterial culture of platelet units and extension of storage to 7 days. Transfusion 2001;41:1S.
33. Zhang WW: Development and application of adenoviral vectors for gene therapy of cancer. Cancer Gene Ther 1999;6:113–138.
34. Onedera M, Nelson DM, Sakiyama Y, et al: Gene therapy for severe combined immunodeficiency caused by adenosine deaminase deficiency: Improved retroviral vectors for clinical trials. Acta Haematol 1999;101:89–96.
35. Jaffe A, Bush A, Geddes DM, Alton EW: Prospects for therapy in cystic fibrosis. Arch Dis Child 1999;80:286–289.
36. Winslow RM: New transfusion strategies: Red cell substitutes. Ann Rev Med 1999;50:337–353.
37. Ketchman EM, Cairns CB: Hemoglobin-based oxygen carriers: Development and clinical potential. Ann Emerg Med 1999;33:326–337.
38. Toy PT: Effectiveness of transfusion audits and practice guidelines. Arch Pathol Lab Med 1994;118:435–437.
39. Toy PT: Audit and education in transfusion medicine. Vox Sang 1996;70:1–5.
40. Petrides M: When less is more: Cost-containment in transfusion medicine. Tranfus Sci 1997;18:603–612.
41. AuBuchon JP: The role of transfusion medicine physicians: A vanishing breed? Arch Pathol Lab Med 1999;123:663–667.
42. Popvsky MA, Triulzi D: The role of the transfusion medicine clinical consultant. Am J Clin Pathol 1996;105:798–801.
43. Laposata M: What many of us are doing or should be doing in clinical pathology: A list of the activities of the pathologist in the clinical laboratory. Am J Clin Pathol 1996;106:571–573.
44. Hocker P, Hartmann T: Management of massive transfusion. Acta Anaesth Scand 1997;111(Suppl):205–207.
45. Crosson JT: Massive transfusion. Clin Lab Med 1996;16:873–882.
46. Van Cott EM, Laposata M: Laboratory evaluation of hypercoagulable states. Hematal Oncol Clin North Am 1998;12:1141–1166.
47. Conjoint Task Force on Clinical Pathology Residency Training Writing Committee: Graylyn conference report: Recommendations for reform of clinical pathology residency training. Am J Clin Pathol 1995;103:127–129.
48. Kirby JE, Laposata M: The nature and extent of training activities in clinical pathology required for effective consultation on the laboratory test selection and interpretation. Arch Pathol Lab Med 1997;121:1163–1167.
49. Hadman DC: The Oregon priority-setting exercise: Quality of life and public policy. Hastings Cent Rep 1991;21(S): 11–16.
50. Hadorn DC: Setting health care priorities in Oregon: Cost effectiveness meets the rule of rescue. JAMA 1991;265:2218–2225.

PART II

Blood Banking

i. Red Blood Cells

Chapter 2

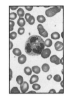

Membrane Blood Group Antigens and Antibodies

Marion E. Reid
Constance M. Westhoff

Erythrocyte blood group antigens are polymorphic, inherited, carbohydrate or protein structures located on the outside surface of the red blood cell (RBC) membrane. Our ability to detect and identify blood group antigens and antibodies has contributed significantly to current safe supportive blood transfusion practice and to the appropriate management of pregnancies at risk for hemolytic disease of the newborn (HDN). Exposure to erythrocytes carrying an antigen lacking on the RBCs of the recipient can elicit an immune response in some individuals. Thus, blood group antigens are clinically important in allogeneic blood transfusions, maternofetal blood group incompatibility, and organ transplantation. By virtue of their relative ease of detection by hemagglutination and generally straightforward mode of inheritance, blood group antigens have been used in genetic, forensic, and anthropologic investigations. The polymorphisms of blood groups have been exploited as a tool to monitor in vivo survival of transfused RBCs and to monitor engraftment of bone marrow transplants. Antigen profiles have been used to predict inheritance of diseases encoded by a gene in close proximity to the gene encoding the blood group antigen. Blood group antigens have also contributed to our understanding of cell membrane structure.

The national standard of practice for blood transfusion in the United States is outlined in the *Standards for Blood Banks and Transfusion Services*, published by the American Association of Blood Banks (AABB).[1] These standards, which were developed by and are continually revised by experts in the field, address all areas of blood collection and transfusion, including donor selection, blood collection, component preparation, donor blood testing, labeling, conditions for storage, transportation and expiration, apheresis, compatibility testing and selection of components, issue and transfusion of blood and components, administration of Rh immune

globulin, transfusion complications, autologous blood, records, quality assurance, antibody identification, bone marrow and peripheral blood progenitor cells, and tissue storage and issue. All hospitals accredited by the AABB must adhere to these standards.

One of the most important clinical concerns in contemporary transfusion medicine occurs with the discovery that a patient requiring transfusion has an unexpected blood group antibody. Although the laboratory can characterize an antibody in terms of specificity, immunoglobulin class and in vitro characteristics, it cannot always predict the antibody's clinical significance. Therefore, when a blood group antibody is detected, an important, although often overlooked, first step is to review all available pertinent patient information (Table 2.1). One can then assess the potential for adverse effects by correlating the serologic information with the patient history and also with historical clinical experience in other patients. A patient who has not been exposed to RBCs by transfusion or pregnancy is unlikely to have a clinically significant alloantibody.

■ Erythrocyte Membrane

The erythrocyte membrane consists of lipids, proteins, and carbohydrates, which interact to form a dynamic and fluid structure. By dry weight, the ratio of protein-to-lipid-to-carbohydrate in the RBC membrane is 49:43:8. The RBC membrane behaves as a semisolid, with elastic and viscous properties that are not observed with simple lipid vesicles. These properties are critical for the RBC to survive in the circulation for approximately 120 days during numerous cycles (approximately 75,000) and passages through narrow veins and sinusoids in the spleen. The RBC accomplishes this goal without intracellular machinery to repair damage. The multiple

Table 2.1   Potentially Useful Information for Problem-Solving in Immunohematology

Available Information	Considerations
Patient demographics	Diagnosis, age, sex, ethnicity, transfusion and/or pregnancy history, drugs, intravenous fluids (lactated Ringer's solution, IVIgG, antilymphocyte globulin), infections, malignancies, hemoglobinopathies, stem cell transplantation
Initial serologic results	ABO, Rh, direct antiglobulin test, phenotype, antibody detection, autologous control, crossmatch
Hematology/chemistry values	Hemoglobin, hematocrit, bilirubin, lactate dehydrogenase, reticulocyte count, haptoglobin, hemoglobinuria, albumin:globulin ratio, red blood cell (RBC) morphology
Sample characteristics	Site and technique of collection, age of sample, anticoagulant, hemolysis, lipemic, color of serum/plasma, agglutinates/aggregates in the sample
Other	Check records in current and previous institutions for antibodies to blood group antigens
Antibody identification	Autologous control, phase of reactivity, potentiator (saline, albumin, low-ionic-strength solution, polyethylene glycol), reaction strength, effect of chemicals on antigen (proteases, thiol reagents), pattern of reactivity (single antibody or mixture of antibodies), characteristics of reactivity (mixed field, rouleaux), hemolysis, preservatives/antibiotics in reagents, use of washed RBCs

connections between the membrane skeleton and the lipid bilayer cause the bilayer to follow the contours of the membrane skeleton. Together, the membrane skeleton and lipid bilayer gives the erythrocyte shape and resilience.[2, 3]

Lipids

The lipids in the RBC membrane form a bilayer with the hydrophobic tails on the inside and the hydrophilic polar head groups to either the outside (extracellular) or the inside (cytoplasmic) surface (Fig. 2.1). The following three types of lipids occur in the RBC membrane: phospholipids (50%), cholesterol (40%), and glycolipids (10%). The arrangement of phospholipids in the bilayer is asymmetrical. The outer leaflet contains predominantly the neutral phospholipids (phosphatidylcholine and sphingomyelin), and the inner leaflet contains predominantly the aminophospholipids (phosphatidylethanolamine and phosphatidylserine). The presence of phosphatidylserine, which is negatively charged, on the inner monolayer results in a significant difference in charge between the two sides of the bilayer. The lipid molecules can diffuse rapidly within their own monolayer, but they rarely "flip-flop," maintaining membrane "sidedness."[2]

Proteins

Peripheral proteins form a meshwork under the lipid bilayer that is called the *membrane skeleton*. This name implies a relatively rigid structure; however, the meshwork is actually fluid and flexible. The RBC membrane skeleton is associated with the lipid bilayer through specific interactions with transmembrane proteins. For example, spectrin interacts with ankyrin, which in turn binds to band 3 (anion exchanger 1 [AE1]), a multi-pass protein; spectrin also binds to protein 4.1, which binds to the single-pass proteins glycophorin C (GPC) and glycophorin D (GPD). Spectrin, glycophorin, and band 3 account for more than 60% of the total membrane protein. Other minor attachment sites probably exist.

Many blood group antigens are carried on transmembrane proteins; however, a few antigens are carried on glycosylphosphatidylinositol (GPI)–linked proteins or on glycolipids (see Fig. 2.1). Some transmembrane proteins interact with other transmembrane proteins (e.g., band 3 and GPA; Kell and Kx; Rh and RhAG) or with lipids (e.g., Rh). A few antigens

are carried on proteins that are adsorbed from the plasma (Lewis and Chido/Rodgers).

Carbohydrates

Carbohydrates are essentially restricted to the extracellular surface of the RBC membrane, where they collectively form a negatively charged environment that is largely responsible for keeping the RBCs from adhering to one another and to the endothelium. The majority of carbohydrates are attached to lipids on ceramide and to proteins by attachment to asparagine (N-linked) or to serine or threonine (O-linked) during passage through the lumen of the Golgi.[4]

The carbohydrates form the *glycocalyx*, a negatively charged barrier approximately 10 Å thick around the outside of the RBC membrane. This barrier can keep immunoglobulin (Ig) G antibodies, particularly those recognizing antigens that reside close to the lipid bilayer, from interacting with the corresponding antigen. Thus, the glycocalyx affects the ability of an IgG antibody to cause direct agglutination; therefore, the distance of an antigen from the lipid bilayer has a greater impact on agglutination than does the number of antigen sites.[5]

■ RBC Blood Group Antigens

Figure 2.1 depicts the membrane components that are known to carry blood group antigens. Some antigens are carbohydrates attached to lipids or to proteins, some are protein, and some require both protein and carbohydrates. Although the blood group antigens do not themselves have a function, the molecules on which they are carried do. The function of proteins carrying blood group antigens has been determined through (1) observation of the morphology of RBCs that lack the protein (Table 2.2), (2) direct experimentation, or (3) comparison of the predicted protein sequence with protein databases to identify similar proteins whose function is known.

Recognition of a blood group antigen begins with discovery of an antibody. When an individual whose RBCs lack an antigen is exposed to RBCs that possess that antigen, the person may mount an immune response and produce an antibody that reacts with the antigen in a recognizable manner. Depending on the characteristics of the antibody and, to some extent, on the number and topology of antigens on the RBC

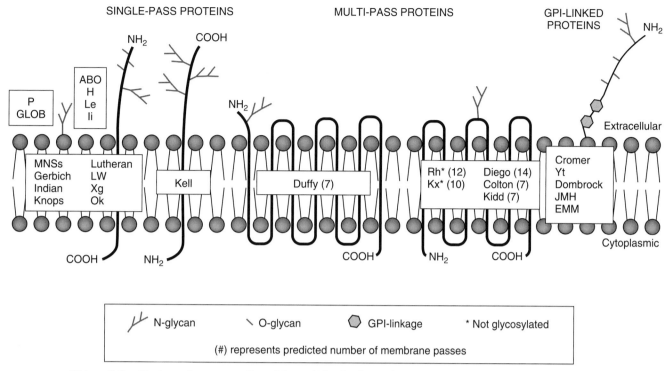

Figure 2.1 Diagram of a cross-section of the red blood cell membrane lipid bilayer and various membrane components that carry blood group antigens. GPI, glycosylphosphatidylinositol.

membrane, the interaction between antibody and antigen may be detected by agglutination, sensitization, or hemolysis. In human blood grouping, most tests involve agglutination, in which clumping of the RBCs serves as the detectable endpoint.[6] Only after an antibody has been produced to a polymorphic marker on an erythrocyte is the corresponding antigen named.

Terminology

A working party on terminology for RBC surface antigens, sanctioned by the International Society for Blood Transfusion (ISBT) has categorized the blood group antigens into four classifications.[7] The genetically discrete blood group systems are summarized in Table 2.3, which gives the name, ISBT system number, chromosome location, gene name, associated antigens, component name, and possible functions for each system. Table 2.4 contains the ISBT name, number, and associated antigens for blood group collections (serologically, biochemically, or genetically related antigens), the series of low-incidence antigens, and the series of high-incidence antigens.

As RBC antigens were discovered, notations were devised to describe them. The terminology used is inconsistent: a single letter (e.g., A, D, K), a symbol with a superscript (e.g., Fy^a, Jk^b, Lu^a) or a numerical notation (e.g., Fy3, Lu4, K12) is used. Even within the same blood group system, antigens have been named with different schemes, resulting in a cumbersome terminology for describing phenotypes. Throughout the discussion of red cell antigens, we use the classic terminology accepted by the ISBT. The use of the same symbol with a different superscript letter (e.g., Fy^a and Fy^b) indicates products of alleles (antithetical antigens).[7]

Inheritance

Most blood group antigens are encoded by genes on autosomes.[8] Most are codominant (e.g., M/N, E/e, K/k, Fy^a/Fy^b), but some appear to be dominant if an antibody to the presumed antithetical antigen has not been discovered (e.g., Ul^a, Cr^a). Some rare phenotypes appear to be inherited in a dominant manner—for example, dominant type Lu(a–b–)—or a recessive manner—for example, recessive type Lu(a–b–).

Table 2.2 Red Blood Cell Morphology and Associated Phenotype

Shape	Clinical Manifestation	Protein	Phenotype
Stomatocyte	Mild hemolytic anemia	Absent Rh or RhAG (Rh50)	Rh_{null}, Rh_{mod}
Elliptocyte	Slightly reduced RBC survival	Absent GPC and GPD	Ge: -2, -3, -4 (Leach)
Acanthocyte	Elevated CPK, muscular choreiform movements, neurologic defects, reduced RBC survival	Absent Kx	McLeod

CPK, creatinine phosphokinase; GP, glycophorin; RBC, red blood cell.

Table 2.3 Genetically Discrete Blood Group Systems

Name	ISBT Number	Chromosome Location	Gene Name ISBT	Gene Name ISGN	Associated Antigens	Component Name	Possible Function
ABO	001	9q34.2	ABO	ABO	A, B, A,B, A$_1$	Carbohydrate	
MNS	002	4q28.2-q31.1	MNS	GYPA, GYPB	M, N, S, s, U, He, Mi^a, Vw +35 more	GPA; GPB	Carrier of sialic acid
P	003	22q11.2-qter	P1	P1	P1	Carbohydrate	
Rh	004	1p36.13-p34.3	RH	RHD, RHCE	D, C, E, c, e, f, C^w, V, G, +36 more	RhCE; RhD	Transport
Lutheran	005	19q13.2	LU	LU	Lu^a, Lu^b, Lu3, Lu4, Au^a, Au^b +12 more	Lutheran glycoprotein; B-CAM	Adhesion
Kell	006	7q33	KEL	KEL	K, k, Kp^a, Kp^b, Ku, Js^a, Js^b +16 more	Kell glycoprotein	Enzymatic
Lewis	007	19p13.3	LE	FUT3	Le^a, Le^b, Le^{ab}, Le^{bh}, ALe^b, BLe^b	Carbohydrate	
Duffy	008	1q22-q23	FY	DARC	Fy^a, Fy^b, Fy3, Fy4, Fy5, Fy6	Fy glycoprotein	Chemokine receptor
Kidd	009	18q11-q12	JK	SLC14A1	Jk^a, Jk^b, Jk3	Kidd glycoprotein	Urea transport
Diego	010	17q21-q22	DI	SLC4A1	Di^a, Di^b, Wr^a, Wr^b, Wd^a, Rb^a +14 more	Band 3	Anion transport
Yt	011	7q22	YT	ACHE	Yt^a, Yt^b	Acetylcholinesterase	Enzymatic
Xg	012	Xp22.32	XG	XG	Xg^a	Xg^a glycoprotein	Adhesion
Scianna	013	1p35-p32	SC	SC	Sc1, Sc2, Sc3	Sc glycoprotein	
Dombrock	014	12p13.2-p12.1	DO	DO	Do^a, Do^b, Gy^a, Hy, Jo^a	Do glycoprotein	Enzymatic
Colton	015	7p14	CO	AQP1	Co^a, Co^b, Co3	Channel-forming integral protein	Water transport
Landsteiner-Wiener	016	19p13.3	LW	LW	LW^a, LW^{ab}, LW^b	LW glycoprotein	Adhesion
Chido/Rodgers	017	6p21.3	CH/RG	C4A, C4B	CH1, CH2, Rg1 +6 more	C4A; C4B	Complement regulation
Hh	018	19q13.3	H	FUT1	H	Carbohydrate	
Kx	019	Xp21.1	XK	XK	Kx	Kx glycoprotein	Transport
Gerbich	020	2q14-q21	GE	GYPC	Ge2, Ge3, Ge4, Wb, Ls^a, An^a, Dh^a	GPC; GPD	Interacts with Protein 4.1
Cromer	021	1q32	CROM	DAF	Cr^a, Tc^a, Tc^b, Tc^c, Dr^a, Es^a, IFC, WES^a, WES^b, UMC	CD55 (DAF)	Complement regulation
Knops	022	1q32	KN	CR1	Kn^a, Kn^b, McC^a, Sl^a, Yk^a	CD35 (CR1)	Complement regulation
Indian	023	11p13	IN	CD44	In^a, In^b	CD44	Adhesion
Ok	024	19pter-p13.2	OK	CD147	Ok^a	CD147	Adhesion
Raph	025	11p15.5	MER2	MER2	MER2	Not defined	

B-CAM, cell adhesion molecule; GP, glycophorin; ISBT, International Society for Blood Transfusion; ISGN, International Society for Gene Nomenclature.

Two antigens, Xg^a and Kx, are encoded by genes on the X chromosome and are inherited in a classic X-linked manner.

Expression

Some blood group antigens are also found on nonerythroid cells. For example, A, B, H, Kn^a (CD35), In^a (CD44), Ok^a (CD147), and Cromer-related antigens (CD55) have a wide tissue distribution.[9, 10]

The ability to culture stem cells and sort erythroid lineages and the availability of monoclonal antibodies have enabled the estimation of the timing of expression of blood group antigens during in vitro erythroid maturation. The blood group antigens appear in the following order: GPC, Kell, RhAG, LW, RhCE, GPA, band 3, RhD, Lutheran, and Duffy.[11, 12]

Maturation

Several blood group antigens are not expressed or are only weakly expressed on fetal RBCs and do not reach adult levels until a person is approximately 2 years of age. Cord RBCs do not express Le^a, Sd^a, Ch, Rg, or AnWj antigens. Antibodies to these antigens are unlikely to cause HDN, because antigen expression is a prerequisite for HDN. Cord RBCs express the

Table 2.4 Other Blood Groups

Name	ISBT* Number	Associated Antigens
Collections		
Cost	205	Cs^a, Cs^b
Ii	207	I, i
Er	208	Er^a, Er^b
Globoside	209	P, P^k, LKE
Unnamed	210	Le^c, Le^d
Series		
Low-incidence antigens	700	By, Chr^a, Bi, Bx^a, Rd, Pt^a + 15 more
High-incidence antigens	901	Vel, Lan, At^a, Jr^a, JMH, Emm, AnWj, Sd^a, Duclos, PEL, ABTI, MAM

*International Society for Blood Transfusion.

following antigens more weakly than adult RBCs: A, B, H, P$_1$, I, Le^b, Lu^a, Lu^b, Yt^a, Vel, Do^a, Do^b, Gy^a, Hy, Jo^a, Xg^a, Kn, and Bg. In contrast, the i and LW antigens are more strongly expressed on cord RBCs. Furthermore, although adults express more LW on D-positive than on D-negative RBCs, cord RBCs express LW antigens equally regardless of D type. This information makes the testing of cord RBCs useful in antibody identification studies.

Molecular Basis

The majority of genes (or gene families) encoding blood group antigens have been cloned and sequenced,[13] and the molecular basis of many blood group antigens has been determined.[14–17] Relevant details are given in Chapters 3 through 5. Information concerning the molecular basis of blood group antigens can also be obtained from the Blood Group Antigen Mutation Database whose website is www.bioc.aecom.yu.edu/bgmut/index.htm

Evolution

It has been known for many years from agglutination with human sera that blood group antigens have homologues in anthropoid apes.[18] The availability of monoclonal antibodies and molecular analysis of the gene homologues from non-human primates have contributed to defining the epitopes of human blood group antigens.[18–22] Additionally, because of the conserved nature of proteins, protein sequence comparisons are contributing to predictions about the function of human proteins (see Table 2.3). The sequencing of the genomes of many model organisms has allowed researchers to make testable inferences about protein function. Blood groups have benefited from this revolution.

◼ **Blood Group Antibodies**

Immunogenicity

Several factors influence the ability to stimulate antibody production, including antigen size, complexity, and dose as well as host HLA genotype and other, as yet unidentified, susceptibility factors. Most carbohydrate-based RBC antigens are T-cell–independent and therefore tend to elicit an IgM response. The protein-based antigens usually are T-cell–dependent and induce an IgM primary response that progresses to IgG.[23] Antigen exposure usually occurs by transfusion of products containing RBCs or during pregnancy (immune antibodies) or by exposure to microbes (apparently, naturally occurring antibodies). Table 2.5 summarizes the usual type of immunoglobulin response and the potential clinical significance, in transfusion or in HDN, of selected blood group antibodies, which are listed in order of clinical significance.[9]

Clinical Significance

Antibodies recognizing antigens in the ABO blood group system are by far the most clinically significant. Others occur

Table 2.5 Characteristics of Some Blood Group Alloantibodies

Antibody Specificity	IgM (Direct)	IgG (Indirect)	Clinical Transfusion Reaction	HDN
ABO	Most	Some	Immediate; mild to severe	Common; mild-moderate
Rh	Some	Most	Immediate/delayed; mild to severe	Common; mild to severe
Kell	Some	Most	Immediate/delayed; mild to severe	Sometimes; mild to severe
Kidd	Few	Most	Immediate/delayed; mild to severe	Rare; mild
Duffy	Rare	Most	Immediate/delayed; mild to severe	Rare; mild
M	Some	Most	Delayed (rare)	Rare; mild
N	Most	Rare	None	None
S	Some	Most	Delayed; mild	Rare; mild to severe
s	Rare	Most	Delayed; mild	Rare; mild to severe
U	Rare	Most	Immediate/delayed; mild to severe	Rare; severe
P1	Most	Rare	None (rare)	None
Lutheran	Some	Most	Delalyed	Rare; mild
Le^a	Most	Few	Immediate (rare)	None
Le^b	Most	Few	None	None
Diego	Some	Most	Delayed; none to severe	Mild to severe
Colton	Rare	Most	Delayed; mild	Rare; mild to severe
Dombrock	Rare	Most	Immediate/delayed; mild to severe	Rare; mild
LW	Rare	Most	Delayed; none to mild	Rare; mild
Yt^a	Rare	Most	Delayed (rare); mild	None
I	Most	Rare	None	None
Ch/Rg	Rare	Most	Anaphylactic (3 cases)	None
JMH	Rare	Most	Delayed (rare)	None
Knops	Rare	Most	None	None
Xg^a	Rare	Most	None	None

in the following order, from the most commonly to the least commonly encountered in transfusion practice: anti-D, anti-K, anti-E, anti-c, anti-Fy^a, anti-C, anti-Jk^a, anti-S, anti-Jk^b. All other clinically significant antibodies occur with an incidence of less than 1% of immunized patients.[24–26] Antibodies that are considered clinically insignificant unless the antibody reacts in tests performed strictly at 37°C are anti-P$_1$, anti-M, anti-N, anti-Lu^a, anti-Le^a, anti-Le^b, and anti-Sd^a. Other clinically insignificant antibodies that react at 37°C in the indirect antiglobulin test (IAT) are those of the Knops and Ch/Rg systems and anti-JMH (Table 2.6).

The incidence of a blood group antibody depends on both the prevalence and the immunogenicity of the antigen. Immunized patients frequently produce multiple antibodies, and the more antibodies present, the more difficult they are to identify.

Detection and Identification

Compatibility testing (testing patient's serum against donor's RBCs) still uses techniques that were described 100 years ago for direct agglutination, and 50 years ago for indirect agglutination. Even today, with our detailed understanding of blood group antigens, we have no single technical procedure able to detect all known blood group antibodies. The hemagglutination technique is simple and inexpensive, does not require sophisticated equipment, and, when done correctly, is sensitive and specific in terms of clinical relevance. Agglutination should be graded according to the strength of reaction, and an

Table 2.6 Clinical Significances of Some Alloantibodies to Blood Group Antigens

Clinically Significant ?	Alloantibodies
Always	A and B
	H in O$_h$
	Rh
	Kell
	Duffy
	Kidd
	Diego
	S, s, U
	P, PP1 P^k
	Vel
Sometimes	At^a
	Colton
	Cromer
	Dombrock
	Gerbich
	Indian
	Jr^a
	JMH
	Lan
	Landsteiner-Wiener
	Scianna
	Yt
Not unless reactive at 37°C	A$_1$
	H
	Le^a
	Lutheran
	M, N
	P1
	Sd^a
Not usually	Chido/Rodgers
	Cost
	Knops
	Le^b
	Xg^a

evaluation of the reaction strength can aid in identification of antibodies, especially when multiple antibodies are present in a serum.[6]

The first blood group antigens to be identified were those that could be agglutinated by the alloantibodies when antigen-positive RBCs were suspended in a saline medium (direct agglutination). This direct agglutination reflects the fact that these antibodies are usually IgM and detect carbohydrate antigens (ABO, P$_1$, Le and H antigens). Although anti-A and anti-B are highly clinically significant, antibodies to the other carbohydrate antigens generally are not.

Most of the other antigens (e.g., Rh, Kell, Duffy, and Kidd) are proteins and are detected by the IAT. This test detects IgG antibodies, complement attached to RBCs, or both. The sensitized RBCs are washed to remove unattached immunoglobulin (which would inhibit the antiglobulin reagent), and anti-human immunoglobulin is added. The specimen is centrifuged and examined for agglutination. The antiglobulin test can be direct or indirect. The "direct" agglutination test is used to detect RBCs sensitized in vivo, such as (1) alloantibodies in transfusion reactions or HDN and (2) autoantibodies in autoimmune hemolytic anemia (AIHA) or cold hemagglutinin disease (CHAD). "Indirect" agglutination is used to detect RBCs sensitized in vitro, for instance, in antigen typing, antibody detection and identification, and crossmatching.

To identify antibodies, serum is tested against RBCs of known phenotype in various techniques. It is sometimes helpful to treat antigen-positive test RBCs with chemical agents and to compare the antibody reactivity in tests against treated and untreated RBCs to aid antibody identification (Table 2.7).[16] Brief, but informative, descriptions of the technical and clinical aspects of most blood group antibodies can be found elsewhere.[6, 27]

■ Locating Antigen-Negative Blood

Once a patient is actively immunized to an RBC antigen and produces a clinically significant alloantibody, the patient is considered immunized for life and must be transfused with antigen-negative RBCs, even if the antibody is no longer detectable. Patients with passively acquired antibody (e.g., neonates and recipients of plasma products, Rh immune globulin, IVIgG) are not actively immunized and must be transfused with antigen-negative RBCs only while the passive antibody is still present. Selection of blood for transfusion of a patient with blood group alloantibodies is the joint responsibility of the staff at the transfusion service, the donor center, and the clinician. Thus, it is very important that there be communication regarding the number of units of RBC products required and the time frame involved. Figure 2.2 is a flow chart that outlines the process for locating blood, and Table 2.8 lists the incidence of donors whose RBCs lack selected antigens.

To locate antigen-negative blood for transfusion, it is not necessary to identify an antibody in the donor blood to a low-incidence antigen detected in the recipient's blood during compatibility testing, because another unit of donor blood is unlikely to be positive for the same uncommon antigen. In contrast, if an antibody to a low-incidence antigen is detected in the serum of a pregnant woman, identification of the antibody, or determination of its reactivity with paternal RBCs,

Table 2.7   Reactivity of Antigen-Positive Red Blood Cells After Treatment with Ficin/Papain or DTT*

Ficin/Papain	DTT (200 mM)	Possible, Antibody Specificity
Negative	Positive	M,N,S,s†; Fyᵃ,Fyᵇ; Ge2,Ge4; Xgᵃ; Ch/Rg
Negative	Negative	Indian; JMH
Positive	Weak	Cromer; Knops (weak in ficin), Lutheran; Dombrock; AnWj; MER2
Variable	Negative	Ytᵃ
Positive	Negative	Kell; LW; Scianna
Positive	Positive	A, B; H; P1; Rh; Lewis; Kidd; Fy3; Diego; Co; Ge3; Okᵃ, I, i; P, LKE; Atᵃ; Csᵃ; Emm; Erᵃ; Jrᵃ; Lan; Vel, Sdᵃ, PEL
Positive	Enhanced	Kx

*DTT, dithiothreitol.
†s variable with ficin/papain.

is required to predict the likelihood and severity of HDN in the baby. Locating blood for exchange transfusion is not difficult, for the reason previously described.

If a patient's serum contains alloantibodies to a high-incidence antigen, blood for transfusion may be very difficult to locate. Whether the investigation is for transfusion purposes or for prediction of HDN, the antibody should be identified. The identification aids in both the assessment of its clinical significance and the location of appropriate blood for transfusion. Family members, in particular siblings, are the first source to investigate for antigen-negative units.

Compatibility Procedures

Most laboratories follow recommendations made by the AABB,[1] and all must comply with regulations of state and federal agencies. Routine approaches involve testing a blood sample from a prospective recipient for ABO and D blood groups and for detection of blood group antibodies. In most cases, no unexpected antibodies are detected, and donor RBCs of appropriate ABO and D blood type are selected for transfusion. A sample of the donor's RBCs may be cross-matched with the patient's serum by means of either an immediate spin procedure or the IAT. Alternatively, the blood can be issued without direct cross-testing if a computer check is performed.[6] Any blood typing problems should be resolved, and when antibodies are detected, they should be identified. Knowing the specificity of an antibody helps (1) establish whether it is likely to be clinically significant and (2) determine the approach necessary to provide an adequate supply of compatible blood. Once an antibody has been identified, antigen-negative RBC products selected for transfusion should be tested with the patient's serum by the IAT.

It is important not to delay surgery or transfusion unnecessarily by attempting to obtain antigen-negative RBCs for patients with clinically insignificant antibodies. Also, in hemolytic anemia due to warm-reactive autoantibodies, compatibility may be difficult to demonstrate. The important issue is to be sure that there are no underlying, clinically significant alloantibodies. This fact can be determined with autologous or homologous autoabsorptions,[6] which require extra time and,

Figure 2.2   Flow chart for locating antigen-negative blood.

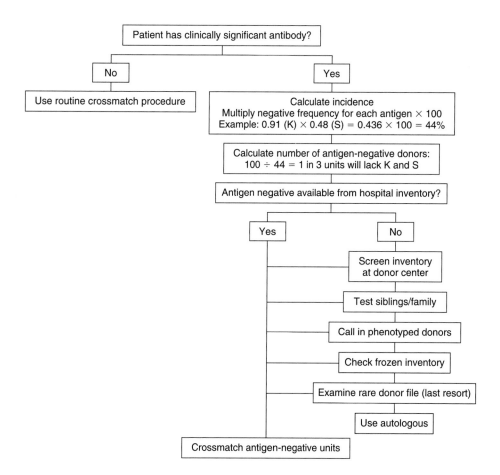

Table 2.8 Antigen Negativity Incidence for Common Polymorphic Antigens*

System	Antigen	Incidence of Antigen Negativity	
		White	Black
Rh	D	.15	.08
	C	.32	.73
	E	.71	.78
	c	.20	.04
	e	.02	.02
	f	.35	.08
	Cw	.98	.99
	V	>.99	.70
	VS	>.99	.73
	CE	<.01	<.01
	cE	.72	.78
	Ce	.32	.73
MNS	M	.22	.26
	N	.30	.25
	S	.48	.69
	s	.11	.06
	M×S×	.15	.19
	M×s×	.01	.02
	N×S×	.1	.16
	Ns×	.06	.02
P	P1	.21	.06
Lewis	Lea	.78	.77
	Leb	.28	.45
Lutheran	Lua	.92	.95
	Lub	<.01	<.01
Kell	K	.91	.98
	k	.002	<.01
	Kpa	.98	>.99
	Kpb	<.01	<.01
	Jsa	>.99	.80
	Jsb	<.001	.01
Duffy	Fya	.34	.90
	Fyb	.17	.77
Kidd	Jka	.23	.08
	Jkb	.26	.51
Dombrock	Doa	.33	.45
	Dob	.18	.11
Colton	Coa	<.01	
	Cob	.90	

*To calculate the incidence of compatible donors, multiply the incidence of antigen-negative donors for each antibody, e.g., the incidence of K×, S×, Jk(a×) donors in the general donor pool is (0.91) × (0.48) × (0.23) = 0.10 in 100, or 1 in 1000.

possibly, the services of an immunohematology reference laboratory. It is helpful to remember that patients without a history of immunization (transfusion or pregnancy) are unlikely to have underlying alloantibodies. However, a patient's transfusion history can be unreliable, because many patients are unaware or forget that they have received transfusions.[28]

■ Choice of Antigen-Negative Blood for Diseases Requiring Long-Term Transfusion Therapy

Transfusion management of patients who require long-term transfusion therapy, in particular patients with sickle cell anemia, has been the subject of heated debates.[29, 30] There is still no consensus as to the best and most practical approach, although the goal is to provide blood with maximal survival. In addition to the traditional practice of providing antigen-negative blood only after the patient has made an antibody, approaches that

have been adopted include: (1) providing phenotype-matched blood after the first antibody is made, (2) providing blood matched for D, C, E, and K antigens, and (3) providing fully antigen-matched blood (i.e., matched for D, C, E, c, e, K, Fya, Fyb, Jka, and Jkb antigens).

Clearly, if the objective is to prevent immunization to blood group antigens, initial phenotype matching is the logical approach; however, this approach does not prevent the production of antibodies to high-incidence antigens, such as U, Jsb, Cra, hrS, and hrB. The decision whether the blood donor community can support this approach lies with the directors of the transfusion service and of the donor center that supplies the blood. Providing phenotypically matched RBC products is logistically difficult and expensive. Although from the patient's perspective it is desirable to be transfused only with phenotype-matched blood, the community may not be able to meet the blood needs of such a patient. Indeed, in some regions, it is a challenge to provide antigen-negative blood to patients who have already made the antibodies.

■ Complications of Transfusion

As previously described, physicians in some locations may choose to provide phenotype-matched blood for patients with sickle cell anemia who undergo long-term transfusion therapy. Because the incidences of antigens differ in various ethnic groups, blood for these patients is most likely to be found among African American donors, whose RBCs more commonly lack C, E, K, S, Fya, Fyb, and Jkb antigens than the RBCs of white donors.[31] However, it is worth noting that RBCs from African American donors are more likely (approximately 1 in 5) to express antigens for which we do not routinely test, such as VS, Jsa, Goa, and DAK.[32] Thus, because all these antigens are immunogenic but are not present on screening cells, it is recommended in this group of patients that blood be crossmatched using the IAT in preference to performing a computer match. This crossmatching approach would prevent a potential transfusion reaction due to antibodies such as anti-VS, anti-Jsa, anti-Goa, and anti-DAK.

Although current pretransfusion practice has drastically reduced the incidence of hemolytic transfusion reactions, they still occur. The single most common cause of a hemolytic transfusion reaction is clerical error. It should be noted that several conditions mimic hemolytic transfusion reactions; they are summarized in Table 2.9. For more details, see Chapter 33 and a review by Beauregard and Blajchman.[33]

The three chapters following this one provide details about specific blood group antigens. Chapter 3 focuses on the ABO system and other carbohydrate antigens. Chapter 4 concentrates on the Rh, Kell, Duffy, and Kidd systems, in which the corresponding antibodies are potentially highly clinically significant. Chapter 5 describes aspects of the other blood groups.

Many World Wide Web (WWW) sites have useful information about blood group systems. Some URL (Uniform Resource Locator) addresses that may be of interest to the reader are as follows:

1. www.bioc.aecom.yu.edu/bgmut/index.htm

   The website of the Blood Group Antigen Mutation Database, a mutation database of gene loci encoding common and rare blood group antigens. Albert Einstein

Table 2.9 Causes of Apparent In Vivo Hemolysis

Immune Causes	ABO incompatibility
	Clinically significant alloantibody
	Anamnestic alloantibody response
	Autoimmune hemolytic anemia
	Cold agglutinin disease
	Hemolytic disease of the newborn
	Drug-induced hemolytic anemia
	Polyagglutination (sepsis T-active plasma)
	Paroxysmal cold hemoglobinuria
	Thrombotic thrombocytopenic hemolytic uremia syndrome (a microangiopathic process)
Nonimmune causes	
Mechanical	Poor sample collection
	Small-bore needle used for infusion
	Excessive pressure during infusion
	Malfunctioning blood warmer
	Donor blood exposed to excessive heat or cold
	Urinary catheter
	Crush trauma
	Prosthetic heart valves
	Aortic stenosis
	March hemoglobinuria
Microbial	Sepsis
	Malaria
	Contamination of donor blood
Chemical	Inappropriate solutions infused
	Drugs infused
	Serum phosphorus <0.2 mg/dL
	Water irrigation of bladder
	Azulfidine
	Dimethyl sulfoxide
	Venom (snake, bee, brown recluse spider)
	Certain herbal preparations, teas, enemas
Inherent red blood cell abnormalities	Paroxysmal nocturnal hemoglobinuria
	Sickle cell anemia
	Spherocytosis
	Hemoglobin H
	Glucose-6-phosphate dehydrogenase deficiency

College of Medicine of Yeshiva University in New York. Provides links to many other sites.

2. www.iccbba.com

   The website of the International Society of Blood Transfusion, with links to information about topics such as ISBT128.

3. www.iccbba.com/page25.htm

   The website for the ISBT Working Party on Terminology for Red Cell Surface Antigens.

4. www.aabb.org

   The website of the American Association of Blood Banks; is interactive and provides links to other sites.

5. www.bbts.org.uk

   The website of the British Blood Transfusion Society.

REFERENCES

1. Standards Committee of American Association of Blood Banks: Standards for Blood Banks and Transfusion Services, 19th ed. Bethesda, MD, American Association of Blood Banks, 1999.
2. Alberts B, Bray D, Lewis J, et al: Molecular Biology of the Cell, 3rd ed. New York, Garland Publishing, 1994.
3. Hoffman R, Benz EJ, Shattil SJ, et al (eds): Hematology: Basic Principles and Practice, 2nd ed. New York, Churchill Livingstone, 1995.
4. Paulson JC, Colley KJ: Glycosyltransferases: Structure, localization, and control of cell type-specific glycosylation. J Biol Chem 1989;264:17615–17618.
5. Anstee DJ, Gardner BG: The direct agglutination of red cells by IgG antibodies is dependent on the position of antigens relative to the lipid bilayer [abstract]. Transf Med 1991;1(Suppl 2):57.
6. Brecher M: Technical Manual, 14th ed. Bethesda, MD, American Association of Blood Banks, 2002.
7. Garratty G, Dzik WH, Issitt PD, et al: Terminology for blood group antigens and genes: Historical origins and guidelines in the new millennium. Transfusion 2000;40:477–489.
8. Reid ME, McManus K, Zelinski T: Chromosome location of genes encoding human blood groups. Transf Med Rev 1998;12:151–161.
9. Mollison PL, Engelfriet CP, Contreras M: Blood Transfusion in Clinical Medicine, 10th ed. Oxford, Blackwell Science, 1997.
10. Anstee DJ, Spring FA: Red cell membrane glycoproteins with a broad tissue distribution. Transf Med Rev 1989;3:13–23.
11. Southcott MJG, Tanner MJ, Anstee DJ: The expression of human blood group antigens during erythropoiesis in a cell culture system. Blood 1999;93:4425–4435.
12. Green CA, Daniels GL: Development of erythroid cell surface markers during in vitro erythropoiesis: A comparison of two methods [abstract]. Transf Med 1999;9(Suppl 1):9.
13. Lögdberg L, Reid ME, Miller JL: Cloning and genetic characterization of blood group carrier molecules and antigens. Transf Med Rev 2002;16:1–10.
14. Avent ND: Human erythrocyte antigen expression: Its molecular bases. Br J Biomed Sci 1997;54:16–37.
15. Issitt PD, Anstee DJ: Applied Blood Group Serology, 4th ed. Durham, NC, Montgomery Scientific Publications, 1998.
16. Reid ME, Lomas-Francis C: The Blood Group Antigen Facts Book. San Diego, Academic Press, 1996.
17. Reid ME, Yazdanbakhsh K: Molecular insights into blood groups and implications for blood transfusions. Curr Opin Hematol 1998;5:93–102.
18. Blancher A, Reid ME, Socha WW: Cross-reactivity of antibodies to human and primate red cell antigens. Transf Med Rev 2000;14:161–179.
19. Salvignol I, Calvas P, Socha WW, et al: Structural analysis of the RH-like blood group gene products in nonhuman primates. Immunogenetics 1995;41:271–281.
20. Huang C-H, Xie S-S, Socha WW, Blumenfeld OO: Sequence diversification and exon inactivation in glycophorin A gene family from chimpanzee to human. J Mol Evol 1995;41:478–486.
21. Xie SS, Huang C-H, Reid ME, et al: The glycophorin A gene family in gorillas: Structure, expression, and comparison with the human and chimpanzee homologues. Biochem Genet 1997;35:59–76.
22. Westhoff CM, Silberstein LE, Wylie DE: Evidence supporting the requirement for two proline residues for expression of the c. Transfusion 2000;40:321–324.
23. Roitt I, Brostoff J, Male D: Immunology, 4th ed. London, Mosby, 1996.
24. Giblett ER: A critique of the theoretical hazard of inter vs. intra-racial transfusion. Transfusion 1961;1:233–238.
25. Giblett ER: Blood group alloantibodies: An assessment of some laboratory practices. Transfusion 1977;4:299–308.
26. Hoeltge GA, Domen RE, Rybicki LA, Schaffer PA: Multiple red cell transfusions and alloimmunization: Experience with 6996 antibodies detected in a total of 159,262 patients from 1985 to 1993. Arch Pathol Lab Med 1995;119:42–45.
27. Reid ME, Øyen R, Marsh WL: Summary of the clinical significance of blood group alloantibodies. Semin Hematol 2000;37:197–216.
28. Regan F, Hewitt P, Vincent B, Nolan A: Do patients know they have been transfused? Vox Sang 1999;76:248–249.
29. Wayne AS, Kevy SV, Nathan DG: Transfusion management of sickle cell disease. Blood 1993;81:1109–1123.
30. Ness PM: To match or not to match: The question for chronically transfused patients with sickle cell anemia. Transfusion 1994;34:558–560.
31. Sosler SD, Jilly BJ, Saporito C, Koshy M: A simple, practical model for reducing alloimmunization in patients with sickle cell disease. Am J Hematol 1993;43:103–106.
32. Sausais L, Øyen R, Rios M, et al: DAK, a low incidence antigen shared by D^{IIIA} and R^N [abstract]. Transfusion 1999;39(Suppl 1):79S.
33. Beauregard P, Blajchman MA: Hemolytic and pseudo-hemolytic transfusion reactions: An overview of the hemolytic transfusion reactions and the clinical conditions that mimic them. Transf Med Rev 1994;8:184–199.

Chapter 3

ABO and Related Antigens

Constance M. Westhoff

Marion E. Reid

This chapter summarizes current knowledge of the blood groups composed of terminal carbohydrate moieties, the ABO, H, Lewis, Ii, and P systems (International Society of Blood Transfusion [ISBT] system or collection numbers given in parentheses). The antigens are the products of the action of glycosyltransferase enzymes, and they share biochemical synthesis pathways and precursor framework oligosaccharide molecules. The antigens are carried on large oligosaccharide chains covalently linked to proteins (glycoproteins), lipids (glycolipids), or both on the red blood cell (RBC). In addition, some are expressed on tissues, and soluble forms can be found in various secretions and excretions.

■ ABO and Hh Systems (ISBT Systems 001 and 018)

History

ABO was the first blood group system to be discovered. In 1900, Landsteiner mixed sera and RBCs from his colleagues and observed agglutination.[1] On the basis of the agglutination pattern, he named the first two blood group antigens A and B, using the first two letters of the alphabet. RBCs not agglutinated by either sera were first called type C but became known as "ohne A" and "ohne B" (*ohne* is German for "without") and finally O. Landsteiner received the Nobel Prize in 1930, 30 years after the discovery of the ABO blood groups.

Unfortunately, transfusion based on agglutination reactions was largely ignored, and surgeons continued performing direct donor-to-patient blood transfusions. This practice provided many opportunities to observe symptoms of severe and fatal hemolytic transfusion reactions. Not until methods were developed to store and preserve blood (1914–1917) did blood transfusion move to the blood bank environment, and World War I saw the first large-scale transfusions based on serologic ABO selection of donors.[2]

Antigens

The ABO antigens were biochemically characterized in the 1950s and 1960s (reviewed in Yamamoto[3]) as carbohydrate structures on glycoproteins and glycolipids. The ABO system consists of four antigens with ISBT numbers—A; B; A,B; and A$_1$—but there are additional subgroups (e.g., A$_2$, A$_3$, A$_X$, A$_{el}$, B$_3$), and Hh is a separate system.[4] The antigens are synthesized in a stepwise fashion by glycosyltransferase enzymes that sequentially add specific monosaccharide sugars in specific linkages to a growing oligosaccharide precursor chain. The terminal sugar determines antigen specificity: an *N*-acetylgalactosamine residue results in expression of A antigen, and a terminal galactose residue is responsible for the B antigen. These structures are similar, differing only in that A antigen has a substituted amino group on carbon 2 (Fig. 3.1). The precursor substrate for A and B antigens is the H antigen (Fig. 3.2). The terminal fucose in α(1,2) linkage to galactose is responsible for H antigen specificity, and large amounts of H are present on group O RBCs, because H is not converted to A or B. Some H antigen precursor also remains on A and B RBCs, listed as follows in descending order of frequency: A$_2$, B, A$_2$B, A$_1$, A$_1$B.

RBC membrane proteins carry well over 2×10^6 A, B, and H antigens (ABH) combined per RBC, and most (80%) are located on the major integral membrane protein, band 3 (anion exchanger 1, or AE1), which is the RBC anion exchanger. In addition, the glucose transporter Rh-associated glycoprotein (RhAG) and aquaporin-1 (Colton) also carry A, B, and H, but in smaller amounts (reviewed in Lowe[5]). A, B, and H antigens are also found in lesser amounts as lipid-linked glycoconjugates associated with the RBC membrane via a ceramide moiety.

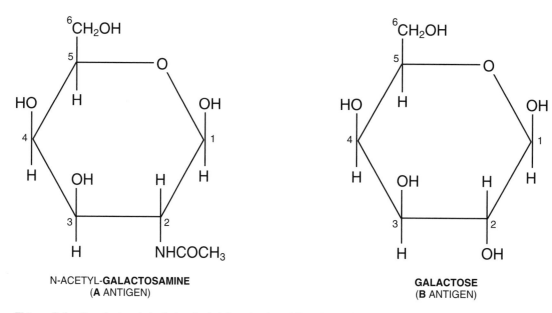

Figure 3.1   Terminal carbohydrates that define the A and B antigens. The terminal galactose residues differ only in that the A antigen has a substituted amino-acetyl group on carbon number two.

After their discovery on RBCs, the ABH antigens were also found on many tissues. Large amounts are expressed on endothelial and epithelial cells of the lung and gut, and the epithelial cells of the urinary and reproductive tracts; hence, they are called *histo–blood group antigens*. ABH antigens are also found in secretions (particularly saliva) and fluids (milk and urine) of 80% of the population who have the secretor (Se) phenotype.[6]

As tissue antigens, ABH are important in solid organ allotransplantation. Recipient antibodies react with antigens on the transplanted organ, and complement activation at the surface of endothelial cells results in rapid destruction and acute rejection.[7] However, successful transplantation across ABO barriers is possible, particularly with blood group A_2 to O, and with current immunosuppressive and pretreatment regimens (reviewed by Rydberg[8]).

The incidence of ABO blood groups differs in populations (Table 3.1).[9] Group B is found twice as frequently in African Americans and Asians as in white persons. Group A subgroups are more common than Group B subgroups, and A_2 has an average incidence of 20% of group A patients.[10] Subgroup A_2 is rare in Asians.

Inherited and Acquired ABH Antigen Variants

Subgroups of A and B have weaker expression of the respective antigens. The difference between A_1 and A_2 is quantitative,

because the number of A antigens is reduced on A_2. The difference is also qualitative, because there are structural differences in the branching of the oligosaccharide chains. The structural difference explains why $A_{subgroup}$ individuals often make anti-A_1. The reagent *Dolichos biflorus* lectin distinguishes A_1 from A_2 and other A subgroups. Acquired B antigen results from the action of bacterial deacetylase, an enzyme that can remove an acetyl group from the A-terminal sugar, *N*-acetylgalactosamine. Galactosamine is similar to galactose, the B-specific terminal residue, and anti-B reagents can cross-react with the deacetylated structure.[11] Acquired B usually occurs in individuals suffering from colon or rectal carcinoma, intestinal obstruction, or infections involving gram-negative bacteria from the gut. It is transient and, because the acquired B develops at the expense of A antigen, the phenotype is found only in group A patients.

A or B antigen expression can weaken in patients with acute leukemia or stress hematopoiesis. Chromosomal deletions and lesions that involve the ABO locus on chromosome 1 can result in the loss of transferase expression in the leukemic cell population. A decrease in A or B antigen expression, when found without a hematologic disorder, can be prognostic of a preleukemic state. In stress hematopoiesis, the higher turnover and early release from the bone marrow results in reduced branching of the carbohydrate chains, causing weakened expression.[12]

Rare "Bombay" phenotype RBCs (first reported in Bombay, India) lack H antigen, and consequently, without H precursor, they also lack A and B antigens. These RBCs type routinely as group O, designated O_h, and the serum contains potent anti-H in addition to anti-A and anti-B.[12, 13]

ABO Genes

In 1959, Watkins and Morgan[14] correctly suggested that the genes for the carbohydrate ABO determinants actually encoded enzymes responsible for the assembly of the subunits. The ABO locus encodes the A and B glycosyltransferases,

Table 3.1   ABO Blood Groups and Incidence

Phenotype	Incidence (%)		
	White	African American	Asian
A_1	34	19	27
A_2	10	8	Rare
B	9	19	25
A_1B	3	3	5
A_2B	1	1	Rare
O	44	49	43

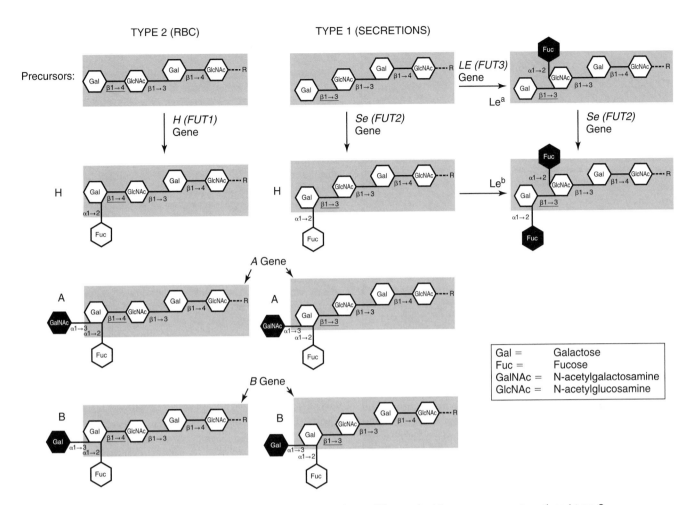

Figure 3.2 Synthesis of A, B, and H, and Lewis antigens. Oligosaccharide precursor core type 1 and type 2 structures differ only in the linkage between the terminal galactose (Gal) and the *N*-acetylglucosamine (GlcNAc), shown underscored. Terminal carbohydrates that define the antigens are shown in *black*.

which were mapped by linkage analysis to chromosome 9q34.[15] Researchers cloned the A-glycosyltransferase in 1990 by exploiting the fact that some tumors have increased expression of ABH antigens and the corresponding glycosyltransferase. Soluble enzyme was isolated from lung tissue for amino acid sequencing,[16] and complementary DNA (cDNA) libraries from gastric carcinoma and colon adenocarcinoma cell lines from individuals with different ABO phenotypes were screened and sequenced to determine the molecular differences among the transferases.[17, 18]

The ABO glycosyltransferase gene contains seven exons and spans approximately 18 to 20 kb.[19] It encodes a 354–amino acid, 41-kD transferase that has a short N-terminal region, a hydrophobic transmembrane segment for retention in the Golgi membrane, and a large C-terminal, catalytically active domain (Fig. 3.3). The glycosyltransferase enzymes are membrane-bound in the lumen of the Golgi,[20] and glycosylation of membrane proteins takes place during transit through the Golgi. Some soluble enzyme is also found in body fluids and plasma and is derived from the membrane-bound enzyme through proteolysis that cleaves the catalytic domain from the membrane-spanning domain.[21]

There are only four amino acid differences between A and B transferase in the catalytic domain. The last two differences,

residues 266 and 268, are primarily responsible for the substrate specificity (see Fig. 3.3).[18] The group O phenotype results from mutations in A or B alleles that cause a loss of glycosyltransferase activity. The most common group O (O$_1$) results from a single nucleotide deletion near the N-terminus of the gene that causes a frameshift mutation and early termination with no active enzyme production. A and B subgroups result from a variety of mutations that cause reduced activity of the glycosyltransferase. The rare B(A) and cis AB phenotypes result from variant glycosyltransferases that, at critical substrate selective positions, have a combination of A- and B-specific residues. For example, in cis AB (Fig. 3.4), the first substitution is identical to that described for the A$_2$ transferase (Leu156), and the second is that found in the B transferase (Ala268).[22] Many other mutations and variations in ABO alleles can cause weak ABO subgroups. Currently, 29 weak subgroup alleles have been reported[23]; however, current information is maintained on the Blood Group Antigen Mutation Database website (www.bioc.aecom.yu.edu/bgmut/abo_common.htm).

For additional information regarding the ABO blood group system, the interested reader is referred to Volume 11 of the journal *Transfusion Medicine*, which is dedicated to the ABO system.[24]

Figure 3.3 Model of the glycosyltransferases and their location in the lumen of the Golgi. Proteolytic cleavage, shown as scissors generates the soluble enzyme found in body fluids and plasma. The *boxed areas* on the A_2 and $O_{(1)}$ glycosyltransferases indicate the altered protein sequence that results from the frameshift gene mutations. (The O truncated enzyme probably does not reach the Golgi membrane.)

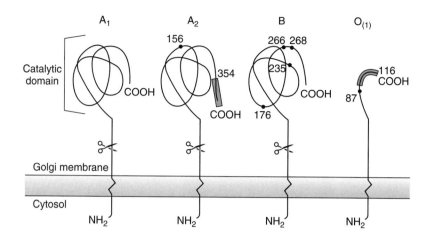

H (*FUT1*) and Secretor (*FUT2*) Genes

The biosynthesis of H antigen found on RBCs and epidermis and that found in secretions involves two different α(1,2)-fucosyltransferase enzymes encoded by two closely linked genes on chromosome 19q13.3,[25] *FUT1* and *FUT2*. These genes are also referred to as the *H* gene and the *Se* (secretor) gene. Both encode enzymes that add an H-specific fucose sugar to a precursor oligosaccharide core structure, but they act on different precursor structures. Four different core structures, all tetrasaccharides (4 sugars) with terminal galactose residues, are found in human cells, and these core structures differ among tissues.[5] Type 1 precursors are found in the acinar cells of salivary glands and the epithelial lining of the pulmonary, gastrointestinal, urinary, and reproductive tracts. Type 2 precursors are expressed by RBCs and other tissues.[5] These precursors are identical except for the terminal galactose linkage (see Fig. 3.2). H antigen is synthesized in RBCs when the *H* gene (*FUT1*)–encoded fucosyltransferase attaches a fucose via an α(1,2) linkage to the terminal galactose of type 2 precursor chains. H antigen in secretions is synthesized when the *Se* (Secretor, *FUT2*) gene–encoded fucosyltransferase attaches a fucose via an α(1,2) linkage to the terminal galactose on type 1 precursor chains in secretory tissues. The A and B glycosyltransferases do not discriminate type 1 or type 2 chains and add *N*-acetylgalactosamine (A) or galactose (B) sugars to H antigens on both (i.e., in secretions and on RBCs) (see Fig. 3.2).

H (*FUT1*) encodes a 365–amino acid, and *Se* (*FUT2*) encodes either a 332– or a 343–amino acid (there are two potential initiator codons) type II transmembrane protein. These genes are similar to A and B transferases in structure. They share 68% identity in a region of 292 amino acids and are clearly homologous. *H* (*FUT1*) is only 9 kb, and the coding region is contained in a single 1.1-kb exon.[26, 27]

Homozygosity for defective *Se* (*FUT2*) is responsible for the nonsecretor (sese) phenotype, which has an incidence of approximately 20%. At least six different mutations that cause loss of enzyme activity have been reported (reviewed in Spitalnik and Spitalnik[28]), and they vary among populations. In white persons, a nonsense mutation at nucleotide G428A (se428) is found, whereas a mutation at se571 is common in Asians, and se849 is found in Taiwanese. In addition, a normally functioning variant, designated *Se¹*, and a variant with reduced enzyme activity, *Se^W*, are found in Asians. (The reduced activity of the *Se^W* fucosyltransferase is responsible for the Le(a+b+) phenotype in Asians; see later.)

The majority of nonsecretors have at least one functional *H* (*FUT1*). The exceptions, who are homozygous for null alleles at both *H* (*FUT1*) and *Se* (*FUT2*) loci, have the Bombay phenotype. Because such people lack H antigen both in secretions and on RBCs, they make potent anti-H and must be transfused with RBCs from other Bombay people. In contrast, para-Bombay individuals are homozygous for null alleles at *H*

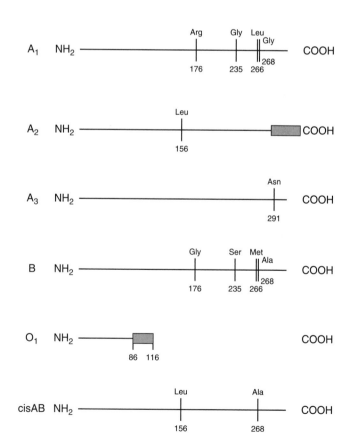

Figure 3.4 Representation of the amino acid sequence differences in the ABO glycosyltransferases. The *grey boxes* on the A_2 and O_1 glycosyltransferases indicate the altered protein sequence that results from the frameshift gene mutations.

Table 3.2 Comparison of H Antigen in Bombay, para-Bombay, and Normal Phenotypes

Phenotype	H Antigen		Predicted Genotype	Antibody
	Blood Cells	Secretion		
Common				
Secretor	H+	Yes	*HH*; *Hh*; *SeSe*; *Sese*	
Nonsecretor	H+	No	*HH*; *Hh*; *sese*	
H-deficient				
Bombay	H–	No	*hh*; *sese*	Anti-H
Para-Bombay	H weak	No	*(H)*; *sese*	Anti-H
Para-Bombay	H weak	Yes	*(H)*;*SeSe*; *Sese*	Anti-HI

(*FUT1*) but have at least one functional *Se* (*FUT2*) allele; they lack H antigen on their RBCs, but have H antigen in secretions (Table 3.2).[5] Those with a para-Bombay phenotype who are nonsecretors have clinically significant anti-H in their serum. More than 20 different mutations in *H* (*FUT1*) have been associated with Bombay and para-Bombay phenotypes (summarized by Costache and associates[29]).

Expression

ABO antigens are not fully developed at birth. Cord and infant RBCs have linear oligosaccharide structures with single termini to which the A, B, and H sugars can be added. Not until a person is approximately 2 to 4 years of age do complex branching oligosaccharide structures appear in the blood, which create additional termini. The antigens are then fully developed (and can accurately be tested for A_1 status) and remain fairly constant throughout life.[30–32] ABO-related hemolytic disease of the newborn (ABO-HDN) is usually mild because of the weaker RBC expression of A and B antigens and also because tissue expression provides additional antigen targets for maternal antibodies. Tissue expression of the ABO antigens varies during fetal development, but they are expressed on endothelial and epithelial cells of most organs and RBCs in 5- to 6-week-old embryos.[33]

A, B, and H antigens may be detected on lymphocytes of people with a secretor (*Se*) gene as a result of adsorption from the plasma as glycolipids. In contrast, platelets also contain A-, B-, and H-transferases, making A, B, and H antigens intrinsic on platelet glycoproteins.[34] Thus, ABO incompatibility can compromise the outcome in platelet transfusions.[10, 10a]

Evolution

The ABH antigens appear earlier on epithelial cells than on blood cells,[35] so they may have, or may have had, functions in early development. ABO antigens appear on the RBCs of nonhuman primates—chimpanzee, gorilla, orangutan, gibbon, baboon, and several species of Old and New World monkeys.[36] Therefore, the ABO polymorphism has been maintained from species to species for more than 37 million years,[37] suggesting that there must be some importance to maintaining variation in ABO types. Primate studies reveal that the oldest common ancestral gene is A and that B alleles have arisen from the ancestral A alleles on at least three independent occasions.[38] However, the nonfunctional O allele has become one of the most common alleles and is even fixed in some South American populations. Nonfunctional or null alleles are expected to remain rare, unless they confer a selective advantage. Why the null allele evolved can only be speculated upon at present, but the presence in group O individuals of natural antibodies against A and B determinants may have offered important protection against bacteria and parasites[38] or even smallpox.[39]

Antibodies

Anti-A and anti-B are found in the sera of individuals who lack the corresponding antigens. They are produced in response to environmental stimulants, such as bacteria, and have therefore been termed "natural" antibodies.[40–42] Antibody production begins after birth, reaching a peak at 5 to 10 years of age and declining with increasing age. The carbohydrate antigens elicit an immune response that is mainly thymus-independent, so the antibodies formed are mostly immunoglobulin M (IgM). IgM antibodies activate complement, which, in conjunction with the high density of ABO antigen sites on RBCs, is responsible for the severe, life-threatening transfusion reactions that may be caused by ABO-incompatible transfusions.

HDN caused by ABO antibodies is usually mild, for the following three reasons: (1) placental transfer is limited to the fraction of IgG anti-A and anti-B found in maternal serum, (2) fetal ABO antigens are not fully developed,[43] and (3) ABO tissue antigens provide additional targets for the antibodies. ABO-HDN is most often seen in non–group O infants of group O mothers, because anti-A, anti-B, and anti-A,B of group O mothers often has a significant IgG component.

Potent anti-H (along with anti-A and anti-B) found in O_h (Bombay) or para-Bombay nonsecretors destroys transfused RBCs of any ABO group, so these individuals must be transfused only with blood of the Bombay phenotype.[44] In contrast, anti-H in non-Bombay individuals is usually IgM and clinically insignificant. Anti-IH is not uncommonly found in patient sera and is usually IgM; compatible blood is easily found among donors of identical ABO type.[10, 45]

Enzyme-Converted O Cells (ECO)

Blood group O is considered the "universal donor" because it can be transfused to patients of all ABO types. Therefore, enzymes that remove terminal carbohydrates from the nonreducing end of carbohydrate chains could be used to remove terminal A and B sugars in order to convert the blood supply to all universal group O units. An enzyme from coffee beans, α-galactosidase, has been the most successful at removing galactose to convert blood group B to group O. RBCs treated in this manner have normal survival when transfused to group B, A, or O recipients.[46] Removal of *N*-acetylgalactosamine to convert group A to group O has been much more problematic, owing to the inaccessibility of the carbohydrates on internal branching chains, especially those found on A_1 cells. Currently, the procedures required to convert B to O, which include exposure to low pH followed by numerous washings, make them impractical for general use, but this is an active area of research.[47, 48]

■ The Lewis System (ISBT System 007)

History

The Lewis system, first reported in 1946 by Mourant,[49] was named after the first patient to make the antibody. What was thought at the time to be the antithetical antigen was found in 1948, and the designations Le[a] and Le[b] were applied at a later time.[13] We now know that these antigens are not antithetical, because they are not products of alternative forms of a single gene. Rather, they result from the sequential action of two fucosyltransferases encoded at independent loci (*LE-FUT3* and *Se-FUT2*).

Antigens

Lewis antigens, unlike antigens of all other blood group systems except Chido/Rodgers, are not intrinsic to the RBC but are synthesized in the intestinal epithelial cells. Lewis antigens circulate in plasma while bound to glycosphingolipids and are passively adsorbed onto RBCs.[50, 51]

There are four Lewis phenotypes—Le(a+b−), Le(a−b+), Le(a−b−) and Le(a+b+). African Americans have a higher incidence of the Le(a−b−) phenotype, and Le(a+b+) is very rare in white persons and African Americans but not uncommon in Asians (Table 3.3).

Le[a] and Le[b] are synthesized in a stepwise manner by two transferase enzymes that add fucose residues only to type 1 chains, which are found in secretions but not in RBCs (see Fig. 3.2). The nature and substrate specificity of the enzymes have been elucidated only recently. The α(1,4)-fucosyltransferase encoded by *LE* (*FUT3*) catalyses the addition of a fucose to carbon 4 of the subterminal *N*-acetylglucosamine (GlcNAc) residue of the type 1 precursor chains, creating the Le[a] structure (see Fig. 3.2). (Note that this transferase cannot act similarly on the type 2 chains found on RBCs, because they already have Gal on carbon 4 of the subterminal GlcNAc, which blocks the acceptor site; this fact explains why the Lewis antigens are not synthesized in RBCs).

The Le[a] structure remains unchanged, resulting in the Le(a+b−) phenotype, unless the individual is a secretor (*Se-FUT2*). In the presence of the α(1,2)-fucosyltransferase encoded by the secretor locus (discussed previously), the Le[a] structure is

converted to Le[b] by the addition of a fucose residue to carbon 2 of the terminal galactose residue on the same chain. Le[b] antigen is synthesized at the expense of Le[a] antigen, resulting in the Le(a−b+) phenotype. This finding explains early observations that (1) individuals with RBCs that typed as Le(b+) were secretors of ABH substance, (2) those with Le(a+) RBCs were nonsecretors, and (3) individuals with Le(a−b−) RBCs could be either secretors or nonsecretors of ABH. Ninety percent of white persons inherit normal *LE* (*FUT3*), and 80% carry a functional *Se* (*FUT2*), accounting for the prevalence of the Le(a−b+) phenotype in the white population (see Table 3.3).[5, 39]

Le(a−b−) arises from homozygous defects in *LE* (*FUT3*), regardless of the *Se* (*FUT2*). Le(a+b+) individuals have weak expression of both Le[a] and Le[b] and are sometimes called "partial secretors." They have reduced α(1,2)-fucosyltransferase activity, and the molecular basis for the phenotype has been determined (see later).

Genes

The gene responsible for Lewis carbohydrates, *LE* (*FUT3*), located on the short arm of chromosome 19 (19p13.3), has been cloned and encodes a 361–amino acid, type II membrane-bound enzyme.[52] It is one of the series of genes, all located on chromosome 19, that encode fucosyltransferases. The long arm of chromosome 19 is the location for both the secretor gene *Se* (*FUT2*)—which not only determines ABH secretor status but also interacts with *LE* (*FUT3*) to synthesize Le[b] antigens—and the *H* gene (*FUT1*)—which is responsible for H antigen on RBCs.

Le(a−b+) individuals have a least one functional *LE* (*FUT3*) and *Se* (*FUT2*), and are secretors of ABH antigens. Le(a+b−) individuals have at least one functional *LE* (*FUT3*), and this phenotype identifies the 20% of individuals with defective *Se* (*FUT2*) (see discussion of the ABO system). Le(a+b+), found in relatively high prevalence in Taiwan, results from inheritance of *Se[w]*, which encodes an amino acid change in the catalytic domain resulting in reduced activity of the enzyme encoded by *Se* (*FUT2*). Le(a−b−) individuals have point mutations in the *LE* (*FUT3*) gene (*le/le*). At least six different defective alleles (*le[1]-le[6]*) have been reported, and mutations at nucleotides 508, 1067, and 202 severely reduce or inactivate the fucosyltransferase (summarized by Spitalnik and Spitalnik[28]). A mutation at nucleotide 59 results in an amino acid change in the transmembrane domain, which does not affect the enzyme activity but may affect the Golgi localization. This mutation is responsible for the paradoxical Le(a−b−) RBC phenotype in people with Lewis antigens in their saliva.[53]

Expression

Lewis antigens are not expressed on cord RBCs. Lewis antigen levels on RBCs are often diminished during pregnancy, possibly due to pregnancy-associated changes in plasma lipoproteins.[54] Lewis antigens are also found on lymphocytes and platelets (secondarily adsorbed from the plasma), on other tissues, including pancreas, stomach, intestine, skeletal muscle, renal cortex, and adrenal glands, and in soluble form in saliva as glycoproteins. Lewis antigens may be of some consequence in renal allografts. Graft survival has been reported to be reduced in patients who lack Lewis antigens, but this issue is controversial.[12] The Le[b] antigen may be a receptor for *Helicobacter pylori,* a feature that could explain the association of gastric ulcers and secretor status.[55, 56]

Table 3.3 Lewis Blood Group Phenotypes and Incidence

Phenotype	Incidence (%)		
	White	African	Asian
Le(a−b+)	72	55	72
Le(a+b−)	22	23	22
Le(a−b−)	6	22	6
Le(a+b+)	Rare	Rare	3

Antibodies

Lewis antibodies are primarily IgM and are usually not clinically significant. Lewis antibodies often complicate antibody identification when multiple antibodies are present, but they are easy to inhibit with saliva (made isotonic) from secretors or with commercially prepared Lewis substance. Lewis antibodies occur in the sera of Le(a–b–) persons and may be naturally occurring.[10]

Rare hemolytic transfusion reactions, due to transfusion of Le(a+) RBCs to recipients with anti-Le[a], have been reported.[57] Because Le(a–) RBCs are found in almost 80% of donors, it is easy to select Le(a–) RBCs for transfusion to recipients with anti-Le[a] when the antibody is reactive at 37°C.[58] Because Lewis antigens are not intrinsic to the RBC membrane and are present in plasma, selection of Le(b–) RBCs is unnecessary for recipients with anti-Le[b], because Lewis antigens in donor plasma readily neutralize Lewis antibodies in transfusion recipients.[50]

The intimate relationship between Lewis and ABH antigens is revealed by antibodies such as anti-Le[bH], which reacts best with O Le(b+) cells. Crossmatching ABO-identical RBCs (rather than O) usually provides compatible blood. Anti-Le[bA] reacts best with A Le(b+) cells. These antibodies are IgM and not clinically significant.

Anti-Le[a] and anti-Le[b] are not known to cause HDN, because they are usually IgM, and because fetal RBCs type as Le(a–b–).[10]

■ The Ii Blood Group Collection (ISBT Collection 207)

History

In 1956, Wiener and colleagues[59] described the I antigen after making an intense study of a particularly severe case of hemolysis, or cold hemagglutinin disease (CHAD or CAD), due to anti-I. They used the symbol I to emphasize the high degree of *i*ndividuality of RBCs failing to react with the patient's serum at room temperature. Because the patient's serum was only weakly reactive in vitro with bovine RBCs, she was transfused with a small volume of bovine RBCs, but an anaphylactic-type reaction discouraged Wiener and colleagues[59] from further attempts to transfuse bovine RBCs.

Antigens

I and i antigens, which are synthesized on RBCs, are subterminal portions of the same carbohydrate chains that carry ABH antigens. Biosynthesis requires the sequential action of β-3-N-acetylglucosaminyltransferase and β-4-galactosyltransferase.[12] I and i are not allelic; rather, they differ in their branching structure. The i antigen, found predominantly on fetal and infant RBCs, is characterized by disaccharide units (Gal-GlcNAc) linked in a straight chain.[60] During the first 2 years of life, many of these linear chains are modified into branched chains,[30] resulting in the appearance of I antigens, found predominantly on adult RBCs. I specificity develops at the expense of i antigens when the branched structures appear.

Gene

The gene responsible for I antigen synthesis is thought to be *IGnt*, which is located on chromosome 6p24. The I locus

has not been unequivocally identified, however, because several genes at different locations have been identified as I branch–forming enzymes.[61] The gene encodes β(1,6)-N-acetylglucosaminyltransferase, a 400–amino acid, type II membrane protein similar in structure to other glycosyltransferases.[62] This enzyme is responsible for the branching synthesis of I antigen and so is probably developmentally regulated. The adult i phenotype is associated with a Gly348Glu or Arg383His mutation, or a gene deletion.[61]

Expression

Adult RBCs express predominantly I antigens and little or no i antigen, whereas newborn infant RBCs have strong expression of i antigens and small amounts of I antigen.[63] Adult RBCs vary in the amount of I antigen. I and i can also be found on lymphocytes and platelets. The I and i antigens are referred to by some as "histo-blood group antigens" because, like ABH antigens, they are not restricted to RBCs but are found on most cells and in various body fluids.[12] Many conditions that result in stress hematopoiesis result in altered I and i antigen expression; typically, I expression is weakened but i expression is enhanced.

Antibodies

The sera of all individuals contain anti-I as a common autoantibody that is reactive at or below room temperature and is usually benign. These autoantibodies are commonly referred to as *cold agglutinins*. If the autoantibody is reactive at room temperature, problems in compatibility testing may result, but prewarming components and testing at 37°C easily circumvents them.[64] Even in patients undergoing hypothermia during surgical procedures, there are no reports of anti-I causing RBC destruction. Alloanti-I made by the rare i adult phenotype is clinically significant and causes destruction of transfused I+ RBCs.

In contrast, CHAD is characterized by high titers of monoclonal anti-I antibodies, which cause in vivo hemolysis and hemolytic anemia. These pathologic autoantibodies often react at 30°C in albumin and can fix complement.[65] The autologous circulating RBCs of a patient with CHAD are often strongly coated with complement component C3d, making them relatively resistant to destruction. In contrast, when donor RBCs are transfused to a patient with CHAD, they may be rapidly destroyed by circulating antibody. If transfusion cannot be avoided, donor RBCs should be transfused through a blood warmer.[10]

The titer and thermal range of anti-I are often increased after infection with *Mycoplasma pneumoniae*.[11] Approximately 50% of patients with infectious mononucleosis may have transient anti-i in their sera, but less than 1% have hemolysis.[66] Transient autoanti-i can occur in patients with lymphoproliferative disorders (e.g., Hodgkin's disease).

■ The P System (ISBT System 003) and GLOB Collection (ISBT Collection 209)

History

The P blood group system was first discovered by Landsteiner and Levine[67] in 1927 after they injected rabbits with human RBCs. The first antigen discovered in this system appeared to be present on all human RBCs. It was named the P antigen because this was the first letter after M, N and O, which had already been used. This antigen, present in 79% of white people, was renamed P₁; according to current ISBT terminology, however, the name is now written as P1, whereas P_1 denotes the P1+ phenotype.[4, 13] This chapter uses the more familiar P_1 terminology. Other related antigens P, P^k, and LKE have been assigned to the GLOB collection because, although they are related biochemically to the P_1 antigen, their genetic association is still unclear. The P system glycosyltransferase genes are the last of the carbohydrate blood group transferases to be cloned.

Antigens

The P_1, P, and P^k blood group antigens are defined by sugars added to precursor glycosphingolipids and are not found on glycoproteins. Biosynthesis occurs by the sequential addition of monosaccharides to a precursor substrate catalyzed by glycosyltransferases. Two pathways are involved in the production of these antigens from a common precursor, galactose β(1,4)-glucose-ceramide, also called lactosylceramide (Fig. 3.5). In one pathway, lactosylceramide is converted to P^k (also called CD77), an antigen of very high incidence that is the precursor structure for synthesis of P. P is produced by the action of a second enzyme, and P antigen is found on all RBCs except the rare p and P^k phenotypes.

P antigen is a cellular receptor for the B19 parvovirus, which causes fifth disease, a common childhood illness, and occasionally can cause more severe disorders of erythropoiesis. The virus causes both transient aplastic crises in patients with underlying hemolysis and anemia in immunocompromised patients.[68] Individuals with the p phenotype lack both P and P^k and are naturally resistant to parvovirus B19 infection. P^k (CD77) is present on epithelial cells and immature B cells in the germinal center and is a receptor molecule for Shiga-like toxins from *Escherichia coli* 0157.[69] LKE antigen is formed when two additional carbohydrate residues (galactose and sialic acid) are added to P (see Fig. 3.5).

Table 3.4 P Blood Group System Phenotypes and Incidence

Phenotypes	Incidence (%)		Antigens
	Caucasians	African Americans	
P_1	79	94	P_1, P, P^{k*}
P_2	21	6	P, P^{k*}
P_1^k	Very rare	Very rare	P_1, P^k
P_2^k	Very rare	Very rare	P^k
P	Very rare	Very rare	None

P^{k*} is difficult to detect on these cells because it is converted to P.

In the second pathway, lactosylceramide is converted to P_1 antigen. The biochemical pathway is not completely established, and whether the same α(1–4)-galactosyltransferase gene is responsible for synthesis of both P^k and P_1 antigens is debated.

Reports have suggested that P_1 antigen is a receptor for uropathogenic strains of *E. coli* and that P_1 on urinary tract tissue allows the bacteria to bind to and ascend the urinary tract more easily.[39]

The RBC phenotypes that carry various combinations of these antigens are shown in Table 3.4.

P_1 and P_2 phenotypes are common. Among white persons, 21% are P_1-negative, but the incidence of P_1-negative people is greater in Southeast Asian populations; 80% of Cambodians and Vietnamese are P_1-negative. The "null" phenotype is p.

Genes

The cloning of the *a4Gal-T* transferase gene from the chromosome 22 region, where P_1 is linked, revealed that this gene actually encodes P^k synthetase activity.[70] The p phenotype is due to alterations and mutations in this *a4Gal-T* transferase gene.[71] The molecular basis of the P1 blood group polymorphism is as yet unknown.

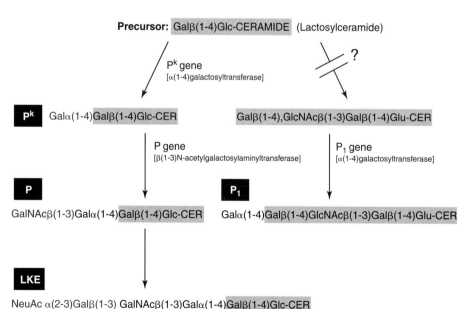

Figure 3.5 Biosynthesis of the P_1, P^k, P, and LKE antigens. Glc, glucose; CER, ceramide.

Expression

P_1 antigen is considerably weaker in children than in adults, and its expression does not reach adult level until 7 years of age. However, P_1 antigen is more strongly expressed on fetal RBCs than on neonatal RBCs, and P_1 expression weakens as the fetus ages. RBCs from different people show variation in the strength of the P_1 antigen, which can be seen during analysis of panel results in the identification of anti-P_1. P_1 and P are also expressed on lymphocytes, granulocytes, and monocytes.[12]

P_1 antigens are expressed in a wide variety of organisms, including bacteria, nematodes, earthworms, liver flukes, pigeons, and tapeworms.[12]

Antibodies

P_1-negative individuals frequently produce anti-P_1. This cold-reactive IgM antibody does not cross the placenta and has rarely been reported to cause hemolysis in vivo.[72] Like Lewis antibodies, anti-P_1 can often complicate antibody identification when multiple antibodies are present. However, anti-P_1 antibodies are easily neutralized with commercially prepared P_1 substance. Hydatid cyst fluid, *Echinococcus* cyst fluid, or pigeon egg white may be used. Anti-P^k is also neutralized by these substances.

Persons with the very rare p phenotype lack P_1, P and P^k antigens and may produce anti-P,P_1,P^k (anti-Tj^a), a potent hemolytic IgM antibody that can cause immediate hemolytic transfusion reactions.[10,13] In women with the p, P_1^k, or P_2^k phenotypes, cytotoxic IgM and IgG3 antibodies directed against P antigens, P^k antigens, or both are associated with a higher than normal rate of spontaneous abortions.[12,73]

Autoanti-P, the Donath-Landsteiner autoantibody, is found in patients with paroxysmal cold hemoglobinuria (PCH) and in some patients with acquired immune hemolytic anemia.[74] The autoantibody, complement-fixing IgG, is a biphasic hemolysin that binds to RBCs in the cold and then hemolyzes them when warmed. Thus, the patient's serum causes hemolysis of RBCs that have been first incubated in melting ice and then incubated at 37°C.[75] This antibody should be considered when the patient has hemoglobinuria and C3 alone is present on the RBCs. Transfusion is seldom required in PCH, because the anemia is usually transient. P-negative blood is rare, and P-positive blood has been used successfully for transfusion in patients with severe anemia.[10]

■ Summary

Despite the clinical relevance, especially of the ABO blood groups, the physiologic function of the carbohydrate antigens is unclear. The fact that some microbes and parasites use the carbohydrate blood group determinants as receptors certainly may contribute to their variation but does not shed light on their function. Specific interactions between cells might involve the blood group portions of cell surface glycoconjugates. Certainly, the carbohydrate structures on RBCs are important to impart the net negative charge on the membrane, keeping RBCs from adhering to one another and to the extracellular matrix. However, at present, the specific function of these carbohydrate molecules is unknown.

REFERENCES

1. Landsteiner K: Zur Kenntnis der antifermentativen, lytischen und agglutinierenden Wirkungen des Blutserums und der Lymphe. Zbl Bakt 1900;27:357.
2. Hess JR, Schmidt PJ: The first blood banker: Oswald Hope Robertson. Transfusion 2000;40:110–113.
3. Yamamoto F: Molecular genetics of the ABO histo-blood group system. Vox Sang 1995;69:1–7.
4. Daniels GL, Anstee DJ, Cartron J-P, et al: Blood group terminology 1995: ISBT working party on terminology for red cell surface antigens. Vox Sang 1995;69:265–279.
5. Lowe JB: The blood group-specific human glycosyltransferases. Baillieres Clin Haematol 1993;6:465–492.
6. Clausen H, Hakomori S: ABH and related histo-blood group antigens: Immunochemical differences in carrier isotypes and their distribution. Vox Sang 1989;56:1–20.
7. Platt JL, Bach FH: The barrier to xenotransplantation. Transplantation 1991;52:937–947.
8. Rydberg L: ABO-incompatibility in solid organ transplantation. Transfus Med 2001;11:325–342.
9. Wallace ME, Gibbs FL (eds): Blood Group Systems: ABH and Lewis. Arlington, VA, American Association of Blood Banks, 1986.
10. Mollison PL, Engelfriet CP, Contreras M: Blood Transfusion in Clinical Medicine, 10th ed. Oxford, Blackwell Science, 1997.
10a. Curtis BR, Edwards JT, Hessner MJ, et al: Blood group A and B antigens are strongly expressed on platelets of some individuals. Blood 96:1574–1581.
11. Gerbal A, Maslet C, Salmon C: Immunological aspects of the acquired B antigen. Vox Sang 1975;28:398–403.
12. Daniels G: Human Blood Groups. Oxford, Blackwell Science, 1995.
13. Race RR, Sanger R: Blood Groups in Man, 6th ed. Oxford, Blackwell Scientific, 1975.
14. Watkins WM, Morgan WTJ: Possible genetical pathways for the biosynthesis of blood group mucopolysaccharides. Vox Sang 1959;4:97–119.
15. Ferguson-Smith MA, Aitken DA, Turleau C, de Grouchy J: Localisation of the human ABO: Np-1: AK-1 linkage group by regional assignment of AK-1 to 9q34. Hum Genet 1976;34:35–43.
16. Clausen H, White T, Takio K, et al: Isolation to homogeneity and partial characterization of a histo-blood group A defined Fucα1→2Galα1→3-N-acetylgalactosaminyltransferase from human lung tissue. J Biol Chem 1990;265:1139–1145.
17. Yamamoto F, Clausen H, White T, et al: Molecular genetic basis of the histo-blood group ABO system. Nature 1990;345:229–235.
18. Yamamoto F, Hakomori S: Sugar-nucleotide donor specificity of histo-blood group A and B transferases is based on amino acid substitutions. J Biol Chem 1990;265:19257–19262.
19. Yamamoto F, McNeill PD, Hakomori S: Genomic organization of human histo-blood group ABO genes. Glycobiology 1995;5:51–58.
20. Paulson JC, Colley KJ: Glycosyltransferases: Structure, localization, and control of cell type-specific glycosylation. J Biol Chem 1989;264:17615–17618.
21. Watkins WM: Biochemistry and genetics of the ABO, Lewis, and P blood group systems. Adv Hum Genet 1980;10:1–136.
22. Yamamoto F-I: Review: Recent progress in the molecular genetic study of the histo-blood group ABO system. Immunohematology 1994;10:1–7.
23. Olsson ML, Irshaid NM, Hosseini-Maaf B, et al: Genomic analysis of clinical samples with serologic ABO blood grouping discrepancies: Identification of 15 novel A and B subgroup alleles. Blood 2001;98:1585–1593.
24. Commemoration of the centenary of the discovery of the ABO blood group system. Transfus Med 2001;11: number 4 pp. 243–351.
25. Ball SP, Tongue N, Gibaud A, et al: The human chromosome 19 linkage group FUT1 (H), FUT2 (SE), LE, LU, PEPD, C3, APOC2, D19S7 and D19S9. Ann Hum Genet 1991;55:225–233.
26. Kelly RJ, Rouquier S, Giorgi D, et al: Sequence and expression of a candidate for the human secretor blood group α(1,2)-fucosyltransferase gene (FUT2). J Biol Chem 1995;270:4640–4649.
27. Larsen RD, Ernst LK, Nair RP, Lowe JB: Molecular cloning, sequence, and expression of a human GDP-L-fucose:beta-D-galactoside 2-alpha-L-fucosyltransferase cDNA that can form the H blood group antigen. Proc Natl Acad Sci U S A 1990;87:6674–6678.

28. Spitalnik PF, Spitalnik SL: Human blood group antigens and antibodies. Part 1: Carbohydrate determinants. In Hoffman R, Benz EJ, Shattil SJ, et al (eds): Hematology: Basic Principles and Practice. Philadelphia, Churchill Livingstone, 2000, pp 2188–2196.

29. Costache M, Cailleau A, Fernandez-Mateos P, et al: Advances in molecular genetics of alpha-2- and alpha-3/4-fucosyltransferases. Transfus Clin Biol 1997;4:367–382.

30. Hakomori S: Blood group ABH and Ii antigens of human erythrocytes: Chemistry, polymorphism, and their developmental change. Semin Hematol 1981;18:39–62.

31. Witebsky E, Engasser LM: Blood groups and subgroups of the newborn. I: The A factor of the newborn. J Immunol 1949;61:171.

32. Watanabe K, Hakomori S: Status of blood group carbohydrate chains in ontogenesis and oncogenesis. J Exp Med 1976;144:644–653.

33. Szulman AE: The histological distribution of the blood group substances in man as disclosed by immunofluorescence. IV: The ABH antigens in embryos at the fifth week post fertilization. Hum Pathol 1971;2:575–585.

34. Cartron J-P, Mulet C, Bauvois B, et al: ABH and Lewis glycosyltransferases in human red cells, lymphocytes and platelets. Rev Fr Transfus 1980;23:271–282.

35. Hakomori S, Kobata EA: Blood group antigens. In Sela M (ed): The Antigens, vol 2. San Diego, Academic Press, 1975, pp 79–140.

36. Moor-Jankowski J, Wiener AS, Rogers CR: Human blood group factors in non-human primates. Nature 1964;202:663–665.

37. Martinko JM, Vincek V, Klein D, Klein J: Primate ABO glycosyltransferases: Evidence for trans-species evolution. Immunogenetics 1993;37:274–278.

38. Saitou N, Yamamoto F: Evolution of primate ABO blood group genes and their homologous genes. Mol Biol Evol 1997;14:399–411.

39. Issitt PD, Anstee DJ: Applied Blood Group Serology, 4th ed. Durham, NC, Montgomery Scientific, 1998.

40. Springer GF, Horton RE, Forbes M: Origin of anti-human blood group B agglutinins in white leghorn chicks. J Exp Med 1959;110:221.

41. Thomsen O: Immunisierung von Menschen mit Antigenem Gruppenfremden Blute. Z Rassenphysiol 1930;2:105.

42. Baumgarten A, Kruchok AH, Weirich F: High frequency of IgG anti-A and -B antibody in old age. Vox Sang 1976;30:253–260.

43. Romans DG, Tilley CA, Dorrington KJ: Monogamous bivalency of IgG antibodies. I: Deficiency of branched ABHI-active oligosaccharide chains on red cells of infants causes the weak antiglobulin reactions in hemolytic disease of the newborn due to ABO incompatibility. J Immunol 1980;124:2807–2811.

44. Davey RJ, Tourault MA, Holland PV: The clinical significance of anti-H in an individual with the O$_h$ (Bombay) phenotype. Transfusion 1978;18:738–742.

45. Vengelen-Tyler V: Technical Manual, 13th ed. Bethesda, MD, American Association of Blood Banks, 1999.

46. Goldstein J, Siviglia G, Hurst R, et al: Group B erythrocytes enzymatically converted to group O survive normally in A, B, and O individuals. Science 1982;215:168–170.

47. Lenny LL, Hurst R, Goldstein J, Galbraith RA: Transfusions to group O subjects of 2 units of red cells enzymatically converted from group B to group O. Transfusion 1994;34:209–214.

48. Lenny LL, Hurst R, Zhu A, et al: Multiple-unit and second transfusions of red cells enzymatically converted from group B to group O: Report on the end of Phase 1 trials. Transfusion 1995;35:899–902.

49. Mourant AE: A "new" human blood group antigen of frequent occurrence. Nature 1946;158:237–238.

50. Sneath JS, Sneath PHA: Transformation of the Lewis groups of human red cells. Nature 1955;176:172.

51. Marcus DM, Cass LE: Glycosphingolipids with Lewis blood group activity: Uptake by human erythrocytes. Science 1969;164:553–555.

52. Kukowska-Latallo JF, Larsen RD, Nair RP, Lowe JB: A cloned human cDNA determines expression of a mouse state-specific embryonic antigen and the Lewis blood group α(1,3/1,4)-fucosyltransferase. Genes Dev 1990;4:1288–1303.

53. Mollicone R, Reguigne I, Kelly RJ, et al: Molecular basis for Lewis alpha(1,3/1,4)-fucosyltransferase gene deficiency (FUT3) found in Lewis-negative Indonesian pedigrees. J Biol Chem 1994;269:20987–20994.

54. Hammar L, Mansson S, Rohr T, et al: Lewis phenotype of erythrocytes and Le^b-active glycolipid in serum of pregnant women. Vox Sang 1981;40:27–33.

55. Boren T, Falk P, Roth KA, et al: Attachment of *Helicobacter pylori* to human gastric epithelium mediated by blood group antigens. Science 1993;262:1892–1895.

56. Clyne M, Drumm B: Absence of effect of Lewis A and Lewis B expression on adherence of *Helicobacter pylori* to human gastric cells. Gastroenterology 1997;113:72–80.

57. Waheed A, Kennedy MS, Gerhan S, Senhauser DA: Transfusion significance of Lewis system antibodies. Am J Clin Pathol 1981;76:294–298.

58. Issitt PD: Antibodies reactive at 30°C, room temperature and below. In American Association of Blood Banks: Clinically Significant and Insignificant Antibodies. Washington, DC, American Association of Blood Banks, 1979, pp 13–28.

59. Wiener AS, Unger LJ, Cohen L, Feldman J: Type-specific cold auto-antibodies as a cause of acquired hemolytic anemia and hemolytic transfusion reactions: Biologic test with bovine red cells. Ann Intern Med 1956;44:221–240.

60. Feizi T: The blood group Ii system: A carbohydrate antigen system defined by naturally monoclonal or oligoclonal autoantibodies of man. Immunol Commun 1981;10:127–156.

61. Yu L-C, Twu Y-C, Chang C-Y, Lin M: Molecular basis of the adult i phenotype and the gene responsible for the expression of the human blood group I antigen. Blood 2001;98:3840–3845.

62. Bierhuizen MF, Mattei MG, Fukuda M: Expression of the developmental I antigen by a cloned human cDNA encoding a member of a beta-1,6-N-acetylglucosaminyltransferase gene family. Genes Dev 1993;7:468–478.

63. Marsh WL: Anti-i: A cold antibody defining the Ii relationship in human red cells. Br J Haematol 1961;7:200–208.

64. Issitt PD, Jackson VA: Useful modifications and variations of technics in work on I system antibodies. Vox Sang 1968;15:152–153.

65. Garratty G, Petz LD, Hoops JK: The correlation of cold agglutinin titrations in saline and albumin with haemolytic anaemia. Br J Haematol 1977;35:587–595.

66. Worlledge SM, Dacie JV: Haemolytic and other anaemias in infectious mononucleosis. In Carter RL, Penman HG (eds): Infectious Mononucleosis. Oxford, Blackwell Scientific, 1969, pp 82–89.

67. Landsteiner K, Levine P: Further observations on individual differences of human blood. Proc Soc Exp Biol Med 1927;24:941.

68. Luban NL: Human parvoviruses: Implications for transfusion medicine [review]. Transfusion 1994;34:821–827.

69. Karmali MA: Infection by verocytotoxin-producing *Escherichia coli*. Clin Microbiol Rev 1989;2:15–38.

70. Steffensen R, Carlier K, Wiels J, et al: Cloning and expression of the histo-blood group P^k UDP-galactose:Ga1β-4G1cβ1-cer α1, 4-galactosyltransferase: Molecular genetic basis of the p phenotype. J Biol Chem 2000;275:16723–16729.

71. Furukawa K, Iwamura K, Uchikawa M, et al: Molecular basis for the p phenotype: Identification of distinct and multiple mutations in the alpha 1,4-galactosyltransferase gene in Swedish and Japanese individuals. J Biol Chem 2000;275:37752–37756.

72. Chandeysson PL, Flye MW, Simpkins SM, Holland PV: Delayed hemolytic transfusion reaction caused by anti-P$_1$ antibody. Transfusion 1981;21:77–82.

73. Levine P: Comments on hemolytic disease of newborn due to anti-PP$_1$P^k (anti-Tj^a). Transfusion 1977;17:573–578.

74. Levine P, Celano MJ, Falkowski F: The specificity of the antibody in paroxysmal cold hemoglobinuria. Transfusion 1963;3:278.

75. Petz LD, Garratty G: Acquired Immune Hemolytic Anemias. New York, Churchill Livingstone, 1980

Chapter 4

Rh, Kell, Duffy, and Kidd Blood Group Systems

Constance M. Westhoff
Marion E. Reid

This chapter summarizes four clinically significant blood group systems that are defined by protein polymorphisms. The proteins that carry these blood group antigens were difficult to isolate because they are integral membrane proteins present as minor components of the total red blood cell (RBC) protein. Biochemical techniques developed in the 1970s and 1980s enabled their purification and partial amino acid sequencing. In the 1990s, the protein sequence data were used to construct nucleic acid probes for amplification and screening of bone marrow cDNA libraries to isolate the genes. In the last decade, there has been a considerable increase in the amount of information about these blood group antigens; principally, the development and use of the polymerase chain reaction (PCR) has resulted in the rapid elucidation of the molecular basis for the antigens and phenotypes.

■ Rh Blood Group System

History

The Rh system is second only to the ABO system in importance in transfusion medicine. The reason is that Rh antigens, especially D, are highly immunogenic and can cause hemolytic disease of the newborn (HDN) and severe transfusion reactions. HDN was first described by a French midwife in 1609 in a set of twins, of whom one was hydropic and stillborn, and the other was jaundiced and died of kernicterus.[1,2] In 1939, Levine and Stetson[3] described a woman who delivered a stillborn fetus and suffered a severe hemolytic reaction when transfused with blood from her husband. Her serum agglutinated the RBCs of her husband and 80 of 104 ABO-compatible donors. Subsequently, in 1941, Levine and colleagues[4] correctly concluded that the mother had been immunized by the fetus, which carried an antigen inherited from the father, and suggested that the cause of the erythroblastosis fetalis was maternal antibody in the fetal circulation. Attempts to immunize rabbits against this new antigen were not successful.[1] Levine and colleagues did not name the antigen.[5]

Meanwhile, Landsteiner and Wiener, in an effort to discover additional blood groups, injected rabbits and guinea pigs with rhesus monkey RBCs. The antiserum agglutinated not only rhesus cells but also the RBCs of 85% of a group of white subjects from New York, whom the researchers called "Rh positive"; the remaining 15% were "Rh negative."[1] Because the "anti-Rhesus" appeared to have reactivity indistinguishable from the maternal antibody reported by Levine and Stetson, the antigen responsible for HDN was named "Rh." Later it was realized that the rabbit antiserum was not recognizing the same antigen but was detecting an antigen found in greater amounts on Rh-positive than on Rh-negative RBCs.[6] This antigen was named LW for Landsteiner and Wiener,[1] and the original human specificity became known as anti-D.

As early as 1941, it was obvious that Rh was not a simple single antigen system. Fisher named the C and c antigens (A and B had been used for ABO) on the basis of the reactivity of two antibodies that recognized antithetical antigens, and used the next letters of the alphabet, D and E, to define antigens recognized by two additional antibodies.[1] Anti-e, which recognized the e antigen, was identified in 1945.[7]

Nomenclature

The Rh system has long been acknowledged as one of the most complex blood group systems because of its large number of antigens (45) and the heterogeneity of its antibodies. The introduction of two different Rh nomenclatures reflected the differences in opinion concerning the number of genes that encoded these antigens. The Fisher-Race nomenclature

Table 4.1 Nomenclature and Incidence for Rh Haplotypes

Haplotype Based on Antigens Present	Shorthand for Haplotype	Incidence (%)		
		White	African American	Asian
DCe	R_1	42	17	70
DcE	R_2	14	11	21
Dce	R_0	4	44	3
DCE	R_z	< 0.01	< 0.01	1
ce	r	37	26	3
Ce	r′	2	2	2
cE	r″	1	< 0.01	< 0.01
CE	r^y	< 0.01	< 0.01	< 0.01

was based on the premise that three closely linked genes, C/c, E/e, and D, were responsible, whereas the Wiener nomenclature (Rh-Hr) was based on the belief that a single gene encoded one "agglutinogen" that carried several blood group factors.

Even though neither theory was correct (there are two genes, *RHD* and *RHCE*, correctly proposed by Tippett[8]), the Fisher-Race designation (CDE) for haplotypes is often preferred for written communication, and a modified version of Wiener's nomenclature (the original form is nearly obsolete) is preferred for spoken communication (Table 4.1). A capital "R" indicates that D is present, and a lowercase "r" (or "little r") indicates that it is not. The C or c and E or e Rh antigens carried with D are represented by subscripts: 1 for Ce (R_1), 2 for cE (R_2), 0 for ce (R_0), and Z for CE (R_z). The CcEe antigens present without D (r) are represented by superscript symbols: "prime" for Ce (r′), "double-prime" for cE (r″) and "y" for CE (r^y) (see Table 4.1). The "R" versus "r" terminology allows one to convey the common Rh antigens present on one chromosome in a single term (a phenotype). Dashes are used to represent missing antigens of the rare deletion (or CE-depleted) phenotypes; for example, D—lacks C/c and E/e antigens.

In 1962, Rosenfield and associates[9] introduced numerical designations for the Rh antigens to more accurately represent the serologic data, to be free of genetic interpretation, and to be more compatible for computer use (Table 4.2). However this numerical nomenclature, with a few exceptions (Rh17, Rh32, Rh33), is not widely used in the clinical laboratory.

Proteins

Despite the clinical importance of the Rh blood groups, the RBC membrane proteins that carry them were identified only in the late 1980s.[10, 11] The extremely hydrophobic nature of these multi-pass transmembrane proteins made the biochemical isolation difficult and limited progress in their characterization until the genes were cloned.

The Rh proteins, designated RhD and RhCE, are 417–amino acid, nonglycosylated proteins; one carries the D antigen, and the other carries various combinations of the CE antigens (ce, cE, Ce, or CE).[12–14] RhD differs from RhCE by 32 to 35 amino acids (depending on which form of RhCE is present), and both are predicted to span the membrane 12 times. They migrate in SDS-PAGE (sodium dodecyl sulfate—polyacrylamide gel electrophoresis) gels with an approximate molecular weight ratio (M_r) of 30,000 to 32,000, and hence are referred to as the *Rh30 proteins*. They are covalently linked to fatty acids (palmitate) in the lipid bilayer.[15]

Table 4.2 Rosenfield Numerical Terminology for Rh Antigen

Numerical Term	ISBT Symbol
Rh1	D
Rh2	C
Rh3	E
Rh4	c
Rh5	e
Rh6	ce or f
Rh7	Ce
Rh8	C^W
Rh9	C^X
Rh10	V
Rh11	E^W
Rh12*	G
Rh17	Hr_0†
Rh18	Hr
Rh19	hr^s
Rh20	VS
Rh21	C^G
Rh22	CE
Rh23*	D^W
Rh26	c-like
Rh27	cE
Rh28	hr^H
Rh29	Rh29
Rh30	Go^a
Rh31	hr^B
Rh32	Rh32‡
Rh33	Rh33§
Rh34	Hr^B‖
Rh35	Rh35‖
Rh36	Be^a
Rh37	Evans
Rh39	Rh39
Rh40	Tar
Rh41	Rh41
Rh42	Rh42
Rh43	Crawford
Rh44	Nou
Rh45	Riv
Rh46	Sec
Rh47	Dav
Rh48	JAL
Rh49	STEM
Rh50	FPTT
Rh51	MAR
Rh52	BARC

*Rh13 through Rh16, Rh24, and Rh25 are obsolete.

†High-incidence antigen; the antibody is made by D––/D– and similar phenotypes.

‡Low-incidence antigen expressed by $\bar{R}^N$ and DBT phenotypes.

§Originally described on R_0^{Har} phenotype, but also found on $\bar{R}^N$, and D^{Vla} (C)–, R_0^{JOH}, and R_1^{Lisa}.

‖Low-incidence antigen on D(C)(e) cells.

ISBT, International Society for Blood Transfusion.

A 409–amino acid glycosylated protein that coprecipitates with the Rh30 proteins and migrates with an approximate M_r of 40,000 to 100,000 is called RhAG (Rh-associated glycoprotein) or Rh50 glycoprotein to reflect its apparent molecular weight.[16] RhAG (Rh50) shares 37% amino acid identity with the Rh30 proteins and has the same predicted membrane topology. RhAG is not polymorphic and does not carry Rh antigens. It is important for targeting the Rh30 proteins to the membrane, because mutations in, or lack of expression of, RhAG results in a lack of Rh antigen expression (Rh_{null}), or a marked reduction of Rh antigen expression (Rh_{mod}).[17] RhAG has one N-glycan chain that also carries ABO and Ii specificities (Fig. 4.1).

Rh-Core Complex

Rh and RhAG proteins are associated in the membrane, possibly as a tetramer consisting of two molecules of each as a core complex.[18] Evidence that other proteins interact with this Rh-core complex comes from observations that Rh_{null} RBCs have reduced expression of CD47 (an integrin-associated protein) and of glycophorin B (a sialoglycoprotein that carries S or s and U antigens). Rh_{null} RBCs also lack LW, a glycoprotein of approximate M_r 42,000 that belongs to the family of intercellular adhesion molecules. It has been shown that the presence of band 3 (the anion exchanger) enhanced the expression of the Rh antigens in transfected cells, suggesting that band 3 may also be associated with the Rh-core complex.[19] The Rh-core complex may also be linked to the membrane skeleton,[17] but which proteins it might be linked to is not known.

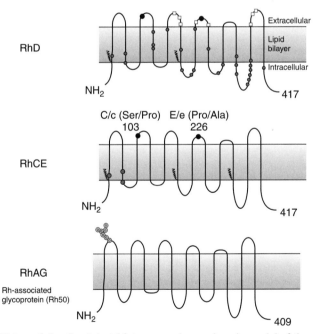

Figure 4.1 Predicted 12-transmembrane domain model of the RhD, RhCE, and RhAG proteins in the red blood cell membrane. The amino acid differences between RhD and RhCE are shown as symbols. The eight extracellular differences between RhD and RhCE are indicated as *open boxes*. The *zigzag lines* represent the location of possible palmitoylation sites. Positions 103 and 226 in RhCE that are critical for C/c and E/e expression, respectively, are indicated as *black circles*. The N-glycan on the first extracellular loop of the Rh-associated glycoprotein is indicated by the *branched structure*.

Genes

Two genes, designated *RHD* and *RHCE*, encode the Rh proteins. Rh-positive individuals have both genes, whereas most Rh-negative white people have only the *RHCE* gene.[20] The genes are 97% identical. Each gene has 10 exons and is the result of a gene duplication on chromosome 1p34-p36.[21] A comprehensive diagram of the intron-exon structure of *RHD* and *RHCE* can be found in the review by Avent and Reid.[22]

The single gene, *RHAG*, located at chromosome 6p11-p21.1 encodes RhAG. *RHAG* is 47% identical to the *RH* genes and also has 10 exons.[16, 23]

Antigens

As previously described, the major Rh antigens are D, C, c, E, and e. The many other Rh antigens (see Table 4.2) define compound antigens in *cis*, for example, f (ce), Ce, and CE, low-incidence antigens arising from partial D hybrid proteins (D[w], Go[a], BARC, etc.), high-incidence antigens, and other variant antigens. The molecular bases of most Rh antigens have been determined.

Studies to estimate the number of D, C/c, and E/e antigen sites on RBCs found differences between Rh phenotypes. The number of D antigens ranges from 10,000 on Dce/ce RBCs to 33,000 on DcE/DcE. The number of C, c, and e antigens per RBC varies from 8500 to 85,000.[6] Because we now know that C or c and E or e are carried on the same protein, their numbers should be equivalent. The equivalency was not always demonstrated in these studies, reflecting the inherent difficulty in the use of radiolabeled polyclonal antiserum to estimate antigen numbers. Results of tests with monoclonal antibodies to high-incidence Rh antigens suggest that the total number of Rh proteins (Rh30) per RBC is 100,000 to 200,000. The number of RhAG (Rh50) is also estimated to be 100,000 to 200,000,[24] consistent with predictions that Rh and RhAG are present in the membrane as a tetramer of two molecules of each.[18]

D Antigen

Rh-positive and *Rh-negative* refer to the presence and absence, respectively, of the D antigen, which is the most immunogenic of the Rh antigens. The Rh-negative (D-negative) phenotype occurs in 15% to 17% of white persons but is not common in other ethnic populations. The absence of D in people of European descent is primarily the result of deletion of the entire RHD gene and occurred on a Dce (R_0) haplotype because the allele most often carried with the deletion is ce. However, rare D-negative white persons carry an RHD gene that is not expressed because of a premature stop codon,[25] a 4–base pair (bp) insertion at the intron 3/exon 4 junction,[26] point mutations, or RHD/CE hybrids.[27, 28] Most of these are associated with the uncommon Ce (r′) or cE (r″) haplotypes.

D-negative phenotypes in Asian or African persons, however, are most often caused by inactive or silent *RHD* rather than a complete gene deletion. Asian D-negative individuals occur with a frequency of less than 1%, and most carry mutant *RHD* genes associated with *Ce*,[29] indicating that the gene mutations probably originated on a DCe (R_1) haplotype. Only 3% to 7% of South African black persons are D-negative, but 66% of this group have *RHD* genes that contain a 37-bp internal duplication,[30] which results in a premature stop codon. The 37-bp insert *RHD*-pseudogene was also found in 24% of

ORIGIN OF THE COMMON RHCE GENES

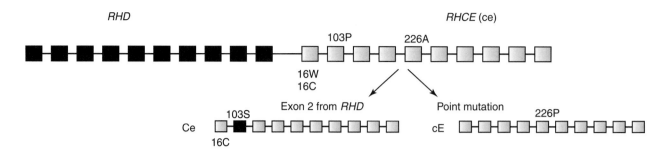

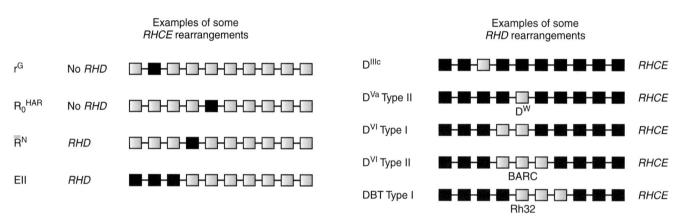

Figure 4.2 *Top panel,* Diagram of the *RHD* and *RHCE* genes indicating the changes that resulted in the common RhCE polymorphisms. The shared exon 2 of *RHD* and *RHCE* (shown as a *black box*) explains the expression of G antigen on RhCe and RhD proteins. *Bottom panel,* Examples of some *RHCE* and *RHD* rearrangements.

D-negative African Americans. In addition, 15% of the D-negative phenotypes in Africans result from a hybrid *RHD-CE-D^s* gene characterized by expression of VS, weak C and e, and no D antigen.[30] Only 18% of D-negative Africans and 54% of D-negative African Americans completely lack *RHD*.

This information is important to the design of PCR-based methods to predict the D status of a fetus at risk for HDN. The population being tested and the different molecular events responsible for D-negative phenotypes must be considered. Testing of samples from the parents limits the possibility of misinterpretation.

WEAK D (FORMERLY KNOWN AS D^u)

An estimated 0.2% to 1% of white persons (and a greater number of African Americans) have reduced expression of the D antigen, which is characterized serologically as failure of the RBCs to agglutinate directly with anti-D typing reagents and requires the use of the indirect antiglobulin test for detection. The number of samples classified as *weak D* depends on the characteristics of the typing reagent. These weak D antigens were previously referred to as *D^u*, a term that has been abolished. The molecular basis of weak D expression is heterogeneous. A transcription defect was seen in one individual,[31] and in others, the transcript level was normal.[32]

In a larger study of samples from Germany, Wagner and colleagues[33] were able to associate the presence of point mutations in *RHD* transcripts with weak D expression. More

than 70% of the samples had a Val270Gly amino acid change, but a total of 16 different mutations, clustered in four regions of the RhD protein, were found. These mutations cause amino acid changes predicted to be intracellular or in the transmembrane regions of RhD and not on the outer surface of the RBC.[33] This study suggests that the mutations do affect the efficiency of insertion and, therefore, the quantity of RhD protein in the membrane but do not affect D epitopes.

The majority of individuals with a weak D phenotype can safely receive D-positive blood and do not make anti-D. However, two weak D types (type 4.2.2 and type 15) have been reported to make anti-D.[34] These weak D then, would more accurately be classified as partial-Ds (described later); however, their reactivity with current anti-D typing sera leads to their classification as weak D. The serologic differentiation of weak D from partial D is not unequivocal. Importantly, donor center typing procedures must detect and label weak D RBC components as "D-positive."

A very weak form of D (D_el), detected by absorption and elution of anti-D, has a high incidence in Hong Kong Chinese and Japanese persons. It results from a deletion that encompasses exon 9 of *RHD*.[35]

PARTIAL D ANTIGENS (D CATEGORIES OR D MOSAICS)

The D antigen has long been described as a "mosaic" on the basis of the observation that some Rh-positive individuals make alloanti-D when exposed to normal D antigen. It was hypothesized that the RBCs of these individuals lack some part of RhD and that they can produce antibodies to the missing portion. Molecular analysis has shown that this hypothesis is correct, but what was not predicted is that the missing portions of *RHD* are replaced by corresponding portions of *RHCE* (Fig. 4.2).[22, 36] Some replacements involve entire exons, and the novel sequence of amino acids generates new antigens (D^W, BARC, Rh32, etc.) (Table 4.3). In addition, several exon rearrangements can give rise to the same partial D category (e.g., D^{VI} can result from type I, II, or III rearrangements see Fig. 4.2). Other partial D antigens result from multiple amino acid conversions between *RHCE* and *RHD*, and some are the result of single point mutations in *RHD* (D^{VII}, DMH, DFW) (see Table 4.3). These point mutations are predicted to be located on an extracellular loop or portion of the RhD protein, in contrast to the weak D antigens already described, which are predicted to have mutations located in cytoplasmic or transmembrane regions. Individuals with partial D antigens can make anti-D and therefore ideally should receive D-negative donor blood. In practice, however, most are typed as D-positive and are recognized only after they have made anti-D.

ELEVATED D

Several phenotypes, including D—, Dc— and DC^w—, have an elevated expression of D antigen and no, weak, and variant CE antigens, respectively.[6] They are caused by replacement of portions of *RHCE* by *RHD*,[22, 36] analogous to the partial D rearrangements already described. The additional *RHD* sequences in *RHCE* along with a normal *RHD* may explain the enhanced D and accounts for the reduced or missing CE antigens. Immunized people with these CE-depleted phenotypes make anti-Rh17.

C/c and E/e Antigens

There are four major allelic forms of *RHCE*: ce, Ce, cE, and CE.[14] C and c differ by four amino acids: Cys16Trp (cysteine at residue 16 replaced by tryptophan) encoded by exon 1, and Ile60Leu, Ser68Asn, and Ser103Pro encoded by exon 2. Only residue 103 is predicted to be extracellular; it is located on the second loop of RhCE (see Fig. 4.1). The amino acids encoded

by exon 2 of *RHC* are identical to those encoded by exon 2 of *RHD*. At the genomic level, *RHce* appears to have arisen from transfer of exon 2 from *RHD* into *RHce* (see Fig. 4.2). The shared exon 2 explains the expression of the G antigen on both RhD and RhC proteins.

E and e differ by one amino acid, Pro226Ala. This polymorphism, predicted to reside on the fourth extracellular loop of the protein (see Fig. 4.1), is encoded by exon 5. A single point mutation in *RHce* resulted in *RHcE* (see Fig. 4.2).[14, 37]

C^W and C^X antigens result from single amino acid changes, encoded by exon 1, which are predicted to be located on the first extracellular loop of the RhCE protein.[38]

The antigens V and VS are expressed on RBCs of more than 30% of black persons. They are the result of a Leu245Val substitution located in the predicted eighth transmembrane segment of Rhce.[39] The close location of the e antigen, Ala226 on the fourth extracellular loop, suggests that Leu245Val causes a local conformation change responsible for the weakened expression of e antigen in many black persons who are V and VS positive. The V–VS+ phenotype results from a Gly336Cys change on the 245Val background.[40]

Other modifications of *RHCE*, which are uncommon, are the hybrids D^{HAR}, r^G, R^N and several E/e variants (see Fig. 4.2). D^{HAR} (R$_0^{Har}$), which is found in individuals of German ancestry, has been found more frequently since implementation of monoclonal anti-D for routine typing. The RBCs may type as Rh-positive with monoclonal anti-D, whereas reactions with polyclonal anti-D (including the weak D test) are negative. These individuals have only one D-specific exon (exon 5) and should be treated as Rh-negative for transfusion and Rh immune globulin prophylaxis. R^N RBCs are found in people of African origin and type as e-weak (or negative) with polyclonal reagents, but are indistinguishable from "normal" e-positive RBCs with some monoclonal anti-e. The E variants, EI, EII, and EIII, result either from a point mutation (EI) or from gene conversion events that lead to replacement of several extracellular RhcE amino acids with RhD residues (EII and EIII) and loss of some E epitope expression.[41] Category EIV RBCs, which have an amino acid substitution in an intracellular domain, do not lack E epitopes but have reduced E expression.[42]

Table 4.3   Molecular Basis of Some Rh Antigens, Partial D, and Unusual Phenotypes

Molecular Basis		Gene	Phenotype/Antigen
Single point mutations		*RHD*	Partial D: DMH; D^{VII}; D+G–; DFW; DHR; D^{Va}; D^{HMi}; DNU; D^{II}; DNB
			Weak D (previously called D^u)
		RHCE	C^X; C^W; Rh:–26; E type I, IV; V+VS+
Multiple mutations (gene conversions)		*RHD*	Partial D: D^{IIIa}; D^{IVa}; D^{Va}; DFR type I
		RHCE	E type III
Rearranged gene(s)	*RHD*	*RHD-CE-D*	Partial D: D^{IIIb}; D^{IIIc}; D^{IVb}; D^{Va}; D^{VI}; DFR type II; DBT r''^{G}; (Ce)Ce; (C)ce^{s}VS+V–
	RHCE	*RHCE-D-CE*	R$_0^{Har}$; r^G; R^N
		RHD-CE	E type II
	RHD: RHCE	*RHD-CE: RHCE-D*	DC^W–
		RHD: RHCE-D-CE	D––; D••; Dc–
		RHD: RHD-CE	D••
		RHCE-D: RHD-CE	D••

An e variant results from deletion of the codon for Arg229, which is close to the Ala226 residue associated with normal e expression.[43] Variant expression of e is also associated with the presence of a Cys residue instead of Trp at position 16 in the Rhce protein.[44] The very rare RH:-26 results from a Gly96Ser transmembrane amino acid change that abolishes Rh26 and weakens c expression.[45]

In summary, Rh antigen expression is affected not only by changes in extracellular amino acids but also, and significantly, by intracellular changes, highlighting the conformational nature of these blood group antigens and complicating attempts to map the Rh epitopes to specific amino acid residues.

Rh$_{null}$

Rh$_{null}$ individuals, who lack expression of all Rh antigens, suffer from a compensated hemolytic anemia and have variable degrees of spherocytosis, stomatocytosis, and increased RBC osmotic fragility.[46] The phenotype is very rare, occurring on two different genetic backgrounds; the "regulator" type, caused by a "suppressor gene" at an unlinked locus (previously referred to as X^0r), and the "amorph" type, which maps to the *RH* locus. It is now clear that in the regulator type of Rh$_{null}$, the suppression of Rh is caused by a lack of, or a mutant, RhAG protein. Regulator type RBCs express no Rh and no RhAG proteins. The amorph type of Rh$_{null}$ results from mutations in *RHCE* on a deleted *RHD* background.[47] Amorph type RBCs express no Rh protein and have reduced (20% of normal) RhAG.

Antibodies

Most Rh antibodies are immunoglobulin G (IgG), subclasses IgG1 and IgG3 (IgG2 and IgG4 have also been detected), and some sera have an IgM component.[48] Rh antibodies do not activate complement, although two rare exceptions have been reported. The lack of complement activation by Rh antibodies is thought to be due to the distance between antigens, but is probably due to a lack of mobility.[6] Reactivity of Rh antibodies is enhanced by enzyme treatment of the test RBCs, and most react optimally at 37°C.

Anti-D can cause severe transfusion reactions and severe HDN. Approximately 80% to 85% of D-negative persons make anti-D after exposure to D-positive RBCs. The lack of response in 15% may be due to antigen dose, recipient HLA-DR alleles, and other as yet unknown genetic factors. Anti-D was the most common Rh antibody, but its incidence has greatly diminished with the prophylactic use of Rh immune globulin for prevention of HDN. ABO incompatibility between the mother and the fetus has a partial protective effect against immunization to D; this finding suggested the rationale for development of Rh immune globulin.[48]

Anti-c, clinically the most important Rh antibody after anti-D, may cause severe HDN. Anti-C, -E, and -e do not often cause HDN, and when they do, it is usually mild.[6, 48]

Autoantibodies to high-incidence Rh antigens often occur in the sera of patients with warm autoimmune hemolytic anemia and in some cases of drug-induced autoimmune hemolytic anemia. These autoantibodies are nonreactive with Rh$_{null}$ cells.[49]

Monoclonal anti-D, made by immortalizing human B lymphocytes in vitro with Epstein-Barr virus, is available. Most monoclonal anti-D does not react with partial D^{VI} cells; therefore, anti-D for typing reagents is usually a blend of various monoclonals (or monoclonal and polyclonal). Monoclonal anti-D has not yet been tested clinically for its ability to prevent immunization after pregnancy but has been shown to suppress D immunization in D-negative male volunteers.[50]

Expression

Northern blot analysis indicated that Rh and RhAG messenger RNA (mRNA) are restricted to cells of erythroid and myeloid lineage, but reverse transcriptase–polymerase chain reaction (RT-PCR) found Rh mRNA splicing isoforms in B and T lymphocytes and monocytes.[51] The significance of this observation is not yet known. During erythropoiesis, RhAG appears early (on CD34+ progenitors) but the Rh proteins appear later—RhCE first, followed by RhD.[52]

Evolution

The *RH* genes arose from an early duplication of the erythrocyte *RHAG* gene. *RH* and *RHAG* have been investigated in nonhuman primates[53, 54] and rodents,[55–57] and most, with the exception of gorillas and chimpanzees, have a *RHAG* and only one *RH* gene. The *RH* gene duplicated in some common ancestor of gorillas, chimpanzees, and humans, leading to *RHCE* and *RHD*. Chimpanzees and some gorillas have three *RH* genes, indicating that a third duplication has taken place in these species.

Function

The predicted membrane structures of Rh and RhAG suggest that they are transport proteins, and the analysis of their amino acid sequence reveals distant similarity to ammonium (NH_4^+) transporters in bacteria, fungi, and plants.[58] Indirect evidence for ammonium transport comes from yeast complementation experiments[59] and direct evidence comes from uptake of ammonium by RhAG when expressed in *Xenopus* oocytes.[60] Rh and RhAG homologues have been found in many organisms, including the sponge *(Geodia)*, the slime mold *(Dictyostelium)*, the fruit fly *(Drosophila)*, and the frog *(Xenopus)* (summarized by Huang and colleagues[61]), indicating that they are conserved throughout evolution. Additionally, the expression of nonerythroid Rh and RhAG homologues in kidney, testis, brain, and liver[62, 63] suggests that they have a related function in other tissues.

Summary

The molecular basis of many of the Rh antigens has now been elucidated. The revelation that RhD and RhCE proteins differ by 35 amino acids explains why D antigen is so immunogenic. In addition, exchanges between *RHD* and *RHCE*, mainly by gene conversion, have generated many Rh polymorphisms. The proximity of the two genes on the same chromosome probably affords greater opportunity for exchange. This finding finally explains the myriad of antigens observed in the Rh blood group system and gives interesting insight into the evolutionary history of duplicated genes and the interactions that can take place between them.

■ The Kell and Kx System

History

The Kell blood group system was discovered in 1946, just a few weeks after the introduction of the antiglobulin test.

The RBCs from a newborn baby who was thought to be suffering from HDN gave a positive reaction in the direct antiglobulin test.[64] The serum of the mother reacted with RBCs from her husband, her older child, and 9% of random donors. The system was named from Kelleher, the mother's surname, and the antigen is referred to as K (synonyms: Kell, K1). Three years later, the more common antigen, k (synonyms: Cellano, K2), which has a high incidence in all populations, was identified through the typing of large numbers of RBC samples with an antibody that had also caused a mild case of HDN.[65] The Kell system remained a simple two-antigen system until 1957, when the antithetical Kp^a and Kp^b antigens were reported, as was the K$_0$ (Kell$_{null}$) phenotype.[6] Subsequently, the number of Kell antigens has grown to 23, making Kell one of the most polymorphic blood group systems known.

Proteins

The Kell protein is a type II glycoprotein with an approximate M$_r$ of 93,000. It has a 665–amino acid carboxyl terminal extracellular domain, a single 20–amino acid transmembrane domain, and a 47–amino acid N-terminal cytoplasmic domain.[66] The protein has five N-glycosylation sites and 15 extracellular cysteine residues that cause folding through the formation of multiple intrachain disulfide bonds (Fig. 4.3). This explains why Kell blood group antigens are inactivated when RBCs are treated with reducing agents, such as dithiothreitol (DTT) and aminoethylisothiouronium bromide (AET), which disrupt disulfide bonds.[67] All Kell system antigens are carried on this glycoprotein, which is present at 3500 to 17,000 copies per RBC.[68, 69] All but two (Js^a and Js^b) of the Kell antigens are localized in the N-terminal half of the protein before residue 550, strongly suggesting that the C-terminal domain does not tolerate change and is functionally important. Indeed, the Kell glycoprotein is a zinc endopeptidase (see later), and the C-terminus contains a zinc-binding domain that is the catalytic site.[70, 71]

Kx is a 444–amino acid, 37-kD protein that is linked by a disulfide bond to the Kell protein.[17] Kx is predicted to span the membrane 10 times (see Fig. 4.3), is not glycosylated, and may be a membrane transport protein. RBCs lacking Kx have the McLeod phenotype, which is characterized by a marked reduction of Kell antigens, acanthocytosis, and reduced in vivo RBC survival.

Genes

The *KEL* gene has been localized on chromosome 7q33. It consists of 19 exons spanning approximately 21.5 kb.[72, 73] The Kell antigens result from nucleotide mutations that cause single amino acid substitutions in the protein (Table 4.4). The lack of Kell antigens, K$_0$, is caused by several different molecular defects, including nucleotide deletion, defective splicing, premature stop codons, and amino acid substitutions.[71, 74, 75]

The *XK* gene is on the short arm of the X chromosome at Xp21.[76] *XK* has three exons, and mutations cause the McLeod syndrome which, because the gene is X-linked, affects males. Carrier females, because of X-chromosome inactivation, have two populations of RBCs (one of the McLeod phenotype and one normal), and the proportion varies from 5% McLeod: 95% normal to 85% McLeod: 15% normal.[77, 78]

McLeod Syndrome

When testing medical students in 1961, Allen and coworkers[79] found that one of the students, Mr. McLeod, had RBCs with very weak expression of Kell antigens. It is now evident that he lacked Kx, which is important for expression of Kell, and that lack of Kx is the basis for the McLeod syndrome. Males with the McLeod syndrome have muscular and neurologic defects, including skeletal muscle wasting, elevated serum creatine phosphokinase, psychopathology, seizures with basal ganglia degeneration, and cardiomyopathy.[70, 80] Most symptoms develop after the fourth decade of life. The syndrome is very rare. Approximately 60 males have been identified, and all but 2 have been white; however,

Figure 4.3 Kell and Kx proteins. Kell is a single-pass protein, but Kx is predicted to span the red blood cell membrane 10 times. Kell and Kx are linked by a disulfide bond, shown as –S—. The amino acids that are responsible for the more common Kell antigens are shown. The N-glycosylation sites are shown as Y. The *hollow Y* represents the N-glycosylation site that is not present on the K (K1) protein.

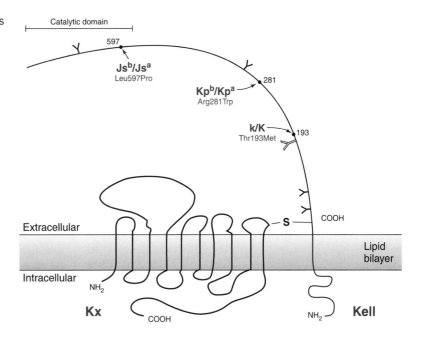

Table 4.4 Molecular Basis of Antigens in the Kell Blood Group System

Antigen	Amino Acid	Position
k(K2)	Threonine	193
K(K1)	Methionine	
Kp^a(K3)	Tryptophan	281
Kp^b(K4)	Arginine	
Kp^c(K21)	Glutamine	
Js^a(K6)	Proline	597
Js^b(K7)	Leucine	
K11	Valine	302
K17	Alanine	
K14	Arginine	180
K24	Proline	
Ul^a	Glutamic acid→Valine	494

Table 4.5 Kell Phenotypes and Incidence

	Incidence (%)	
Phenotype	White	African American
K–k+	91	98
K+k+	8.8	2
K+k–	0.2	Rare
Kp(a+b–)	Rare	0
Kp(a–b+)	97.7	100
Kp(a+b+)	2.3	Rare
Kp(a–b–c+)	0.32 Japanese	0
Js(a+b–)	0	1
Js(a–b+)	100	80
Js(a+b+)	Rare	19
K11	High incidence	
K17	Low incidence	
K14	High incidence	
K24	Low incidence	
Ul^a	Low incidence (2.6% in Finns, 0.46% in Japanese)	

because of the plethora of symptoms, the syndrome is probably underdiagnosed.

Fifteen different mutations in the *XK* gene were found in a study of 17 families and involve major and minor deletions, point mutations, and splice site or frameshift mutations that result in the absence or truncation of Kx protein.[17, 80] At one time, chronic granulomatous disease (CGD) was thought to be related to the McLeod syndrome, but the gene controlling CGD is near the *XK* gene on the X chromosome, and the small minority of patients with CGD who have the McLeod phenotype have X-chromosome deletions encompassing both genes.[6, 81]

Antigens

The Kell system consists of five sets of high-incidence and low-incidence antigens, as follows (the names of the high-incidence antigens appear in **boldface**:

- K and **k**
- Kp^a, **Kp^b**, and Kp^c
- Jsa and **Js^b**
- **K11** and K17
- **K14** and K24

In addition, 11 independently expressed antigens, 3 low-incidence (Ul^a; K23; VLAN), and 9 high-incidence (Ku; Km; K12; K13; K16; K18; K19; K22; Tou), have been identified. The null phenotype, K$_0$, lacks Kell antigens, and Kell$_{mod}$ phenotypes have a weak expression of Kell antigens.

Kell antigens show population variations (Table 4.5). K has an incidence of 9% in white persons but is much less common in people of other ethnic backgrounds.[1, 82] Kp^a and K17 are also mainly found in white persons. Js^a is almost exclusively found in African Americans, with an incidence of 20%. Ul^a is found in Finnish and Japanese persons.[1, 82]

The molecular basis of most of the Kell antigens has been determined (see Table 4.4).[71, 83] The K methionine substitution disrupts a glycosylation consensus sequence so that K has one less N-glycan than k.[84] Js^a and Js^b are located within a cluster of cysteine residues,[85] a finding that explains why they are more susceptible than other Kell antigens to treatment with reducing agents.[86] No Kell haplotype has been found to express more than one low-incidence Kell antigen, not because of structural constraints, but because multiple expression would require more than one mutation encoding a recognized Kell system antigen to occur in the same gene.[87]

Weaker expression of Kell antigens is found when RBCs carry Kp^a in *cis*.[88–90] Weak expression of Kell antigens can be inherited, or acquired and transient. Inherited weak expression occurs when the Kell-associated Kx protein is absent (McLeod phenotype), when glycophorins C and D are absent (Leach phenotype), or when a portion of the extracellular domain of glycophorin C and D, specifically exon 3, is deleted (some Gerbich-negative phenotypes).[90, 91] Transient depression of Kell system antigens has been associated with the presence of autoantibodies mimicking alloantibodies in autoimmune hemolytic anemia and with microbial infections. Kell expression was reduced in two cases of idiopathic thrombocytopenic purpura (ITP) but returned to normal after remission.[6]

Antibodies

Kell antigens are highly immunogenic, and anti-K is common. However, because more than 90% of donors are K-negative, it is not difficult to find compatible blood for patients with anti-K. The other Kell system antibodies are less common but are also usually IgG, and they have caused transfusion reactions and HDN or neonatal anemia. In HDN due to Kell antibodies, neither maternal antibody titers nor amniotic bilirubin levels are good predictors of the severity of the disease. Reports demonstrate that Kell antigens are expressed very early during erythropoiesis[52] and that Kell antibodies can cause suppression of erythropoiesis in vitro.[92] This finding suggests that the low level of bilirubin observed, in the presence of neonatal anemia, is due to Kell antibodies that bind to erythroid progenitors and exert effects before hemoglobinization.

Anti-Ku is the antibody made by immunized K$_0$ individuals, and Ku represents the high-incidence or "total-Kell" antigen. McLeod males with CGD make anti-Kx+Km; this antibody reacts strongly with K$_0$ cells, weaker with RBCs of common Kell phenotype, and not at all with McLeod phenotype RBCs. Anti-Km, made by McLeod persons who do not have CGD, reacts with RBCs of common Kell phenotypes but not with K$_0$ or McLeod RBCs, suggesting that it detects one or more epitopes requiring both the Kell and Kx proteins. One case has been reported of a McLeod male without CGD who made an apparent anti-Kx without the presence of anti-Km.[81]

Expression

Kell system antigens appear to be erythroid-specific and are expressed very early during erythropoiesis.[52] Kx mRNA is found in muscle, heart, brain, and hematopoietic tissue.[17]

Evolution

Primate RBCs express the k antigen but not the K antigen, indicating that the K mutation appeared in human lineage. Chimpanzees are Js(a+b−),[93] and Js[a] is also present on RBCs from Old World monkeys,[94] suggesting that Js[b] also arose after human speciation. Kell protein is not found on immunoblots of RBCs from sheep, goat, cattle, rabbit, horse, mouse, donkey, cat, dog, or rat.[95]

Function

The Kell glycoprotein has similarity with the M13 or neprilysin family of zinc endopeptidases that cleave a variety of physiologically active peptides. One member of this family, endothelin-converting enzyme 1 (ECE-1), is a membrane-bound metalloprotease that catalyzes the proteolytic activation of big endothelin-1 (big ET-1).[96] Like ECE-1, Kell protein can proteolytically cleave endothelins, specifically big ET-3 to generate ET-3, which is a potent vasoconstrictor.[97] ET-3 is also involved in the development of the enteric nervous system and in migration of neural crest–derived cells. The biologic role of the endothelins is not yet completely elucidated, but they act on two G protein–coupled receptors, ET_A and ET_B, which are found on many cells. Kell$_{null}$ individuals, who lack Kell protein, do not have any obvious defect, so they do not immediately give insight into the biologic function of the Kell protein. This lack of defect in K$_{null}$ people may be because other enzymes probably also cleave ET-3,[97] and determining whether Kell$_{null}$ individuals have abnormal levels of plasma endothelins is an active area of investigation.

◼ Duffy (Fy) Blood Group System

History

The Duffy (Fy[a]) blood group antigen was first reported in 1950 by Cutbush and associates,[98] who described the reactivity of an antibody found in a hemophiliac male who had received multiple transfusions. This blood group system bears the patient's surname, Duffy, the last two letters of which provide the abbreviated nomenclature (Fy). Fy[b] was found 1 year later.[99] In 1975, Fy was identified as the receptor for the malarial parasite *Plasmodium vivax*.[100] This discovery explained the predominance of the Fy(a–b–) (Fy$_{null}$) phenotype, which confers resistance to malarial invasion, in persons originating from West Africa.

Proteins

The Fy protein is a transmembrane glycoprotein of 35 to 43 kD consisting of a glycosylated amino-terminal region, which protrudes from the membrane and has seven transmembrane-spanning domains (Fig. 4.4).[101, 102] In 1993, it was realized that Fy was the erythrocyte chemokine receptor that could bind interleukin-8 and monocyte chemotactic peptide-1 (MCP-1).[103] The cloning of the *FY* gene[104] confirmed that it belongs to the conserved family of chemokine receptors.

Gene

The *FY* gene is located on the long arm of chromosome 1q22-q23[105] and spans 1.5 kb. The gene, which has only two exons, contains two ATG codons. The upstream exon contains the major start site.[106, 107] The same two-exon organization is also found in genes for other chemokine receptors.[108]

Antigens

The Fy[a] and Fy[b] antigens are encoded by two allelic forms of the gene, designated *FYA* and *FYB*, and are responsible for the Fy(a+b–), Fy(a–b+) and Fy(a+b+) phenotypes.[107, 109] They differ by a single amino acid located on the extracellular domain (see Fig. 4.4).

Fy[x], which is a weak expression of Fy[b], is found in white persons and is due to a single mutation in the *FYB* gene.[110, 111] The amino acid change, which is located in the first intracellular cytoplasmic loop, is associated with a decrease in the amount of protein in the membrane and results in diminished expression of Fy[b], Fy3, and Fy6 antigens as well as reduced binding of chemokine.[108, 112, 113]

Figure 4.4 The predicted seven-transmembrane domain structure of the Duffy protein. The amino acid change responsible for the Fy[a]/Fy[b] polymorphism, the mutation responsible for Fy[x] glycosylation sites, and the regions where Fy3 and Fy6 map are indicated.

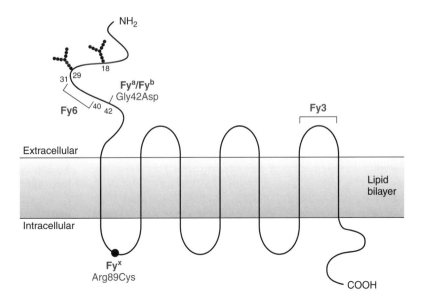

Fy3, as determined with one monoclonal anti-Fy3, is located on the third extracellular loop,[114] whereas Fy6 maps to the amino-terminal loop of the protein. The aspartic acid at amino acid 25 and glutamic acid at 26 are critical for anti-Fy6 binding.[115]

The Fy(a–b–) phenotype found in African Americans is caused by a mutation in the promoter region of *FYB* (T to C at position –46), which disrupts a binding site for the erythroid transcription factor GATA-1 and results in the loss of Fy expression on RBCs.[116, 117] The Fy protein has also been found on endothelial cells (see later). Because the erythroid promoter controls expression only in erythroid cells, expression of Fy proteins on endothelium is normal in these Fy(a–b–). All African persons with a mutated GATA sequence to date have been shown to carry *FYB*; therefore, Fy[b] is expressed on their nonerythroid tissues. This finding explains why Fy(a–b–) individuals make anti-Fy[a] but not anti-Fy[b].[118] It also is relevant in the selection of antigen-matched units for Fy(a–b–) patients with sickle cell disease, because they would *not* be expected to make anti-Fy[b] on stimulation with Fy[b] donor units. The *FYA* allele with a mutated GATA sequence has been found in Papua New Guinea.[119]

The Fy(a–b–) phenotype in white persons is very rare (Table 4.6).[1] One propositus, an Australian (AZ) woman, appears to be homozygous for a 14-bp deletion in *FYA*, which introduces a stop codon in the protein[120]; a Cree Indian female (Ye), a white female (NE), and a Lebanese Jewish male (AA) carry different Trp to stop codon mutations.[121] Because these mutations would result in a truncated protein, these people would not be expected to express endothelial or erythroid Fy protein. All four people made anti-Fy3.

There are 13,000 to 14,000 Fy antigen sites per RBC,[122] and Fy[a], Fy[b], and Fy6 antigens are sensitive to proteolytic enzyme treatment of antigen-positive RBCs, although Fy3 is resistant.

Antibodies

Fy antigens are estimated to be 40 times less immunogenic than K antigens, and most Fy antibodies arise from stimulation by blood transfusion. They are mostly IgG, subclass IgG1, and only rarely are IgM. Anti-Fy[b] is less common than anti-Fy[a], and Fy antibodies are often found in sera with other antibodies. Anti-Fy3 is made by rare white Fy(a–b–) individuals.[6] Anti-Fy6 is a mouse monoclonal antibody.[108]

Expression

Duffy mRNA is present in kidney, spleen, heart, lung, muscle, duodenum, pancreas, placenta, and brain.[104, 108] Cells responsible for Fy expression in these tissues are the endothelial

Table 4.6 Duffy Phenotypes and Incidence

Phenotype	Incidence (%)				
	Caucasians	Blacks	Chinese	Japanese	Thai
Fy(a+b–)	17	9	90.8	81.5	69
Fy(a–b+)	34	22	0.3	0.9	3
Fy(a+b+)	49	1	8.9	17.6	28
Fy(a–b–)*	Rare	68	0	0	0
Fy[x]	1.4	0	0	0	0

*Fy(a–b–), incidence in Israeli Arabs 25%; Israeli Jews, 4%.

cells lining postcapillary venules,[123–125] except in the brain, where expression is localized to the Purkinje cell neurons.[126, 127] The same polypeptide is expressed in endothelial cells and RBCs, but in brain, a larger, 8.5-kb mRNA is present. The function of Fy on neurons is an area of active investigation.

In the fetus, Fy antigens can be detected at 6 to 7 weeks of gestation and are well developed at birth.[1] The expression of these antigens was found to occur late during erythropoiesis and RBC maturation.[52]

Evolution

RBCs of monkeys and apes react with anti-Fy[b], and the conserved GT repeat sequences in the 3' flanking region of the gene both suggest that *FYB* was the ancestral gene.[128, 129] The first human divergence occurred when a mutation in the erythroid promoter region of *FYB* resulted in the loss of Fy[b] expression on RBCs. This mutation conferred resistance to malaria infection in regions where *P. vivax* was endemic and selected for the high proportion of Fy(a–b–) in populations of African ancestry. Later, a single nucleotide change in the *FYB* gene caused the *FYA* polymorphism in people of European and Asian ancestry. Fy has been cloned from several nonhuman primates, including chimpanzees, squirrel monkeys, and rhesus monkeys, and from cows, pigs, rabbits, and mice.[108]

Function

The importance of Fy as a receptor for the malarial parasite *P. vivax* is well established, but its biologic role as a chemokine receptor on RBCs, endothelial cells, and brain is not yet clear. The chemokine receptors are a family of proteins that are receptors on target cells for the binding of chemokines. Chemokines are so named because they are *cytokines* that are *chemotactic* (cause cell migration), and their receptors are an active area of investigation.[130] Chemokine receptors have been found principally on lymphocytes, where they are coupled to G-proteins and activate intracellular signaling pathways that regulate cell migration into tissues. Unlike other chemokine receptors, Fy does not have a conserved amino acid DRY-motif in the second extracellular loop, and cells transfected with Fy and stimulation with chemokines do not mobilize free calcium.[101] Also, Fy can bind chemokines from both the CXC (IL-8, MGSA) and the CC (RANTES, MCP-1, MIP-1) classes of chemokines.[108] These features have led investigators to hypothesize that it may act as a scavenger or sink for excess chemokine release into the circulation.[131, 132] If the function of Fy on RBCs is to scavenge excess chemokine, it may be that Fy(a–b–) individuals would be more susceptible to septic shock[125] or to cardiac damage after infarction. Renal allografts have been reported to have shorter survival in African American Fy(a–b–) recipients,[133] and Fy has been shown to be upregulated in the kidney during renal injury.[134]

Abundant expression of Fy on high endothelial venules and sinusoids in the spleen,[125] which is a site central to chemokine-induced leukocyte trafficking, suggests a role in leukocyte migration into the tissues. Fy is also similar to the receptor for endothelins (ET$_B$), vasoactive proteins that strongly influence vascular biology and that may also be mitogenic.[108]

■ The Kidd Blood Group System

History

The Kidd blood group system was discovered in 1951, when a "new" antibody in the serum of Mrs. Kidd (who also had anti-K) caused HDN in her sixth child. Jk came from the initials of the baby (John Kidd), because K had been used previously for Kell.[135] Anti-Jk[b] was found 2 years later in the serum of a woman who had a transfusion reaction (she also had anti-Fy[a]).[136] Kidd system antibodies are characteristically found in sera with other blood group antibodies, suggesting that Kidd antigens are not particularly immunogenic. However, Kidd antibodies induce a rapid and robust anamnestic response that is responsible for their reputation for causing severe delayed hemolytic transfusion reactions.

Proteins

The Kidd glycoprotein has an approximate M_r of 46,000 to 60,000 and is predicted to span the membrane ten times. The third extracellular loop is large and carries an N-glycan at Asn211 (Fig. 4.5). The protein has ten cysteine residues, but only one is predicted to be extracellular, a fact that explains why the antigens are not sensitive to disulfide reagents. There is internal homology between the N-terminal and C-terminal halves of the protein, with each containing an LP box (LPXXTXPF) characteristic of urea transporters.[137] Isolation of the Kidd protein from RBCs was elusive, and cloning of the Kidd gene was accomplished with primers complementary to the rabbit kidney urea transporter. A clone isolated from a human bone marrow library with the PCR product was confirmed by in vitro transcription-translation to encode a protein that carried Kidd blood group antigens.[138]

Gene

The Kidd blood group gene (*HUT11* or *SLC14A1*) is located at chromosome 18q11-q12.[139, 140] The *HUT11* gene has 11 exons and spans approximately 30 kb. Two alternative polyadenylation sites generate transcripts of 4.4 and 2.0 kb, which appear to be used equally. Exons 4 to 11 encode the mature protein.[17, 141]

Table 4.7 Kidd Phenotypes and Incidence

	Incidence(%)		
Phenotype	White	African	Asian
Jk(a+b−)	26.3	51.5	23.2
Jk(a−b+)	23.4	8.1	26.8
Jk(a+b+)	50.3	40.8	49.1
Jk(a−b−)	Rare	Rare	0.9 (Polynesian)

Antigens

Two antigens, Jk[a] and Jk[b], are responsible for the three common phenotypes—Jk(a+b−), Jk(a−b+) and Jk(a+b+). The two antigens are found with similar frequency in white persons but show large differences in other ethnic groups (Table 4.7).[1] The Jk(a−b−) phenotype is rare but occurs with greater incidence in Asian and Polynesian people.

The Jk[a] and Jk[b] polymorphism is located on the fourth extracellular loop and is caused by a single amino acid substitution (see Fig. 4.5).[142] The null phenotype has been reported to arise on the following two genetic backgrounds: homozygous inheritance of a silent allele and inheritance of a dominant inhibitor gene, *In(Jk)*, which is unlinked to *JK (HUT11)*.[1] The silent alleles were found to have acceptor or donor splice site mutations that cause skipping of exon 6 or exon 7.[141, 143] In Finnish persons, a single point mutation (Ser291Pro) was the only change associated with silencing of the expression of Jk[b].[143] The unlinked dominant inhibitor gene has not yet been identified.

The Jk3 antigen ("total Jk") is found on RBCs that are positive for Jk[a], Jk[b], or both, but the specific amino acid residues responsible for Jk3 are unknown. There are approximately 14,000 Jk[a] antigen sites on Jk(a+b−) RBCs.[122]

Antibodies

Neither anti-Jk[a] or anti-Jk[b] is common, and anti-Jk[b] is found less often than anti-Jk[a]. Once a Kidd antibody is identified, compatible blood is not difficult to find, because 25% of donors are negative for each antigen. Unfortunately, Kidd antibodies are often found in sera that contain other alloantibodies,

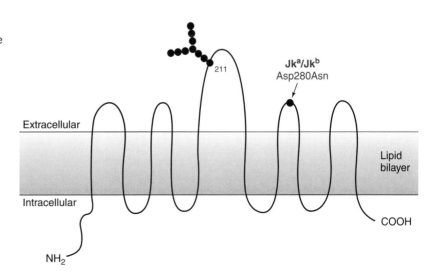

Figure 4.5 Predicted 10-transmembrane domain structure of the Kidd/urea transporter. The polymorphism responsible for the Kidd antigens and the site for the N-glycan are indicated.

so the situation is often more complicated. In addition, the antibodies are known to cause delayed hemolytic transfusion reactions (DHTRs) and are responsible for at least one third of all cases of DHTRs.[48] The antibodies often decrease in titer, react only with cells that are from persons homozygous for the antigen (the dosage phenomenon), or may escape detection altogether in the sensitized patient's serum before transfusion. If the patient is transfused with antigen-positive RBCs, an anamnestic response results, with an increase in the antibody titer and hemolysis of the transfused RBCs.[48]

Because Kidd antibodies are mainly IgG, it was assumed that they must activate complement to cause such prompt RBC destruction. Kidd antibodies can be partially IgM, however, and the minor IgM component may be responsible for the pattern of destruction of incompatible RBCs in DHTRs. This theory is based on evidence that serum fractions containing only IgG anti-Jk^a do not bind complement.[144] Kidd antibodies only rarely cause HDN, and if they do, it is typically not severe. Anti-Jk^a has occasionally been found as an autoantibody, and the concurrent, temporary suppression of antigen expression has also been reported.[48] Anti-Jk3, sometimes referred to as anti-Jk^{ab}, is produced by Jk(a–b–) individuals and reacts with RBCs that are positive for Jk^a, Jk^b, or both.[145]

Expression

In the fetus, Kidd antigens can be detected at 11 weeks of gestation and are well developed at birth.[6] Immunohistochemical and in situ hybridization have shown that Kidd/HUT11 is also expressed on endothelial cells of vasa recta in the medulla of the human kidney.[17]

Evolution

Expression of RBC Kidd antigens has not been investigated in nonhuman primates, but the human RBC Kidd protein is clearly a member of a family of urea transporters, which have homologues in the human kidney and in nonhuman primates.

Function

A first clue to the function of Kidd came from the observation in 1982 that the RBCs of a male of Samoan descent were resistant to lysis in 2M urea, which was being used to lyse RBCs for platelet counting.[146] His RBCs were Jk(a–b–), and subsequent investigations revealed that movement of urea into Jk(a–b–) RBCs was equivalent to passive diffusion, in contrast to RBCs with normal Kidd antigens, with rapid urea influx. Fast urea transport in human RBCs is thought to be advantageous for RBC osmotic stability in the kidney, especially during transit through the vasa recta from the papilla to the iso-osmotic renal cortex.[147] Urea transport in the kidney contributes to urinary concentration and water preservation. Two types of urea transporters have now been characterized, vasopressin-sensitive transporters and constitutive transporters. The Kidd/HUT11 in RBCs and kidney medulla is a constitutive transporter. A vasopressin-sensitive transporter, HUT2, which is expressed in the collecting ducts of the kidney, has 62% sequence identity with Kidd/HUT11. *HUT2* is also located on chromosome 18q12, suggesting that both transporters evolved from an ancestral gene duplication.[148] Jk$_{null}$ individuals do not suffer a clinical syndrome except for a reduced capacity to concentrate urine,[149] suggesting that other mechanisms or other gene family members, like *HUT2*, can compensate for the missing Kidd/HUT11 protein.

■ Summary

The last decade has witnessed the rapid elucidation of the molecular basis for the various blood group antigens and phenotypes. In the next decade, research focus is turned to determination of the structure and function of the proteins carrying these blood group antigens. Null individuals ("natural knockouts"), persons who lack the antigens and the proteins that carry them, exist for all four of these blood group systems. Reminiscent of what is being found in many genetically engineered knockout mice, most of the individuals with null phenotypes do not have serious or any obvious defects. This observation is consistent with growing evidence that many genes have evolved as members of larger gene families, which appear to have overlapping abilities to substitute for the disrupted gene family member. Evidence is accumulating that genes encoding blood group proteins are also members of larger gene families. The mouse homologues of some of these blood group genes have been cloned, and knockout mice are being generated to study them. This process may aid in the further elucidation of the structure and function of the molecules carrying blood group antigens.

REFERENCES

1. Race RR, Sanger R: Blood Groups in Man, 6th ed. Oxford, Blackwell Scientific, 1975.
2. Bowman JM: RhD hemolytic disease of the newborn [editorial; comment]. N Engl J Med 1998;339:1775–1777.
3. Levine P, Stetson RE: An unusual case of intragroup agglutination. JAMA 1939;113:126–127.
4. Levine P, Burnham L, Katzin EM, Vogel P: The role of iso-immunization in the pathogenesis of erythroblastosis fetalis. Am J Obstet Gynecol 1941;42:925–937.
5. Rosenfield RE: Who discovered Rh? A personal glimpse of the Levine-Wiener argument. Transfusion 1989;29:355–357.
6. Daniels G: Human Blood Groups. Oxford: Blackwell Science, 1995.
7. Mourant AE: A new rhesus antibody. Nature 1945;155:542.
8. Tippett P: A speculative model for the Rh blood groups. Ann Hum Genet 1986;50:241–247.
9. Rosenfield RE, Allen FH Jr, Swisher SN, Kochwa S: A review of Rh serology and presentation of a new terminology. Transfusion 1962;2:287–312.
10. Agre P, Saboori AM, Asimos A, Smith BL: Purification and partial characterization of the M_r 30,000 integral membrane protein associated with the erythrocyte Rh(D) antigen. J Biol Chem 1987;262:17497–17503.
11. Bloy C, Blanchard D, Dahr W, et al: Determination of the N-terminal sequence of human red cell Rh(D) polypeptide and demonstration that the Rh(D), (c), and (E) antigens are carried by distinct polypeptide chains. Blood 1988;72:661–666.
12. Arce MA, Thompson ES, Wagner S, et al: Molecular cloning of RhD cDNA derived from a gene present in RhD-positive, but not RhD-negative individuals. Blood 1993;82:651–655.
13. Chérif-Zahar B, Bloy C, Le Van Kim C, et al: Molecular cloning and protein structure of a human blood group Rh polypeptide. Proc Natl Acad Sci USA 1990;87:6243–6247.
14. Simsek S, de Jong CA, Cuijpers HT, et al: Sequence analysis of cDNA derived from reticulocyte mRNAs coding for Rh polypeptides and demonstration of E/e and C/c polymorphisms. Vox Sang 1994;67:203–209.
15. Hartel-Schenk S, Agre P: Mammalian red cell membrane Rh polypeptides are selectively palmitoylated subunits of a macromolecular complex. J Biol Chem 1992;267:5569–5574.
16. Ridgwell K, Spurr NK, Laguda B, et al: Isolation of cDNA clones for a 50 kDa glycoprotein of the human erythrocyte membrane associated with Rh (rhesus) blood-group antigen expression. Biochem J 1992;287:223–228.

17. Russo DC, Qyen R, Powell VI, et al: First example of anti-Kx in a person with the McLeod phenotype and without chronic granulomatous disease. Transfusion 2000;40:1371–1375.

18. Eyers SA, Ridgwell K, Mawby WJ, Tanner MJ: Topology and organization of human Rh (rhesus) blood group-related polypeptides. J Biol Chem 1994;269:6417–6423.

19. Beckmann R, Smythe JS, Anstee DJ, Tanner MJA: Functional cell surface expression of band 3, the human red blood cell anion exchange protein (AE1), in K562 erythroleukemia cells: Band 3 enhances the cell surface reactivity of Rh antigens. Blood 1998;92:4428–4438.

20. Colin Y, Chérif-Zahar B, Le Van Kim C, et al: Genetic basis of the RhD-positive and RhD-negative blood group polymorphism as determined by Southern analysis. Blood 1991;78:2747–2752.

21. Chérif-Zahar B, Mattei MG, Le Van Kim C, et al: Localization of the human Rh blood group gene structure to chromosome region 1p34.3-1p36.1 by in situ hybridization. Hum Genet 1991;86:398–400.

22. Avent ND, Reid ME: The Rh blood group system: A review. Blood 2000;95:375–387.

23. Huang C-H: The human Rh50 glycoprotein gene—structural organization and associated splicing defect resulting in Rh_{null} disease. J Biol Chem 1998;273:2207–2213.

24. Chérif-Zahar B, Raynal V, Gane P, et al: Candidate gene acting as a suppressor of the RH locus in most cases of Rh-deficiency. Nature Genet 1996;12:168–173.

25. Avent ND, Martin PG, Armstrong-Fisher SS, et al: Evidence of genetic diversity underlying Rh D⁻, weak D (Dᵘ), and partial D phenotypes as determined by multiplex polymerase chain reaction analysis of the RHD gene. Blood 1997;89:2568–2577.

26. Andrews KT, Wolter LC, Saul A, Hyland CA: The RhD- trait in a white patient with the RhCCee phenotype attributed to a four-nucleotide deletion in the RHD gene. Blood 1998;92:1839–1840.

27. Huang C-H: Alteration of RH gene structure and expression in human dCCee and DCᵂ- red blood cells: Phenotypic homozygosity versus genotypic heterozygosity. Blood 1996;88:2326–2333.

28. Wagner FF, Frohmajer A, Flegel WA: RHD positive haplotypes in D negative Europeans. BMC Genetics 2001;2:10.

29. Okuda H, Kawano M, Iwamoto S, et al: The RHD gene is highly detectable in RhD-negative Japanese donors. J Clin Invest 1997;100:373–379.

30. Singleton BK, Green CA, Avent ND, et al: The presence of an RHD pseudogene containing a 37 base pair duplication and a nonsense mutation in Africans with the RhD-negative blood group phenotype. Blood 2000;95:12–18.

31. Rouillac C, Gane P, Cartron J, et al: Molecular basis of the altered antigenic expression of RhD in weak D (Dᵘ) and RhC/e in Rᴺ phenotypes. Blood 1996;87:4853–4861.

32. Beckers EAM, Faas BH, Ligthart P, et al: Lower antigen site density and weak D immunogenicity cannot be explained by structural genomic abnormalities or regulatory defects of the RHD gene. Transfusion 1997;37:616–623.

33. Wagner FF, Gassner C, Müller TH, et al: Molecular basis of weak D phenotypes. Blood 1999;93:385–393.

34. Wagner FF, Frohmajer A, Ladewig B, et al: Weak D alleles express distinct phenotypes. Blood 2000;95:2699–2708.

35. Chang JG, Wang JC, Yang TY, et al: Human Rh_{Del} is caused by a deletion of 1,013 bp between introns 8 and 9 including exon 9 of RHD gene. Blood 1998;92:2602–2604.

36. Huang C-H: Molecular insights into the Rh protein family and associated antigens. Curr Opin Hematol 1997;4:94–103.

37. Mouro I, Colin Y, Chérif-Zahar B, et al: Molecular genetic basis of the human Rhesus blood group system. Nature Genet 1993;5:62–65.

38. Mouro I, Colin Y, Sistonen P, et al: Molecular basis of the RhCᵂ (Rh8) and RhCˣ (Rh9) blood group specificities. Blood 1995;86:1196–1201.

39. Faas BHW, Beckers EAM, Wildoer P, et al: Molecular background of VS and weak C expression in blacks. Transfusion 1997;37:38–44.

40. Daniels GL, Faas BHW, Green CA, et al: The VS and V blood group polymorphisms in Africans: A serological and molecular analysis. Transfusion 1998;38:951–958.

41. Noizat-Pirenne F, Mouro I, Gane P, et al: Heterogeneity of blood group RhE variants revealed by serological analysis and molecular alteration of the RHCE gene and transcript. Br J Haematol 1998;103:429–436.

42. Noizat-Pirenne F, Mouro I, Roussel M, et al: The molecular basis of a D (C) (E) complex probably associated with the RH35 low frequency antigen [abstract]. Transfusion 1999;39(Suppl):103S.

43. Huang C-H, Reid ME, Chen Y, Novaretti M: Deletion of Arg229 in RhCE polypeptide alters expression of RhE and CE-associated Rh6 [abstract]. Blood 1997;90(Suppl 1):272a.

44. Westhoff CM, Silberstein LE, Wylie DE, et al: 16Cys encoded by the RHce gene is associated with altered expression of the e antigen and is frequent in the R_0 haplotype. Br J Haematol 2001;113:666–671.

45. Faas BHW, Ligthart PC, Lomas-Francis C, et al: Involvement of Gly96 in the formation of the Rh26 epitope. Transfusion 1997;37:1123–1130.

46. Ballas SK, Clark MR, Mohandas N, et al: Red cell membrane and cation deficiency in Rh null syndrome. Blood 1989;63:1046–1055.

47. Huang C-H, Chen Y, Reid ME, Seidl C: Rh_{null} disease: The amorph type results from a novel double mutation in RhCe gene on D-negative background. Blood 1998;92:664–671.

48. Mollison PL, Engelfriet CP, Contreras M: Blood Transfusion in Clinical Medicine, 10th ed. Oxford, Blackwell Science, 1997.

49. Petz LD, Garratty G: Acquired Immune Hemolytic Anemias. New York, Churchill Livingstone, 1980.

50. Kumpel BM, Goodrick MJ, Pamphilon DH, et al: Human Rh D monoclonal antibodies (BRAD-3 and BRAD-5) cause accelerated clearance of Rh D⁺ red blood cells and suppression of Rh D immunization in Rh D⁻ volunteers. Blood 1995;86:1701–1709.

51. Kajii E, Umenishi F, Nakauchi H, Ikemoto S: Expression of Rh blood group gene transcripts in human leukocytes. Biochem Biophys Res Commun 1994;202:1497–1504.

52. Southcott MJG, Tanner MJ, Anstee DJ: The expression of human blood group antigens during erythropoiesis in a cell culture system. Blood 1999;93:4425–4435.

53. Westhoff CM, Wylie DE: Investigation of the human Rh blood group system in nonhuman primates and other species with serologic and Southern blot analysis. J Mol Evol 1994;39:87–92.

54. Salvignol I, Calvas P, Socha WW, et al: Structural analysis of the RH-like blood group gene products in nonhuman primates. Immunogenetics 1995;41:271–281.

55. Westhoff CM, Schultze A, From A, et al: Characterization of the mouse RH blood group gene. Genomics 1999;57:451–454.

56. Blancher A, Klein J, Socha WW (eds): Molecular Biology and Evolution of Blood Group and MHC Antigens in Primates. Berlin, Springer-Verlag, 1997.

57. Kitano T, Sumiyama K, Shiroishi T, Saitou N: Conserved evolution of the Rh50 gene compared to its homologous Rh blood group gene. Biochem Biophys Res Commun 1998;249:78–85.

58. Marini AM, Urrestarazu A, Beauwens R, André B: The Rh (rhesus) blood group polypeptides are related to NH₄⁺ transporters. Trends Biochem Sci 1997;22:460–461.

59. Marini AM, Matassi G, Raynal V, et al: The human rhesus-associated RhAG protein and a kidney homologue promote ammonium transport in yeast. Nature Genet 2000;26:341–344.

60. Westhoff CM, Ferreri-Jacobia M, Mak Don-On, Foskett JK: Identification of the erythrocyte Rh blood group glycoprotein as a mammalian ammonium transporter. J Biol Chem 2002;277:12499–12502.

61. Huang C-H, Liu PZ, Cheng JG: Molecular biology and genetics of the Rh blood group system. Semin Hematol 2000;37:150–165.

62. Liu Z, Peng J, Mo R, et al: Rh type B glycoprotein is a new member of the Rh superfamily and a putative ammonia transporter in mammals. J Biol Chem 2001;276:1424–1433.

63. Liu Z, Chen Y, Mo R, et al: Characterization of human RhCG and mouse Rhcg as novel nonerythroid Rh glycoprotein homologues predominantly expressed in kidney and testis. J Biol Chem 2000;275:25641–25651.

64. Coombs RRA, Mourant AE, Race RR: In-vivo isosensitization of red cells in babies with haemolytic disease. Lancet 1946;i:264–266.

65. Levine P, Backer M, Wigod M, Ponder R: A new human hereditary blood property (Cellano) present in 99.8% of all bloods. Science 1949;109:464–466.

66. Lee S, Zambas ED, Marsh WL, Redman CM: Molecular cloning and primary structure of Kell blood group protein. Proc Natl Acad Sci USA 1991;88:6353–6357.

67. Advani H, Zamor J, Judd WJ, et al: Inactivation of Kell blood group antigens by 2-aminoethylisothiouronium bromide. Br J Haematol 1982;51:107–115.

68. Hughes-Jones NC, Gardner B: The Kell system: Studies with radiolabeled anti-K. Vox Sang 1971;21:154–158.

69. Masouredis SP, Sudora E, Mohan LC, Victoria EJ: Immunoelectron microscopy of Kell and Cellano antigens on red cell ghosts. Haematologia 1980;13:59–64.

70. Marsh WL, Redman CM: The Kell blood group system: A review. Transfusion 1990;30:158–167.

71. Lee S: Molecular basis of Kell blood group phenotypes. Vox Sang 1997;73:1–11.

72. Lee S, Zambas ED, Marsh WL, Redman CM: The human Kell blood group gene maps to chromosome 7q33 and its expression is restricted to erythroid cells. Blood 1993;81:2804–2809.

73. Lee S, Zambas E, Green ED, Redman C: Organization of the gene encoding the human Kell blood group protein. Blood 1995;85:1364–1370.

74. Lee S, Russo DC Reiner AP, et al: Molecular defects underlying the Kell null phenotype. J Biol Chem 2001;276:27281–27289.

75. Yu LC, Twu YC, Chang CY, Lin M: Molecular basis of the Kell-null phenotype: A mutation at the splice site of human KEL gene abolishes the expression of Kell blood group antigens. J Biol Chem 2001;276:10247–10252.

76. Bertelson CJ, Pogo AO, Chaudhuri A, et al: Localization of the McLeod locus (XK) within Xp21 by deletion analysis. Am J Hum Genet 1988;42:703–711.

77. Marsh WL, Redman CM: Recent developments in the Kell blood group system. Transfus Med Rev 1987;1:4–20.

78. Øyen R, Reid ME, Rubinstein P, Ralph H: A method to detect McLeod phenotype red blood cells. Immunohematology 1996;12:160–163.

79. Allen FH, Krabbe SMR, Corcoran PA: A new phenotype (McLeod) in the Kell blood group system. Vox Sang 1961;6:555–560.

80. Danek A, Rubio JP, Rampoldi L, et al: McLeod neuroacanthocytosis: Genotype and phenotype. Ann Neurol 2001;50:755–764.

81. Russo DC, Lee S, Reid ME, Redman C: Point mutations causing the McLeod phenotype. Transfusion 2002;42:287–293.

82. Reid ME, Lomas-Francis C: The Blood Group Antigen Facts Book. San Diego, Academic Press, 1996.

83. Lee S, Wu X, Son S, et al: Point mutations characterize KEL10, the KEL3, KEL4, and KEL21 alleles, and the KEL17 and KEL11 alleles. Transfusion 1996;36:490–494.

84. Lee S, Wu X, Reid ME, et al: Molecular basis of the Kell (K1) phenotype. Blood 1995;85:912–916.

85. Lee S, Wu X, Reid ME, Redman C: Molecular basis of the K:6, −7 [Js(a+b−)] phenotype in the Kell blood group system. Transfusion 1995;35:822–825.

86. Branch DR, Muensch HA, Sy Siok Hian AL, Petz LD: Disulfide bonds are a requirement for Kell and Cartwright (Yt^a) blood group antigen integrity. Br J Haematol 1983;54:573–578.

87. Yazdanbakhsh K, Lee S, Yu Q, Reid ME: Identification of a defect in the intracellular trafficking of a Kell blood group variant. Blood 1999;94:310–318.

88. Allen FH Jr, Lewis SJ, Fudenberg H: Studies of anti-Kp^b, a new antibody in the Kell blood group system. Vox Sang 1958;3:1–13.

89. Allen FH, Lewis SJ: Kp^a (Penney), a new antigen in the Kell blood group system. Vox Sang 1957;2:81–87.

90. Øyen R, Halverson GR, Reid ME: Review: Conditions causing weak expression of Kell system antigens. Immunohematology 1997;13:75–79.

91. Anstee DJ: Blood group-active surface molecules of the human red blood cell. Vox Sang 1990;58:1–20.

92. Vaughan JI, Warwick R, Letsky E, et al: Erythropoietic suppression in fetal anemia because of Kell alloimmunization. Am J Obstet Gynecol 1994;171:247–252.

93. Redman CM, Lee S, ten Huinink D, et al: Comparison of human and chimpanzee Kell blood group systems. Transfusion 1989;29:486–490.

94. Blancher A, Reid ME, Socha WW: Cross-reactivity of antibodies to human and primate red cell antigens. Transfus Med Rev 2000;14:161–179.

95. Jaber A, Loirat MJ, Willem C, et al: Characterization of murine monoclonal antibodies directed against the Kell blood group glycoprotein. Br J Haematol 1991;79:311–315.

96. Xu D, Emoto N, Giaid A, et al: ECE-1: A membrane-bound metalloprotease that catalyzes the proteolytic activation of big endothelin-1. Cell 1994;78:473–485.

97. Lee S, Lin M, Mele A, et al: Proteolytic processing of big endothelin-3 by the Kell blood group protein. Blood 1999;94:1440–1450.

98. Cutbush M, Mollison PI, Parkin DM: A new human blood group. Nature 1950;165:188.

99. Ikin EW, Mourant AE, Pettenkofer HJ, Blumenthal G: Discovery of the expected haemagglutinin anti-Fy^b. Nature 1951;168:1077–1078.

100. Miller LH, Mason SJ, Dvorak JA, et al: Erythrocyte receptors for (Plasmodium knowlesi) malaria: Duffy blood group determinants. Science 1975;189:561–563.

101. Neote K, Mak JY, Kolakowski LF Jr, Schall TJ: Functional and biochemical analysis of the cloned Duffy antigen: Identity with the red blood cell chemokine receptor. Blood 1994;84:44–52.

102. Chaudhuri A, Zbrzezna V, Johnson C, et al: Purification and characterization of an erythrocyte membrane protein complex carrying Duffy blood group antigenicity. Possible receptor for Plasmodium vivax and Plasmodium knowlesi malaria parasite. J Biol Chem 1989;264:13770–13774.

103. Horuk R, Colby TJ, Darbonne WC, et al: The human erythrocyte inflammatory peptide (chemokine) receptor: Biochemical characterization, solubilization, and development of a binding assay for the soluble receptor. Biochemistry 1993;32:5733–5738.

104. Chaudhuri A, Polyakova J, Zbrzezna V, et al: Cloning of glycoprotein D cDNA, which encodes the major subunit of the Duffy blood group system and the receptor for the Plasmodium vivax malaria parasite. Proc Natl Acad Sci U S A 1993;90:10793–10797.

105. Mathew S, Chaudhuri A, Murty VV, Pogo AO: Confirmation of Duffy blood group antigen locus (FY) at 1q22–>23 by fluorescence in situ hybridization. Cytogenet Cell Genet 1994;67:68.

106. Iwamoto S, Li J, Omi T, et al: Identification of a novel exon and spliced form of Duffy mRNA that is the predominant transcript in both erythroid and postcapillary venule endothelium. Blood 1996;87:378–385.

107. Iwamoto S, Omi T, Kajii E, Ikemoto S: Genomic organization of the glycophorin D gene: Duffy blood group Fy^a/Fy^b alloantigen system is associated with a polymorphism at the 44-amino acid residue. Blood 1995;85:622–626.

108. Hadley TJ, Peiper SC: From malaria to chemokine receptor: The emerging physiologic role of the Duffy blood group antigen. Blood 1997;89:3077–3091.

109. Tournamille C, Le Van Kim C, Gane P, et al: Molecular basis and PCR-DNA typing of the Fy^a/Fy^b blood group polymorphism. Hum Genet 1995;95:407–410.

110. Parasol N, Reid M, Rios M, et al: A novel mutation in the coding sequence of the FY*B allele of the Duffy chemokine receptor gene is associated with an altered erythrocyte phenotype. Blood 1998;92:2237–2243.

111. Olsson ML, Smythe JS, Hansson C, et al: The Fy^x phenotype is associated with a missense mutation in the Fy^b allele predicting Arg89Cys in the Duffy glycoprotein. Br J Haematol 1998;103:1184–1191.

112. Tournamille C, Le Van Kim C, Gane P, et al: Arg89Cys substitution results in very low membrane expression of the Duffy antigen/receptor for chemokines in Fy^x individuals (erratum in 95:2753). Blood 1998;92:2147–2156.

113. Yazdanbakhsh K, Øyen R, Yu Q, et al: High level, stable expression of blood group antigens in a heterologous system. Am J Hematol 2000;63:114–124.

114. Lu ZH, Wang ZX, Horuk R, et al: The promiscuous chemokine binding profile of the Duffy antigen/receptor for chemokines is primarily localized to sequences in the amino-terminal domain. J Biol Chem 1995;270:26239–26245.

115. Wasniowska K, Blanchard D, Janvier D, et al: Identification of the Fy6 epitope recognized by two monoclonal antibodies in the N-terminal extracellular portion of the Duffy antigen receptor for chemokines. Mol Immunol 1996;33:917–923.

116. Tournamille C, Colin Y, Cartron JP, Le Van Kim C: Disruption of a GATA motif in the Duffy gene promoter abolishes erythroid gene expression in Duffy-negative individuals. Nature Genet 1995;10:224–228.

117. Iwamoto S, Li J, Sugimoto N, et al: Characterization of the Duffy gene promoter: Evidence for tissue-specific abolishment of expression in Fy(a−b−) of black individuals. Biochem Biophys Res Commun 1996;222:852–859.

118. Le Pennec PY, Rouger P, Klein MT, et al: Study of anti-Fya in five black Fy(a−b−) patients. Vox Sang 1987;52:246–249.

119. Zimmerman PA, Woolley I, Masinde GL, et al: Emergence of FY*A^{null} in a Plasmodium vivax-endemic region of Papua New Guinea. Proc Natl Acad Sci USA 1999;96:13973–13977.

120. Mallinson G, Soo KS, Schall TJ, et al: Mutations in the erythrocyte chemokine receptor (Duffy) gene: The molecular basis of the Fy^a/Fy^b antigens and identification of a deletion in the Duffy gene of an apparently healthy individual with the Fy(a−b−) phenotype. Br J Haematol 1995;90:823–829.

121. Rios M, Chaudhuri A, Mallinson G, et al: New genotypes in Fy(a−b−) individuals: Nonsense mutations (Trp to stop) in the coding sequence of either *FYA* or *FYB*. Br J Haematol 2000;108:448–454.

122. Masouredis SP, Sudora E, Mahan L, Victoria EJ: Quantitative immunoferritin microscopy of Fy^a, Fy^b, Jk^a, U, and Di^b antigen site numbers on human red cells. Blood 1980;56:969–977.

123. Hadley TJ, Lu ZH, Wasniowska K, et al: Postcapillary venule endothelial cells in kidney express a multispecific chemokine receptor that is structurally and functionally identical to the erythroid isoform, which is the Duffy blood group antigen. J Clin Invest 1994;94:985–991.

124. Peiper SC, Wang ZX, Neote K, et al: The Duffy antigen/receptor for chemokines (DARC) is expressed in endothelial cells of Duffy negative individuals who lack the erythrocyte receptor. J Exp Med 1995;181:1311–1317.

125. Chaudhuri A, Nielsen S, Elkjaer ML, et al: Detection of Duffy antigen in the plasma membranes and caveolae of vascular endothelial and epithelial cells of nonerythroid organs. Blood 1997;89:701–712.

126. Horuk R, Martin A, Hesselgesser J, et al: The Duffy antigen receptor for chemokines: Structural analysis and expression in the brain. J Leukocyte Biol 1996;59:29–38.

127. Horuk R, Martin AW, Wang Z, et al: Expression of chemokine receptors by subsets of neurons in the central nervous system. J Immunol 1997;158:2882–2890.

128. Li J, Iwamoto S, Sugimoto N, et al: Dinucleotide repeat in the 3′ flanking region provides a clue to the molecular evolution of the Duffy gene. Hum Genet 1997;99:573–577.

129. Chaudhuri A, Polyakova J, Zbrzezna V, Pogo O: The coding sequence of Duffy blood group gene in humans and simians: Restriction fragment length polymorphism, antibody and malarial parasite specificities, and expression in nonerythroid tissues in Duffy-negative individuals. Blood 1995;85:615–621.

130. Luster AD: Chemokines—chemotactic cytokines that mediate inflammation. N Engl J Med 1998;338:436–445.

131. Tilg H, Shapiro L, Atkins MB, et al: Induction of circulating and erythrocyte-bound IL-8 by IL-2 immunotherapy and suppression of its *in vitro* production by IL-1 receptor antagonist and soluble tumor necrosis factor receptor (p75) chimera. J Immunol 1993;151:3299–3307.

132. de Winter RJ, Manten A, de Jong YP, et al: Interleukin 8 released after acute myocardial infarction is mainly bound to erythrocytes. Heart 1997;78:598–602.

133. Danoff TM, Hallows KR, Burns JE, et al: Influence of the Duffy blood group on renal allograft survival in African-Americans [abstract]. J Am Soc Nephrol 1998;9:670A.

134. Liu X-H, Hadley TJ, Xu L, et al: Up-regulation of Duffy antigen receptor expression in children with renal disease. Kidney Int 1999;55:1491–1500.

135. Allen FH, Diamond LK, Niedziela B: A new blood-group antigen. Nature 1951;167:482.

136. Plaut G, Ikin EW, Mourant AE, et al: A new blood group antibody, anti-Jk^b. Nature 1953;171:431.

137. Rousselet G, Ripoche P, Bailly P: Tandem sequence repeats in urea transporters: Identification of a urea transporter signature sequence. Am J Physiol 1996;270:F554–F555.

138. Olivès B, Neau P, Bailly P, et al: Cloning and functional expression of a urea transporter from human bone marrow cells. J Biol Chem 1994;269:31649–31652.

139. Geitvik GA, Hoyheim B, Gedde-Dahl T, et al: The Kidd (*JK*) blood group locus assigned to chromosome 18 by close linkage to a DNA-RFLP. Hum Genet 1987;77:205–209.

140. Leppert M, Ferrell R, Kambok MI, et al: Linkage of the polymorphic protein markers *F13B*, *CIS*, *CIR* and blood group antigen Kidd in CEPH reference families [abstract]. Cytogenet Cell Genet 1987;46:647.

141. Lucien N, Sidoux-Walter F, Olivès B, et al: Characterization of the gene encoding the human Kidd blood group/urea transporter protein: Evidence for splice site mutations in Jk$_{null}$ individuals. J Biol Chem 1998;273:12973–12980.

142. Olivès B, Merriman M, Bailly P, et al: The molecular basis of the Kidd blood group polymorphism and its lack of association with type 1 diabetes susceptibility. Hum Mol Genet 1997;6:1017–1020.

143. Irshaid NM, Henry SM, Olsson ML: Genomic characterization of the Kidd blood group gene:different molecular basis of the Jk(a−b−) phenotype in Polynesians and Finns. Transfusion 2000;40:69–74.

144. Yates J, Howell P, Overfield J, et al: IgG Kidd antibodies are unlikely to fix complement [abstract]. Transfus Med 1996;6(Suppl 2):29.

145. Pinkerton FJ, Mermod LE, Liles BA, et al: The phenotype Jk(a−b−) in the Kidd blood group system. Vox Sang 1959;4:155–160.

146. Heaton DC, McLoughlin K: Jk(a−b−) red blood cells resist urea lysis. Transfusion 1982;22:70–71.

147. Macey RI, Yousef LW: Osmotic stability of red cells in renal circulation requires rapid urea transport. Am J Physiol 1988;254:C669–C674.

148. Martial S, Olivès B, Abrami L, et al: Functional differentiation of the human red blood cell and kidney urea transporters. Am J Physiol Renal Fluid Electrolyte Physiol 1996;271:F1264–F1268.

149. Sands JM, Gargus JJ, Frohlich O, et al: Urinary concentrating ability in patients with Jk(a−b−) blood type who lack carrier-mediated urea transport. J Am Soc Nephrol 1992;2:1689–1696.

Chapter 5

Other Blood Group Systems and Antigens

Marion E. Reid
Constance M. Westhoff

This chapter provides information for the 16 blood group systems not covered in Chapters 3 and 4. The systems are discussed here in the order of their ISBT numbers (see Table 2.3). Antibodies to antigens in these systems are less common than those described in the preceding chapters, and information regarding their general clinical significance is summarized in Tables 2.5 and 2.6.

The red blood cell (RBC) membrane components carrying the antigens of 13 of the systems described in this chapter are depicted in Figure 5.1. The carrier proteins of the Sc and RAPH systems are not shown in this figure, because their structure remains unknown. The antigens of the Chido/Rodgers system are adsorbed onto the RBC, and are not integral membrane components, and thus they also are not included in Figure 5.1.

■ The MNS System (ISBT System 002)

History

The MNS system, discovered in 1927, was the second blood group system to be recognized. The first two antigens, M and N, were named from the second and fifth letters of the word *immune*, because the corresponding antibodies were produced through immunization of rabbits with human RBCs, and it was thought that the first letter, I, might be confused with the number 1.[1, 2] The S antigen, the next to be identified, was named from the city (*S*ydney) where the first anti-S was discovered.[3] When the antithetical antigen was identified, the logical name s was used. The name for the high-incidence antigen U was derived from the "almost *universal* distribution of the new blood factor."[4] Many of the other antigens were named after the original family in which an antigen-positive neonate suffered from hemolytic disease of the newborn (HDN).

Gene, Protein, and Antigens

MNS antigens are carried on glycophorin (GP) A and GPB, which are encoded by homologous genes (respectively, *GYPA* and *GYPB*) on chromosome 4q28-q31.[5] *GYPA* has seven exons, and *GYPB* has five exons and one pseudo-exon. A third homologous gene, *GYPE*, completes this glycophorin gene family, but it is not clear whether the product of *GYPE* is expressed on the RBC membrane. The glycophorin gene cluster encompasses approximately 330 kb in the following order: *GYPA, GYPB, GYPE.*[6]

GPA and GPB are homologous single-pass membrane sialoglycoproteins oriented with their N-termini to the exterior of the RBC. GPA has 15 potential sites for O-glycans, one N-glycan, and an approximate M_r of 43,000 on sodium dodecyl sulfate–polyacrylamide gel electrophoresis (SDS-PAGE); there are approximately 1,000,000 copies of GPA per RBC. GPB has 11 potential sites for O-glycans, no N-glycan, an approximate M_r of 25,000 on SDS-PAGE, and there are approximately 200,000 copies per RBC.[7, 8]

M and N antigens are carried on alternative forms of GPA and are the result of amino acid substitutions at residues 1 and 5. The M antigen has Ser at position 1 and Gly at position 5, whereas the N antigen has Leu at position 1 and Glu at position 5. The first 26 amino acids of the N form of GPA are identical to GPB. Anti-N reagents prepared for use in the clinical setting are formulated to detect the N antigen on GPA but not the N on GPB ('N').[9–13] Using these reagents, human RBCs type as M+N−, M−N+, or M+N+.

S and s antigens are carried on alternative forms of GPB. At amino acid residue 29, Met is critical for the S antigen, and Thr for the s antigen. Both antigens also involve the amino acids at residues 25, 28, 34, and 35.[14] Persons who

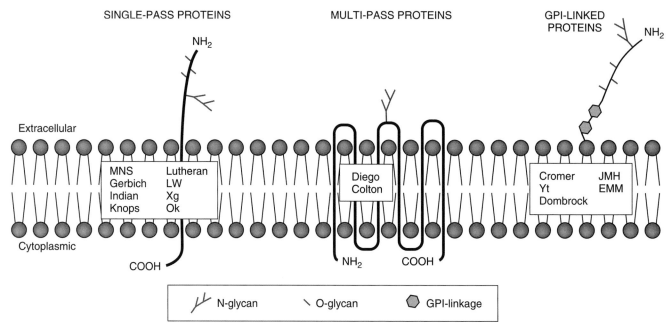

Figure 5.1   Diagram of the red blood cell membrane illustrates the type of membrane components that carry the blood group antigens described in Chapter 5. The figure does not show components carrying Chido/Rodgers antigens, because they are not integral membrane components, or Sc and RAPH blood group systems, most of the components carrying the blood group collections, and high- and low-incidence antigens, because their structure is unknown.

are S–s–, usually blacks, may be negative for the high-incidence antigen U owing to a deletion of or an altered form of *GYPB*.[15–17] Because M/N and S/s are on homologous proteins that are encoded by adjacent genes, they are inherited en bloc, accounting for linkage dysequilibrium between the antigens (Table 5.1).

The MNS blood group system is highly polymorphic, with 43 antigens.[18–20] Many of the antigens are uncommon, resulting from an amino acid substitution or multiple rearrangements between *GYPA* and *GYPB* (Table 5.2).[15] Low-incidence antigens in the MNS blood group system are as follows, in alphabetical order: Cl^a, DANE, Dantu, ERIK, Far, HAG, He, Hil, Hop, Hut, MARS, M^e, M^g, Mi^a, MINY, Mit, Mt^a, Mur, MUT, M^v, Nob, Ny^a, Or, Os^a Ri^a, s^D, SAT, St^a, TSEN, Vr, Vw.[7] The rare null phenotypes of this system— En(a–), which lacks MN antigens; U–, which lacks S$_s$ antigens;

and M^{k}M^k, which lacks all MNS antigens—most often result from gene deletions.[8] Some antigens that are associated with the MNS system, but which are not numbered by the International Society of Blood Transfusion (ISBT) Working Party on Terminology for Red Cell Surface Antigens, are a consequence of altered glycosylation at residues 2, 3, and 4 of GPA. They include Tm, Sj, M$_1$, Can, Sext, and Hu.[21]

Antibodies

Anti-M and anti-N antibodies are usually cold-reactive, clinically insignificant antibodies that are naturally occurring, that is, present in persons who have not been previously transfused or pregnant. Anti-M can be immunoglobulin (Ig) M or IgG (mostly cold-reactive), but anti-N are mostly IgM and rarely IgG. Reactivity of anti-M is often enhanced by acidification of the serum, whereas anti-N are more specific at alkaline pH. Technical problems with these antibodies can usually be avoided if the test is performed strictly at 37°C.

Anti-M is more common than anti-N. Anti-M is common in antenatal patients (even when the fetus is M-negative); however, there are few reports of potent IgG anti-M that is active at 37°C and causes HDN. If a rare example of anti-M, reactive at 37°C, is identified, the patient should be transfused with M-negative blood as a precaution. Anti-N is not known to cause hemolytic transfusion reactions or HDN; therefore, selection of N-negative blood for transfusion of patients with the antibody is not necessary. It should be noted, however, that rare examples of anti-N, which are compatible only with N–U– RBCs, may be clinically significant.[22]

In contrast, antibodies to S, s, and U usually occur after stimulation and are capable of causing hemolytic transfusion reactions and HDN.[23] Antigen-negative blood should be

Table 5.1   Incidence of Various MNS Phenotypes

	Percentage	
Phenotype	Whites	Blacks
M+N–S+s–	6	2
M+N–S+s+	14	7
M+N–S–s+	10	16
M+N+S+s–	4	2
M+N+S+s+	22	13
M+N+S–s+	23	33
M–N+S+s–	1	2
M–N+S+s+	6	5
M–N+S–s+	15	19
M+N–S–s–	0	0.4
M+N+S–s–	0	0.4
M–N+S–s–	0	0.7

Table 5.2 Hybrid Glycophorin Molecules, Phenotype Symbol, and Associated Low-Incidence Antigens

Molecular Basis	Glycophorin	Phenotype Symbol	Associated Novel Antigens
GYP(A-B)	GP(A-B)	GP.MEP(En[a–]UK)	None known
		GP.Hil(Mi.V)	Hil, MINY
		GP.JL(Mi.XI)	TSEN, MINY
		GP.TK	SAT
GYP(B-A)	GP(B-A)	GP.Sch(M^r)	St^a
		GP.Dantu	Dantu
GYP(A-ψB-A)	GP(A-B-A)	GP.Vw(Mi.I)	Vw
		GP.Hut(Mi.II)	Hut, MUT
		GP.Nob(Mi.VII)	Nob
		GP.Joh(Mi.VIII)	Nob, Hop
		GP.Dane(Mi.IX)	Mur, DANE
GYP(A-ψB-A)*	Gp(A-A)	GP.Zan(M^z)	St^a
GYP(A-ψB-A-B)	Gp(B-A-B)	GP.Mur(Mi.III)	Mur, MUT, Hil, MINY
		GP.Bun(Mi.VI)	Mur, MUT, Hop, Hil, MINY
		GP.HF(Mi.X)	MUT, Hil, MINY
		GP.Hop(Mi.IV)	Mur, MUT, Hop, TSEN, MINY
GYPA nucleotide substitution*	GPA (t1)	GP.EBH	ERIK
	GP(A-A) (t2)	GP.EBH	St^a

*Genes that result in more than 1 transcript (t).
ψ, pseudo exon.

selected for transfusion of persons with these antibodies. Most anti-S and anti-s are IgG antibodies shown to be reactive on the indirect antiglobulin test (IAT). However, IgM anti-S exist and are more common than IgM anti-s. Anti-U is IgG, reacts on the IAT, and can cause severe transfusion reactions or severe HDN.

Human sera often contain antibodies against one or more of the MNS system antigens, particularly antibodies directed at the low-incidence antigens, but the source of the stimulation is usually unknown.[23] These antibody specificities are often not separable by absorption or elution, and they recognize amino acid sequences common to more than one antigenic determinant. Antibodies to low-incidence antigens in the MNS system may be IgG or IgM. The corresponding antigens are well-developed on RBCs from newborn babies, and the antibodies may cause HDN. Almost all random donors are compatible, and there is no difficulty in finding blood for transfusion.

Anti-En^a is an umbrella term for immune antibodies that react with high-incidence determinants along GPA. The reactivity of anti-En^a in serologic tests using protease-treated RBCs depends on the location of the specific antigen on GPA. En^a antibodies are usually IgG, react on the IAT, and may cause transfusion reactions or HDN.[7, 22] It is difficult, if not impossible, to find compatible donor blood for patients with these antibodies. Siblings of such patients should be tested for compatibility, and patients urged to donate blood for long term cryogenic storage when their clinical state permits.

Expression

Antigens in the MNS system are expressed on RBCs from newborns. GPA and GPB are expressed in renal endothelium and epithelium.[24, 25] Expression of GPA and GPB in erythroid tissues occurs early in erythroid differentiation, but the associated antigens are detectable only later in erythroid development.[8, 26]

Evolution

GPA and the MN antigens are found on RBCs of all anthropoid apes (chimpanzee, gorillas, orangutan, and gibbon) and Old World monkeys, but GPB has been found only in humans and the anthropoid apes. Only humans have S and s antigens. The glycophorin gene duplication that generated GPA and GPB is not present in gibbon or orangutans and probably occurred in a common ancestor of anthropoid apes.[27]

Function

GPA (synonym, MIRL II) may function as a complement regulator[28] and is a receptor for bacteria, viruses, and malaria parasites.[9, 29, 30] It is a chaperone for band 3 transport to the RBC membrane and is the major component contributing to the negatively charged RBC glycocalyx,[8, 31] which may contribute anti-adhesion properties.[32–34] Rare GPA and GPB null phenotypes: En(a–), U–, and M^{k}M^k have RBCs that survive normally and people with these rare phenotypes have no apparent health defects.[8]

■ The Lutheran System (ISBT System 005)

History

Anti-Lu^a was first found in 1946 in the serum of a patient who had received multiple transfusions, and it agglutinated 8% of random samples.[35] The system should have been named Lutteran, after the name of the donor of the Lu(a+) RBCs; however, the hand-written label on the blood sample from the original donor was misread.

Gene, Protein, and Antigens

Lutheran (LU), along with *Secretor*, provided the first example of autosomal linkage in humans, the first example of autosomal crossing over, and the first indication that crossing over in humans is more common in females than in males.[36, 37]

The *LU* gene, located on chromosome 19q13.2-q13.3, consists of 15 exons distributed over approximately 12 kb of DNA. *LU* encodes the Lutheran (Lu) glycoprotein and a spliced form of the glycoprotein, B-cell adhesion molecule (CAM). Lu glycoprotein passes through the RBC membrane once with the N-terminus oriented to the extracellular surface. The protein is predicted to have five disulfide-bonded, extracellular, Ig superfamily (IgSF) domains (two variable-region sets and three constant-region sets).[38] The Lu glycoprotein has five sites for N-glycans and is O-glycosylated and has an approximate M_r of 85,000 on SDS-PAGE; there are 1500 to 4000 copies per RBC.[39, 40] The minor isoform (B-CAM) has an approximate M_r of 78,000, because it lacks the cytoplasmic tail and has an increased expression on epithelial cancer cells.[38, 41]

The Lutheran system consists of four pairs of antigens (Lu^a/Lu^b; Lu6/Lu9; Lu8/Lu14; Au^a/Au^b) and 10 independent antigens. The Lu^a antigen is present in 5% of blacks and 8% of whites, and the antithetical antigen, Lu^b, is present in more than 99% of random blood samples.[7] Only Lu9 and Lu14 are low-incidence antigens; the others are either polymorphic (Lu^a, Au^a, Au^b) or of high incidence (Lu^b, Lu3, Lu4, Lu5, Lu6, Lu7, Lu8, Lu11, Lu12, Lu13, Lu16, Lu17, and Lu20). The molecular basis of Lu^a/Lu^b is His77Arg, and that of Au^a/Au^b is Thr539Ala.[42, 43]

The Lu^a and Lu^b antigens, and most of the other Lutheran antigens, are resistant to treatment by papain, ficin, sialidase, and low concentrations (50 mM) of dithiothreitol (DTT), and are sensitive to treatment by trypsin and α-chymotrypsin.[7]

Lutheran-null phenotypes have at least three genetic backgrounds. The original Lu(a–b–) phenotype was discovered by the proposita herself when her own RBCs were not agglutinated by anti-Lu^a or anti-Lu^b.[44] Later, it was shown that these RBCs had weak expression of Lutheran antigens and that this Lu(a–b–) phenotype is inherited in a dominant manner.[44] The presence of an inhibitor gene, unlinked to *LU* and named *In(Lu)* (inhibitor of Lutheran),[45] was proposed, and it is now known that the presence of *In(Lu)* is associated with reduced expression of CD44.[46, 47] *In(Lu)* is also associated with a weak expression of P$_1$, AnWj, In^b, i, and MER2 blood group antigens.[48] The Lu(a–b–) phenotype can also arise from recessive and X-linked inheritance[44] (Table 5.3).

Antibodies

Antibodies in this system are rarely encountered because the antigens are not highly immunogenic (see Table 2.5).[23] Anti-Lu^a are usually IgG and reactive on the IAT, but they may be IgM and may directly agglutinate Lu(a+) RBCs, giving characteristic stringy agglutinates surrounded by unagglutinated RBCs. Anti-Lu^a has not been implicated in transfusion reactions and has rarely caused mild HDN. Anti-Au^a and anti-Au^b are rare, usually found in sera that

contain other antibodies. They are IgG, react on the IAT, and can cause mild transfusion reactions, but neither has caused HDN.

Several Lutheran antibodies are directed at antigens of high incidence; the one most frequently encountered is anti-Lu^b. Lu^b antibodies are IgG and react by the IAT, but can occasionally be IgM. Anti-Lu^b can cause mild transfusion reactions and has rarely caused mild HDN. Lu(b–) blood should be used for transfusion, but only about 1 in 500 donors are Lu(b–). Anti-Lu3 is found only in the serum of immunized people of the rare recessive Lu(a–b–) phenotype. The antibody is usually IgG, is reactive on the IAT, and may cause a delayed transfusion reaction or HDN. Blood with the Lu(a–b–) phenotype should be used for transfusion of patients with these antibodies.

Antibodies to other high-incidence Lutheran antigens, usually weak IgG antibodies, have not been reported to cause HDN. With the exception of one example of anti-Lu6, which was shown to destroy transfused Lu6 RBCs, these specificities have not caused transfusion reactions. If a patient has formed a Lutheran antibody directed at a high-incidence antigen, it is important to test for compatible siblings and encourage the patient to donate blood for long-term storage when clinical status permits. Anti-Lu9 and anti-Lu14 define low-incidence antigens that have not been reported to cause transfusion reactions or HDN.[7] Most randomly collected blood is antigen-negative and compatible.

Expression

Lutheran antigens are expressed weakly on cord RBCs. The antigens are present in various tissues, including brain, heart, kidney, liver, lung, pancreas, placenta, and skeletal muscle.[38]

Function

The protein carrying Lutheran antigens has sequence homology with intracellular adhesion molecules (ICAMs) that are characterized by binding to the integrin lymphocyte function-related antigen (LFA-1). Although the function of the Lutheran glycoprotein is not fully defined, its involvement in cell-to-cell and cell-to-substrate adhesion is probable. The nature of the extracellular and cytoplasmic domains suggests receptor and signal-transduction functions. Lutheran glycoproteins bind laminin, a major component of basement membranes.[49] On RBCs, Lutheran glycoprotein may be involved in the adherence of RBCs to vascular endothelial cells and in vaso-occlusion that is characteristic of sickle cell disease.[50]

■ Diego System (ISBT System 010)

History

The Diego blood group system was named after the producer of the first example of anti-Di^a. The antibody, which had

Table 5.3 Characteristics of Lu(a–b–) Phenotypes

Lu(a–b–) Phenotype	Lutheran Antigens	Make Anti-Lu3	CD44	CDw75	I/i Antigen
Recessive	Absent	Yes	Normal	Normal	Normal/normal
Dominant	Weak	No	Weak (25%–39% of normal)	Strong	Normal/weak
X-linked	Weak	No	Normal	Absent	Weak/strong

caused HDN in a Venezuelan baby, was reported in detail in 1955. Anti-Di[b] was described in 1967, and for many years, the system consisted of two antithetical antigens, Di[a] and Di[b].[22] The finding that Di[a] and Di[b] are carried on band 3, the anion exchanger (AE1),[51, 52] was the beginning of the expansion of the Diego system. In 1995, Bruce and colleagues[52, 53] located the Wr[a] and Wr[b] antigens on band 3. Since then, many low-incidence antigens have been assigned to this system, which now consists of 18 antigens.[20, 54, 55]

Gene, Protein, and Antigens

The gene encoding band 3 and, thus, the Diego antigens is *SLC4A1* (solute carrier family 4, anion exchanger member 1; synonyms: *DI*; *AE1*; *EPB-3*). *SLC4A1* consists of 20 exons distributed over 18 kb of DNA and is located on chromosome 17q12-q21.[56, 57] There are more than 1,000,000 copies of band 3 in the RBC membrane, making it the most abundant integral RBC protein. The glycoprotein passes through the RBC membrane multiple times and has both the N-terminus and the C-terminus oriented to the cytoplasm. Band 3 has one large N-glycan, on the fourth extracellular loop, with repeating lactosaminyl groups that accounts for the broad banding pattern of approximate M_r 95,000 to 105,000 on SDS-PAGE. The N-glycan carries A, B, H, I, and i blood group activity.[58]

The Di[a]/Di[b] polymorphism is located on the last extracellular loop and is defined by Pro854 (Di[b]) or Leu854 (Di[a]).[52] The Di[a] antigen is rare in most populations but is polymorphic in people of Mongoloid ancestry. The incidence in South American Indians may be as high as 54%, and 10% to 12% of Native Americans are Di(a+).[59] The incidence of Di[b] is generally greater than 99.9%; however, the incidence of Di[b] among Native Americans is reduced to 96% and is likely to be lower in those populations with a high incidence of Di[a]. The Wr[a]/Wr[b] polymorphism is located on the fourth extracellular loop, close to the insertion into the RBC membrane, and is defined by Lys658 (Wr[b]) or Glu658 (Wr[a]); however, for expression, the Wr[b] antigen also requires the presence of normal GPA.[53, 60, 61]

The other antigens in the Diego system—Wd[a], Rb[a], WARR, ELO, Wu, Bp[a], Mo[a], Hg[a], Vg[a], Sw[a], BOW, NFLD, Jn[a] and KREP[20]—are of low incidence and are each associated with a single point mutation.[54, 55] The antigens are resistant to treatment of RBCs by proteolytic enzymes, sialidase, DTT, chloroquine, and acid.[7]

Antibodies

Diego antibodies are usually IgG that react on the IAT and do not bind complement. These antibodies have caused transfusion reactions (usually delayed) and HDN.[7, 62]

Expression

Diego antigens are expressed on RBCs of newborns. Band 3, in addition to its presence on RBCs, has been found in the intercalated cells of the distal and collecting tubules of the kidney and on granulocytes.[58]

Evolution

A variant form of band 3, Memphis I (56Glu), has a faster migration on SDS-PAGE than the more common form (56Lys). Evidence suggests that the primordial gene encodes 56Glu and that 56Lys is the result of a more recent mutation.[63]

Function

Band 3 exchanges anions (HCO_3^-/Cl^-) across the RBC membrane. In addition, band 3 has a structural role through the interaction of its N-terminal domain with ankyrin, band 4.2, and band 4.1 in the RBC membrane skeleton.[57, 58] An altered form of band 3, with a deletion of amino acid residues 400 through 408, is present in ovalocytes of Southeast Asian people and causes the RBCs to be rigid.[64–66] Numerous mutations exist in the predicted cytoplasmic or transmembrane domains of band 3 and give rise to hereditary spherocytosis, congenital acanthocytosis, and distal renal tubular acidosis.[55, 67]

■ Yt Blood Group System (ISBT System 011)

History

The Yt system was named in 1956,[68] the last letter of the antibody producer's name, Cartwright, being used because the other letters of the name were already in use. The logic was that if all the other letters had been used, "Why not t?," or "Why t?" (Yt) (M. Pickles, personal communication, 1999).

Gene, Protein, and Antigens

ACHE encodes acetylcholinesterase (AChE), a glycosylphosphatidylinositol-linked (GPI-linked) glycoprotein that exists as a dimer in the RBC membrane.[69] The gene is located on chromosome 7q22 and consists of six exons.[7, 70, 71] Alternative splicing results in different domains at the C-terminus of AChE. AChE glycoprotein has N-glycans and O-glycans and an approximate M_r of 160,000 (72,000 monomer) on SDS-PAGE; there are 10,000 copies per RBC.[7, 69]

Yt[a] and Yt[b] antigens are antithetical and a consequence of an amino acid substitution on AChE, His353Asn (originally numbered 322).[72] Yt[a] occurs with an incidence of more than 99% in random blood samples. Yt[b] has an incidence of 8% in most populations, but of 20% or higher in Israelis.[73]

The antigens are sensitive to treatment of RBCs by papain, ficin, α-chymotrypsin, and DTT but resistant to treatment by trypsin, sialidase, chloroquine, and acid.[7]

Antibodies

Yt antibodies usually are IgG, are reactive on IAT, and do not bind complement. These antibodies have caused delayed transfusion reactions but not HDN.

Expression

AChE is expressed on hematopoietic and innervated tissue (including brain and muscle).[74, 75] The antigens are expressed weakly on RBCs of newborns and are absent from RBCs of people with paroxysmal nocturnal hemoglobinuria (PNH) III.[76]

Evolution

A form of AChE has been found in the electric fish *Torpedo californica*.[77]

Function

AChE is a well-characterized enzyme that hydrolyses acetylcholine and is an essential component of cholinergic neurotransmission.[74] The role of AChE in RBCs is unknown,[78] but the molecule is enzymatically active.[69]

■ Xg Blood Group System (ISBT System 012)

History

Anti-Xg^a, discovered in 1962, detects an antigen encoded by a locus on the X chromosome. The "X" was used because of the association with the X chromosome, and the g stood for *G*rand Rapids, Michigan, the home of the male patient who had received multiple transfusions and who made the first anti-Xg^a.[79] Xg^a has been useful in linkage studies involving the X chromosome and in sex chromosome aneuploidy, in which an abnormal number of X chromosomes occurs.[59]

Gene, Protein, and Antigens

The gene encoding Xg^a has been cloned and is located at Xp22.32; it is not subject to X-inactivation. The first three of the ten exons of *XG* are situated in the pseudoautosomal region of the X chromosome; exons 4 through 10 are X-specific; hence the alternative name *PBDX* (pseudoautosomal boundary divided on X) for *XG*.[80]

The Xg glycoprotein passes through the membrane once with the amino-terminus to the outside of the RBC. N-glycans are not present, but there are 16 potential sites for O-glycans, and the protein has numerous proline residues. On SDS-PAGE, Xg has a M$_r$ of 22,000 to 29,000, and there are approximately 9000 copies per RBC.[7] The molecular basis that distinguishes Xg(a+) from Xg(a−) has not been determined. Xg glycoprotein has 48% identity with the CD99 glycoprotein.[80] Because an altered form of CD99 in a person with alloanti-CD99 has been described, the ISBT Working Party assigned CD99 the number XG2 (012.002).[81]

The incidence of Xg^a differs in males (65.6%) and females (88.7%), and there is a phenotypic association between the expression of Xg^a and CD99 (formerly known as 12E7 antigen) (Table 5.4). The Xg^a antigen is sensitive to treatment of RBCs by proteolytic enzymes but resistant to treatment by sialidase and DTT.[7]

Antibodies

Anti-Xg^a is usually IgG that is reactive on the IAT and may bind complement. Some anti-Xg^a are apparently naturally occurring. These antibodies have not caused transfusion reactions or HDN.[7]

Expression

The antigen is expressed weakly on RBCs of newborns. Xg is expressed on fibroblasts as well as on fetal liver, spleen, thymus, and adrenal glands and on adult bone marrow.[80]

Evolution

Xg^a is on the RBCs of some gibbons (*Hylobates lar*). RBCs of other great apes, various monkeys (including baboons), mice, and dogs are Xg(a−).[59]

Table 5.4   Phenotype Relationship of Xg^a and 12E7[CD99] Antigens

Sex	Xg^a	CD99 Expression
Male	Positive	High
	Negative	High or low
Female	Positive	High
	Weak positive	High
	Negative	Low

Function

The role of the protein carrying Xg^a in RBCs is unknown, but Xg is homologous with CD99 (formerly known as 12E7 protein).[82] CD99 has been implicated in cell-to-cell adhesion events[83, 84] and is expressed on human RBCs, all leukocyte lineages, and all other human tissue tested.

■ Scianna Blood Group System (ISBT System 013)

History

The Scianna system was named after the first antibody producer. The first example of anti-Sc1 (initially called anti-Sm) was reported in 1962. The antithetical antigen, Sc2, was originally called Bu^a.[59]

Gene, Protein, and Antigens

The gene encoding Sc antigens, which is located on chromosome 1p36.2-p22.1, has not been cloned; thus, little is known about the glycoprotein. Biochemical analysis indicates that the Sc glycoprotein has at least one N-glycan, one or more disulfide bonds, and an approximate M$_r$ of 60,000 to 68,000 on SDS-PAGE. The number of copies per RBC and the molecular basis of the antigens have not been determined.[85]

The high-incidence antigen Sc1 (incidence ≈99.9%) is antithetical to the low-incidence antigen Sc2 (1%). Sc1, Sc2, and the high-incidence antigen Sc3 are lacking on RBCs of the very rare null phenotype Sc:−1,−2,−3. The antigens are resistant to treatment of RBCs by papain, ficin, trypsin, α-chymotrypsin, sialidase, acid, and 50 mM of DTT, but sensitive to treatment of RBCs with 200 mM of DTT.[7]

Antibodies

Scianna antibodies are usually IgG reactive on the IAT, and some bind complement. These antibodies have not caused transfusion reactions, and although they have caused cord RBCs to be positive in the direct antiglobulin test (DAT), they have not caused HDN. Several examples of autoanti-Sc1 have been reported, some reactive in tests using patient serum but not plasma. Autoanti-Sc3-like antibodies have been described in one patient with lymphoma and in one patient with Hodgkin's disease whose RBCs had suppressed Sc antigens.[7]

Expression

The Sc antigens are expressed on RBCs of newborns.

■ Dombrock Blood Group System (ISBT System 014)

History

The first antibody of the Dombrock system, anti-Do^a, was identified in 1965 in the serum of Mrs. Dombrock. Anti-Do^b was found in 1973. In 1995, it was realized that the Gregory-negative phenotype was the null of the Dombrock system.[86]

Gene, Protein, and Antigens

The Dombrock antigens are carried on a mono-ADP-ribosyl-transferase (ART4), encoded by the *DO* gene.[87] The gene, located at chromosome 12p13.2-p12.1,[88] is composed of three exons distributed over 14 kb.[87, 89, 90]

The glycoprotein has an approximate M_r of 47,000 to 58,000 on SDS-PAGE and is attached to the RBC membrane via a GPI anchor.[76] The number of copies per RBC is not known.

The incidence of each Dombrock phenotype and the association of Gregory (Gy^a), Holley (Hy), and Joseph (Jo^a) phenotypes with Do^a and Do^b are summarized in Table 5.5. Although three nucleotide substitutions are associated with the various *DO* alleles, the amino acid substitutions associated with expression of the antigens are as follows: Do^a/Do^b, Asn265Asp;[87] Hy+/Hy−, Gly108Val; and Jo(a+)/Jo(a−), Thr117Ile.[91] The Gy(a−) phenotype arises from different molecular backgrounds—donor and acceptor splice site mutations, nonsense mutation, and deletion of eight nucleotides.[92–94] The antigens are resistant to treatment of RBCs by ficin, papain, sialidase, 50 mM of DTT, and acid, weakened by treatment with α-chymotrypsin, and sensitive to treatment by trypsin and 200 mM of DTT.[7]

Antibodies

Do^a and Do^b antigens are poor immunogens, and anti-Do^a and anti-Do^b are rarely found as single specificities. In contrast, Gy^a is immunogenic. Antibodies in the Do system are usually IgG reactive on the IAT and do not bind complement. These antibodies have caused delayed transfusion reactions and a positive DAT result but no clinical HDN. Anti-Do^a and anti-Do^b are notorious for disappearing in vivo.[62]

Expression

The Dombrock antigens are expressed on RBCs of newborns but are absent from PNH III RBCs.[76]

■ Colton Blood Group System (ISBT System 015)

History

The Colton system, named after the first producer of anti-Co^a, was reported in 1967.

Gene, Protein, and Antigens

The Colton blood group antigens are carried on the water transport protein, known as channel-forming integral protein (CHIP-1) or aquaporin-1 (AQP-1).[95] The gene (*AQP1* or *CO*) encoding the Colton glycoprotein has been cloned and is on chromosome 7q14. It comprises four exons distributed over 17 kb.

The glycoprotein passes through the RBC membrane multiple times, has cytoplasmic N- and C-termini, and is N-glycosylated. The N-glycan carries A, B, H, I, and i blood group activity. On SDS-PAGE, the Colton glycoprotein has an approximate M_r of 28,000 in the unglycosylated form and 40,000 to 60,000 in the glycosylated form.[95] There are 120,000 to 160,000 molecules of CHIP-1 arranged in tetramers on the RBC membrane.[7]

The Colton blood group system consists of three antigens, Co^a, Co^b, and Co3. Co^a has an incidence of 99.9%, its antithetical antigen Co^b has an incidence of 10%, and Co3 is present on all RBCs except those of the very rare null phenotype Co(a−b−). Only four Co(a−b−) propositi are reported, all of which were found because of the presence of anti-Co3 in their sera. The Co(a−b−) phenotype arises from various molecular backgrounds, including exon deletion, missense mutations, and a single nucleotide insertion.[96–98]

The amino acid substitution responsible for the Co^a/Co^b polymorphism is on the first extracellular loop of CHIP-1 and results from an Ala45Val substitution.[99] The antigens are resistant to treatment of RBCs by proteases, sialidase, DTT, and acid.[7]

Antibodies

Antibodies in the Co system are usually IgG reactive on the IAT, and some bind complement. The antibodies have caused delayed transfusion reactions and HDN.[62]

Expression

The Co antigens are expressed on RBCs of newborns. CHIP-1 is strongly expressed in the kidney on the apical surface of proximal tubules, the basolateral membrane subpopulation of collecting ducts in the cortex, and the descending tubules in the medulla, as well as on liver bile ducts, gallbladder, brain, lung, eye epithelium, cornea, lens, choroid plexus, hepatobiliary epithelia, and capillary endothelium.[95, 100]

Evolution

A murine homologue of the *AQP* gene has been described.[101]

Function

The function of CHIP-1 is to transport water. CHIP-1 accounts for 80% of water reabsorption in kidneys. CHIP-1 may enable RBCs to rehydrate rapidly after shrinking in the hypertonic environment of the renal medulla.[102] Apparently healthy propositi with the Co(a−b−) phenotype and CHIP-1 deficiency have RBCs with an 80% reduction in the ability to transport water.[96]

■ LW Blood Group System (ISBT System 016)

History

In 1940, Landsteiner and Wiener[103] produced an antibody by injecting rabbits and guinea pigs with RBCs from rhesus

Table 5.5 Dombrock Phenotypes and Their Incidences (in Percentage)

Phenotype	Do^a	Do^b	Gy^a	Hy	Jo^a	Whites	Blacks
Do(a+b−)	+	0	+	+	+	18	11
Do(a+b+)	+	+	+	+	+	49	44
Do(a−b+)	0	+	+	+	+	33	45
Gy(a−)	0	0	0	0	0	Rare	0
Hy−	0	weak	weak	0	0	0	Rare
Jo(a−)	weak	0/weak	+	weak	0	0	Rare

monkeys; they named the antibody Rh after rhesus monkey. A few years later, it was shown that the animal anti-Rh were different from the human Rh antibody (i.e., anti-D); thus, the animal anti-Rh was renamed anti-LW in honor of Landsteiner and Wiener.

The historical terminology LW_1, LW_2, LW_3, and LW_4 to describe phenotypes was changed when the antithetical relationship of the antigen defined by anti-Ne[a] (now called anti-LW[b]) and that defined by anti-LW made by LW_3 people (now called anti-LW[a]) was recognized.[7, 104]

Gene, Protein, and Antigens

The protein carrying LW antigens is homologous to the ICAMs and is a member of the IgSF.[105] The gene (LW) encoding the LW glycoprotein has been cloned; it consists of three exons distributed over 2.65 kb of DNA on chromosome 19.

The LW glycoprotein passes through the RBC membrane once, and the N-terminal extracellular region is organized into two IgSF domains.[105] LW glycoprotein has an approximate M_r of 37,000 to 43,000 on SDS-PAGE, has three pairs of cysteine residues and four potential N-glycan sites, and is O-glycosylated.

LW[a] is a common antigen, whereas LW[b] has an incidence of less than 1% in most Europeans (but is found in 6% of Finns and in 8% of Estonians). RBCs with the Rh_{null} phenotype lack LW antigens and type LW(a–b–). The LW[ab] antigen was originally defined by the alloantibody made by the only genetically LW(a–b–) person. There is a phenotypic relationship between LW and the D antigen of the Rh system; D-positive RBCs have stronger expression of LW antigen than D-negative RBCs, and the expression of LW is stronger on cord RBCs than on RBCs from adults.[106]

The LW[a]/LW[b] polymorphism is due to the amino acid substitution Gln70Arg.[107] LW antigens require intramolecular disulfide bonds and the presence of divalent cations, notably Mg^{2+}, for expression.[108] The antigens are resistant to treatment of RBCs by ficin, papain, trypsin, α-chymotrypsin (but may be weakened), sialidase, and acid; they are sensitive to treatment of RBCs by pronase and DTT. These features are helpful in the differentiation of anti-LW from anti-D, because the D antigen is resistant to pronase and DTT treatment.[7]

The LW gene of the only genetic LW(a–b–) person has a 10-deletion and a premature stop codon in the first exon.[109]

Transient loss of LW antigens from the RBC has been described in pregnancy and in patients with diseases, particularly Hodgkin's disease, lymphoma, leukemia, sarcoma, and other forms of malignancy. Such loss of LW antigens is usually associated with the production of LW antibodies.[110]

Antibodies

Antibodies in the LW system are IgM and IgG that are reactive at room temperature or on the IAT and do not bind complement. They have occasionally caused mild delayed transfusion reactions and mild HDN. Autoanti-LW are common in patients with transient depression of LW antigens and can appear to be alloantibodies.[62]

Expression

The LW antigens are expressed on RBCs of newborns in equal amounts regardless of D type. In contrast, D-positive RBCs of adults express more LW than D-negative RBCs.

Evolution

LW antigen has been detected on RBCs of all primate species tested, including chimpanzee, gorilla, orangutan, and a variety of species of monkeys. LW has not been detected on RBCs of nonprimate species, such as mouse, rat, rabbit, sheep, goat, horse, and cattle.[111]

Function

LW glycoprotein is an ICAM that binds to CD11/CD18 leukocyte integrins.[112] It is a possible marker for lymphocyte maturation or differentiation, but its function on RBCs is not clear.

■ Chido/Rodgers Blood Group System (ISBT System 017)

History

Antigens in the Chido/Rodgers system were named after the first antibody producers, Ch for Chido and Rg for Rodgers. Anti-Ch was first described in 1967, and when anti-Rg was reported in 1976, there were obvious similarities between them. Although the Ch and Rg antigens are readily detected on RBCs and were given blood group system status, later work revealed that Ch and Rg antigens are located on the fourth component of complement (C4), which becomes bound to RBCs from the plasma.

Gene, Protein, and Antigens

In the complement activation through the classical pathway, C4 becomes bound to the RBC membrane and undergoes further cleavage; ultimately, a tryptic fragment, C4d, remains on the RBC. This C4d glycoprotein carries the Ch/Rg blood group antigens. Electrophoresis identified the following two isoforms of C4: C4B, the slower-migrating molecule, expresses Ch antigens, and C4A, the faster molecule, expresses Rg antigens.[113] C4A and C4B are not the products of alleles, but are encoded by genes at two very closely linked loci located at chromosome 6p21.3. Silent alleles are relatively common at each locus. C4A and C4B have been cloned, and each consists of 41 exons and is 22 kb long, although a shorter form of C4B exists. C4A and C4B glycoproteins are 99% identical in their amino acid sequences.

The Chido/Rodgers blood group system contains nine antigens. Some or all of the antigens may be expressed by a particular phenotype. Ch1 to Ch6, Rg1, and Rg2 have frequencies greater than 90%. The WH antigen has an incidence of about 15%. The various antigens are associated with amino acid differences in eight residues.[114, 115] The antigens are stable in stored serum or plasma, and the phenotypes of this system are most accurately defined in plasma by hemagglutination inhibition tests.[7]

The antigens are sensitive to treatment of RBCs by proteases and resistant to treatment by sialidase, DTT, and acid. RBCs coated with C4 (+C3) through the use of low-ionic strength 10% sucrose solution give enhanced reactivity with anti-Ch and anti-Rg; this feature has been used to aid identification of antibodies.[7]

Antibodies

Antibodies in the Ch/Rg system are usually IgG reacting by the IAT, do not activate complement, and are considered benign and nebulous. There can be considerable variation in the reaction strength obtained with different RBC samples. Although these antibodies do not generally cause transfusion reactions, they have caused anaphylactic reactions.[116] The antibodies have not caused HDN. Anti-Ch and anti-Rg are neutralized in the test tube or in the circulation by plasma from Ch-positive and Rg-positive persons, respectively.

Expression

Ch/Rg antigens are absent or weakly expressed on RBCs of newborns. They are weakly expressed on RBCs of some people with the dominant Lu(a−b−) phenotype and on GPA-deficient (i.e., sialidase-deficient) RBCs. Indeed, it is not possible to coat sialidase-deficient RBCs with C4 in vitro through the 10% sucrose technique.[117]

Function

C4A binds preferentially to proteins, and C4B to carbohydrates. C4B binds more effectively to the RBC surface (through sialic acid) and thus is more effective at promoting hemolysis. A single amino acid substitution, Asp1106His, converts the functional activity of C4B to C4A, whereas Cys1102Ser affects hemolytic activity and IgG binding.[118]

Inherited low levels of C4 may be a predisposing factor for diseases such as insulin-dependent diabetes and autoimmune chronic active hepatitis. Specific C4 allotypes and null genes have been associated with numerous autoimmune disorders, including Graves disease and rheumatoid arthritis. Lack of C4B (Ch−) bestows greater susceptibility to bacterial meningitis on children. Lack of C4A (Rg−) results in a predisposition for systemic lupus erythematosus (SLE).[118]

■ Gerbich Blood Group System (ISBT System 020)

History

The Gerbich system was named in 1960 after Mrs. Gerbich, the first antibody producer.

Gene, Protein, and Antigens

The three high-incidence antigens (Ge2, Ge3, and Ge4) and four low-incidence antigens (Wb, Ls^a, An^a, and Dh^a) of the Gerbich blood group system are carried on GPC, GPD, or both. The two glycoproteins are products of the *GYPC* gene.[119] The gene, located at chromosome 2q14-q21, consists of four exons. The smaller GPD polypeptide is generated by the use of alternative translation initiation sites. On SDS-PAGE, GPC has an approximate M_r of 40,000; it has one N-glycan and 13 sites for O-glycans. GPD has an approximate M_r of 30,000, no N-glycan, and 8 sites for O-glycans. There are approximately 135,000 copies of GPC and 50,000 copies of GPD per RBC. GPC and GPD pass through the RBC membrane once with their N-terminus oriented to the outside of the membrane.

Ge2 is located on the N-terminus of GPD; Ge3 is located between amino acid residues 40 and 50 on GPC and between residues 19 and 28 on GPD; and Ge4 is located at the N-terminus of GPC. Of the four low-incidence antigens, three (Wb, An^a, Dh^a) are the result of an amino

acid substitution, and one (Ls^a) is created by a novel amino acid sequence derived from a duplication of exon 3 and encoded by nucleotides at the exon 3 to exon 3 junction.[119]

Except in Papua New Guinea, Gerbich-negative RBCs are seldom found. The three Gerbich-negative phenotypes are as follows: Ge:−2,3,4 (the Yus phenotype), Ge:−2,−3,4 (the Gerbich phenotype), and Ge:−2,−3,−4 (the Leach phenotype). The Leach phenotype is the null of the Gerbich system. The PL type (the original propositus) arises from a deletion of exons 3 and 4 of *GYPC*. The LN type is caused by a deletion of nucleotide 134, changing Pro45Arg of GPC, a frameshift mutation, and a premature stop codon. The Gerbich phenotype is due to a deletion of exon 3, and the Yus phenotype is due to a deletion of exon 2 of *GYPC*.[119-123] The Yus and Gerbich phenotypes have been found in diverse populations, but in the Melanesians of Papua New Guinea only the Gerbich type has been found.[119] The Leach phenotype has been restricted to people of Northern European extraction.

Ge2 and Ge4 are sensitive to treatment of RBCs by ficin, papain, and trypsin; Ge3 is sensitive to trypsin but resistant to ficin and papain; and all antigens are resistant to treatment of RBCs with α-chymotrypsin, DTT, and acid.[7]

Antibodies

The antibodies may be immune or naturally occurring. Most are IgG and are reactive on the IAT, and some of these bind complement; some antibodies may be IgM. Although some antibodies have caused delayed transfusion reactions, others have been benign. Clinical HDN due to these antibodies has not been reported, but the antibodies have been eluted from cord RBCs that tested positive on DAT. Antibodies to the high-incidence Gerbich antigens are rare; the least rare specificity is anti-Ge2, which can be produced by any of the three Gerbich-negative phenotypes. Clinically significant autoanti-Ge have been reported. Because Ge-negative donors are rare, it is important to test siblings of Ge-negative patients for compatibility, and to urge such patients to donate blood for long-term storage.[62]

Antibodies to low-incidence antigens in the Ge blood group system are rare, and RBCs from almost all random donors are compatible; there is no difficulty in finding blood for transfusion of patients with these antibodies. One brief report implicated anti-Ls^a in HDN,[124] but there are no reports of HDN due to anti-Wb, anti-An^a, or anti-Dh^a.

Expression

Ge antigens are expressed on RBCs of newborns. Gerbich antigens are weak on protein 4.1-deficient RBCs because the membranes of such cells have reduced levels of GPC and GPD. The majority of RBC samples with Leach or Gerbich phenotypes have a weak expression of Kell blood group system antigens. GPC and GPD are expressed on erythroblasts and fetal liver and in several nonerythroid tissues, including kidney, brain cerebellum, and ileum.[7]

Function

GPC and GPD are possibly involved in RBC membrane integrity via interaction with protein 4.1. Both glycophorins are markedly reduced in protein 4.1-deficient RBCs.[125]

■ Cromer Blood Group System (ISBT System 021)

History

The Cromer system was named after the first antibody producer, Mrs. Cromer. When the antibody was first identified in 1965, it was believed to be anti-Go[b]; later, however, it was recognized as a new specificity, and in 1975, it was renamed anti-Cr[a].

Gene, Protein, and Antigens

Blood group antigens in the Cromer system are carried on the complement regulatory protein, decay-accelerating factor (DAF, CD55). The *DAF* gene, located at chromosome 1q32, is one of a group of genes known as the regulation of complement activation (RCA) cluster. The gene spans approximately 40 kb and comprises 11 exons.[126] The DAF glycoprotein is arranged into four extracellular short consensus repeat (SCR) domains, each with about 60 amino acid residues, and is attached to the RBC membrane through GPI linkage. On SDS-PAGE, DAF has an approximate M_r of 64,000 to 73,000 (reduced) and 60,000 to 70,000 (nonreduced). One N-glycan and 15 O-glycans are present on each glycoprotein, and there are 20,000 copies of DAF per RBC.[127]

Cromer is a system of 11 antigens with two sets of antithetical antigens, Tc[a]/Tc[b]/Tc[c] and WES[a]/ WES[b]. Eight of the antigens (Cr[a], Tc[a], Dr[a], Es[a], IFC, WES[b], UMC, and GUTI) are of high incidence, and three (Tc[b], Tc[c], and WES[a]) are of low incidence. These antigens are lacking from the Cromer null phenotype, the Inab phenotype. The amino acids required for expression of all the antigens have been determined; with the exception of Dr[a], all are due to a single amino acid change.[128, 129] In the Dr(a–) phenotype, the level of expression of DAF, and therefore of all Cromer system antigens, is greatly reduced. The Cr(a–) phenotype is the least rare of the negative phenotypes, and with the exception of one Spanish-American woman, all people with Cr(a–) RBCs are black. Most of the other phenotypes are exceedingly rare.

Cromer antigens are resistant to treatment of RBCs by ficin, papain, trypsin, 50 mM of DTT, sialidase, and acid, are sensitive to α-chymotrypsin, and are weakened by 200 mM of DTT.[7]

Antibodies

Antibodies in the Cromer system are usually IgG, are reactive on the IAT, and do not bind complement. The antibodies have caused mild delayed transfusion reactions but not HDN. When a patient's antibody is directed at a high-incidence antigen, it is important to test siblings in the quest for compatible blood and to urge the patient to donate blood for long-term storage when clinical status permits.[62]

Expression

The Cromer antigens are expressed on RBCs of newborns. DAF is preferentially expressed on the apical surface of trophoblasts and may protect the conceptus from antibody-mediated hemolysis.[130] DAF is not expressed on RBCs from patients with PNH III. Dr(a–) variant RBCs express inherited Cromer antigens very weakly.

Cromer antigens are present in the plasma and urine of people with the corresponding antigen on their RBCs. This soluble form of the antigens can be used for hemagglutination inhibition tests, although the urine requires prior concentration.[131]

Function

DAF prevents assembly and accelerates the decay of C3 and C5 convertases, decreasing the deposition of C3 on the RBC surface and thereby reducing complement-mediated hemolysis.[127]

Five of the six known people with the Inab phenotype have intestinal disorders. Dr[a] is the receptor for uropathogenic *Escherichia coli.*[7]

■ Knops Blood Group System (ISBT System 022)

History

The antigens Kn[a], Kn[b], McC[a], Sl[a], and Yk[a] had long been grouped together for serologic reasons. In 1991, the Knops blood group system was established when these antigens were shown to be on complement receptor 1 (CR1). The system was named after Mrs. Knops, the first antibody producer.

Gene, Protein, and Antigens

Knops antigens are encoded by various forms of *CR1.*[132] Like *DAF*, the *CR1* gene is located within the regulation of complement activation cluster on chromosome 1q32. *CR1* has four allotypes, A, B, C, and D. The most common allotypes are A (82%) and B (18%); the other two are rare.

CR1 (CD35) is an unusual protein with 30 short consensus repeat domains. SDS-PAGE reveals the approximate M_r of the CR1 allotypes as follows: 190,000 (C allotype), 220,000 (A allotype), 250,000 (B allotype), and 280,000 (D allotype). Of 20 potential N-glycan sites, only 6 to 8 are usually occupied; there are four cysteine residues. Each RBC contains 20 to 1500 copies of CR1. The CR1 glycoprotein passes through the RBC membrane once with its N-terminus toward the extracellular surface. The molecular basis of the McC[a]/McC[b] polymorphism is associated with a Lys1590Glu missense mutation, and the Sl[a]/Vil polymorphism with an Arg1601Gly missense mutation.[133] The antigens are weakened by treatment of RBCs with ficin and papain, are sensitive to treatment by trypsin, α-chymotrypsin, and 200 mM of DTT, and are resistant to sialidase, 50 mM of DTT, and acid.[7]

With the exception of the low-incidence antigen Kn[b], the antigens in this system are fairly common and have a similar prevalence (>90%) in different populations; however, Sl[a] is present on RBCs of 98% of whites but on only 60% of blacks.

Typing for Knops system antigens can be challenging because of the low level of expression on the RBCs of some people as well as the lack of potent antisera. Disease processes causing CR1 deficiency and, therefore, weak expression of Knops system antigens can lead to false-negative results. Furthermore, the low level of expression can lead to variable results in tests on different samples from the same patient.

Antibodies

Antibodies in the Knops system are usually IgG and reactive on the IAT, and they do not bind complement. The antibodies do not cause transfusion reactions or HDN, and once identified, they can be ignored for clinical purposes. Identification may be complicated by the fluctuation of antigen expression on RBCs. Anti-Kn[a] is the most common antibody in white persons, and anti-Sl[a] is the most common in black persons.[22]

Expression

The Knops antigens are weakly expressed on RBCs of newborns, RBCs with the dominant Lu(a–b–) phenotype, and RBCs of patients with autoimmune diseases. CR1 is present on B cells, a subset of T cells, monocytes, macrophages, neutrophils, eosinophils, glomerular podocytes, and splenic follicular dendritic cells.[134]

Function

CR1 has an inhibitory effect on complement activation by both the classical and alternative pathways. CR1 binds C3b and C4b, thereby mediating phagocytosis by neutrophils and monocytes. RBC CR1 is important in the processing of immune complexes, binding them for transport to the liver and spleen for removal from the circulation. The presence of CR1 on other blood cells and tissues suggests that it has multiple functions.[132] The CR1 copy number per RBC (and thus antigen strength) is reduced in SLE, cold hemagglutinin disease (CHAD), PNH, hemolytic anemia, insulin-dependent diabetes mellitus, acquired immunodeficiency syndrome, some malignant tumors, and any condition associated with increased clearance of immune complexes.

CR1, and the Sl[a] antigen in particular, may act as a receptor for the malarial parasite *Plasmodium falciparum*, and thus, the Sl(a–) phenotype may provide selective advantage.[135]

■ Indian Blood Group System (ISBT System 023)

History

The In[a] antigen, reported in 1973, is on RBCs from 4% of Indians from Bombay. This blood group system was named because of its association with India.

Gene, Protein, and Antigens

In[a] and In[b], the antigens of the Indian system, are carried on CD44 (synonyms: In(Lu)-related p80; HUTCH-1; H-CAM; GP90[HERMES], Pgp-1; ECRMIII; Ly-24; p85).[136] The *CD44* gene is located at chromosome 11p13 and consists of at least 19 exons, 10 of which are variably spliced. The CD44 glycoprotein passes through the RBC membrane once, and the extracellular N-terminus has six cysteine residues, six N-glycan sites, four chondroitin sulfate sites, and potential sites for O-glycans. There are 2000 to 5000 copies of CD44 per RBC. SDS-PAGE shows that CD44 has an approximate M_r of 80,000 when reduced. The In[a]/In[b] polymorphism is due to Pro46Arg on CD44.[137] In[b] is a common antigen, and In[a] is rare in white persons but has an incidence of 4% in Indians, 10% in Iranians, and nearly 12% in Arabs. The antigens are sensitive to treatment of RBCs by proteases and DTT but resistant to treatment with sialidase and acid.[7]

The In(a–b–) phenotype was described in a patient with a novel form of congenital dyserythropoietic anemia (CDA) and CD44 deficiency,[138] but it was not possible to ascertain whether the phenotype was genetically determined or related to the patient's hematologic disorder. The RBCs of the patient

also typed AnWj– and Co(a–b–) and had a reduced level of LW[ab] expression.

Antibodies

Antibodies in the Indian system are usually IgG and reactive on the IAT, and they do not bind complement. Some antibodies may directly agglutinate RBCs, but the reactivity is greatly enhanced by the IAT. These antibodies have caused decreased RBC survival and a positive DAT result in the neonate, but not HDN. A severe, delayed, hemolytic transfusion reaction due to anti-In[b] has been reported.[139]

Expression

Indian antigens are weakly expressed on cord RBCs as well as on RBCs from people with the dominant Lu(a–b–) phenotype and from pregnant women. CD44 is expressed on neutrophils, lymphocytes, monocytes, brain, breast, colon epithelium, gastric tissue, heart, kidney, liver, lung, placenta, skin, spleen, thymus and fibroblasts.

Joint fluid from patients with inflammatory synovitis has higher than normal levels of soluble CD44.[138] The serum CD44 value is elevated in some patients with lymphoma.

Function

CD44 has a diverse range of biologic functions involving cell–cell and cell–matrix interactions in cells other than RBCs.[136] It is an adhesion molecule in lymphocytes, monocytes, and some tumor cells. CD44 binds to hyaluronate and other components of the extracellular matrix and is also involved in immune stimulation as well as signaling between cells.[140]

■ Ok Blood Group System (ISBT System 024)

History

Anti-Ok[a] was first identified in 1979 in the serum of a Japanese woman (Mrs. Okbutso) who had received a transfusion, and was therefore named after her. After the identification of the gene encoding the Ok protein, the Ok[a] antigen attained system status in 1999.[20]

Gene, Protein, and Antigens

The Ok[a] blood group antigen is carried on CD147 and is encoded by the *OK* gene at 19pter-p13.2. CD147 (synonyms: extracellular matrix metalloproteinase inducer (EMMPRIN); M6; OX-47; CE9; basigin; gp42; neurothelin; HT7; 5A11) is an N-glycosylated glycoprotein that passes through the RBC membrane once with its N-terminus to the extracellular surface. It is also a member of the IgSF. On SDS-PAGE, CD147 is shown to have an approximate M_r of 35,000 to 69,000. The Ok[a] polymorphism is due to an amino acid substitution at residue 92 [Glu for Ok(a+) and Lys for Ok(a–)].[141, 142] Ok[a] is resistant to treatment of RBCs by proteases, sialidase, DTT, and acid.[7] The eight known Ok(a–) probands are Japanese.

Antibodies

The original example of anti-Ok[a] is IgG and is reactive on the IAT; it does not bind complement. This antibody caused reduced cell survival but not HDN. Only one other example of human anti-Ok[a] is known.

Expression

The Ok^a antigen on RBCs is well-developed at birth. CD147 has a broad expression pattern in both hematopoietic and nonhematopoietic tissues and is upregulated on activated lymphocytes and monocytes.[143, 144]

Evolution

The Ok^a antigen is on RBCs from gorillas and chimpanzees but not on RBCs from rhesus monkeys, baboons, and marmosets.[141] Homologues of the Ok^a glycoprotein have been found in the rat (OX-47 or CE9), mouse (basigin), rabbit, and chicken (neurothelin or HT7).[143]

Function

Human CD147 on tumor cells is thought to bind an unknown ligand on fibroblasts, which stimulates their production of collagenase and other extracellular matrix metalloproteinases, thus enhancing tumor cell invasion and metastasis.[145] In studies with CD147 knockout mice, RBCs were apparently not compromised. CD147 may be involved in the function of the blood-brain barrier[146] and lymphocyte inactivation.[147]

■ RAPH Blood Group System (ISBT System 025)

History

A new polymorphism on RBCs was originally defined by monoclonal antibodies (1D12, 2F7) and called MER2 (M for monoclonal; ER for Eleanor Roosevelt, the name of the laboratory producing the antibodies). Later, the polymorphism was also recognized by human polyclonal antibodies, and when the MER2 antigen attained system status in 1999, the system was named RAPH after the first patient to make the specificity.

Gene, Protein, and Antigens

The MER2 antigen is encoded by a gene located on chromosome 11p15, but it has not been cloned, and the molecular basis of the antigen is not known. Ninety-two percent of English blood donors are MER2-positive, and 8% are MER2-negative. The antigen strength varies among different RBC samples. The antigen is resistant to treatment of RBCs by papain, ficin, and sialidase but sensitive to treatment by trypsin, α-chymotrypsin, and DTT.[7]

Antibodies

The three examples of human anti-MER2 (anti-RAPH) are IgG and reactive on the IAT, and two of the three antibodies bind complement. These antibodies have not caused HDN nor transfusion reactions; indeed, two siblings with the antibody have received numerous crossmatch-incompatible RBC transfusions without problems. The three antibody producers were Indian Jews.[148]

Expression

The antigen is expressed on RBCs of newborns. MER2 is expressed on fibroblasts, and its expression may be reduced on Lu(a–b–) RBCs of persons with the *In(Lu)* gene.

Function

All three people (two probands) with anti-MER2 (anti-RAPH) had renal failure requiring dialysis. It is possible that the protein carrying the MER2 antigen is required for normal kidney function.[148]

■ Other Antigens

Table 2.4 lists antigens that are not included in blood group systems. Three of the blood group collections are carbohydrate antigens (Ii, GLOB, Unnamed). Antigens of the Ii and GLOB collections are discussed in Chapter 3. The other two (Cost, Er) are presumed to be protein antigens, and the antibodies to antigens in these systems are generally not clinically significant. Antigens in the 700 series of low-incidence antigens occur in less than 1% of most populations and have no known alleles. Antibodies to many of these low-incidence antigens have caused HDN.[7] Antigens in the 901 series of high-incidence antigens occur in more than 90% of people, have no known alleles, and cannot be placed in a blood group system or collection. Antibodies to Vel, Lan, At^a, Jr^a, AnWj, PEL, ABTI, and MAM can cause HDN and transfusion reactions.[7, 20] Finding blood for the patients with any of the antibodies to these antigens can be difficult, and the patient should be encouraged to predeposit autologous units for long-term frozen storage. JMH and EMM are carried on GPI-linked proteins, and antibodies to these antigens are of little clinical concern.

REFERENCES

1. Landsteiner K, Levine P: A new agglutinable factor differentiating human blood. Proc Soc Exp Biol Med 1927;24:600–603.
2. Levine P: A review of Landsteiner's contributions to human blood groups. Transfusion 1961;1:45–52.
3. Garratty G, Dzik WH, Issitt PD, et al: Terminology for blood group antigens and genes: Historical origins and guidelines in the new millennium. Transfusion 2000;40:477–489.
4. Wiener AS, Unger LF, Gordon EG: Fatal hemolytic transfusion reaction caused by sensitization to a new blood factor U. JAMA 1953;153:1444–1446.
5. Rahuel C, London J, d'Auriol L, et al: Characterization of cDNA clones for human glycophorin A: Use for gene localization and for analysis of normal or glycophorin-A–deficient (Finnish type) genomic DNA. Eur J Biochem 1988;172:147–153.
6. Vignal A, London J, Rahuel C, Cartron J-P: Promoter sequence and chromosomal organization of the genes encoding glycophorins A, B and E. Gene 1990;95:289–293.
7. Reid ME, Lomas-Francis C: The Blood Group Antigen Facts Book. San Diego, Academic Press, 1996.
8. Chasis JA, Mohandas N: Red blood cell glycophorins. Blood 1992;80:1869–1879.
9. Dahr W: Immunochemistry of sialoglycoproteins in human red blood cell membranes. In Vengelen-Tyler V, Judd WJ (eds): Recent Advances in Blood Group Biochemistry. Arlington, VA, American Association of Blood Banks, 1986, pp 23–65.
10. Fukuda M: Molecular genetics of the glycophorin A gene cluster. Semin Hematol 1993;30:138–151.
11. Anstee DJ, Spring FA, Parsons SF, et al: Molecular background of human blood group antigens. In Hackel E, Tippett P (eds): Human Genetics 1994: A Revolution in Full Swing. Bethesda, MD, American Association of Blood Banks, 1994, pp 1–52.
12. Blanchard D: Human red cell glycophorins: Biochemical and antigenic properties. Transfus Med Rev 1990;4:170–186.
13. Reid ME: Some concepts relating to the molecular genetic basis of certain MNS blood group antigens. Transfus Med 1994;4:99–111.
14. Dahr W, Gielen W, Beyreuther K, Krüger J: Structure of the Ss blood group antigens. I: Isolation of Ss-active glycopeptides and differentiation of the antigens by modification of methionine. Hoppe Seylers Z Physiol Chem 1980;361:145–152.
15. Huang C-H, Blumenfeld OO: MNSs blood groups and major glycophorins: Molecular basis for allelic variation. In Cartron J-P, Rouger P (eds): Molecular Basis of Human Blood Group Antigens. New York, Plenum Press, 1995, pp 153–188.

16. Storry JR, Reid ME: Characterization of antibodies produced by S-s-individuals. Transfusion 1996;36:512–516.
17. Greenwalt TJ, Sasaki T, Sanger R, et al: An allele of the S(s) blood group genes. Proc Natl Acad Sci U S A 1954;40:1126–1129.
18. Daniels GL, Anstee DJ, Cartron J-P, et al: Blood group terminology 1995: ISBT working party on terminology for red cell surface antigens. Vox Sang 1995;69:265–279.
19. Daniels GL, Anstee DJ, Cartron JP, et al: Terminology for red cell surface antigens—Makuhari report. Vox Sang 1996;71:246–248.
20. Daniels GL, Anstee DJ, Cartron JP, et al: Terminology for red cell surface antigens—Oslo report. Vox Sang 1999;77:52–57.
21. Dahr W, Knuppertz G, Beyreuther K, et al: Studies on the structures of the Tm, Sj, M1, Can, Sext and Hu blood group antigens. Biol Chem Hoppe Seyler 1991;372:573–584.
22. Issitt PD, Anstee DJ: Applied Blood Group Serology, 4th ed. Durham, NC, Montgomery Scientific, 1998.
23. Mollison PL, Engelfriet CP, Contreras M: Blood Transfusion in Clinical Medicine, 9th ed. Oxford, Blackwell Science, 1993.
24. Harvey J, Parsons SF, Anstee DJ, Bradley BA: Evidence for the occurrence of human erythrocyte membrane sialoglycoproteins in human kidney endothelial cells. Vox Sang 1988;55:104–108.
25. Anstee DJ, Holmes CH, Judson PA, Tanner MJA: The use of monoclonal antibodies to determine the distribution of red cell surface proteins on cells and tissues. In Agre PC, Cartron J-P (eds): Protein Blood Group Antigens of the Human Red Cell: Structure, Function, and Clinical Significance. Baltimore, Johns Hopkins University, 1992, pp 170–181.
26. Southcott MJG, Tanner MJ, Anstee DJ: The expression of human blood group antigens during erythropoiesis in a cell culture system. Blood 1999;93:4425–4435.
27. Blancher A, Reid ME, Socha WW: Cross-reactivity of antibodies to human and primate red cell antigens. Transfus Med Rev 2000;14:161–179.
28. Tomita A, Radike EL, Parker CJ: Isolation of erythrocyte membrane inhibitor of reactive lysis type II: Identification as glycophorin A. J Immunol 1993;151:3308–3323.
29. Hadley TJ, Miller LH, Haynes JD: Recognition of red cells by malaria parasites: The role of erythrocyte-binding proteins. Transfus Med Rev 1991;5:108–113.
30. Miller LH: Impact of malaria on genetic polymorphism and genetic diseases in Africans and African Americans. Proc Natl Acad Sci U S A 1994;91:2415–2419.
31. Jentoft N: Why are proteins O-glycosylated? Trends Biochem Sci 1990;15:291–294.
32. Groves JD, Tanner MJ: The effects of glycophorin A on the expression of the human red cell anion transporter (band 3) in Xenopus oocytes. J Membr Biol 1994;140:81–88.
33. Groves JD, Tanner MJ: Role of N-glycosylation in the expression of human band 3-mediated anion transport. Mol Membr Biol 1994;11:31–38.
34. Groves JD, Tanner MJ: Glycophorin A facilitates the expression of human band 3-mediated anion transport in Xenopus oocytes. J Biol Chem 1992;267:22163–22170.
35. Callender STE, Race RR: A serological and genetical study of multiple antibodies formed in response to blood transfusion by a patient with lupus erythematosus diffusus. Ann Eugen 1946;13:102.
36. Cook PJL: The Lutheran-secretor recombination fraction in man: A possible sex-difference. Ann Hum Genet 1965;28:393–401.
37. Mohr J: A search for linkage between the Lutheran blood group and other hereditary characters. Acta Path Microbiol Scand 1951;28:80–96.
38. Parsons SF, Mallinson G, Holmes CH, et al: The Lutheran blood group glycoprotein, another member of the immunoglobulin superfamily, is widely expressed in human tissues and is developmentally regulated in human liver. Proc Natl Acad Sci U S A 1995;92:5496–5500.
39. Parsons SF, Mallinson G, Judson PA, et al: Evidence that the Lu^b blood group antigen is located on red cell membrane glycoproteins of 85 and 78 kd. Transfusion 1987;27:61–63.
40. Anstee DJ: Blood group-active surface molecules of the human red blood cell. Vox Sang 1990;58:1–20.
41. Rahuel C, Kim CL, Mattei MG, et al: A unique gene encodes spliceoforms of the B-cell adhesion molecule cell surface glycoprotein of epithelial cancer and of the Lutheran blood group glycoprotein. Blood 1996;88:1865–1872.
42. El Nemer W, Rahuel C, Colin Y, et al: Organization of the human LU gene and molecular basis of the Lu^a/Lu^b blood group polymorphism. Blood 1997;89:4608–4616.
43. Parsons SF, Mallinson G, Daniels GL, et al: Use of domain-deletion mutants to locate Lutheran blood group antigens to each of the five immunoglobulin superfamily domains of the Lutheran glycoprotein: Elucidation of the molecular basis of the Lu^a/Lu^b and the Au^a/Au^b polymorphisms. Blood 1997;89:4219–4225.
44. Crawford MN: The Lutheran blood group system: Serology and genetics. In Pierce SR, Macpherson CR (eds): Blood Group Systems: Duffy, Kidd and Lutheran. Arlington, VA, American Association of Blood Banks, 1988, pp 93–117.
45. Taliano V, Guevin RM, Tippett P: The genetics of a dominant inhibitor of the Lutheran antigens. Vox Sang 1973;24:42–47.
46. Telen MJ, Eisenbarth GS, Haynes BF: Human erythrocyte antigens: Regulation of expression of a novel erythrocyte surface antigen by the inhibitor Lutheran In(Lu) gene. J Clin Invest 1983;71:1878–1886.
47. Spring FA, Dalchau R, Daniels GL, et al: The In^a and In^b blood group antigens are located on a glycoprotein of 80,000 MW (the CDw44 glycoprotein) whose expression is influenced by the In(Lu) gene. Immunology 1988;64:37–43.
48. Poole J: The Lutheran blood group system—1991 [review]. Immunohematology 1992;8:1–8.
49. El Nemer W, Gane P, Colin Y, et al: The Lutheran blood group glycoproteins, the erythroid receptors for laminin, are adhesion molecules. J Biol Chem 1998;273:16686–16693.
50. Udani M, Zen Q, Cottman M, et al: Basal cell adhesion molecule Lutheran protein—the receptor critical for sickle cell adhesion to laminin. J Clin Invest 1998;101:2550–2558.
51. Spring FA, Bruce LJ, Anstee DJ, Tanner MJ: A red cell band 3 variant with altered stilbene disulphonate binding is associated with the Diego (Di^a) blood group antigen. Biochem J 1992;288:713–716.
52. Bruce LJ, Anstee DJ, Spring FA, Tanner MJ: Band 3 Memphis variant II: Altered stilbene disulfonate binding and the Diego (Di^a) blood group antigen are associated with the human erythrocyte band 3 mutation Pro^{854}→Leu. J Biol Chem 1994;269:16155–16158.
53. Bruce LJ, Ring SM, Anstee DJ, et al: Changes in the blood group Wright antigens are associated with a mutation at amino acid 658 in human erythrocyte band 3: A site of interaction between band 3 and glycophorin A under certain conditions. Blood 1995;85:541–547.
54. Zelinski T: Erythrocyte band 3 antigens and the Diego blood group system. Transfus Med Rev 1998;12:36–45.
55. Jarolim P, Rubin HL, Zakova D, et al: Characterization of seven low incidence blood group antigens carried by erythrocyte band 3 protein. Blood 1998;92:4836–4843.
56. Zelinski T, Coghlan G, White L, Philipps S: The Diego blood group locus is located on chromosome 17q. Genomics 1993;17:665–666.
57. Tanner MJ: Molecular and cellular biology of the erythrocyte anion exchanger (AE1). Semin Hematol 1993;30:34–57.
58. Tanner MJA: The structure and function of band 3 (AE1): Recent developments. Mol Membr Biol 1997;14:155–165.
59. Race RR, Sanger R: Blood Groups in Man, 6th ed. Oxford, Blackwell Scientific, 1975.
60. Blumenfeld OO, Huang C-H, Xie SS, Blancher A: The MNSs blood group system: Molecular biology of glycophorins in humans and nonhuman primates. In Blancher A, Klein J, Socha WW (eds): Molecular Biology and Evolution of Blood Group and MHC Antigens in Primates. Berlin, Springer-Verlag, 1997, pp 113–146.
61. Reid ME: Contribution of MNS to the study of glycophorin A and glycophorin B. Immunohematology 1999;15:5–9.
62. Reid ME, Øyen R, Marsh WL: Summary of the clinical significance of blood group alloantibodies. Semin Hematol 2000;37:197–216.
63. Palatnik M, Simoes ML, Alves ZM, Laranjeira NS: The 60 and 63 kDa proteolytic peptides of the red cell membrane band-3 protein: Their prevalence in human and non-human primates. Hum Genet 1990;86:126–130.
64. Jarolim P, Palek J, Amato D, et al: Deletion in erythrocyte band 3 gene in malaria-resistant Southeast Asian ovalocytosis. Proc Natl Acad Sci U S A 1991;88:11022–11026.
65. Tanner MJ, Bruce L, Martin PG, et al: Melanesian hereditary ovalocytes have a deletion in red cell band 3. Blood 1991;78:2785–2786.
66. Schofield AE, Reardon DM, Tanner MJ: Defective anion transport activity of the abnormal band 3 in hereditary ovalocytic red blood cells. Nature 1992;355:836–838.
67. Jarolim P, Shayakul C, Prabakaran D, et al: Autosomal dominant distal renal tubular acidosis is associated in three families with heterozygosity for the R589H mutation in the AE1 (band 3) Cl$^-$/HCO$_3^-$ exchanger. J Biol Chem 1998;273:6380–6388.

68. Eaton BR, Morton JA, Pickles MM, White KE: A new antibody, anti-Yt^a, characterizing a blood group of high incidence. Br J Haematol 1956;2:333–341.

69. Spring FA, Gardner B, Anstee DJ: Evidence that the antigens of the Yt blood group system are located on human erythrocyte acetylcholinesterase. Blood 1992;80:2136–2141.

70. Coghlan G, Kaita H, Belcher E, et al: Evidence for genetic linkage between the *KEL* and *YT* blood group loci. Vox Sang 1989;57:88–89.

71. Getman DK, Eubanks JH, Camp S, et al: The human gene encoding acetylcholinesterase is located on the long arm of chromosome 7. Am J Hum Genet 1992;51:170–177.

72. Bartels CF, Zelinski T, Lockridge O: Mutation at codon 322 in the human acetylcholinesterase (ACHE) gene accounts for YT blood group polymorphism. Am J Hum Genet 1993;52:928–936.

73. Levene C, Bar-Shany S, Manny N, et al: The Yt blood groups in Israeli Jews, Arabs, and Druse. Transfusion 1987;27:471–474.

74. Taylor P: The cholinesterases. J Biol Chem 1991;266:4025–4028.

75. Li Y, Camp S, Rachinsky TL, et al: Gene structure of mammalian acetylcholinesterase: Alternative exons dictate tissue-specific expression. J Biol Chem 1991;266:23083–23090.

76. Telen MJ, Rosse WF, Parker CJ, et al: Evidence that several high-frequency human blood group antigens reside on phosphatidylinositol-linked erythrocyte membrane proteins. Blood 1990;75:1404–1407.

77. Sussman JL, Harel M, Frolow F, et al: Atomic structure of acetylcholinesterase from *Torpedo californica*: A prototypic acetylcholine-binding protein. Science 1991;253:872–879.

78. Lawson AA, Barr RD: Acetylcholinesterase in red blood cells. Am J Hematol 1987;26:101–111.

79. Mann JD, Cahan A, Gelb AG, et al: A sex-linked blood group. Lancet 1962;1:8–10.

80. Ellis NA, Tippett P, Petty A, et al: *PBDX* is the *XG* blood group gene. Nature 1994;8:285–290.

81. Daniels GL, Anstee DJ, Cartron JP, et al: International Society of Blood Transfusion working party on terminology for red cell surface antigens: Vienna report. Vox Sang 2001;80:193–197.

82. Schlossman SF, Bounsell L, Gilks W, et al: CD antigens 1993. Blood 1994;83:879–880.

83. Tippett P, Ellis NA: The Xg blood group system: A review. Transfus Med Rev 1998;12:233–257.

84. Gelin C, Aubrit F, Phalipon A, et al: The E2 antigen, a 32 kd glycoprotein involved in T-cell adhesion processes, is the MIC2 gene product. EMBO J 1989;8:3253–3259.

85. Spring FA, Herron R, Rowe G: An erythrocyte glycoprotein of apparent M$_r$ 60,000 expresses the Sc1 and Sc2 antigens. Vox Sang 1990;58:122–125.

86. Banks JA, Hemming N, Poole J: Evidence that the Gy^a, Hy and Jo^a antigens belong to the Dombrock blood group system. Vox Sang 1995;68:177–182.

87. Gubin AN, Njoroge JM, Wojda U, et al: Identification of the Dombrock blood group glycoprotein as a polymorphic member of the ADP-ribosyltransferase gene family. Blood 2000;96:2621–2627.

88. Eiberg H, Mohr J: Dombrock blood group (*DO*): Assignment to chromosome 12p. Hum Genet 1996;98:518–521.

89. Koch-Nolte F, Haag F, Braren R, et al: Two novel human members of an emerging mammalian gene family related to mono-ADP-ribosylating bacterial toxins [erratum published in Genomics 1999 Jan 1;55(1):130]. Genomics 1997;39:370–376.

90. Erratum (to Koch-Nolte F, et al, in Genomics, 39:370–376, 1997). Genomics 2002;55:130.

91. Rios M, Hue-Roye K, Øyen R, et al: Insights into the Holley-negative and Joseph-negative phenotypes. Transfusion 2002; (in press).

92. Rios M, Hue-Roye K, Lee AH, et al: DNA analysis for the Dombrock polymorphism. Transfusion 2001;41:1143–1146.

93. Bailly P, Lucien N, Celton JL, et al: A short deletion within the blood group Dombrock locus causing a Do$_{null}$ phenotype (abstract). Transfus Clin Biol 2001;8 (Suppl 1):167s.

94. Rios M, Storry JR, Hue-Roye K, et al: Two new molecular bases for the Dombrock null phenotype. Br J Haematol 2002;117:765–767.

95. Preston GM, Agre P: Isolation of the cDNA for erythrocyte integral membrane protein of 28 kilodaltons: Member of an ancient channel family. Proc Natl Acad Sci U S A 1991;88:11110–11114.

96. Preston GM, Smith BL, Zeidel ML, et al: Mutations in *aquaporin-1* in phenotypically normal humans without functional CHIP water channels. Science 1994;265:1585–1587.

97. Chretien S, Catron JP: A single mutation inside the NPA motif of aquaporin-1 found in a Colton-null phenotype [letter]. Blood 1999;93:4021–4023.

98. Joshi SR, Wagner FF, Vasantha K, et al: An *AQP1* null allele in an Indian woman with Co (a–b–) phenotype and high-titer anti-Co3 associated with mild HDN. Transfusion 2001;41:1273–1278.

99. Smith BL, Preston GM, Spring FA, et al: Human red cell aquaporin CHIP. I: Molecular characterization of ABH and Colton blood group antigens. J Clin Invest 1994;94:1043–1049.

100. King LS, Agre P: Pathophysiology of the aquaporin water channels. Annu Rev Physiol 1996;58:619–648.

101. Moon C, Williams JB, Preston GM, et al: The mouse aquaporin-1 gene. Genomics 1995;30:354–357.

102. Smith BL, Baumgarten R, Nielsen S, et al: Concurrent expression of erythroid and renal aquaporin CHIP and appearance of water channel activity in perinatal rats. J Clin Invest 1993;92:2035–2041.

103. Landsteiner K, Wiener AS: An agglutinable factor in human blood recognized by immune sera for rhesus blood. Proc Soc Exp Biol Med 1940;43:223.

104. Sistonen P, Tippett P: A 'new' allele giving further insight into the LW blood group system. Vox Sang 1982;42:252–255.

105. Bailly P, Hermand P, Callebaut I, et al: The LW blood group glycoprotein is homologous to intercellular adhesion molecules. Proc Natl Acad Sci U S A 1994;91:5306–5310.

106. Mallinson G, Martin PG, Anstee DJ, et al: Identification and partial characterization of the human erythrocyte membrane component(s) that express the antigens of the LW blood-group system. Biochem J 1986;234:649–652.

107. Hermand P, Gane P, Mattei MG, et al: Molecular basis and expression of the LW^a/LW^b blood group polymorphism. Blood 1995;86:1590–1594.

108. Bloy C, Hermand P, Blanchard D, et al: Surface orientation and antigen properties of Rh and LW polypeptides of the human erythrocyte membrane. J Biol Chem 1990;265:21482–21487.

109. Hermand P, Le Pennec PY, Rouger P, et al: Characterization of the gene encoding the human LW blood group protein in LW$^+$ and LW$^-$ phenotypes. Blood 1996;87:2962–2967.

110. Giles CM: The LW blood group: A review. Immunol Commun 1980;9:225–242.

111. Shaw MA: Monoclonal anti-LWab and anti-D reagents recognize a number of different epitopes: Use of red cells of non-human primates. J Immunogenet 1986;13:377–386.

112. Bailly P, Tontti E, Hermand P, et al: The red cell LW blood group protein is an intercellular adhesion molecule which binds to CD11/CD18 leukocyte integrins. Eur J Immunol 1995;25:3316–3320.

113. O'Neill GJ, Yang SY, Tegoli J, et al: Chido and Rodgers blood groups are distinct antigenic components of human complement C4. Nature 273;273:668–670.

114. Yu CY, Campbell RD, Porter RR: A structural model for the location of the Rodgers and the Chido antigenic determinants and their correlation with the human complement component C4A/C4B isotypes. Immunogenetics 1988;27:399–405.

115. Giles CM, Jones JW: A new antigenic determinant for C4 of relatively low frequency. Immunogenetics 1987;26:392–394.

116. Westhoff CM, Sipherd BD, Wylie DE, Toalson LD: Severe anaphylactic reactions following transfusions of platelets to a patient with anti-Ch. Transfusion 1992;32:576–579.

117. Tippett P, Storry JR, Walker PS, et al: Glycophorin A-deficient red cells may have a weak expression of C4-bound Ch and Rg antigens. Immunohematology 1996;12:4–7.

118. Moulds JM: Association of blood group antigens with immunologically important proteins. In Garratty G (ed): Immunobiology of Transfusion Medicine. New York, Marcel Dekker, 1994, pp 273–297.

119. Reid ME, Spring FA: Molecular basis of glycophorin C variants and their associated blood group antigens. Transfus Med 1994;4:139–149.

120. Colin Y, Rahuel C, London J, et al: Isolation of cDNA clones and complete amino acid sequence of human erythrocyte glycophorin C. J Biol Chem 1986;261:229–233.

121. Chang S, Reid ME, Conboy J, et al: Molecular characterization of erythrocyte glycophorin C variants [abstract]. Blood 1989;74(Suppl 1):11a.

122. Telen MJ, Le Van Kim C, Chung A, et al: Molecular basis for elliptocytosis associated with glycophorin C and D deficiency in the Leach phenotype. Blood 1991;78:1603–1606.

123. Winardi R, Reid M, Conboy J, Mohandas N: Molecular analysis of glycophorin C deficiency in human erythrocytes. Blood 1993;81:2799–2803.

124. Sistonen P: Some notions on clinical significance of anti-Ls[a] and independence of *Ls* from Colton, Kell, and Lewis blood group loci [abstract]. XIX Congress of ISBT, 1986;652.

125. Alloisio N, Morle L, Bachir D, et al: Red cell membrane sialoglycoprotein β in homozygous and heterozygous 4.1(−) hereditary elliptocytosis. Biochim Biophys Acta 1985;816:57–62.

126. Post TW, Arce MA, Liszewski MK, et al: Structure of the gene for human complement protein decay accelerating factor. J Immunol 1990;144:740–744.

127. Lublin DM, Atkinson JP: Decay-accelerating factor: Biochemistry, molecular biology and function. Annu Rev Immunol 1989;7:35–58.

128. Telen MJ, Rao N, Udani M, et al: Molecular mapping of the Cromer blood group Cr[a] and Tc[a] epitopes of decay accelerating factor: Toward the use of recombinant antigens in immunohematology. Blood 1994;84:3205–3211.

129. Lublin DM, Kompelli S, Storry JR, Reid ME: Molecular basis of Cromer blood group antigens. Transfusion 2000;40:208–213.

130. Holmes CH, Simpson KL, Wainwright SD, et al: Preferential expression of the complement regulatory protein decay accelerating factor at the fetomaternal interface during human pregnancy. J Immunol 1990;144:3099–3105.

131. Daniels GL, Okubo Y, Yamaguchi H, et al: UMC, another Cromer-related blood group antigen. Transfusion 1989;29:794–797.

132. Ahearn JM, Fearon DT: Structure and function of the complement receptors, CR1 (CD35) and CR2 (CD21). Adv Immunol 1989;46:183–219.

133. Moulds JM, Zimmerman PA, Doumbo OK, et al: Molecular identification of Knops blood group polymorphisms found in long homologous region D of complement receptor 1. Blood 2001;97:2879–2885.

134. Rao N, Ferguson DJ, Lee SF, Telen MJ: Identification of human erythrocyte blood group antigens on the C3b/C4b receptor. J Immunol 1991;146:3502–3507.

135. Rowe JA, Moulds JM, Newbold CI, Miller LH: *P-falciparum* rosetting mediated by a parasite-variant erythrocyte membrane protein and complement-receptor 1. Nature 1997;388:292–295.

136. Telen MJ, Ferguson DJ: Relationship of Inb antigen to other antigens on In(Lu)-related p80. Vox Sang 1990;58:118–121.

137. Telen MJ, Udani M, Washington MK, et al: A blood group-related polymorphism of CD44 abolishes a hyaluronan-binding consensus sequence without preventing hyaluronan binding. J Biol Chem 1996;271:7147–7153.

138. Parsons SF, Jones J, Anstee DJ, et al: A novel form of congenital dyserythropoietic anemia associated with deficiency of erythroid CD44 and a unique blood group phenotype [In(a−b−), Co(a−b−)]. Blood 1994;83:860–868.

139. Joshi SR: Immediate haemolytic transfusion reaction due to anti-In[b]. Vox Sang 1992;63:232–233.

140. Goldstein LA, Zhou DFH, Picker LJ, et al: A human lymphocyte homing receptor, the Hermes antigen, is related to cartilage proteoglycan core and link proteins. Cell 1989;56:1063–1072.

141. Williams BP, Daniels GL, Pym B, et al: Biochemical and genetic analysis of the OK[a] blood group antigen. Immunogenetics 1988;27:322–329.

142. Spring FA, Holmes CH, Simpson KL, et al: The Ok[a] blood group antigen is a marker for the M6 leukocyte activation antigen, the human homolog of OX-47 antigen, basigin and neurothelin, an immunoglobulin superfamily molecule that is widely expressed in human cells and tissues. Eur J Immunol 1997;27:891–897.

143. Kasinrerk W, Fiebiger E, Stefanova I, et al: Human leukocyte activation antigen M6, a member of the Ig superfamily, is the species homologue of rat OX-47, mouse basigin, and chicken HT7 molecule. J Immunol 1992;149:847–854.

144. Anstee DJ, Spring FA: Red cell membrane glycoproteins with a broad tissue distribution. Transfus Med Rev 1989;3:13–23.

145. Biswas C, Zhang Y, DeCastro R, et al: The human tumor cell-derived collagenase stimulatory factor (renamed EMMPRIN) is a member of the immunoglobulin superfamily. Cancer Res 1995;55:434–439.

146. Seulberger H, Unger CM, Risau W: HT7, neurothelin, basigin, gp42 and OX-47—many names for one developmentally regulated immunoglobulin-like surface glycoprotein on blood-brain barrier endothelium, epithelial tissue barriers and neurons. Neurosci Lett 1992;140:93–97.

147. Ghebrehiwet B, Lu PD, Zhang W, et al: Identification of functional domains on gC1Q-R, a cell surface protein that binds to the globular "heads" of C1Q, using monoclonal antibodies and synthetic peptides. Hybridoma 1996;15:333–342.

148. Daniels GL, Levene C, Berrebi A, et al: Human alloantibodies detecting a red cell antigen apparently identical to MER2. Vox Sang 1988;55:161–164.

ii. Platelet Antigens

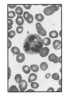

Chapter 6

Human Platelet Antigens

Thomas J. Kunicki
Diane J. Nugent

■ Platelet Membrane Glycoproteins

Among the variety of glycoproteins on the human platelet surface, there are several that contribute to the immunogenic makeup of the platelet (Table 6.1).

Integrins

The integrins are membrane glycoprotein heterodimers, each consisting of noncovalently associated α and β subunits.[1] The specificity of an integrin is dictated in large part by the identity of its α subunit, even though ligand binding per se may occur within a significant portion of the β subunit. The number of possible αβ combinations is apparently limited, however, and selective pairing in humans between 17 α and 8 β subunits has led to the discovery of 23 different integrins. These ubiquitous receptors mediate a wide range of cell adhesion events that are important to every fundamental

area of human biology, including embryonal development, immunocompetence, wound healing, and hemostasis. Two platelet membrane receptors that figure prominently in the antigenic profile of platelets, the cohesion receptor $\alpha_{IIb}\beta_3$ and the collagen receptor $\alpha_2\beta_1$, are integrins.

The Platelet Cohesion Receptor, Integrin $\alpha_{IIb}\beta_3$

The numerically predominant platelet integrin $\alpha_{IIb}\beta_3$, initially designated glycoprotein (GP) IIb-IIIa, mediates the common cohesive pathway that results from platelet activation in vivo (i.e., platelet aggregation supported by the binding of adhesive proteins such as fibrinogen and von Willebrand factor [vWF]). The α subunit of this integrin, α_{IIb}, is synthesized exclusively by megakaryocytes. Consequently, $\alpha_{IIb}\beta_3$ is a unique marker for platelets or cell lines with a megakaryocytic phenotype. Glanzmann thrombasthenia (GT) is an inherited disorder of platelet function characterized by an inability of platelets to bind fibrinogen and undergo agonist-induced aggregation.[2] The molecular defect in this disease involves either a quantitative or a qualitative abnormality of $\alpha_{IIb}\beta_3$. The $\alpha_{IIb}\beta_3$ heterodimer complex is depicted schematically in Figure 6.1.

The Platelet Collagen Receptor, Integrin $\alpha_2\beta_1$

Another integrin that contributes significantly to platelet function is the collagen receptor $\alpha_2\beta_1$ (GPIa-IIa).[3] This integrin plays a fundamental role in adhesion of blood platelets to both fibrillar (types I, II, III, and V) and nonfibrillar (types IV, VI, VII, and VIII) collagens.[4-7] Unlike α_{IIb}, the α_2 subunit is a single-chain molecule[8]; like several other integrin α subunits, it contains an additional 129-amino-acid segment known as the I-domain (Fig. 6.2). Inherited platelet deficiencies of the α_2 subunit have been described, and patients with these abnormalities exhibit chronic mucocutaneous bleeding and

Table 6.1 Functional Properties of Selected Membrane Glycoprotein (GP) Complexes

GP	Alternative Names	Receptor Function	Protein Ligands
Ib-IX-V	—	Adhesion	vWF
$\alpha_{IIb}\beta_3$	GPIIb-IIIa, CD41/CD61	Adhesion	Fibrinogen
		Cohesion	Fibrinogen
			Fibronectin
			Vitronectin
			vWF
$\alpha_2\beta_1$	GPIa-IIa, VLA-2, CD49b/CD29	Adhesion	Collagen
$\alpha_5\beta_1$	GPIc-IIa, VLA-5, CD49e/CD29	Adhesion	Fibronectin
$\alpha_6\beta_1$	GPIc'-IIa, VLA-6, CD49f/CD29	Adhesion	Laminin

vWF, von Willebrand factor; VLA, very late activation (antigen); CD, cell differentiation (antigen).

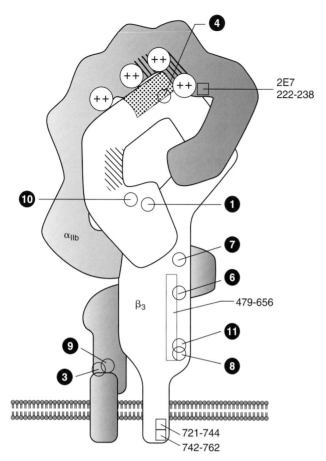

Figure 6.1 Schematic diagram of the integrin $\alpha_{IIb}\beta_3$. The α_{IIb} and β_3 subunits form a noncovalently associated heterodimer. The hatched area of α_{IIb} represents the decapeptide recognition site. On β_3, the stippled region represents the RGD recognition site; the hatched region, an alternative fibrinogen recognition site. Divalent cations (positively charged spheres) are required for both complex integrity and ligand binding. In this and subsequent figures, the locations of the polymorphisms that give rise to alloantigens are indicated by a black circle within which is the corresponding human platelet-specific alloantigen (HPA) designation, as described in Table 6.3. Regions that contain autoantigenic determinants are indicated by boxed areas and include two sequences on the cytoplasmic tail of β_3 (residues 721 through 762), a portion of the cysteine-rich domain of β_3 (479 through 656) and the discreet epitope 2E7 located at residues 222 through 238 of α_{IIb}.

prolonged bleeding times.[9, 10] More importantly, the expression of $\alpha_2\beta_1$ on platelets differs markedly among normal subjects and depends on the inheritance of multiple alleles of the α_2 gene.[11, 12] Although the levels of the integrins $\alpha_5\beta_1$ or $\alpha_{IIb}\beta_3$ and the GPIb-IX-V complex on platelets (molecules per platelet) certainly vary from one individual to the next,[11, 13] these differences never exceed a fraction of the mean population level. On the other hand, the number of $\alpha_2\beta_1$ molecules per platelet varies as much as fivefold and correlates precisely with quantitative measurements of platelet adhesion to type I or type III collagen.[11]

Regulation of $\alpha_2\beta_1$ expression could certainly modulate the antigenicity of this membrane receptor. It is also possible that similar factors influence expression of other platelet integrins, including $\alpha_{IIb}\beta_3$, but the extent to which that occurs remains to be determined.

The Receptor Complex GPIb-IX-V

The adhesion receptor complex Ib-IX-V[14, 15] is a heptamer composed of one molecule of glycoprotein V (GPV) associated with two molecules of each of three separate gene products, glycoproteins Ibα, Ibβ, and IX—(2) Ibα: (2)Ibβ: (2) IX: (1)V (Fig. 6.3).[16] This complex is a receptor for vWF and the initial mediator of transient platelet contact and attachment to the vessel wall under essentially all conditions of flow or shear stress. The vWF binding site on the complex is located within the amino-terminal domain of GPIbα.[15, 17, 18] The Bernard-Soulier syndrome is an inherited disorder of platelet function characterized by defective platelet adhesion to subendothelium and a quantitative or qualitative defect in the Ib-IX-V complex caused by mutations in genes encoding either the GPIbα or the GPIX component.[19–21]

Platelet Glycolipids

Glycolipids play an important role in the structural and functional characteristics of the platelet membrane, as in all cell types. Less is known about platelet glycolipid structure and immunogenicity compared with the platelet glycoproteins, but important contributions have been made in this area, permitting the identification of a number of immunogenic glycolipid components of the membrane (Table 6.2).[22] The predominant glycolipid on human platelets is lactosyl ceramide, representing 64% of the neutral glycolipids. Other neutral glycolipids include trihexosyl ceramide, glycosyl ceramide, and globoside. The principal fatty acids

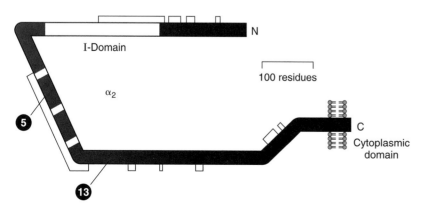

Figure 6.2 Schematic diagram of the α_2 subunit, which belongs to the subfamily of a subunits that are single-chain molecules with an additional I-domain (*large open bar*) sequence. Three putative calcium-binding repeats are indicated (*small open bars*), as are the sites of the alloantigenic HPA-5 and HPA-13bW polymorphisms. The locations of disulfide bonds (*thin lines*) are hypothetical.

Figure 6.3 Schematic diagram of the GPIb-IX-V complex. GPIb is composed of a heavy chain (Ibα) and a light chain (Ibβ) linked by a disulfide bond (S–S). The Ib molecule is noncovalently associated with GPIX. All three polypeptides span the membrane, are glycosylated (*open diamonds or circles*), and contain repetitive leucine-rich glycoprotein sequences (*open areas*). Two each of Ibα, Ibβ, and IX are associated with one molecule of V. In the case of Ibα, von Willebrand factor binds at the amino-terminal region (N) of the molecule, and five additional O-glycosylated repeats generate a carbohydrate-rich (macroglycopeptide) carboxyl region (C). The positions of the Ibα polymorphism that gives rise to the HPA-2 alloantigen system and the tandem 13-amino-acid repeats (*) are indicated. Also shown is the HPA-12bW polymorphism on GPIbβ.

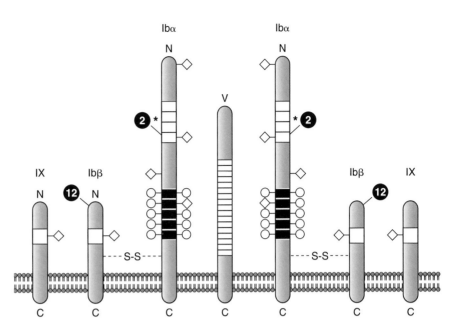

associated with these neutral glycolipids are behenic acid (22:0), arachiditic acid (20:0), and lignoceric acid (24:0). Ganglioside I (identified as hematoside or GM3) represents 92% of the acidic glycolipids, and ganglioside II represents 5% of the platelet acidic glycolipid composition.

■ Alloantigens

The proliferation of serologically defined alloantigens on platelet glycoproteins has led to the development of a consensus nomenclature, in which each of the alloantigens is prefixed by the letters HPA, for human platelet antigen[23, 24] (Table 6.3). These polymorphisms really define a limited number of allelic variants (Table 6.4), and it is important to understand the molecular basis for distinguishing the allelic variants of each immunogenic glycoprotein.[25]

Two clinically significant syndromes are the direct result of sensitization to platelet-specific alloantigens: neonatal alloimmune thrombocytopenic purpura (NATP) and post-transfusion purpura (PTP).

Neonatal Alloimmune Thrombocytopenia and Post-transfusion Purpura

NATP is caused by maternal sensitization to paternal allo-antigens on fetal platelets (Table 6.5). However, only a fraction of women who are negative for the platelet antigen in question deliver infants affected with NATP. For example, in the Western world, responsiveness to HPA-1a is the most common cause of NATP, yet the frequency of homozygous

Table 6.2 Glycolipid Antigens of Platelets

Cardiolipin (CL)
Lactosylceramide
Glycosphingolipids (GSL)
Acidic: sulfatides/gangliosides
  Monogalactosyl sulfatide (16/6 idiotype)
Neutral: globotriosyl ceramide
  Globotetraosyl ceramide

HPA-1b mothers in the general Caucasian population is 2% and estimates of the incidence of NATP are no greater than 0.05%. A key to understanding this discrepancy lies in the finding that responsiveness to HPA-1a shows a human leukocyte antigen (HLA) restriction.[26–28] HPA-1a and HPA-1b are defined by the Leu33/Pro33 β₃ polymorphism.[29–33] Individuals who are homozygous for Pro33 (homozygous HPA-1b) and responsive to the predominant HPA-1a antigen are almost exclusively HLA-DRB3*0101[27] or -DQB1*02.[34, 35] In the case of HLA-DRB3*0101, the calculated risk factor is 141, a risk level equivalent to that of the hallmark of HLA restriction in autoimmune disease, ankylosing spondylitis and HLA-B27.[35] In contrast, responsiveness of homozygous HPA-1a individuals to the HPA-1b allele is not linked to HLA.[35, 36] T cells are the likely candidates for providing HLA restriction in this case. In one case of NATP, Maslanka and colleagues[35] provided elegant evidence that T cells that share CDR3 motifs are stimulated by peptides containing the same Leu33 polymorphism that is recognized by anti-HPA-1a alloantibodies. In the case of another, less frequent antigen, HPA-6b, there appears to be an association between responsiveness and the major histocompatability complex (MHC) genes HLA-DRB1*1501, -DQA1*0102, or -DQB1*0602.[37]

Responsiveness to HPA-1a is not the sole cause of NATP. In a large study of 348 cases of clinically suspected NATP,[38] 78% of serologically confirmed cases were caused by anti-HPA-1a and 19% by anti-HPA-5b. All other specificities accounted for no more than 5% of cases. In reports from other laboratories, the association of NATP with other alloantigens, such as HPA-3a, HPA-3b, HPA-1b, or HPA-2b, has been noted but is rare.[39–42] Obviously, differences in allelic gene frequencies among racial or ethnic populations has an important impact on the frequency of responsiveness to a particular alloantigen. Table 6.6 summarizes some of the known variation in allelic gene frequencies in various world populations. For example, in the Japanese population, anti-HPA-1a has never been shown to be involved in NATP, and antibodies specific for HPA-4b play a dominant clinical role.[43] This is probably because the gene frequency for the

Table 6.3 Human Platelet-Specific Alloantigens

Glycoprotein	Class	HPA-	Synonym	Nucleotide	Amino Acid	NATP	PTP	Ref
α_{IIb}	Public	3a	Bak^a Lek^a	T_{2622}	Ile843	+	+	66
		3b	Bak^b	G_{2622}	Ser843	?	+	
	Private	9bW	Max^a	A_{2603}	Met837	+	–	83
				G_{2603}	Val837			
β_3	Public	1a	Pl^{A1} Zw^a	T_{196}	Leu33	++	++	30
		1b	Pl^{A2} Zw^b	C_{196}	Pro33	+	+	
		4a	Pen^a Yuk^b	G_{526}	Arg143	+	+	70
		4b	Pen^b Yuk^a	A_{526}	Gln143	+	–	
	Private	6bW	Tu^a Ca^a	A_{1564}	Gln489	+	–	79
				G_{1564}	Arg489			
		7bW	Mo^a	G_{1317}	Ala407	+	–	200
				C_{1317}	Pro407			
		8bW	Sr^a	T_{2004}	Cys636	+	–	201
				C_{2004}	Arg636			
		10bW	La^a	A_{281}	Gln62	+	–	84
				G_{281}	Arg62			
		11bW	Gro^a	A_{1996}	His633	+	–	202
				G_{1996}	Arg633			
			Oe^a			+	–	88
			Va^a			+	–	89
α_2	Public	5a	Br^b Zav^b Hc^a	G_{1648}	Glu505	+	–	203
		5b	Br^a Zav^a Hc^b	A_{1648}	Lys505	++	+	
	Private	13bW	Sit^a	T_{2531}	Met799			204
				C_{2531}	Thr799			
GP Ibα	Public	2a	Ko^b Sib^b	C_{524}	Thr145	–	–	205
		2b	Ko^a Sib^a	T_{524}	Met145	+	?	
	Private		Pe^a					90
GP Ibβ	Private	12bW	Iy^a	A_{141}	Glu15	+	–	206
				G_{141}	Gly15			
GPV	Private		Pl^T					91
CD109	Public		Gov^a			+	?	207
			Gov^b			+	–	

Public, gene frequency >0.02 (Western population); private, gene frequency <0.02 (Western population); NATP, presence in neonatal alloimmune thrombocytopenic purpura; PTP, presence in post-transfusion purpura.

Table 6.4 Alloantigenic Alleles of Platelet Membrane Glycoproteins

Glycoprotein	Alleles	Gene Frequency*	HPA- Determinants
Integrin subunit α_2	Glu^{505} Thr^{799}	0.92	5a
	Lys^{505} Thr^{799}	0.08	5b
	Glu^{505} **Met^{799}**	<0.01	5a; 13bW (Sit^a)
GP Ibα	Thr^{145}	0.93	2a
	Met^{145}	0.07	2b
GP Ibβ	Gly^{15}	0.998	—
	Glu^{15}	0.002	12bW (Iy^a)
Integrin subunit α_{IIb}	Val^{837}, **Ile^{843}**	0.61	3a
	Val^{837}, **Ser^{843}**	0.39	3b
	Met^{837}, Ser^{843}	0.003	3b, 9bW (Max^a)
Integrin subunit β_3	Leu^{33}, Arg^{62}, Arg^{143}, Pro^{407}, Arg^{489}, Arg^{633}, Arg^{636}	0.85	1a, 4a
	Pro^{33}, Arg^{62}, Arg^{143}, Pro^{407}, Arg^{489}, Arg^{633}, Arg^{636}	0.15	**1b**, 4a
	Leu^{33}, Arg^{62}, **Gln^{143}**, Pro^{407}, Arg^{489}, Arg^{633}, Arg^{636}	<0.001	1a, **4b**
	Leu^{33}, Arg^{62}, Arg^{143}, Pro^{407}, **Gln^{489}**, Arg^{633}, Arg^{636}	0.003	1a, 4a, **6bW**
	Leu^{33}, Arg^{62}, Arg^{143}, **Ala^{407}**, Arg^{489}, Arg^{633}, Arg^{636}	0.001	1a, 4a, **7bW**
	Leu^{33}, Arg^{62}, Arg^{143}, Pro^{407}, Arg^{489}, Arg^{633}, **Cys^{636}**	<0.001	1a, 4a, **8bW**
	Leu^{33}, **Gln^{62}**, Arg^{143}, Pro^{407}, Arg^{489}, Arg^{633}, Arg^{636}	<0.001	1a, 4a, **10bW**
	Leu^{33}, Arg^{62}, Arg^{143}, Pro^{407}, Arg^{489}, **His^{633}**, Arg^{636}	<0.001	1a, 4a, **11bW**

*Gene frequencies are for Caucasian populations.

HPA-1b allele among the Japanese (0.02) is much lower than that found in Western populations (0.15). Conversely, the gene frequency of the HPA-4b allele in Japan (0.0083) is higher than that observed in Western populations (<0.001).

PTP occurs 7 to 10 days after an immunogenic blood (platelet) transfusion (see Table 6.5). It most often affects previously nontransfused, multiparous women. As with NATP, there is an increased risk for development of PTP among

Table 6.5   Alloimmune Thrombocytopenias

Neonatal Alloimmune Thrombocytopenic Purpura (NATP)

Incidence: 1 per 3000 in a retrospective study, 1 per 2200 births in a prospective study
Maternal antibodies produced against paternal antigens on fetal platelets
Similar to erythroblastosis fetalis, except that 50% of cases occur during first pregnancy
Most frequently implicated antigens are HPA-1a and HPA-5b (United States and Europe)
In the case of responsiveness to HPA-1a, there is a high-risk association with HLA-DRB3*0101 or -DQB1*02
In the case of responsiveness to HPA-6b, there is an increased association with HLA-DRB1*1501, -DQA1*0102, or -DQB1*0602

Post-transfusion Purpura (PTP)

Almost all reported patients (>95%) have been women previously sensitized by pregnancy or transfusion
Thrombocytopenia usually occurs 1 wk after transfusion
Homozygous HPA-1b individuals account for a majority of cases (>60%)
High-risk association with HLA-DRB3*0101 or -DQB1*02
Enigmatically, the recipient's antigen-negative platelets are destroyed by autologous antibody

Table 6.6   Gene Frequencies of the Major Alloantigenic Alleles in Various World Populations

HPA-Designation	Population (Ref. Nos.)							
	Western (208–210)	Japan (211)	Amerindian (212)	Black (212)	Korea (213)	African American (213)	Finn (214)	Thai (215)
1a	0.85	0.998	>0.993	0.885	0.995		0.86	>0.998
1b	0.15	0.002	<0.007	0.115	0.005		0.14	<0.002
2a	0.93	0.835	0.058	0.852		0.82	0.91	0.917
2b	0.07	0.165	0.042	0.148		0.18	0.09	0.083
3a	0.61						0.59	0.37
3b	0.39						0.41	0.63
4a	0.998	0.989						0.991
4b	0.002	0.011						0.009
5a	0.92					0.79	0.95	0.973
5b	0.08					0.21	0.05	0.027

HLA-DR3-positive individuals, and HPA-1a is the antigen most often implicated (in Western populations).[26, 44]

The exact mechanism by which the recipient's antigen-negative platelets are cleared from the circulation in PTP is not yet fully understood. Proposed mechanisms include the following: (1) during the first phase of PTP, the recipient develops antibodies that recognize "framework" determinants (conserved protein structures surrounding the specific polymorphic sites), and these react with each of the allelic forms of the antigen; (2) recipient antibodies form immune complexes with soluble antigens from donor platelets, and these interact with autologous platelets via an Fc receptor-dependent mechanism; and (3) soluble antigen from the transfused product is adsorbed onto recipient platelets, rendering them passively positive for the antigen in question. Platelet membrane microparticles are known to be a constituent of fresh frozen plasma and platelet concentrates.[45] It is conceivable that the $\alpha_{IIb}\beta_3$ complex could become adsorbed onto neighboring platelets via this process.

HPA-1b platelets had been reported to become HPA-1a-positive when incubated with plasma from HPA-1a-positive individuals.[46–48] Although this passive transfer of soluble antigen has been proposed as a mechanism for clearance of the recipient platelets in PTP, Ehmann and colleagues[49] contend that this finding is an in vitro artifact. They provided evidence in patients with PTP for the presence of immune complexes composed of donor antigen and recipient antibody.

At this time, there is a lack of conclusive evidence to support or refute any one of the proposed mechanisms for the pathology of PTP.

Immunochemistry of Platelet Alloantigens

By convention, the designation HPA has been assigned to alloantigen systems in which the precise polymorphism that accounts for the serologic difference between alleles has been identified. Five diallelic systems (HPA-1 through -5) are well established (see Table 6.3), and eight low-frequency antigens (HPA-6bW through -13bW) are now recognized. Three additional low-frequency antigens remain to be precisely localized. Of the sixteen, nine are expressed by the integrin β_3 subunit (HPA-1, -4, -6bW, -7bW, -8bW, -10bW, and -11bW, plus Oe^a and Va^a); two are localized on the integrin α_{IIb} subunit (HPA-3 and -9bW); two are found on the integrin α_2 subunit (HPA-5 and -13bW); two are expressed by the GPIbα (HPA-2 and Pe^a); and one is expressed by GPIbβ (HPA-12bW).

HPA-1. The HPA-1 alloantigen system is defined by the Leu33/Pro33 polymorphism, which, according to the disulfide bonding scheme proposed by Calvete and associates,[33] is enclosed within a small, 13-amino-acid loop formed by the pairing of Cys26 with Cys38. This region of the molecule is held proximal to the distal cysteine-rich region in the middle of β_3 by a long-range disulfide bond linking Cys5 and Cys435.[50] The importance of the three-dimensional structure imposed by the Cys26–Cys38 disulfide bond constraint to expression of the HPA-1 determinants is evidenced by the fact that linear peptides corresponding to the $\beta_3(26-38)$ sequence are not antigenic.[51] Moreover, in this structure, the antigens are not lost after denaturation of β_3 in ionic detergents, but they are immediately destroyed on subsequent disulfide bond reduction. The complex structure of the β_3 molecule and the sensitivity of the determinants to this structure is the likely explanation for the observed heterogeneity in binding properties of anti-HPA-1a alloantibodies.[52, 53] Although all alloantibodies bind to the denatured molecule or to recombinant amino-terminal segments of the molecule expressed in *Escherichia coli*,[54, 55] a subset of antibodies appear to require presentation of the antigenic loop within a more native environment (e.g., the nondenatured molecule).[52, 53]

Anti-HPA-1a antibodies inhibit clot retraction and also inhibit platelet aggregation, presumably because they block the binding of fibrinogen.[56, 57] Ryu and colleagues[58] reported that there is a dose-dependent stimulation versus inhibition of fibrinogen binding induced by anti-HPA-1a. A similar effect has been attributed to other platelet inhibitors, particularly the disintegrins, arginine-glycine-aspartate (RGD) peptides, and certain snake venoms.[59]

Genetic differences in $\alpha_{IIb}\beta_3$ may influence the development of arterial thromboses, because this integrin plays such a critical role in platelet thrombus formation. When comparing Chinese hamster ovary and human kidney embryonal 293 cells transfected with either the HPA-1a or HPA-1b forms of the β_3 subunit together with an identical α_{IIb} subunit, Vijayan and coworkers[60] observed no difference in soluble fibrinogen binding or adhesion to immobilized fibronectin. However, significantly more HPA-1b cells adhered to immobilized fibrinogen in an $\alpha_{IIb}\beta_3$-dependent manner. Because of this and additional observations, it was concluded that the HPA-1b polymorphism alters integrin-mediated functions of adhesion, spreading, actin cytoskeleton rearrangement, and clot retraction.

HPA-2. Two previously described polymorphisms of the Ib-IX-V complex, termed Ko and Sib, are now known to be reflections of two linked polymorphisms, one of which defines the diallelic system, HPA-2.[61-65] In the GPIbα sequence, a Thr/Met polymorphism at residue 145 is associated with HPA-2a and HPA-2b epitopes, respectively (see Fig. 6.3).

HPA-3. The HPA-3 system is associated with an Ile843/Ser843 polymorphism of α_{IIb} (Fig. 6.4).[66] In addition,

Take and associates[67] reported that the binding of certain anti-HPA-3a antisera to α_{IIb} is decreased after desialation of α_{IIb}, raising the possibility that glycosylation of α_{IIb} may contribute to or influence the expression of the HPA-3 epitopes. Moreover, anti-HPA-3 alloantibodies do not bind to the precursor form of the α_{IIb} molecule, pro-α_{IIb}.[66] Therefore, O-glycosylation at the polymorphic Ser843 may influence specificity or accessibility of HPA-3 determinants.

At this time, there has not yet appeared any report concerning the effect of antibodies specific for HPA-3a antigens on fibrinogen binding, platelet aggregation, or clot retraction. Because the α_{IIb} molecule is expressed only on platelets, megakaryocytes, and cells with a megakaryocyte lineage, the HPA-3 epitopes are not found on other cells types, as noted previously.

HPA-4. Another diallelic human alloantigen system, known as Pen (or Yuk), is found on β_3 and is associated with an Arg185/Gln186 polymorphism.[57, 68-70] Given the proximity of the Pen polymorphism to the RGD binding domain (residues 109–171) of β_3, it is not surprising that anti-HPA-4a antibodies completely inhibit aggregation of HPA-4a homozygous platelets.[57]

Other cells that express β_3 as the β subunit of the vitronectin receptor, including endothelial cells, fibroblasts, and smooth muscle cells, also express HPA-1 and HPA-4 epitopes.[71-74] This could contribute to the complexity of the clinical symptoms in alloimmune-mediated thrombocytopenia. At this time, little is known about the involvement of tissues other than platelets in these conditions.

HPA-5. The HPA-5 system is located on the integrin subunit α_2 (see Fig. 6.2).[75, 76] The detection of this system was facilitated by the development of a highly sensitive murine monoclonal antibody–based monoclonal antibody immobilization of platelet antigen (MAIPA) assay.[77] Like the preceding alloantigenic systems, the HPA-5 system is diallelic. Roughly 200 to 2000 copies of α_2 are present on the surface of normal platelets, and each α_2 molecule expresses a single HPA-5 epitope.[75] The integrin α_2 is distributed on a wide variety of cells, but nothing is currently known about the antigenicity of the HPA-5 determinants on receptors expressed by cell types other than platelets.

HPA-6bW. This alloantigen, originally known as Ca^a or Tu^a, is defined by β_3 Gln489 resulting from the substitution of alanine at base pair 1564 (A$_{1564}$).[78-80]

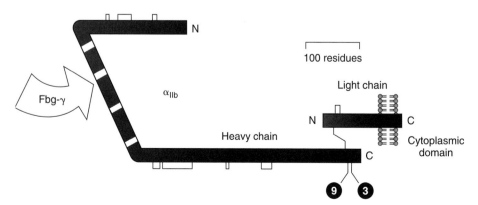

Figure 6.4 Schematic diagram of the α_{IIb} subunit. This subunit is composed of two chains linked by a single interchain disulfide bond. The light chain is a transmembrane molecule. The open areas represent four putative divalent cation (calcium)-binding repeats, and the location of the binding site for the fibrinogen γ-chain carboxy dodecapeptide (Fbg-γ) is indicated by a large arrow. The positions of the HPA-3 and the HPA-9bW polymorphisms are indicated. C, carboxyl terminal; N, amino terminal.

HPA-7bW and HPA-8bW. Two novel alloantigens have been localized to β_3.[81, 82] The alloantigen HPA-8bW is classified as a private alloantigen because it appears to be inherited within a single family or family group but is not expressed by the general population. The unique feature of the HPA-8bW polymorphism is that it is associated with an Arg636Cys substitution and thereby results in an additional unpaired cysteine residue.[81] Since the initial characterization of this alloantigen, it has been accepted that all cysteine residues in β_3 are involved in disulfide bridges. Despite the addition of this new sulfhydryl group, the HPA-8bW-positive β_3 subunit still associates with α_{IIb} and contributes to an expressed $\alpha_{IIb}\beta_3$ complex without apparent impairment of function. The alloantigen HPA-7bW is produced by a cytosine-to-guanine substitution at base pair 1317 of β_3, which results in replacement of Pro407 by Ala407.[82] HPA-7bW is a very low-frequency alloantigen and has been detected in only 1 of 450 random donors outside of the family of the initial patient.

HPA-9bW. Originally named Max^a, HPA-9bW is the second determinant to be localized to the integrin α_{IIb} subunit. It is defined by the Met837 replacement.[83]

HPA-10bW. Initially named La^a, the HPA-10bW determinant is defined by the β_3 Gln62 substitution.[84]

HPA-11bW. The private antigen HPA-11bW (Gro^a) is defined by the β_3 substitution His633 (A$_{1996}$).[85]

HPA-12bW. Initially designated Ly^a, the HPA-12bW determinant is found in 1 of 249 unrelated German donors and is defined by the GPIbβ substitution Glu15 (A$_{141}$).[24]

HPA-13bW. The substitution Met799 (T$_{2531}$) in integrin subunit α_2 creates the alloantigenic HPA-13bW determinant, originally known as Sit^a.[24]

Gov. The alloantigenic polymorphism, Gov, is uniquely expressed by a different protein receptor. Kelton and associates[86] initially described the Gov system, which is now known to be carried by the 175-kD glycosyl phosphatidyl-inositol-anchored glycoprotein CD109. Alloantibodies defining each of two alleles (Gov^a and Gov^b) were detected in two patients who had received multiple platelet transfusions[86] and, more recently, in three patients who had developed NATP.[87] The genotypic frequencies in the Canadian population are 81% for Gov^a and 75% for Gov^b.

Additional Suspected Alloantigens. Four additional alloantigens have been serologically defined (see Table 6.3), but their precise polymorphic residues or structures have not yet been identified. Two of these alloantigens, the low-frequency antigens Oe^a and Va^a,[88, 89] are associated with the integrin β_3 subunit. Another, Pe^a, is localized to GPIbα.[90] The last, known as Pl^T, was implicated in a single case of NATP and was localized to GPV by immunoblot assay.[91]

■ Isoantibodies

Isoantibodies are produced against an epitope that is expressed by all normal individuals and is not polymorphic. In the area of human platelet immunology, a classic example of isoimmunization occurs when a patient with an inherited deficiency of a membrane glycoprotein is subjected to multiple platelet transfusions in order to correct a bleeding diathesis. GT and Bernard-Soulier syndrome are such inherited disorders, wherein the individual either lacks or expresses an altered form of $\alpha_{IIb}\beta_3$ (GT) or Ib-IX-V (Bernard-Soulier syndrome). Isoantibodies developed by transfused patients do not distinguish any of the allelic forms of the glycoproteins (such as HPA-3 or HPA-1 alloantigens on $\alpha_{IIb}\beta_3$) but react with the platelets of all normal persons tested. Because the immunized individual does not express the platelet glycoprotein that carries the epitope in question, these antibodies do not bind to their own platelets.

Isoantibodies in Glanzmann Thrombasthenia

Several cases have been documented in which patients with GT have produced antibodies specific for α_{IIb}, β_3, or the $\alpha_{IIb}\beta_3$ complex.[92–96] Our research group has defined an idiotype (OG) that is associated at high frequency with isoantibodies specific for the integrin subunit β_3 that are generated by GT patients.[94, 97–99] Rabbit polyclonal anti-OG idiotype was shown to bind to immunoglobulin G (IgG) specific for $\alpha_{IIb}\beta_3$ obtained from 11 nonrelated GT patients, including an unrelated patient "ES" studied by Coller and colleagues,[93] all of whom had developed isoantibodies of very similar specificity. On the other hand, anti-OG did not recognize $\alpha_{IIb}\beta_3$-specific antibodies produced by other unrelated GT patients, whose isoantibodies had specificities distinct from that of the OG isoantibody. Moreover, anti-OG did not recognize $\alpha_{IIb}\beta_3$-specific antibodies developed by any patients with idiopathic thrombocytopenic purpura (ITP) or by six representative patients with alloimmune thrombocytopenias; in addition, anti-OG never bound to IgG from nonimmunized control individuals.

Anti-OG binds to selected protein ligands of $\alpha_{IIb}\beta_3$, namely fibrinogen, vitronectin, and vWF, but not to other known protein ligands such as fibronectin or type I collagen. The epitopes recognized by anti-OG on these three adhesive proteins are either very similar or identical, because each protein can inhibit the binding of anti-OG to any of the others. The epitope on fibrinogen is recognized by anti-OG resides in the Bβ chain and is probably contained within the first 42 amino acids from the amino terminal.[100] Because OG IgG inhibits fibrinogen binding to $\alpha_{IIb}\beta_3$, the specificity of the OG idiotype defines a novel binding motif for the integrin $\alpha_{IIb}\beta_3$ that is shared by fibrinogen, vitronectin, and vWF but is distinct from previously described RGD-containing sites on the fibrinogen Aα chain or the fibrinogen γ chain carboxyl-terminal decapeptide site. Moskowitz and coworkers[100] employed specific proteolytic forms of fibrinogen to confirm that the epitope recognized by anti-OG 2 is located within Bβ 1 through 42. This represents an excellent example of molecular mimicry, in which an antigen-selected, IgG inhibitor of $\alpha_{IIb}\beta_3$ function shares a novel recognition sequence common to three physiologic protein ligands of that receptor.

Isoantibodies in Bernard-Soulier Syndrome

Because Bernard-Soulier syndrome is less frequently encountered than GT, it follows that isoantibodies produced in conjunction with this syndrome are also less frequently encountered. In the only clearcut case of such an isoantibody,[101] the isolated IgG impaired both normal platelet adhesion to subendothelial elements and in vitro aggregation in response to ristocetin and bovine factor VIII.

■ Autoantigens

Autoimmune (or idiopathic) thrombocytopenia (AITP or ITP) is the most frequently encountered form of immune thrombocytopenia.[102, 103] This disorder can be classified as acute or chronic on the basis of the duration of the thrombocytopenia, the chronic form persisting longer than 6 to 12 months. The acute, self-limited form occurs predominantly in children, often after a viral illness or immunization, and affects boys and girls with equal frequency. The chronic form is mainly an adult illness and affects twice as many women as men. Life-threatening bleeding occurs in up to 1% of patients with ITP. The reason that some patients sustain severe hemorrhagic complications and others do not remains unexplained, but because of differences in the clinical expression of chronic and acute ITP it has been theorized that the mechanisms of disease for each form are different.

Recent data suggest that cytokine dysregulation may lead to autoimmune thrombocytopenia, although the true etiology of AITP remains unknown.

Glycoproteins as Autoantigens

The integrin $\alpha_{IIb}\beta_3$ was the first platelet membrane component to be identified as a dominant antigen in patients with chronic ITP,[104] and subsequent studies from several laboratories confirmed the important contribution of this receptor to the autoantigenic makeup of the human platelet.[77, 105–110]

Attempts to further localize autoepitopes on either integrin subunit have been more successful with regard to β_3. Early on, Kekomaki and associates[110] defined a prominent autoantigenic region as the 33-kD chymotryptic fragment of β_3 located within the cysteine-rich region of β_3 (Fig. 6.5), which was bound by both plasma autoantibodies and autoantibody eluted from patients' platelets. Fujisawa and colleagues[111–113] subsequently determined that plasma autoantibodies in 5 of 13 patients with chronic ITP bound to

peptides representing β_3 residues 721 through 744 or 742 through 762, the carboxyl-terminal region of β_3 that is presumed to be located in the cytoplasm of the platelet, whereas autoantibodies eluted from the platelets of other ITP patients bound to other areas of β_3 within the extracellular domain (perhaps identical to the 33-kD region defined by Kekomaki and associates[110]). Most importantly, they determined that certain platelet-associated autoantibodies bound preferentially to cation-dependent conformational antigens on the $\alpha_{IIb}\beta_3$ complex.[113]

More recently, additional autoantigenic epitopes have been identified on the β_3 subunit. Nardi and colleagues[114] identified the peptide β_3(49–66) as a site that is bound by a majority of affinity-purified antibodies isolated from serum immune complexes of immunologic thrombocytopenic patients infected with the human immunodeficiency virus (HIV-1). This is not a peptide that is bound by serum IgG antibodies from control subjects or from patients with the classic form of ITP. Using random peptide bacteriophage display libraries, Bowditch and associates[115] determined that plasma antibody eluates from one ITP patient bound to two distinct hexapeptides, and the binding to one of these could be inhibited by the sequence β_3(734–739).

Plasma antibody eluates from patients were used[115] to select for phage displaying autoantibody-reactive peptides; they identified anti-$\alpha_{IIb}\beta_3$ antibody-specific phage encoding the peptide sequences Arg-Glu-Lys-Ala-Lys-Trp (REKAKW) and Pro-Val-Val-Trp-Lys-Asn (PVVWKN) and the hexapeptide sequence Arg-Glu-Leu-Leu-Lys-Met. Each phage showed saturable dose-dependent binding to immobilized autoantibody, and binding could be blocked with purified $\alpha_{IIb}\beta_3$. The binding of plasma autoantibody to the phage encoding REKAKW was blocked by a synthetic peptide derived from the β_3 cytoplasmic tail; however, binding to PVVWKN was not. Using sequential overlapping peptides from the β_3 cytoplasmic region, an epitope was localized to the sequence Arg-Ala-Arg-Ala-Lys-Trp, at β_3(734–739).

Autoantibodies reactive with α_{IIb} were identified in two patients with chronic ITP,[108, 109] and in one of those patients the antibody was subsequently shown to react with a

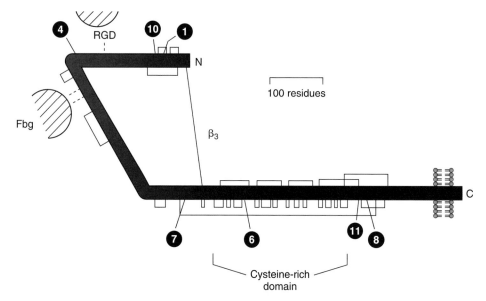

Figure 6.5 Schematic diagram of the β_3 subunit. The β_3 subunit is a single-chain, transmembrane molecule. Twenty-eight intrachain disulfide bonds are present, at least one of which is thought to bring the amino-terminal domain (N) proximal to the cysteine-rich domain at the carboxy (C) third of the molecule. The approximate positions of RGD and fibrinogen (Fbg) binding sites are indicated. The locations of the HPA-1, -4, -6bW, -7bW, -8bW, -10bW, and -11bW polymorphisms are indicated by a black circle within which is the numerical alloantigen designation.

chymotryptic, 65-kD, carboxyl-terminal fragment of the α_{IIb} heavy chain[109] (see Fig. 6.4).

Further work by this group[116] made use of a similar technique to map an autoepitope on α_{IIb}. They used a filamentous phage library that displays random peptides, 11 amino acids in length and flanked on each side by a cysteine, to identify peptide sequences recognized by an anti-platelet autoantibody that blocked fibrinogen binding to $\alpha_{IIb}\beta_3$. Phage from individual colonies, after the fourth purification, were tested for binding to the autoantibody. A phage expressing the sequence CTGRVPLGFEDLC exhibited saturable dose-dependent binding to immobilized autoantibody. This binding could be blocked by purified $\alpha_{IIb}\beta_3$ and α_{IIb} but not by β_3. The peptide amino acid sequence has partial identity with amino acids 4 through 10 and 31 through 35 on α_{IIb}. This work suggests that the autoantibody is binding on the first 35 amino acids of α_{IIb} and infers that region of α_{IIb} is critical for ligand binding.

Ethylenediaminetetraacetic acid (EDTA)-dependent autoantibodies represent a special category of autoantibodies that are adsorbed by autologous platelets when whole blood is drawn in EDTA.[117] In one case of EDTA-dependent "pseudothrombocytopenia," an IgM antibody was shown to bind to α_{IIb} by immunoblot assay and crossed immunoelectrophoresis.[118]

Finally, it should be remembered that, although most autoantibodies apparently induce thrombocytopenia, a minority can induce platelet dysfunction without an increase in platelet clearance.[119, 120] The proportion of the two types of autoantibody, that which leads to platelet clearance and that which blocks platelet function, may be a very important factor controlling the unpredictable clinical severity of ITP.

The $\alpha_{IIb}\beta_3$ integrin is not the only integrin implicated as an antigen target for human autoantibodies. Serum IgG autoantibodies specific for integrin subunit α_2 were identified in a unique case of autoimmune platelet dysfunction after myasthenia gravis.[121] This autoantibody inhibited aggregation of normal platelets induced by collagen or wheat germ agglutinin. This is the first case in which autoantibodies to GPIa were associated with a chronic hemorrhagic disorder, and this study provides strong indirect support for a role of this integrin in hemostasis in vivo.

Autoantibodies to components of the Ib-IX-V complex are also frequently encountered in adult chronic ITP.[122] He and colleagues[123] have made progress in the localization of selected autoantigenic epitopes on the GPIb molecule. Epitopes were most frequently found on a recombinant fragment of Ibα corresponding to residues 240 through 485, and next most often on a fragment representing residues 1 through 247. Among those antibodies reactive with the former sequence, further epitope mapping identified the dominant determinant as the 9-amino-acid sequence, TKEQTTFPP (residues 333 through 341).[123] In some cases in which autoantibody to Ib-IX was detected, the clinical presentation proved to be particularly severe and refractory to therapy.[124] One case of "pseudo–Bernard-Soulier syndrome" (dysfunction of the Ib-IX-V receptor complex) was reported to be caused by an autoantibody to Ib.[125] Finally, in a subset of childhood ITP, that associated with *Varicella zoster* infection, the GPV component of this receptor was found to be the dominant target of serum autoantibodies that did not crossreact with viral antigens.[126] At the same time, in another group of children with this disease, it was found that serum antibodies

specific for viral antigens can crossreact with normal platelet antigens and may thus contribute to platelet clearance.[127]

It was hoped that the antigenic targets in acute and chronic forms of ITP might be different, so that antigen identity might one day be used as an early indicator of clinical outcome. However, investigators have demonstrated that autoantibody specificity in chronic versus acute ITP is quite similar, particularly in children.[128, 129] Nonetheless, a distinction between antigen specificity and an acute versus chronic course in ITP may yet be found in the early stages of the autoimmune response. Clearly, prospective studies aimed at answering this question are still warranted.

How large is the autoepitope repertoire on a given glycoprotein antigen? The answer to this important question will affect the feasibility of developing therapeutic and diagnostic measures based on epitope specificity. Because the autoantibodies that react with a given epitope are likely to share idiotypes, one can approach this question from two angles—analyzing the epitope repertoire, analyzing the idiotype repertoire, or both. Two studies have addressed the extent of the autoantigen repertoire on $\alpha_{IIb}\beta_3$ by analyzing the competitive binding between human autoantibodies and murine monoclonal antibodies.[130, 131] However, the results were conflicting, and the data from this limited number of studies remain insufficient to judge the size of the autoepitope repertoire on $\alpha_{IIb}\beta_3$. Additional analyses aimed at epitope localization are necessary, and perhaps novel approaches will expedite this task. One such novel approach is the development of human monoclonal autoantibodies specific for $\alpha_{IIb}\beta_3$ and other platelet glycoproteins.

Human monoclonal antibodies are an alternative tool in the search for glycoprotein epitopes that are autoimmunogenic in humans. The first human monoclonal antibody against a platelet glycoprotein, developed by Nugent and colleagues,[132] was derived from an individual with ITP producing an antibody against β_3. This human monoclonal antibody detects a neoantigen associated with β_3 that is expressed only on stored or thrombin-activated platelets. A number of human monoclonal autoantibodies specific for the heavy chain of GPIb were generated from the lymphocytes of an ITP patient with serum autoantibody specific for Ib.[133] The heavy chain variable-region genes of four of these antibodies were sequenced and were found to be markedly homologous to human immunoglobulin, germ-line, heavy chain variable-region genes.[133] Most recently, another human monoclonal autoantibody was produced that is specific for the heavy chain of α_{IIb}.[134] The epitope recognized by this antibody (2E7) was identified as a contiguous amino acid sequence at residues 231 to 238 with an immunodominant tryptophan residue at position 235 (see Fig. 6.4).[135] This is the first time that the precise epitope on α_{IIb} or β_3 recognized by a human antibody has been identified.

From the foregoing analysis, it is clear that further studies are required to determine the extent to which the production of human autoantibodies to platelet glycoproteins is clonally restricted. Given a selected number of idiotypes related to autoimmunity to $\alpha_{IIb}\beta_3$, one could potentially use the anti-idiotype to modulate immunization to $\alpha_{IIb}\beta_3$. Along these lines, it has been reported that intravenous immunoglobulin (IVIG), which is routinely used to reverse acute thrombocytopenia in ITP, may contain anti-idiotype directed to idiotypes of autoantibody but not alloantibodies that recognize $\alpha_{IIb}\beta_3$.[136]

Nugent[124] defined a DM idiotype that is characteristic of human autoantibodies that are specific for the Ib heavy chain. This latter study clearly suggests that the repertoire of idiotypes expressed by human autoantibodies specific for membrane glycoproteins, such as those of the human platelet, will be narrowly defined and, therefore, amenable to study.

Glycolipids as Antigens

A number of reports have implicated cardiolipin, lactosyl ceramide, and other glycosphingolipids (GSLs) as autoantigenic targets[137–143] (see Table 6.2). van Vliet and colleagues[141] analyzed the binding of serum IgG/IgM antibodies from 30 ITP patients to platelet GSLs separated by high-performance thin-layer chromatography. Acidic GSLs, namely sulfatides and gangliosides, were identified as the major targets of serum autoantibodies. Thirteen of the 30 sera, including 5 with anti-cardiolipin antibodies, had antibodies that bound to sulfatides, whereas 4 sera showed antibody binding to gangliosides. Koerner and associates[137] employed a more efficient phase partition separation of acidic GSLs from neutral GSLs and were able to demonstrate that serum antibodies specific for neutral GSLs were more characteristic of ITP. Two classes of GSL autoantigens were defined: those associated with general autoimmunity, which were detected in the sera of patients with either systemic lupus erythematosus (SLE) or ITP, and those peculiar to platelet-specific autoimmunity, which were detected only in the sera of ITP patients. Two GSL forms belong to the platelet-specific group, but they are present in minute amounts, and further characterization awaits large-scale purification. Fifty percent (6/12) of patients with ITP had serum IgG or IgM antibodies that bound these platelet-specific GSLs. Sera from none of 10 patients with nonimmune thrombocytopenia, none of 10 patients with SLE, and only 1 of 18 normal subjects gave positive reactions with the platelet-specific GSL group. The general GSL antigen group includes globotriaosyl ceramide, globotetraosyl ceramide, and a third unidentified neutral GSL. Antigens in the general group were bound by IgG or IgM antibodies in the sera of 10 of 10 patients with SLE, 8 of 12 patients with ITP, none of 10 patients with nonimmune thrombocytopenia, and none of 18 control subjects. These findings provide compelling support for a role of neutral GSLs as antigenic targets in selected cases of ITP.

Animal Models of Idiopathic Thrombocytopenic Purpura

Many investigators have searched in animals for clinical correlates of human ITP. These attempts have been largely unsuccessful, but an exception may have evolved from concerted studies in dogs. As pointed out in a series of reports by Lewis and Meyers,[144] there is now substantial evidence that ITP in dogs and ITP in humans are clinically analogous syndromes. In 32 cases of canine ITP, increased platelet-bound IgG was detected in a majority of the animals,[30] and immunoglobulin eluted from the platelets of 11 of 19 affected dogs bound to homologous normal canine platelets.[144] Furthermore, immunoglobulin specific for integrin subunits α_{IIb} or β_3, or both, was detected in sera of 4 of 17 dogs tested. The authors concluded that, in canine ITP, immunoglobulin bound to the surface of platelets is directed against host antigens, and the target antigen is frequently $\alpha_{IIb}\beta_3$. Given the similarities between these findings and the cumulative experience with human ITP, the canine model may prove to be

a valuable tool to further understanding of the pathogenesis of the autoimmune response to platelet antigens.

Immunoregulatory Dysfunction

It is likely that immunomodulatory therapy will be feasible in autoimmune-mediated thrombocytopenia because of the excellent response of AITP to the intravenous infusion of high-dose immunoglobulin and the demonstration of anti-idiotype antibodies in these preparations.[136, 145] It is generally agreed that Fc blockade plays a major role in the success of IVIG infusions, given that a rise in platelet count is obtained in most patients regardless of age or etiology of the autoantibody. There is also increasing evidence that treatment alters T-cell subsets and may produce alterations in cytokine production.[146] Several reports of cytokine response to therapy have appeared, but there is a lack of evidence documenting in vivo changes in cytokine messenger RNA expression or serum cytokine levels. Because many of these immunoregulatory effects may take place in the microenvironment of the spleen or bone marrow, the reported in vitro changes in circulating cell subsets or cytokine production should be interpreted with optimistic caution.

T-Lymphocyte and Cytokine Studies in AITP

Many investigators have examined defects involving T cells or an abnormal dominance of one of the T-helper subsets, Th1 or Th2, and their associated cytokines in autoimmune disease. As yet, no clear T-cell pattern has been established in AITP, nor is there any published information on the presence or absence of Th3 subsets in AITP. Perhaps this reflects the heterogeneous nature of AITP and suggests that the T-cell dysregulation may evolve in different directions depending on the age or gender of the patient and the nature of the underlying environmental or viral triggers.

Given the importance of the T-cell receptor (TCR) in other autoimmune diseases, it is not surprising that initial studies by Ware and coworkers[147, 148] focused on utilization of TCR-$\gamma\delta$. In 11 children with acute ITP and 19 children with chronic ITP, they observed increased numbers of TCR-$\gamma\delta$-positive T lymphocytes. In those patients with the highest elevations (TCR-$\gamma\delta$+/CD3+ percentage ranging from 37.8% to 48.1% at initial evaluation), the expanded cell population exclusively expressed the surface $V_\delta2/V_\gamma9$ heterodimer. Analysis of the nucleotide sequences used by these TCR-$\gamma\delta$+ cells demonstrated a diverse set of VDJC gene segment rearrangements, suggesting a superantigen response. There was a close correlation between the number of TCR-$\gamma\delta$+ cells and the degree of thrombocytopenia in each patient, but no specific platelet-reactive T-cell clones were isolated from that group. Eight T-cell clones were isolated that showed in vitro proliferation against allogeneic platelets from two children with chronic ITP and elevated numbers of $V_\beta8+T$ cells.[148] Four of seven positive clones also exhibited measurable interleukin-2 (IL-2) secretion after platelet stimulation, providing further evidence for T-cell reactivity. These results provided the first evidence that patients with ITP may have platelet-reactive T lymphocytes identifiable at the clonal level, supporting the hypothesis that autoreactive peripheral T lymphocytes in AITP may mediate or participate in the pathogenesis of this disorder.

Using the common AITP target antigen $\alpha_{IIb}\beta_3$, Kuwana and associates[149] extended these T-cell studies to examine in vitro production of antibody to this platelet glycoprotein by peripheral blood mononuclear cells (PBMCs). T-cell proliferative responses to platelet membrane $\alpha_{IIb}\beta_3$ were examined in 14 patients with chronic ITP, 7 patients with SLE with or without thrombocytopenia, and 10 healthy donors. Although peripheral blood T cells from all subjects failed to respond to the protein complex in its native state, chemically reduced $\alpha_{IIb}\beta_3$ stimulated T cells from three ITP patients and one SLE patient with thrombocytopenia, and tryptic peptides of $\alpha_{IIb}\beta_3$ stimulated T cells from almost all subjects. Characterization of the T-cell response induced by modified $\alpha_{IIb}\beta_3$ showed that the response was restricted by HLA-DR. Responsive T cells had a CD4+ phenotype, and the proliferation was accelerated only in ITP patients, suggesting in vivo activation of these T cells. IgG anti-$\alpha_{IIb}\beta_3$ synthesis by PBMCs in culture could be induced using modified $\alpha_{IIb}\beta_3$ as antigen, but only with PBMCs from ITP patients who had already demonstrated platelet-associated anti-$\alpha_{IIb}\beta_3$ antibody. Anti-$\alpha_{IIb}\beta_3$ antibody produced in these media was absorbed by normal platelets. None of the PBMC cultures from healthy donors contained significant amounts of IgG anti-$\alpha_{IIb}\beta_3$ antibody, but *all* of them showed T-cell proliferation in response to trypsin-digested $\alpha_{IIb}\beta_3$. The authors concluded that CD4+ and HLA-DR–restricted T cells reactive to $\alpha_{IIb}\beta_3$ are involved in the production of anti-platelet autoantibody in ITP patients and are involved in the pathogenesis of chronic ITP.

Comparable T-cell proliferation by healthy donors in response to $\alpha_{IIb}\beta_3$ had been described 2 years before Kuwana's experiments by Filion and colleagues.[150] Their study documented the presence of autoreactive T cells specific for $\alpha_{IIb}\beta_3$ in the periphery of healthy individuals (N = 25). Using an in vitro T-cell proliferation assay, they showed that activation of these specific $\alpha_{IIb}\beta_3$-autoreactive TCR-$\alpha\beta$+ CD4+ CD8– T cells required internalization and processing of the $\alpha_{IIb}\beta_3$ by antigen-presenting cells and its presentation by HLA-DR class II molecules in the presence of exogenous IL-2. This implies that certain autoreactive T cells that respond to platelet membrane antigens are not necessarily eliminated through intrathymic deletion. The persistence of platelet-reactive T cells in the periphery of healthy individuals suggests that there must be a tightly regulated cellular network to keep these autoreactive T-cell clones in check.

Regulatory cells are also involved in the immunoglobulin idiotypic network to limit the expansion of pathologic forms of anti-platelet antibody. Pooled immunoglobulin (IVIG) from healthy donors contains antibodies reactive with idiotypes expressed by natural autoantibodies, disease-related autoantibodies, or B-cell surface immunoglobulins. IVIG also contains antibodies reactive with the idiotype, framework, and constant regions of the β chain of the TCR. Therefore, it is not surprising that infusion of IVIG modulates synthesis and release of cytokines. Kazatchkine and associates[151, 152] proposed that the immunoregulatory effect of IVIG in autoimmune disease depends on the selection of the recipient's immune repertoires by the variable-region (V_H or V_L) specificities of the infused immunoglobulins. Mehta and Badakere[153] observed that immunoglobulins (IVIG or anti-D immunoglobulin preparations) or their Fab fragments inhibited the binding of anti-platelet autoantibodies to normal platelets, whereas Fc regions derived from them were ineffective. The fact that IVIG is rich in these regulatory elements

suggests that normal individuals employ these repertoires to maintain self-tolerance and suppress autoreactive T- or B-cell activity.

Antiplatelet autoantibodies are frequently associated with collagen vascular disease (e.g., SLE, thyroiditis, Evan syndrome, primary biliary cirrhosis). They are also manifested in states of congenital or acquired immune dysfunction, including common variable dysgammaglobulinemia, DiGeorge syndrome, autoimmune lymphoproliferative syndrome, pregnancy, and infection by HIV or Epstein-Barr virus. To address the reasons why platelet antigens are such common targets for autoreactive antibodies, researchers are beginning to examine the role of the platelet itself in the triggering of AITP. It is now clear that the activated platelet shares many of the costimulatory receptors commonly found on lymphocytes (CD40L, CD80) and monocytes (CD14).[154, 155] In an activated state, the platelet itself might substitute for the accessory cells that trigger autoantibody production, temporarily bypassing the tightly regulated T- and B-cell idiotypic network. Semple and colleagues[154] found that a significant proportion of children with acute (80%), chronic (71%), or chronic-complex (55%) AITP had circulating platelets that expressed HLA-DR, in contrast to normal controls and patients with nonimmune thrombocytopenia. HLA-DR was variably coexpressed on distinct smaller- and larger-sized platelet populations with CD41, CD45, CD14, CD80, and/or glycophorin molecules. In normal healthy individuals, platelets express only MHC class I molecules. The authors hypothesized that HLA-DR expression on these young platelets may play a role in the triggering or perpetuation of AITP.

In the pediatric age group, patients appear to have a Th1 type of cytokine response, with very low IL-4 and IL-6 and increased levels of IL-2, interferon-γ, and tumor necrosis factor-β (TNF-β).[156, 157] Adult chronic AITP, immune thrombocytopenia associated with malignancy, and the autoimmunity/lymphoproliferation syndrome with defects in the Fas apoptosis pathway are characterized by increased levels of IL-10, -11, -6, and -13.[157–161] Studies by Zimmerman and associates[162] and by Bussel and colleagues[163] compared changes in T-cell subsets and cytokine production in response to IVIG versus WinRho (anti-D). Zimmerman's group found that IVIG and dexamethasone induced an alteration of T-lymphocyte subsets and suppression of in vitro T-lymphocyte proliferation.[162] Although it was equally effective in the treatment of AITP in children, they found that anti-D caused significantly less inhibition than did IVIG or dexamethasone. Anti-D did not affect T-lymphocyte subsets (including the TCR variable β repertoire); in vitro T-lymphocyte proliferation to mitogens, recall antigens, or IL-2; in vitro IgG synthesis induced by pokeweed mitogen; or T-lymphocyte cytokine messenger RNA levels.

Bussel and coworkers[163] compared the changes in cytokine levels after treatment with IVIG and anti-D in thrombocytopenic adults without HIV infection. Patients were treated with either IVIG or anti-D. IL-6, IL-10, monocyte chemoattractant protein-1 (MCP-1), and TNF-α were measured in duplicate on each sample using an enzyme immunosorbent assay (ELISA) technique. Compared with baseline levels, there was an increase in three of four cytokines 2 hours after administration of anti-D, with MCP-1 reaching the highest levels; only TNF-α failed to change significantly from baseline. After IVIG administration, there was a significant increase in IL-10 at 4 hours and in MCP-1 at 1 day after therapy; no changes were seen in IL-6 or TNF-α. The authors hypothesized that the early increase in these macrophage-synthesized cytokines with anti-D demonstrates the substantial interaction of antibody-coated red blood cells with macrophages. The differences compared with IVIG treatment presumably occur because anti-D creates a large model immune complex of hundreds of antibodies on each red blood cell. Both IVIG and anti-D result in decreased splenic clearance of antibody-coated platelets, but each has additional effects that may be tailored to the AITP population. Immune therapy that may disrupt the pathologic production of autoantibody has also been initiated using humanized monoclonal antibodies to CD40L or other accessory molecules.[164, 165] Early results in adult patients with refractory AITP appear promising but remain to be substantiated in large-scale clinical studies.

Drug-Induced Immune Thrombocytopenia

Antibody-mediated thrombocytopenia can result from the administration of many and diverse drugs. A number of different mechanisms may be responsible for the pathogenesis of this family of thrombocytopenic disorders, and Aster has classified five types.[166] First, certain drugs, acting as haptens, may bind covalently to platelet membrane glycoproteins in vivo and stimulate the production of drug (hapten)-dependent antibodies that bind to the drug-membrane protein targets. Second, drugs such as quinidine, quinine, and sulfonamide antibiotics may induce the production of antibodies that bind to membrane glycoproteins only when the drug (or one of its metabolites) is present. Third, certain drugs may trigger the production of true autoantibodies capable of binding to cell-membrane glycoproteins in the absence of drug. Fourth, antibodies may be induced that react with drug–protein complexes. An example is heparin-induced immune thrombocytopenia (HIT), in which the primary pathogenetic mechanism results from antibodies specific for heparin–platelet factor 4 (PF4) complexes. In HIT, the exact mechanisms by which these complexes cause platelet destruction and, in some patients, thrombosis remain to be determined. Fifth, thrombocytopenia in patients treated with inhibitors of the platelet fibrinogen receptor $\alpha_{IIb}\beta_3$ (ligand mimetics) may result from antibodies specific for ligand-induced binding sites (LIBS) induced by the binding of these mimetics to the receptor.

Quinine/Quinidine Purpura

Although drug-induced thrombocytopenia (DITP) may be a complication of therapy involving a variety of drugs, it is most frequently seen in the United States with the administration of quinine or quinidine.[167] It has been proposed that the following criteria must be met before an individual can be considered to have DITP: (1) the patient is not thrombocytopenic before administration of the drug; (2) thrombocytopenia occurs after drug ingestion and begins to reverse shortly after cessation of drug; (3) thrombocytopenia does not recur after cessation of drug treatment; and (4) all other causes of thrombocytopenia are ruled out.[168]

The exact mechanism for platelet clearance is not yet certain. However, cumulative evidence now favors a mechanism whereby the drug induces the expression of a neoantigen on the platelet surface[169–174] that is recognized by circulating

antibodies only in the presence of the drug. The observation that platelets from patients with Bernard-Soulier syndrome (who lack Ib-IX-V) failed to lyse in the presence of drug-dependent antibody, specific drug, and complement, was the first indication that a specific platelet antigen is recognized by such antibodies.[174] This finding led other laboratories to confirm that purified Ib-IX competes for drug plus antibody and is therefore likely to contain the antigenic epitope in question. Evidence of direct binding of such antibodies to Ib-IX was first provided by Chong and associates,[172] and Berndt and colleagues[171] established that the complex of both Ib and IX is probably required for maximum antigen expression. Integrin $\alpha_{IIb}\beta_3$ is also a dominant target for many quinine- and quinidine-dependent antibodies.[175, 176] Continued study of the drug-dependent autoimmune phenomena and their relation to platelets is warranted, with particular attention to a comparison of the clinical significance of drug-dependent autoantibodies that bind to either Ib-IX or $\alpha_{IIb}\beta_3$.

Chong and associates[176] used a panel of murine monoclonal antibodies in competitive binding assays to map the domains on Ib-IX-V that were bound by drug-dependent antibodies from 12 patients with DITP. The combined data showed that one quinine-dependent antibody binds to an epitope on the amino-terminal portion of Ibα, and five other quinine-dependent antibodies recognize a complex-specific epitope proximal to the membrane-associated region of Ib-IX. Each of six quinidine-dependent antibodies contained two specificities, one for the same Ib-IX complex epitope described previously, and the other for IX alone. Additional observations were that antibodies reactive with Ib-IX were more predominant (12/12 patients) than those binding $\alpha_{IIb}\beta_3$ (3/12 patients), and that antibodies specific for Ib-IX-V were present in titers 8- to 32-fold higher than the corresponding $\alpha_{IIb}\beta_3$-binding antibodies in the same patient samples. In each case, the antibodies that bound to Ib-IX-V were distinct from those that recognized $\alpha_{IIb}\beta_3$. The specificity of quinine- and quinidine-dependent antibodies for a conformation-sensitive epitope or epitopes on the GPIX component of the complex was confirmed by Lopez and coworkers[177] using monoclonal antibody inhibition assays.

Regions of $\alpha_{IIb}\beta_3$ that bind to quinine- or quinidine-dependent antibodies were further localized by Visentin and associates.[178] Of 13 patient sera containing such antibodies, 10 were reactive with both Ib-IX and $\alpha_{IIb}\beta_3$, 2 reacted with Ib-IX alone, and 1 reacted with $\alpha_{IIb}\beta_3$ alone. Again, in those sera in which both specificities were identified, the anti-Ib-IX-V antibodies were distinct from those that bound to $\alpha_{IIb}\beta_3$. Seven sera containing anti-$\alpha_{IIb}\beta_3$ antibodies were further characterized: three bound only to the $\alpha_{IIb}\beta_3$ complex, one bound to α_{IIb} alone, and three bound to β_3 alone. Those that recognized β_3 alone were found to bind to epitopes on the major 61-kD chymotryptic fragment of β_3 that are resistant to deglycosylation with endo-H. In the case of sulfonamide-induced immune thrombocytopenia,[179] the causative antibodies are almost exclusively specific for calcium-dependent (complex-specific) epitopes on the integrin $\alpha_{IIb}\beta_3$.

One additional intriguing aspect of certain cases of DITP is worthy of mention, because it may have an important bearing on the general understanding of the autoimmune response to platelets. Based on anecdotal evidence, it has been suspected that some cases of chronic ITP[122] are initiated in clinical situations that, from all appearances, could be classified as DITP. The only difference is that selected autoantibodies persist long after exposure to the insulting drug. Direct evidence to support of this contention was obtained by Nieminen and Kekomaki.[180] They found that those DITP patients with Ib-IX-specific antibodies, despite a very intense and acute thrombocytopenia, recovered promptly after drug removal. On the other hand, DITP patients with more prolonged thrombocytopenia and persistently elevated platelet immunoglobulin (>1 month after drug removal) had antibodies that reacted with additional target antigens, including integrin $\alpha_{IIb}\beta_3$. To better understand the pathogenesis of both DITP and classic ITP, it may become important in the future to distinguish between the acute but readily reversible clinical situation that we accept as DITP and the more complex disease situation that is initiated by drug exposure and evolves into a more classic form of ITP.

Heparin-Induced Immune Thrombocytopenia

HIT is a life-threatening condition that results in thrombocytopenia and can be associated with thrombosis.[181–184] In contrast to quinine- or quinidine-dependent antibodies, the actual binding of heparin-dependent antibodies (HDA) to the platelet surface appears to be of very low affinity.[181] It has also been determined that HDAs differ from other forms of drug-dependent antibodies in that they can often be *activating*, causing not only thrombocytopenia but also heparin-dependent platelet aggregation, thromboxane synthesis, and granule release that can be quantitated by preloading the platelets with [14C] serotonin. The effects of HIT, therefore, are exacerbated by serious thrombotic complications. Approximately 30% of these patients die, and an additional 20% develop vascular occlusions that result in gangrene and subsequent amputation.[185]

Although the precise mechanism of HDA binding to platelets eluded investigators for many years, it was generally accepted that the activating properties of HDAs must be mediated by Fc-dependent binding to platelets. In this regard, Kelton and colleagues[182] showed that the platelet release reaction induced by HDAs could be blocked by pretreatment of the platelets with human or goat IgG Fc fragments. Adelman and associates[186] showed that the Fab regions of HDA alone are not sufficient to cause platelet activation. Chong and associates[187] showed that purified rabbit IgG and its Fc, but not Fab, fragments markedly inhibit platelet aggregation induced by HDAs, and a number of groups observed that the monoclonal anti-Fc receptor antibody, IV.3, can block platelet activation by HDAs.[182, 188]

Subsequent findings from several study groups have led to the consensus that the dominant pathologic factor in HIT is circulating antibody specific for a complex of heparin and PF4, a basic chemokine that is normally stored in a releasable protein pool within the platelet α-granules.[189–193] It is now accepted that heparin-PF4 complexes, which are detected in 85% of patients with HIT,[194] can bind to the membrane of platelets[190, 195, 196] or endothelial cells.[190] In those cases in which the HDAs are IgG, the Fc portion can crosslink to the platelet FcγRIIA receptor, inducing platelet activation, release, aggregation, and thrombosis.[190, 192, 193, 197] However, HIT can also be associated with antibodies of IgM and IgA isotypes,[198] in which case the FcμR of lymphocytes or the FcαR of monocytes and neutrophils, as well as complement activation, may play a role in the pathology of this disorder.

It is now generally accepted that one of the major stimuli for the thrombosis associated with HIT is the Fc receptor–mediated, immune complex–dependent activation of platelets. In support of this theory, Warkentin and colleagues[184] pointed out that this mechanism probably involves and is complicated by the propensity of these immune complexes to generate procoagulant platelet-derived microparticles.

Alternative protein targets may be involved in selected cases of HIT. For example, in 9 of 15 patients with HIT who lacked detectable antibodies to heparin-PF4 complexes, Amiral and coworkers[199] found evidence of autoantibodies specific for the chemokines neutrophil-activating peptide-2 (NAP-2) or IL-8. PF4 is about 60% homologous to NAP-2 and 40% homologous to IL-8, leading to the proposal that HIT involving these proteins could proceed along a mechanism similar to that invoked for PF4.

REFERENCES

1. Hynes RO: Integrins: Versatility, modulation, and signaling in cell adhesion. Cell 1992;69:11–25.
2. George JN, Caen JP, Nurden AT: Glanzmann's thrombasthenia: The spectrum of clinical disease. Blood 1990;75:1383–1395.
3. Kunicki TJ, Nugent DJ, Staats SJ, et al: The human fibroblast class II extracellular matrix receptor mediates platelet adhesion to collagen and is identical to the platelet glycoprotein Ia-IIa complex. J Biol Chem 1988;263:4516–4519.
4. Kunicki TJ, Nurden AT, Pidard D, et al: Characterization of human platelet glycoprotein antigens giving rise to individual immunoprecipitates in crossed immunoelectrophoresis. Blood 1981;58:1190–1197.
5. Pischel KD, Bluestein HG, Woods VL: Platelet glycoprotein Ia, Ic, and IIa are physicochemically indistinguishable from the very late activation antigens adhesion-related proteins of lymphocytes and other cell types. J Clin Invest 1988;81:505–513.
6. Takada Y, Wayner EA, Carter WG, Hemler ME: Extracellular matrix receptors, ECMRII and ECMRI, for collagen and fibronectin correspond to VLA-2 and VLA-3 in the VLA family of heterodimers. J Cell Biochem 1988;37:385–393.
7. Saelman EUM, Nieuwenhuis HK, Hese KM, et al: Platelet adhesion to collagen types I through VIII under conditions of stasis and flow is mediated by GPIa/IIa (alpha 2 beta 1 integrin). Blood 1994;83:1244–1250.
8. Takada Y, Hemler ME: The primary structure of the VLA-2/collagen receptor alpha 2 subunit (platelet GPIa): Homology to other integrins and the presence of a possible collagen-binding domain. J Cell Biol 1989;109:397–407.
9. Nieuwenhuis HK, Akkerman JWN, Houdijk WPM, Sixma JJ: Human blood platelets showing no response to collagen fail to express surface glycoprotein Ia. Nature 1985;318:470–472.
10. Kehrel B, Balleisen L, Kokott R, et al: Deficiency of intact thrombospondin and membrane glycoprotein Ia in platelets with defective collagen-induced aggregation and spontaneous loss of disorder. Blood 1988;71:1074–1078.
11. Kunicki TJ, Orchekowski R, Annis D, Honda Y: Variability of integrin alpha 2 beta 1 activity on human platelets. Blood 1993;82:2693–2703.
12. Kritzik M, Savage B, Nugent DJ, et al: Nucleotide polymorphisms in the alpha 2 gene define multiple alleles which are associated with differences in platelet alpha 2 beta 1. Blood 1998;92:2382–2388.
13. Montgomery RR, Kunicki TJ, Taves C, et al: Diagnosis of Bernard-Soulier syndrome and Glanzmann's thrombasthenia with a monoclonal assay on whole blood. J Clin Invest 1983;71:385–389.
14. Lopez JA, Chung DW, Fujikawa K, et al: Cloning of the alpha chain of human platelet glycoprotein Ib: A transmembrane protein with homology to leucine-rich alpha 2-glycoprotein. Proc Natl Acad Sci U S A 1987;84:5615–5619.
15. Titani K, Takio K, Handa M, Ruggeri ZM: Amino acid sequence of the von Willebrand factor-binding domain of platelet membrane glycoprotein Ib. Proc Natl Acad Sci U S A 1987;84:5610–5614.

16. Modderman PW, Admiraal LG, Sonnenberg A, et al: Glycoproteins V and Ib-IX form a noncovalent complex in the platelet membrane. J Biol Chem 1992;267:364–369.

17. Vicente V, Houghten RA, Ruggeri ZM: Identification of a site in the alpha chain of platelet glycoprotein Ib that participates in von Willebrand factor binding. J Biol Chem 1990;265:274–280.

18. Ruggeri ZM, Zimmerman TS, Russell S, et al: von Willebrand factor binding to platelet glycoprotein Ib complex. Methods Enzymol 1992;215:263–275.

19. Drouin J, McGregor JL, Parmentier S, et al: Residual amounts of glycoprotein Ib concomitant with near-absence of glycoprotein IX in platelets of Bernard-Soulier patients. Blood 1988;72:1086–1088.

20. Ware J, Russell SR, Vicente V, et al: Nonsense mutation in the glycoprotein Ib-alpha coding sequence associated with Bernard-Soulier syndrome. Proc Natl Acad Sci U S A 1990;87:2026–2030.

21. Roth GJ: Molecular defects in the Bernard-Soulier syndrome: Assessment of receptor genes, transcripts and proteins. C R Acad Sci III 1996;319:819–826.

22. Schick PK: Platelet glycolipids. In Kunicki TJ, George JN (eds): Platelet Immunobiology: Molecular and Clinical Aspects. Philadelphia: JB Lippincott, 1989, pp 31–43.

23. von dem Borne AEGKr: Nomenclature of platelet antigen systems. Br J Haematol 1990;74:239–240.

24. Santoso S, Kiefel V: Human platelet-specific alloantigens: Update. Vox Sang 1998;74:249–253.

25. Newman PJ, McFarland JG, Aster RH: The alloimmune thrombocytopenias. In Loscalzo J, Scharf AI (eds): Thrombosis and Hemorrhage. Baltimore, William & Wilkins, 1998, pp 599–615.

26. Reznikoff-Etievant MF, Dangu C, Lobet R: HLA-B8 antigen and anti-Pl[A1] alloimmunization. Tissue Antigens 1981;18:66–68.

27. Valentin N, Vergracht A, Bignon JD, et al: HLA-Drw52a is involved in alloimmunization against PL-A1 antigen. Hum Immunol 1990;27:73–79.

28. Reznikoff-Etievant MF, Muller JY, Julien F, et al: An immune response gene linked to MHC in man. Tissue Antigens 1981;22:312.

29. Kunicki TJ, Aster RH: Isolation and immunologic characterization of the human platelet alloantigen, PlA1. Mol Immunol 1979;16:353–360.

30. Newman PJ, Derbes RS, Aster RH: The human platelet alloantigens, PLA1 and PLA2, are associated with a leucine33/proline33 amino acid polymorphism in membrane glycoprotein IIIa, and are distinguishable by DNA typing. J Clin Invest 1989;83:1778–1781.

31. Bowditch RD, Tani PH, Halloran CE, et al: Localization of a Pl[A1] epitope to the amino terminal 66 residues of platelet glycoprotein IIIa. Blood 1992;79:559–562.

32. Goldberger A, Kolodziej M, Poncz M, et al: Effect of single amino acid substitutions on the formation of the PlA and Bak alloantigenic epitopes. Blood 1991;78:681–687.

33. Calvete JJ, Henschen A, Gonzalez-Rodriguez J: Assignment of disulphide bonds in human platelet GPIIIa: A disulphide pattern for the beta-subunits of the integrin family. Biochem J 1991;274:63–71.

34. L'Abbé D, Tremblay L, Filion M, et al: Alloimmunization to platelet antigen HPA-1a (Pl[A1]) is strongly associated with both HLA-DRB3*0101 and HLA-DQB1*0201. Hum Immunol 1992;34:107–114.

35. Maslanka K, Yassai M, Gorski J: Molecular identification of T cells that respond in a primary bulk culture to a peptide derived from a platelet glycoprotein implicated in neonatal alloimmune thrombocytopenia. J Clin Invest 1996;98:1802–1808.

36. Kuijpers RW, von dem Borne AE, Kifel V, et al: Leucine 33-proline 33 substitution in human platelet glycoprotein IIIa determines HLA-DRw52a (Dw24) association of the immune response against HPA-1a (Zwa/PlA1) and HPA-1b (Zwb/PlA2). Hum Immunol 1992;34:253–256.

37. Westman P, Hashemi-Tavoularis S, Blanchette V, et al: Material DRB1*1501, DQA1*0102, DQB1*0602 haplotype in fetomaternal alloimmunization against human platelet alloantigen HPA-6b (GPIIIa-Gln489). Tissue Antigens 1997;50:113–118.

38. Mueller-Eckhardt C, Kiefel V, Grubert A, et al: 348 cases of suspected neonatal alloimmune thrombocytopenia. Lancet 1989;1:363–366.

39. von dem Borne A, von Riesz E, Verheugt F, et al: Bak[a], a new platelet-specific antigen involved in neonatal alloimmune thrombocytopenia. Vox Sang 1980;39:113–120.

40. McGrath K, Minchinton R, Cunningham I, Ayberk H: Platelet anti-Bak[b] antibody associated with neonatal alloimmune thrombocytopenia. Vox Sang 1989;57:182–184.

41. Mueller-Eckhardt C, Becker T, Weishet M, et al: Neonatal alloimmune thrombocytopenia due to fetomaternal Zw[b] in compatibility. Vox Sang 1986;50:94–96.

42. Grenet P, Dausset J, Dugas M, et al: Purpura thrombopenique neonatal avec isoimmunisation foeto-maternelle anti-Ko[a]. Arch Fr Pediatr 1965;22:1165–1174.

43. Shibata Y, Matsuda I, Miyaji T, Ichikawa Y: Yuk[a], a new platelet antigen involved in two cases of neonatal alloimmune thrombocytopenia. Vox Sang 1986;50:177–180.

44. Mueller-Eckhardt C: HLA-B8 antigen and anti-Pl[A1] alloimmunization. Tissue Antigens 1982;19:154–158.

45. George JN, Pickett EB, Heinz R: Platelet membrane microparticles in blood bank fresh frozen plasma and cryoprecipitate. Blood 1987;68:307–309.

46. Waraejcka D, Janson M, Aster RH: The Pl[A1] antigen, but not HLA antigens, can be acquired by platelets from plasma. Blood 1985;66:109a.

47. Kickler TS, Ness PM, Herman JH, Bell WR: Studies on the pathophysiology of posttransfusion purpura. Blood 1986;68:347.

48. Dancis A, Ehmann C, Ferzinger R, et al: Studies on the mechanisms of Pl[A1] post-transfusion purpura (PTP). Blood 1986;68:106a.

49. Ehmann WC, Dancis A, Ferzinger R, et al: Post-transfusion purpura: Evidence that conversion of Pl[A1] negative platelets to the Pl[A1] positive phenotype is an in vitro artifact. Blood 1987;70:339a.

50. Beer J, Coller BS: Evidence that platelet glycoprotein IIIa has a large disulfide-bonded loop that is susceptible to proteolytic cleavage. J Biol Chem 1989;264:17564–17573.

51. Flug F, Espinola R, Liu L-X, et al: A 13-mer peptide straddling the leucine[33]/proline[33] polymorphism in glycoprotein IIIa does not define the PL[A1] epitope. Blood 1991;77:1964–1969.

52. Honda S, Honda Y, Ruan C, Kunicki TJ: The impact of three-dimensional structure on the expression of Pl[A1] alloantigens on human integrin beta 3. Blood 1995;86:234–242.

53. Valentin N, Visentin GP, Newman PJ: Involvement of the cysteine-rich domain of glycoprotein IIIa in the expression of the human platelet alloantigen, Pl[A1]: Evidence for heterogeneity in the humoral response. Blood 1995;85:3028–3033.

54. Bowditch RD, Tani P, McMillan R: Reactivity of autoantibodies from chronic ITP patients with recombinant glycoprotein IIIa peptides. Br J Haematol 1995;91:178–184.

55. Barron-Casella EA, Kickler TS, Rogers OC, Casella JF: Expression and purification of functional recombinant epitopes for the platelet antigens, Pl[A1] and Pl[A2]. Blood 1994;84:1157–1163.

56. Van Leeuwen E, Leeksma O, van Mourik J, et al: Effect of the binding of antiZw[a] antibodies on platelet function. Vox Sang 1984;47:280–289.

57. Furihata K, Nugent DJ, Bissonette A, et al: On the association of the platelet-specific alloantigen, Pen[a], with glycoprotein IIIa: Evidence for heterogeneity of glycoprotein IIIa. J Clin Invest 1987;80:1624–1630.

58. Ryu T, Davis JM, Schwartz KA: Dose-dependent platelet stimulation and inhibition induced by anti-PlA1 IgG. J Lab Clin Med 1990;116:91–99.

59. Du X, Plow EF, Frelinger AL III, et al: Ligands "activate" integrin alpha IIb beta 3 (platelet GPIIb-IIIa). Cell 1991;65:409–416.

60. Vijayan KV, Goldschmidt-Clermont PJ, Roos C, Bray PF: The P1(A2) polymorphism of integrin beta(3) enhances outside-in signaling and adhesive functions. J Clin Invest 2000;105:793–802.

61. Saji H, Maruya E, Fujii H, et al: New platelet antigen, Sib[a], involved in platelet transfusion refractoriness in a Japanese man. Vox Sang 1989;56:283–287.

62. van der Weerdt CM, van de Wiel-Dorfmeyer H, Engelfriet CP, van Loghem JJ: A new platelet antigen. In Proceedings of the 8th Congress of the European Society of Haematology. Basel: S Karger, 1961, p 379.

63. Dausset J, Berg P: Un novel exemple d'anticorps anti-plaquetaire Ko. Vox Sang 1963;8:341–3417.

64. Ware J, Russell S, Ruggeri ZM: Genetic basis for the molecular polymorphisms of platelet glycoprotein Ib-alpha. Thromb Haemost 1991;65:347a.

65. Kuijpers RWAM, Faber NM, Cuypers HTM, et al: NH[2]-Terminal globular domain of human platelet glycoprotein Ib-alpha has a methionine[145]/threonine[145] amino acid polymorphism, which is associated with the HPA-2 (Ko) alloantigens. J Clin Invest 1992;89:381–384.

66. Lyman S, Aster RH, Visentin GP, Newman PJ: Polymorphism of human platelet membrane glycoprotein IIb associated with the Bak^a/Bak^b alloantigen system. Blood 1990;75:2343–2348.

67. Take H, Tomiyama Y, Shibata Y, et al: Demonstration of the heterogeneity of epitopes of the platelet-specific alloantigen, Baka. Br J Haematol 1990;76:395–400.

68. Santoso S, Shibata Y, Kiefel V, et al: Identification of Yuk(b) alloantigen on platelet glycoprotein IIIa. Thromb Haemost 1987;58:197.

69. Wang L, Juji T, Shibata Y, et al: Sequence variation of human platelet membrane glycoprotein IIIa associated with the Yuk^a/Yuk^b alloantigen system. Proc Japan Acad 1991;67:102–106.

70. Wang R, Furihata K, McFarland JG, et al: An amino acid polymorphism within the RGD binding domain of platelet membrane glycoprotein IIIa is responsible for the formation of the Pen^a/Pen^b alloantigen system. J Clin Invest 1992;90:2038–2043.

71. Newman PJ, Kawai Y, Montgomery RR, Kunicki TJ: Synthesis by cultured human umbilical vein endothelial cells of two proteins structurally and immunologically related to platelet membrane glycoproteins IIb and IIIa. J Cell Biol 1986;103:81–86.

72. Giltay JC, Leeksma OC, Von dem Borne AEG, and van Mourik JA: Alloantigenic composition of the endothelial vitronectin receptor. Blood 1988;72:230–233.

73. Kawai Y, Montgomery RR, Furihata K, Kunicki TJ: Expression of platelet alloantigens on human endothelial cells and HEL cells [abstract]. Thromb Haemost 1987;58:4.

74. Giltay JC, Brinkman H-JM, Von dem Borne AEGK, van Mourik JA: Expression of the alloantigen Zw^a (or Pl^{A1}) on human vascular smooth muscle cells and foreskin fibroblasts: A study on normal individuals and a patient with Glanzmann's thrombasthenia. Blood 1989;74:965–970.

75. Kiefel V, Santoso S, Katzmann B, Mueller-Eckhart C: The Br^a/Br^b alloantigen system on human platelets. Blood 1989;73:2219–2223.

76. Woods VL Jr, Pischel KD, Avery ED, Bluestein HG: Antigenic polymorphism of human very late activation protein-2 (platelet glycoprotein Ia-IIa): Platelet alloantigen Hc^a. J Clin Invest 1989;83:978–985.

77. Kiefel V, Santoso S, Weisheit M, Mueller-Eckhardt C: Monoclonal antibody-specific immobilization of platelet antigens (MAIPA): A new tool for the identification of platelet-reactive antibodies. Blood 1987;70:1732–1733.

78. McFarland JG, Blanchette V, Collins J, et al: Neonatal alloimmune thrombocytopenia due to a new platelet-specific alloantibody. Blood 1993;81:3318–3323.

79. Wang R, McFarland JG, Kekomaki R, Newman PJ: Amino acid 489 is encoded by a mutational "hot spot" on the beta 3 integrin chain: The CA/TU human platelet alloantigen system. Blood 1993;82:3386–3391.

80. Kekomaki R, Jouhikainen T, Ollikainen J, et al: A new platelet alloantigen, Tu^a, on glycoprotein IIIa associated with neonatal alloimmune thrombocytopenia in two families. Br J Haematol 1993;83:306–310.

81. Santoso S, Newman P, Kalb R, et al: An unpaired cysteine residue is involved in epitope formation but has no influence on platelet GPIIIa expression and function. Blood 1992;80:128A.

82. Kuijpers RWAM, Simsek S, Faber NM, et al: Single point mutation in human glycoprotein IIIa is associated with a new platelet-specific alloantigen (Mo) involved in neonatal alloimmune thrombocytopenia. Blood 1993;81:70–76.

83. Noris P, Simsek S, De Bruijne-Admiraal LG, et al: Max^a, a new low-frequency platelet-specific antigen localized on glycoprotein IIb, is associated with neonatal alloimmune thrombocytopenia. Blood 1995;86:1019–1026.

84. Peyruchaud O, Bourre F, Morel-Kopp M-C, et al: HPA-10w^b (La^a): Genetic determination of a new platelet-specific alloantigen on glycoprotein IIIa and its expression in COS-7 cells. Blood 1997;89:2422–2428.

85. Simsek S, Vlekke ABJ, Kuijpers RWAM, et al: A new private platelet antigen, Gro^a, localized on glycoprotein IIIa, involved in neonatal alloimmune thrombocytopenia. Vox Sang 1994;67:302–306.

86. Kelton JG, Smith JW, Horsewood P, et al: Gov$^{a/b}$ alloantigen system on human platelets. Blood 1990;75:2172–2176.

87. Bordin JO, Kelton JG, Warner MN, et al: Maternal immunization to Gov system alloantigens on human platelets. Transfusion 1997;37:823–828.

88. Kroll H, Santoso S, Bohringer M, et al: Neonatal alloimmune thrombocytopenia caused by immunization against Oe^a, a new low frequency alloantigen on platelet glycoprotein IIIa [abstract]. Blood 1995;86:540a–540a.

89. Kekomaki R, Raivio P, Kero P: A new low-frequency platelet alloantigen, Va^a, on glycoprotein IIb/IIIa associated with neonatal alloimmune thrombocytopenia. Transfus Med 1992;2:27–33.

90. Kekomaki R, Partanen J, Pitkanen S, et al: Glycoprotein Ib/IX-specific alloimmunization in an HPA 2b-homozygous mother in association with neonatal thrombocytopenia. Thromb Haemost 1993;69(Suppl):997.

91. Beardsley DS, Ho JS, Moulton T. PI^T: A new platelet specific antigen on glycoprotein V. Blood 1987;70:347a.

92. Degos L, Dautigny A, Brouet JC, et al: A molecular defect in thrombasthenic platelets. J Clin Invest 1975;56:236–242.

93. Coller BS, Peershke EIB, Seligsohn U, et al: Studies on the binding of an alloimmune and two murine monoclonal antibodies to the platelet glycoprotein IIb-IIIa complex receptor. J Lab Clin Med 1986;107:384–396.

94. Kunicki TJ, Furihata K, Bull B, Nugent D: The immunogenicity of platelet membrane glycoproteins. Transfus Med Rev 1987;1:21–33.

95. Nurden AT, Jallu V, Hourdille P, et al: Evidence for multiple antibodies in the sera of two patients with immune thrombocytopenia of different origins. Thromb Haemost 1989;62:565.

96. Bierling P, Fromont P, Elbez A, et al: Early immunization against platelet glycoprotein IIIa in a newborn Glanzmann type I patient. Vox Sang 1988;55:109.

97. Gruel Y, Nugent DJ, Kunicki TJ: Molecular specificity of anti IIb/IIIa human antibodies. Semin Thromb Hemost 1995;21:60–67.

98. Gruel Y, Brojer E, Nugent DJ, Kunicki TJ: Further characterization of the thrombasthenia-related idiotype OG: Anti-idiotype defines a novel epitope(s) shared by fibrinogen B beta chain, vitronectin and von Willebrand factor and required for binding to beta 3. J Exp Med 1995;180:2259–2267.

99. Ishida F, Gruel Y, Brojer E, et al: Repertoire cloning of a human IgG inhibitor of alpha IIb beta 3 function: The OG idiotype. Mol Immunol 1995;32:613–622.

100. Moskowitz KA, Scudder LE, Coller BS: Fibrinogen lacking the B beta-chain 1 amino acids supports platelet adhesion, aggregation, and GPIIb/IIIa (alpha IIb beta 3) receptor redistribution and helps to localize the epitope of an anti-GPIIIa antiidiotypic antibody [abstract]. Blood 1995;86(Suppl):247a.

101. Tobelem G, Levy-Toledano S, Bredoux R, et al: New approach to determination of specific functions of platelet membrane sites. Nature 1976;263:427–429.

102. Karpatkin S: 1985. Autoimmune thrombocytopenic purpura. Semin Hematol 1985;22:260–288.

103. Beardsley DS: Platelet autoantigens. In Kunicki TJ, George JN (eds): Platelet Immunobiology: Molecular and Clinical Aspects. Philadelphia: JB Lippincott, 1989, p 121.

104. Van Leeuwen EF, van der Ven JTM, Engelfriet CP, von dem Borne AEGKr: Specificity of autoantibodies in autoimmune thrombocytopenia. Blood 1982;59:23–29.

105. Woods VL, Oh EH, Mason D, McMillan R: Autoantibodies against the platelets glycoprotein IIb/IIIa complex in patients with chronic ITP. Blood 1984;63:368–375.

106. Beardsley DS, Spiegel JE, Jacobs MM, et al: Platelet membrane glycoprotein IIIa contains target antigens that bind anti-platelet antibodies in immune thrombocytopenias. J Clin Invest 1984;74:1701–1707.

107. McMillan R, Tani P, Millard F, et al: Platelet-associated and plasma anti-glycoprotein autoantibodies in chronic ITP. Blood 1987;70:1040–1045.

108. Tomiyama Y, Kurata Y, Mizutani H, et al: Platelet glycoprotein IIb as a target antigen in two patients with chronic idiopathic thrombocytopenic purpura. Br J Haematol 1987;66:535–538.

109. Tomiyama Y, Kurata Y, Shibata Y, et al: Immunochemical characterization of an autoantigen on platelet glycoprotein IIb in chronic ITP: Comparison with the Bak^a alloantigen. Br J Haematol 1989;71:76–83.

110. Kekomaki R, Dawson B, McFarland J, Kunicki TJ: Localization of human platelet autoantigens to the cysteine-rich region of glycoprotein IIIa. J Clin Invest 1991;88:847–854.

111. Fujisawa K, O'Toole TE, Tani P, et al: Autoantibodies to the presumptive cytoplasmic domain of platelet glycoprotein IIb-IIIa in patients with chronic immune thrombocytopenic purpura. Blood 1991;77:2207–2213.

112. Fujisawa K, Tani P, O'Toole TE, et al: Different specificities of platelet-associated and plasma autoantibodies to platelet GPIIb-IIIa in patients with chronic immune thrombocytopenic purpura. Blood 1992;79:1441–1446.

113. Fujisawa K, Tani P, McMillan R: Platelet-associated antibody to glycoprotein IIb/IIIa from chronic immune thrombocytopenic purpura patients often binds to divalent cation-dependent antigens. Blood 1993;81:1284–1289.

114. Nardi MA, Liu LX, Karpatkin S: GPIIIa-(49-66) is a major pathophysiologically relevant antigenic determinant for anti-platelet GPIIIa of HIV-1-related immunologic thrombocytopenia. Proc Natl Acad Sci U S A 1997;94:7589–7594.

115. Bowditch RD, Tani P, Fong KC, McMillan R: Characterization of autoantigenic epitopes on platelet glycoprotein IIb/IIIa using random peptide libraries. Blood 1996;12:4579–4584.

116. Escher R, Vogel M, Miescher S, et al: Recombinant anti-GPIIb/IIIa autoantibodies inhibit binding of fibrinogen to GPIIb/IIIa. Blood 1999;94(Suppl):450a.

117. Von dem Borne AEGK, van der Lelie J, Vos JJE, et al: Antibodies against cryptantigens of platelets. In Decary F, Rock G (eds): Platelet Serology: Research Progress and Clinical Implications. Basel: S Karger, 1986, p 33.

118. van Vliet H, Kappers-Klunne M, Abels J: Pseudothrombocytopenia: A cold antibody against platelet glycoprotein GPIIb. Br J Haematol 1986;62:501–511.

119. Niessner H, Clemetson KJ, Panzer S, et al: Acquired thrombasthenia due to GPIIb/IIIa-specific platelet autoantibodies. Blood 1986;68:571–576.

120. Balduini C, Grignani G, Sinigaglia F, et al: Severe platelet dysfunction in a patient with autoantibodies against membrane glycoproteins IIb/IIIa. Haemostasis 1987;7:98–104.

121. Deckmyn H, Chew SL, Vermylen L: Lack of platelet response to collagen associated with an autoantibody against glycoprotein Ia: A novel cause of acquired qualitative platelet dysfunction. Thromb Haemost 1990;64:74–79.

122. Szatkowski NS, Kunicki TJ, Aster RH: Identification of glycoprotein Ib as a target for autoantibody in idiopathic (autoimmune) thrombocytopenic purpura. Blood 1986;67:310–315.

123. He R, Reid DM, Jones CE, Shulman NR: Extracellular epitopes of platelet glycoprotein Ib-alpha reactive with serum antibodies from patients with chronic idiopathic thrombocytopenic purpura. Blood 1995;86:3789–3796.

124. Nugent DJ: Human monoclonal antibodies in the characterization of platelet antigens. In Kunicki TJ, George JN (eds): Platelet Immunobiology: Molecular and Clinical Aspects. Philadelphia: JB Lippincott, 1989, pp 273–290.

125. Devine DV, Curie MS, Rosse WF, Greenberg CS: Pseudo-Bernard-Soulier syndrome: Thrombocytopenia caused by autoantibody to platelet glycoprotein Ib. Blood 1987;70:428–431.

126. Mayer JL, Beardsley DS: Varicella-associated thrombocytopenia: Autoantibodies against platelet surface glycoprotein V. Pediatr Res 1996;40:615–619.

127. Wright JF, Blanchette VS, Wang H, et al: Characterization of platelet-reactive antibodies in children with varicella-associated acute immune thrombocytopenic purpura (ITP). Br J Haematol 1996;95:145–152.

128. Berchtold P, McMillan R, Tani P, et al: Autoantibodies against platelet membrane glycoproteins in children with acute and chronic immune thrombocytopenic purpura. Blood 1989;74:1600–1602.

129. Winiarski J: IgG and IgM antibodies to platelet membrane glycoprotein antigens in acute childhood idiopathic thrombocytopenic purpura. Br J Haematol 1989;73:88–92.

130. Varon D, Karpatkin S: A monoclonal antiplatelet antibody with decreased reactivity for autoimmune thrombocytopenic platelets. Proc Natl Acad Sci U S A 1983;80:6992–6995.

131. Tsubakio T, Tani P, Woods VL, McMillan R: Autoantibodies against platelet GPIIb/IIIa in chronic ITP react with different epitopes. Br J Haematol 1987;67:345–348.

132. Nugent DJ, Kunicki TJ, Berglund C, Bernstein ID: A human monoclonal autoantibody recognizes a neoantigen on glycoprotein IIIA expressed on stored and activated platelets. Blood 1987;70:16–22.

133. Hiraiwa A, Nugent DJ, Milner EB: Sequence analysis of monoclonal antibodies derived from a patient with idiopathic thrombocytopenic purpura. Autoimmunity 1990;8:107–113.

134. Kunicki TJ, Furihata K, Kekomaki R, et al: A human monoclonal autoantibody specific for human platelet glycoprotein IIb (integrin alpha IIb) heavy chain. Hum Antibodies Hybridomas 1990;1:83–95.

135. Kunicki TJ, Plow EF, Kekomaki R, Nugent DJ: A human monoclonal autoantibody 2E7 is specific for a peptide sequence of platelet glycoprotein IIb: Localization of the epitope to IIb231–238 with an immunodominant Trp-235. J Autoimmun 1991;4:415–431.

136. Berchtold P, Dale GL, Tani P, McMillan R: Inhibition of autoantibody binding to platelet glycoprotein IIb/IIIa by anti-idiotypic antibodies in intravenous immunoglobulin. Blood 1989;74:2414–2417.

137. Koerner TAW, Weinfeld HM, Bullard LSB, Williams LCJ: Antibodies against platelet glycosphingolipids: Detection in serum by quantitative HPTLC-autoradiography and association with autoimmune and alloimmune processes. Blood 1989;74:274–284.

138. Harris EN, Asherson RA, Gharavi AE, et al: Thrombocytopenia in SLE and related autoimmune disorders: Association with anticardiolipin antibodies. Br J Haematol 1985;59:227–230.

139. Harris EN, Gharavi AE, Hegde U, et al: Anticardiolipin antibodies in autoimmune thrombocytopenic purpura. Br J Haematol 1985;59:231–234.

140. Kaise S, Yasuda T, Kasukawa R, et al: Antiglycolipid antibodies in normal and pathologic human sera and synovial fluids. Vox Sang 1985;49:292–300.

141. Van Vliet HHDM, Kappers-Klunne MC, van der Hel JWB, Abels J: Antibodies against glycosphingolipids in sera of patients with idiopathic thrombocytopenic purpura. Br J Haematol 1987;67:103–108.

142. dePosba NK, Pfueller SL: Characterization of platelet components to which antiplatelet IgG antibodies bind in idiopathic thrombocytopenic purpura [abstract]. Clin Exp Pharmacol Physiol 1982;9:532.

143. Weinfeld HM, Williams LCJ, Koerner TAW: Detection and frequency of platelet antibodies with glycolipid specificity. Transfusion 1986;26:583.

144. Lewis DC, Meyers KM: Studies of platelet-bound and serum platelet-bindable immunoglobulins in dogs with idiopathic thrombocytopenic purpura. Exp Hematol 1996;24:696–701.

145. Imbach P, Barandun S, d'Apuzzo V: High-dose intravenous gammaglobulin for idiopathic thrombocytopenic purpura in childhood. Lancet 1981;1:1228–1230.

146. Tsubakio T, Kurata Y: Alteration of T cell subsets and immunoglobulin synthesis in vitro during high-dose gammaglobulin therapy in patients with idiopathic thrombocytopenic purpura. Blood 1983;74:697–702.

147. Ware RE, Howard TA: Elevated numbers of gamma-delta (gamma detla+) T lymphocytes in children with immune thrombocytopenic purpura. J Clin Immunol 1994;14:247.

148. Ware RE, Howard TA: Phenotypic and clonal analysis of T lymphocytes in childhood immune thrombocytopenic purpura. Blood 1993;82:2137–2142.

149. Kuwana M, Kaburaki J, Ikeda Y: Autoreactive T cells to platelet GPIb-IIIa in immune thrombocytopenic purpura: Role in production of anti-platelet autoantibody. J Clin Invest 1998;102:1393–1402.

150. Filion MC, Proulx C, Bradley AJ, et al: Presence in peripheral blood of healthy individuals of autoreactive T cells to a membrane antigen present on bone marrow-derived cells. Blood 1996;88:2144–2150.

151. Mouthon L, Kaveri S, Kazatchkine M: Immune modulating effects of intravenous immunoglobulin (IVIg) in autoimmune diseases. Transfus Sci 1994;15:393–408.

152. Lacroix-Desmazes S, Mouthon L, Spalter SH, et al: Immunoglobulins and the regulation of autoimmunity through the immune network. Clin Exp Rheumatol 1996;15(Suppl):S9–S15.

153. Mehta YS, Badakere SS: In-vitro inhibition of antiplatelet autoantibodies by intravenous immunoglobulins and Rh immunoglobulins. J Postgrad Med 1996;42:46–49.

154. Semple JW, Milev Y, Cosgrave D, et al: Differences in serum cytokine levels in acute and chronic autoimmune thrombocytopenic purpura: Relationship to platelet phenotype and antiplatelet T-cell reactivity. Blood 1996;87:4245–4254.

155. Nugent D, Berman M, Imfeld K, et al: Depressed IL-4 levels in children with acute and chronic immune thrombocytopenia (ITP). FASEB 1998;12:A609.

156. Garcia-Suarez J, Prieto A, Reyes E, et al: Abnormal gamma IFN and alpha TNF secretion in purified CD2+ cells from autoimmune thrombocytopenic purpura (ATP) patients: Their implication in the clinical course of the disease. Am J Hematol 1995;49:271–276.

157. Andersson J: Cytokines in idiopathic thrombocytopenic purpura (ITP). Acta Paediatr 1998;424(Suppl):61–64.

158. Dianzani U, Bragardo M, DiFranco D, et al: Deficiency of the Fas apoptosis pathway without Fas gene mutations in pediatric patients with autoimmunity/lymphoproliferation. Blood 1997;89:2871–2879.

159. Crossley AR, Dickinson AM, Proctor SJ, Dalvert JE: Effects of interferon-alpha therapy on immune parameters in immune thrombocytopenic purpura. Autoimmunity 1996;24:81–100.

160. Lazarus AH, Joy T, Crow AR: Analysis of transmembrane signaling and T cell defects associated with idiopathic thrombocytopenic purpura ITP. Acta Paediatr 1998;424(Suppl):21–25.

161. Erduran E, Aslan Y, Aliyazicioglu Y, et al: Plasma soluble interleukin-2 receptor levels in patients with idiopathic thrombocytopenic purpura. Am J Hematol 1998;57:119–123.

162. Zimmerman SA, Malinoski FJ, Ware RE: Immunologic effects of anti-D (WinRho-SD) in children with immune thrombocytopenic purpura. Am J Hematol 1998;57:131–138.

163. Bussel J, Heddle N, Richards C, Woloski M: MCP-1, IL-10, IL-6 and TNF-alpha levels in patients with ITP before and after iv anti-D and IVIG treatments. Blood 1999;94:15a–15a.

164. George J, Raskob G, Bussel J, et al: Safety and effect on platelet count of repeated doses of monoclonal antibody to CD40 ligand in patients with chronic ITP. Blood 1999;94(Suppl):19a.

165. Bussel J, Wissert M, Oates B, et al: Humanized monoclonal anti-CD40 ligand antibody (Hu5c8) rescue therapy of 15 adults with severe chronic refractory ITP. Blood 1999;94:646a–646a.

166. Aster RH: Drug-induced immune thrombocytopenia: An overview of pathogenesis. Semin Hematol 1999;36:2–6.

167. Shulman NR: Immunoreactions involving platelets: I. A steric and kinetic model for formation of a complex from a human antibody, quinidine as a haptene, and platelets; and for fixation of complement by the complex. J Exp Med 1975;107:665–690.

168. Hackett T, Kelton JG, Powers P: Drug-induced platelet destruction. Semin Thromb Hemost 1982;8:116–137.

169. Van Leeuwen EF, Engelfriet CP, Von dem Borne AEG Jr: Studies on quinine and quinidine-dependent antibodies against platelets and their reaction with platelets in the Bernard-Soulier syndrome. Br J Haematol 1982;51:551–560.

170. Pfueller SL, de Posbo NK, Bilston RA: Platelets deficient in glycoprotein I have normal Fc receptor expression. Br J Haematol 1984;56:607–615.

171. Berndt MC, Chong BH, Bull HA, et al: Molecular characterization of quinine/quinidine drug-dependent antibody platelet interaction using monoclonal antibodies. Blood 1985;66:1292–1301.

172. Chong BH, Berndt MC, Koutts J, Castaldi PA: Quinidine-induced thrombocytopenia and leukopenia: Demonstration and characterization of distinct antiplatelet and antileukocyte antibodies. Blood 1983;62:1218–1223.

173. Christie DJ, Muller PC, Aster RH: Fab-mediated binding of drug-dependent antibodies to platelets in quinidine- and quinine-induced thrombocytopenia. J Clin Invest 1985;75:310–314.

174. Kunicki TJ, Johnson MM, Aster RH: Absence of the platelet receptor for drug-dependent antibodies in the Bernard-Soulier syndrome. J Clin Invest 1978;62:716–719.

175. Christie DJ, Mullen PC, Aster RH: Quinine- and quinidine platelet antibodies can react with GPIIb/IIIa. Br J Haematol 1987;67:213–219.

176. Chong BH, Du X, Berndt MC, et al: Characterization of the binding domains on platelet glycoproteins Ib-IX and IIb-IIIa complexes for the quinine/quinidine-dependent antibodies. Blood 1991;77:2190–2199.

177. Lopez JA, Li CQ, Weisman S, Chambers M: The glycoprotein Ib-IX complex-specific monoclonal antibody SZ1 binds to a conformation-sensitive epitope on glycoprotein IX: Implications for the target antigen of quinine/quinidine-dependent autoantibodies. Blood 1995;85:1254–1258.

178. Visentin GP, Newman PJ, Aster RH: Characteristics of quinine- and quinidine-induced antibodies specific for platelet glycoproteins IIb and IIIa. Blood 1991;77:2668–2676.

179. Curtis BR, McFarland JG, Wu G-G, et al: Antibodies in sulfonamide-induced immune thrombocytopenia recognize calcium-dependent epitopes on the glycoprotein IIb/IIIa complex. Blood 1994;84:176–183.

180. Nieminen U, Kekomäki R: Quinidine-induced thrombocytopenic purpura: Clinical presentation in relation to drug-dependent and drug-independent platelet antibodies. Br J Haematol 1992;80:77–82.

181. Lynch DM, Howe SE: Heparin-associated thrombocytopenia: Antibody binding specificity to platelet antigens. Blood 1985;66:1176.

182. Kelton JG, Sheridan D, Santos A, et al: Heparin-induced thrombocytopenia: Laboratory studies. Blood 1988;72:925–930.

183. Chong BH: Heparin-induced thrombocytopenia. Br J Haematol 1995;89:431–439.

184. Warkentin TE, Hayward CP, Boshkov LK, et al: Sera from patients with heparin-induced thrombocytopenia generate platelet-derived microparticles with procoagulant activity: An explanation for the thrombotic complications of heparin-induced thrombocytopenia. Blood 1994;84:3691–3699.

185. Berndt MC, Chong BH, Andrews RK: Biochemistry of drug-dependent platelet autoantigens. In Kunicki TJ, George JN (eds): Immunobiology. Philadelphia: JB Lippincott, 1989, pp 132–147.

186. Adelman B, Sobel M, Fujimura Y, et al: Heparin-associated thrombocytopenia: Observations on the mechanism of platelet aggregation. J Lab Clin Med 1989;113:204–210.

187. Chong BH, Castaldi PA, Berndt MC: Heparin-induced thrombocytopenia: Effects of rabbit IgG and its Fab and Fc fragments on antibody-heparin-platelet interaction. Thromb Res 1989;55:291–295.

188. Chong BH, Fawaz I, Chesterman CN, Berndt MC: Heparin-induced thrombocytopenia: Mechanism of interaction of the heparin-dependent antibody with platelets. Br J Haematol 1989;73:235–240.

189. Amiral J, Bridey F, Dreyfus M, et al: Platelet factor 4 complexed to heparin is the target for antibodies generated in heparin-induced thrombocytopenia. Thromb Haemost 1992;68:95–96.

190. Visentin GP, Ford SE, Scott JP, Aster RH: Antibodies from patients with heparin-induced thrombocytopenia/thrombosis are specific for platelet factor 4 complexed with heparin or bound to endothelial cells. J Clin Invest 1994;93:81–88.

191. Greinacher A, Potzsch B, Amiral J, et al: Heparin-associated thrombocytopenia: Isolation of the antibody and characterization of a multimolecular PF4-heparin complex as the major antigen. Thromb Haemost 1994;71:247–251.

192. Kelton JG, Smith JW, Warkentin TE, et al: Immunoglobulin G from patients with heparin-induced thrombocytopenia binds to a complex of heparin and platelet factor 4. Blood 1994;83:3232–3239.

193. Amiral J, Bridey F, Wolf M, et al: Antibodies to macromolecular platelet factor 4-heparin complexes in heparin-induced thrombocytopenia: A study of 44 cases. Thromb Haemost 1995;73:21–28.

194. Greinacher A, Amiral J, Dummel V, et al: Laboratory diagnosis of heparin-associated thrombocytopenia and comparison of platelet aggregation test, heparin-induced platelet activation test, and platelet factor 4/heparin enzyme-linked immunosorbent assay. Transfusion 1994;34:381–385.

195. Arepally G, Reynolds C, Tomaski A, et al: Comparison of PF4/heparin ELISA assay with 14C-serotonin release assay in the diagnosis of heparin induced thrombocytopenia. Am J Clin Pathol 1995;104:648–654.

196. Greinacher A, Michels I, Liebenhoff U, et al: Heparin associated thrombocytopenia: Immune complexes are attached to the platelet membrane by the negative charge of highly sulphated oligosaccharides. Br J Haematol 1993;84:711–716.

197. Newman PM, Chong BH: Heparin-induced thrombocytopenia: New evidence for the dynamic binding of purified anti-PF4-heparin antibodies to platelets and the resultant platelet activation. Blood 2000;96:182–187.

198. Amiral J, Wolf M, Fischer AM, et al: Pathogenicity of IgA and/or IgM antibodies to heparin-PF4 complexes in patients with heparin-induced thrombocytopenia. Br J Haematol 1996;92:954–959.

199. Amiral J, Marfaing-Koka M, Wolf M, et al: Presence of autoantibodies to interleukin-8 or neutrophil-activating peptide-2 in patients with heparin-associated thrombocytopenia. Blood 1996;88:410–416.

200. Kuijpers RWAM, Simsek S, Faber NM, et al: Single point mutation in human glycoprotein IIIa is associated with a new platelet-specific alloantigen (Mo) involved in neonatal alloimmune thrombocytopenia. Blood 1993;81:70–76.

201. Santoso S, Kalb R, Kiefel V, et al: A point mutation leads to an unpaired cysteine residue and a molecular weight polymorphism of a functional platelet beta 3 integrin subunit: The Sra alloantigen system of GPIIIa. J Biol Chem 1994;269:8439–8444.

202. Simsek S, Folman C, Van der Schoot CE, et al: The Arg633His substitution responsible for the platelet antigen Gro^a unravelled by SSCP analysis and direct sequencing. Br J Haematol 1997;97:330–335.

203. Santoso S, Kalb R, Walka V, et al: The human platelet alloantigens Br(a) and Br(b) are associated with a single amino acid polymorphism on glycoprotein Ia (integrin subunit alpha-2). J Clin Invest 1993;92:2427–2432.

204. Santoso S, Amrhein J, Sachs U, et al: A mutational hot spot Thr$_{799}$Met on the α_2 integrin subunit leads to the formation of new human platelet alloantigen Sit[a] and affects collagen-induced aggregation. Blood 1997;90:261a–261a.

205. Kuijpers R, Faber NM, Cuypers HTM, et al: The N-terminal globular domain of human platelet glycoprotein Iba has a methionine[145]/threonine[145] amino-acid polymorphism, which is associated with the HPA-2 (Ko) alloantigens. J Clin Invest 1992;89:381–384.

206. Sachs UJH, Kiefel V, Bohringer M, et al: Single amino acid substitution in human platelet glycoprotein Ib beta is responsible for the formation of the platelet-specific alloantigen Iy[a]. Blood 2000;95:1849–1855.

207. Smith JW, Hayward CPM, Horsewood P, et al: Characterization and localization of the Gov[a/b] alloantigens to the glycosylphosphatidylinositol-anchored protein CDw109 on human platelets. Blood 1995;86:2807–2814.

208. Warkentin TE, Smith JW: The alloimmune thrombocytopenic syndromes. Transfus Med Rev 1997;11:296–307.

209. Holensteiner A, Walchshofer S, Adler A, et al: Human platelet antigen gene frequencies in the Austrian population. Haemostasis 1995;25:133–136.

210. Newman PJ, Valentin N: Human platelet alloantigens: Recent findings, new perspectives. Thromb Haemost 1995;74:234–239.

211. Tanaka S, Ohnoki S, Shibata H, et al: Gene frequencies of human platelet antigens on glycoprotein IIIa in Japanese. Transfusion 1996;36:813–817.

212. Corvas DT, Delgado M, Zeitune MM, et al: Gene frequencies of the HPA-1 and HPA-2 platelet antigen alleles among the Amerindians. Vox Sang 1997;73:182–184.

213. Kim HO, Jin Y, Kickler TS, et al: Gene frequencies of the five major human platelet antigens in African American, white and Korean populations. Transfusion 1995;35:863–867.

214. Kekomaki S, Partanen J, Kekomaki R: Platelet alloantigens HPA-1, -2, -3, -5 and -6b in Finns. Transfus Med 1995;5:193–198.

215. Urwijitaroon Y, Barusrux S, Romphruk A, Puapairoj C. Frequency of human platelet antigens among blood donors in northeastern Thailand. Transfusion 1995;35:868–870.

iii. Leukocyte Antigens

Chapter 7

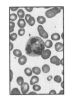

HLA and Granulocyte Antigens

Glenn E. Rodey

◼ HLA and Neutrophil Antigens

The exchange of tissue between outbred members of the same species inevitably exposes systems of alloantigens. Transplantation antigens were first recognized during the early 1900s by tumor biologists.[1] These investigators, who tried to propagate spontaneous murine tumors by transplanting the cells from affected animals into healthy outbred animals, were unsuccessful because the transplanted tissue was invariably rejected. The pioneering investigations of this phenomenon by George Snell and Peter Gorer led to the recognition of the major histocompatibility complex (MHC) in mice, termed H-2.[2-4] The closely linked H-2 genes encode a series of molecules that are responsible for rejection of any cells bearing incompatible H-2 molecules. The human leukocyte antigen (HLA) complex is the equivalent MHC in humans. Neutrophil-specific alloantigens, identified through pregnancy, were recognized as a cause of transient neonatal neutropenia. This chapter briefly reviews the structure and function of these alloantigen systems and their clinical relevance to hematopoietic stem cell transplantation, pregnancy, and blood transfusion.

◼ HLA Genes

The HLA genetic complex, which is the most polymorphic system known, is a series of closely linked genes located on the short arm of chromosome 6. The region spans a distance of about 4000 kilobases (kb). The complex contains more than 250 loci (genes and pseudogenes), of which some 21 are directly related to transplantation.[5] The loci code for over 900 class I and class II alleles. Figure 7.1 shows the specific regions and some of the common HLA loci.

Nomenclature

Two HLA nomenclatures are currently used: an older list of specificities based on immunological techniques such as serology or in vitro mixed leukocyte culture reactions and a newer molecular nomenclature based on specific nucleotide sequences of alleles.

Immunological Nomenclature

The current immunological nomenclature, shown in Table 7.1,[6] is based on the following system (e.g., HLA-B44). HLA- refers to the MHC. This is followed by a capital letter to indicate the specific segregant series (e.g., A, B, C, DR, DQ, and DP). The capital letter is followed by a number that designates the specificity. Historically, specificities for the A and B loci are numbered together in their order of discovery. However, numerics for the other segregant series start with number one. Specificities that were considered to be provisional, that is, had not received an official designation by the World Health Organization (WHO) nomenclature committee, were previously preceded by a small "w." This letter is no longer used for that purpose. However, it is retained in the nomenclature in four circumstances. To prevent possible confusion between HLA-C locus specificities and complement components, the prefix w is permanently retained. DP and Dw specificities also retain the w to indicate that both sequences were originally defined by cellular techniques. Finally, the public specificities, Bw4 and Bw6, retain the w to indicate that they are epitopes rather than allelic gene products (see "Antigenic Structure of HLA Molecules").

A modification of this nomenclature is the use of a three- or four-number sequence, such as HLA-A210 or B2708, to indicate a specific allele that can be identified serologically,

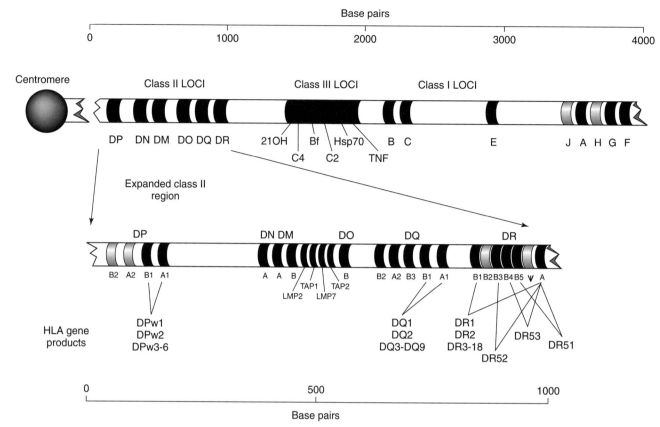

Figure 7.1 Simplified map of the human leukocyte antigen (HLA) genetic complex. The lower DNA segment is an expansion of the class II region to demonstrate the paired α and β chain relationships. (Adapted from Rodey GE: HLA antigen and antibody system. In Hoffman R, Benz EJ Jr, Shattil SJ, et al [eds]: Hematology. Basic Principles and Practice, 2d ed. New York, Churchill Livingston, 1995, p 142.)

usually by a monoclonal antibody. It should be mentioned that the serologically defined specificities are based on the detection of epitopes rather than on specific alleles. Anti-HLA-A2 antisera, for example, were originally thought to detect a specific allele. However, the specificity actually comprises more than 30 distinct A2 alleles.

Sequence-Defined Allelic Nomenclature

This nomenclature, first recommended in 1987 by the WHO nomenclature committee,[7] defines HLA alleles on the basis of documented HLA nucleotide sequences. In this nomenclature, for example, HLA-A*0201, "HLA-" designates the MHC and a capital letter indicates the segregant series. The "*" indicates that the nomenclature is based on DNA analysis. The numeric representing a specific allele in this nomenclature is usually four digits as noted, but it can be up to seven digits long and may include a capital letter suffix such as N (null allele) or L (low expression), for example, HLA-A*2402102L. The first two digits indicate the allele's relationship to a serologically defined specificity (A24). The second two digits indicate the specific allele (*2402). A fifth digit indicates that two or more alleles have been identified with a single nucleotide difference that does not lead to an amino acid difference (*24021 versus 24022). The sixth and seventh digits indicate that a polymorphism exists in the noncoding region of an allele. The allelic variant containing the noncoding polymorphism is indicated by

"02" in these positions, and the normal allelic variant is given the "01" designation (*2402101 versus *2402202L, indicating low expression).

The resolution of DNA-based HLA typing can vary from antigen level to allele level, depending on the primers and technique used. If the procedure does not discriminate between molecular variants of HLA-A2, for example, it is appropriate to assign the result as HLA-A*02. A complete listing of WHO HLA nomenclature is periodically published in the journals *Human Immunology*, *Tissue Antigens*, and *The European Journal of Immunogenetics*. Monthly updates of the current list (1998) are also published in these journals.

Structure of the HLA Genetic Complex

The HLA complex is divided into the class I, class II, and class III regions (see Fig. 7.1) to indicate the general locations of loci. The class I region spans about 2000 kb and contains loci for the α chains of the classical HLA-A, -B, and -C molecules and the nonclassical HLA-E, -F, and -G molecules. The region also contains a number of class I pseudogenes and various non-HLA genes of known and unknown function. The locus encoding β₂-microglobulin, the light chain of HLA class I molecules, is on chromosome 15.[8] The class II region contains the loci for both the α and β chains of the class II molecules, HLA-DR, -DQ, -DP, -DM, and -DO. The DR, DQ, and DP molecules are expressed on the

Table 7.1 Listing of Serologically Definable HLA Specificities

A	B		C	DR	DQ	DP
A1	B5	B50(21)	Cw1	DR1	DQ1	DPw1
A2	B7	B51(5)	Cw2	DR103	DQ2	DPw2
A203	B703	B5102	Cw3	DR2	DQ3	DPw3
A210	B8	B5103	Cw4	DR3	DQ4	DPw4
A3	B12	B52(5)	Cw5	DR4	DQ5(1)	DPw5
A9	B13	B53	Cw6	DR5	DQ6(1)	DPw6
A10	B14	B54(22)	Cw7	DR6	DQ7(3)	
A11	B15	B55(22)	Cw8	DR7	DQ8(3)	
A19	B16	B56(22)	Cw9(w3)	DR8	DQ9(3)	
A23(9)	B17	B57(17)	Cw10(w3)	DR9		
A24(9)	B18	B58(17)		DR10		
A2403	B21	B59		DR11(5)		
A25(10)	B22	B60(40)		DR12(5)		
A26(10)	B27	B61(40)		DR13(6)		
A28	B2708	B62(15)		DR14(6)		
A29(19)	B35	B63(15)		DR1403		
A30(19)	B37	B64(14)		DR1404		
A31(19)	B38(16)	B65(14)		DR15(2)		
A32(19)	B39(16)	B67		DR16(2)		
A33(19)	B3901	B70		DR17(3)		
A34(10)	B3902	B71(70)		DR18(3)		
A36	B40	B72(70)				
A43	B4005	B73		DR51		
A66(10)	B41	B75(15)				
A68(28)	B42	B76(15)		DR52		
A69(28)	B44(12)	B77(15)				
A74(19)	B45(12)	B78		DR53		
A80	B46	B81				
	B47					
	B48	Bw4				
	B49(21)	Bw6				

Data from Bodmer JG, Marsh SGE, Albert ED, et al: Nomenclature for factors of the HLA system, 1998. Tissue Antigens 1999;54:407.

cell membranes, whereas DM and DO are intracellular molecules. The region also contains genes (*TAP1*, *TAP2*, *LMP2*, and *LMP*) that play an important role in providing peptides for loading into class I molecules.[9, 10] A common denominator for these and the class I and II genes is that all are inducible by interferon-γ.

The class III region lies between the class I and II regions and contains some genes that may be indirectly involved in MHC function and others that have no obvious direct relationship to MHC function. They include the structural genes for the complement components factor B, C2, and C4; MICA and MICB; tumor necrosis factor β; and CYP21, the gene coding for 21-hydroxylase.

Inheritance and Expression of HLA Genes

HLA genes are inherited as autosomal codominant traits. The frequency of null or low-expression alleles is low: 2% for class I A, B, and C loci and 0% for DRB1 and DQ.[6] Because the loci within the HLA complex are closely linked, the recombination rates between HLA-A, -B, -C, -DR, and -DQ are only about 1.5% to 2.0%. Thus, parental HLA haplotypes are normally inherited en bloc. In a family with one or more siblings, the statistical probabilities that a sibling will have a genotypic HLA-identical sibling or a sibling who shares no haplotypes are each 25%.

Certain combinations of genes occur in HLA haplotypes more frequently than expected on the basis of the gene frequencies. This phenomenon is called linkage disequilibrium (LD).[11] The HLA genes that may be found in LD are not the same in different ethnic or racial groups. The frequency of HLA genes and the patterns of LD reflect the combinations of HLA gene products that evolved in different geographical areas as an adaptation to the types of pathogens specific for those areas. LD may hold together combinations of HLA class I and II genes that had particularly good survival benefits for the population. LD significantly affects the clinical use of matching in transplantation and transfusion. Patients with common haplotypes are more likely to find HLA-compatible unrelated donors within a population with similar ethnic or racial backgrounds. In contrast, patients with HLA genes that are not held together by LD have a proportionately more difficult time in finding compatible donors. Table 7.2 lists some common haplotypes found in different populations in the United States. The information was obtained from the National Marrow Donor Program database through a link with the ASHI website (www.swmed.edu/home_pages_ASHI/prepr/mori_abd.htm).

The distribution of HLA class I and II on different types of cells varies according to the tissue. In general, class I and II molecules can be expressed on virtually all nucleated cells, especially during inflammatory responses or stimulation with interferon-γ.[12] In resting cells, such as hepatocytes and myocytes, minimal expression occurs. Both class I and class II are constitutively expressed on many differentiating nucleated hematopoietic cells. They are not expressed on stem cells or mature erythrocytes. However, remnant class I expression can occur on young reticulocytes, accounting for the Bg "red cell" antigen system.[13] Platelets and resting T cells express only class I antigens, but class II molecules are also expressed on activated T cells.

Table 7.2   Common Haplotypes Found in American Ethnic or Racial Groups

Rank	Hyplotype (% frequency)*			
	African	Asian	Caucasian	Latin
1	A30,B42,DR3 (1.67)	A33,B58,DR3 (1.58)	A1,B8,DR3 (5.18)	A2,B35,DR8 (1.76)
2	A1,B8,DR3 (1.25)	A33,B44,DR6 (1.46)	A3,B7,DR2 (2.63)	A29,B44,DR7 (1.71)
3	A3,B7,DR2 (0.76)	A24,B52,DR2 (1.38)	A2,B44,DR4 (2.15)	A1,B8,DR3 (1.67)
4	A2,B44,DR4 (0.65)	A2,B46,DR9 (1.35)	A2,B7,DR2 (1.80)	A2,B35,DR4 (1.29)
5	33,B53,DR8 (0.63)	A33,B47,DR7 (1.34)	A29,B44,DR7 (1.47)	A3,B7,DR2 (1.19)

*Haplotype frequency in the specific population.
From the National Marrow Donor Program (NMDP) internet site (see text).

■ HLA Gene Products

Functions of HLA Gene Products

The primary function of MHC molecules eluded investigators for more than 20 years after their discovery as transplantation antigens. In 1969, McDevitt and Chinitz[14] reported that the genetic control of murine antibody responses to simple protein antigens, previously observed by Green and colleagues,[15] was controlled by genetic factors located in the H-2 system. This gave rise to the concept that the MHC contained immune response (Ir) genes. Three years later, Kindred and Shreffler[16] discovered that cooperation between helper T cells and B cells required H-2 compatibility. In 1974, Zinkernagel and Doherty[17] demonstrated a similar requirement for H-2 compatibility between antiviral cytotoxic T lymphocytes (CTL) and their virus-infected target cells for effective cytotoxicity. These early studies led to the subsequent discovery that MHC molecules, together with specific peptides, serve as the T-cell receptor ligand. Antigen presentation to T cells and the closely related T-cell receptor repertoire in the thymus appear to be the major biological function of MHC molecules (for reviews, see references 18 to 21).

MHC molecules serve two and possibly three additional functions. Class I molecules are recognition targets for natural killer (NK) cell inhibitory receptors.[22–26] NK cells, part of the innate immune system, lack antigen-specific T-cell receptors, and the activation of NK cells occurs through relatively nonselective receptors. To prevent activation and killing of normal cells, multiple inhibitory receptors have evolved on NK cells,[27] most of which recognize epitopes of class I molecules. In contrast to normal cells, many virus-infected cells and tumor cells lack HLA expression and are functionally invisible to T cells. NK cells are able to kill these cells because their inhibitory receptors are not activated.

Specialized HLA molecules encoded by the HLA-E and -G loci play an important role in preventing immunological injury to the fetus during pregnancy.[28, 29] The trophoblastic tissues of the placenta lack classical HLA class I and II molecules, preventing recognition of fetus-derived alloantigens by T cells. However, NK cells would be activated under these conditions. To counterbalance this potential threat, evolution has provided specialized HLA molecules that are not recognized by T cells but inhibit NK cell activation. HLA-E is apparently loaded with a peptide derived from the leader sequence of HLA-G. This complex activates an inhibitory receptor, CD49/NKG2A, present on the trophoblastic cell membranes.

Finally, a growing number of studies indicate that MHC genes and gene products may be involved in mating preference, specifically preferential selection of MHC-disparate mates. Boyse and his colleagues originally reported this observation in the 1970s,[30–32] and later studies in humans seem to support the concept.[33, 34] The proposed mechanism responsible for the phenomenon is that MHC molecules or the peptides carried by the molecules are converted into aromatic compounds by bacteria in sweat and urine. It has also been suggested that the type of colonial bacteria present in an individual and responsible for the production of specific aromatics may be partly determined by the HLA genotype.

The Physical Structure of HLA Gene Products

Class I and II molecules are glycoproteins composed of two dissimilar protein chains (heterodimers). The four chains belong to the immunoglobulin superfamily. Although the peptide chains for each class of molecules are different, the overall three-dimensional configuration of the molecules is similar.

HLA class I molecules contain an α (heavy) protein chain with a molecular weight of approximately 45,000, which is noncovalently associated with β_2-microglobulin (light), a nonpolymorphic protein of molecular weight 12,000. The α chain amino acids are folded into three distinct regions called the α1, α2, and α3 domains. All significant polymorphisms detected by serological and cellular techniques reside in the α1 and α2 domains.[35] Early structural models of class I molecules indicated that both the α1 and α2 domains contained stretches of amino acid sequences that were arranged into helical structures rather than the more usual sheets typical of globular proteins. The significance of this observation was not appreciated until the landmark studies of Bjorkman and colleagues[36, 37] elucidated the three-dimensional structure of HLA-A2. The α1 and α2 domains form a platform overlain by the two helical structures to create the peptide binding site. This groove accommodates processed peptides for presentation to T-cell receptors.

Class II molecules also consist of two distinct glycoprotein chains, α and β, of molecular weight approximately 28,000 and 33,000. Amino acids in each chain are folded into two domains. In contrast to those of class I molecules, both class II chains are transmembrane proteins. Within 6 years after the discovery of the HLA class I structure, the crystalline structure of the class II molecule DRI was demonstrated and showed an overall structure similar to that of class I.[38]

The high degree of polymorphism found in both class I and II molecules is restricted to specific, hypervariable regions of the HLA molecule that are located along the regions that form the peptide groove.[39, 40] The remaining portions of the molecules are relatively conserved, reflecting structural constraints imposed by the functions of the molecules in antigen presentation and cellular interactions.

Functional Differences Between Class I and Class II Molecules

Even though they are structurally homologous, class I and II molecules have significant functional differences. Class I molecules contain a binding site in the α3 domain that selectively accommodates the CD8 accessory molecule.[41] Class II has an analogous binding site that accommodates the CD4 accessory molecule.[42] This feature partly explains why T cell receptors of CD4+ T cells and CD8+ T cells preferentially bind to class II and class I molecules, respectively. A major difference between the two types of HLA molecules is the origin of peptides and the site in which the peptides are loaded. The distinctive peptide loading pathways are called the endogenous and the exogenous pathways.

The Endogenous Pathway

Peptides presented by class I MHC molecules originate mainly from proteins found in the cytosol.[21] Most are derived from self-proteins under normal circumstances. Endogenous peptides are also derived from viral proteins and tumor-associated proteins. Peptides from phagocytosed microbial antigens and other endocytosed material can also gain access to newly synthesized class I molecules by leakage into the cytosol.[43] This may constitute a minor component of the endogenous pathway. Evolution appears to have provided the endogenous pathway and class I MHC molecules as a mechanism to survey the internal environment of the cell for antigens from replicating organs and from mutated self-proteins that would otherwise escape recognition by antibody or other extracellular immune mechanisms.

Class I molecules must bind peptides within the endoplasmic reticulum. Otherwise, the physical association of the class I heavy chain with β2-microglobulin is unstable. Until the time that peptides are loaded into their peptide grooves, class I molecules are stabilized by a complex series of cofactors that include two calcium-dependent chaperones and the protein tapasin.[44-46] The newly formed HLA heavy chain first associates with calnexin. When β2-microglobulin associates with the heavy chain, calnexin dissociates and calreticulin binds. During this time, tapasin also associates with the class I–calreticulin complex. The complex then binds to MHC-encoded transporter associated with antigen processing molecules (TAP1-TAP2 heterodimer) through the class I molecule. TAP1 molecules insert through the endoplasmic reticulum membrane.

Endogenous peptides that will be transported through TAP molecules are derived from proteins that are degraded into a series of peptides through the action of cytosolic proteasomes. Two proteins, LMP2 and LMP7, that are involved in this process are encoded in the class II region of HLA.[10, 21] Because proteasomes contain multiple protease enzymes, a variety of different peptides may be obtained from the same protein. The class I molecules ultimately select the appropriate peptides on the basis of anchor residues and affinity. If no peptides meet the criteria for binding after a period of time, the class I molecules are released and possibly reutilized. This process produces peptides derived from class I or class II that can be loaded and presented by other HLA molecules, which has clinical relevance in allotransplantation.

Peptides transported into the endoplasmic reticulum insert into the peptide groove of the docked class I molecules. Stable trimeric complexes are then transported to the plasma membrane and expressed on the membrane surface.

Exogenous Pathway

Foreign proteins derived from the external environment are taken up by specialized antigen-presenting cells (APCs) by either mass pinocytosis (dendritic cells), phagocytosis (macrophages), or receptor-mediated endocytosis (B cells). The antigen-containing vacuoles fuse with lysosomes and with endosomes that are rich in class II molecules (MHC class II peptide-loading compartments or MIICs).[47, 48] The proteins undergo limited proteolysis to provide a source of exogenously derived peptides. Concurrently, MHC class II molecules are assembled in the endoplasmic reticulum. Early class II molecules contain a third chain, in addition to α and β, called the invariant chain (Ii). Nonamer complexes containing three Ii, three α, and three β chains form and are transported to MIIC.[49] The Ii chains serve several important functions in the exogenous pathway.[50-52] They occupy the peptide-binding groove and prevent endogenously derived peptides from binding to the newly assembled class II molecules. They also stabilize new class II molecules. Finally, they contain amino acid sequences that target the traffic of the molecular complex to MIICs.

Upon entry into MIICs, most of the invariant chain is degraded, leaving only the small portion that is bound in the peptide groove (called class II–associated Ii chain, or CLIP). The nonclassical class II molecule HLA-DM facilitates the process of unloading CLIP and of loading specific endogenous peptide into classical HLA class II molecules.[53-56] HLA-DM expression and Ii expression are coregulated with the classical class II genes. DM is largely absent from the cell membrane but accumulates in MIICs.[57] DM molecules do not bind peptides within their own peptide grooves. The role of DM in peptide loading is to function as a chaperone for class II molecules that are empty or loaded with low-stability peptides. Class II molecules are susceptible to denaturation during this period, and DM molecules prevent this until a high-stability peptide is loaded. The DM molecule then dissociates from the stable peptide-MHC trimer, which is then transported to the plasma membrane and is expressed on its surface. Lymphocytes and thymic epithelial cell MIICs contain an additional class II molecule called HLA-DO. DO, which is inducible by interferon-γ, apparently competitively inhibits DM chaperone function, but the reason for this is still unclear.[58, 59]

Antigenic Structure of HLA Molecules

The minimum structural unit that can be recognized by a B-cell or T-cell receptor is called an antigenic determinant or *epitope*. Epitopes that differ among individual members of the same species are referred to as *alloepitopes*. Protein epitopes may be as small as 6 to 15 amino acids.[60] Because the polymorphic regions of HLA molecules may contain more than 200 amino acids, it is not surprising that they contain multiple alloepitopes that are capable of inducing humoral and cellular responses following alloimmunization. HLA alloepitopes are defined with well-characterized, operationally monospecific alloantibodies or cloned T lymphocytes. Serologically definable epitopes are located principally on and around the exposed portions of the peptide groove. The epitopes recognized by T cells are less precisely mapped, but many are probably distinct from the serologically defined epitopes. High-frequency public alloepitopes do not occur in class II DRB1 and DQB1 gene products, so the following discussion focuses on the antigenic structure of class I, A and B locus alleles.

Serologically defined epitopes have been divided into two general types.[61] Epitopes that occur only on a single related group of gene products, such as the HLA-A2 allelic variants, are referred to as private or group-specific epitopes. HLA antisera, functionally specific for private specificities, were originally extremely important for defining and discriminating the products of different HLA genes. Other HLA antibodies that react with more than one gene product, for example, anti-HLA-A2,28,9, detect shared or cross-reactive epitopes termed public epitopes. Many of the public epitopes are widely distributed among different HLA molecules. Antibodies to public epitopes have been used to categorize HLA gene products into major cross-reactive groups (CREGs). The current significance of public epitopes, however, is their clinical relevance for patients awaiting transplants or requiring repetitive platelet transfusions. A single alloantibody directed against a public epitope can have devastating consequences for potential transplant recipients or patients who require repetitive platelet transfusions.

The HLA-Bw4 and Bw6 specificities are good examples of high-frequency public epitopes. These two specificities were originally thought to define a diallelic locus closely linked to but distinct from HLA. All individuals type positively for Bw4, Bw6, or both Bw4 and Bw6. Sequential immunoprecipitation studies subsequently demonstrated that

Bw4 and Bw6 are alternative public epitopes present on all HLA-B molecules as well as on HLA-A23, 24, 25, and 32.[39, 62] Table 7.3 is a summary of the major CREGs, the public epitopes that are the basis for the CREGs, and the probable positions of the epitopes on the HLA molecule.

The terms *cross-reactive groups* and *public epitopes* are often used interchangeably, but they are not always synonymous. A single public epitope accounts for all of the observed cross-reactivity in three major CREGs (4C, 6C, and 12C). In others, such as the A2 CREG and the B7 CREG, three public epitopes contribute to serological cross-reactivity in each group.[63, 64] Donor selection for highly sensitized thrombocytopenic patients, based on matching for CREGs or for public epitopes, is discussed further in the following.

■ HLA Humoral Alloimmunization

Humoral HLA alloimmunization may occur after the introduction of an allogeneic tissue into a recipient. This event is the result of pregnancy, organ or tissue transplantation, or repetitive transfusion of blood products. Sometimes the production of HLA antibodies is transient, disappearing after 1 to 4 months.[65, 66] This commonly occurs after limited blood transfusions in a previously nonimmune individual. In other circumstances, especially after pregnancies or previous transplants, HLA alloantibodies can persist for years in the apparent absence of new immunizing events. Retention of antigen in lymphoid tissues may be a common cause of persistent HLA antibodies.[67, 68] However, additional, but unknown, factors determine whether an HLA alloantibody response persists or declines. The search for these factors continues to be a subject of active investigation.

Table 7.3 The Major HLA Class I, Serologically Defined, Cross-Reactive Groups and Associated Public Epitopes

Major Cross-Reactive Groups (CREGs) 1C,10C,2C (2,28p, 2,9,28p, 2,17p), 5C (5p, 21p), 7C (7p, 22p, 27p, 40p), 8C, 12C, 4C, 6C	
CREGs	**Publics**
1C=A1,3,9 (23,24),11,29,30,31,36,80	Three to four, poorly defined
10C=A10 (25,26,34,66),1,28 (68,69),32,33,43,74	10,28,33p (**10p**)
2C=A2,9 (23,24),28 (68,69),17 (B57,58)	2,28,9p (**9p**)
	2,28p (**28p**)
	2,17p (**17p**)
5C=B5 (51,52),15 (62,63,75,76,77,78),17 (57,58),18,	5,35,53,18,70 (**5p**)
21 (49,50),35,46,53,70 (71,72),73,4005	all 5C (**21p**)
7C=B7,8,13,22 (54,55,56),27,	7,27,42,46,54,55,56p (**22p**)
40 (60,61),41,42,47,48,59,67,81,82	7,13,27,60,61,47p (**27p**)
	7,8,41,42,48,60,81p (**7p**)
	7,60,48 (**40p**)
8C=8,14 (64,65),16 (38,39),18,59,67	Probably one, poorly-defined
12C=B12 (44,45),13,21 (49,50),37,40 (60,61),41,47	Probably one
4C=23,24,25,32 (Aw4),Bw4	Bw4 (**4C**)
6C=Bw6	Bw6 (**6C**)

Possible Epitope Locations

1C=Several possibilities
10C=**10p** (RNTRN 62–66)
2C=**28p** (TTKH 142–145); **9p** (127K); **17p** (GETRK 62–66)
5C=**5p** (ASPRT 41–45); **21p** (not clear)
7C=**7p** (DKLE 177–180); **22p** (YKAQA 67–71); **27p** (E 163); **40p** (K178)
8C=not clear
12C=(TSPRK 41–45)
4C=**Bw4** (TALR or NALR 80–83)
6C=**Bw6** (NLRG 80–83)

HLA alloimmunization does not always lead to the production of immune effector responses. Normally, only 25% to 30% of individuals who undergo primary alloimmunization through pregnancy, transplantation, or donor-specific transfusions produce HLA antibodies. Why up to 75% of alloimmunized patients do not produce antibodies is still unclear, although induction of donor-specific hyposensitization is one possibility. The production of HLA antibodies by B cells is T cell dependent. In primary immune responses, T cells, activated by interaction with dendritic cells bearing the appropriate HLA peptide, are induced to express CD40 ligand as well as cytokines that are critical for B-cell activation and differentiation.[69] The activated T cells can then interact with antigen-specific B cells through interactions between CD40 and CD40 ligand. To interact effectively, the T cell and B cell must have specificity for epitopes shared by the same protein molecule, although they may recognize different epitopes.

The processing and recognition of alloantigens in the setting of transplantation or transfusion occur through two distinct pathways, called the direct and indirect allorecognition pathways. The direct pathway can be defined operationally as antigen presentation by allogeneic APCs, whereas the indirect pathway is antigen presentation by self-APCs (Fig. 7.2). Direct allorecognition is generally an early and vigorous response caused by the combined major and minor histincompatibilities presented by allogeneic APCs (APCs of donor origin in organ transplantation or of recipient origin in acute graft-versus-host disease). Generally, the direct response involves the activation of a large number of T-cell clones. The estimated precursor frequencies involved in direct recognition may be as high as 0.5%.[70, 71] Because the allogeneic APCs are also a major target of the direct response, they are eventually eliminated. Thus, direct alloimmune responses are usually self-limited. Indirect allorecognition, although less vigorous in most cases, is not self-limited and may persist for years.

In organ transplantation, the probable cause of indirect recognition is alloantigens shed from the graft and then processed by the recipient's APCs as exogenous antigens. The activatable T-cell precursor frequencies for a discrete alloantigen would be similar to those for other nominal antigens such as tetanus toxoid, approximately 0.01%.[70] However, multiple alloantigen incompatibilities would cause a cumulative increase in precursor frequencies and a potential increase in severity of the rejection process. Indirect pathway allorecognition may play a significant mechanism in the pathogenesis of chronic allograft rejection and possibly chronic graft-versus-host disease.[72, 73]

■ HLA Typing, Crossmatching, and Antibody Screening Procedures

Complement-dependent cytotoxicity (CDC) has traditionally been used for HLA typing, crossmatching, and antibody detection.[74] DNA-based HLA typing became available to clinical laboratories in the early 1990s, and it is increasingly used as the major typing procedure.[75, 76] DNA-based HLA typing is comparable to CDC in cost, labor, and time and is significantly more accurate. All current DNA typing assays utilize the polymerase chain reaction (PCR) to amplify the genes of interest. Three commonly used procedures involve sequence-specific primers (PCR-SSP), sequence-specific oligonucleotide probes (PCR-SSO), and sequence-based typing (PCR-SBT).

PCR-SSP uses multiple primer pairs that discriminate many of the known alleles of a specific locus, such as the A locus. The amplicon is then subjected to denaturing agarose gel electrophoresis. This assay is useful for laboratories with relatively low work volumes. PCR-SBT is often used to supplement SSP when the primer combinations cannot distinguish between two alleles. The major rate-limiting factor for PCR-SSP as volume increases is the requirement for increasing numbers of electrophoresis units and thermal cyclers (the multiple primer pairs are usually amplified individually). With higher work volumes or large-volume typing of donor registries, PCR-SSO is usually required. In this assay, locus-specific primers, such as A, B, C, DRB1, and DQB1, are used for amplification. This requires no more than 8 to 10 amplification tubes, compared with as many as 96 for some PCR-SSP kits. The amplicon and specific probes are hybridized, and the hybridization is usually visualized by enzyme-dependent colorimetric techniques.

Two versions of PCR-SSO are currently used, depending on the volume of samples. For batch testing, usually 35 to 50 samples per run, each nylon membrane is dotted with a specific probe, which is bound to the membrane by ultraviolet B irradiation or chemicals. Individual patient's samples are then dotted on the membranes and allowed to hybridize with the probe. The number of probes determines the number

PATHWAYS OF ALLOANTIGEN RECOGNITION

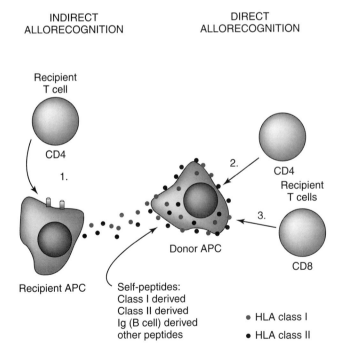

INDIRECT
ALLORECOGNITION

DIRECT
ALLORECOGNITION

Recipient
T cell

CD4

1.

2.

CD4
Recipient
T cells

3.

Donor APC

CD8

Recipient APC

Self-peptides:
Class I derived
Class II derived
Ig (B cell) derived
other peptides

● HLA class I
● HLA class II

Figure 7.2 Cartoon depicting two direct allorecognition pathways (CD4 and CD8) and the indirect pathway (CD4). Antigens are processed and presented by donor or recipient antigen-presenting cells (APCs). This example is based on a solid-organ transplant in which the direct pathway utilizes donor-origin APCs and the direct pathway recipient APCs. HLA, human leukocyte antigen; Ig, immunoglobulin.

of membranes utilized for each batch of samples. The technique is referred to as *dot blotting*. For smaller sample numbers and faster turnaround times, a modified technique involving *reverse dot blots* or *reverse line probes* is used, in which a patient's amplified DNA is applied to a membrane or to tubes, followed by addition of individual probes.

HLA antibody screening and analysis procedures that employ solid-phase immunoassays are now available to clinical laboratories. The assays use HLA class I or class II antigens that have been purified from cells of HLA-typed individuals. The purified antigen preparations are used to coat the wells of microtiter plates (enzyme-linked immunosorbent assay) or to coat microparticles that can be analyzed in a flow cytometer. It should be noted that the HLA molecules are not individually purified. The preparations are analogous in composition to the combined class I or II molecules present on a cell except that they are presumably free of non-HLA molecules. This technology, when fully validated, will almost certainly replace the antiglobulin-augmented CDC (AHG-CDC) test for routine screening and analysis.

Finally, crossmatching by AHG-CDC or CDC is increasingly supplemented with indirect binding assays such as those available with sensitive agglutination kits or flow cytometry.[77] Crossmatching is especially valuable for selecting platelet donors when HLA-typed donor panels are not available or confirming that a product has been correctly chosen.

■ Applications of HLA Testing in Transplantation and Transfusion

The major application of HLA testing in the fields of hematology-oncology and transfusion medicine is in selection of donors for allogeneic hematopoietic stem cell transplantation (HSCT). When unrelated donors became available through the National Marrow Donor Program (NMDP) and other registries, the need for allele-level HLA typing increased. In fact, unrelated HSCT has been a major driving force for the development of low-cost, high-resolution typing techniques. Provision of HLA-compatible single-donor platelet transfusions for highly HLA-sensitized thrombocytopenic patients is an additional but less common important clinical application of HLA testing.

Hematopoietic Stem Cell Transplantation

Identification of a suitable donor is one of the first steps in the complex process of HSCT when transplantation is determined to be the best treatment for a patient. The search always begins within the family, specifically looking for genotypic HLA-identical siblings. When siblings are available for a patient, the statistical probability that one of the siblings is genotypically HLA identical is 25%. If none is available, other available family members, such as parents, aunts, and uncles, are HLA typed to determine whether fortuitously shared haplotypes or haplotypes with a single mismatch occur within the family. The probability of finding compatible, nonsibling related donors varies among different populations, depending on the relative genetic homogeneity of the population. For example, recurring haplotypes that are common in Dutch, Vietnamese, or Finnish populations, to name a few, increase the likelihood of finding HLA-compatible nonsibling family members.[78] The overall chance of finding an HLA-compatible family member in the United States is approximately

33%.[79] Low-resolution typing by serology or equivalent DNA-based procedures is usually adequate to select donors from within a family if all four parental haplotypes are clearly distinguishable within the family. If assignment of haplotypes is ambiguous because of shared parental antigens or apparent homozygosity in a parent, higher resolution typing may be warranted to resolve the ambiguity.

When a suitable donor cannot be found within the family, a search is initiated through the NMDP or other national registries for an acceptable donor.[80] Before initiation of a formal search, the patient's HLA-DRB1 alleles should be identified using high-resolution, DNA-based typing. As previously noted, in the selection of related donors ethnicity-specific haplotypes are common, and this becomes even more apparent when allele-level matching is performed. Thus, the best opportunity to find a compatible unrelated donor for a patient is to search among potential donors of similar genetic or ethnic background. Some of the most difficult matching searches are for patients whose parents each came from a distinct ethnic background because one of the haplotypes is usually uncommon in potential donors searched for either ethnic population (see Table 7.2).

Criteria for determining an acceptable HLA match or mismatch when using unrelated donor stem cells are still evolving and will be influenced by other developing technologies of immunosuppression and management. Intuitively, it would make sense to match alleles at all of the HLA loci, mimicking as much as possible the HLA-identical sibling. Practically, this is not often possible. Currently, the NMDP requires, at a minimum, that a prospective recipient is typed by low-resolution (antigen-level) HLA-A, -B, -DQ, and -DR51, -52, or -53 typing and high-resolution (allele-level) HLA-DRB1 typing. New studies indicate that class I incompatibility at the allele level may be an equally important determinant of graft-versus-host disease.[81] A retrospective study of NMDP transplants is in progress to answer this important question. The role of allele-level DQ matching[82] in HSCT is still controversial. It has been particularly difficult to study the relative roles of DQ and DRB1 allelic incompatibility independently because of the strong linkage that exists between the two loci.

Platelet Transfusion

Thrombocytopenic patients who receive repetitive blood or platelet transfusions may become immunized to alloantigens present on the platelet membranes. The major alloantigen systems of platelets include platelet-specific, ABO system, and HLA class I antigens. The most common cause of immunological refractoriness to platelet transfusion is alloimmunization to HLA antigens. Most of the described platelet-specific antigen systems are encoded by loci with two major alleles (diallelic), and one of the alleles is expressed in the population at high frequency. For example, the phenotypic frequency of the HPA-1 (P1^{A1}) gene is about 97%.[83] These antigens are quite immunogenic and can induce antibodies that destroy transfused platelets. However, they are not a major cause of platelet refractoriness simply because the number of potentially incompatible patients is small.

Routine use of leukoreduced blood products has significantly decreased the overall rate of HLA alloimmunization from as high as 50% to 15% to 20% of multiply transfused patients.[66] Many of the patients who are alloimmunized or become alloimmunized after blood product transfusions are multiparous women, and it is probable that there will always be a low percentage of patients who are alloimmunized to HLA despite the use of filters or ultraviolet irradiation of platelet products.

No single strategy has emerged among transfusion centers for provision of HLA-compatible platelet transfusions to immunologically refractory thrombocytopenic patients. Patients who are immunologically refractory generally have a few broadly reactive antibodies against public epitopes of HLA class I molecules.[84–86] Hence, the effort of a blood center to provide the best matched product is often in vain because best matched usually means one or two incompatibilities. In patients with broadly reactive antibodies that react with up to 90% of donors, the odds of the best matched product providing effective hemostasis are extremely low (see the following).

Two general approaches can be employed to provide compatible single-donor platelets to refractory thrombocytopenic patients. One approach is to crossmatch every prospective donor with the patient's serum and select only crossmatch-negative donors. Platelets from crossmatch-negative donors are effective in 70% to 80% of cases.[87–90] Moreover, HLA typing is not required if crossmatching is the only criterion for donor selection. However, crossmatching alone is not always practical. Many of the alloimmunized patients have HLA antibodies that react with more than 90% of the random population. For a patient reactive with 95% of the population, a minimum of 20 donors would have to be crossmatched to find one who is compatible. Thus, both crossmatching and HLA-based selection have a role in the treatment of immunologically refractory patients. The most cost-effective method depends on the degree of sensitization of the patient, the availability of HLA-typed platelet donors, and the skill of the HLA laboratory in identifying HLA antibody specificities.

The literature describing the results of crossmatch studies for platelet transfusion in relation to techniques and choice of donor target cells is confusing and occasionally misleading. Intuitively, one would choose platelets as the logical target cell because they bear both HLA class I and platelet-specific targets. However, the density of HLA class I antigens on lymphocytes is much higher than on platelets, making lymphocytes more sensitive targets for HLA class I antibody detection. Because the major cause of platelet refractoriness is HLA antibody, the lymphocyte is a more suitable target for detecting HLA antibodies. Unfortunately, lymphocyte crossmatching is reported to be less predictive of good platelet transfusion responses than platelet crossmatching because virtually all of the comparative studies chose the least sensitive lymphocytotoxic crossmatch assay (CDC) and compared it with one of the most sensitive clinical platelet assays (indirect binding). Thus, many low-level HLA antibodies have been called platelet-specific antibodies because CDC reactivity was negative.

A second approach is to select donors on the basis of HLA types supplemented with knowledge of HLA antibody specificities the refractory patient has developed (Table 7.4). Donors matched for HLA private and public epitopes would be ideal, but such donors are rarely available because of HLA polymorphism. Matching donors for the 9 major CREGs or 15 major public epitopes greatly extends the use of the donor file and provides a reasonable number of compatible donors because most of the antibodies responsible for HLA refractoriness are directed against the public epitopes.

When matched products are no longer available, donor selection is based on *selective mismatching*, that is, choosing HLA antigen mismatches to which the patient is not yet alloimmunized. For example, a patient with antibodies reactive with 95% of donors has potentially 100 compatible donors available in a donor file of 2000. The challenge is knowing how to identify the compatible donors without resorting to wholesale crossmatching. Knowledge of the HLA specificity of antibodies in the patient's serum is critical for the rational selection of mismatched donors. A patient with a defined antibody to the Bw6 public epitope, for example,

Table 7.4   Search Strategy for Potential HLA-Typed Platelet Donors That Includes Analyses of Public Epitopes and Antibodies to Public Epitopes

Data Needed for Search

Recipient phenotype (based on private epitopes): A1,3,B8,27
Recipient phenotype (based on public epitopes); 1C,–,7C,8C,4C,6C (see Table 7.3)
Recipient serum analysis: anti-2C (A2,28,9,B17) HLA antibodies detected
  Prioritized donor search
    HLA match
    HLA compatible*
    HLA public match[†]
    Permissible mismatch[‡]
    Random crossmatching

Acceptable Donor Phenotype(s) for:

HLA match: A1,3,B8,27
HLA compatible: Any donor with one or two blanks in the phenotype, e.g., A1,–;B8,–
HLA public match: Any donor with no public epitope incompatibilities
Permissible mismatch: Any donor lacking the 2C public epitope
Random crossmatching: Any crossmatch-negative donor[§]

*Platelet donor has "blanks" in phenotype because of either homozygosity or rare HLA alleles.
[†]Donor phenotype usually contains mismatched private epitopes, previously referred to as cross-reactive mismatching.
[‡]Selection requires careful analysis of recipient serum for HLA alloantibodies.
[§]No evidence of donor-specific HLA or platelet antibodies in recipient serum.
HLA, human leukocyte antigin.

requires a donor who is Bw6 negative. Providing reasonably accurate HLA specificity analysis requires use of either the AHG-CDC or newer solid-phase immunoassays. Standard CDC and indirect binding to platelets are not sufficiently sensitive procedures. Software-based HLA specificity analysis programs that are supplied with the commercial immunoassays must be interpreted with caution as they are not always accurate, especially in highly reactive antisera. The user must know how to assess the reactivity patterns manually under these conditions.

Finally, immunologically refractory patients who do not achieve good responses to platelets from donors selected by all available criteria may be alloimmunized to non-HLA antigens. For these patients, crossmatching is the best method of selection and donor platelets might be the most appropriate crossmatch target cell because platelet-specific antigens might also be detected.

■ Neutrophil Antigens and Antibodies

Antibodies against neutrophil-associated polymorphic antigens are responsible for transfusion reactions and several neutropenic disorders. The definitions of neutrophil-specific and HLA alloantibodies are historically and etiologically interwoven. Both were originally detected by leukoagglutination techniques, and both types of antibodies were induced as a consequence of alloimmunization by repetitive blood transfusion or pregnancy.[91-94] Thus, neutrophil-specific alloantisera often contained HLA alloantibodies as well. Lalezari and colleagues[95] defined one of the first neutrophil-specific antigen systems in a neonate with transient neutropenia and clearly separated it from HLA.

Antibody-mediated neutropenias and transfusion reactions caused by neutrophil-associated antibodies are relatively uncommon. Some immunologically mediated neutrophil syndromes can be fatal, but they are potentially preventable with appropriate screening programs. Unfortunately, the cost of performing these labor-intensive procedures is high. This high cost, a general lack of good reagents for many specificities, and the inherent biological variation of neutrophils as antibody targets currently preclude routine neutrophil antibody screening of blood donors or expectant mothers. New PCR-based assays and direct sequencing of molecules that bear the neutrophil-associated epitopes have accelerated the genetic definition of these specificities. Detection of many

antineutrophil antibodies is becoming more cost-effective as solid-phase immunoassays and flow cytometric procedures are employed. Therefore, routine screening of high-risk patients could be possible in the next few years.

Neutrophil Alloantigens

Neutrophil-specific antigens were first recognized as a cause of self-limited neutropenia in neonates. Maternal antibodies, developed as a consequence of incompatible fetal neutrophil antigens, were then passively transferred to the neonate. The alloepitopes responsible for the neutrophil-associated specificities are located on several distinct membrane proteins, which are discussed in the following. Several neutrophil specificities are not discussed because they are incompletely characterized or antisera are not available for study. These include ND1, NE1, and NC1 (the latter subsequently was shown to be identical to NA2).

Nomenclature

A standardized nomenclature was agreed upon and recommended by the Granulocyte Antigen Working Party of the International Society of Blood Transfusion and is summarized in Table 7.5.[95] Two discrete segregant series of neutrophil-specific antigens have been described: NA and NB. Three alleles are recognized for the NA series (NA1, NA2, and SH) and two for the NB series (NB1, NB2). NA antigens have been identified as epitopes located on the Fc γ receptor IIIb (FcγRIIIb) of the neutrophil.[96, 97] However, the location of the NB antigens is still not known. Additional antigen systems that are shared by neutrophils and other leukocytes include MART and OND, which are found on CD11b and CD11a components, respectively, of β_2 integrins.[98, 99] Also, a poorly characterized group (5c), reported by van Rood and colleagues[100] during the 1960s, is found on leukocytes.[101] HLA, ABO, and Ii are other widely distributed antigens that are also found on neutrophils. The density of HLA molecules on neutrophils is fairly low, so they are not a good target choice for detecting HLA antibodies. The approximate phenotypic frequencies of the antigens are NA1, 46%; NA2, 88%; SH, 5%; NB1, 97%; and NB2, 32%. There are reports describing individuals who express NA1, NA2, and SH, suggesting that in some individuals SH may not be an allele of the NA series but a product of a locus closely linked to NA1, perhaps through gene duplication.[102]

Table 7.5 Human Neutrophil Antigen Nomenclature

Antigen System	Antigen	Location	Previous Name	Alleles	Frequency (%)		
					Whites	Asians	Blacks
HNA-1	HNA-1a	FcγRIIIb	NA1	FCGR3B*1	58	89	68
	HNA-1b	FcγRIIIb	NA2	FCGR3B*2	88	51	78
	HNA-1c	FcγRIIIb	SH	FCGR3B*3	5	ND	38
HNA-2	HNA-2a	gp50–64	NB1	Not defined	97	88–99	ND
HNA-3	HNA-3a	gp70–95	5b	Not defined	97		
HNA-4	HNA-4a	CD11b	MART	CD11B*1	99		
HNA-5	HNA-5a	CD11a	OND	CD11A*1	96		

ND, not determined.
Modified from Bux J: Nomenclature of granulocyte alloantigens. ISBT Working Party on Platelet and Granulocyte Serology, Granulocyte Antigen Working Party. International Society of Blood Transfusion. Transfusion 1999;39:662.

The Neutrophil Fc γ Receptor (NA1, NA2, SH)

The NA series of antigens are epitopes that occur on the neutrophil FcγRIIIb. This low-affinity receptor binds the Fc region of immunoglobulin G (IgG) molecules that are complexed to specific antigens or other immunoglobulins. FcγRIIIb does not bind native monomeric IgG with significant affinity. The molecules are glycosyl phosphatidylinositol (GPI)-anchored glycoproteins that are shed into plasma during neutrophil activation or apoptosis.[103] The locus encoding this gene product is located on chromosome 1. Structurally, it is a member of the Ig superfamily of glycoproteins. Allelic gene products bearing the NA1 or NA2 serologically defined epitopes differ by five nucleotides and also differ in molecular weight because of glycosylation differences. FcγRIIIb is also called CD16. Approximately 0.1% of European caucasoids do not express FcgRIIIb and, predictably, do not express the NA1 or NA2 specificities.[104, 105] The phenotype is referred to as NA null. A third serologically defined specificity, SH, located on the FcγRIIIb molecule has been described and confirmed. It is thought to represent a molecular variant of the NA2-bearing FcγRIIIb.[97]

β₂ Integrins (MART and LAN)

Integrins are a large family of adhesion receptors.[106] The receptors and their ligands are essential for effective trafficking of neutrophils out of the circulation and into sites of inflammation. Each integrin is a heterodimer of two noncovalently associated proteins, α and β. There are approximately 11 distinct α chains and five distinct β chains. Different combinations of the α and β chains provide about 15 distinct integrins. MART is an epitope on the α (CD11a) chain of CD11a/CD18 (the LFA-I molecule). OND is an epitope on the α chain (CD11b) of the CD11b/CD18 (complement receptor 3 or CR3 receptor) whose ligands are C3bi, factor X, and fibrinogen. Phenotypic frequencies of the epitopes are shown in Table 7.5

■ Methods of Alloantibody Detection

The most common current techniques for detecting neutrophil and granulocyte alloantibodies are leukoagglutination (NA1, NA2, NB1, SH, MART, OND, and 5b) and indirect immunofluorescence (all but 5b).[107] A newer procedure that is becoming more widely available is monoclonal antibody immobilization of granulocyte antigen.[108] In general, the detection of neutrophil-specific antigens and alloantibodies is still performed primarily in reference laboratories.

■ Clinical Applications of Granulocyte Antigens and Antibodies

The major clinical applications of granulocyte antigen and alloantibody detection are in cases of neonatal neutropenia and in transfusion-related acute lung injury (TRALI). Both conditions are uncommon but potentially fatal.

Alloimmune Neonatal Neutropenia

Alloimmune neonatal neutropenia (ANN) is caused by maternal alloantibodies induced by incompatible neutrophil-specific antigens of the fetus.[94, 109–111] The most common causes of ANN are antibodies directed against NA1 (34%), NB1 (13%), and NA2 (12%). The neonate has a specific deficiency of mature neutrophils because these antigens are not expressed on neutrophil precursors. Neutropenia lasts for 2 weeks to as long as 6 months, depending on how quickly the antibodies are eliminated. The etiologic diagnosis is based on typing neutrophil-specific antigens in mother and child and identifying a specific antibody in the mother's blood.

Febrile Transfusion Reactions and Granulocyte Transfusions

Febrile transfusion reactions were not uncommon when blood transfusions were given as whole blood. Febrile reactions can have multiple etiologies. They may be caused by the release of proinflammatory cytokines into the plasma of stored blood products,[112, 113] may be components of allergic reactions, and may be a consequence of HLA or other alloantibodies against antigens of the transfused product.[113, 113a] The occurrence of febrile reactions has been significantly reduced through the routine use of packed red blood cells and leukoreduced blood products.

Granulocyte transfusions are still given to selected patients with neutropenia because of impaired bone marrow production, often as a result of HSCT. In these circumstances, it is critical that patients are tested for the presence of HLA- and granulocyte-specific antibodies. The presence of incompatibilities can cause febrile reactions, TRALI, and poor incremental responses to the product.

Transfusion-Related Acute Lung Injury

This uncommon but potentially fatal reaction is usually due to the presence of a high-titer, antileukocyte antibody in donor plasma. The specificity of antibodies includes HLA and most of the specificities described in Table 7.5.[114–117] The syndrome is characterized by the onset of acute respiratory distress related to pulmonary edema caused by acute inflammatory reactions within the lung. The occurrence of this type of reaction has prompted several investigators to recommend routine screening of multiparous blood donors for anti-HLA and antineutrophil antibodies. The cost of such screening, however, is prohibitive in most centers. Alternatively, multiparous blood donor products could be used for preparing only blood products that do not contain significant amounts of plasma.

REFERENCES

1. Little CC: The genetics of tumor transplantation. In Snell GD (ed): Biology of the Laboratory Mouse. Philadelphia, Blakiston, 1941; pp 106–111.
2. Gorer PA: The detection of antigenic differences in mouse erythrocytes by employment of immune sera. Br J Exp Pathol 1936;17:42.
3. Snell GD: Methods for the study of histocompatibility genes. Genetics 1948;49:87.
4. Gorer PA, Lyman S, Snell GD: Studies on the genetic and antigenic basis of tumor transplant linkage between a histocompatibility gene and "fused" in mice. Proc R Soc Lond 1948;135:499.
5. Campbell RD, Trowsdale J: Map of the human MHC. Immunol Today 1993;14:349.
6. Bodmer JG, Marsh SGE, Albert ED, et al: Nomenclature for factors of the HLA system, 1998. Tissue Antigens 1999;53:407.
7. Bodmer WF, Albert E, Bodmer JG, et al: Nomenclature for factors of the HLA system, 1987. In Dupont B (ed): Immunobiology of HLA. New York, Springer-Verlag, 1989, p 72.
8. Goodfellow PW, Jones EA, van Hegringen J, et al: The β-2 microglobulin gene is in chromosome 15 and not in the HL-A region. Nature 1975;254:267.
9. Trowsdale J, Hanson I, Mockridge I, et al: Sequences encoded in the class 11 region of the MHC related to the "ABC" superfamily of transporters. Nature 1990;348:741.

10. Glynne R, Powis SH, Beck S, et al: A proteasome-related gene between the two ABC transporter loci in the class II region of the human MHC. Nature 1991;353:357.

11. Whitehead AS, Truedsson L, Schneider PM, et al: The distribution of human C4 DNA variants in relation to major histocompatibility complex alleles and extended haplotypes. Hum Immunol 1988;21:23.

12. Skoskiewicz MJ, Colvin RB, Schneeberger EE, Russell PS: Widespread and selective induction of major histocompatibility complex–determined antigens in vivo by γ-interferon. J Exp Med 1985;162:645.

13. Morton JA, Pickles MM, Sutton L: The correlation of Bga blood group with the HLA-A7 leukocyte group: demonstration of antigenic sites on red cells and leukocytes. Vox Sang 1971;17:536.

14. McDevitt HO, Chinitz A: Genetic control of the antibody response: relationship between immune response and histocompatibility (H-2) type. Science 1969;163:1207.

15. Green I, Paul WE, Benacerraf B: Genetic control of immunological responsiveness in guinea pigs to 2,4 dinitrophenol conjugates of poly-L-arginine, protamine, and poly-L-ornithine. Proc Natl Acad Sci USA 1969;64:1095.

16. Kindred B, Shreffler DC: H-2 dependence of co-operation between T and B cells in vivo. J Immunol 1972;109:940.

17. Zinkernagel RM, Doherty PC: Restriction of in vitro T cell–mediated cytotoxicity in lymphocytic choriomeningitis within a syngeneic or semiallogeneic system. Nature 1974;48:701.

18. Sebzda E, Mariathasan S, Ohteki T, et al: Selection of the T cell repertoire. Annu Rev Immunol 1999;17:829.

19. Rammensee H-G, Bachmann J, Stevanovic S: MHC Ligands and Peptide Motifs. Austin, Tex, Landes Bioscience, 1997.

20. Watts C: Capture and processing of exogenous antigens for presentation on MHC molecules. Annu Rev Immunol 1997;15:821.

21. Pamer E, Cresswell P: Mechanisms of MHC class I–restricted antigen processing. Annu Rev Immunol 1998;16:323.

22. Ljunggren HG, Karre K: In search of the "missing self": MHC molecules and NK recognition. Immunol Today 1990;11:7.

23. Lanier L: NK cell receptors. Annu Rev Immunol 1998;6:359.

24. Shimizu Y, DeMars R: Demonstration by class I gene transfer that reduced susceptibility of human cells to natural killer cell–mediated lysis is inversely correlated with HLA class I antigen expression. Eur J Immunol 1989;19:447.

25. Storkus WJ, Howell DN, Salter RD, et al: NK susceptibility varies inversely with target cell class I HLA antigen expression. J Immunol 1987;138:657.

26. Storkus WJ, Alexander J, Payne JA, et al: Reversal of natural killing susceptibility in target cells expressing transfected class I HLA genes. Proc Natl Acad Sci USA 1989;86:2361.

27. Vyas Y, Selvakumar A, Steffens U, Dupont B: Multiple transcripts of the killer cell immunoglobulin-like receptor family, KIR3DL1 (NKB1), are expressed by natural killer cells of a single individual. Tissue Antigens 1998;52:510.

28. Lano M, Lee N, Navarro F, et al: HLA-E bound peptides influence recognition by inhibitory and triggering CD94/NKG2 receptors: preferential response to an HLA-G–derived nonamer. Eur J Immunol 1998;28:2854.

29. Leibson PJ: Cytotoxic lymphocyte recognition of HLA-E: utilizing a nonclassical window to peer into classical MHC. Immunity 1998;9:289.

30. Yamazaki K, Boyse EA, Mike V, et al: Control of mating preferences in mice by genes in the major histocompatibility complex. J Exp Med 1976;144:1324.

31. Yamazaki M, Yamazaki K, Beauchamp GK, et al: Distinctive urinary odors governed by the major histocompatibility locus of the mouse. Proc Natl Acad Sci USA 1981;78:5815.

32. Penn D, Potts W: How do major histocompatibility complex genes influence odor and mating preferences? Adv Immunol 1999;69:411.

33. Wedekind C, Seebeck T, Bettens F, Paepke A: MHC-dependent mate preferences in humans. Proc R Soc Lond B Biol Sci 1995;360:245.

34. Wedekind C, Furi S: Body odour preferences in men and women: do they aim for specific MHC combinations or simply heterozygosity? Proc R Soc Lond B Biol Sci 1997;264:1471.

35. Parham P, Lomen CE, Lawlor DA, et al: Nature of polymorphism in HLA-A, -B, and -C molecules. Proc Natl Acad Sci USA 1988;85:4005.

36. Bjorkman PJ, Saper MA, Samraoui B, et al: Structure of the HLA class I histocompatibility antigen, HLA-A2. Nature 1987;329:506.

37. Bjorkman PJ, Saper MA, Samraoui B, et al: The foreign antigen binding site and T cell recognition regions of class I histocompatibility antigens. Nature 1987;329:512.

38. Brown JH, Jardetzky TS, Gorga JC, et al: Three-dimensional structure of the human class II histocompatibility antigen HLA-DR1. Nature 1993;364:33.

39. Mason PM, Parham P: HLA class I region sequences, 1998. Tissue Antigens 1998;51:417.

40. Marsh SGE: HLA class II region sequences, 1998. Tissue Antigens 1998;51:467.

41. Rosenstein Y, Ratnofsky S, Burakoff SJ, Herrmann SH: Direct evidence for binding of CD8 to HLA class I antigens. J Exp Med 1989;169:149.

42. Doyle C, Strominger JL: Interaction between CD4 and class II MHC molecules mediates cell adhesion. Nature 1988;330:256.

43. Pfeifer JD, Wick MJ, Roberts RL, et al: Phagocytic processing of bacterial antigens for class I MHC presentation to T cells. Nature 1993;361:359.

44. David V, Hochstenbach F, Ragagopalan S, Brenner MB: Interaction with newly synthesized and retained proteins in the endoplasmic reticulum suggests a chaperone function for human integral membrane protein IP90 (calnexin). J Biol Chem 1993;268:9585.

45. Vassilakos A, Cohen-Doyle MF, Peterson PA, et al: The molecular chaperone calnexin facilitates folding and assembly of class I histocompatibility molecules. EMBO J 1996;15:1495.

46. Sadasivan B, Lehner PJ, Ortmann B, et al: Roles for calreticulin and a novel glycoprotein, tapasin, in the interaction of MHC class I molecules with TAP. Immunity 1996;5:103.

47. Peters PJ, Neefjes JJ, Oorschot V, et al: Segregation of MHC class II molecules from MHC class I molecules in the Golgi complex for transport to lysosomal compartments. Nature 1991;349:669.

48. Pieters J, Horstmann H, Bakke O, et al: Intracellular transport and localization of major histocompatibility complex class II molecules and associated invariant chain. J Cell Biol 1991;115:1213.

49. Lamb CA, Cresswell P: Assembly and transport properties of invariant chain trimers and HLA-DR–invariant chain complexes. J Immunol 1992;148:3478.

50. Cresswell P: Invariant chain structure and MHC class II function. Cell 1996;84:505.

51. Riberdy JM, Newcomb JR, Surman MJ, et al: HLA-DR molecules from an antigen-processing mutant cell line are associated with invariant chain peptides. Nature 1992;360:474.

52. Romagnoli P, Germain RN: The CLIP region of invariant chain plays a critical role in regulating major histocompatibility complex class II folding, transport, and peptide occupancy. J Exp Med 1994; 180:1107.

53. Morris P, Shaman J, Attaya M, et al: An essential role for HLA-DM in antigen presentation by class II major histocompatibility molecules. Nature 1994;368:551.

54. Denzin LK, Robbins NF, Carboy-Newcomb C, Cresswell P: Assembly and intracellular transport of HLA-DM and correction of the class II antigen-processing defect in T2 cells. Immunity 1994;1:595.

55. Denzin LK, Cresswell P: HLA-DM induces CLIP dissociation from MHC class II alpha beta dimers and facilitates peptide loading. Cell 1995;82:155.

56. Sloan VS, Cameron P, Porter G, et al: Mediation by HLA-DM of dissociation of peptides from HLA-DR. Nature 1995;375:802.

57. Sanderson F, Kleijmeer MJ, Kelly A, et al: Accumulation of HLA-DM, a regulator of antigen presentation, in MHC class II compartments. Science 1994;266:1566.

58. Liljedahl M, Kuwana T, Fung-Leung WP, et al: HLA-DO is a lysosomal resident which requires an association with HLA-DM for efficient intracellular transport. EMBO J 1996;15:4817.

59. Denzin LK, Sant'Angelo DB, Hammond C, et al: Negative regulation by DO of MHC class II–restricted antigen processing. Science 1997;278:106.

60. Schlossman SF, Yaron A, Ben-Efraim S, Sober HA: Immunogenicity of a series of α, N-DNP-L lysines. Biochemistry 1967;4:168.

61. Rodey GE, Fuller TC: Public epitopes and the antigenic structure of HLA molecules. Crit Rev Immunol 1987;7:229.

62. Wan AM, Ennis P, Parham P, Holmes N: The primary structure of HLA-A32 suggests a region involved in formation of the Bw4/Bw6 epitopes. J Immunol 1986;137:3671.

63. Fuller AA, Trevithick JE, Rodey GE, et al: Topographic map of the HLA-A2 CREG epitopes using human alloantibody probes. Hum Immunol 1990;28:284.

64. Fuller AA, Rodey GE, Parham P, Fuller TC: Epitope map of the HLA-B7 CREG using affinity-purified human alloantibody probes. Hum Immunol 1990;28:306.

65. Scornik JC, Ireland JE, Howard RJ, Pfaff WW: Assessment of the risk for broad sensitization by blood transfusions. Transplantation 1984;37:249.

66. Slichter S, Schiffer C, McFarland J, et al: Trial to reduce alloimmunization to platelet transfusion (TRAP): a controlled, prospective comparison of leukocyte-reduction, UV-B-irradiation, and single donor apheresis products to control random pooled platelets. N Engl J Med 1998;337:1861.

67. Gray D, Skarvall H: B cell memory is short-lived in the absence of antigen. Nature 1988;360:336.

68. Szakal AK, Kosco MH, Tew JG: Microanatomy of lymphoid tissue during humoral immune responses: structure function relationships. Annu Rev Immunol 1989;7:91.

69. Germain RN: Antigen processing and presentation. In Paul WE (ed): Fundamental Immunology. Philadelphia, Lippincott-Raven, 1999, p 27.

70. van Oers MHJ, Pinkster J, Zeijlemaker WP: Quantification of antigen-reactive cells among human T lymphocytes. Eur J Immunol 1978;8:477.

71. Singal DP: Quantitative studies of alloantigen-reactive human lymphocytes in primary and secondary MLC. Hum Immunol 1980;1:67.

72. Fangmann J, Dalchau R, Fabre JW: Rejection of skin allografts by indirect allorecognition of donor class I major histocompatibility complex peptides. J Exp Med 1992;175:1521.

73. Benichou G: Direct and indirect antigen recognition: the pathways to allograft immune rejection. Front Biosci 1999;4:476.

74. Terasaki PI, McClelland JD: Microdroplet assay of human serum cytotoxins. Nature 1964;204:998.

75. Olerup O, Zetterquist H: HLA-DR typing by PCR amplification with sequence-specific primers (PCR-SSP) in 2 hours: an alternative to serological DR typing in clinical practice including donor-recipient matching in cadaveric transplantation. Tissue Antigens 1992;39:225.

76. Mach B, Tiercy J-M: Genotypic typing of HLA class II: from the bench to the bedside. Hum Immunol 1991;30:278.

77. Lazda VA, Pollak R, Mozes MF, Jonasson O: The relationship between flow cytometer crossmatch results and subsequent rejection episodes in cadaver renal allograft recipients. Transplantation 1988;45:562.

78. Partanen J, Koskimies S: HLA DQ and DP locus mismatches and their effect on MLC in HLA class I- and DRB1-matched unrelated patient/donor pairs waiting for allogeneic bone-marrow transplantation. Scand J Immunol 1994;39:301.

79. Beatty PG, Mori M, Milford E: Impact of racial genetic polymorphism on the probability of finding an HLA-matched donor. Transplantation 1995;60:778.

80. Beatty PG, Kollman C, Howe CW: Unrelated-donor marrow transplants: the experience of the National Marrow Donor Program. Clin Transpl 1995;4:271.

81. Sasazuki T, Juji T, Morishima Y, et al: Effect of matching of class I HLA alleles on clinical outcome after transplantation of hematopoietic stem cells from an unrelated donor. Japan Marrow Donor Program. N Engl J Med 1998;339:1177.

82. Petersdorf EW, Longton GM, Anasetti C, et al: Definition of HLA-DQ as a transplantation antigen. Proc Natl Acad Sci USA 1996;93:15358.

83. Kunicki TJ: Human platelet antigens. In Hoffman R, Benz EJ, Shattil SJ, et al (eds): Hematology. Basic Principles and Practice. New York, Churchill Livingstone, 1995, p 1961.

84. Lobo PI: Development of anti-HLA antibodies following renal transplantation—their characteristics and natural history. Tissue Antigens 1982;19:356.

85. Oldfather JW, Anderson CB, Phelan DL, et al: Prediction of crossmatch outcome in highly sensitized patients based on the identification of serum HLA antibodies. Transplantation 1986;43:267.

86. Rodey GE, Neylan JF, Whelchel JD, et al: The epitope specificity of HLA class I alloantibodies. I. Frequency analysis of antibodies to private versus public specificities in potential transplant recipients. Hum Immunol 1994;39:272.

87. Freedman J, Hooi C, Garvey MB: Prospective platelet crossmatching for selection of random compatible donors. Br J Haematol 1984;56:9.

88. MacPherson BR, Hammond PB, Maniscalco CA: Alloimmunization to public HLA antigens in multi-transfused platelet recipients. Ann Clin Lab Sci 1986;16:38.

89. Kickler TS, Nedd PM, Braine HG: Platelet crossmatching. A direct approach to the selection of platelet transfusions for the alloimmunized thrombocytopenic patient. Am J Clin Pathol 1988;90:69.

90. Rachel JM, Summers TC, Sinor LT, Plapp FV: Use of a solid phase red cell adherence method for pretransfusion platelet compatibility testing. Am J Clin Pathol 1988;90:63.

91. Dausset J, Nenna A: Présence d'une leuco-agglutinine dans le sérum d'un cas d'agranulocytose chronique. C R Soc Biol 1952;146:1539.

92. Moeschlin S, Wagner K: Agranulocytosis due to the occurrence of leukocyte agglutinins (pyramidon and cold agglutinins). Acta Haematol 1952;8:29.

93. Payne R, Rolfs MR: Fetomaternal leukocyte incompatibility. J Clin Invest 1958;37:1756.

94. van Rood JJ, van Leeuwen A, Ernisse JG: Leukocyte antibodies in sera of pregnant women. Vox Sang 1959;4:427.

95. Lalezari P, Nuasbaum M, Gelman S, Spaet TH: Neonatal neutropenia due to maternal isoimmunization. Blood 1960;15:236.

96. Bux J: Nomenclature of granulocyte alloantigens. ISBT Working Party on Platelet and Granulocyte Serology, Granulocyte Antigen Working Party. International Society of Blood Transfusion. Transfusion 1999;39:662.

97. Ory PA, Clark MR, Kwoh EE, et al: Sequences of complementary DNAs that encode NA1 and NA2 forms of Fc receptor III on human neutrophils. J Clin Invest 1989;84:1688.

98. Bux J, Stein EL, Bierling P, et al: Characterization of a new alloantigen (SH) on the human neutrophil Fcγ receptor IIIb. Blood 1997;89:1027.

99. Kline WE, Press C, Clay M, et al: Three sera defining a new granulocyte-monocyte-T-lymphocyte antigen. Vox Sang 1986;50:181.

100. Simsek S, van den Schoot CE, Daams M, et al: Molecular characterization of antigenic polymorphisms (Ond^a and Mart^a) of the β_2 family recognized by human leukocyte alloantisera. Blood 1996;88:1350.

101. van Leeuwen A, Eernise JG, van Rood JJ: A new leukocyte group with two alleles: leukocyte group five. Vox Sang 1964;9:431.

102. Lalezari F, Bernard GE: Identification of a specific leukocyte antigen, another presumed example of 5b. Transfusion 1965;5:135.

103. Koene HR, Kleijer M, Roos D, et al: Fc gamma RIIIB gene duplication: evidence for presence and expression of three distinct Fc gamma RIIIB genes in NA(1+,2+)SH(+) individuals. Blood 1998;91:673.

104. Huizinga TWJ, Shoot E, van der Jost G, et al: PI-linked receptor FcRIII is released on stimulation of neutrophils. Nature 1988;333:667.

105. Frormont P, Bettaieb A, Skouri H, et al: Frequency of the PMN-FcRIII deficiency in the French population and its involvement in the development of neonatal alloimmune neutropenia. Blood 1992;79:2131.

106. Flesch BK, Achtert G, Bauer F, Neppert J: The NA "null" phenotype of a young man is caused by an Fc gammaRIIB gene deficiency while the products of the neighboring Fc gammaRIIA and Fc gammaRIIIA genes are present. Ann Hematol 1998;76:215.

107. Bluestone JA, Khattri R, van Seventer GA: Accessory molecules. In Paul WE (ed): Fundamental Immunology. Philadelphia, Lippincott-Raven, 1999, p 449.

108. Verheugt FWA, Von dem Borne AE, Decary F, Engelfriet CP: The detection of granulocyte alloantibodies with an indirect immunofluorescence test. Br J Haematol 1977;36:533.

109. Bux J, Kober B, Kiefel V, Mueller-Eckhardt C: Analysis of granulocyte reactive antibodies using an immunoassay based upon monoclonal-antibody-specific immobilization of granulocyte antigens. Transfus Med 1993;3:157.

110. Lalezari P, Bernard GE: An isologous antigen-antibody reaction with human neutrophils related to neonatal neutropenia. J Clin Invest 1966;45:1741.

111. Lalezari P, Murphy GB, Allen FH: NB1, a new neutrophil antigen involved in the pathogenesis of neonatal neutropenia. J Clin Invest 1971;50:1108.

112. Levine DH, Madyastha P, Wade R, Levkoff AH: Neonatal isoimmune neutropenia. Pediatr Res 1981;15:296a.

113. Federowicz I, Barren BB, Anderson JW, et al: Characterization of reactions after transfusion of exclusively pre-storage leukoreduced cellular blood components. Transfusion 1996;36:21.

113a. Brubaker DB: Clinical significance of white cell antibodies in febrile nonhemolytic transfusion reactions. Transfusion 1990; 8:733.

114. Densmore TL, Goodnough LT, Ali S, et al: Prevalence of HLA sensitization in female apheresis donors. Transfusion 1999;39:103.

115. Bux J, Becker F, Seeger W, et al: Transfusion-related acute lung injury due to HLA-A2–specific antibodies in recipient and NBl-specific antibodies in donor blood. Br J Haematol 1996;93:707.

116. Santamaria A, Moya F, Martinez C, et al: Transfusion-related acute lung injury associated with an NA1-specific antigranulocyte antibody. Haematologica 1998;83:951.

117. Van Buren NL, Stroncek DF, Clay ME, et al: Transfusion-related acute lung injury caused by an NB2 granulocyte-specific antibody in a patient with thrombotic thrombocytopenic purpura. Transfusion 1990;30:42.

Chapter 8

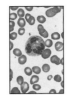

Blood Donation

Alfred J. Grindon
Bruce Newman

■ Donor Recruitment

Background

Approximately 8 million volunteers donate 1.6 times a year in the United States, producing 12.6 million units of whole blood. Of that total, almost 2% represent units that are directed for a specific recipient and 5% are autologous.[1] Of the total collected, approximately 11.5 million units of red blood cells are transfused.

There is a regular loss of donors from the donor pool. To keep the units collected constant, these lost donors must be replaced with first-time donors or the remaining donors must donate more frequently. The number of units from first-time donors typically ranges from 15% to 25% of the total. The number of potential first-time donors must be greater than the number of units actually drawn, tested, and placed into production because first-time donors are roughly twice as likely to have disqualifying medical conditions as regular donors.[2] Unit losses are greater when a unit is tested with a new infectious disease test or a new health history question is added to the donor screening system.

Generally, 60% of the adult population is eligible to give blood.[3] At present, it is estimated that 3% of the population of a given community donates 1.6 times within a given year. Annual blood donations, then, numerically represent about 5% of the total population. Because an increase of donations from 5% to 6% would increase the available blood by 20% and essentially eliminate the potential of blood shortages, an important goal is to determine the best systems for donor recruitment, donor retention, or increasing donation frequency.

Donor Recruitment

Ideally, immediately after collection, blood donors would schedule (and then keep) their next donation appointment.

This goal is not often realized. Many interrelated elements go into donor recruitment and retention, such as having a pleasant donation experience with recognition and thanks from the collection staff. However, recruitment professionals continue to seek the elements that have the most significant impact.

Survey work done in the 1970s showed that almost 50% of eligible donors had given blood in the past,[4] suggesting that there is no great need to educate the public about either the need for blood or the mechanics or ease of being a blood donor. Furthermore, approximately 25% of eligible donors had given blood within the past 4 years.[4] The two most important reasons these donors gave for dropping from the register of active donors were that blood donation was no longer convenient and that they were not personally asked to donate. Because donor retention is generally thought to be easier to achieve than recruitment of new donors, how might we address these issues?

Convenience is typically addressed by collecting at the school, business, or industry rather than having donors recruited to come to a fixed site. Alternatively, self-contained mobile units, typically of four- to six-bed capacity, can be sent for small donor groups. Despite the fact that it is generally more cost-effective to use fixed sites and donation hours at fixed sites can often be arranged to make donation more convenient, it has been found that collection in the evening or on weekends at a fixed site is less effective than collection at the workplace with the support of the employer. Intensive telerecruitment of repeat blood donors is usually necessary for a fixed site to be successful.

A typical successful method of donor recruitment is to have the center recruiter approach the leader of a business, school, or community (typically through volunteer blood center board members) and ask to have that group sponsor a blood drive. A senior executive is asked to chair the program by providing a personal message of support, hosting employee rallies, and designating an employee in each work group to serve as a recruiter. This employee should recruit each coworker in his or her group face to face, provide a specific appointment time for the donor, and remind the potential donor the day before or the day of the blood drive. The successful drive is followed by some sort of recognition of the organizers and donors by the company. When followed, these steps have almost always produced a successful and predictable blood drive. The challenges are obtaining donor group agreement to have a rally, finding sufficient employee recruiters, and having donors arrive at their scheduled time rather than having all donors arrive, for instance, at the lunch hour.

Donor Motivation

One approach to the recruitment of volunteer donors has been the concept of *individual responsibility*: patients and their families or friends are responsible for the procurement or replacement of transfused blood. Individuals could meet this responsibility either by seeing that blood was replaced by family or friends after transfusion or by giving regularly at the workplace, thereby ensuring the availability of blood for themselves and their families by accumulating blood "credits." Although this system required cumbersome tracking of blood credits, the major concern was that it sometimes put pressure to donate or replace blood on those least able to give. Subsequently, it was recognized that this pressure to replace blood was likely to increase first-time donors, who have higher deferral rates, higher unsuccessful phlebotomy rates, and higher positive test rates. A formal individual responsibility system has not been used in most parts of the United States for some years.

The current prevailing philosophy is one of *community responsibility*: everyone who can should give for the benefit of the community, and blood is available to anyone in need without the recipient incurring a recruitment burden.

Clearly, paying donors has been a successful motivator. However, with the growing recognition in the 1970s that paid donors had a greater likelihood of transmitting disease,[5] the use of blood from paid donors essentially ceased. This trend was reinforced when the Food and Drug Administration (FDA) in its Code of Federal Regulations (CFR) required blood to be labeled as either "volunteer" or "paid," the latter to indicate "a person who receives monetary payment for a blood donation."[6] A few small U.S. blood collection facilities today continue to pay donors, but these organizations have demonstrated that their donors have an infectious disease marker frequency similar to that of volunteer donors[7] and may have special procedures in place to use only repeat donors. Although payment has become an anomaly in whole blood or component collection, it is used regularly for the recruitment of donors of source plasma, intended for further manufacture into derivatives. Because the pooled plasma from these donations is subjected to procedures such as pasteurization, there is less concern about the potentially increased risk for infectious disease transmission from these derivatives as a result of using paid donors. Countries that have elected to have a volunteer plasma program have struggled, usually unsuccessfully, to meet their needs.[8]

If direct payment or blood insurance plans are not used, what serves to motivate blood donors? One would like to determine, if possible, why donors give so that they can be recruited and retained more effectively.[9] On the other hand, motivators must be minimal so that they do not serve to recruit those who should not give because their blood could be more dangerous to a recipient.

The issue of donor motivation has been an area of concern to the FDA and the American Association of Blood Banks (AABB). The CFR, in its definition of paid and volunteer donors,[6] states that "Benefits, such as time off from work, membership in blood assurance programs and cancellation of non-replacement fees that are not readily convertible to cash, do not constitute payment within the meaning of this paragraph."

The AABB has listed the items that its membership felt represented compensation or inducements, those that did not, and the strategies for which general agreement could not be reached (Table 8.1).[10] Where gifts or items of recognition are given, it is best, to the extent possible, to give them for coming to the blood drive and not as a condition of donation.

Another potential inappropriate motivation not under the control of the blood center, but intrinsic to the donation process, is donation to obtain a test result, particularly for antibodies to the human immunodeficiency virus (HIV): 3.2% of surveyed donors stated that they had done so in the previous 12 months.[11] The concern that some individuals donate blood at the time newly developed tests are put into place ("magnet effect") has been shown to be unfounded, at least for HIV p24 antigen testing.[12] Nevertheless, it remains important for at-risk individuals to have access to confidential or anonymous testing at facilities other than the blood center.

■ Blood Collection

Background

Blood donation is accomplished by a series of processes to ensure, to the extent possible, that both the donor's and the recipient's health is protected. Proven benefit to donors is limited to discovery of treatable abnormalities despite, for instance, the controversial hypothesis that donation, by depletion of iron stores, improves cardiovascular status.[13, 14] Therefore, the risk to these volunteers must be kept to an absolute minimum.

Donation is conducted under specific rules found in the CFR as well as in guidelines and memoranda published from time to time by the FDA. In addition, the AABB *Standards for Blood Banks and Transfusion Services* (Standards)[15] provides requirements for collection that address these protections and are keyed to federal publications. Many states and municipalities also have their own regulations, often by referral to the Standards. These regulations are constantly changing: the Standards, the AABB (www.aabb.org), and the FDA (www.fda.gov/cber) are reasonable sources to ensure currency. Requirements for donor qualification in current AABB Standards[15] are shown in Table 8.2.

Collection Site

The collection site must be appropriate for collection. It should be pleasant and must meet standards of current Good Manufacturing Practices[16] for cleanliness and capability of

Table 8.1 Acceptable and Unacceptable Donor Compensation or Inducements

Unacceptable Compensation or Inducements

Cash payment or cash equivalent
Lottery tickets
Discounts on merchandise
Valuable* merchandise
Tax deduction
Reduction in fees for premarital screening tests in association with a blood donation
Community service credits for parolees
Alternative sentencing or judicial sentence reduction
Credit toward raising grades for high school or college students
Raffle tickets for valuable* items

Items Not Considered Payment or Inducement

Employer's customary compensation (paid time off) to an employee in order to donate blood
Tokens or prizes that are not of such value as to motivate a potential donor to conceal detrimental medical
  background and that are made available to all potential donors
Recognition items for donation milestones (e.g., gallon donor pins)

Practices Where General Agreement Could Not Be Reached

Blood assurance benefits to the donor or others
Cancellation, discount, or refund of the blood replacement or deposit fee
Free supplemental laboratory screening or diagnostic testing
Time off from work unrelated to that directly involving donations
Tickets to events

*One that could induce donation by an individual who, if acting upon personal motivation alone, would not give blood.

Table 8.2 AABB Standards: Requirements for Donor Qualification. Reference Standard 5.4.1A—Requirements for Allogeneic Donor Qualification

Item No.	Category	Criteria
1	Age	≥17 years or applicable state law
2	Whole Blood Volume Collected	Maximum of 10.5 mL/kg of donor weight, including samples, and blood collection container shall be cleared for volume collected
3	Donation Interval	8 weeks after whole blood donation (Standard 5.6.7.1 applies) 16 weeks after two-unit red cell collection 4 weeks after infrequent apheresis ≥2 days after plasma-, platelet-, or leukapheresis (See exceptions in Standard 5.5)
4	Blood Pressure	≤180 mm Hg systolic ≤100 mm Hg diastolic
5	Pulse	50–100, without pathologic irregularities <50 acceptable if an otherwise healthy athlete
6	Temperature	≤37.5 C (99.5 F) if measured orally, or equivalent if measured by another method
7	Hemoglobin/Hematocrit	≥12.5 g/dL/≥38%; blood obtained by earlobe puncture shall not be used for this determination
8	Drug Therapy	Medication evaluation: Finasteride (Proscar, Propecia), isotretinoin (Accutane)—Defer 1 month after receipt of last dose Acitretin (Soriatane)—Defer 3 years Etretinate (Tegison)—Defer indefinitely Ingestion of aspirin–containing medications or those that irreversibly inhibit platelet function within 36 hours of donation precludes use of donor as sole source of platelets
9a	Medical History General health	The donor shall be free of major organ disease (heart, liver, lungs), cancer, or abnormal bleeding tendency, unless determined suitable by blood bank medical director
9b	Pregnancy	Defer if routine donation.
9c	Receipt of blood, component, or other human tissue	Family history of CJD[1] or receipt of tissue or tissue derivatives (dura mater, pituitary growth hormones of human origin)—Defer indefinitely. Receipt of blood, components, human tissue, or clotting factor concentrates-Defer for 12 months
9d	Immunizations and vaccinations	Receipt of toxoids, or synthetic or killed viral, bacterial, or rickettsial vaccines if donor is symptom-free and afebrile—No deferral [Anthrax, cholera, diphtheria, hepatitis A, hepatitis B, influenza, Lyme disease, paratyphoid, pertussis, plague, pneumococcal polysaccharide, polio (injection), rabies (no exposure), Rocky Mountain spotted fever, tetanus, typhoid (by injection)] Receipt of live attenuated viral and bacterial vaccines—2-week deferral measles (rubeola), mumps, polio (oral), typhoid (oral), yellow fever

(continued)

Table 8.2 AABB Standards: Requirements for Donor Qualification. Reference Standard 5.4.1A—Requirements for Allogeneic Donor Qualification (Continued)

Item No.	Category	Criteria
		Receipt of live attenuated viral and bacterial vaccines—4-week deferral 　German measles (rubella), chicken pox (*Varicella zoster*) Receipt of other vaccines—12-month deferral 　Hepatitis B immune globulin (HBIG), unlicensed vaccines
9e	Infectious diseases	Defer indefinitely: History of viral hepatitis after 11th birthday Confirmed positive test for HBsAg Repeatedly reactive test for anti-HBc on more than one occasion Present or past clinical or laboratory evidence of infection with HCV, HTLV, or HIV or as excluded by current FDA regulations and recommendations for the prevention of HIV transmission by blood and components Donated the only unit of blood or component that resulted in the apparent transmission of hepatitis, HIV, HTLV A history of babesiosis or Chagas' disease Evidence of or obvious stigmata of parenteral drug use Use of a needle to administer nonprescription drugs Donors recommended for indefinite deferral for risk of vCJD, as defined in most recent FDA guideline 12-month deferral from the time of: Application of a tattoo Mucous membrane exposure to blood Nonsterile skin penetration with instruments or equipment contaminated with blood or body fluids other than the donor's own Residing in the household and/or having sexual contact with an individual with symptomatic HBV or unspecified viral hepatitis or a confirmed positive test for HBsAg Sexual contact with an individual with HIV infection or at high risk of HIV injection[2,3] Incarceration in a correctional institution (including jails and prisons) for more than 72 consecutive hours Completion of therapy for treatment of syphilis or gonorrhea or a reactive screening test for syphilis in the absence of a negative confirmatory test. History of syphilis or gonorrhea
9f	Malaria	Prospective donors who have had a diagnosis of malaria shall be deferred for 3 years after becoming asymptomatic. Immigrants, refugees, or citizens coming from a country in which malaria is considered endemic by the Malaria Branch, Centers for Disease Control and Prevention,[5] US Department of Health and Human Services, may be accepted 3 years after departure from the area if they have been free from unexplained symptoms suggestive of malaria. Residents of countries in which malaria is not endemic but who have been in an area in which malaria is considered to be endemic may be accepted 12 months after departing that area.[4] However, they shall have been free of unexplained symptoms suggestive of malaria, irrespective of the receipt of antimalarial prophylaxis. Donations from which only the frozen plasma is to be used shall be exempt from these restrictions.
10	At Risk	Evaluation: Prospective donors shall be questioned and appropriately deferred if behavior is suggestive of high risk for HIV infection.[2] Alcohol intoxication or obvious stigmata of alcohol habituation. Lesions on the skin at the venipuncture site.

[1]FDA Guidance for Industry dated November 23, 1999 "Revised Precautionary Measures to Reduce the Possible Risk of Transmission of Creutzfeldt-Jakob Disease (CJD) and New Variant Creutzfeldt-Jakob Disease (nvCJD) by Blood and Blood Products."
[2]FDA Memorandum dated April 23, 1992 "Revised Recommendation for the Prevention of Human Immunodeficiency Virus (HIV) Transmission by Blood and Blood Products."
[3]FDA Memorandum dated December 11, 1996 "Interim Recommendations for Deferral of Donors at Increased Risk for HIV-1 Group 0 Infection."
[4]The Department of Defense has recommended a 24-month deferral. Department of Defense Memorandum dated October 14, 1999 "Deferral of Service Members Stationed in Possible Malaria Areas in the Republic of Korea," and February 28, 2001 update.
[5]www.cdc.gov/travel

being cleaned and decontaminated, ventilation, space, and temperature.

■ Donor Health Screening

General Principles

In order to allow careful comparison of donor health history and infectious disease marker reactivity with previous records from the donor, accurate donor identification is essential. Many collection facilities now request photographic identification of donors to facilitate accurate identification and this comparison. Some organizations use a hand-held or portable computer to screen donors to prevent early whole blood donation (before 8 weeks) and to detect donors with previously identified deferral factors such as positive tests, high-risk behaviors for infectious diseases, and other deferrable medical conditions.[17]

After registration, the blood donor is provided with explanatory information about the blood donation process. This information generally covers the screening process and phlebotomy, potential donation-related complications, reasons for self-deferral, notification process for positive postdonation tests, how donor confidentiality is preserved, and a warning not to donate for test results. This reading material should be in language simple enough that all literate donors can comprehend it.[18]

The donor then answers a series of questions designed to maximize safety for both the donor and recipient and ensure a potent product. In most organizations, the donor completes a written questionnaire answering "Yes/No" questions. A nurse or technician, acting as a health historian, evaluates the questionnaire and obtains follow-up information based on the donor's answers. Other options are for the staff to ask some or all of the questions[19] or for donors to use a computer.[20] These methods may differ in the accuracy of the answers obtained. Some reports have suggested that use of a computer may increase reports of high-risk behavioral activity because the donors are less intimidated.[20]

The questions must address the requirements of the CFR[21] and Standards.[15] The AABB has a uniform questionnaire that fulfills these requirements and, if unchanged, can be used by any collection organization with assurance of regulatory compliance[22] (Table 8.3). The CFR and Standards provide some general guidelines for blood donor suitability, but every collection organization must develop a comprehensive approach to donor suitability that addresses hundreds of diseases, conditions, and behaviors.[23] Unfortunately, necessary data are not available to allow knowledgeable decisions for many diseases and conditions, and informed opinions must be used. In some cases, guidelines or regulations are medically illogical but must be followed to ensure regulatory compliance.[23]

Donor Health History and Donor Safety

The age of consent for blood donation may be different from the driving age or voting age, and these differences may vary from state to state. However, most states permit blood donation at age 17. There is no upper age limit. Blood donors must be in relatively good health. After a standard blood donation, the blood volume lost is mostly replaced within a few hours and completely replaced within 48 to 72 hours. Assuming adequate iron stores, the red blood cells are replaced within 3 to 5 weeks. Allogeneic blood donation is limited to once every 8 weeks to ensure a safety margin for replacement of the red blood cells and to allow time for absorption of dietary iron sufficient to prevent the development of iron deficiency. Iron deficiency is rarely a problem for men but is common among women, who often have marginal iron stores as a result of menstrual blood loss.

Open-ended questions may be used to ask about the donor's overall health, whether the donor, is under the care of a health professional, and whether the donor has any medical conditions not addressed by another question. These questions are designed to cast a wide net to find conditions that may affect donor or recipient safety. Specific questions address cardiac pain, lung disease, liver disease, blood diseases, pregnancy, and history of cancer. Whereas donors with some medical problems are not permitted to donate until the condition has resolved, donors with controlled hypertension and diabetes can donate, as can most donors with arthritis, thyroid disease, and heart disease. Medications themselves rarely affect donor safety, but the reason for taking the medication may be a donor safety issue. For example, taking a coronary vasodilator may indicate ongoing angina and preclude donation.

A donor must also have adequate weight to undergo routine donor phlebotomy. This information is most commonly collected by history, not by weighing the donor. Standards allows donation of 10.5 mL of whole blood for every kilogram of donor weight.[15] Thus, a donor who weighs 50 kg cannot donate more than 525 mL of whole blood, including samples for testing.

Donor Health History and Recipient Safety

Most of the health history questions are designed to protect the blood recipient from infectious diseases. Donors currently ill with infections are deferred until they recover. Donors are deferred if they have a history of serious blood-borne infections with a tendency toward chronicity, such as HIV, viral hepatitis B and C, or a history of a positive marker for these agents. Because hepatitis A does not involve a prolonged carrier state and childhood hepatitis is most likely to have been hepatitis A, it is reasonable to accept for donation prospective donors who have a history of hepatitis before age 11. Donors who know that they have antibody to hepatitis B surface antigen (HBsAg) are accepted because such individuals are immune and not infectious. Donors with known antibody to hepatitis B core antigen (anti-HBcAg) are deferred because this antibody may be present without surface antigen in an infectious donor early in the course of the disease and because anti-HBcAg may serve as a surrogate marker for other infectious diseases, such as non-A, non-B, non-C hepatitis or retroviral agents that are as yet uncharacterized.

Donors with a history of other infections such as babesiosis and Chagas disease are permanently deferred. Donors with malaria are deferred for 3 years if no symptoms recur, and those who travel to an area in which malaria is endemic are deferred for 12 months from the date of return. Some behaviors have been associated with increased risk for HIV or hepatitis infection, such as intravenous drug use and prostitution, and require indefinite deferral.[24] Behaviors such as visiting a prostitute or having sexual contact with an intravenous drug user require a 12-month deferral.

Some deferral periods are controversial. The current indefinite deferral for "male-to-male sex, even once, since 1977" is thought by some to be unreasonable.[25] As another example, variant Creutzfeldt-Jakob disease has not been demonstrated to be transmitted by transfusion. However, because transmission is a theoretical possibility, potential donors who have spent a cumulative 3 months in the United Kingdom (UK) between 1980 and 1996 (the period when bovine spongiform encephalopathy [BSE], or "mad cow" disease, was at its peak) are indefinitely deferred, as are potential donors who spent a cumulative 6 months on European military bases. Further, those who have spent a cumulative 5 years in European countries other than the UK, or received a blood transfusion in the UK from 1980 to the present, are also deferred.[26]

Exposure to blood requires a 12-month deferral. Such blood exposures may occur through a blood transfusion, tattoo, human bite, accidental needlestick, nonsterile ear or body piercing, or acupuncture. Donors who are vaccinated with killed viruses are generally acceptable for blood donation, but donors vaccinated with live-attenuated viruses are deferred for 2 weeks (e.g., measles, mumps) or 4 weeks (e.g., German measles). Donors who are vaccinated with experimental vaccines or vaccinated for exposure to hepatitis B or rabies are deferred for 12 months, the former because of the uncertain nature of the vaccine and the latter because of risk of disease rather than the vaccine itself.

Table 8.3   Uniform Donor History Questions

The following information was current as of June 2002. As the 14th edition of the *Technical Manual* went to press, the Food and Drug Administration was in the process of reviewing a new questionnaire, prepared by an inter-organizational task force. For the most current Uniform Donor History Questionnaire, consult the AABB web site, www.aabb.org.

1. Have you ever donated or attempted to donate blood using a different (or another) name here or anywhere else?
2. In the past 8 weeks, have you given blood, plasma, or platelets here or anywhere else?
3. Have you for any reason been deferred or refused as a blood donor or told not to donate?
4. Are you feeling well and healthy today?
5. In the past 12 months, have you been under a doctor's care or had a major illness or surgery?
6. Have you ever had chest pain, heart disease, or recent or severe respiratory disease?
7. Have you ever had cancer, a blood disease, or a bleeding problem?
8. Have you ever had yellow jaundice, liver disease, viral hepatitis, or a positive test for hepatitis?
9. Have you ever had malaria, Chagas' disease, or babesiosis?
10. A. Have you ever taken etretinate (Tegison) for psoriasis?
    B. In the past 3 years, have you taken acitretin (Soriatane)?
    C. In the past 36 hours, have you taken aspirin, or anything that has aspirin in it?
    D. In the past month, have you taken isotretinoin (Accutane) or finasteride (Proscar) (Propecia)?
    E. In the past 4 weeks, have you taken any pills or medications?
       1. Since 1980, have you ever injected bovine (beef) insulin?
11. In the past 4 weeks, have you had any shots or vaccinations?
12. In the past 12 months, have you been given rabies shots?
13. Female donors: In the past 6 weeks, have you been pregnant or are you pregnant now?
14. A. In the past 3 years, have you been outside the United States or Canada?
    B. Since 1980, have you ever lived in, or traveled to Europe?
       1. If the donor answers no, then go to question 15.
       2. If the donor answers yes, then ask
          a. From 1980 through 1996, did you spend time that adds up to 3 months or more in the UK (England, Northern Ireland, Scotland, Wales, the Isle of Man, the Channel Islands, Gibraltar, or the Falkland Islands)?
          b. Since 1980, have you received a transfusion of blood, platelets, plasma, cryoprecipitate, or granulocytes in the UK (England, Northern Ireland, Scotland, Wales, the Isle of Man, the Channel Islands, Gibraltar, or the Falkland Islands)?
          c. Since 1980, have you spent time that adds up to 5 years or more in France?
    C. From 1980 through 1996, were you a member of the US military, a civilian military employee or a dependent of a member of the US military?
       1. If the donor answers no, then go to question 15.
       2. If the donor answers yes, then ask either a. or b.
          a. Did you spend a total time of 6 months or more associated with a military base in any of the following countries: Belgium, The Netherlands, Germany, Spain, Portugal, Turkey, Italy, or Greece?
          b. From 1980 through 1996, did you spend a total time of 6 months or more associated with a military base in Belgium, The Netherlands, or Germany?
15. A. Have you ever received growth hormone made from human pituitary glands?
    B. Have you received a dura mater (or brain covering) graft?
    C. Have any of your blood relatives had Creutzfeldt-Jakob disease?
16. In the past 12 months, have you had close contact with a person with yellow jaundice or viral hepatitis, or have you been given Hepatitis B Immune Globulin (HBIG)?
17. In the past 12 months, have you taken (snorted) cocaine through your nose?
18. In the past 12 months, have you received blood or had an organ or tissue transplant or graft?
19. In the past 17 months, have you had a tattoo applied, ear or skin piercing, acupuncture, or come into contact with someone else's blood?
20. A. In the past 12 months, have you had a positive test for syphilis?
    B. In the past 12 months, have you had or been treated for syphilis or gonorrhea?
21. In the past 12 months, have you given money or drugs to anyone to have sex with you?
22. A. At any time since 1977, have you taken money or drugs for sex?
    B. In the past 12 months, have you had sex, even once, with anyone who has taken money or drugs for sex?
23. A. Have you ever used a needle, even once, to take drugs that were not prescribed by a doctor?
    B. In the past 12 months, have you had sex, even once, with anyone who has used a needle to take drugs not prescribed by a doctor?
24. Male Donors: Have you had sex with another male, even once, since 1977?
25. Female donors: In the past 12 months, have you had sex with a male who has had sex, even once, since 1977 with another male?

(Continued)

Table 8.3 Uniform Donor History Questions (*Continued*)

26. A. Have you ever taken clotting factor concentrates for a bleeding problem, such as hemophilia?
    B. In the past 12 months, have you had sex, even once, with someone who has taken clotting factor concentrates for a bleeding problem such as hemophilia?
27. A. Do you have AIDS or have you had a positive test for the AIDS virus?
    B. In the past 12 months, have you had sex, even once, with someone who has AIDS or has had a positive test for the AIDS virus?
28. Are you giving blood because you want to be tested for HIV or the AIDS virus?
29. Do you understand that if you have the AIDS virus, you can give it to someone else, even though you may feel well and have a negative AIDS test?
30. A. Were you born in, have you lived in, or have you traveled to any African country since 1977?
    B. When you traveled to <country(ies)> did you receive a blood transfusion or any other medical treatment with a product made from blood?
    C. Have you had sexual contact with anyone who was born in or lived in any African country since 1977?
31. In the past 12 months, have you been in jail or prison?
32. Have you read and understood all the donor information presented to you, and have all of your questions been answered?

Most medications used by donors are acceptable for blood recipients, but a few are not because they are cytotoxic (e.g., cyclophosphamide), cause congenital anomalies (e.g., finasteride, isotretinoin, acitretin, etretinate),[15] or are associated with infections (e.g., human pituitary-derived growth hormone). In other cases, the medication, such as an antibiotic, signifies an infection that requires a deferral. A few questions are designed to ensure a quality product. Some donors with a history of a clotting factor, platelet, or red blood cell disorder are deferred because one or more of their blood components may be defective. Some donors treated for these disorders may also have a problem resulting from the treatment; persons with severe hemophilia treated in the past with pooled factor VIII may have a high incidence of hepatitis.

Donor Physical Examination

The physical examination consists of evaluation of the donor's pulse rate and rhythm, blood pressure, and temperature and inspection of the donor's potential venipuncture sites. The donor's pulse must be regular and between 50 and 100 beats per minute. Athletic donors with a pulse rate below 50 can be accepted. The donor's blood pressure must be less than 180/100 on the day of donation; blood pressure medications are acceptable. A donor temperature less than 99.6°F protects both the donor and the recipient. An elevated temperature signifies the potential for transmission of an infectious agent to a patient. Screening the donor's arms for infection, scars, or lesions at the venipuncture site indicative of intravenous drug abuse protects the recipient from infectious agents.

Hemoglobin

To ensure that blood is not drawn from anemic donors, the Standards and the CFR require that donors have a hemoglobin of 12.5 g/dL or greater (Standards allows a hematocrit of 38% or higher). Neither specifies a sampling method, or test method or provides for differences depending on gender or altitude. Since ear lobe sampling gives a hematocrit value that is 4.5 to 7 percentage points higher on average than sampling venous blood,[27, 28] these higher values allow collection from donors whose venous hematocrit is, in fact, below 38%. In some cases, donors with true hematocrits below 30% have been accepted on the basis of ear stick blood samples.[29] Standards now states that blood obtained by earlobe puncture shall not be used for this determination.

Depletion of iron stores in frequent blood donors has been a cause of concern. Symptoms of iron deficiency anemia generally do not appear until the hemoglobin falls to less than 9 g/dL. Therefore, predonation screening of donors to ensure adequate hemoglobin levels would protect against iron deficiency disease, although not against depletion of iron stores. Some have suggested that donations from women be limited to less frequent intervals to limit iron depletion. Others have proposed specific testing for adequacy of iron stores (e.g., transferrin), and still others have proposed newer forms of oral iron supplementation, less toxic to children, for frequent blood donors, particularly menstruating women.[30] A public health concern with the last proposal is the potential masking of a gastrointestinal malignancy. On the other hand, some have suggested a lower hemoglobin standard for women because the normal range for women extends below 12.5 g/dL.[31] This policy would increase the number of acceptable donors but potentially increase the likelihood of iron depletion in women.

Many facilities use the tendency of a drop of blood to sink in copper sulfate solution as a simple and inexpensive hemoglobin screen. A drop of blood with a hemoglobin level of 12.5 g/dL sinks in a copper sulfate solution with a specific gravity of 1.053. If the hemoglobin in the drop of blood is below 12.5 g/dL, the drop does not sink.[32] Most centers follow a failed copper sulfate test with a microhematocrit; approximately half of the donors with a failed copper sulfate test have a microhematocrit of 38% or greater.[36] This combination is generally the basis for accepting donors whose hemoglobin is acceptable without falsely accepting anemic donors.

Although designed for donor and recipient safety, the physical examination can also serve a public health function because significant treatable hypertension, arrhythmias, or anemia may be detected.

Confidential Unit Exclusion

It is important to provide an opportunity for donors who may be under pressure to donate to let the collection facility know that their blood should not be used for transfusion. Many centers provide an opportunity for donors to exclude their units confidentially at the time of collection by *confidential unit exclusion* (CUE). In addition, centers can provide a confidential telephone number for call-back should the donor remember additional information that might affect the safety of the unit.

When CUE was first used, the marker frequency of CUE positive units was significantly higher than those of donors not selecting CUE.[33] Further, as many as 20% of donors found to be positive for anti-HIV used CUE. Today, these marker frequency differences are not as great (except in repeated users of CUE) and may represent prevalence rather than incidence.[34, 35] Further, up to half of CUE indications can be the result of donor error.[36, 37] For this reason, most centers using CUE destroy the unit but continue to allow the donor to donate blood.

After the interview, physical examination, hemoglobin screen, and CUE procedure, the donor is asked to sign that he or she has read and understood the written material provided, has answered all the questions truthfully, understands the risks of blood donation including the potential for a donor reaction, and gives consent for the collection of the blood, its testing, and its use. Unfortunately, many experienced donors merely skim the written material because they feel that they know the information or want to move quickly through the process. Further, a donor mail survey suggested that 1.9% of donors do not provide an accurate history and would have been deferred had correct answers been provided. Indeed, the same survey indicated that 0.4% of donors had not informed the health historian of an infectious disease risk factor occurring in the previous 3 months.[38] The steps in determination of donor suitability are shown in Figure 8.1.

■ Collection Process

Blood collection techniques are designed to ensure the safety and efficacy of the product obtained. These techniques begin with a reaffirmation of the donor's identity, often by asking the donor to state his or her full name and other identifiers to the phlebotomist holding the donor history information. A number uniquely identifying the unit to be collected is placed on the bag, the form containing the donor history and physical examination results, and tubes to be collected for testing. At the time of actual collection, these numbers are checked to ensure that they all match.

The phlebotomist then inflates a blood pressure cuff to a pressure somewhat above venous pressure (or uses a tourniquet), finds an appropriate vein, and cleans the skin thoroughly. The cleaning is usually performed in two steps[39]: a prolonged scrub with a soap solution and a final cleaning with an iodine compound, usually polyvinylpyrrolidone (PVP-iodine). The blood is collected into a bag placed in a scale device, which allows the exact amount (usually 450 or 500 mL) to be drawn. It is agitated during collection, either manually or with an automated device, to ensure adequate mixing with the anticoagulant-preservative solution.

When the collection is complete, the tubing is sealed between the bag and the donor. Typically, the bag is separated, pilot tubes are filled from the donor tubing, the needle is removed, and pressure is applied to the donor's arm. After a few minutes, an appropriate bandage is applied and the donor is escorted to a refreshment area, where liquids are given under observation to ensure that no harm comes to the donor if a vasovagal reaction occurs. The collection tubing attached to the bag is stripped toward the bag to ensure that the blood in this tubing is thoroughly mixed with anticoagulant, and the tubing is then sealed into segments.

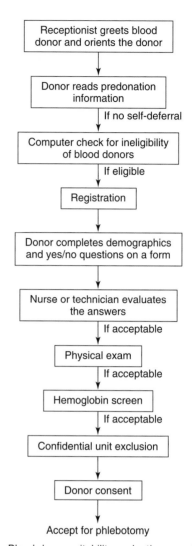

Figure 8.1   Blood donor suitability evaluation: one typical flow.

Before donors leave the center, they should receive postdonation information describing the need to drink liquids, permissible activity levels, care of the venipuncture site, and a telephone number to call if the donor becomes ill or recollects or wishes to change health history information.

■ Adverse Reactions and Injuries after Donation

Phlebotomy may cause soreness and local tissue injury at the venipuncture site. Postphlebotomy bruising is the most common adverse event (Table 8.4). Two studies of outpatient phlebotomy suggest an incidence of bruising of approximately 9% to 16%.[40, 41] A frank hematoma is much less common—0.3% at the donation site and 0.05% additional reported by the donor later. Bruising, soreness, and hematomas generally resolve within 2 weeks.

Vasovagal donor reaction is the most common systemic event,[42–45] occurring in 2% to 3% of donors. Vasovagal reactions are 5 to 10 times more frequent in younger persons (8% to 11%) than in older, experienced donors (1% to 1.5%).[46] Besides youth, additional predisposing factors include first-time donor status,[44, 45, 47] lower weight,[44, 45, 47, 48] and history of a previous reaction.[49, 50] There is clearly also a

Table 8.4 Classification and Frequency of Adverse Donor Reactions and Injuries

Reaction	Frequency (%)
Vasovagal reaction	2–3
Vasovagal reaction with syncope	0.08–0.34[52]
Angina, myocardial infarction, stroke	0.0005[43]
Local injury	
Hematoma (time of donation)	0.3
Hematoma (after donation)	0.05
Bruise (follow-up on blood samples)	9–16[41,42]
Arterial puncture (reported)	0.001–0.01[52]
Arterial pseudoaneurysm	Rare
Arteriovenous fistula	Very rare
Compartment syndrome	Very rare
Local needle injury	0.016[62]
Local irritation or allergy to tape or antiseptic solution	0.5 (estimate)
Local infection at venipuncture site	0.0005 (estimate)
Thrombophlebitis or phlebitis	0.001–0.002 (estimate)

Estimates based on unpublished interviews with collection staff, Detroit Red Cross.

psychological component because a vasovagal reaction can occur before phlebotomy or after observing other donors who fainted ("epidemic" fainting).

Vasovagal donor reactions develop suddenly, during or immediately after phlebotomy. Common early symptoms and signs are lightheadedness, weakness, pallor, nausea, hypotension, and diaphoresis.

Approximately 5% of vasovagal reactions progress to loss of consciousness (syncope). Syncopal rates vary among blood centers, ranging from 0.08% to 0.34% of donors.[52] In contrast to nonsyncopal vasovagal reactions, syncopal reactions are more likely to occur after phlebotomy—about 60% occur at the refreshment table and 12% occur after the donor has left the collection site. Thirty to 45 percent of the syncopal reactions include involuntary tetany or tonic-clonic convulsive movements.[51] These usually last less than 30 seconds; 20% may last longer, up to a minute or two. A few donors may have associated urinary incontinence. Tetany can rarely occur without syncope as a result of prolonged hyperventilation leading to hypocapnia and reduced ionized calcium.

Severe vasovagal reactions may resemble shock clinically, except that the pulse is slow rather than fast. The blood pressure is extremely low, and the donor becomes pale or (rarely) cyanotic. Severe reactions are treated by withdrawing the needle to avoid injury if convulsive movements occur, ensuring airway adequacy, and elevating the donor's legs to increase blood flow to the heart. It is also common practice to use cold neck compresses or ammonium salts to stimulate the donor. Treatment with intravenous fluids or medications is unnecessary. Some centers keep tongue protectors available, but damage to the tongue from convulsive movements is rare. The typical time for recovery from a vasovagal reaction is 5 to 30 minutes. For prolonged or recurrent reactions, it may be prudent to transfer the donor to an emergency room for further monitoring. The donor who has had a reaction should be advised that these reactions may recur within the next several hours, and extra caution should be used in driving or operating heavy machinery. Donors with multiple or severe reactions might be discouraged from attempting to give blood again in the near future.

The main risk associated with a vasovagal reaction is the trauma suffered during a fall in a sudden syncopal episode. Fractures and other significant injuries have been reported.[42] Severe vasovagal reactions can be prevented to some degree by experienced staff who keep donors' minds occupied and who are alert for early symptoms so that the reaction can be stopped.[52, 53] Donors who hyperventilate with loss of carbon dioxide can develop respiratory alkalosis, which can cause symptoms of hypocalcemia or potentiate a vasovagal reaction.[54] Increasing carbon dioxide retention by having such a donor rebreathe into a paper bag may reverse alkalosis and relieve these symptoms.

Donors who have severe vasovagal reactions recover spontaneously. No reports of deaths caused by blood donation–related vasovagal reaction appear in the medical literature, although there are reports of cardiac arrest in patients after venipuncture for blood sample collection.[55, 56]

Other local injuries and reactions are much less common (see Table 8.2). Arterial punctures are rare.[51] The most common finding is a rapid phlebotomy, with blood that is usually bright red in color. A pulsating needle is sometimes present. Upon recognition, the phlebotomy should be stopped and pressure should be applied for at least 10 minutes. Because the thick arterial wall does not collapse, there is a risk that the puncture hole will not close. This is unusual, but it may lead to brachial artery pseudoaneurysm[57, 58] or, rarely, an arterial-venous fistula[59] or a compartment syndrome.[60] All three complications require surgical repair.

Approximately 1 in every 6000 blood donors reports symptoms consistent with a neurologic needle injury.[61, 62] Symptoms may include pain and paresthesias at the venipuncture site extending into the donor's hand, fingers, or shoulder area. The injury may reflect direct trauma from a needle or pressure from a hematoma or both. A hematoma is present in approximately 25% of cases.[61] Recovery is often seen in a few days (40%), and 70% recover completely within 30 days. The remaining 30% take as long as 9 months to recover. A few donors have a small area of persistent numbness even after 9 months. Rarely, significant permanent neurologic damage occurs.[61]

Manufacturers of adhesive tape, bactericidal solutions, and gauze are required to test their products for irritation and sensitization properties by standard techniques before FDA approval and release. Nonetheless, contact allergic reactions occur. Alternative solutions can be used for those with allergic reactions to iodine-containing products, and arm wrapping can be performed to avoid skin contact with tape.

Serious systemic reactions after blood donation, such as myocardial infarction and cerebral vascular accident, occur but are quite rare. These reactions may be coincidental events.[42] In the initial U.S. experience with blood donation during World War II, eight such serious events occurred in 7 million blood donations.[42] Six of these eight donors would not have been eligible to donate by the current Standards.

■ Processing and Labeling of Donor Blood

Samples of donor blood, carefully linked to the unit itself, are tested to determine ABO group and Rh type. Although only blood from donors with a history of transfusion or pregnancy must be tested for the presence of unexpected antibodies, blood centers find it easier to test all donors for such antibodies. In addition, all donor blood is tested to determine its potential for transmission of well-characterized infectious diseases. Required tests include serologic tests for syphilis, HBsAg, anti-HBcAg, anti-HIV type 1 and 2, anti-human T-cell lymphotropic virus type I and II, anti-hepatitis C virus (HCV), and the p24 antigen of HIV. Although nucleic acid amplification testing (NAT) for HIV and HCV is not now required, it has become almost universal in the United States. When NAT is performed for HIV, HIV p24 antigen testing is not required. Only if these tests are nonreactive is blood released for transfusion.

In addition, the donor's identifying characteristics (name, birth date, address, and social security number) are compared with a registry of previous donors deferred because of health history or infectious disease markers. Such comparative systems are relatively sophisticated, using algorithms to ensure that a donor is not incorrectly accepted despite a change of, for instance, a letter in the donor's last name. Donor deferral registries are required to be kept by the collecting facility and checked before the blood is labeled for distribution to transfusion services.[63] There is currently no requirement for a national registry, although larger blood systems maintain a registry across all their collecting facilities.

■ Special Blood Donation Considerations

Despite continual reduction of the risk of transfusion-transmitted disease, the public retains an exaggerated fear of disease transmission[64] and seeks to reduce that minute risk further using approaches such as autologous and directed donation.

Autologous Donation

For many years, patients have given blood before an operative procedure to be used for themselves. This approach received a major impetus with the recognition of the risk of transfusion-transmitted HIV infection in the mid-1980s. The advantages of using autologous blood are reduction of the risk of transfusion-transmitted diseases and avoidance of sensitization to allogeneic blood–related antigens and transfusion-related immune modulation. These advantages accrue to the extent that the use of allogeneic blood can be reduced or avoided completely.

The disadvantages are the logistics and cost of collection of the units of blood preoperatively, with the assurance that these units arrive at the hospital and are used before allogeneic units are used, and the fact that, as a group, patients are less suited to blood donation than are volunteer donors. As the risk of transfusion-transmitted disease is reduced with new or improved testing, the advantages of autologous donation are dramatically reduced. Such donations may still be useful for patients who are expected to use several units of blood and are relatively young and otherwise in good health, but for many others the process is not cost-effective as measured by traditional cost-benefit approaches.[65] Furthermore, the frequency of a severe donor reaction requiring hospitalization, although quite low, is significantly higher in autologous donors than in allogeneic donors (1 in 17,000 vs. 1 in 200,000).[66] Because the

---

Box 8.1   Clinical Controversies: Autologous Donations

Pro: No risk of transfusion-transmitted viral disease.
        No risk of sensitization, immunomodulation, and other non-infectious adverse effects.
        Psychologically comforting to patient.
        In some states, availability required by law.

Con: Minimal real reduction in risk of transfusion-transmitted disease, as testing improves.
        Greater likelihood of error, since procedure nonroutine.
        Although risk of severe donor reaction remains small, risk greater for autologous than for allogeneic donor.
        Real risk of recipient transfusion reaction remains.
        Cost efficacy poor, unless patient has long life expectancy and is anticipated to use several units.

I feel that there is little scientific justification for autologous donation today. Therefore, it is reasonable to insist that potential autologous donors have no donation risk greater than for allogeneic donation.

---

advantage of autologous donation is so minimal, even a slight increase in donor risk is unacceptable. Thus, centers should not hesitate to defer autologous donors who are at high risk for an adverse event, such as those with significant arteriosclerotic heart disease or symptomatic aortic stenosis (see Box 8.1).

If an autologous donation is not used by the intended patient, it is almost always discarded, even if the donor meets all allogeneic criteria. Such units are from patients (rather than donors), who have a higher infectious disease marker frequency than regular allogeneic donors.[67] Standards does not allow the routine use of such blood (crossover) by a nonautologous recipient.

Criteria of acceptability for autologous donation are somewhat different from those for allogeneic donation. Because this blood is not used for recipients other than the autologous recipient, there are no concerns about viral or parasitic transfusion-transmitted diseases, and these questions in the donor history can be eliminated. There is concern, however, about donor bacterial infections and subsequent bacterial proliferation upon blood storage. If drawn at a blood center, the blood should be fully tested; if positive markers for infectious disease are found, the blood must be labeled to indicate a biohazard risk, and if it is found to be positive for HIV or hepatitis B virus, the attending physician and the hospital's transfusion service medical director must agree to the use of the blood. These testing procedures are not currently required if the blood is collected by the transfusing hospital.

Because there is benefit to autologous donors and patients, current safety standards for allogeneic donors can be modified. For instance, the donor can donate every 72 hours (and typically no less than 72 hours before surgery) rather than at an interval of at least 56 days as required for allogeneic donation. In practice, most autologous donors donate weekly; for surgery requiring several units of blood, this is best accomplished by beginning 4 to 6 weeks beforehand. Similarly, the required donor hemoglobin level is lowered from 12.5 to 11 g/dL, a level sufficient to ensure that transfusion preoperatively will not be required. In some cases, the donor is given supplemental iron or erythropoietin to allow removal of required amounts of blood without development of anemia.[68]

Directed Donations

Blood centers have for some time allowed blood from one individual to be designated for or directed to another. Some patients and families of patients about to receive a transfusion have been unwilling to obtain blood from the general supply and have sought blood designated for them from family and friends. Although this practice sometimes enhances the patient's emotional well-being, there is no evidence that blood from such self-selected donors is safer than the volunteer supply. There have been concerns that some directed donors are under pressure to give and may misrepresent historical data that would otherwise lead to deferral. Although the infectious disease marker frequency is higher in directed donors, this higher seroprevalence is to a large extent related to the demographic and first-time donor status of this group.[69] Blood from directed donors not used for the intended recipient may be crossed over into the general inventory.

The provision of such blood for a specific patient is expensive because it is time-consuming and logistically difficult. Further, the process can be frustrating for patients and donors because the expected donor may be deferred, may have an unsuccessful collection, may have positive test results, or may be incompatible with the recipient (see Box 8.2). However, there may be some clinical situations in which this practice is reasonable. For instance, a neonate needing regular small-volume transfusions for a limited period of time may be well served by limiting donor exposure, with repeated transfusions from the same directed donor.[70] Here, although the donor would be giving more frequently than every 8 weeks, the slight donor risk is compensated by the limitation of donor exposures for the recipient.

Similarly, one can use a small group of donors for chronically transfused patients with sickle cell anemia or thalassemia[71] or provide patient-specific products, such as platelets from a sibling for a recipient refractory to random platelets, or human platelet antigen 1a (HPA-1a) (Pl^{A1})–negative maternal platelets to a thrombocytopenic infant whose serum contains maternal anti-HPA-1a. In these special situations, the benefit to the recipient may outweigh the additional donor risk incurred by modification of established standards for allogeneic blood donors.

Donors with Hemochromatosis

Hereditary hemochromatosis is a disease of genetic origin, characterized in the homozygous state by an abnormal increase in iron absorption resulting in storage of iron in organs and subsequent organ failure. The heart, liver, and pancreas may be affected, with congestive heart failure, cirrhosis, and diabetes. The disease is treated by phlebotomy, more aggressively during an initial period of iron removal and then regularly thereafter for maintenance of iron stores. Except for extensive iron absorption and storage, these affected patients are normal until iron storage damage is seen relatively late in the course of their disease.

Whereas the CFR currently requires that blood obtained from therapeutic phlebotomies, if used for allogeneic transfusion, be labeled with the donor's disease and that blood not be drawn more frequently than every 56 days, the FDA has stated that it will consider exemptions to these regulations.[72] The requesting facility must not charge for the therapeutic phlebotomy for these patients, whether the blood is used or not. Some centers, in the United States and elsewhere, have for years used blood collected from these donors in the chronic maintenance phase of phlebotomy treatment if they meet other allogeneic criteria. Some patients with hemochromatosis have been regular blood donors, unrecognized by the blood center as having the disease.[73] It is likely that the use of these patients as donors will not add significantly to the blood supply because of the low penetrance of this condition[74] (see Box 8.3).

■ Apheresis Donation

Collection of Two Units of Red Blood Cells

Continuous flow techniques can be used for the collection of red blood cells with other blood components.[75] Alternatively, two units of red blood cells can be collected at

---

Box 8.2 Clinical Controversies: Directed Donations

Pro: Psychological relief for patient.
Possibility of safer unit (as defined by infectious disease marker frequency) if careful and well-informed donor selection performed.

Con: Expensive, logistically difficult.
Most directed donors selected to include family and friends, few data showing increased safety (based on marker frequency).
Process itself, because nonroutine, may be less safe.

I feel that this process does not add to patients' safety but will continue because of public demand.

Box 8.3 Clinical Controversies: Use of Patients with Hemochromatosis as Blood Donors (Assuming No Therapeutic Phlebotomy Fee)

Pro: May add donors and units to the blood supply.
Blood center serves as a community health care provider.
Provides good public relations.
No additional risk shown for donor or recipient.

Con: New units added may be minimal and more costly.
Units probably need to be collected only at locations offering therapeutic phlebotomy.
Theoretical minimal recipient risk, because motivation is donor health rather than altruism.

I feel that although risk is minimal, cost (primarily loss of therapeutic phlebotomy revenues) may be significant and units few. Could be used effectively at minimal cost in a smaller center or in a facility not now charging for therapeutic phlebotomy.

one sitting. This approach is conceptually attractive: presenting donors whose ABO groups are known could be directed to plasmapheresis if group AB and to double red blood cell collection if group O, alleviating group-specific shortages of these two components.[76] In addition, units of rare phenotype or autologous units could be more readily collected. Although the volume removed is comparable to that of a whole blood collection, the removal of twice the usual amount of red blood cells means that donor criteria are necessarily more stringent.

The FDA requires an interdonation interval of 16 weeks.[77] Currently, donors must have a precollection hemoglobin of 13.3 g/dL (or a hematocrit of 40%).[78] Standards adds that "the volume of red cells removed…shall not…result in a donor hematocrit less than 30% or hemoglobin less than 10 g/dL after volume replacement."[15] In addition, because of concern about the extracorporeal volumes during the collection, men must be at least 5 feet 1 inch in height and have a measured weight of at least 130 pounds. The comparable figures for women are 5 feet 5 inches and 150 pounds.[77] Recommendations for two-unit collection from autologous donors are comparable: a hemoglobin of 12 g/dL (or hematocrit of 36%) and a weight of 130 pounds. Two-unit collections are obtained using a single-needle procedure, taking about 45 minutes. Most donors who qualify have been willing to participate in this program because it eliminates the visit for the second donation.

Adverse Effects

The primary adverse effect is a mild citrate reaction.[79] Although a perceived reduced exercise capacity was noted in one of eight donors,[80] there is no statistical difference between these donors and whole blood donors in postdonation fatigue, lightheadedness, and nausea.[81]

Plateletpheresis

Plateletpheresis offers the advantage of obtaining an adult dose of platelets from a single donor and the opportunity to produce a product that is consistently leukoreduced. The benefits of having a single donor exposure per dose include a reduced likelihood of septic transfusion reactions (1 of 19,519 transfusions compared with 6 of 10,219 transfusions of whole blood–derived platelets),[82] reduced infectious disease risk, and a product that can be human leukocyte antigen (HLA)–matched or crossmatched for alloimmunized, refractory patients. As infectious disease testing becomes more sensitive (or when platelets undergo a viral inactivation process) and filtration leukoreduction is more regularly used for whole blood–derived platelets, the benefits of apheresis platelets become less clear except as a supplement for insufficient numbers of whole blood–derived platelets and the treatment of alloimmunized platelet recipients.

Donor Recruitment

Because platelet apheresis donation often requires two venipunctures and takes 1 to 2 hours rather than the usual 7 to 8 minutes for a whole blood donation, recruitment of these donors is typically somewhat different than that of whole blood donors. Often, these donors are recruited from the ranks of repeat whole blood donors by use of informational material distributed at blood drives or by direct telephone recruitment. Some centers have made a practice of HLA typing these

donors in order to have a readily available pool of donors to treat alloimmunized patients refractory to random platelets. The advent of platelet crossmatching techniques and the reduction in the frequency of development of alloimmunization have made the availability of a large HLA-typed donor pool less necessary.

The frequent plateletpheresis donor is more likely to be older, male, white, and have achieved a higher educational level than a whole blood donor. The incidence of infectious disease markers in apheresis donors is similar to that in repeat whole blood donors.[83]

Collection

Apheresis donors must meet all the health history, physical, and laboratory requirements of allogeneic whole blood donors (unless the apheresis component is expected to be of particular value to a recipient and the donation is approved by the medical director). Plateletpheresis donors should not have taken aspirin-containing medication within the preceding 36 hours because aspirin inhibits cyclooxygenase-1, blocking the generation of thromboxane A_2. This blockage inhibits the platelet release reaction and renders the donated platelets less effective, particularly when the donor is the sole source of platelets for the recipient. As two large veins are often required, adequate venous access is important. Platelet products may be collected from these donors by apheresis at 2-day intervals but not more than twice weekly or 24 times yearly.[15] If they are collected at intervals of less than 4 weeks, the donor platelet count must be shown to be at least 150,000/μL before commencing collection. This count may be a precount or a precollection or postcollection count from a previous procedure. In addition, red blood cell losses must not exceed the loss of red blood cells permitted by whole blood collection for any 8-week period as well as in the preceding 12 months. Plasma losses must be less than 1 L (1.2 L for persons weighing more than 80 kg) every 7 days, with a maximum of 15 L in 12 months.

Current cell separator devices have been designed to allow the collection of substantially more than the minimum numbers of platelets (75% of units obtained by plateletpheresis must have at least 3×10^{11} platelets)[15] with a white cell content adequate to meet leukoreduction standards. The resulting products can be issued as leukoreduced without further filtration. Because large numbers of platelets can be obtained from some donors, there has been an increasing tendency to split the resulting product into two or even three transfusion doses. Although such doses meet product standards (3×10^{11} is required for each split product),[15] there is some controversy about the appropriate dose for a typical adult or even how such a dose should be determined. If a dose should produce an increment (in a nonrefractory patient) that minimizes the risk of spontaneous bleeding and it is desirable that that increment be maintained for 48 hours (to allow transfusion no more frequently than every other day), an appropriate dose could be 4×10^{11} to 4.5×10^{11}. With this dosage guideline, far fewer products could be split.

Adverse Effects

Donors of plateletpheresis products have risks of untoward reactions similar to those of donors of whole blood. As these donors tend to be older and repeat donors and the donation is isovolemic, the frequency of vasovagal reactions tends to be lower. These donors may experience symptoms of hypocalcemia, related to the infusion of citrate as part of the procedure. The symptoms most commonly include lightheadedness and perioral and peripheral paresthesias and are readily treated by ingestion of calcium-containing antacid tablets. If the donor's symptoms are not relieved by this simple approach, the citrate reinfusion rate can be slowed or the procedure stopped. Other than mild citrate reactions, adverse events are seen with an overall frequency of 2.18% (428 of 19,611 donations from 17 centers).[84] The most common adverse events are related to the venipuncture, with a frequency of 1.30%; a palpable hematoma accounted for 88% of these. The risk of a hematoma is higher for a plateletpheresis procedure than for a whole blood donation (0.3% for the latter; see Table 8.2).

Frequencies of all adverse events are nearly threefold higher in donors undergoing an apheresis donation for the first time. Vasovagal reactions, for instance, range from 2.0% in first-time to 0.5% in repeat donations.[88a] Other procedure-related problems (red blood cell hemolysis, air emboli, clots, and leaks) have been reported but are extremely rare with current machine hardware and software and trained operators. Although the preceding multicenter data (collected for the Hemapheresis Committee of the AABB)[84] are useful as an overall analysis of adverse events in apheresis donors, the results were quite variable from center to center. Some hospital-based centers recruit family members, many of whom would not have been previous whole blood donors. Whereas adverse events are generally less frequent with apheresis donations, hospital-based programs may have a higher frequency of serious adverse events. One such program with an overall frequency of adverse events of 0.81% had 0.24% (47 of 19,736 procedures) serious events.[85] Seven of these 47 donors required transfer to an emergency department.

The removal of large numbers of platelets in a plateletpheresis procedure causes a drop in the peripheral blood platelet count of $30,000/\mu L$[86] to $50,000/\mu L$[87] on average, with recovery in a few days. Repeated frequent plateletpheresis may cause a gradual decrease to unacceptably low levels, requiring temporary cessation of donation. The platelet count usually recovers in these donors over several months without treatment. Donors who continue to exhibit thrombocytopenia even with monthly apheresis procedures need to have their interdonation interval prolonged or stop serving as apheresis donors.

Lymphocytes have a density similar to that of heavier platelets. Intensive plateletpheresis removes large numbers of lymphocytes and depletes long-lived T lymphocytes, in theory leading to immune dysfunction. However, although reduction in lymphocytes has been seen, no clinical risk has been observed in healthy donors.[89]

Granulocytapheresis

Granulocytes have been collected by apheresis techniques for more than 30 years. When transfused to a neutropenic recipient in large doses, they provide a neutrophil increment in the recipient peripheral blood and migrate to a site of infection. Efficacy, in terms of survival of patients, has been more difficult to demonstrate. Data for both dogs[90] and humans[91] indicate that efficacy is dose related; however, the doses that could be obtained from donors before the avail-

ability of granulocyte colony-stimulating factor (G-CSF) were marginally effective. This fact, coupled with significant recipient pulmonary reactions, improved antibiotic therapy, and recognition of the adverse effects of leukocyte alloimmunization, led to less frequent use of granulocytes.

Because G-CSF, particularly with concomitant administration of corticosteroid, can allow the collection of almost four times more granulocytes than was possible with steroid alone,[92] interest in granulocyte transfusion has been renewed. Granulocytes from G-CSF–treated donors produce a significant increment in granulocytopenic recipients, have somewhat prolonged survival, and migrate effectively to sites of infection.[93] Unfortunately, G-CSF can currently be used for stimulation of normal donors before granulocytapheresis only as an Investigational New Drug. When G-CSF in approved for this purpose, it will be widely used. Although anecdotal results of large-dose granulocyte transfusions have been encouraging, there are as yet no conclusive studies regarding the effect of such transfusions on the survival of infected neutropenic recipients.

Donor Recruitment

Recruitment of granulocyte donors is a particular challenge because collection of adequate adult doses usually requires the use of corticosteroid before the collection. In the future, G-CSF injection may become part of routine granulocyte collections as well. There can be regular symptoms associated with these medications. Hospital-based programs have traditionally used members of the patient's family as donors. Here, the discomfort of the medication and the procedure is often readily tolerated because the procedure provides an outlet for the need to help. For community blood centers, the collective experience with the use of corticosteroid suggests that sufficient numbers of donors can be recruited to meet needs for these products: 60% of regular plateletpheresis donors at one center agreed to undergo granulocytapheresis, and 98% of these donors stated that they would be willing to participate again.[93] Because recipient antibodies to HLA and granulocyte-specific antigens can cause transfusion reactions and render the transfused granulocytes less effective,[94, 95] a large pool of well-characterized donors may be necessary. As granulocytes are contaminated with large numbers of red blood cells, ABO-compatible donors are also required.

Collection Procedure

In order to achieve the maximal granulocyte yield, the donor should be given G-CSF and corticosteroid and the product collected using a red blood cell sedimenting agent according to the cell separator manufacturer's protocol. G-CSF has been used widely to stimulate granulocyte production after chemotherapeutic marrow ablation and to stimulate peripheral blood progenitor cell production for transplantation. When given to volunteers as a single subcutaneous dose, it causes a marked release of marginated granulocytes from the spleen into the peripheral blood during the first few hours.[96] Steroid administration increases the number of circulating granulocytes by releasing cells from storage and marginal pools.

Dosage and timing of premedication have varied. G-CSF is typically given in doses of 5 to 10 $\mu g/kg$ subcutaneously, usually 12 hours before the collection procedure. Corticosteroids are given as prednisone or dexamethasone, the latter given as a dose of 8 to 12 mg, depending on the donor's weight, between 4 and 12 hours before the procedure. A uniform dose of 450 μg of G-CSF coupled with 8 mg of dexamethasone, both given 12 hours before, has been shown to be as effective as larger doses.[97]

Because the density of granulocytes is only slightly lower than that of red blood cells, it has been difficult to provide clean centrifugal separation without the use of a rouleaux-inducing agent to enhance red blood cell sedimentation. Hetastarch is most widely used for this purpose, but both 6% hetastarch and 10% pentastarch are in current use. In a controlled clinical trial, steroid-stimulated donors undergoing procedures with both sedimenting agents had a greater granulocyte yield with hetastarch ($2.3 \pm 0.67 \times 10^{10}$ vs. $1.4 \pm 0.76 \times 10^{10}$ for pentastarch).[98] However, hetastarch accumulates more readily in the extravascular space and is less rapidly cleared. This persistence can be a problem for family donors who may be subjected to repeated granulocytapheresis over several days because the transient plasma expansion can cause localized edema, headache, and other symptoms of fluid retention. The total product dose given to a donor should be monitored; it may be possible to reduce the dose for a given donor from one procedure to the next. This problem is not significant for volunteer donors giving infrequently, and there is less of a problem for donors undergoing repeated granulocytapheresis with pentastarch. Although traces of hetastarch may be detected in the donor years later, the small amounts present have not been shown to have clinical significance. Premedication with G-CSF and dexamethasone and collection with the use of hetastarch provides a product with a granulocyte yield of $7.25 \pm 1.54 \times 10^{10}$, compared with yields with dexamethasone alone of $2.16 \pm 0.71 \times 10^{10}$.[98]

Adverse Effects

The adverse effects of plateletpheresis procedures can also be seen with granulocytapheresis. In addition, there are potential unique reactions with granulocytapheresis because of the drugs and sedimenting agents used. A single dose of corticosteroid has minimal side effects, but insomnia or flushing has been reported in up to 25% of donors.[92] Donors participating regularly in a granulocytapheresis program (or family members undergoing repeated granulocytapheresis) probably should not have diseases exacerbated by prolonged use of corticosteroid, such as peptic ulcer, diabetes mellitus, hypertension, or glaucoma. With the administration of a single dose of G-CSF and dexamethasone, 72% of donors exhibit side effects; these are commonly mild bone pain (41%) and headaches (30%), both readily relieved by analgesics, and insomnia (30%).[93] In addition to the fluid retention effects of the starches, hetastarch may rarely cause local allergic reactions.

Plasmapheresis

Plasma can be obtained as a by-product of the collection of whole blood, directly by apheresis, or concurrently with other apheresis procedures. If separated and frozen shortly after collection, it can be considered fresh frozen plasma (FFP). If FFP time limits are exceeded, the plasma, still frozen, may be considered recovered plasma. Such plasma is sent for pooling and fractionation into plasma derivatives. Plasma can also be collected concurrently with other apheresis procedures (typically plateletpheresis). Finally, plasma can

be obtained directly by plasmapheresis. This procedure is performed by blood centers for specific types of FFP, such as group AB, generally in short supply. In addition, it is performed by commercial firms providing "source" plasma, so called because it is not used for direct transfusion but is the primary source of material pooled for fractionation into plasma derivatives.

Source plasma procurement has its own specific set of regulatory requirements designed to protect the donor from overly aggressive plasmapheresis. No more than 1000 mL of whole blood (1200 mL for donors weighing at least 80 kg) may be obtained (with at least the red blood cells returned to the donor) every 2 days, and no more than 2000 mL of whole blood (2400 mL for donors at least 80 kg) may be obtained within a 7-day period.[99] Collection of plasma at these frequencies requires periodic physical examination by a physician and periodic determination of serum protein levels.

For donors undergoing regular but less frequent plasmapheresis, such as regular plasma collection concurrent with plateletpheresis, the FDA guidelines for "infrequent plasmapheresis"[100] allow collection at an interval of 4 weeks or greater, if donors meet whole blood criteria, to an annual maximum of 12 L (14.4 L if at least 80 kg).

■ Staff Safety

Safety is always a concern for staff working with blood donors. In the donor area, attention should be paid to the use of needles, lancets, and microhematocrit tubes. Staff safeguards in this area have had increasing regulatory surveillance.[101] Although needles always require careful use, filling pilot tubes can be particularly dangerous. Devices are available to accomplish this task with minimal risk. Needles are also available with retractable covers to facilitate staff safety. Lancets and the platforms used with some types of disposable lancets must be handled with care. Glass microhematocrit tubes can break and puncture skin when pressed into the clay sealing substance. All these devices need to be disposed of in a "sharps" container, typically a box with sturdy sides. Workers preparing segments from the plastic tubing of the blood bag need to be protected from breakage and spraying of blood from these segments at the time of sealing.

When dealing with patients, it is necessary to use universal precautions (including the use of gloves by phlebotomists), both for staff protection and for prevention of disease transmission to other patients. For blood center employees in contact with patients (for instance, during therapeutic apheresis, during therapeutic phlebotomy, or with autologous donors) the same precautions are necessary. However, volunteer blood donors have a much lower prevalence of transfusion-transmitted disease than patients, and although gloves should be made available for all collection staff who wish to use them, wearing gloves is required for staff protection only if the staff member is in training or has abraded or eczematous skin. The safety of exposure to the blood of volunteer donors has been shown by the low frequency of disease markers in the collection staff.[102]

Staff working in a blood center must be encouraged to receive hepatitis B vaccine and its administration or refusal documented.[103] Further, if significant blood exposure (such as through a needlestick) occurs, the employee should be counseled immediately and offered prophylaxis for HIV infection.[104] Because postexposure prophylaxis (PEP) should begin within 2 hours of exposure, if the offer to treat is accepted, treatment cannot be postponed until test results are available. Although PEP for potential HIV transmission should be offered, it is reasonable for the counselor to recommend that the offer *not* be accepted for exposure to volunteer donor blood.[105] For exposure to patients' blood, PEP should be used until test results are available.

Treatment for other transfusion-transmitted diseases is less time sensitive and can await testing of the donor or seroconversion of the staff member. If the donor is found to be HBsAg positive and the staff member is not immune to hepatitis B, hepatitis B immune globulin and vaccine can be given.[103]

REFERENCES

1. Sullivan MT, Wallace EL, Umana WO, Schreiber GB: Trends in the collection and transfusion of blood in the United States, 1987–1997 [abstract]. Transfusion 1999;39(Suppl):1S
2. General Accounting Office: Blood Supply: Availability of Blood (GAO/HEHS-99-187R). Washington, DC: U.S. General Accounting Office, September 20, 1999.
3. Linden JV, Gregorio DI, Kalish RI: An estimate of blood donor eligibility in the general population. Vox Sang 1988;54:96–100.
4. Drake AW, Finkelstein SN, Sapolsky HM: The American Blood Supply. Cambridge, Mass, MIT Press, 1982, pp 87–94.
5. Eastlund T: Monetary blood donation incentives and the risk of transfusion-transmitted infection. Transfusion 1998;38:874–882.
6. Code of Federal Regulations, 21 CFR 606.121(c)(5). Washington, DC, U.S. Government Printing Office, 2000.
7. Strauss RG: Blood donations, safety, and incentives. Transfusion 2001;41:165–167.
8. Barker LF, Westphal RG: Voluntary, nonremunerated blood donation: still a world health goal? Transfusion 1998;38:803–806.
9. Piliavin JA: Why do they give the gift of life? A review of research on blood donors since 1977. Transfusion 1990;30:444–459.
10. Wallas CH, Lipton KS: Donor Incentives (Association Bulletin 94-6). Bethesda, Md. American Association of Blood Banks, 1994.
11. Williams AE, Thompson RA, Kleinman SH: Characterization of active blood donors who recently donated blood primarily to receive an HIV test [abstract]. Transfusion 1995;35(Suppl):42S.
12. Busch M, Stramer S: The efficiency of HIV p24 antigen screening of US blood donors: projections versus reality. Infus Ther Transfus Med 1998;25:194–197.
13. Sullivan JL: Iron and the sex differences in heart disease risk. Lancet 1981;1:1293–1294.
14. Meyers DG: The iron hypothesis: does iron play a role in atherosclerosis? Transfusion 2000;40:1023–1029.
15. Menitove J (ed): Standards for Blood Banks and Transfusion Services, 21st ed. Bethesda, Md, American Association of Blood Banks, 2000.
16. Code of Federal Regulations, 21 CFR 606.40. Washington, DC, U.S. Government Printing Office, 2000.
17. Grindon AJ, Norrell S, Robertson WR, et al: Predonation determination of donor eligibility [abstract]. Transfusion 1995;35(Suppl):72S.
18. Mayo DJ, Rose AM, Matchett SE, et al: Screening potential blood donors at risk for human immunodeficiency virus. Transfusion 1991;31:466–474.
19. Silvergleid AJ, Leparc GF, Schmidt PJ: Impact of explicit questions about high-risk activities on donor attitudes and donor deferral patterns: results in two community blood centers. Transfusion 1989;29:362–364.
20. Zuck TF, Cumming PD, Wallace EL: Computer-assisted audiovisual health history self-interviewing. Results of the pilot study of the Hoxworth Quality Donor System. Transfusion 2001;41:1469–1474.
21. Code of Federal Regulations, 21 CFR 640.3. Washington, DC, U.S. Government Printing Office, 2000.
22. Uniform Donor History Question (June 2002). In Brecher ME (ed): Technical Manual, 14th ed. Bethesda, Md, American Association of Blood Banks, 2002, pp 102–103.
23. Newman B: Blood donor suitability and allogeneic whole blood donation. Transfusion Medicine Review 2001;15:234–244.
24. FDA Memorandum: Revised Recommendations for the Prevention of Human Immunodeficiency Virus (HIV) Transmission by Blood and Blood Products. Bethesda, Md, Food and Drug Administration, April 23, 1992.

25. Murphy JL: Criteria for screening blood donors: science or politics? JAMA 1997;278:289.
26. Guidance for Industry Revised Preventive Measure to Reduce the Possible Risk of Transmission of Creutzfeldt-Jakob Disease and Variant Creutzfeldt-Jakob Disease by Blood and Blood Products. US Department of HHS, Food and Drug administration, Center for Biologics Evaluation and Research, January 2002.
27. Coburn TJ, Miller WV, Parrill WD: Unacceptable variability of hemoglobin estimation on samples obtained from ear punctures. Transfusion 1977;17:265–268.
28. Avoy DR, Canuel ML, Otton BM, et al: Hemoglobin screening in prospective blood donors: a comparison of methods. Transfusion 1977;17:261–264.
29. Newman B: Very anemic donors pass copper sulfate screening test [letter]. Transfusion 1997;37:670–671.
30. International Forum: How much blood, relative to his body weight, can a donor give over a certain period, without a continuous deviation of iron metabolism in the direction of iron deficiency? Vox Sang 1981;41:336–343.
31. U.S. Public Health Service: CDC criteria for anemia in children and childbearing-aged women. MMWR Morb Mortal Wkly Rep 1989;38:400–404.
32. Cable RG: Hemoglobin determination in blood donors. Transfus Med Rev 1995;9:131–144.
33. Nusbacher J, Chiavetta J, Naiman R, et al: Evaluation of a confidential method of excluding blood donors exposed to human immunodeficiency virus. Transfusion 1986;26:539–541.
34. Peterson LR, Lackritz E, Lewis WF, et al: The effectiveness of the confidential unit exclusion option. Transfusion 1994;34:865–869.
35. Korelitz JJ, Williams AE, Busch MP, et al: Demographic characteristics and prevalence of serologic markers among donors who use the confidential unit exclusion process: the Retrovirus Epidemiology Donor Study. Transfusion 1994;34:870–876.
36. Kean CA, Hsueh Y, Querrin JJ, et al: A study of confidential unit exclusion. Transfusion 1990;30:707–709.
37. Kessler D, Valinsky JE, Bianco C: Sensitivity and specificity of confidential unit exclusion (CUE)—does it work? [abstract] Transfusion 1993;33(Suppl):35S.
38. Williams AE, Thomson RA, Schreiber GB, et al: Estimates of infectious disease risk factors in US blood donors. JAMA 1997;277:967–972.
39. Vengelen-Tyler V (ed): Technical Manual, 13th ed. Bethesda, Md. American Association of Blood Banks, 1999, pp 713–714.
40. Galena HJ: Complications occurring from diagnostic venipuncture. J Fam Pract 1992;34:582–584.
41. Howanitz PJ, Cembrowski GS, Bachner P: Laboratory phlebotomy. College of American Pathology Q-probe study of patient satisfaction and complication in 23,783 patients. Arch Pathol Lab Med 1991;115:867–872.
42. Boynton MH, Taylor ES: Complications arising in donors in a mass blood procurement project. Am J Med Sci 1945;209:421–436.
43. Fainting in blood donors. A report to the Medical Research Council prepared by a subcommittee of the Blood Transfusion Research Committee. Br Med J 1944;1:279–283.
44. Tomasulo PA, Anderson AJ, Paluso MB, et al: A study of criteria for blood donor deferral. Transfusion 1980;20:511–518.
45. Kasprisin DO, Glynn SH, Taylor F, et al: Moderate and severe reactions in blood donors. Transfusion 1992;32:23–26.
46. Khan W, Newman B: Comparison of donor reaction rates in high-school, college, and general blood drives [abstract]. Transfusion 1999;39(Suppl):31S.
47. Trouern-Trend J, Cable R, Badon S, et al: Vasovagal reaction in blood donors: influence of gender, age, donation status, weight, blood pressure, and pulse. A case-controlled multicenter study. Transfusion 1999;39:316–320.
48. Poles FC, Boycott M: Syncope in blood donors. Lancet 1942;2:531–535.
49. Maloney WC, Lonnergan LR, McClintock JK, et al: Syncope in blood donors. N Engl J Med 1946;234:114–118.
50. Brown H, McCormack P: An analysis of vasomotor phenomena (faints) occurring in blood donors. Br Med J 1942;1:1–5.
51. Newman B: Donor reactions and injuries from whole blood donations. Transfus Med Rev 1997;11:64–75.
52. Williams GE: Syncopal reactions in blood donors. Br Med J 1942;1:783–786.
53. Ogata H, Iinuma N, Nagashima K, et al: Vasovagal reactions in blood donors. Transfusion 1980;20:679–683.
54. McHenry LC, Fazekas JF, Sullivan JF: Cerebral hemodynamics of syncope. Am J Med Sci 1961;241:173.

55. Engel GL: Psychologic stress, vasodepressor (vasovagal) syncope, and sudden death. Ann Intern Med 1978;89:403–412.

56. Tizes R: Cardiac arrest following routine venipuncture. JAMA 1976;236:1846–1847.

57. Newman B: Arterial punctures in whole blood donors. Transfusion 2001;41:1390–1392.

58. Kumar S, Agnihotri SK, Khanna SK: Brachial artery pseudoaneurysm following blood donation. Transfusion 1995;35:791.

59. Lung J, Wilson S: Development of arteriovenous fistula following blood donation. Transfusion 1971;11:145–146.

60. Gibble J, Ness P, Anderson G, Conry-Cantilena C: Compartment syndrome and hand amputation after whole blood phlebotomy: report of a case [abstract]. Transfusion 1999;39(Suppl):30S.

61. Newman BH, Waxman DA: Blood donation–related neurologic needle injury: evaluation of 2 years' worth of data from a large blood center. Transfusion 1996;36:213–215.

62. Berry PR, Wallis WE: Venipuncture nerve injuries. Lancet 1977;1:1236–1237.

63. Sherwood WC: Donor deferral registries. Transfus Med Rev 1993;7:121–128.

64. Finucane ML, Slovic P, Mertz CK: Public perception of the risk of blood transfusion. Transfusion 2000;40:1017–1022.

65. Etchason J, Petz L, Keeler E, et al: The cost-effectiveness of preoperative autologous blood donations. N Engl J Med 1995;332:719–724.

66. Popovsky MA, Whitaker B, Arnold N: Severe outcomes to allogeneic and autologous blood donation: frequency and characterization. Transfusion 1995;35:734–737.

67. Grossman BJ, Stewart NC, Grindon AJ: Increased risk of a positive test for antibody to hepatitis B core antigen (anti-HBc) in autologous blood donors. Transfusion 1988;28:283–285.

68. Goodnough LT, Monk TG, Andriole GL: Erythropoietin therapy. N Engl J Med 1997;336:933–938.

69. Williams AE, Wu Y, Klineman SH: The declining use and comparative seroprevalence of directed whole blood donations [abstract]. Transfusion 2000;40(Suppl):5S.

70. Strauss RG, Barnes A, Blanchette VS, et al: Directed and limited-exposure blood donations for infants and children. Transfusion 1990;30:68–72.

71. Hare VW, Liles BA, Crandall LW, Nufer CN: "Partners for Life"—a safer therapy for chronically transfused children [abstract]. Transfusion 1994;34(Suppl):92S.

72. Guidance for Industry (Draft): Variances for Blood Collection from Individuals with Hereditary Hemochromatosis. Bethesda, Md, Food and Drug Administration, Center for Biologics Evaluation and Research, December 20, 2000.

73. Sanchez AM, Schreiber GB, Glynn SA, et al: Unreported deferrable risk and frequency of hemochromatosis and polycythemia in blood donors [abstract]. Transfusion 1999;39(Suppl):1S.

74. Beutler E, Felitti VJ, Koziol JA, et al: Penetrance of 845G-A (C282Y) HFE hereditary haemochromatosis mutation in the USA. Lancet 2002;359:211–2118.

75. Elfath MD, Whitley P, Jacobson MJ, et al: Evaluation of an automated system for the collection of packed RBCs, platelets, and plasma. Transfusion 2000;40:1214–1222.

76. Shi PA, Ness PM: Two-unit red cell apheresis and its potential advantages over traditional whole-blood donation. Transfusion 1999;39:218–225.

77. Guidance for Industry: Recommendations for Collecting Red Blood Cells by Automated Apheresis Methods. Bethesda, Md. Food and Drug Administration, Center for Biologics Evaluation and Research, January 30, 2001.

78. MCS+ for RBC Apheresis: Owner's Operating and Maintenance Manual for Use with Software Revision E. PN 39220-00, Revision F. Braintree, MA, Haemonetics Corporation, January 1998.

79. Schmidt AL, Randels J, Wieland M, et al: Collection of 2 unit autologous or allogeneic red blood cells by apheresis using Haemonetics MCS+ [abstract]. J Clin Apheresis 1997;12:41.

80. Sherman LA, Lippmann MB, Ahmed P, et al: Effect on cardiovascular function and iron metabolism of the acute removal of 2 units of red cells. Transfusion 1994;34:573–577.

81. Axelrod FB, Catton P, Beeler SA: A comparison of post donation reactions in 2 unit automated red cell apheresis collection using the Haemonetics MCS+ with 1 unit manual whole blood collection in autologous donors [abstract]. Transfusion 1995;35(Suppl):65S.

82. Morrow JF, Braine HG, Kickler TS, et al: Septic reactions to platelet transfusions. JAMA 1991;266:555–558.

83. Glynn SA, Schreiber GB, Busch MP, et al: Demographic characteristics, unreported risk behaviors, and the prevalence and incidence of viral infections: a comparison of apheresis and whole blood donation. Transfusion 1998;38:350–358.

84. McLeod BC, Price TH, Owen H, et al: Frequency of immediate adverse effects associated with apheresis donation. Transfusion 1998;38:938–943.

85. Despotis GJ, Goodnough LT, Dynis M, et al: Adverse events in platelet apheresis donors: a multivariate analysis in a hospital-based program. Vox Sang 1999;77(1):24–32.

86. Simon TL, Sierra ER, Ferdinando B, et al: Collection of platelets with a new cell separator and their storage in a citrate-plasticized container. Transfusion 1991;31:335–339.

87. Katz AJ, Genco PV, Blumberg N, et al: Platelet collection and transfusion using the Fenwal CS-3000 cell separator. Transfusion 1981;21:560–563.

88. Lazarus EF, Browning J, Norman et al: Sustained decreases in platelet count associated with multiple, regular plateletphere donations. Transfusion 2001;41:756–761.

89. McCullough J: Introduction to apheresis donations including history and general principles. In McLeod BC, Price TH, Drew MJ (eds): Apheresis: Principles and Practice. Bethesda, Md. American Association of Blood Banks, 1997, p 40.

90. Applebaum FR, Bowles CA, Makuch RW, et al: Granulocyte transfusion therapy of experimental *Pseudomonas* septicemia: study of cell dose and collection technique. Blood 1978;52:323–331.

91. Strauss RG: Therapeutic granulocyte transfusions in 1993. Blood 1993;81:1675–1678.

92. Leitman SF, Oblitas JM: Optimization of granulocytapheresis mobilization regimens using granulocyte colony stimulating factor (G-CSF) and dexamethasone [abstract]. Transfusion 1997;37(Suppl):67S.

93. Price TH, Bowden RA, Boeckh M, et al: Phase I/II trial of neutrophil transfusions from donors stimulated with G-CSF and dexamethasone for treatment of patients with infections in hematopoietic stem cell transplantation. Blood 2000;95:3302–3309.

94. McCullough J, Clay ME, Hurd D, et al: Effect of leukocyte antibodies and HLA matching on the intravascular recovery, survival, and tissue localization of 111-indium labeled granulocytes. Blood 1986;67:522–528.

95. Adkins DR, Goodnough LT, Shenoy S, et al: Effect of leukocyte compatibility on neutrophil increment after transfusion of granulocyte colony-stimulating factor–mobilized prophylactic granulocyte transfusions and on clinical outcomes after stem cell transplantation. Blood 2000;95:3605–3612.

96. Lord LI, Bronchud MH, Owens S, et al: The kinetics of human granulopoiesis following treatment with granulocyte colony-stimulating factor in vivo. Proc Natl Acad Sci USA 1989;86:9499–9503.

97. Liles WC, Rodger E, Dale DC: Combined administration of G-CSF and dexamethasone for the mobilization of granulocytes in normal donors: optimization of dosing. Transfusion 2000;40:643–644.

98. Lee J-H, Leitman SF, Klein HG: A controlled comparison of the efficacy of hetastarch and pentastarch in granulocyte collections by centrifugal leukapheresis. Blood 1995;86:4662–4666.

99. Code of Federal Regulations, 21 CFR 640.60. Washington, DC, U.S. Government Printing Office, 2000.

100. FDA Memorandum: Revision of FDA Memorandum of August 27, 1982: Requirements for Infrequent Plasmapheresis Donors. Bethesda, Md. Food and Drug Administration, March 10, 1995.

101. Occupational Safety and Health Administration: Occupational exposure to bloodborne pathogens; needlesticks and other sharps injuries; final rule. Fed Regist 2001;66:5317–5325.

102. Page PL: Risk of hepatitis B exposure in regional blood services. Transfusion 1987;27:242–244.

103. Centers for Disease Control: Updated U.S. Public Health Service Guidelines for the Management of Occupational Exposures to HBV, HCV, and HIV and Recommendations for Postexposure Prophylaxis. MMWR Recomm Rep 2001;50(RR-11):1–52.

104. Code of Federal Regulations, 29 CFR 1910.1030. Washington, DC, U.S. Government Printing Office, 2000.

105. Grindon AJ, Keelan LT, Lenes BA: HIV post-exposure prophylaxis for blood center healthcare workers [abstract]. Transfusion 1998;38(Suppl):109S.

Chapter 9

Lookback Investigations and Product Recall/Withdrawal

Alfred J. Grindon

■ Product-Related Notifications

Notifications about suspect components or derivatives from a blood collection facility to a hospital transfusion service (called, in regulatory parlance, the *firm* and the *consignee*, respectively) may be grouped into three general categories: recalls, market withdrawals, and lookbacks. In both recalls and market withdrawals, the center discovers information after the component was distributed that indicates that the product did not meet required standards for distribution when it was sent to the hospital. If the deviation from the standard was the result of an error in the collection or processing of the unit by the collecting facility, in violation of the laws administered by the United States Food and Drug Administration (FDA), especially violations of current Good Manufacturing Practices, "and against which the agency would initiate legal action,"[1] the process is called a *biologic recall.* Although this action can be undertaken by the FDA, it is almost always performed by the blood banking community in a voluntary fashion.[2] If large multiunit recalls are excluded, the more common blood center recalls occur typically at an approximate rate of 1 in 5000 components distributed.[3]

If the information comes after collection, but does not result from an actionable violation, the action taken is considered a *market withdrawal.* For the blood center, this usually represents information provided by a blood donor or a third party after donation that, if known at the time of donation, would have led to deferral of the donor. Blood component–related market withdrawals occur with approximately the same frequency as recalls.[4]

■ SQuIPP

In deciding whether postdistribution information warrants recall or withdrawal, it is helpful to consider *SQuIPP,* an

Table 9.1 SQuIPP

Use SQuIPP to help determine whether a product needs to be recalled or withdrawn

Safety: does the product have a greater potential than usual for harmful effects?

Quality: does the product conform to preestablished specifications or standards?

Identity: is the identity of the final product and its labeling certain?

Purity: is the product free of extraneous contaminating matter?

Potency: can the product produce the desired effect?

acronym for safety, quality, identity, purity, and potency (Table 9.1). Any deviation from established procedures or deferral criteria that would lead to reduced *safety* in the product (i.e., greater potential for harmful effects) generally leads to withdrawal or recall. For instance, a presenting donor may state that he received a tattoo 4 months earlier, before a donation 3 months ago. Because donors with tattoos represent a group that may have a greater risk of carrying transfusion-transmissible disease, donors with recent tattoos are deferred. Had the center known of the tattoo at the time of the earlier donation, the donor would have been deferred; therefore, components distributed from the donation 3 months ago must be withdrawn.

Quality represents conformance of a product or process with preestablished specifications or standards. If it is discovered after the release of a leukoreduced component that the leukoreduction quality control for that component failed, then the component must be recalled.

Identity indicates the need to ensure that the identification of the donor, the unit, and its components is certain throughout the collection, processing, and labeling steps. For instance, if a unit of red blood cells, acceptable in every other way, is stated on the label to be negative for K1 when it is not, the unit is "misbranded," and it could be harmful to a recipient whose serum contains anti-K1.

Purity deals with freedom from extraneous contaminating matter in a product. If, after a recipient febrile transfusion reaction, the residue from a unit of Platelets is cultured and is found to contain microorganisms, the other components from that collection should be withdrawn, because they may also have been contaminated.

Potency represents the ability of a product to produce the desired effect. Here, it typically indicates a failure of quality control. The findings that fewer than 75% of Platelets units have 5.5×10^{10} platelets and that red blood cell recovery after leukoreduction of red blood cells is less than the required amount represent a loss of potency. If these products had been distributed, they would have led to a recall.

■ Action Taken by the Center

When the collecting facility discovers that a product that does not meet SQuIPP criteria has been released, staff members must work rapidly to notify the receiving transfusion service. For in-date products that may still be in the hospital inventory, this notification is done typically by telephone, to allow immediate quarantine of the suspect product, followed by written notification. The center must also quarantine any in-date products in its inventory. Because adverse information is typically obtained at the time of a subsequent attempted donation, platelet and red blood cell components are usually outdated, but frozen plasma, frozen red blood cells, and cryoprecipitate may still be in the center or hospital inventory. The center in-date inventory must be identified and quarantined quickly. Hospitals must be notified of in-date components as soon as possible, with written notification following soon afterward. When the hospital returns suspect components, the center usually destroys them or corrects the underlying problem with appropriate documentation. If the postdonation information would lead to donor deferral in the future, the center must place the donor in the deferral registry and must notify the donor of this action, to prevent collection and distribution of potential future donations. The center must document its actions and must seek from the consignee information regarding the final disposition of components.

Recalls must also be reported to the FDA. They are subsequently classified by FDA as follows: class I, "reasonable probability [of] serious health consequences"; class II, "temporary or medically reversible adverse health consequences"; class III, "not likely to cause adverse health consequences."[1] These recalls are then reported publicly several months later.[3]

■ Action Taken by the Hospital

When notified that products are being recalled or withdrawn, the hospital must act immediately to quarantine any such products in the inventory. The hospital must ensure that proper steps are taken and documented. When products have been transfused (75% of recalls in one hospital were found to be for components already transfused),[4] the hospital transfusion service must consider carefully the appropriate steps to take, in concert with hospital administration and risk management. For some recalls or withdrawals, no further action may be necessary. For instance, when a unit that was incorrectly labeled as K1 negative was subsequently transfused to a recipient who had no anti-K1, no clinician or patient notification would be needed, merely a note for the record of the facts. For other situations, the transfusion service may wish to notify the clinician but advise him or her that patient notification is probably unnecessary. For instance, red blood cells from a donor who had traveled to a malarial area and that were transfused 6 months earlier would have caused transfusion-induced malaria within 50 days of transfusion, and if no febrile disease developed, these red blood cells would represent no additional risk.[5] Finally, in some cases, the patient should be notified, particularly when there is some risk of infectious disease transmission, so that investigation, counseling, and treatment can be considered. Patient notification may be required, for instance, for possible transmission of human immunodeficiency virus (HIV) or hepatitis C virus (HCV).[6] In each case in which a component has been transfused, the transfusion service must balance the evidence that an infectious agent was transmitted through transfusion, the potential benefit to the recipient of receiving this information, and the potential harm to the recipient when no diagnostic test exists that can resolve whether such transmission has occurred.[7] If the transfusion service physician finds the information sent to be insufficient, sometimes more information can be obtained from the blood center. Fortunately, most recall and market withdrawal notifications have little clinical significance.[4, 8]

■ Lookback

When a donor unit is found to be positive for an infectious disease marker, several actions must be taken by the collecting blood center. Obviously, the implicated unit must be destroyed, and this disposition must be recorded. In addition, donor-related actions are required (notification, counseling, and placement in a donor deferral registry), and action often must be taken with regard to previous units donated by that donor.

Donor Notification and Counseling

A donor who is found by history to be at risk of carrying a transfusion-transmissible disease is often given printed information at the blood drive. This material should describe the donor's placement in a donor deferral system and the period of time of this deferral. If after successful donation the donor is discovered to be positive for an infectious disease marker, the donor must be notified of the test results and the medical significance of these results, must be given information about the implicated disease (often in the form of a "fact sheet" about the particular disease), and must be advised whether medical care should be sought. Further, the donor should be told whether he or she is now and will remain in the future ineligible to give blood. Finally, if the donor is placed into a donor deferral registry, the donor must be informed of this fact. All this information should be conveyed in readily understandable language (i.e., at an eighth grade reading level). In some situations, face-to-face counseling is preferred. To ensure that the donor understands the consequences of the test result, not only with regard to potential deferral from subsequent donation but also in terms of the availability of and need for treatment and the steps to reduce the risk of transmitting the disease to others, this notification process has become more rigorous. The standards of the American Association of Blood Banks require donor education, counseling, and referral, as appropriate.[9] For test deferrals, the FDA requires "...reasonable attempts to notify the donor within 8 weeks ..."[10]

Previous Units: Lookback

For most diseases, *prevalence*, measured for transfusion-transmitted diseases by an infectious disease marker, typically an antibody, is usually of less concern for blood safety than *incidence,* or the new acquisition and development of disease, because blood with a marker indicating prevalence is discarded. For a newly acquired viral agent, the concern is about the *window period*, defined as the time between donor infection and the appearance of detectable markers of disease. The window period may be conveniently divided into two parts: an eclipse period, when the agent is undergoing proliferation in host tissue but is not present in sufficient numbers in the blood to be infectious,[11] and the subsequent infectious period, when circulating virus can be transmitted by the blood. The goal of test improvement has been to increase sensitivity to the extent that the infectious window period is reduced as much as possible. Because an infectious window period still exists, and may have been longer in the past, when a donor is found to have a newly acquired antibody marker of an infectious disease, the more recent previously seronegative donations of that donor must be regarded as suspect.[12] The risk of a previous donation's transmitting disease depends on the incidence of the disease and on the length of the infectious window period, the latter a function of the sensitivity of the test used. For HIV or HCV, using nucleic acid amplification testing, the infectious window period may be a few days at most.[11] Notification of recipients of previously donated seronegative units is important, so that the recipients may be tested and, if they are positive for the agent, counseled and treated appropriately.

Actions by the Center and the Hospital

The blood center must identify previously donated units at risk from the implicated donor and must determine the components made from these units and the consignees to whom these components were shipped. The center must then notify the hospital of the situation and must obtain information about the final disposition of the components. If in-date components from such units may be available, the consignee should be notified as soon as possible after the detection of a repeat reactive screening test.

The specifics vary by disease: For HIV and human T-cell leukemia/lymphoma virus (HTLV), the center searches for the first seronegative (or untested) unit previously donated and for all units donated for at least 1 year before that donation.[13] The center must identify all components made from the suspect units and must determine where they were sent. If any in-date components exist, these must be identified and quarantined if they are in the center. If these components have been distributed, the consignees of such components should be notified within a few days of the positive test result. The hospital, in turn, must ensure that the patient is notified (typically through the clinician, but, if necessary, by the hospital directly) within a few weeks. For HIV, even if the patient is

deceased, the patient's next of kin must be notified.[13] For HTLV, in contrast, the clinician can make the decision not to notify the patient or recipient, if the decision is warranted clinically. Both the center and the hospital must document notification attempts.

For HCV lookback on a donor found to be seropositive, the same process is used: the center must identify units 12 months before the last seronegative unit, locate the consignees of components made from those units and shipped to the consignee, and notify the consignee within 45 days of the repeat reactive donation. The consignee must ensure that the patient is notified of the need for HCV testing and of the availability of testing and counseling. There must be documentation of three attempts to notify the recipient within 12 weeks of notification by the center.[13]

A massive retrospective HCV lookback of units donated between 1990 and 1999 and on which lookback had not already been performed was begun in 1999 and was completed by 2001. This *targeted* (identification of specific blood recipients) lookback process may not be very cost-effective. One estimate is that of approximately 300,000 recipients to be notified, perhaps only 5 to 10,000 will be living and will have newly recognized infections, and 1500 will benefit from therapy.[14] Interim data from the United States Centers for Disease Control and Prevention corroborate these numbers: only about 0.5% of recipients will be found to have newly recognized infections.[15] Despite the inefficiency of the targeted lookback process, no compelling evidence indicates that general notification of all blood recipients will be effective[16]; many of those recipients identified by targeted lookback would not otherwise be identified and treated.

REFERENCES

1. CFR 7.1–7.59. Washington, DC, United States Government Printing Office, 1997.
2. Bozzo T: Blood component recalls. Transfusion 39:439–441, 1999.
3. Ramsey G, Sherman L: Blood component recalls in the United States. Transfusion 39:473–478, 1999.
4. Ramsey G, Fryxell LM, Russell DL, Sherman LA: Three-year hospital experience with a system for tracking blood supplier notifications about blood products. Transfusion 38(Suppl):123S, 1998.
5. Guerrero IC, Weniger BC, Schultz MG: Transfusion malaria in the United States, 1972–1981. Ann Intern Med 99:221–226, 1983.
6. United States Food and Drug Administration: Current good manufacturing practices for blood and blood components: Notification of consignees receiving blood and components at increased risk for transmitting HIV infection. Final rule: HHS docket No.91N-0152. Fed Reg 61:47413–47474, 1996.
7. Smith DM, Lipton KS: Association Bulletin 97-3: Consignee/Recipient Notification Guidelines. Bethesda, MD, American Association of Blood Banks, 1997.
8. Grindon AJ, Harris SL, Roback JD, et al: Low patient risk from market withdrawn (MW) blood components. Transfusion 39(Suppl):125S, 1999.
9. Menitove JE (ed): Standards for Blood Banks and Transfusion Services, 21st ed. Bethesda, MD, American Association of Blood Banks, 2002, p 5.2.2
10. United States Food and Drug Administration: General requirements for blood, blood components, and blood derivatives: Notification of deferred donors. Final rule. Fed Reg 66:112;31166, 2001.
11. Murthy KK, Henrard DR, Eichberg JW, et al: Redefining the HIV-infectious window period in the chimpanzee model: Evidence to suggest that viral nucleic acid testing can prevent blood-borne transmission. Transfusion 39:688–693, 1999.
12. Ward JW, Holmberg SD, Allen JR, et al: Transmission of human immunodeficiency virus (HIV) by blood transfusion screened as negative for HIV antibody. N Engl J Med 318:473–478, 1988.

13. United States Food and Drug Administration: Current good manufacturing practices for blood and blood components: Notification of consignees and transfusion recipients receiving blood and blood components at increased risk of transmitting HCV infection ("lookback"). Proposed rule. Fed Reg 65:69377–69416, 2000.

14. AuBuchon JP: Public health, public trust, and public decision making: making hepatitis C virus lookback work. Transfusion 39:123–127, 1999.

15. Culver DH, Alter MJ, Mullan RJ, Margolis HS: Evaluation of the effectiveness of targeted lookback for HCV infection in the United States: Interim results. Transfusion 40:1176–1181, 2000.

16. Zuck T: Cited in Busch MP: Let's look at human immunodeficiency virus look-back before leaping into hepatitis C look-back. Transfusion 31:655–661, 1991.

Chapter 10

Quality Improvement and Control

Richard J. Benjamin

■ Quality

Quality, "a degree of excellence" or "superiority of kind,"[1] is an ephemeral attribute that is difficult to define quantitatively. The patient's view of quality of service bears little relationship to the "documented free of defect" approach taken by regulatory agencies. Consequently, blood bank professionals find themselves held to quality standards set by a variety of agencies that tend to have different foci. For example, the Joint Commission for Accreditation of Healthcare Organizations (JCAHO) focuses on service aspects, examining components of the transfusion service involved in ordering, processing, and transfusion of blood. At the other extreme, the Food and Drug Administration (FDA) concentrates on the quality of the end product and applies pharmaceutical industry standards to the collection, testing, and provision of safe blood. Over the years, these complementary but frequently overlapping approaches have led to the need for transfusion services to maintain sophisticated compliance programs to maintain accreditation. An understanding of the manner in which this environment developed facilitates comprehension for the uninitiated.

■ Regulatory Background

Blood products are viewed as both biologics and drugs,[2] and blood banks have been subject to license and inspection since May 1946 under the provisions of the Public Health Service (PHS) Act.[3] In 1972, responsibility for blood components was transferred from the National Institutes of Health (NIH) to the FDA, which published Current Good Manufacturing Practices (cGMPs) for blood and blood components[4] in November 1975, specifically designed to regulate the blood industry. These regulations were intended to ensure uniform blood component production throughout the United States and gave the FDA authority to regulate and inspect both licensed and unlicensed blood banks. Nevertheless, it was the epidemic of acquired immunodeficiency syndrome (AIDS) in the 1980s that highlighted the public health risk of transfusion and spurred the regulatory agencies to focus heavily on the safety of transfusion.

All establishments that collect, process, or transfuse blood components are required to register with the FDA.[5] This entails an annual submission of a list of products and processes performed. Establishments that manufacture and transport products over state lines are further required to license both their establishment and the individual products manufactured before commencing operations. All registered facilities are subject to biennial inspections to ensure that the blood produced is safe, effective, free of adulteration, and appropriately labeled. The FDA has considered the regulation of facilities that manufacture cellular and tissue-based therapeutics, including hematopoietic stem cells derived from blood, umbilical cord blood, and bone marrow.[6] As a first step to regulation, the FDA now requires registration of facilities engaged in processing such cells. Licensed establishments had to register by April 2001, and nonlicensed facilities must undertake registration by January 2003. The intent of these requirements is clear. The FDA intends to regulate novel and established cellular and tissue-based therapeutic products in a fashion analogous to the regulation of drugs and blood products.

Beginning in 1980, the FDA and the Health Care Financing Administration (HCFA) began coordinating visits to unlicensed blood banks according to a memorandum of understanding.[7] This agreement resulted in HCFA taking over inspection responsibility for a significant number of transfusion services that store and issue blood products manufactured elsewhere. Transfusion services that do not collect or process blood (even autologous blood) and that are approved by HCFA for Medicare reimbursement are exempt from registration with the FDA under this agreement. Currently, the FDA inspects only manufacturers of blood and components, including those collected for autologous use. However, the FDA reserves the right to inspect nonregistered transfusion services where there are indications of noncompliance with the cGMPs.

Blood banks and transfusion services also test blood (e.g., ABO and Rh typing, viral marker testing) and are therefore subject to the Clinical Laboratory Improvement Amendments[8, 9] (CLIA 1988), which set standards for good laboratory practices. Responsibility for ensuring compliance with CLIA is also assigned to the HCFA. This is achieved during biennial inspections by the JCAHO, an accrediting agency with deemed status from HCFA.

Many states in the United States also require registration of blood banks and transfusion services and have annual reporting requirements for adverse events and for transfusion and collection statistics. Requirements for reporting and inspections vary from state to state.

Finally, professional bodies such as the American Association of Blood Banks (AABB),[10] the College of American Pathologists (CAP),[11] and the Foundation for Accreditation of Hematopoietic Cell Therapy (FAHCT)[12] publish lists of voluntary standards to which many institutions subscribe. Annual inspections are undertaken to ensure compliance. These voluntary standards are intended to allow the profession to inspect and regulate its own practices outside the punitive environment of federal and state regulation. Accreditation by these agencies has yet to preclude inspection by the FDA or JCAHO.

■ Blood Transfusion as a Service

The purpose of quality assurance is to provide high-quality care of patients and to ensure safe, effective blood products. The focus of the JCAHO regulatory effort is predominantly on service issues related to the quality of care of patients. JCAHO guidelines and biennial inspections therefore ensure that hospitals have systems in place for reviewing blood utilization, including (1) ordering; (2) distribution, handling, and dispensing; (3) administration; and (4) the effects of transfusion. Oversight of these reviews is the responsibility of a hospital transfusion committee composed of members from departments that use blood, the clinical laboratories, blood bank, nursing, and administration.[13, 14] In this view, transfusion is a cooperative effort that requires quality assessment and documented improvement exercises that are performed continuously, according to objective guidelines used to monitor performance. Specific aspects that may be subject to audit and review include the adequacy of the blood supply, the use and wastage of autologous blood, mislabeling of patients' specimens, turnaround time from ordering to transfusion for immediate and routine orders, and the documentation of patients' identification and vital signs at the time of transfusion. Further important aspects are investigations of transfusion reactions, the appropriateness of blood orders, the use of intraoperative blood salvage equipment, and the use and maintenance of blood warmers.

Table 10.1   Examples of Criteria for Blood Component Administration in Adults

Red blood cells
  Symptomatic anemia in a normovolemic patient
  Acute loss of > 15% of blood volume or evidence of inadequate O_2 delivery
  Hematocrit < 27% in a chronically transfused patient
  Hematocrit < 30% in patient with severe cardiac or pulmonary dysfunction

Platelets
  Platelet count < 10,000/μL in a stable patient without bleeding risk factors
  Platelet count < 20,000/μL in a stable patient with risk factors for bleeding
  Platelet count < 50,000/μL for impending surgery or invasive procedure
  Bleeding in patient with qualitative platelet defect regardless of cause

Fresh frozen plasma
  PT and/or PTT > 1.5 normal value in patient undergoing surgery, an invasive procedure, or active bleeding
  To reverse coumadin overdose in a bleeding patient
  Bleeding after transfusion of more than one blood volume or signs of disseminated intravascular coagulation
  For plasma exchange in patients with thrombotic thrombocytopenic purpura

Cryoprecipitate
  Prevention or treatment of bleeding in patients with dysfibrinogenemia
  Prevention or treatment of bleeding in patients with fibrinogen < 100 mg/dL

Transfusion guidelines and criteria for using specific products vary between institutions and are developed by the transfusion committee with reference to criteria published in peer-reviewed journals. Examples are shown in Table 10.1. Such practice guidelines are not intended to serve as medical indications for transfusion; rather, they set limits outside which the ordering physician should be required to provide additional justification. Review of appropriateness of blood use is an important function of the transfusion committee, and there is a requirement that 5% of all transfusions be audited on a quarterly basis. Review may take one of three forms:

1. Prospective review, in which the physician is required to provide an indication for each transfusion. This is assessed by the blood bank technologist, who determines whether the appropriate criteria are met. If not, the physician is asked to provide further justification for the specific order. If transfusion is urgent, the blood product may be released and the follow-up information obtained retrospectively.

2. Concurrent review, which requires transfusions to be assessed within 24 hours of issue, while the patient is still in the hospital and the indications are still fresh in the memory of the physician. Both concurrent and prospective review provide opportunities to educate medical staff with respect to appropriate use of transfusions.

3. Retrospective review, which is undertaken some time after transfusion. This type of review is less effective. Trends in transfusion practice may be documented, although less educational benefit is gained.

Overall, the purpose of blood utilization review is to provide opportunities to identify areas that need quality improvement. The emphasis is as much on ensuring that blood is available and used when it is needed as it is on preventing waste of a limited resource and unnecessary exposure of patients to the risks of transfusion.

■ Blood as a Drug

Blood components are drugs from the point of view of the FDA because their use is meant to produce therapeutic benefit for the patient.[15] Establishments that collect blood (even autologous products) are viewed as pharmaceutical manufacturers. This approach raises significant practical issues. The principles of cGMP for drugs, as laid out in the Code of Federal Regulations (CFR)[16] and described in the following, are based on the concepts of continuous process control and lot release of products. In this view, blood donors are analogous to sources of raw material and donor testing is simply quality control of incoming supplies. Furthermore, each blood product is a unique lot and therefore requires individual lot release, whereas with drugs a batch of drug may be released. With blood products, quality control of each lot is not usually feasible. For this reason more emphasis is placed on quality assurance of overall processes rather than testing each product for quality parameters, such as volume, weight, hematocrit, and leukocyte content.

The FDA clearly recognizes the unique nature of blood products as both blood and biologics and has promulgated a second series of regulations, specific for blood,[4] that complement those in the 21 CFR 211 series. The underlying principle of regulatory control of blood products is that by enforcing strict quality assurance of manufacturing processes, the statutory agencies hope to ensure the quality of individual blood products. Nevertheless, the advances in the field of blood safety, including the development of new tests (e.g., nucleic acid testing) and processes (e.g., leukoreduction), outstrip the ability of the federal government to promulgate law. Consequently, the industry relies on a series of guidelines and notices from the FDA that supplement the CFR and create many standards for the industry.

■ The Principles of cGMP

The concept of cGMPs is founded on the need to demonstrate control of all aspects of a manufacturing process, with documentation of all variables. This control should allow any single product to be tracked from donor to recipient and all regents, facilities, and personnel to be traced so that any deviations may be fully identified, investigated, and rectified. Tight control of the manufacturing process, combined with suitable in-process quality control procedures and regular quality assurance exercises, serves to ensure the potency, efficacy, and purity of the final product.

The statutes promulgated in 21 CFR 211[16] cover all aspects of manufacture, including personnel, buildings and facilities, equipment, components and containers, packaging, labeling, storage, holding and distribution, records, production and process controls, and salvaged products. Central to this philosophy is the need to document all procedures in standards of practice (SOP) and to qualify all facilities, equipment, and components by validation before use. A key role is ascribed to the quality control unit, which has overall responsibility for the release of final products.

■ Continuous Quality Improvement

Continuous quality improvement (CQI) is based on the premise that, despite the utmost care, processes and systems cannot be designed to be perfect, essentially because it is not possible to predict all eventualities. It is therefore necessary to implement an evolutionary refining process to detect deviations and to put in place appropriate corrective actions (Fig. 10.1). The FDA requires that establishments have in place procedures for thoroughly searching for signs of deviations in processes. These may become apparent during validation of a new process, during quality control (QC) and quality assurance (QA) audits, or through occurrences such as

Figure 10.1 Continuous quality improvement.

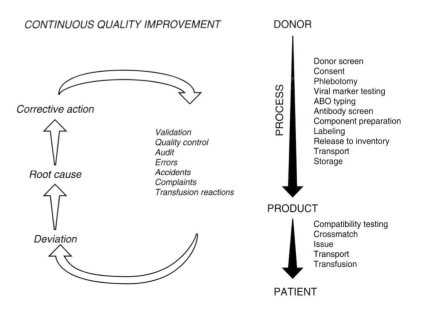

errors, accidents, complaints, and transfusion reactions. Establishments must have systems in place to investigate such deviations, to determine their root cause, and to put in place corrective action. Central to this concept is the idea that staff and customers must be encouraged to report deviations; indeed, they should be encouraged to search actively for mistakes without fear of retribution. This view recognizes deviations as opportunities to improve and to provide better services. Well-designed processes performed by well-trained staff should ideally not allow deviations. When they occur, the assumption is that they are due to problems with the system rather than individual mistakes. Indeed, a no-liability atmosphere promotes reporting and ultimately leads to systemic quality improvement.

■ The Role of the Quality Assurance Unit

Ensuring the safety of blood products requires the implementation of effective control over manufacturing processes and systems. In 1995 the FDA published guidelines that require blood establishments to develop written QA programs with an emphasis on error prevention rather than retrospective detection.[17] QA is the sum of activities planned and performed to provide confidence that all systems and their elements that influence the quality of a product are functioning as expected and can be relied upon. QA functions include QC procedures and audits as well as ensuring that standards are in place for facilities, personnel, procedures, equipment, testing, and record keeping.

All blood establishments are required to have a QA function, either as a QA unit in large establishments or a single individual in small transfusion services. Whatever the size, the QA unit is required to be separate from the management of production and to report directly to the responsible head or the designated qualified person in charge of the operation. The QA unit has final responsibility for the quality of products released and must have the power to stop production and release of product if it deems necessary.

Major responsibilities of the QA unit include the following:

1. Standard operating procedures

   Development of written procedures is a fundamental component of cGMP that promotes an environment with minimal variation. Ensuring that SOPs exist and that they accurately describe each procedure is a basic function of the QA unit. Each SOP must be reviewed, be signed, and be indexed in a master copy of SOPs. SOPs must be available to employees who perform the tasks. SOPs must be updated promptly to reflect changes in processes, and these modifications must be appropriately documented. SOPs must exist for QA unit activities that define its role in reviewing, approving, and authorizing all SOPs.

2. Training and education

   The QA unit should assist in developing, reviewing, and approving training and educational programs for all personnel. This responsibility includes new employee orientation; cGMP, SOP, and QA training; as well as technical, supervisory, managerial, and computer system training. The QA unit is ultimately responsible for ensuring that personnel are appropriately qualified and trained to perform their tasks. Written documentation of training must be on file.

3. Competence evaluation

   The QA unit should implement a formal regular competence evaluation program to ensure that staff maintain the skills to perform their tasks. This program should include direct observation of performance of routine and QC procedures, review of worksheets, preventive maintenance records, and written tests to assess theory and knowledge of SOPs. Remedial action and retraining should be documented in the personnel records.

4. Proficiency testing

   The QA unit should review and monitor proficiency testing procedures and results to ensure adequate evaluation of test methods, equipment, and personnel competence. Proficiency testing should be performed by the same personnel who perform the tasks routinely and should include backup or alternative testing (e.g., manual procedures performed during computer downtime). There should also be a written plan for remedial action in the case of unsuccessful proficiency testing performance.

5. Validation

   The QA unit is responsible for ensuring that validation protocols are designed prospectively, performed, and evaluated and that written validation reports are prepared. Although validation of test methods is a standard practice in the clinical laboratory, the extension of these principles to manufacturing processes, computer systems, and facilities poses unique challenges. Validation requires documented evidence to demonstrate that the system is performing as designed with the expected degree of accuracy and reproducibility. Complaints, errors, accidents, and problems at critical control points should be reviewed to determine the need for revalidation, according to the FDA's Guideline on General Principles of Validation.[18]

6. Equipment and computers

   Equipment in particular should undergo installation qualification by the establishment (not the manufacturer). This is a form of validation that establishes "confidence that process equipment and ancillary systems are capable of consistently operating within established limits and tolerances." There should be written procedures for equipment qualification, validation, maintenance, calibration, and monitoring. A major piece of equipment that is easily overlooked in the blood bank is the computer-based information system. The FDA has recognized that computers play a central role in practically all blood bank processes and that the risk of deviation caused by computer errors is high. For this reason, blood bank information systems are considered medical devices in their own right and are directly regulated by the Center for Biologics Evaluation and Research (CBER) at the FDA, requiring 510(k) approval before being marketed. This places a unique burden on the manufacturers of blood bank software to demonstrate good software engineering practices and to document and validate all aspects of their systems.

Furthermore, blood establishments are required to validate all aspects of software on site, an exhaustive process that is described in a dedicated guideline from the FDA.[19] As with other processes in the blood bank, there must be a system in place to document complaints and problems with computer software and hardware, with documented investigation, root cause analysis, and corrective actions. New versions of software require revalidation. Many institutions find that they require a dedicated computer person to perform these tasks despite the purchase of commercial software systems. The situation for homegrown computer programs has been less clear historically, as these are not for commercial sale. Homegrown systems may be utilized without preapproval, but the FDA has made it clear that they expect the same standards to apply to homegrown computer system design as to commercial vendors. Although they do not routinely inspect the manufacturers of homegrown systems, they enforce the full weight of the law should major deficiencies in the computer system become apparent during routine blood bank inspection.

7. Error/accident reports, complaints, and adverse reactions

   Licensed establishments are required to report to CBER all errors and accidents that affect the safety, potency, identity, or purity of a blood product. The FDA has announced that nonlicensed establishments have to report similar occurrences if the product has left the control of the establishment by the time the occurrence is detected.[20] It is the role of the QA unit to investigate all complaints, errors, and accidents to determine whether there is a need to report each occurrence. Similarly, all adverse reactions must be fully investigated and documented, and recalls and withdrawals must be handled according to established procedures. In particular, transfusion reactions must be fully investigated, and in cases of suspected bacterial contamination, a full review of manufacturing procedures must be undertaken. Fatalities that are related to either the donation process or the receipt of blood products are reportable within 24 hours to a special hot line at the FDA. This has to be followed within a week by a full written report describing the occurrence and its subsequent investigation. This, in turn, usually triggers a focused FDA inspection.

   As outlined earlier, an essential element of CQI is feedback into the QA system of knowledge acquired through investigation of complaints, errors, accidents, or adverse reactions. This is seen as a vital source of information on which continuous quality improvement efforts can be focused through a system of corrective actions and fine-tuning of existing processes.

8. Records management

   The QA unit is responsible for ensuring that all records, including computer records, are adequately stored and held for the appropriate periods as defined by the FDA. Systems of storage, especially computerized systems, must be fully validated and reviewed as necessary to ensure completeness.

9. Lot release procedures

   Each component released by a blood establishment represents one lot of product and bears a lot number, usually the unit number assigned at the time of collection. QA procedures must ensure that all records pertaining to manufacture are reviewed for accuracy, completeness, and compliance with existing standards before release. A second person should review the significant steps. Labeling procedures especially are considered critical control points and must be tightly controlled.

10. QA audits

   A QA audit is one mechanism for evaluating the effectiveness of the total quality system. Comprehensive audits should be conducted periodically in accordance with written procedures and should consist of a review of a statistically significant number of records. On occasion, focused audits may be conducted when quality problems have been identified or to monitor a particular critical control point. Individuals conducting audits must have sufficient knowledge and expertise in the process under review but must not be responsible for the processes being audited. There should be a written report documenting audit procedures and results, which should include a review by the responsible head or other designated qualified person to evaluate the results of the audit so that suitable corrective action can be implemented. QA audits should be constructed using a systems approach and may include review of donor suitability, blood collection, manufacturing, product testing, storage and distribution, lot release, and computers. QA audits should evaluate critical control points and key elements in each system, and each establishment should customize its audits for its own systems.

■ Conclusion

Quality management in transfusion medicine is a formalized process that is required by law. Quality is also a mind-set that accepts only the best and works hard to improve, despite cost constraints, shortages in the skilled workforce, evolving technology, and a growing regulatory burden. Despite the appearance that progress in safety accrues in infinitesimally small increments, it is now clear that, along with refinements in donor screening and viral marker testing, the implementation of cGMP principles in the blood bank and improved clinical practice are responsible for the safety revolution that has occurred in blood transfusion.

REFERENCES

1. Webster's 9th New Collegiate Dictionary. Springfield, Mass, Merriam-Webster Inc, 1991.
2. Federal Food, Drug and Cosmetic Act. Title 21 USC Sec 201 (Amended by FDA Modernization Act of 1997).
3. Public Health Service Act, Biologic products. Title 42 USC Sec 262 (revised annually).
4. Code of Federal Regulations. Title 21 CFR 606. Washington, DC, US Government Printing Office, 2000 (revised annually).
5. Department of Health and Human Services, Food and Drug Administration, Office of Regulatory Affairs: FDA Compliance Policy Guide. Registration of Blood Banks and Other Firms Collecting, Manufacturing, Preparing and Processing Human Blood or Blood

Products. Bethesda, Md, Food and Drug Administration, 2000, Sec 230.110.

6. Human cells, tissues and cellular and tissue-based products; establishment registration and listing. 21 CFR 207, 807 and 1271. Fed Regist 2001;66:5447.

7. Department of Health and Human Services, Food and Drug Administration: FDA Compliance Policy Guide. Memorandum of Understanding 1980: 7155e.03 Chapter 55e. Bethesda, Md, Food and Drug Administration, 1980.

8. Department of Health and Human Services: Medicare, Medicaid and CLIA programs: regulations implementing the Clinical Laboratory Improvement Amendments of 1988 (CLIA 1988). Fed Regist 1992;57:7002.

9. Code of Federal Regulations. Title 42 CFR 493.1. Washington, DC, US Government Printing Office, 2000 (revised annually).

10. Menitove JE (ed): Standards for Blood Banks and Transfusion Services, 19th ed. Bethesda, Md, American Association of Blood Banks, 1999.

11. How to Inspect the Transfusion Medicine Laboratory. Chicago, College of American Pathologists, 1999.

12. Foundation for Accreditation of Hematopoietic Cell Therapy: Standards (1995). Omaha, Nebr, Author, 1995.

13. Silberstein LE, Kruskall MS, Stehling LC, et al: Strategies for the review of transfusion practices. JAMA 1989;262:1993–1997.

14. Stehling L, Luban NLC, Anderson KC, et al: Guidelines for blood utilization review. Transfusion 1994;34:438–448.

15. Department of Health and Human Services, Food and Drug Administration, Office of Regulatory Affairs: FDA Compliance Policy Guide. Human Blood and Blood Products as Drugs (CPG 7134.02). Bethesda, Md, Food and Drug Administration, 1996, Sec 230.120.

16. Code of Federal Regulations. Title 21 CFR 211. Washington, DC, US Government Printing Office, 2000 (revised annually).

17. Department of Health and Human Services, Center for Biologics Evaluation and Research: Guideline for Quality Assurance in Blood Establishments (Docket no 91N-0450), 1995.

18. Department of Health and Human Services, Center for Drugs and Biologics, Center for Devices and Radiological Health: Guideline on General Principles of Process Validation. Rockville, Md, Division of Manufacturing and Product Quality, 1987.

19. Department of Health and Human Services, Center for Biologics Evaluation and Research: Draft Guideline for the Validation of Blood Establishment Computer Systems (Docket no 93N-0394). Office of Communication, Training and Manufacturers Assistance, 1993.

20. Department of Health and Human Services, Food and Drug Administration: Biological products: reporting of biological product deviations in manufacturing. Fed Regist 2000;65:66621.

Chapter 11

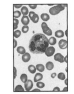

Component Preparation and Storage

Mary Beth Allen

The process of transfusion therapy begins with the collection of a volume of blood by either whole blood donation or an apheresis collection procedure. Whole blood is drawn and can subsequently be separated into its constituents: packed red blood cells, plasma, white cells, and platelets. This division of whole blood into separate parts, or *component preparation*, accomplishes several objectives. First, it enables blood products to be transfused selectively according to specific patients' needs. Second, by increasing the number of transfusable products per volunteer donation, it maximizes the number of transfusion recipients who benefit from this valuable community resource. And lastly, component preparation enables blood collection agencies to maximize their financial return associated with the expense of each blood collection procedure. In this chapter, we explore the fundamental technical principles of this process known as component preparation. The clinical aspects of component transfusion therapy are addressed in separate chapters in this text.

■ Collection

Whole Blood

Whole blood collections may be performed at 8-week intervals and consist of no more than 10.5 mL per kilogram of donor body weight.[1] The donor may not be pregnant, should be at least 17 years of age, and should meet healthy donor requirements for temperature, blood pressure, pulse rate, and hemoglobin or hematocrit.[2] Donors taking medications or those with heart, liver, or lung disease or a history of cancer or abnormal bleeding should be excluded or evaluated by a medical director.[3]

Donors must be evaluated for at-risk behavior, including evidence of alcohol or drug use and histories of sexually transmitted diseases.[4] Recipients of transfusions of blood or blood components, blood derivatives, human tissue or tissue derivatives, immunizations, or vaccines must be deferred for the recommended intervals specified by the relevant regulatory agencies.[5] Likewise, individuals with histories of exposures to viral diseases, malaria, and protozoan diseases, such as Chagas disease or babesiosis, should be deferred for the recommended intervals.[6]

Collecting facilities must provide donors with educational materials regarding the risks of infectious diseases transmitted by transfusion, including acquired immunodeficiency syndrome,[7] so that they may understand the potential consequences for recipients if they donate in spite of known risk factors. The information must be conveyed in a manner that can be readily understood by the donor, and donors must be provided an opportunity to ask questions regarding the educational materials.[7] Written informed consent must be obtained before collection and should be consistent with applicable law. The informed consent should contain an explanation of the significant risks of the collection procedure in language that is understandable to the donor.[8] Donors may be offered the option of *unit exclusion* after donation, which is a mechanism to indicate that the donated unit should not be transfused to patients. If unit exclusion is offered, it should be provided in a manner that ensures confidentiality[9] to the donor. Donors should also be encouraged to provide *postdonation information* regarding development of symptoms of illness immediately after donation or the recollection of relevant donor history that was not disclosed at the time of donation.

Apheresis

Apheresis donor requirements are defined by the frequency of donations. *Infrequent* donations are collections performed at greater than 4-week intervals; *frequent* donations are collections performed at less than 4-week intervals. Donor requirements for infrequent donations are the same as for whole blood donors.[10] Frequent donors must comply with the Food and Drug Administration (FDA) requirements for donor testing and physical examination.[11] As with whole blood donors, informed consent must be obtained and documented.

Donors must be carefully observed by trained personnel during the apheresis procedure. In the event of unexpected adverse donor reaction, immediate assistance must be available to apheresis personnel and appropriate medical care must be provided to the donor.

Care must be taken to ensure that repeated donations do not result in cumulative depletion of the donor. For example, donors undergoing frequent plateletpheresis must maintain a minimum platelet count of 150,000/µL.[12] Removal of plasma during frequent plasmapheresis may not exceed the amount approved by the FDA.[13] Similarly, red blood cell losses during consecutive apheresis procedures during any 8-week or 12-month period may not exceed the volume allowed for whole blood collections.[14]

Therapeutic apheresis procedures may be performed to facilitate removal of a specific constituent, such as plasma or white blood cells. All therapeutic procedures must be requested by the patient's attending physician and should be deemed appropriate by the apheresis department medical director. As with all donation procedures, appropriate information should be provided to the patient and informed consent obtained, and appropriate medical care should be provided as needed.[15] Blood or blood components collected during therapeutic apheresis procedures may not be used for transfusion and should be discarded in a manner consistent with the department's policies for medical waste management.

Anticoagulants

Several anticoagulant-preservatives are currently approved by the FDA for storage of blood and blood components. These include citrate, phosphate, and dextrose (CPD) and CP2D, which have a 21-day storage limit for red blood cells maintained at 1 to 6°C. Blood collected in citrate, phosphate, dextrose, and adenine (CPDA-1) may be stored for 35 days if maintained at 1 to 6°C.[16] The purpose of all these anticoagulants is to support metabolic activity of the red blood cells, maintain an anticoagulated state, and minimize the effects of degradation during storage. Table 11.1 illustrates the content of the anticoagulant-preservative solutions.[17] Citrate, provided by trisodium citrate and citric acid, maintains the anticoagulated state through chelation of calcium,

thereby inhibiting the calcium-dependent steps of the coagulation cascade. Dextrose and adenine support synthesis of adenosine triphosphate (ATP) by the stored red blood cells, and sodium phosphate serves as a buffer to minimize the effects of decreasing pH in the stored product.

Additive systems, such as AS-1, AS-3, and AS-5, enable red blood cell storage to extend to 42 days at 1 to 6°C.[18] Additive collection systems consist of a primary collection bag containing anticoagulant-preservative and attached satellite bags, one of which is empty and is eventually used to contain separated plasma. The other satellite bag contains the additive solution, which must be added to the anticoagulated red blood cells within 72 hours after collection. Additive solutions, in addition to extending the shelf life of the red blood cell product, result in a packed red blood cell product with a hematocrit of approximately 60%, which improves flow rate and facilitates rapid administration of the product. Composition of the additive solutions is illustrated in Table 11.2.[19]

The biochemical changes that occur during storage are known as *storage lesions*. These are represented in Table 11.3.[20] Storage lesions typically do not have clinically significant consequences in transfused recipients; however, special care may be warranted for pediatric and neonatal recipients.[21]

Rejuvenation of red blood cells stored in CPD or CPDA-1 solutions can be accomplished through addition of a solution containing pyruvate, inosine, phosphate, and adenine.[22] The rejuvenation solution may be added either during storage or up to 3 days after expiration of the red blood cells.[23] Rejuvenated red blood cells may be glycerolized and frozen for extended storage.[24] However, all rejuvenated red blood cells should be washed prior to infusion to remove the potentially toxic inosine.

Blood should be collected into a sterile container that contains appropriate anticoagulant solution. The collection should begin with a single venipuncture causing minimal trauma to tissues. The contents of the container should be mixed frequently and thoroughly. Commercially available collection sets contain 63 mL of anticoagulant-preservative, which results in a solution-to-blood ratio of 1.4:10.[25]

The standard collection volume is 450 mL ± 45 mL of blood or 405 to 495 mL. Low-volume collections of 300 to 404 mL may be used for red blood cell transfusions if appropriately labeled but may not be used for the manufacture of components.[26] Collection should be completed within 15 minutes to ensure optimal component quality.[27] Sterility of the products should be maintained by use of sterile solutions and disposables and proper use of aseptic technique. Products collected in an integral or *closed* system may be maintained for the recommended storage periods for that component. However, if the system is entered or *open*, components have a

Table 11.1 Content of Anticoagulant-Preservative Solutions (g/L)

Component	ACD-A	CPD	CP2D	CPDA-1
Trisodium citrate	22.00	26.30	26.30	26.30
Citric acid	8.00	3.27	3.27	3.27
Dextrose	24.50	25.50	51.10	31.90
Monobasic sodium phosphate		2.22	2.22	2.22
Adenine				0.275

ACD, acid-citrate-dextrose; CPD, citrate, phosphate, and dextrose; CPDA-1, citrate, phosphate, dextrose, and adenine.

Table 11.2 Content of Additive Solutions (mM)

Component	AS-1 (Adsol)	AS-3 (Nutricel)	AS-5 (Optisol)
Dextrose	111.00	55.50	45.50
Adenine	2.00	2.22	2.22
Monobasic sodium phosphate	0.00	23.00	0.00
Mannitol	41.20	0.00	45.40
Sodium chloride	154.00	70.00	150.00

Table 11.3   Biochemical Changes of Stored Red Blood Cells

Variable	CPD		CPDA-1				AS-1*	AS-3†	AS-5*
	Whole Blood		Whole Blood	Red Blood Cells	Whole Blood	Red Blood Cells	Red Blood Cells	Red Blood Cells	Red Blood Cells
Days of storage	0	21	0	0	35	35	42	42	42
% Viable cells (24 hours post-transfusion)	100	80	100	100	79	71	76(64–85)	84	80
pH (measured at 37°C)	7.20	6.84	7.60	7.55	6.98	6.71	6.6	6.5	6.5
ATP (% of initial value)	100	86	100	100	56(±16)	45(±12)	60	59	68.5
2,3-DPG (% of initial value)	100	44	100	100	<10	<10	<5	<10	<5
Plasma K$^+$ (mmol/L)	3.9	21	4.20	5.10	27.30	78.50‡	50	46	45.6
Plasma hemoglobin (mg/L)	17	191	82	78	461	658.0‡	N/A	386	N/A
% Hemolysis	N/A	N/A	N/A	N/A	N/A	N/A	0.5	0.9	0.6

*Based on information supplied by the manufacturer.
†From Simon, et al.[4]
‡ Values for plasma hemoglobin and potassium concentrations may appear somewhat high in 35-day stored RBC units; the total plasma in these units is only about 70 mL.
From American Association of Blood Banks: Technical Manual, 14th ed. Bethesda, Md, AABB, 2002.

shortened shelf life of 24 hours for components stored at 1 to 6°C or 4 hours for components stored at 20 to 24°C.[28] Sterile connection devices may be utilized to facilitate component manufacture while maintaining maximal shelf life for the products.

Allogeneic Donor Testing

Testing of allogeneic donor blood should include determination of the donor's ABO group and Rh type. The ABO should be determined by testing the donor's cells with reagent anti-A and anti-B (forward type) and by testing the donor's serum or plasma for expected isoagglutinins against known Al and B red blood cells (reverse type). The forward typing must be consistent with the reverse typing. Any discrepancies must be resolved before release of the donor unit.[29] The Rh type should be determined using anti-D. If initial anti-D testing is negative, a test for weakened D antigen should be performed. Positive reactions in either the D typing or the weak D testing require that the unit be labeled "Rh POSITIVE." Only units from donors testing negative for both D and weak D may be labeled as "Rh NEGATIVE." ABORh determinations must always be performed from a specific donor unit; historical ABORh types from previous donations may not be used to label the current unit.[30]

Donations should also be tested for unexpected serum antibodies to red blood cell antigen if the donor has a history of previous transfusion or pregnancy or other potentially sensitizing event. The antibody screen should be performed by a method or technology capable of detecting clinically significant antibodies.[31]

Donations must also be tested to prevent transmission of infectious diseases to recipients. The testing currently required includes hepatitis B surface antigen, hepatitis B core antibody, anti–human T-cell leukemia/lymphoma virus type I (HTLV-I), anti–HTLV-II, human immunodeficiency virus type 1 (HIV-1) antigen, anti–HIV-1, anti–HIV-2, anti–hepatitis C virus, and syphilis.[32] Chapter 12 offers an in-depth discussion of infectious diseases potentially transmitted by transfusion. Positive results for any of the preceding infectious disease tests preclude the distribution of the donor product except in the case of approved emergency release. Untested units must be clearly labeled to indicate

their status. Emergency-released units subsequently found to test positive require appropriate, immediate notification of physicians.

Donors found positive on any of the preceding tests for infectious diseases should be notified by the collection facility's medical director in keeping with standard operating procedures and regulatory requirements. The collecting facility must also have in place a mechanism, consistent with FDA requirements,[33] for quarantine and disposition of units previously collected from donors who are repeatedly reactive for any of the preceding infectious disease tests and for notification of the recipients of those products when appropriate.[34]

■ Component Preparation

Whole Blood

Whole blood products are the transfusion therapy equivalent of whole blood circulating in vivo. Whole blood is composed of red blood cells, white blood cells, platelets, and plasma. Whole blood has limited clinical indications and is appropriate only when replacement of both blood volume and red blood cell mass is required, as in cases of massive blood loss. Trauma services have largely replaced whole blood transfusions with readily available sterile intravenous solutions in conjunction with units of packed red blood cells. Indeed, whole blood units now serve primarily as the source material for blood component products.

Red Blood Cells

Red blood cells are obtained by either sedimentation or centrifugation of whole blood, followed by removal of the plasma portion. The resulting packed red blood cell products should have a hematocrit less than or equal to 80%.[35] Red blood cells are indicated for replacement of red blood cell mass and for restoration of oxygen-carrying capacity. Red blood cells retain the original expiration date of the parent whole blood product, provided the plasma removal has been performed in an integral or closed system. If the container system has been entered in any way, the system is referred to as *open*, and the expiration must be shortened to 24 hours from the time the unit was entered[36] to protect against bacterial contamination.

Red blood cells are frequently modified to address specific transfusion requirements for patients. Common modifications include washing (removal of plasma proteins to protect against allergic transfusion reactions), irradiation (exposure to radioactive sources to prevent graft-versus-host disease in immunocompromised recipients), and leukoreduction (removal of white blood cells to prevent alloimmunization and viral disease transmission and to reduce the occurrence of febrile transfusion reactions). Each of these common product modifications is discussed in detail in subsequent chapters of this text.

Frozen Red Blood Cells

Less common, although still important, modifications include freezing, deglycerolization, and rejuvenation of red blood cells. Freezing of red blood cells is normally undertaken to preserve units with rare phenotypes or autologous units intended for future use. Red blood cells must be carefully managed during the freezing process to maintain post-thaw viability. The first requirement for successful red blood cell freezing is careful control of the rate of freezing. Freezing at a rate slower than 10°C/min results in water outside the red blood cell freezing before water inside the red blood cell. This creates an osmotic gradient, causing intracellular water to migrate outside the cell membrane and resulting in a dehydrated red blood cell. Conversely, red blood cells that are frozen too quickly form intracellular ice crystals, which may damage the cellular construction of the red blood cell. Therefore, a balance between cellular dehydration and intracellular ice crystal damage must be achieved by carefully controlling the rate of freezing.[37]

The second critical aspect of red blood cell freezing is the use of cryoprotective agents. Cryoprotective agents are of two types: penetrating and nonpenetrating. Penetrating agents, such as glycerol and dimethyl sulfoxide (DMSO), are small molecules capable of passing through the red blood cell membrane into the intracellular space. There, they form a protective osmotic barrier that prevents the escape of water into the extracellular space, thereby preventing cellular dehydration. High concentrations of these penetrating cryoprotectants have been shown to prevent ice crystal formation.[38] Of these two common cryoprotectants, glycerol is relatively pharmacologically inert and is therefore frequently used for red blood cell preservation. DMSO, however, is a powerful solvent and may have adverse effects if residual amounts are transfused to recipients. Special care should be exercised when preparing or infusing products using DMSO as the cryoprotective agent.

Nonpenetrating cryoprotective agents, such as hydroxyethyl starch (HES), are molecules too large to pass through the red blood cell membrane. They protect cell viability by vitrification, or formation of a noncrystalline shell around the exterior of the red blood cell,[39] which inhibits intracellular dehydration. Of all these cryoprotective agents, high-concentration glycerol is most commonly utilized in freezing of red blood cells.

Red blood cells are normally frozen within 6 days of collection[40] except when rejuvenated. Once frozen, units may be stored at −65°C for up to 10 years, in compliance with FDA licensure for the product Red Blood Cells, Frozen and current standards of the American Association of Blood Banks (AABB). However, units of extremely rare phenotypes may be maintained in frozen storage for extended periods if the need for extended storage is appropriately documented by the facility's medical director. Units have been successfully transfused after 21 years in storage.[41]

Deglycerolized Red Blood Cells

Upon removal from frozen storage, the frozen red blood cell units must be thawed and washed to remove the cryoprotective agents. There are multiple procedures for cryoprotectant removal, but most use a principle of multiple washes with a series of solutions of decreasing osmolarity. This gradual removal of cryoprotectant is essential to prevent hemolysis of the red blood cell product and to return it to a transfusable state of osmotic equilibrium.

Frozen (deglycerolized) red blood cells are comparable to fresh, liquid red blood cells. The frozen (deglycerolized) red blood cells have had plasma, anticoagulant, and most of their platelets and white blood cells removed by the freezing-deglycerolization process. Therefore, deglycerolized red blood cells may be indicated for use in immunoglobulin A (IgA)–deficient patients with clinically significant anti-IgA antibodies and for patients with severe reactions to transfused plasma proteins.[42] Modern leukoreduction filters, however, are more efficient at white blood cell removal than deglycerolization and therefore are a better component choice for prevention of recurrent febrile transfusion reactions, transmission of cytomegalovirus (CMV), and alloimmunization against human leukocyte antigen (HLA) in recipients. Freezing and deglycerolization do not remove all viable lymphocytes and therefore should not be substituted for irradiation for prevention of graft-versus-host disease.

Rejuvenated Red Blood Cells

Rejuvenated red blood cells are red blood cells treated by a solution containing pyruvate, inosine, phosphate, and adenine, which restores 2,3-diphosphoglycerate and ATP to at least normal levels.[43] Rejuvenation may take place during storage and up to 3 days after the expiration date.[44] The rejuvenated unit may then be glycerolized and frozen for prolonged storage or stored at 1 to 6°C if used within 24 hours.[45] If rejuvenated units are used in a liquid state, they must be washed to remove the rejuvenation solution because inosine may cause adverse effects if transfused.

Platelets

Platelet concentrates are platelet products separated from centrifuged whole blood and must contain 5.5×10^{10} platelets in at least 75% of the products prepared by the facility.[46] Quality control of the platelet counts should be performed at maximal storage time or at the time of use on a minimum of four products per month. Platelets should be prepared within 8 hours of collection from whole blood that has not been stored at temperatures below 20 to 24°C.[47] The platelets should be suspended in an adequate volume of plasma to maintain a minimum pH of 6.2 by the end of their allowable shelf life.[48] Platelet products should be inspected visually before transfusion; products showing excessive platelet aggregation should not be used for transfusion purposes. Platelets are used to support patients whose own platelets are either insufficient in number or functionally inadequate to maintain normal hemostasis. Clinical aspects of platelet transfusion are described in Chapters 17 and 31.

The current shelf life for platelet concentrates is 5 days from the day of collection. Platelet viability is markedly affected by storage conditions, and suboptimal conditions may contribute to a degradation of platelet morphology known as platelet storage lesion. Optimal storage parameters include (1) maintenance at temperatures between 20 and 24°C, (2) constant, gentle agitation to prevent aggregation, (3) an adequate volume of plasma to maintain the pH at 6.2 or above, (4) appropriate anticoagulant-preservative solution to maintain platelet metabolism, and (5) storage in a plastic container with sufficient surface area to support adequate oxygen exchange.[49]

Apheresis collection may also be used to produce platelet products known as single-donor platelets or plateletphereses. Because large numbers of platelets can be harvested from a single donor by apheresis, these products are frequently used to minimize the number of donor exposures to patients requiring frequent platelet transfusions. Plateletpheresis donors should meet all apheresis donor requirements; however, donation may be more frequent than whole blood donation. Plateletpheresis donors may donate at intervals of at least 48 hours and not more frequently than twice a month or 24 times per year.[50]

Plateletpheresis products must contain at least 3.0×10^{11} platelets in at least 75% of the products tested.[51] As with platelet concentrates, pH should be maintained at a minimum of 6.2 during the product's shelf life. Plateletpheresis products with robust platelet counts may be divided or *split* into two individual products, provided each product contains a minimum of 3.0×10^{11} platelets in each container.[52] All other requirements for storage and shelf life are the same as for platelet concentrates manufactured from whole blood.

Granulocytes

Granulocyte products are suspensions of granulocytes in donor plasma, prepared by apheresis. Granulocyte components must contain a minimum of 1.0×10^{10} granulocytes in 75% of the products tested.[53] Clinical relevance of granulocytes is described in detail in Chapter 18. Generally, granulocytes are transfused to patients with reversible neutropenia and gram-negative sepsis unresponsive to antibiotic therapy.[54] Granulocyte therapy has not been universally effective in adults, but the response to granulocyte transfusion in infants has been more successful. For adults, daily doses for several consecutive days are normally recommended to ensure optimal benefit.

Collection of a product containing 1.0×10^{10} granulocytes requires pretreatment of the donor with HES, corticosteroids, or growth factors. HES is a sedimenting agent that promotes rouleaux of red blood cells. These aggregated red blood cells sediment much more effectively than untreated red blood cells during apheresis centrifugation, allowing more effective separation of the granulocytes from the underlying band of red blood cells. HES has a circulating half-life of 24 to 29 hours, but residual HES can be detected for as long as 1 year after administration.[55] Facilities that administer HES prior to granulocyte apheresis should have written policies regarding maximum allowable doses of sedimenting agents that may be administered to any single donor over a period of time.

Corticosteroids may also be administered to facilitate granulocyte recovery in the apheresis product. Corticosteroids such as hydrocortisone, prednisone, methyl prednisone, or dexamethasone promote release of granulocytes from the storage pool into circulation. Again, the collection facility should have written procedures regarding the recommended dosing schedule for corticosteroid pretreatment. Care should

be taken to identify donors with preexisting medical conditions that might be adversely affected by administration of corticosteroids.[56]

Growth factors, such as granulocyte colony-stimulating factor (G-CSF) or granulocyte-macrophage colony-stimulating factor (GM-CSF), may also facilitate recovery of granulocytes. Administration of GM-CSF has been shown to increase recovery of granulocytes to 10×10^{10} per apheresis collection and appears to be well tolerated by both donor and product recipient.[57] Administration of any enhancing agent should require specific permission for the drug or sedimenting agent in the donor's informed consent for the leukapheresis procedure.

Laboratory testing for granulocyte products should include ABORh, antibody screen, and infectious disease testing. Because of their high red blood cell content, granulocytes should be ABO compatible with the intended recipient. Compatibility testing must be performed if the granulocyte unit contains more than 2 mL of packed red blood cells.[58] Granulocyte products should be transfused as quickly as possible after collection for maximum granulocyte viability. This may necessitate performing laboratory testing concurrently with the collection or obtaining emergency release approval from the patient's attending physician for administration prior to completion of testing.

Fresh Frozen Plasma

Fresh frozen plasma (FFP) components are prepared by separating plasma from red blood cells of a single donor and storing the plasma at −18°C. The separation must occur within 8 hours of collection if collected in CPD, CP2D, or CPDA-1 anticoagulant. If acid-citrate-dextrose (ACD) anticoagulant is used, the separation must take place within 6 hours of collection.[59] Plasma may be collected by either whole blood donation or apheresis. When stored at −18°C or below, FFP has a shelf life of 1 year. If not utilized within 12 months, the product can be relabeled as "plasma" and stored for an additional 4 years.[60]

Plasma is the liquid portion of whole blood, which contains water, electrolytes, albumin, globulin, clotting factors, and other plasma proteins. Its principal purpose is to correct coagulation factor deficiencies in patients, and it occasionally serves as a replacement fluid for patients undergoing therapeutic plasma exchanges. Clinical applications of plasma products are described in Chapter 14. Prompt freezing after collection preserves the labile coagulation factors V and VIII. Rapid freezing of the FFP unit itself can be accomplished in dry-ice ethanol or dry-ice antifreeze baths (using protective overwrap layers), between layers of dry ice, in specially designed blast freezers, or in regular biochemical freezers at −65°C or less.[61] It is advisable to freeze products in a manner that makes it easy to detect whether the product has been thawed and subsequently refrozen, such as indenting the product with a tube or rubber band or freezing flat to produce an air bubble in the side of the product. Any thawing with subsequent refreezing would eliminate these telltale marks from the products.

Plasma, Liquid Plasma, Cryoprecipitate-Reduced Plasma, Recovered Plasma, and Source Plasma

Plasma components may be created by separation of the plasma portion from the red blood cells at any time during shelf life and up to 5 days after the whole blood expiration date.[62]

This plasma may be labeled as "liquid plasma" and stored at 1 to 6°C for a maximum of 5 days after the whole blood expiration or may be labeled as "plasma" and stored at −18°C or below for up to 5 years.[63] These plasma and liquid plasma components differ from FFP mainly by their lack of labile coagulation factors and by exhibiting higher levels of potassium and ammonia as a result of extended storage with degrading red blood cells. If cryoprecipitate was originally removed from the whole blood collection, the residual plasma product must be labeled to indicate so. Cryoprecipitate-reduced plasma is sometimes used as a replacement fluid for patients with thrombotic thrombocytopenic purpura undergoing therapeutic plasma exchange.

There are limited clinical indications for plasma and liquid plasma products. However, these products are commonly converted to an unlicensed product known as "recovered plasma" and sold to fractionators for manufacture of blood product derivatives such as albumin and immune globulins.[64] Collection facilities that provide the unlicensed recovered plasma product to manufacturers are required by the FDA to have a "short supply agreement" with the manufacturer.[65] Plasma collected by apheresis that is intended for further manufacture into blood derivatives is labeled "source plasma." Like recovered plasma, it has no expiration date and requires retention of records for an indefinite period of time.

Cryoprecipitate

Cryoprecipitated antihemophilic factor (Cryo) is the cold-insoluble portion of plasma processed from FFP by thawing the FFP unit at 1 to 6°C.[66] The cryoprecipitate is then promptly centrifuged, separated from the plasma, and then refrozen within 1 hour.[67] All cryoprecipitate components should contain a minimum of 150 mg of fibrinogen and 80 IU of coagulation factor VIII.[68] Cryoprecipitate is transfused primarily as a source of replacement fibrinogen. Cryoprecipitates are stored at −18°C or lower for a period of 1 year.[69] Cryoprecipitates may be thawed at 30 to 37°C and pooled into a single product for infusion within 4 hours[70] or may be pooled before freezing and stored at −18°C for up to 1 year. These pooled products are known as cryoprecipitated antihemophylic factor pooled and must be labeled with the number of units contained in the pool, volume of saline used in pooling, and instructions to use within 4 hours after thawing.[71] Appropriate quality control and record keeping for the pooled products should be maintained.

■ Labeling, Storage, and Shipping

Labeling

The labeling process should conform to the most recent version of the U.S. industry consensus standard for the uniform labeling of blood and blood components using International Society for Blood Transfusion (ISBT) 128 or the 1985 FDA uniform labeling guideline.[72] Labels should be firmly affixed to the container and contain clear, eye-readable information. Information may also be barcoded or machine readable, and any manual handwritten corrections should be in legible, indelible, moisture-proof ink.[73] The labeling process must include a second verification that the ABO, Rh, expiration date, and component labels have been appropriately attached to the container. Products must be uniquely labeled using a numeric or alphanumeric system so that any product can be identified and traced from its origin to its final disposition. Original unique identifying numbers affixed by the collecting facility may not be removed or obscured. Any intermediate facility that affixes an additional identifying label on the product must include its facility name on the additional label. A maximum of two unique identifiers may be visible on a product at any given time. If multiple intermediary facilities attach labels to the product, some identifying numbers from intermediary facilities may need to be obliterated; however, the original unit number affixed by the collection facility must remain intact.[74]

Labeling at the time of collection or component preparation must include the following information: the name of the product, a unique numeric or alphanumeric identifier, the type of anticoagulant (except for washed, frozen, deglycerolized, or rejuvenated red blood cells), the approximate volume collected from the donor, names of any sedimenting agents, and identification of the facility performing the collection or modification.[75]

Prior to final labeling, the product and all associated records and tests must be reviewed for acceptability. Acceptability criteria must be defined, and each product must be reviewed to verify that it meets those criteria. Donor records must be reviewed for comparison of previous and current ABO group and Rh type, when possible, and for any indications that the donor is unsuitable. Discrepancies in any testing or acceptability criteria must be resolved before release of the product. Unacceptable testing results or acceptability criteria should trigger a mechanism to quarantine the product immediately and safeguard against its release for transfusion.[76] The final label before distribution to the transfusing facility should contain the following information: temperature of storage, expiration date and (when appropriate) time, identification of facility, ABO group and Rh type, specificity of unexpected red blood cell antibodies (except for cryoprecipitate or washed, frozen, deglycerolized, or rejuvenated red blood cells), and indication of autologous, volunteer, or paid donor, where applicable. The label must also contain instructions to the transfusionist, which include "See circular of information for the use of human blood and blood components," "Properly identify intended recipient," "This product may transmit infectious agents," and "Caution: Federal law prohibits dispensing without a prescription" or "Rx only."[77]

Special product qualities or modifications may require specific labeling. For example, products that have been irradiated must be labeled with the appropriate component name as well as identification of the facility performing the irradiation. Cellular components that are seronegative for CMV must be labeled as such if transfused to patients requiring CMV-seronegative products. Likewise, leukocyte-reduced products must be appropriately labeled. Pooled products must be labeled with the following additional information: the name of the pooled component, final volume, name of the facility performing the modification, a unique numeric or alphanumeric identification number for the pool, the number of units contained in the pool, and the ABO group and Rh type of products in the pool.[78]

Storage

Storage of blood and blood products should be designed to maintain maximum viability in a strictly controlled and secure environment. These designated storage areas may contain only blood, blood components, blood derivatives, donor samples, patients' samples, tissue for transplantation, and related reagent or laboratory supplies.[79] These storage areas must have adequate capacity and air circulation to ensure optimal storage conditions. Requirements for storage of blood products, illustrated in Table 11.4, are defined as those that best preserve blood product viability and safety.[80] Storage devices should have a system for continuous temperature monitoring and recording of temperatures at least every 4 hours. If components are stored at room temperature, outside a controlled storage device, the ambient room temperature should be recorded every 4 hours.

Audible alarm systems should be present on all refrigerators and freezers and set to be activated at a temperature that allows rescue of the blood or blood products before they reach unacceptable temperatures. The audible alarms must be present in an area with sufficient personnel coverage to ensure an immediate response. Alarm systems for liquid nitrogen freezers should be activated when inappropriate levels of liquid nitrogen are reached. Written instructions must specify corrective action to be taken in the event of a storage device failure in order to prevent loss of valuable blood and blood components.[81]

Shipping

As with storage, shipping conditions should be defined that maintain maximum viability of blood and blood components. All blood and blood products should be inspected upon packing and again upon receipt to ensure that the container is intact and the product is normal in appearance. Any product that appears abnormal should not be shipped by the vendor; it should be quarantined and handled according to the facility's standard operating procedure for nonconforming products. Similarly, products that appear abnormal upon receipt should be placed in a segregated storage area, and the nonconformity should be investigated and documented.[82] Upon receipt, all products should be inspected to ensure that the container is undamaged and that labeling of the product is appropriate. If platelet products are shipped, they may not be out of a state of gentle agitation for longer than 24 hours.[83]

■ Pretransfusion Testing

Physician Orders

Requests for transfusion of blood products should originate from the intended recipient's physician. At least two unique identifiers must allow conclusive identification of the intended recipient.[84] These identifiers may include, but are not limited to, information such as the recipient name, medical record number, date of birth, or Social Security number. The request should also clearly specify the type and number of blood products desired. The information contained on the request must exactly correspond to the information on the sample to be used for compatibility testing.

Sample Requirements

Samples used for compatibility testing must be drawn from recipients who have been positively identified at bedside using an identification band system approved by the care facility. The identification band must be present on the recipient's body and contain sufficient information to identify the

recipient positively and uniquely. Blood samples obtained from that patient must be legibly labeled at bedside and should contain at least two unique identifiers, the date of collection, and identification of the person collecting the sample.[85] Information on the request and the patient's sample must be verified for accuracy and completeness by transfusion service personnel prior to testing. Any discrepancies between the information on requests and that on samples should result in generation of new orders and recollection of the sample.

Laboratory Testing

ABO Group

Recipient testing for compatibility includes determinations of the recipient's ABO group and Rh type as well as a screen for antibodies to red blood cell antigens. The recipient's ABO group is determined by testing the recipient's red blood cells with reagent anti-A and anti-B (known as the forward type) and the recipient's cells with reagent A1 and B red blood cell suspensions (known as the reverse type). Any discrepancies between the forward and reverse types should be investigated. If transfusion is necessary before the discrepancy can be resolved, group O donor cells should be transfused.[86]

Rh Type

The recipient's Rh type should be determined using reagent anti-D. Testing for weak D, or Du, is not required for the recipient. Appropriate controls for the D typing should be included as specified in the reagent anti-D manufacturer's insert.

Donor ABO and Rh Confirmatory Typing

The ABO group and Rh type of donor units should be determined by the collection facility and appear on the product label. The transfusion facility is required to confirm the ABO group of all whole blood and red blood cell products before transfusion. Only donor units labeled as Rh negative require confirmatory Rh typing. Confirmatory testing for weak D is not required for donor units.[87] Any discrepancies discovered by confirmatory testing should be reported to the collecting facility and resolved before using the donor product for transfusion.[88]

Antibody Screen

The recipient's sample must be screened for atypical antibodies against red blood cell antigens using a method capable of detecting clinically significant antibodies. The method must include an incubation phase at 37°C, followed by an anti-human globulin (AHG) phase. The cells for antibody screening should be used as individual cell suspensions unless the facility has documentation that equivalent sensitivity can be achieved using pooled screening cells.[89] Control or check cells, coated with IgG, should be used to confirm the AHG phase of testing unless the methodology is an FDA-licensed system that does not require check cells. In that case, the manufacturer's instructions for that methodology should be followed.[90] Positive antibody screens should be investigated to determine whether the reactions are due to clinically significant antibodies. If investigation reveals an antibody that is clinically significant, the transfusion facility must provide appropriate products that enable safe transfusion of the recipient.

Table 11.4 Requirements for Storage, Transportation, and Expiration

Item No.	Components	Storage	Transport	Expiration*	Additional Criteria
1	Whole Blood	1–6°C, unless for room temperature components, then 1–6°C within 8 hours	Cooling toward 1–10°C If intended for room temperature components, approaching (as close as possible to) 20–24°C	ACD/CPD/CP2D: 21 days CPDA-1: 35 days	
2	Whole Blood Irradiated	1–6°C	1–10°C	Original expiration or 28 days from date of irradiation, whichever is sooner	
3	Red Blood Cells	1–6°C	1–10°C	ACD/CPD/CP2D: 21 days CPDA-1: 35 days Additive solution: 42 days Open system: 24 hours	
4	RBCs Deglycerolized	1–6°C	1–10°C	24 hours	
5	RBCs Frozen 40% Glycerol 20% Glycerol	≤ –65°C if 40% Glycerol ≤ –120°C if 20% Glycerol	Maintain frozen state	10 years (A policy shall be developed if rare frozen units are to be retained beyond this time.)	Frozen within 6 days of collection without an additive. Prior to red blood cell expiration if with an additive.
6	RBCs Irradiated	1–6°C	1–10°C	Original expiration or 28 days from date of irradiation, whichever is sooner	
7	RBCs Leukocytes Reduced	1–6°C	1–10°C	ACD/CPD/CP2D: 21 days CPDA-1: 35 days Open system: 24 hours Additive solution: 42 days	
8	RBCs Rejuvenated	1–6°C	1–10°C	24 hours	
9	RBCs Rejuvenated Deglycerolized	1–6°C	1–10°C	24 hours	
10	RBCs Rejuvenated Frozen	≤ –65°C	Maintain frozen state	10 years AS1: 3 years (A policy shall be developed if rare frozen units are to be retained beyond this time.)	
11	RBCs Washed	1–6°C	1–10°C	24 hours	
12	Platelets	20–24°C with continuous gentle agitation	20–24°C (as close as possible to)	24 hours to 5 days, depending on collection system	Maximum time without agitation 24 hours
13	Platelets Irradiated	20–24°C with continuous gentle agitation	20–24°C (as close as possible to)	No change from original expiration date	Maximum time without agitation 24 hours
14	Platelets Leukocytes Reduced	20–24°C with continuous gentle agitation	20–24°C (as close as possible to)	Open system: 4 hours Closed system: No change in expiration	Maximum time without agitation 24 hours

	Component	Storage Temperature	Transport Temperature	Expiration	Special Instructions
15	Platelets Pooled or Open System	20–24°C with continuous gentle agitation	20–24°C (as close as possible to)	4 hours	
16	Platelets Pheresis	20–24°C with continuous gentle agitation	20–24°C (as close as possible to)	24 hours to 5 days, depending on collection system	Maximum time without agitation 24 hours
17	Platelets Pheresis Irradiated	20–24°C with continuous gentle agitation	20–24°C (as close as possible to)	No change from original expiration date	Maximum time without agitation 24 hours
18	Platelets Pheresis Leukocytes Reduced	20–24°C with continuous gentle agitation	20–24°C (as close as possible to)	No change from original expiration date	Maximum time without agitation 24 hours
19	Granulocytes	20–24°C	20–24°C (as close as possible to)	24 hours	Transfuse as soon as possible
20	Granulocytes Irradiated	20–24°C	20–24°C (as close as possible to)	No change from original expiration date	Transfuse as soon as possible
21	Cryoprecipitated AHF	≤−18°C	Maintain frozen state	12 months from original collection	Thaw the FFP at 1–6°C Refreeze cryoprecipitate within 1 hour
22	Cryoprecipitated AHF Thawed	20–24°C	20–24°C (as close as possible to)	Open system or pooled: 4 hours Single unit: 6 hours	Thaw at 30–37°C
23	Fresh Frozen Plasma (FFP) (including donor retested FFP)	≤−18°C or ≤−65°C	Maintain frozen state	≤−18°C: 12 months ≤−65°C: 7 years	Placed in freezer within 8 hours of collection in CPD, CP2D, CPDA-1 or within 6 hours of collection in ACD or as FDA-cleared.
24	FFP Thawed	1–6°C	1–10°C	24 hours	Thaw at 30–37°C or using an FDA-cleared device
25	Plasma Cryoprecipitate Reduced	≤−18°C	Maintain frozen state	12 months from original collection	
26	Plasma Cryoprecipitate Reduced Thawed	1–6°C	1–10°C	24 hours	
27	Plasma Frozen Within 24 Hours of Collection	≤−18°C	Maintain frozen state	12 months from original collection	Placed in freezer within 24 hours of collection
28	Plasma, Frozen Within 24 Hours, Thawed	1–6°C	1–10°C	24 hours	Thaw at 30–37°C or using an FDA-cleared device

(Continued)

Table 11.4 (Continued)

Item No.	Components	Storage	Transport	Expiration*	Additional Criteria
29	Liquid Plasma	1–6°C	1–10°C	5 days after expiration of RBCs	
30	Thawed Plasma	1–6°C	1–10°C	5 days	Closed system
31	Solvent/Detergent-Treated Pooled Plasma	≤–18°C	Maintain frozen state	24 months from manufacture; manufacturer will state expiration date on label	
32	Solvent/Detergent-Treated Pooled Plasma Thawed	20–24°C	20–24°C (as close as possible to)	24 hours	Thaw at 30–37°C or using an FDA-cleared device
33	Recovered Plasma	≤–18°C	≤–18°C	Must be shipped for further manufacture within 12 months	Requires a short supply agreement.[†]
34	Tissue	Conform to source facility's written instructions		Conform to source facility's written instructions	

*If the seal is broken during processing, components stored at 1–6°C shall have an expiration time of 24 hours, and components stored at 20–24°C shall have an expiration time of 4 hours, unless otherwise indicated.
[†]21 CFR 601.22.
From American Association of Blood Banks. Standards for Blood Banks and Transfusion Services, 21st ed. Bethesda, Md, AABB, 2002.

Pretransfusion testing should be performed on samples within 3 days of collection, provided that the intended recipient has been transfused, is pregnant, or experienced some other potentially sensitizing event within the last 3 months. Recipients who have not received transfusions or been otherwise immunologically challenged within 3 months may have samples drawn and tested more than 3 days from the time of transfusion, according to the transfusing facility's standard operating procedure.[91]

Records must also be checked for previous testing results of the intended recipient and any previous results compared with current testing results. The record check must be documented. Data to be compared include ABO and Rh typing within the past 12 months, any difficulty in ABORh typing, previously identified clinically significant antibodies, previous transfusion reactions, and special transfusion requirements.[92] Discrepancies between historical data and current testing should be resolved before transfusion.

Compatibility Testing

Compatibility testing, or crossmatching, involves the intended recipient's serum or plasma combined with a cell suspension prepared from an integral segment attached to the donor unit. The primary purpose of the compatibility test is to detect ABO incompatibilities between donor and recipient. If the recipient currently has a negative antibody screen and no history of clinically significant antibodies, compatibility testing may consist of only an immediate spin phase examination for ABO incompatibility, indicated by agglutination or hemolysis. However, if the recipient's current antibody screen is positive or the recipient has a history of previously identified clinically significant antibodies, the compatibility testing should include an AHG phase.

Massive Transfusion Protocol

Compatibility testing may also be abbreviated if the recipient has received red blood cell transfusions equivalent to his or her total blood volume within a 24-hour time frame. Typically known as a massive transfusion protocol, this procedure acknowledges that standard compatibility testing has limited value when the recipient's own circulating blood volume has been replaced by transfused red blood cell products. Therefore, AHG phase testing provides no greater safety margin for the recipient than immediate spin-only compatibility testing. Massive transfusion protocols should comply with the transfusing facility's standard operating procedure.

Emergency Release Prior to Compatibility Testing

Urgent clinical situations may sometimes require release of blood products before compatibility testing can be completed. In such cases, the attending physician must sign a statement that the clinical situation was sufficiently urgent to require release of blood products before completion of compatibility testing.[93] The transfusion service should provide group O packed red blood cells if the recipient's type is unknown. If the recipient's type has been determined by the transfusing facility, ABO group–specific red blood cells may be issued. These products must be clearly labeled to indicate that compatibility testing has not been completed.[94] Compatibility testing should be completed as quickly as possible after emergency release of products.

Computerized Compatibility Testing

Facilities that have validated their computer systems may use a nonserological technique, known as a computerized crossmatch, to determine compatibility testing. The computerized crossmatch requires that the current recipient sample be tested for ABO group and Rh type and agree with either a previously determined ABO group and Rh type or a second ABO group and Rh type independently determined using the current sample. The computer system must contain the recipient ABO group, Rh type, and antibody screen results as well as donor unit number, product name, donor unit ABO group and Rh type, and the donor unit ABORh confirmation type.[95] There must be a mechanism for verification of data entry prior to transfusion of products, and the system must alert the user to potential ABO discrepancies between donor product and recipient.

Product Selection

ABO Group

Cellular and plasma donor products should be selected on the basis of the intended recipient's ABO group. Whole blood products should be ABO group specific to the recipient; packed red blood cells may be ABO group compatible with the recipient's plasma. Cellular products that contain more than 2 mL of red blood cells, such as granulocytes or plateletpheres, should be ABO group compatible with the recipient's plasma and should undergo compatibility testing.[96] FFP should be ABO compatible with the recipient's red blood cells. Products such as cryoprecipitate, plateletpheresis, and random platelet concentrates should be ABO group compatible with the recipient's red blood cells when feasible. In the event that ABO group–compatible cryoprecipitate or platelet products are not available, the facility should comply with its standard operating procedure that addresses management of the patient after transfusion of substantial volumes of ABO group–incompatible plasma.[97]

Rh Type

Rh-positive recipients may receive either Rh-positive or Rh-negative products; however, the Rh-negative product inventory is typically reserved for use with Rh-negative recipients. Rh-negative recipients should receive Rh-negative cellular products whenever possible to avoid alloimmunization to the D antigen. Transfusion of Rh-positive products to Rh-negative females of childbearing age is of particular concern because of the high probability of alloimmunization and its potential consequence in subsequent pregnancies.[98] Depending on the patient's age and diagnosis, administration of Rh immune globulin may be appropriate and should be evaluated by the transfusion service medical director. Transfusion of Rh-incompatible cellular products should be approved by the facility medical director and comply with the facility's standard operating procedure for management of the patient after transfusion of Rh-incompatible blood products.[99]

Special Circumstances

When recipients are known to have clinically significant antibodies to red blood cell antigens, red blood cell products should be selected that lack the corresponding red blood cell antigens and are compatible as determined by an AHG phase crossmatch method.[100] Exceptions to these guidelines should be approved by the facility medical director.

Patients who have undergone ABO-incompatible bone marrow or stem cell transplantation require transfusion support with products that are compatible with the recipient's ABO group but also support the engrafting cell population. Selection of a product for transfusion depends on whether the recipient-donor combination represents a major or minor incompatibility. Major side incompatibilities, in which the donor cells are incompatible with the recipient's plasma, should be supported with recipient ABO-type red blood cells and donor ABO-type plasma and platelet products. Minor incompatibilities, in which the donor plasma is incompatible with the recipient's red blood cells, should be supported with donor ABO-type red blood cells and recipient ABO-type plasma and platelet products. Transplants that are both major and minor side incompatible should be supported with group O red blood cells and group AB plasma and platelet products. Transfusion support of red blood cell, platelet, and plasma products may convert to the donor's ABO group after the recipient's original red blood cell type and isoagglutinin to donor ABO type are no longer detectable and the direct antiglobulin test is negative.[101]

■ Administration

Patient-Related Issues

Informed Consent

Transfusion of blood products should be prescribed and performed under medical supervision, consistent with state and local regulations. Preparation of the patient should include an informed consent process in which the recipient is provided with sufficient information regarding risks versus benefits of transfusions to be able to make an informed choice regarding transfusion therapy. Informed consent is addressed in detail in Chapter 8.

Recipient Identification and Monitoring

A discussion outlining the transfusion process may help minimize anxiety for the transfusion recipient. Administration of antihistamines before transfusion may minimize common symptoms associated with febrile transfusion reactions. Premedication with antipyretics may mask temperature increases associated with febrile transfusion reactions but may also mask a symptom of serious hemolytic reactions.[102] Premedication before administration of blood products is a medical decision, and the transfusionist should comply with the physician's written orders.

The recipient and the blood product should be positively identified immediately before beginning the transfusion. Positive identification of the recipient at the time of blood product administration is absolutely essential. The single greatest cause of fatal hemolytic transfusion reactions is the administration of ABO-incompatible red blood cells to the wrong recipient.[103] The transfusionist must verify that the information appearing on the blood container label, the attached compatibility record, and the recipient's identification band matches exactly and is appropriate for the recipient. Documentation of this verification process must be maintained.[104] Any information that is affixed to the blood container should remain attached to the product for the duration of the transfusion.

Monitoring of recipients during the transfusion process should comply with the facility's standard operating procedure for administration of blood products. The monitoring should include an appropriate length of time at the onset of blood product administration to allow detection of symptoms of possible transfusion reactions.[105] Transfusion personnel should be aware of symptoms of possible transfusion reactions and the steps to follow when those symptoms are observed in a recipient. Adverse reactions to transfusion are discussed in detail in Chapters 33 to 42. Monitoring also includes documentation of the recipient's vital signs, such as pulse rate, temperature, and blood pressure. The transfusion record must also include the unique donor identification number, date and time of transfusion, identification of the transfusionist, and whether symptoms of transfusion reaction were observed.[106] Significant changes in vital signs should be documented and appropriate care provided as outlined in the facility standard operating procedure.

When the transfusion process is complete, the transfusion record should be included in the recipient's medical record.[107] Caretakers of patients who receive transfusions in an outpatient or home care setting should be provided with written instructions in the event of a suspected transfusion reaction.

Venous Access

Adequate venous access is essential for successful infusion of blood products. Peripheral venous access is preferred whenever possible. Veins in the antecubital fossa are commonly used but limit mobility of the patient's arm for the duration of the infusion process. Veins in the hands, wrists, and feet may also be utilized but must be able to accommodate as a minimum size a 23-gauge, thin-walled needle. Typically, red blood cell administration is accomplished with an 18-gauge or larger needle. Care must be exercised when administering red blood cells through smaller gauge needles to avoid hemolysis of the red blood cells. Use of smaller gauge needles significantly extends the time required for infusion of the total product volume, and care should be exercised to complete product infusion within 4 hours.[108]

If peripheral vein access is unavailable or large volumes of blood products are to be infused over an extended period of time, central venous catheters may be used. Neonatal and pediatric patients require special consideration. Umbilical veins (in newborns) and scalp and foot veins (in infants) may be successfully utilized but typically require the use of smaller gauge needles. Aliquots of appropriate size should be provided to enable infusion over a reasonable time frame in pediatric patients. Care must be exercised when handling small-volume aliquots to prevent hemolysis from too rapid infusion or overwarming of the red blood cells.

Infusion Equipment

Infusion Sets

Blood products should be administered through filters designed to protect recipients from blood clots or particles contained in the blood product, or both.[109] All filters must be utilized according to their manufacturer's instructions. Standard administration sets have in-line filters with pore sizes of 170 to 260 µm, which trap large debris such as blood clots and fibrin strands.

Microaggregate filters, which typically have pore sizes of 20 to 40 μm, trap particles resulting from degenerated platelets and leukocytes. Microaggregate filters were originally designed to prevent adult respiratory distress syndrome (ARDS), in which transfused microaggregates were theorized to contribute to blood microemboli lodging in the recipient's pulmonary circulation. However, subsequent studies have been unable to link use of microaggregate filters with prevention of ARDS. Although routine use of microaggregate filters in low-volume transfusion does not appear beneficial, microaggregate filters can reduce the donor unit leukocyte count to 5×10^8, which should reduce the occurrence of febrile transfusion reactions.[110]

Third-generation or leukocyte reduction filters are capable of decreasing the leukocyte count of each red blood cell product to less than 5×10^6, a level that should protect recipients from HLA alloimmunization and CMV transmission as well as reduce the occurrence of febrile transfusion reactions.[111] Leukoreduction is addressed extensively in Chapter 19. Use of leukoreduction filters has grown steadily and is currently required in several countries outside the United States, including Great Britain and Canada.[112] Leukoreduction of red blood cell products appears to be the developing standard of care in the United States, and major blood product suppliers have announced their intention to move to a universally leukocyte-reduced blood product supply in the near future.[113]

Infusion Solutions

Normal saline (0.9% sodium chloride injection, United States Pharmacopeia) is the preferred solution for administration of blood products. The Circular of Information for the Use of Human Blood and Blood Components[114] permits the use of ABO-compatible plasma, 5% albumin, or plasma protein fraction, with approval of the recipient's physician, for administration of blood products. Other products such as calcium-free isotonic electrolyte solutions may be used, provided that they have been approved for use by the FDA or there is documentation that the addition of the solution to blood products is both safe and efficacious.[115]

Solutions that may not be added to or used for the administration of blood products include all medications, 5% dextrose in water, lactated Ringer solution, and hypotonic sodium chloride solutions.[116] Dextrose and hypotonic solutions may cause swelling and hemolysis of red blood cells, and solutions containing ionized calcium (such as lactated Ringer solution) may reverse the effects of the anticoagulant-preservative solutions and allow formation of small clots.[117]

Warmers

Transfusion of warmed blood products is not routinely necessary; however, patients receiving large-volume or rapid transfusions, especially through central venous catheters, and patients with high-titer cold agglutinins reactive at 37°C may benefit from warmed products.[118] Warming devices may consist of thermostatically controlled water baths, dry heat devices with warming plates, or high-volume countercurrent heat exchangers with water jackets, in which the blood product flows through a plastic chamber surrounded by warm water jackets.[119] Regardless of the device configuration, AABB standards require that the blood products reach no more than 42°C.[120] Devices must be FDA approved and should be equipped with a visible thermometer and an audible alarm that is activated before reaching the 42°C upper limit.[121] Use of microwaves, warming blankets, hot tap water, or other uncontrolled mechanisms to warm blood products is inappropriate and may result in hemolysis of red blood cells.

Infusion Control Devices

Mechanical infusion control devices help regulate the infusion of blood products. They may be either controllers, which use gravity alone for delivery of the blood product, or pumps, which apply positive pressure to the product to control the delivery rate. Pumps may use a mechanical screw drive mechanism to propel a syringe plunger or peristaltic roller pumps or piston cassette-diaphragm pumps to apply pressure to the administration tubing.[122] Variables such as the rate of infusion, amount of pressure, needle size, and even age and temperature of the blood product itself may contribute to the potential for hemolysis of red blood cell products and should be considered when using infusion control devices. Use of infusion devices should always be consistent with the specific manufacturer's instructions as well as the facility's standard operating procedures.

Pressure Devices

Rapid infusion of blood products is sometimes necessary in emergency and operative settings. Pressure devices may be used to speed delivery of blood products in these critical circumstances. Pressurized infusion is typically accomplished by manually squeezing the blood product or by placing the product inside a pressure bag or pressure cuff. These pressure devices are then inflated, which exerts pressure on the blood product container, thereby increasing the flow rate. Pressures in excess of 300 mm Hg may rupture the seams of the blood product container or cause hemolysis as the red blood cells are forced through the needle lumen. Pressure devices should always be used with an 18-gauge or larger administration needle to minimize the possibility of red blood cell hemolysis.[123] Pressure devices are not recommended for use with leukocyte reduction filters.

REFERENCES

1. Menitove J (ed): 5.4.1A Standards for Blood Banks and Transfusion Services, 21st ed. Bethesda, Md, American Association of Blood Banks, 2002, p 64.
2. Menitove J (ed): 5.4.1A Standards for Blood Banks and Transfusion Services, 21st ed. Bethesda, Md, American Association of Blood Banks, 2002, pp 64–65.
3. Menitove J (ed): 5.4.1A Standards for Blood Banks and Transfusion Services, 21st ed. Bethesda, Md, American Association of Blood Banks, 2002, p 65.
4. Menitove J (ed): 5.4.1A Standards for Blood Banks and Transfusion Services, 21st ed. Bethesda, Md, American Association of Blood Banks, 2002, pp 64–66.
5. Menitove J (ed): 5.4.1A 9d Standards for Blood Banks and Transfusion Services, 21st ed. Bethesda, Md, American Association of Blood Banks, 2002, p 65.
6. Menitove J (ed): 5.4.1A 10e Standards for Blood Banks and Transfusion Services, 21st ed. Bethesda, Md, American Association of Blood Banks, 2002, pp 65–66.
7. Food and Drug Administration: Memorandum: Revised Recommendations for the Prevention of Human Immunodeficiency Virus (HIV) Transmission by Blood and Blood Products. April 23, 1992. Rockville, Md, Congressional and Consumer Affairs, 1992.
8. Menitove J (ed): 5.4.2.1 Standards for Blood Banks and Transfusion Services, 21st ed. Bethesda, Md, American Association of Blood Banks, 2002, p 18.

9. Menitove J (ed): 5.4.2 Standards for Blood Banks and Transfusion Services, 21st ed. Bethesda, Md, American Association of Blood Banks, 2002, p 18.

10. Menitove J (ed): 5.5.1 Standards for Blood Banks and Transfusion Services, 21st ed. Bethesda, Md, American Association of Blood Banks, 2002, p 20.

11. Food and Drug Administration: Memorandum: Revision of FDA Memorandum of August 27, 1982: Requirements for Infrequent Plasmapheresis Donors. March 10, 1995. Rockville, Md, Congressional and Consumer Affairs, 1995.

12. Menitove J (ed): 5.5.3.5 Standards for Blood Banks and Transfusion Services, 21st ed. Bethesda, Md, American Association of Blood Banks, 2002, p 22.

13. Food and Drug Administration: Memorandum: Revision of FDA Memorandum of August 27, 1982: Requirements for Infrequent Plasmapheresis Donors. March 10, 1995. Rockville, Md, Congressional and Consumer Affairs, 1995.

14. Food and Drug Administration: Memorandum: Donor Deferral Due to Red Blood Cell Loss During Collection of Source Plasma by Automated Plasmapheresis. December 4, 1995. Rockville, Md, Congressional and Consumer Affairs, 1995.

15. Menitove J (ed): Standards for Blood Banks and Transfusion Services, 21st ed. Bethesda, Md, American Association of Blood Banks, 2002, pp 18–20.

16. Code of Federal Regulations, 21 CFR 610.53(C). Washington, DC, U.S. Government Printing Office, 1998 (revised annually).

17. Vengelen-Tyler V (ed): Technical Manual, 14th ed. Bethesda, Md, American Association of Blood Banks, 2002, Table 8–1, p162.

18. Code of Federal Regulations, 21 CFR 610.53(C). Washington, DC, U.S. Government Printing Office, 1998 (revised annually).

19. Vengelen-Tyler V (ed): Technical Manual, 14th ed. Bethesda, Md, American Association of Blood Banks, 2002, Table 8–2, p163.

20. Vengelen-Tyler V (ed): Technical Manual, 14th ed. Bethesda, Md, American Association of Blood Banks, 2002, Table 8–3, p171.

21. Simon TL, Marcus CS, Myhre BA, Nelson EJ: Effects of AS-3 nutrient-additive solution on 42 and 49 days of storage of red cells. Transfusion 1987;27:178–182.

22. Beutler E: Red cell metabolism and storage. In Anderson KC, Ness PM (eds): Scientific Basis of Transfusion Medicine. Philadelphia, WB Saunders, 1994, pp 188–202.

23. Menitove J (ed): 5.7.5.3 Standards for Blood Banks and Transfusion Services, 21st ed. Bethesda, Md, American Association of Blood Banks, 2002, p 31.

24. Menitove J (ed): 5.7.5.4 Standards for Blood Banks and Transfusion Services, 21st ed. Bethesda, Md, American Association of Blood Banks, 2002, p 32.

25. Menitove J (ed): 5.6.4 Standards for Blood Banks and Transfusion Services, 21st ed. Bethesda, Md, American Association of Blood Banks, 2002, p 24.

26. Vengelen-Tyler V (ed): Technical Manual, 14th ed. Bethesda, Md, American Association of Blood Banks, 2002, p 162.

27. Huh YO, Lichtiger B, Giacco GG, et al: Effect of donation time on platelet concentrates and fresh-frozen plasma. Vox Sang 1989;56:21–24.

28. Menitove J (ed): 5.1.8A Standards for Blood Banks and Transfusion Services, 21st ed. Bethesda, Md, American Association of Blood Banks, 2002, pp 59–63.

29. Menitove J (ed): 5.8.1 Standards for Blood Banks and Transfusion Services, 21st ed. Bethesda, Md, American Association of Blood Banks, 2002, p 36.

30. Menitove J (ed): 5.8 Standards for Blood Banks and Transfusion Services, 21st ed. Bethesda, Md, American Association of Blood Banks, 2002, p 36.

31. Menitove J (ed): 5.8.3.2 Standards for Blood Banks and Transfusion Services, 21st ed. Bethesda, Md, American Association of Blood Banks, 2002, p 37.

32. Menitove J (ed): 5.8.4 Standards for Blood Banks and Transfusion Services, 21st ed. Bethesda, Md, American Association of Blood Banks, 2002, p 37.

33. Food and Drug Administration: Memorandum: FDA Recommendations Concerning Testing for Antibody to Hepatitis B Core Antigen (Anti-HBc). September 10, 1991. Rockville, Md, Congressional and Consumer Affairs, 1991.
Food and Drug Administration: Memorandum: Recommendations for Donor Screening with a Licensed Test for HIV-1 Antigen. August 8, 1995. Rockville, Md, Congressional and Consumer Affairs, 1995.

Food and Drug Administration: Memorandum: Additional Recommendations for Donor Screening with a Licensed Test for HIV-a Antigen. March 14, 1996. Rockville, Md, Congressional and Consumer Affairs, 1996.
Food and Drug Administration: Memorandum: Recommendations for the Quarantine and Disposition of Units from Prior Collections from Donors with Repeatedly Reactive Screening Tests for Hepatitis B Virus (HBV), Hepatitis C Virus (HCV) and Human T-Lymphotropic Virus Type I (HTLV-I). July 19, 1996. Rockville, Md, Congressional and Consumer Affairs, 1996.
Food and Drug Administration: Memorandum: Interim Recommendations for Deferral of Donors at Increased Risk for HIV-I Group O Infection. December 11, 1996. Rockville, Md, Congressional and Consumer Affairs, 1996.
Food and Drug Administration Guidance for Industry: Donor Screening for Antibodies to HTLV-II. August 1997.

34. Food and Drug Administration Guidance for Industry: Current Good Manufacturing Practice for Blood and Blood Components: (1) Quarantine and Disposition of Units from Prior Collections from Donors with Repeatedly Reactive Screening Tests for Antibody to Hepatitis Virus (Anti-HCV); (2) Supplemental Testing, and the Notification of Consignees and Blood Recipients of Donor Test Results for Anti-HCV. September, 1998.

35. Menitove J (ed): 5.7.51 Standards for Blood Banks and Transfusion Services, 21st ed. Bethesda, Md, American Association of Blood Banks, 2002, p 14.

36. Menitove J (ed): 5.1.8A Standards for Blood Banks and Transfusion Services, 21st ed. Bethesda, Md, American Association of Blood Banks, 2002, p 59.

37. Vengelen-Tyler V (ed): Technical Manual, 14th ed. Bethesda, Md, American Association of Blood Banks, 2002, p 179.

38. Meryman HT, Hornblower M: A method for freezing and washing RBCs using a high glycerol concentration. Transfusion 1972;12:145–156.

39. Vengelen-Tyler V (ed): Technical Manual, 14th ed. Bethesda, Md, American Association of Blood Banks, 2002, p 176.

40. Menitove J (ed): 5.7.5.2 Standards for Blood Banks and Transfusion Services, 19th ed. Bethesda, Md, American Association of Blood Banks, 2002, p 31.

41. Valeri CR, Pivacek LE, Gray AD, et al: The safety and therapeutic effectiveness of human red cells stored at 8°C for as long as 21 years. Transfusion 1989;29:429–437.

42. Vengelen-Tyler V (ed): Technical Manual, 13th ed. Bethesda, Md, American Association of Blood Banks, 1999, p 181.

43. Menitove J (ed): 5.7.5.3 Standards for Blood Banks and Transfusion Services, 21st ed. Bethesda, Md, American Association of Blood Banks, 2002, p 31.

44. Menitove J (ed): 5.7.5 Standards for Blood Banks and Transfusion Services, 21st ed. Bethesda, Md, American Association of Blood Banks, 2002, p 31.

45. Menitove J (ed): 5.7.5.2 Standards for Blood Banks and Transfusion Services, 21st ed. Bethesda, Md, American Association of Blood Banks, 2002, p 31.

46. Menitove J (ed): 5.7.5.15 Standards for Blood Banks and Transfusion Services, 21st ed. Bethesda, Md, American Association of Blood Banks, 2002, p 35.

47. Vengelen-Tyler V (ed): Technical Manual, 14th ed. Bethesda, Md, American Association of Blood Banks, 2002, p 168.

48. Menitove J (ed): 5.7.5.15.1 Standards for Blood Banks and Transfusion Services, 21st ed. Bethesda, Md, American Association of Blood Banks, 2002, p 35.

49. Vengelen-Tyler V (ed): Technical Manual, 14th ed. Bethesda, Md, American Association of Blood Banks, 2002, p 168.

50. Menitove J (ed): 5.6.6 Standards for Blood Banks and Transfusion Services, 21st ed. Bethesda, Md, American Association of Blood Banks, 2002, p 18.

51. Menitove J (ed): Standards for Blood Banks and Transfusion Services, 21st ed. Bethesda, Md, American Association of Blood Banks, 2002, p 35.

52. Menitove J (ed): 5.7.5.18 Standards for Blood Banks and Transfusion Services, 21st ed. Bethesda, Md, American Association of Blood Banks, 2002, p 35.

53. Menitove J (ed): 5.7.5.20 Standards for Blood Banks and Transfusion Services, 21st ed. Bethesda, Md, American Association of Blood Banks, 2002, p 36.

54. Vengelen-Tyler V (ed): Technical Manual, 13th ed. Bethesda, Md, American Association of Blood Banks, 1999, pp 174–175.
55. Vengelen-Tyler V (ed): Technical Manual, 13th ed. Bethesda, Md, American Association of Blood Banks, 1999, p 134.
56. Vengelen-Tyler V (ed): Technical Manual, 13th ed. Bethesda, Md, American Association of Blood Banks, 1999, p 134.
57. Bensinger WI, Prie TH, Dale DC, et al: The effects of daily recombinant human granulocyte colony-stimulating factor administration on normal granulocyte donors undergoing leukapheresis. Blood 1993;81:1883–1888.
58. Menitove J (ed): 5.14.5 Standards for Blood Banks and Transfusion Services, 21st ed. Bethesda, Md, American Association of Blood Banks, 2002, p 47.
59. Menitove J (ed): 5.6 Standards for Blood Banks and Transfusion Services, 21st ed. Bethesda, Md, American Association of Blood Banks, 2002, p 23.
60. Vengelen-Tyler V (ed): Technical Manual, 14th ed. Bethesda, Md, American Association of Blood Banks, 2002, p 166.
61. Vengelen-Tyler V (ed): Technical Manual, 14th ed. Bethesda, Md, American Association of Blood Banks, 2002, p 165.
62. Vengelen-Tyler V (ed): Technical Manual, 14th ed. Bethesda, Md, American Association of Blood Banks, 2002, p 166.
63. Vengelen-Tyler V (ed): Technical Manual, 14th ed. Bethesda, Md, American Association of Blood Banks, 2002, p 166.
64. Vengelen-Tyler V (ed): Technical Manual, 14th ed. Bethesda, Md, American Association of Blood Banks, 2002, p 167.
65. Code of Federal Regulations, 21 CFR 601.22. Washington, DC, U.S. Government Printing Office, 1998 (revised annually)
66. Menitove J (ed): 5.1.8A-21 Standards for Blood Banks and Transfusion Services, 21st ed. Bethesda, Md, American Association of Blood Banks, 2002, p 62.
67. Menitove J (ed): 5.7.5.14 Standards for Blood Banks and Transfusion Services, 21st ed. Bethesda, Md, American Association of Blood Banks, 2002, p 34.
68. Menitove J (ed): 5.7.5.10.1 Standards for Blood Banks and Transfusion Services, 21st ed. Bethesda, Md, American Association of Blood Banks, 2002, pp 33–34.
69. Menitove J (ed): 5.7.5.10.1 Standards for Blood Banks and Transfusion Services, 21st ed. Bethesda, Md, American Association of Blood Banks, 2002, p 62.
70. Menitove J (ed): 5.1.8A-22 Standards for Blood Banks and Transfusion Services, 21st ed. Bethesda, Md, American Association of Blood Banks, 2002, p 62.
71. Vengelen-Tyler V (ed): Technical Manual, 14th ed. Bethesda, Md, American Association of Blood Banks, 2002, p 168.
72. Menitove J (ed): 5.1.6.3 Standards for Blood Banks and Transfusion Services, 21st ed. Bethesda, Md, American Association of Blood Banks, 2002, p 11.
73. Menitove J (ed): 5.1.6.3 Standards for Blood Banks and Transfusion Services, 21st ed. Bethesda, Md, American Association of Blood Banks, 2002, pp 11–12.
74. Menitove J (ed): 5.1.6.5.1 Standards for Blood Banks and Transfusion Services, 21st ed. Bethesda, Md, American Association of Blood Banks, 2002, p 12.
75. Menitove J (ed): 5.1.6A, 1–7 Standards for Blood Banks and Transfusion Services, 21st ed. Bethesda, Md, American Association of Blood Banks, 2002, p 56.
76. Menitove J (ed): 5.9 Standards for Blood Banks and Transfusion Services, 21st ed. Bethesda, Md, American Association of Blood Banks, 2002, p 40.
77. Menitove J (ed): 5.1.6A,12 Standards for Blood Banks and Transfusion Services, 21st ed. Bethesda, Md, American Association of Blood Banks, 2002, p 56.
78. Menitove J (ed): 5.1.6A, 15–16 Standards for Blood Banks and Transfusion Services, 21st ed. Bethesda, Md, American Association of Blood Banks, 2002, p 56.
79. Menitove J (ed): 5.1.8A Standards for Blood Banks and Transfusion Services, 21st ed. Bethesda, Md, American Association of Blood Banks, 2002, p 59.
80. Menitove J (ed): 5.1.8A Standards for Blood Banks and Transfusion Services, 21st ed. Bethesda, Md, American Association of Blood Banks, 2002, pp 60–61.
81. Menitove J (ed): 3.4.4 Standards for Blood Banks and Transfusion Services, 21st ed. Bethesda, Md, American Association of Blood Banks, 2002, p 5.
82. Menitove J (ed): 5.1.8.2 Standards for Blood Banks and Transfusion Services, 21st ed. Bethesda, Md, American Association of Blood Banks, 2002, p 14.
83. Menitove J (ed): 5.1.8A, 12–18 Standards for Blood Banks and Transfusion Services, 21st ed. Bethesda, Md, American Association of Blood Banks, 2002, p 61.
84. Menitove J (ed): 5.11.1 Standards for Blood Banks and Transfusion Services, 21st ed. Bethesda, Md, American Association of Blood Banks, 2002, p 42.
85. Menitove J (ed): 5.11 Standards for Blood Banks and Transfusion Services, 21st ed. Bethesda, Md, American Association of Blood Banks, 2002, p 40.
86. Menitove J (ed): 5.12.1 Standards for Blood Banks and Transfusion Services, 21st ed. Bethesda, Md, American Association of Blood Banks, 2002, p 43.
87. Menitove J (ed): 5.12.2 Standards for Blood Banks and Transfusion Services, 21st ed. Bethesda, Md, American Association of Blood Banks, 2002, p 44.
88. Menitove J (ed): 5.11.7.1 Standards for Blood Banks and Transfusion Services, 21st ed. Bethesda, Md, American Association of Blood Banks, 2002, p 43.
89. Menitove J (ed): 5.12.3 Standards for Blood Banks and Transfusion Services, 21st ed. Bethesda, Md, American Association of Blood Banks, 2002, p 44.
90. Menitove J (ed): 5.12.3.4.1 Standards or Blood Banks and Transfusion Services, 21st ed. Bethesda, Md, American Association of Blood Banks, 2002, p 44.
91. Menitove J (ed): 5.12.3.2 Standards for Blood Banks and Transfusion Services, 21st ed. Bethesda, Md, American Association of Blood Banks, 2002, p 44.
92. Menitove J (ed): 5.12.5 Standards for Blood Banks and Transfusion Services, 21st ed. Bethesda, Md, American Association of Blood Banks, 2002, p 45.
93. Menitove J (ed): 5.17.4 Standards for Blood Banks and Transfusion Services, 21st ed. Bethesda, Md, American Association of Blood Banks, 2002, p 51.
94. Menitove J (ed): 5.17.4.3 Standards for Blood Banks and Transfusion Services, 21st ed. Bethesda, Md, American Association of Blood Banks, 2002, p 52.
95. Menitove J (ed): 5.13.2.2 Standards for Blood Banks and Transfusion Services, 21st ed. Bethesda, Md, American Association of Blood Banks, 2002, p 46.
96. Menitove J (ed): 5.14.5 Standards for Blood Banks and Transfusion Services, 21st ed. Bethesda, Md, American Association of Blood Banks, 2002, p 47.
97. Menitove J (ed): 5.14.4 Standards for Blood Banks and Transfusion Services, 21st ed. Bethesda, Md, American Association of Blood Banks, 2002, p 47.
98. Pollack W, Ascari WQ, Crispen JF, et al. Studies on Rh prophylaxis II: Rh immune prophylaxis after transfusion with Rh-positive blood. Transfusion 1971;11:340–344.
99. Menitove J (ed): 5.14.2.1 Standards for Blood Banks and Transfusion Services, 21st ed. Bethesda, Md, American Association of Blood Banks, 2002, p 47.
100. Menitove J (ed): 5.14.3 Standards for Blood Banks and Transfusion Services, 21st ed. Bethesda, Md, American Association of Blood Banks, 2002, p 47.
101. McCullough J. Collection and use of stem cells; role of transfusion centers in bone marrow transplantation. Vox Sang 1994;67:35–42.
102. Vengelen-Tyler V (ed): Technical Manual, 14th ed. Bethesda, Md, American Association of Blood Banks, 2002, p 486. 585–586
103. Sazama K. Reports of 355 transfusion-associated deaths:1976–1985. Transfusion 1990;30:583–590.
104. Menitove J (ed): 5.17.2.1 Standards for Blood Banks and Transfusion Services, 21st ed. Bethesda, Md, American Association of Blood Banks, 2002, p 51.
105. Menitove J (ed): 5.18.6 Standards for Blood Banks and Transfusion Services, 21st ed. Bethesda, Md, American Association of Blood Banks, 2002, p 53.
106. Menitove J (ed): 5.18.5 Standards for Blood Banks and Transfusion Services, 21st ed. Bethesda, Md, American Association of Blood Banks, 2002, p 53.

107. Menitove J (ed): 5.18 Standards for Blood Banks and Transfusion Services, 21st ed. Bethesda, Md, American Association of Blood Banks, 2002, pp 52–53.

108. Menitove J (ed): 5.18.1–10 Standards for Blood Banks and Transfusion Services, 21st ed. Bethesda, Md, American Association of Blood Banks, 2002, pp 52–54.

109. Vengelen-Tyler V (ed): Technical Manual, 14th ed. Bethesda, Md, American Association of Blood Banks, 2002, p 490.

110. Vengelen-Tyler V (ed): Technical Manual, 12th ed. Bethesda, Md, American Association of Blood Banks, 1996, p 487.

111. Vengelen-Tyler V (ed): Technical Manual, 14th ed. Bethesda, Md, American Association of Blood Banks, 2002, p 491.

112. BloodLink BC, Provincial Blood Coordinating Office, British Columbia: Blood Matters, Vol 2, No 1, January 2000.

113. BPAC recommends universal leukoreduction on September 18, 1998. AABB Weekly Report, Vol 4, No 36, September 25, 1998.

114. American Association of Blood Banks, America's Blood Centers, and American Red Cross Circular of Information for the Use of Human Blood and Blood Components, January 1999.

115. Menitove J (ed): 5.18.9 Standards for Blood Banks and Transfusion Services, 21st ed. Bethesda, Md, American Association of Blood Banks, 2002, p 54.

116. Menitove J (ed): 5.18 Standards for Blood Banks and Transfusion Services, 21st ed. Bethesda, Md, American Association of Blood Banks, 2002, pp 53–54.

117. Menitove J (ed): 5.18.9 Standards for Blood Banks and Transfusion Services, 21st ed. Bethesda, Md, American Association of Blood Banks, 2002.

118. Iserson KV, Huestis DW: Blood warming: current applications and techniques. Transfusion 1991;31:558–571.

119. Vengelen-Tyler V (ed): Technical Manual, 14th ed. Bethesda, Md, American Association of Blood Banks, 2002, p 492.

120. Menitove J (ed): 3.5 Standards for Blood Banks and Transfusion Services, 21st ed. Bethesda, Md, American Association of Blood Banks, 2002, p 6.

121. Menitove J (ed): 3.5.1 Standards for Blood Banks and Transfusion Services, 21st ed. Bethesda, Md, American Association of Blood Banks, 2002, p 6.

122. Menitove J (ed): 5.18 Standards for Blood Banks and Transfusion Services, 21st ed. Bethesda, Md, American Association of Blood Banks, 2002, p 52.

123. Menitove J (ed): 5.18.8 Standards for Blood Banks and Transfusion Services, 21st ed. Bethesda, Md, American Association of Blood Banks, 2002, p 53.

Chapter 12

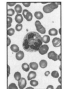

Infectious Disease Testing

Roger Y. Dodd

■ Brief Historical Review

The risk of disease transmission by blood transfusion is extremely low, particularly in the developed nations. This is a consequence of a number of interlocking safety measures, including the selection of safe populations from which donors are drawn, careful donor questioning, laboratory testing, record keeping, and the use of quality systems and good manufacturing practices. These approaches have evolved over the years, and perhaps the most change has been seen in the area of blood testing. Indeed, blood collectors have now added nucleic acid amplification techniques to the battery of tests directed toward the safety of the blood supply. Transmission of known agents has almost been eliminated, but residual fear of the unknown, fueled by a continuing stream of newly emerging or newly recognized microbes, continues.

Although some form of blood transfusion has been used for well over a century, organized approaches did not really commence until the 1940s. At that time, the transmissibility of syphilis by this route was recognized and testing (albeit using nonspecific methods) was implemented. However, viral hepatitis was the biggest unresolved concern from the 1940s to about 1970. Clinical hepatitis was recognized as an almost inevitable consequence of transfusion, but little could be done to prevent it. The greatest benefits during that time were derived from epidemiological studies that established the increased infection risk attributable to commercial donors and prisoners. There were also a number of attempts to use liver function tests to screen blood donors for risk of hepatitis transmission, but none of the tests was broadly adopted.

In 1965, Blumberg and colleagues[1] described the Australia antigen, mistakenly identifying it as an allotypic protein.[2] Subsequently, the antigen was recognized as a component of the hepatitis B virus (HBV), fortuitously produced in considerable excess during both acute and chronic infection. This discovery underlies the entire history of specific serological testing for transfusion-transmissible infections. Between 1969 and 1972, all blood collecting establishments in the United States adopted some form of testing for hepatitis B surface antigen (HBsAg) using agar gel diffusion, counterelectrophoresis, or rheophoresis. Subsequently, Ling and Overby[3] reported on a radioimmunoassay for HBsAg, and this was rapidly adopted. Interestingly, the insensitive gel precipitation methods seemed to affect only about 20% of post-transfusion hepatitis and the frequency of radioimmunoassay-positive samples was about fivefold greater. A brief period of hope that the transfusion hepatitis problem was solved rapidly terminated in disillusion when it was found that most of the additional reactive results were false positive and that post-transfusion hepatitis continued to occur. As a result of the observations on specificity of the radioimmunoassay, confirmatory testing was implemented. Recognition of the hepatitis A virus and development of diagnostic tests for infection with this virus led to the definition of most cases of residual post-transfusion hepatitis as non-A, non-B (NANB).[4]

Extensive studies were performed to characterize the agent or agents of NANB hepatitis but without any real success until 1989.[5] Many attempts were also made to identify donor characteristics that might be used for screening. As a result of two of these studies, recommendations were made to screen donors for elevated levels of alanine aminotransferase (ALT) in the serum and a small number of institutions adopted this measure around 1982.[6, 7] Continuing studies also implicated antibodies to the hepatitis B core antigen (anti-HBc) as another surrogate for NANB infectivity.[8, 9]

Further measures to reduce the incidence of post-transfusion NANB hepatitis were largely set aside as a result of the emergence of the acquired immunodeficiency syndrome (AIDS) and recognition of its transmissibility by blood components and plasma fractions between 1981 and 1984. Although the potential value of the anti-HBc test as a surrogate for AIDS infectivity was discussed, this approach was adopted in only a limited number of blood establishments. Recognition of the human immunodeficiency virus (HIV) as the infectious agent of AIDS by Gallo and Montagnier and their colleagues[10, 11] led to the rapid development and introduction of screening tests for antibodies to the virus. Testing started in March 1985. Because of the persistent nature of HIV infection, the presence of antibodies to HIV was closely linked to infectivity and it is now clear that the introduction of this test played a major role in the almost total elimination of transfusion-transmitted HIV and AIDS. A problem with the exclusive use of anti-HIV as an infection marker is the fact that, early in infection, infectious virus can circulate before the appearance of detectable levels of antibody. Thus, there has been a continuing process of improvement of antibody tests and implementation of additional tests in order to reduce the length of this infectious window period and thus to reduce risk. Not only have antibody tests become much more sensitive, but also tests for HIV p24 antigen and now for HIV RNA have been introduced.

The first human retrovirus to be recognized was the human T-lymphotropic retrovirus type I (HTLV-I).[12] This virus is an oncovirus, and its epidemiology is characterized by extreme geographic clustering in Japan, the Caribbean, and parts of Africa. Clinical outcomes of infection with this virus are relatively uncommon but include the serious T-cell lymphoma/leukemia and a neurological disease called HTLV-associated myelopathy, otherwise termed tropical spastic paraparesis. Subsequently, a closely related virus, HTLV-II, was characterized. Its epidemiology is less well defined, but it appears to be naturally endemic in certain indigenous populations in the Americas and also circulates among injection drug users. The first serological tests to be developed were designed to detect antibodies to HTLV-I, but as a result of cross-reactivity, they also identified the majority of HTLV-II infections. Epidemiologic studies in the U.S. donor population revealed a 0.025% prevalence of anti-HTLV,[13] and

this figure, along with the potentially serious outcomes of infection (which had been shown to occur through transfusion), led to the implementation of donor testing in 1988.

During the same period, there was a reevaluation of the severity of long-term outcomes of NANB hepatitis. As a result of this and of a heightened awareness of blood safety, blood establishments adopted testing for both elevated ALT levels and anti-HBc in the expectation that these tests together might reduce the incidence of transfusion-transmitted NANB hepatitis by about 60%.[8, 9] This projection turned out to be quite accurate. The most important advance in management of NANB was the cloning of a portion of the genome of a virus termed hepatitis C virus. This permitted the development of a test for antibodies to the virus based on peptides expressed from the viral genome. Use of this test revealed that almost all NANB hepatitis was due to hepatitis C. The first-generation test was implemented for donor screening in 1989 to 1990. Subsequently, with the expression of additional peptides, versions 2.0 and 3.0 of the test were successively implemented, with consequent gains in sensitivity. Nevertheless, there continues to be a significant infectious window period, and nucleic acid amplification tests for HCV have also been implemented.

■ Approach to Testing

Blood, blood components, and plasma products are classified as Biologics in the United States. By extension, tests used in the preparation of blood are also classified as Biologics and, as such, are regulated by the U.S. Food and Drug Administration (FDA). This licensure involves extensive clinical trials and stringent regulatory oversight. However, these procedures are somewhat cumbersome and involve considerable resource utilization by manufacturers and regulators. As a consequence, the selection of available tests in the United States may differ from that in other parts of the world. A listing of FDA-licensed tests may be found on the FDA website: http://www.fda.gov/cber/products/testkits.htm. It should be noted that some of these tests may no longer be available. Typical results of the use of these tests in a large voluntary donor population are presented in Table 12.1.

Table 12.1 Results of Confirmatory Testing Among Voluntary Blood Donors, American Red Cross 1996–1997 ($n = 3.27 \times 10^6$)

Marker	Number (%) EIA Repeat Reactive*		Number (%)[†] Positive		Number (%) Negative		Number (%) Indeterminate	
			Number (%) of EIA Repeat Reactive Samples with Confirmatory Results of					
Anti-HIV	2660	(0.082)	208	(7.8)	1245	(46.8)	1207	(45.4)
HIV-1 p24 Antigen[‡]	1625	(0.024)	134	(8.2)	NA		1491[§]	(91.8)
Anti-HTLV-1	3581	(0.11)	323	(9.0)	692	(19.3)	2566	(71.7)
Anti-HCV (3.0)	6032	(0.19)	3397	(56.3)	1423	(23.6)	1212	(20.1)
HBsAg	1456	(0.045)	1001	(68.8)	455	(31.2)	NA	

*Percentage figure is percentage of all donations found repeat reactive in screening test.
[†]The percentage is the positive predictive value of the test.
[‡]Denominator for HIV p24 antigen is approximately 6.75×10^6.
[§]Includes 57 false positives (RNA and follow-up negative), 73 with anti-HIV, and a final yield of 4 anti-HIV negative, RNA positive window case donations.
EIA, enzyme immunoassay; HBsAg, hepatitis B surface antigen; HCV, hepatitis C virus; HIV, human immunodeficiency virus; HTLV, human T-lymphotropic virus.

There is a broad commonality in the implementation of all tests used to ensure the safety of blood and blood components. Every donation is tested, and current requirements in the United States are that the test be performed on a sample drawn at the time of donation. With the exception of testing for viral nucleic acids, which is described later, there are three phases of the testing. Each sample is tested singly; nonreactive results are considered to be negative for the marker, and the corresponding blood unit (and its components) may be issued for transfusion. If the result is reactive, the sample is retested in duplicate. If both of the repeated test results are nonreactive, the sample is classified as negative and the unit or its components are released. However, if one or both of the repeated results are reactive, the sample is classified as repeatedly reactive and the blood unit cannot be issued for transfusion. This practice was initiated when it was recognized that radioimmunoassays (and subsequently enzyme immunoassays [EIAs]) were subject to nonrepeatable reactive results related to minor contamination with the labeled conjugate.

The final phase of testing is the application of confirmatory or supplementary tests, largely intended to ensure that the donor is properly advised about the significance of the screening test results. Although imperfect, this phase of testing markedly improves the accuracy of donor notification and counseling. In certain circumstances, these additional tests may also be used to support reentry of donors whose screening test results are definitively false positive. In some countries, a second screening test is used in place of different technology. In the United States, it has proved effective to use this second EIA strategy to reduce the number of confirmatory tests that have to be performed.[14] The strategy requires that the two EIA tests have essentially the same sensitivity. Despite the use of supplementary or confirmatory testing, the general rule in the United States is that a donor is indefinitely deferred on the basis of a repeatedly reactive screening test result.

There are some exceptions to this generalized algorithm. For example, there is no supplementary or confirmatory test for antibodies to the HBc antigen. In this case, a donor is not permanently deferred until he or she is found to be repeatedly reactive on a second occasion. Somewhat similarly, a donor does not need to be deferred the first time a test for anti-HTLV-I or -II is repeatedly reactive, provided the supplementary test result is nonreactive or indeterminate. When testing for elevated levels of ALT was implemented, deferral policies were also developed on the basis of the level of ALT or the finding of elevated levels on multiple occasions, or both.

Starting in 1999, blood collection establishments in the United States implemented nucleic acid amplification testing (NAT) for HCV and HIV RNA in donor samples. This testing was performed on small (i.e., 16 or 24) pools of samples. In some cases, primary testing was performed using a multiplex system.[15] Consequently, the testing algorithms differ significantly from those outlined previously. A second round of testing is used to resolve pools, followed, in some cases, by another test to differentiate HIV from HCV. In addition, a second, different NAT test is used to confirm or support the results of the primary test. Initially, all NAT for donor blood in the United States was performed under Investigational New Drug (IND) protocols, but one test was

Table 12.2 Results of Nucleic Acid Testing for HIV and/or HCV RNA, United States, 1999–2000

Agent	Gen-Probe		Roche Molecular Systems	
	HIV	HCV	HIV	HCV
Tested	11.04×10^6	11.04×10^6	1.6×10^6	4.8×10^6
Positive	3	43	1	19
Rate per million	0.27	3.9	0.63	4.0

HCV, hepatitis C virus; HIV, human immunodeficiency virus.
Data derived from reference 16.

licensed in February 2002. Table 12.2 outlines the results of NAT for the U.S. blood donor population as of the end of 2000.[16]

Infectious disease testing is not static; there is continuing improvement in four broad areas. First, individual tests are being modified to ensure improved sensitivity and specificity. This is perhaps best exemplified by the rapid progression of anti-HCV tests from version 1.0 to version 3.0. Second, the formats of the tests and the nature of the automated instrument systems are also subject to change and improvement. In some cases these changes improve the performance characteristics of the tests, but they also reduce the need for human intervention and improve adherence to the requirements of good manufacturing practice. Third, a better understanding of the early (window) phase of infection has led to the addition of new test methods for some agents. For example, the measures for HIV now include a test for antibodies to the virus, a test for soluble viral antigen, and a test for viral nucleic acids. In addition, a number of tests are supplemented to detect additional strains or subtypes of a given agent. Fourth, continuing concern about blood safety is likely to lead to the implementation of tests for other agents including imported diseases such as Chagas' disease[17] and emerging infections such as babesiosis.

■ Window Period

At least until the late 1980s, the serologic tests in use were considered to have adequate sensitivity for detecting well-established, chronic infection. Comparison of detection rates among first-time and repeat donors generally revealed that about 50% of all confirmed positive test results were found among first-time donors, although they contributed only 20% of all donations. Concern about the continued occurrence of transfusion-transmitted HIV infection led to much closer evaluation of the risk of infectivity during the early phases of infection, particularly the viremic but antibody-negative window period. Indeed, in a study by Petersen and colleagues,[18] HIV infectivity was demonstrated in one in five seronegative donations collected from individuals who were HIV antibody positive at their next donation. Mathematical modeling showed that the period of such infectivity averaged 45 days as of 1990.[18]

Knowledge of the length of the window period and of the incidence of new infection in the donor population also permitted estimation of the residual risk of infection from transfusion. The availability of closely spaced sequential samples from commercial plasma donors permitted careful characterization of the window period and of the impact of additional tests. These studies showed that as the sensitivity of antibody tests was increased, the HIV window period was reduced to about 22 days.[19] The impact of addition of tests for the HIV-1 p24 antigen and HIV RNA was also estimated.[19] Similarly, the dynamics of early infection with HCV and HBV are now well defined.[20] Although data in 2001 suggested that the benefits of NAT were consistent with projections,[21] this was not the case for HIV-1 p24 antigen, which was detected much less frequently than anticipated. It is possible that because the HIV antigen peak corresponds with the symptomatic phase of early acute HIV infection, the affected donors feel unwell and are less likely to present for donation.

■ Tests by Agent

Hepatitis B Virus

The primary means for the detection of hepatitis B infectivity is the test for HBsAg. This antigen is the first serological marker to appear during acute HBV infection, and it persists during active, chronic infection. It is produced in the cytoplasm of HBV-infected cells. It is often present in the serum at high levels, even up to micrograms per milliliter. It represents the viral coat and is found in the serum or plasma in the form of self-assembled spheres and tubules 22 nm in diameter. It is readily detected by simple sandwich-type immunoassays using animal antibodies to HBsAg (anti-HBs) as a solid-phase capture reagent and a conjugated anti-HBs as a probe. Conventional assays use either a bead or a microplate well as the solid phase, but tests (particularly automated ones) are increasingly based on microparticle substrates. Similarly, enzyme conjugates and chromogenic detection methods are being replaced by chemiluminescent labels.

Currently available tests have an analytic sensitivity on the order of 0.5 ng/mL with a range of 0.08 to 0.7 ng/mL. The epidemiologic sensitivity and specificity of the test are high. Nevertheless, because the prevalence of positive HBsAg findings in the donor population is quite low, the positive predictive value of the test is low. Thus, as with any other donor screening test, any repeatedly reactive finding should be confirmed before the donor is notified. Manufacturers of HBsAg test kits also provide confirmatory reagents, consisting of specific antibodies to HBsAg. The test is repeated in the presence of the antibody and a control test is also run using a normal serum. If the added antibody inhibits the test signal by 50% or more relative to the control, the reactive result is considered to be confirmed as positive. There are some additional steps to be taken in specified circumstances (such as a strong primary test result). It should be noted that very weak reactive signals may also give false-positive results in this confirmatory procedure.

As indicated earlier, testing for anti-HBc was introduced in the United States in 1986 to 1987. It was originally used to screen for NANB hepatitis infectivity as a result of some epidemiologic correlation between HBV and HCV infection, but this use is no longer considered valid or appropriate. In fact, anti-HBc testing was licensed by the FDA as an additional measure to improve safety with respect to HBV. The core antigen is actually the viral capsid, and antibodies appear early in infection but after HBsAg. Originally, it was hypothesized that anti-HBc was the only marker detectable during a window period after the decline of HBsAg and before the appearance of the corresponding protective antibody (anti-HBs). Current test methods are so sensitive that this is probably no longer true. There are both old and contemporary data suggesting that a minority of donations with anti-HBc as the sole marker of HBV infection may be infectious.[22–25] However, the presence of significant levels of anti-HBs seems to negate the risk of any infectivity through the blood (although not from a transplanted liver).[26] Consequently, in Japan, a country with a high prevalence of HBV infection, donors are tested for HBsAg, anti-HBc, and anti-HBs. All units with detectable HBsAg are discarded, as are those with anti-HBc in the absence of anti-HBs. However, units with both antibodies are used for transfusion.[27]

There are two approaches to anti-HBc testing. The initial test to be developed was an inhibition immunoassay. Although there has been additional development, this procedure is still available. The solid phase has recombinant HBc antigen as a capture reagent and the probe is a labeled, partially purified anti-HBc. The presence of anti-HBc in the test sample inhibits the signal. Perhaps surprisingly, this test has rather poor specificity, in part because of reduction-sensitive interfering molecules in some samples.[28] Newer versions of the test incorporate reductants, which clearly increase the specificity of the test. However, the inhibition procedure is also quite sensitive to technique, and reproducibility is not optimal. A second, direct antiglobulin assay for anti-HBc is also available; it appears to be more specific than the inhibition procedure. There is no formal confirmatory procedure for anti-HBc, but the use of two different tests may help to increase the predictive value of a reactive result.

Other HBV Tests

There are other tests for markers of HBV infection, but, in general, they have little current relevance to transfusion medicine, at least in the United States. As pointed out earlier, tests for anti-HBs are available and a positive result usually (but not always) signifies a resolved infection and the absence of circulating virus.[27] Indeed, the presence of anti-HBs may not signify complete elimination of HBV, as the virus may still be present in the liver; transplanted organs from donors with anti-HBs can result in HBV infection in a susceptible recipient.[26] Anti-HBs testing may be used to identify anti-HBc–reactive donations that are safe for transfusion. There are commercially available tests for immunoglobulin M anti-HBc, and this test is useful for diagnosis of acute HBV infection. Tests for the hepatitis B e antigen are of some value in defining the severity of an infection, but the value of a test for the corresponding antibody (anti-HBe) is less clear.

Amplification tests for hepatitis B DNA are available. Testing of plasma for further manufacture has been implemented using relatively large pools of samples (i.e., 512 to 1200). In addition, testing of blood donations for labile components has been implemented in some countries.[29, 30] It is generally accepted that DNA levels are relatively low during most phases of infection when HBsAg cannot be detected, and the benefit of NAT for HBV DNA is unclear. It is likely that this approach may have more benefit in circumstances where donor testing for anti-HBc is not used.

Hepatitis C Virus

The primary screening and diagnostic test for HCV infection is an antiglobulin EIA for antibodies to the virus. As of the beginning of 2001, only two tests were available in the United States. Both use immobilized, recombinant viral antigens as the capture reagent and an anti-immunoglobulin conjugate as the probe. One test is defined as a version 2.0 test, the other as a version 3.0. Both tests use antigens representing the core and NS3/NS4 regions of the viral genome, and the 3.0 version includes an NS5 peptide. In comparison, the first test to be licensed (termed 1.0) used only a single peptide in the capture reagent. This test, although a considerable advance on surrogate testing, lacked both sensitivity and specificity. Subsequent versions are much improved with respect to both of these characteristics.

One licensed supplementary test for anti-HCV is available in the United States. It is a strip immunoassay consisting of a nitrocellulose paper strip bearing HCV peptides at specified locations. There are also controls to ensure that the test is performed properly and to identify reactions related to antibodies to superoxide dismutase (SOD), a carrier protein for expression of some of the peptides. The strip is exposed to a test sample, and any adherent antibodies are detected and visualized by use of an antiglobulin conjugate and chromogenic substrate. The test is designed to complement the version 3.0 EIA and consequently involves essentially the same peptides. Clearly, the test is designed to dissect out and identify the presence of antibodies to different viral epitopes. In common with the Western blot, this approach has two deficiencies: (1) it is a subjective test, and (2) it does not generate outcomes with unequivocal interpretations. That is, results may be defined as nonreactive, positive, or indeterminate. A positive test is defined on the basis of at least two bands with a density greater than or equal to that of the low positive control but in the absence of an SOD band. A negative result is defined as one or more bands with a density less than that of the low positive control. A result is defined as indeterminate if there is only one band with a density greater than or equal to that of the weak positive control or if an SOD band is present, irrespective of other band patterns. An indeterminate result does not clearly establish the presence or absence of current or prior infection with HCV. In testing donors, about 20% of EIA repeat-reactive donations are found to be indeterminate, but only about 1% of these are positive for HCV RNA by polymerase chain reaction (PCR).[31, 32]

At the time of writing, two commercially available NAT procedures are in use for testing donor blood for evidence of HCV infectivity.[33] One is a PCR procedure that is conducted on RNA extracted from pools of 24 plasma samples by standard chemical methods. The other approach uses a transcription-mediated amplification procedure on nucleic acid preparations made by a solid-phase probe-capture method. Both approaches are successful in detecting HCV antibody–nonreactive, RNA-positive window-phase donations. Furthermore, both methods seem to have the same performance characteristics when the different sensitivities of the version 2.0 and 3.0 EIAs are accounted for. HCV RNA levels increase rapidly and reach values of 10^5 to 10^7 copies/mL during the period of about 40 to 50 days before the appearance of detectable HCV antibody. In a review of national experience with NAT, Stramer and colleagues[16] showed that the detection rate for HCV RNA was about 1 in every 260,000 seronegative donations.

Accepted testing algorithms for blood donor screening differ somewhat from those for diagnosis or screening of the

general population in-as-much as the NAT procedures have not been formally accepted as part of the confirmatory process for donors. This is discussed in more detail in Chapter 38.

HIV

As a direct result of the discovery of HIV, the causative agent of AIDS, the first tests for antibodies to this virus were licensed for donor screening in early 1985. All of the initial tests were antiglobulin EIA procedures using viral lysate as the solid-phase capture reagent and enzyme-conjugated antiglobulins as the probe. Early results using one of these procedures nationwide revealed that the prevalence of seropositive donations was 0.038%.[34] Tests for antibodies to HIV have been continuously upgraded. There have been two major changes. First, in 1992 the FDA required that blood donor testing should include a means of detecting infection with HIV-2. This was achieved by the development of combination ("combo") tests designed to identify antibodies to both viruses in the same test. Second, and in some cases as a means of satisfying this requirement, some of the tests evolved to a direct test in which both the capture reagent and the labeled probe were viral peptides (usually prepared by recombinant techniques). These approaches led to much increased sensitivity, cutting the seronegative window period by as much as 23 days.[35] As a result of careful and intensive approaches to donor selection and questioning and of continued testing, fewer than 1 in 25,000 donations are confirmed positive for anti-HIV.

Two tests are licensed for confirmatory or supplemental testing for anti-HIV. The one more commonly used is the Western blot, essentially a research test that was reported in the earliest publication on HIV antibody testing.[36] Also approved for use is an indirect immunofluorescence procedure. The Western blot is similar to the strip immunoassay already mentioned in that it identifies the presence of antibodies to individual viral components. The blot procedure involves separation of viral components by electrophoresis on polyacrylamide gel, followed by transfer (blotting) to a nitrocellulose paper. A strip of the paper is exposed to a test sample, and adherent antibodies are detected and visualized by use of an appropriate conjugated antiglobulin.

A number of attempts have been made to define an effective set of interpretive criteria for the HIV blot, but none has been fully effective.[37–41] The criterion in current use was developed by the Centers for Disease Control and Prevention and the Association of State and Territorial Public Health Laboratory Directors. A positive finding is defined as the presence of at least two of the following bands at an intensity equal to or greater than that of the weak positive control: p24, gp41, and gp120/160. A blot with no visible bands is considered to be negative, and any other band pattern is interpreted as indeterminate (even if the bands are nonviral).[42] In fact, the current approved criterion may lead to false-positive outcomes in as many as 10% of donor samples with a positive blot interpretation.[43] Indeterminate outcomes are frequent; in the American Red Cross system, only 7.8% of EIA repeatedly reactive samples are found to be positive on the blot, 46.8% are negative, and 45.4% are indeterminate. Essentially all of the indeterminate group are unrelated to HIV infection, but current recommendations permit them to be resolved only on the basis of follow-up. A clear advantage of the immunofluorescence alternative method is the much lower frequency of indeterminate results. The interpretation of HIV antibody test results is complicated by the requirement to evaluate EIA repeatedly reactive samples for evidence of HIV-2 infection using a second test based on a viral lysate. There are no licensed supplemental tests for HIV-2, and some individuals may be inappropriately notified that they have been infected with HIV-2 despite its extreme rarity in the U.S. donor population.

The inability to detect HIV in the infectious window period has engendered considerable concern since 1985. As pointed out earlier, the sensitivity of antibody tests has been improved so that the window period has been halved. Nevertheless, the risk is still unacceptable. Although it was known that the soluble HIV-1 p24 antigen could be detected during the window period, an extensive study published in 1990 did not suggest that implementation of the antigen test for screening would have any appreciable yield.[44] Subsequently, the issue was reevaluated and antigen testing was implemented in 1996. Despite predictions that approximately 5 to 10 antigen-positive, antibody-negative donations would be identified each year, the actual detection frequency has been only 1 in 4 million to 9 million donations.[33] Although licensed tests for HIV-1 p24 antigen are accompanied by an immunologic blocking test for confirmation, this test itself generates false-positive results, so the actual status of a donor may be truly defined only by follow-up. A further problem with the HIV-1 p24 antigen test is that the FDA does not permit a negative interpretation; results can be defined only as positive, indeterminate, or invalid.

As is the case for HCV, NAT has been implemented under IND protocols for the detection of HIV RNA. The procedures used are those described previously for HCV. As of the end of 2000, three HIV RNA–positive, antibody-negative, antigen-negative samples were detected as a result of testing 12.6 million donations in pools of 16 or 24.[16] This yield is compatible with expectation. It appears that all p24 antigen–positive, antibody-negative samples would be detected by pooled NAT, and it is anticipated that it will be possible to discontinue HIV-1 p24 antigen testing when NAT procedures are licensed for routine use. Studies have shown that HIV RNA levels increase quite rapidly and normally reach 10^4 to 10^6 copies/mL before the appearance of anti-HIV. Again, the results of NAT have not been formally approved as a supplement to the serologic test results, even though such information would be of clear relevance in notifying and counseling seropositive donors.

HTLV

Although HTLV-I was the first human retrovirus to be identified, donor testing was not initiated until 1988. Seroprevalence studies indicated that approximately 0.025% of the donor population had evidence of infection with the virus.[13] In actuality, as a result of the strong sequence and antigenic homologies, the tests originally developed to detect antibodies to HTLV-I were also able to detect many (perhaps most) infections with HTLV-II. The viruses differ epidemiologically. There are insufficient data to determine the extent to which their pathologic outcomes differ.

Tests for antibodies to HTLV-I and HTLV-II are generally similar to the earliest tests for HIV antibodies. That is, they rely on a viral lysate as the capture reagent and adherent donor antibodies are identified with an antiglobulin conjugate. In 1998, the FDA required that blood donations be additionally evaluated for the presence of antibodies to HTLV-II using a test formally approved for that purpose. This required the development of tests that included specific HTLV-II–derived antigens, and manufacturers developed combo tests for this purpose. Consequently, available tests are identified as tests for the detection of HTLV-I/HTLV-II antibodies.

There are no licensed confirmatory or supplemental tests for the EIA procedures. Western blot tests are commercially available for use under research or IND protocols, but their performance characteristics are far from optimal. In fact, in the American Red Cross system, only 9% of EIA repeatedly reactive samples are positive by blot, 19.3% are negative, and the remaining 71.7% are indeterminate.[32] Some have used radioimmunoprecipitation to supplement these procedures, but this technique is more complex and arduous than the Western blot. A final problem is that additional tests may be required to differentiate HTLV-I and HTLV-II infections. A specific viral peptide–supplemented blot is designed to differentiate these two infections, but it is not readily available to blood collectors. It is, however, reasonable to ask whether there is any clear medical benefit to differentiating these viruses; notification policy does not differ greatly.[45] NAT is available experimentally, but it appears unlikely to be adopted for screening donations.

Syphilis

Although (or perhaps because) testing for syphilis was the first procedure to be implemented for blood safety, it is now the least understood and least justified test in use. The nature and properties of serologic tests for syphilis are described in much greater detail elsewhere.[46] Initially, donor testing was undertaken using nontreponemal tests, such as the rapid plasma reagin (RPR) test. Although these tests were markedly nonspecific, they had the advantage of identifying primarily active or recent infections. Over the past 5 to 10 years, most blood collection agencies have adopted treponemal tests, mainly because they are adaptable to use on automated instruments, including those routinely used for blood typing. Treponemal tests generally indicate current and distant infection even after successful treatment. Repeatedly reactive screening test results are generally confirmed or supplemented by the use of fluorescent treponemal antibody tests, treponemal EIA tests, or nontreponemal tests. The frequency of reactive screening test results among Red Cross donations is about 0.18%. Of these, about 46% are confirmed by a fluorescent treponemal antibody absorption (FTA-ABS) test. Among the confirmed samples, 23% are RPR reactive. Even so, only about 50% of donors with an FTA-ABS–confirmed positive result report a past history of syphilis.

Evolving data suggest that few if any donors who test positive for syphilis antibodies have detectable *Treponema pallidum* DNA or RNA in their circulation.[47] In contrast, many individuals identified through sexually transmitted disease clinics are clearly bacteremic. The FDA has indicated its willingness to evaluate data with a view to reconsidering the need to continue routine syphilis testing for blood donors. It should be noted that, although a history of syphilis results in a 1-year deferral because of concerns that active syphilis might correlate with increased risk for HIV, there is no evidence that a positive test result for syphilis has any meaningful association with window-phase HIV infection.[48]

Cytomegalovirus

Cytomegalovirus (CMV) infection is usually relatively benign, but it can have profound and life-threatening effects on persons with a compromised immune response, including low-birth-weight infants. The virus is ubiquitous, and seroprevalence rates of 50% or more are common among adult populations. For many years, the use of CMV-seronegative blood components has been recommended for particular groups of patients at risk for serious CMV disease.[49, 50] It has been suggested that the use of leukoreduced components may similarly protect these vulnerable groups. Nevertheless, CMV testing continues to be used.[51] Both particle agglutination and EIA tests are available. Seronegative products are labeled as such, but there is no corresponding labeling of seropositive products, which are freely used for recipients who are not considered to be at risk. There is no program for donor notification or deferral for reactive CMV antibody tests. The performance characteristics of tests may differ, and there is no definitive "gold standard." Even the use of nucleic acid amplification techniques has generated results that are not always readily interpreted, perhaps as a consequence of interlaboratory variation in testing.

Surrogate Tests

The usual approach to testing blood for transfusion is to apply a test that identifies a specific marker of the infectious agent concerned. Serologic tests depend on the detection of circulating antigens or antibodies, and NAT methods provide direct detection of the pathogen's RNA or DNA. However, NANB hepatitis and AIDS were recognized as transfusion-transmissible diseases before any specific markers had been identified. In these cases, surrogate tests were considered or implemented. In the case of NANB, key studies clearly documented an association between elevated ALT levels in donors and the development of NANB in the recipients of the donations. Somewhat surprisingly, subsequent analysis showed a similar but nonoverlapping relationship between donor anti-HBc and recipient NANB. Although it was widely recognized that these tests were neither specific nor sensitive for NANB, they were projected to reduce the incidence of such posttransfusion infection by up to 60% and testing for both markers was introduced during 1986 to 1987. Such projections were subsequently validated when tests for anti-HCV came into use.[52]

During the early years of the AIDS epidemic, it was recognized that individuals with the disease were often reactive for anti-HBc. However, a relationship between anti-HBc in donors and transmission of AIDS to recipients was understandably not demonstrable. Some blood centers, particularly in the San Francisco Bay area, implemented anti-HBc testing as a surrogate.[23, 53] Further expansion of this measure was overtaken by the recognition of HIV and by the anticipated availability of a specific test. Other measures based on some of the clinical characteristics of AIDS, such as changed T-cell subset ratios, were proposed as surrogates and implemented in at least one location.[54]

Surrogate tests are inevitably less than satisfactory, usually failing to demonstrate adequate sensitivity or specificity. However, it should be recognized that perceptions have changed materially over the past two decades and there is little doubt that surrogate tests would be seriously considered in the future. One example is the potential use of surrogate markers as a means of identifying individuals in the early stages of disease attributable to transmissible spongiform encephalopathies.

■ Donor and Product Management

Testing is a key component of blood safety. Consequently, components are managed very conservatively with respect to test results. As pointed out earlier, a blood donation is discarded when found to be repeatedly reactive in a test. For the majority of tests, there is also a requirement to identify, retrieve, and quarantine any in–date products from prior donations from the affected donor. This must be achieved within a 3-day time frame but is not necessary if negative confirmatory or supplementary test results are available within this time.

A confirmed positive test result for HIV or HCV in a repeat donor triggers lookback. This process is designed to identify the recipients of prior donations from an individual now found to be seropositive. Such donations may have been in the infectious window period, may have been tested by a less sensitive version of the test, or may have been given before the implementation of the test in question. Lookback may also be triggered by a report that implicates a donor in post-transfusion disease.

Donors with repeatedly reactive test results must be deferred from all further donations, and records must be kept to ensure that they are deferred. Clearly, this process results in loss of many uninfected donors. At the same time, there is little point in continuing to collect blood from an individual who continues to generate false-positive test results, as the donations could not be used. In some circumstances a false-positive test result is not repeated, and so-called reentry algorithms have been developed to permit continued donation. These algorithms generally apply only to donors with repeatedly reactive screening test results that are negative in a licensed confirmatory or supplemental test. After a suitable waiting period, the donor must test nonreactive on screening and supplemental or confirmatory tests before being permitted to give blood again. Acceptable reentry protocols are published by the FDA.

REFERENCES

1. Blumberg BS, Alter HJ, Visnich S: A 'new' antigen in leukemia sera. JAMA 1965;191:541–546.
2. Blumberg BS, Gerstley BJS, Hungerford DA, et al: A serum antigen (Australia antigen) in Down's syndrome, leukemia and hepatitis. Ann Intern Med 1967;66:924–931.
3. Ling CM, Overby LR: Prevalence of hepatitis B virus antigen as revealed by direct radioimmune assay with 125-I-antibody. J Immunol 1972;109:834–841.
4. Feinstone SM, Kapikian AZ, Purcell RH, et al: Transfusion-associated hepatitis not due to viral hepatitis type A or B. N Engl J Med 1975;292:767–770.
5. Choo Q-L, Kuo G, Weiner AJ, et al: Isolation of a cDNA clone derived from a blood-borne non-A, non-B viral hepatitis genome. Science 1989;244:359–362.
6. Alter HJ, Purcell RH, Holland PV, et al: Donor transaminase and recipient hepatitis. Impact on blood transfusion services. JAMA 1981;246:630–634.
7. Aach RD, Szmuness W, Mosley JW, et al: Serum alanine aminotransferase of donors in relation to the risk of non-A, non-B hepatitis in recipients. The Transfusion-Transmitted Viruses Study. N Engl J Med 1981;304:989–994.
8. Stevens CE, Aach RD, Hollinger FB, et al: Hepatitis B virus antibody in blood donors and the occurrence of non-A, non-B hepatitis in

transfusion recipients. An analysis of the Transmission-Transmitted Viruses Study. Ann Intern Med 1984;101:733–738.

9. Koziol DE, Holland PV, Alling DW, et al: Antibody to hepatitis B core antigen as a paradoxical marker for non-A, non-B hepatitis agents in donated blood. Ann Intern Med 1986;104:488–495.

10. Barre-Sinoussi F, Chermann J-C, Rey F, et al: Isolation of a T-lymphotropic retrovirus from a patient at risk for acquired immune deficiency syndrome (AIDS). Science 1983;220:868–871.

11. Gallo RC, Salahuddin SZ, Popovic M, et al: Frequent detection and isolation of cytopathic retroviruses (HTLV-III) from patients with AIDS and at risk for AIDS. Science 1984;224:500–503.

12. Poiesz BJ, Ruscetti FW, Gazdar AF, et al: Detection and isolation of type C retrovirus particles from fresh and cultured lymphocytes of a patient with cutaneous T-cell lymphoma. Proc Natl Acad Sci USA 1980;77:7415–7419.

13. Williams AE, Fang CT, Slamon DJ, et al: Seroprevalence and epidemiological correlates of HTLV-1 infection in U.S. blood donors. Science 1988;240:643–646.

14. Stramer SL, Layug L, Trenbeath J, et al: Use of a second EIA in an HTLV-I/HTLV-II algorithm [abstract]. Transfusion 1998;38(Suppl):81S.

15. Stramer SL: Nucleic acid testing for transfusion-transmissible agents. Curr Opin Hematol 2000;7:387–391.

16. Stramer SL, Caglioti S, Strong DM: NAT of the United States and Canadian blood supply. Transfusion 2000;40:1165–1168.

17. Leiby DA, Read EJ, Lenes BA, et al: Seroepidemiology of *Trypanosoma cruzi*, etiologic agent of Chagas' disease, in US blood donors. J Infect Dis 1997;176:1047–1052.

18. Petersen LR, Satten GA, Dodd R, et al: Duration of time from onset of human immunodeficiency virus type 1 infectiousness to development of detectable antibody. Transfusion 1994;34:283–289.

19. Schreiber GB, Busch MP, Kleinman SH, Korelitz JJ: The risk of transfusion-transmitted viral infections. N Engl J Med 1996;334:1685–1690.

20. Busch MP: HIV, HBV and HCV: new developments related to transfusion safety. Vox Sang 2000;78:253–256.

21. Dodd RY, Aberle-Grasse JM, Stramer SL, ARCNET Program: The yield of nucleic acid testing (NAT) for HIV and HCV RNA in a population of U.S. voluntary donors: relationship to contemporary measures of incidence [abstract]. Transfusion 2000;40(10S):1S.

22. Huang YY, Yang SS, Wu CH, et al: Impact of screening blood donors for hepatitis C antibody on posttransfusion hepatitis: a prospective study with a second-generation anti-hepatitis C virus assay. Transfusion 1994;34:661–665.

23. Dodd RY, Popovsky MA: Antibodies to hepatitis B core antigen and the infectivity of the blood supply. Scientific Section Coordinating Committee. Transfusion 1991;31:443–449.

24. Caspari G, Gerlich WH: Virus safety of blood and plasma products in Germany--state of knowledge and open problems. Infusionsther Transfusionsmed 2000;27:286–295.

25. Allain JP, Hewitt PE, Tedder RS, Williamson LM: Evidence that anti-HBc but not HBV DNA testing may prevent some HBV transmission by transfusion. Br J Haematol 1999;107:186–195.

26. Dodson SF, Issa S, Araya V, et al: Infectivity of hepatic allografts with antibodies to hepatitis B virus. Transplantation 1997;64:1582–1584.

27. Marusawa H, Uemoto S, Hijikata M, et al: Latent hepatitis B virus infection in healthy individuals with antibodies to hepatitis B core antigen. Hepatology 2000;31:488–495.

28. Cheng Y, Dubovoy N, Hayes-Rogers ME, et al: Detection of IgM to hepatitis B core antigen in a reductant containing, chemiluminescence assay. J Immunol Methods 1999;230:29–35.

29. Cardoso MD, Koerner K, Kubanek B: PCR screening in the routine of blood banking of the German Red Cross Blood Transfusion Service of Baden-Wurttemberg. Infusionsther Transfusionsmed 1998;25:116–120.

30. Roth WK, Weber M, Seifried E: Feasibility and efficacy of routine PCR screening of blood donations for hepatitis C virus, hepatitis B virus, and HIV-1 in a blood-bank setting. Lancet 1999;353:359–363.

31. Dow BC, Buchanan I, Munro H, et al: Relevance of RIBA-3 supplementary test to HCV PCR positivity and genotypes for HCV confirmation of blood donors. J Med Virol 1996;49:132–136.

32. Dodd RY, Stramer SL: Indeterminate results in blood donor testing: what you don't know can hurt you. Transfus Med Rev 2000;14:151–160.

33. Stramer SL, Caglioti S, Strong DM: NAT of the United States and Canadian blood supply. Transfusion 2000;40:1165–1168.

34. Schorr JB, Berkowitz A, Cumming PD, et al: Prevalence of HTLV-III antibody in American blood donors. N Engl J Med 1985;313:384–385.

35. Busch MP, Lee LLL, Satten GA, et al: Time course of detection of viral and serologic markers preceding human immunodeficiency virus type 1 seroconversion: implications for screening of blood and tissue donors. Transfusion 1995;35:91–97.

36. Sarngadharan MG, Popovic M, Bruch L, et al: Antibodies reactive with human T-lymphotropic retroviruses (HTLV-III) in the serum of patients with AIDS. Science 1984;224:506–508.

37. Dodd RY, Fang CT: The Western immunoblot procedure for HIV antibodies and its interpretation. Arch Pathol Lab Med 1990;114:240–245.

38. Dock NL, Kleinman SH, Rayfield MA, et al: Human immunodeficiency virus infection and indeterminate Western blot patterns: prospective studies in a low prevalence population. Arch Intern Med 1991;151:525–530.

39. Kleinman S, Busch MP, Hall L, et al: False-positive HIV-1 test results in a low-risk screening setting of voluntary blood donation. JAMA 1998;280:1080–1085.

40. Mortimer PP: The fallibility of HIV western blot. Lancet 1991;337:286–287.

41. Sayre KR, Dodd RY, Tegtmeier G, et al: False-positive human immunodeficiency virus type 1 Western blot tests in noninfected blood donors. Transfusion 1996;36:45–52.

42. Interpretation and use of the Western blot assay for serodiagnosis of human immunodeficiency virus type 1 infections. MMWR Morb Mortal Wkly Rep 1989;38(Suppl 7):1–7.

43. Aberle-Grasse J, Dodd RY, Layug L: Impact on human immunodeficiency virus type 1 (HIV-1) seroprevalence of the change in HIV-1 Western blot criteria. Transfusion 1997;37:246–247.

44. Alter HJ, Epstein JS, Swenson SG, et al: Prevalence of human immunodeficiency virus type 1 p24 antigen in U.S. blood donors—an assessment of the efficacy of testing in donor screening. N Engl J Med 1990;323:1312–1317.

45. Khabbaz RF, Fukuda K, Kaplan JE: Guidelines for counseling human T-lymphotropic virus type I (HTLV-I)– and HTLV type II–infected persons. Transfusion 1993;33:694.

46. Larsen SA, Steiner BM, Rudolph AH: Laboratory diagnosis and interpretation of tests for syphilis. Clin Microbiol Rev 1995;8(1):1–21.

47. Orton SL, Liu H, Dodd RY, et al: Prevalence of circulating *Treponema pallidum* DNA and RNA in blood donors with confirmed positive Syphilis tests. Transfusion 2002;42:94–99.

48. Herrera GA, Lackritz EM, Janssen RS, et al: Serologic test for syphilis as a surrogate marker for human immunodeficiency virus infection among United States blood donors. Transfusion 1997;37:836–840.

49. Preiksaitis JK: Indications for the use of cytomegalovirus-seronegative blood products. Transfus Med Rev 1991;5:1–17.

50. Preiksaitis JK: The cytomegalovirus-"safe" blood product: is leukoreduction equivalent to antibody screening? Transfus Med Rev 2000;14:112–136.

51. Blajchman MA, Goldman M, Freedman JJ, Sher GD: Proceedings of a consensus conference: prevention of post-transfusion CMV in the era of universal leukoreduction. Transfus Med Rev 2001;15:1–20.

52. Donahue JG, Muñoz A, Ness PM, et al: The declining risk of post-transfusion hepatitis C virus infection. N Engl J Med 1992;327:369–373.

53. Busch MP, Dodd RY, Lackritz EM, et al: Value and cost-effectiveness of screening blood donors for antibody to hepatitis B core antigen as a way of detecting window-phase human immunodeficiency virus type 1 infections. Transfusion 1997;37:1003–1011.

54. Galel SA, Lifson JD, Engleman EG: Prevention of AIDS transmission through screening of the blood supply. Annu Rev Immunol 1995;13:201–227.

Chapter 13

Packed RBCs and Related Products

Sally A. Campbell-Lee
Paul M. Ness

Landsteiner[1] discovered the ABO system in 1901, more than 100 years ago. Since that time, the development of a safe and effective anticoagulant-preservative solution[2] and the efforts in World War II that led to current methods of organized blood collection[3] have promoted transfusion medicine to an essential aspect of clinical medicine. The appropriate use of red blood cell concentrates (commonly referred to as packed red blood cells, pRBCs) depends on knowledge of the physiology of red blood cell transfusion and the therapeutic options of various component manipulations (Table 13.1). This chapter covers the manufacturing and storage of, and indications for, whole blood, pRBCs, and related products.

■ Collection

In 1997, nearly 12 million units of whole blood were collected in the United States.[4] Whole blood, composed of red blood cells, leukocytes, platelets, and plasma, is collected into a closed, sterile system. The system consists of a phlebotomy needle, integral donor tubing, and several attached polyvinyl resin bags.[5] Within the polyvinyl resin bags is 63 mL of, most commonly, citrate, phosphate, and dextrose (CPD) or citrate, phosphate, dextrose, and adenine (CPDA-1) anticoagulant-preservative, which provides a shelf-life of 35 days when the contents are stored at 4°C. Including the anticoagulant-preservative, the volume of a unit of whole blood is approximately 510 mL (450 mL of blood plus 63 mL of anticoagulant),[6] although many blood centers now collect 500 mL of donor blood. Within 24 hours of collection, the platelets (if refrigerated) and granulocytes are dysfunctional and several coagulation factors are at suboptimal levels.[7] To optimize factor activity and platelet recovery, preparation of fresh frozen plasma (FFP) and platelet concentrates must occur within 8 hours.[8]

One of the problems with the standard method of collecting whole blood is that the amount of anticoagulant-preservative is predetermined but the exact amount of whole blood collected is not. Because of variability in donor hematocrits, different red blood cell masses are collected per unit, resulting in variable red blood cell mass provided per unit transfused.

A more efficient method of collecting red blood cells for transfusion has been developed. Red blood cells may be collected by apheresis, with the unwanted components returned to the donor. Apheresis has become commonplace in the collection of platelet concentrates and granulocytes. Modified apheresis equipment has been used to collect red blood cells and plasma.[9] The MCS+ machine (Haemonetics Corp., Braintree, MA) was developed for red blood cell collection and is now approved by the U.S. Food and Drug Administration (FDA) for two-unit apheresis with automated return of 500 mL of saline to the donor or collection of one unit of red blood cells and 200 to 550 mL of plasma.[10]

For whole blood collections, a donor must have a hematocrit of at least 38% or a hemoglobin level of 12.5 g/dL and must wait 56 days between donations.[11] The FDA criteria for allogeneic two-unit apheresis red blood cell donation require a minimum hematocrit of 40% or a hemoglobin of 13.3 g/dL with a minimum of 112 days between donation. There are also height and weight requirements to ensure adequate donor red blood cell mass. For men, a minimum height of 5 feet 1 inch and weight of 130 pounds, and for women, 5 feet 5 inches and 150 pounds are required. The red blood cell volumes removed from the donor in two-unit red blood cell apheresis (380 to 500 mL) are comparable to those in whole blood donation (405 to 495 mL). The percentage of total blood volume (8.7% to 10.5%) removed is less than the 15% total blood volume allowed in whole blood donation. Red blood cell apheresis donors do not appear to have more symptomatic anemia than

Table 13.1 pRBC Characteristics and General Indications

Product	Manipulation/Comment	Indications
Whole blood	None	Trauma, massive surgical bleeding
pRBCs, unmodified	Volume reduced	Symptomatic anemia Hemorrhagic shock (with volume expanders)
pRBCs, leukoreduced	White blood cell reduction	Prevent transfusion reactions Reduce alloimmunization Reduce infectious diseases Minimize immunomodulation
pRBCs, washed	Plasma removal	Recurrent severe allergic reactions IgA deficiency with anti-IgA
pRBCs, irradiated	Inactivation of lymphocytes	Prevention of TAGVHD
pRBCs, frozen deglycerolized	Frozen with subsequent deglycerolization/ Facilitates long-term storage	Storage of rare RBC phenotypes Autologous storage
pRBCs, CMV seronegative	Tested and found to be negative serologically/Also applies to leukocytes, platelets, and residual plasma	CMV-negative transplantation Low-birthweight infants CMV-negative pregnant women In utero transfusion

CMV, cytomegalovirus; IgA, immunoglobulin A; RBC, red blood cell; TAGVHD, transfusion-associated graft-versus-host disease.

whole blood donors, and the most common reactions are attributable to citrate toxicity.[11]

The quality of apheresis-collected red blood cells is comparable to that of manually collected red blood cells. In a study by Holme and colleagues,[10] both one-unit and two-unit red blood cell apheresis was performed using the MCS+ with CPD or CP2D preservative. After resuspension in AS-3 additive and storage for 42 days at 4°C, the apheresis units had slightly less hemolysis, lower supernatant potassium levels, and better tolerance for osmotic shock than manually collected units, with no difference in red blood cell adenosine triphosphate (ATP) or 24-hour percent recovery after autologous transfusion.

■ Red Blood Cell Products

Whole Blood

Although whole blood is rarely used, there are certain clinical situations in which it might be preferable to pRBCs. Whole blood can correct combined deficits in oxygen-carrying capacity and blood volume. Whole blood is thus potentially indicated in trauma and massive surgical bleeding when the blood type of the patient has been determined. This approach minimizes the use of red blood cells and plasma from different donors, thus decreasing the risk of transfusion-transmitted infectious disease. In addition, one study demonstrated that a unit of fresh whole blood has a hemostatic effect equivalent to that of 8 to 10 platelet units[12]; this effect appears to be diminished after storage of the blood at 4°C for a period as short as 5 hours,[13] which makes whole blood impractical as a source of platelets.

Although fresh whole blood can be useful for patients who require both oxygen-carrying capacity and volume, adequate inventories are difficult to maintain. Most cases requiring whole blood involve trauma, emergency cardiovascular surgery, or liver transplantation, which can be difficult to predict. In addition, the community need for platelets and plasma must be considered. Therefore, although some have argued that whole blood should be used more often, even for certain elective surgeries most trauma centers continue to manage their cases with pRBCs.[14]

Instead of whole blood, pRBCs and one of several volume expanders can increase oxygen-carrying capacity and volume.

Volume can be replaced with crystalloid, which is not only sterile but also economical, in the setting of mild to moderate blood loss. With more massive transfusion, colloid oncotic pressure may have to be enhanced; colloid solutions such as albumin are preferred to plasma as there is no risk of transfusion-transmitted infectious disease. A study of patients massively transfused (defined as 10 or more units of red blood cell concentrates in 24 hours) and given crystalloid demonstrated that significant thrombocytopenia developed after 20 units of pRBCs. Significant prolongation of the prothrombin and partial thromboplastin times occurred after transfusion of 12 pRBCs.[15] Whether these laboratory values are actually associated with abnormal clinical bleeding deserves investigation.

Plasma is rarely indicated during massive transfusion unless there is a well-documented coagulopathy, as in liver failure or disseminated intravascular coagulation.[16] In some cases of trauma or cardiac surgery, platelet concentrates may be indicated as well to treat microvascular bleeding secondary to dilutional thrombocytopenia or platelet dysfunction secondary to bypass. When a pool of six random units or a single donor apheresis unit of platelets is given, at least 300 mL of plasma is also infused, eliminating the need for concomitant administration of FFP.

pRBCs

pRBCs are manufactured by removal of the majority of plasma from a unit of whole blood. pRBCs have a volume of approximately 250 to 300 mL and a hematocrit of 65% to 80%. pRBCs prepared without further modifications contain white blood cells, platelets, and residual plasma. Transfusion of pRBCs is indicated in the treatment of anemia with symptomatic deficits of oxygen-carrying capacity and hemorrhagic shock when administered with volume expanders. One unit of pRBCs should raise the hemoglobin of an average adult by 1 g/dL and the hematocrit by 3%. For pediatric patients, the usual dose given is 3 mL/kg to raise the hemoglobin by 1 g/dL and the hematocrit by 3%.

Preservation and Storage

The ability of transfused red blood cells to deliver oxygen to tissues and survive in the patient's circulation is the best measure of how well the red blood cells were preserved and stored. Survival of transfused red blood cells is acceptable when at least 70% of the transfused red blood cells are present in the circulation for 24 hours.[6] The development of blood preservatives provided a means to store red blood cells to facilitate blood banking with minimally toxic anticoagulants. A long history of clinical development has provided preservative solutions that optimize storage length and in vivo function. The main concerns that have been addressed are glucose, anticoagulation, ATP, and 2,3-diphosphoglycerate (2,3-DPG).

Glucose

Glucose is the main source of fuel for energy-requiring processes to preserve membrane function. Initially, dextrose was added to citrate as an energy source, but carmelization occurred during heat sterilization because of the alkaline pH.[17] The citrate and dextrose were sterilized separately and mixed before the blood was collected. In 1943, Loutit and Mollison[18] added citric acid, creating acid citrate dextrose (ACD) solution. This formulation decreased the pH, allowed sterilization without carmelization, and facilitated storage for up to 21 days. It was also noted that because of the decreased pH, the blood and preservative solution had to be mixed thoroughly during collection to avoid clot formation.[18]

Anticoagulation

Citrate has been used since the early 1900s as a stable, minimally toxic anticoagulant that also has preservative properties.[19] Citrate in preservative solutions also influences intracellular pH and provides buffering.

Citrate is part of the Krebs cycle of respiration and therefore occurs endogenously. It is metabolized by muscle, liver, and renal cortex and stored in bone. In massive transfusion, citrate has been considered to be a cause of cardiac arrhythmia because of its ability to decrease plasma ionized calcium through chelation, although clear evidence of toxicity resulting from hypocalcemia has been difficult to obtain. Citrate is metabolized rapidly, preventing systemic anticoagulation. However, certain conditions may place patients at risk for toxicity. Hypothermia, liver disease, and hypoparathyroidism are conditions in which patients may already have depressed ionized calcium or may not be able to metabolize the citrate rapidly.[20] Newborns without adequate calcium stores and immature livers may also be at risk. Because supplementation with intravenous calcium may be associated with its own toxicities, routine calcium administration is not recommended in massive transfusion.

Adenosine Triphosphate

The ATP content of pRBCs decreases with storage, from 4.18 μmol/g hemoglobin at collection in CPDA-1 to 2.40 μmol/g hemoglobin at 35 days of storage.[21] Changes in red blood cell shape and increased cell fragility have been noted in stored red blood cells.[22] It was not until 1962 that a direct correlation was made between erythrocyte shape and ATP content.[23] The decrease in ATP with storage is associated with a change in erythrocyte shape from biconcave disc to spherocyte as well as a decrease in membrane lipid content and an increase in cell rigidity. Therefore, ATP must be maintained during storage for appropriate post-transfusion survival of red blood cells. The addition of adenine counteracts the loss of adenine groups and allows enough ATP for red blood cell survival.

2,3-Diphosphoglycerate

The concentration of erythrocyte 2,3-DPG in pRBCs also decreases with storage. The decrease is dependent upon pH. In whole blood collected in CPDA-1, the pH decreases from 7.16 to 6.73 over 35 days as a result of lactic acid formation, and the 2,3-DPG concentration decreases markedly from 13.2 to 0.7 μmol/g hemoglobin.[21]

In the red blood cell, the glucose intermediate metabolite 1,3-DPG is transformed to 2,3-DPG by a mutase. The 2,3-DPG is then dephosphorylated to 3-phosphoglycerate by a phosphatase. The phosphatase is inactive at pH levels above 7.2 but is more active at the lower pH in older pRBCs, contributing to the decreased 2,3-DPG levels.[24]

The function of erythrocyte 2,3-DPG is to bind to deoxyhemoglobin and facilitate oxygen transport. When 2,3-DPG binds to deoxyhemoglobin, the deoxyhemoglobin molecule is stabilized and the equilibrium between deoxyhemoglobin and oxyhemoglobin shifts toward deoxyhemoglobin. This interaction shifts the oxygen dissociation curve to the right, decreasing the oxygen affinity of hemoglobin and enhancing oxygen delivery to tissues.[25] Therefore, with decreased 2,3-DPG levels, the oxygen dissociation curve is shifted to the left, decreasing oxygen delivery to tissues.

Although it may be feared that transfused red blood cells beyond a certain date of storage are of limited benefit to the patient, it has been shown that 2,3-DPG is rapidly regenerated by transfused red blood cells, with nearly complete restoration after 1 day. In addition, in hypoxia, lactic acid is produced, decreasing the pH and thus shifting the oxygen dissociation curve back to the right.[26] An increase in cardiac output also occurs with hypoxia, increasing oxygen delivery. Therefore, for most patients requiring transfusion, decreased 2,3-DPG is of little consequence. For the patient who is in shock and cannot increase cardiac output to compensate, the current preservative solutions may not be optimal because there is no added component to slow the decrease in 2,3-DPG levels.

Additive and Rejuvenation Solutions

In 1983 a red blood cell additive solution, Adsol (Fenwal Laboratories), also referred to as AS-1, was approved for use. Adsol consists of adenine (to help maintain ATP during storage), dextrose, saline, and mannitol. It contains 60% more adenine and approximately 2.5 times as much glucose as CPDA-1.[27] The addition of mannitol prevents excessive hemolysis over the storage period.[28] The increased glucose allows an adequate supply of energy for the red blood cells beyond 35 days, and blood stored with Adsol is outdated in 42 days (Table 13.2 and 13.3).[8] This decreases the number of pRBCs lost because of outdating and is helpful in shipping and storing autologous blood.

One of the added benefits of this preservative solution is that the amount of plasma recovered from a unit of whole blood can be maximized. Whole blood is collected into a system of multiple closed bags containing CPD. The whole blood is then centrifuged for separation, and sufficient plasma is removed to raise the hematocrit to approximately 85%. Then 100 mL of Adsol preservative solution is added to the pRBCs, with a resultant hematocrit of 60% to 70%. Because the final hematocrit is about 62%, the Adsol-preserved pRBCs are less viscous. The lower viscosity results in potentially faster flow rates, which are beneficial in emergency situations.[29] A second commonly used additive solution, AS-3, contains sodium

Table 13.2 42-Day Poststorage pRBC Characteristics after Resuspension in AS-3

Characteristic	Prestorage	Poststorage
pH	6.8	6.4
ATP (μmol/g Hb)	4.1	2.9
DPG (μmol/g Hb)	9.0	0.3
Potassium (mEq/L)	2.4	63
Glucose (mg/dL)	608	402
Plasma Hb (mg/dL)	39	372
Hemolysis (%)		0.61

ATP, adenosine triphosphate; DPG, diphosphoglycerate; Hb, hemoglobin; pRBC, packed red blood cell.
Modified from Holme S, Elfath MD, Whitley P: Evaluation of in vivo and in vitro quality of apheresis-collected RBC stored for 42 days. Vox Sang 1998; 75:212–217

chloride, phosphate, adenine, and glucose and is used similarly to AS-1.

Other additive solutions have been investigated. A solution containing adenine, dextrose, mannitol, sodium citrate, ammonium chloride, and inorganic phosphate was studied.[30] Levels of ATP were higher in this test solution, compared with Adsol, over 84 days of storage. 2,3-DPG levels were higher in the test solution, but not significantly, and hemolysis was higher in the Adsol units. It was thought that the higher ATP concentration in the test solution was due to the ammonium or phosphate ions or both.[30] In vivo survival was demonstrated in a second study using a modification of the previous test solution (less ammonium chloride). The 24-hour chromium-51 viability was superior to that of Adsol at 8 or 9 weeks of storage. Preparation for transfusion required removal of supernatant with one washing step.[31] This additive solution appears to be suitable for extending pRBC shelf life, but confirmatory studies are necessary.

Rejuvenation solutions can restore some intracellular ATP and 2,3-DPG lost during storage. The current FDA-licensed solution contains pyruvate, inosine, phosphate, and adenine. This solution may be added only to pRBCs prepared from whole blood collected in CPD or CPDA-1. It may be added at any point between 3 days after collection and 3 days after expiration. This solution is not intended for intravenous use, and pRBCs must be washed before administration or used when thawing frozen units.[8] Rejuvenation of units stored in AS-1 or AS-3 has also been studied.[32] In one experiment, rejuvenation of the AS-1 and AS-3 pRBCs resulted in above normal levels of ATP after one treatment but suboptimal

levels of 2,3-DPG. A second treatment raised the 2,3-DPG levels to normal. The authors suggested that this may be due to the increased adenine in the storage solutions; the conversion of 1,3-DPG to 3-phosphoglycerate is favored, decreasing 1,3-DPG availability to make 2,3-DPG.[32] Currently, only units stored in CPD or CPDA-1 may be used for rejuvenation.

Temperature

Red blood cell concentrates must be stored between 1 and 6°C.[8] Storage at this temperature slows red blood cell metabolism and facilitates extended storage in blood banks. Liquid blood storage in CPDA-1 allows a shelf life of up to 35 days. Even at 4°C, significant chemical changes take place during the storage period that may have clinical consequences for some patients. These changes are collectively known as the *storage lesion*.

There is no clinically significant change in the plasma levels of sodium and chloride. However, the plasma potassium increases nearly eightfold over 28 days.[33] At a temperature of 4°C, the sodium-potassium pump is essentially nonfunctional and intracellular and extracellular levels gradually equilibrate. In addition, the hemolysis that occurs during the storage period results in increased potassium in the supernatant. However, because the total volume of plasma in pRBCs is low (approximately 70 mL), the total potassium burden is only about 5.5 mEq at product expiration. Therefore, the potassium load is rarely a clinical problem except in the setting of preexisting hyperkalemia and renal failure or for very sick neonates. In these situations, fresher units of red blood cells or washed red blood cells may be used.

Storage Containers

The use of vinyl plastic blood bags and tubing in transfusion medicine is advantageous in the collection, processing, storage, and dispensing of blood components. In the early 1970s, however, there were reports about the potential toxicity of blood stored in bags with di(2-ethylhexyl)phthalate (DEHP). DEHP, the chemical that allows the vinyl plastic to be pliable, is referred to as a plasticizer. DEHP is added in large quantities to the plastic, approximately 40% by weight. It is not bound to the plastic but is dissolved in it. As a result, DEHP can leak into blood stored in the container and be transfused along with the blood. In 1970, Jaeger and Rubin[34] reported that 5 to 7 mg of DEHP could be isolated per 100 mL of blood. In addition, two patients were found to have DEHP at levels ranging from 0.069 to 0.270 mg per gram dry weight

Table 13.3 pRBC Storage and Additive Solutions

Substance Content (mmol/unit)	ACD-A*	CPDA-1*	CPD*	CP2D*	Adsol (AS-1)[†]	Nutri-cell (AS-3)[†]
Citrate	5.3	6.6	6.6	6.6	—	0.2
Phosphate	—	1.0	1.3	1.3		
Glucose	9.4	10.1	8.1	16.3	11.1	5.5
Adenine	—	0.128	—	—	0.21	0.22
NaCl	—	—	—	—	15.4	7.0
Na_2HPO_4	—	—	—	—	—	1.9
Na_3 citrate	—	—	—	—	—	1.9
Mannitol	—	—	—	—	4.1	—
pH	6.9	7.1	7.1	7.1	—	—
Volume (mL) per unit blood	67.5	63	63	63	100	100

*pRBC storage solutions.
[†]pRBC additive solutions.
From Hogman CF: Preparation and preservation of red cells. Vox Sang 1998;74(Suppl 2):177.

of tissue. Concern over the potential toxic effects of DEHP in humans has fueled a great deal of research and much debate. DEHP, identified as a carcinogen in rats and mice,[35] is ubiquitous in the environment. It caused a form of shock lung leading to death when administered to rats in intravenous form,[36] caused testicular atrophy in rats given dietary doses,[37] and led to lung injury in dogs and baboons transfused with stored blood.[38]

Because of an association with hepatomegaly, DEHP has also been linked to potential hepatocarcinogenicity. Hepatomegaly has been shown to be caused by proliferation of cellular organelles called peroxisomes. Peroxisomes are involved in the β-oxidation of fatty acids, producing hydrogen peroxide, which has been suggested to be the causative agent in the carcinogenicity of DEHP.[39] With all of this information, however, no direct causal link has been established between DEHP and cancer in humans.

On the other hand, the search for alternatives to DEHP has identified potential benefits for red blood cell storage. Because of the concerns about toxicity, alternative materials for blood storage containers have been under investigation for some time. A study comparing another plastic, poly-(ethylene-co-ethyl acrylate) (EEA), with polyvinyl chloride (PVC) containing DEHP[40] found that blood stored in EEA containers had higher plasma hemoglobin and greater susceptibility to osmotic lysis than blood stored in PVC containers. When DEHP was added to EEA containers, blood stored in EEA containers without DEHP had greater red blood cell osmotic fragility than blood in EEA with DEHP or PVC containers.

PVC plasticized with butyryl-*n*-trihexyl-citrate (BTHC) has been introduced in place of DEHP. Use of BTHC has not become widespread. Less BTHC than DEHP leaches into the bag contents, and there is excellent 24-hour post-transfusion red blood cell recovery with minimal hemolysis.[41]

Frozen Red Blood Cell Concentrates

Red blood cells can be frozen for long-term storage, up to 10 years, and probably longer for certain indications.[8] After pRBCs are prepared from whole blood, they are treated with glycerol as a cryoprotective agent. Because glycerol binds water, the formation of ice spicules from the solvent water within the unit, which would damage the red blood cells, is prevented.[42] Another theory concerning the efficacy of glycerol is that it prevents cellular hypotonicity or hypertonicity, which may enhance cell lysis. The blood of donors who have sickle cell trait is unsuitable for freezing because hemolysis occurs during routine deglycerolization.[43]

There are three methods of freezing red blood cells,[44] the most common one in the United States being the high-glycerol (40% to 50%) method. A low-glycerol method exists, but it has several disadvantages—liquid nitrogen must be used for storage, and the metal containers in which the plastic blood bags are placed before freezing can cause explosions if the liquid nitrogen leaks.[45] With a third method, agglomeration, the cells are deglycerolized with a low-ionic-strength saline solution. The cells clump and sediment in the bag, after which the supernatant is removed and the cells are washed.[46]

When the glycerol solution has been added, the cells are frozen and stored at −65°C or below in a suitable freezer or in liquid nitrogen with a gas phase temperature below −120°C.[8] In order to be transfused, the cells must be thawed and deglycerolized. One of the initial drawbacks of the high-glycerol

method was that the procedure of thawing and removing the glycerol had many practical limitations. A simpler method of processing these cells for transfusion was developed by Meryman and Hornblower.[46] Their method requires only two cycles of centrifugation, washing with saline, and resuspension with isotonic saline containing glucose.

The remaining product contains few white cells or platelets, and 99.9% of the plasma is removed by the extensive washing during processing.[47] More than 90% of the donor's red blood cells are recovered.[48] The 24-hour post-transfusion survival has been shown to be 85% to 90%.[49]

Post-transfusion survival and oxygen carrying capacity of red blood cells are impacted by the amount of time spent between donation, refrigeration, and freezing.[42] Frozen cells have been shown to maintain prefreezing ATP and 2,3-DPG levels. The standard is to freeze within 6 days of collection, before these factors become significantly depleted. When it is necessary to freeze older units, rejuvenation with a solution containing pyruvate, glucose, phosphate, and adenine can be used.[50]

The major advantage of frozen red blood cells is that rare blood types, such as (Oh) Bombay, can be stored. Patients with rare phenotypes may make autologous donations that can be frozen for later use. Cells from autologous donors can also be frozen if more units are required than can be collected in the maximum 42-day liquid storage period or if surgery is postponed.

For patients who become alloimmunized to multiple clinically significant red blood cell antigens, frozen red blood cells from donors with rare phenotypes are useful. Among these patients are multiple transfused patients with sickle cell anemia who have multiple alloantibodies. African-Americans frequently lack antigens found on most donor red blood cells from whites. During blood drives targeting the African-American community for the benefit of such patients, it is helpful to phenotype these red blood cells and freeze the more uncommon types.

Because 99.9% of plasma is removed in processing frozen red blood cells, patients who may have adverse events related to plasma components may also benefit from the use of frozen red blood cells. For example, immunoglobulin A (IgA)-deficient patients with anti-IgA antibodies may suffer anaphylactoid reactions when exposed to donor plasma. In the past, patients who had multiple febrile nonhemolytic transfusion reactions that persisted despite removal of the buffy coat and treatment with medications also benefited from the more complete removal of cytokine-laden plasma and the leukoreduction that thawed frozen red blood cells offered. Newer leukocyte reduction techniques have largely replaced this indication. Because of the high cost and cumbersome nature of freeze-thaw procedures, other more routine uses of frozen red blood cells are difficult to justify. If a simpler means of preparation of frozen blood were available that avoided the limitations of the open systems now employed, more widespread use could be envisioned.

Cytomegalovirus-Seronegative Red Blood Cell Concentrates

Cytomegalovirus (CMV) is a double-stranded DNA herpesvirus (human herpesvirus 5) that can be transmitted by transfusion. Forty percent to 100% of adults are seropositive for CMV, depending on socioeconomic status and geographic region.[51] Persistent and latent infection can result, as well as reactivation and reinfection. The first report of transfusion-transmitted CMV described a syndrome seen in patients 3 to 8 weeks after cardiopulmonary bypass. The syndrome consisted of fever, lymphocytosis, and splenomegaly.[52] A congenital syndrome including petechiae, hepatosplenomegaly, jaundice, and microcephaly has also been identified. Postnatal infection in children can cause hepatitis. In immunocompromised adults, infection with CMV can result in interstitial pneumonitis, hepatitis, encephalitis, gastroenteritis, thrombocytopenia, or leukopenia; in certain patients receiving transplants, these conditions are associated with a high fatality rate. In immunocompetent adults, fever and hepatitis may result, but most patients have an asymptomatic mononucleosis.[51]

Transfusion-transmitted CMV is of concern in immunocompromised patients. CMV-seronegative blood is often requested for CMV-negative bone marrow transplant candidates or recipients, in utero transfusions, low-birth-weight premature infants of CMV-negative mothers, CMV-negative pregnant women, and rare cases of human immunodeficiency virus–positive, CMV-negative patients. CMV-negative recipients of solid organ transplants from CMV-negative donors are among the patients who may benefit but in whom the risk of using blood products not tested for CMV is not well established.[48]

CMV is known to be carried by lymphocytes. The sites of latency are thought to include CD34-positive progenitor cells and CD13- and CD14-positive monocytes.[51] Thus, transfusion-transmitted disease can be mitigated by removal of leukocytes in the pRBCs. A study published in 1995 compared bedside leukoreduction and CMV-seronegative blood products in bone marrow transplant recipients and suggested that filtration is an effective alternative to CMV-seronegative blood for the prevention of transfusion-transmitted CMV. A follow-up of 142 bone marrow transplant recipients found that in 62 CMV-seronegative recipients of bone marrow from CMV-seronegative donors, supported with the use of leukocyte-reduced blood products, there was no documented CMV infection.[53] The American Association of Blood Banks (AABB) has suggested that both approaches, leukocyte reduction and the use of CMV-seronegative blood, are equivalent in the prevention of CMV transmission.[54]

Leukocyte-Reduced Red Blood Cell Concentrates

Leukocyte-reduced red blood cells are defined by the AABB as having less than 5×10^8 leukocytes in the final component. Leukocyte-reduced red blood cells have a leukocyte count of less than 5×10^6.[8] Early techniques of leukocyte reduction involved centrifugation, washing with saline, and removal of the buffy coat. A second-generation technique known as the spin-cool-filter method was introduced in the 1980s.[55] This method requires use of 1-week-old red blood cells, which are centrifuged and then cooled for 4 hours to enhance microaggregate formation before passage through a microaggregate filter. Currently, filtration can be performed at the bedside or in the laboratory with attachable filters that reduce leukocytes more than 99.9% with less than 10% depletion of red blood cells.[56]

Leukocyte-reduced red blood cells are indicated primarily in the setting of repeated febrile nonhemolytic transfusion reactions. It was previously thought that these reactions were mediated by antibodies to foreign leukocyte antigens.[57] There is now increasing evidence that cytokines produced by the leukocytes during storage also cause these reactions.[58, 59] Prestorage leukocyte reduction may therefore be helpful in preventing such reactions.

A second indication for leukocyte-reduced red blood cells is the prevention of sensitization to human leukocyte antigens (HLAs) in bone marrow transplant recipients and other patients who require frequent platelet transfusion. The Trial to Reduce Alloimmunization to Platelets (TRAP) study[60] demonstrated a reduction in alloimmunization in acute myelogenous leukemia patients who received leukocyte-reduced blood components. Platelet refractoriness, although low in the control group (16%), was reduced among patients receiving leukocyte-reduced products (7%).

Leukocyte-reduced red blood cells may have another indication. The transfusion of allogeneic blood is thought by many scientists to be immunosuppressive, an effect termed transfusion-related immune modulation (TRIM). Several studies appear to document this effect, but some controversy remains. A correlation between pretransplantation allogeneic red blood cell transfusions and improved renal allograft survival has been known for many years.[61, 62] Initial reports appeared before the availability of cyclosporine and other improvements in immunosuppression that made this phenomenon less clinically relevant. However, a subsequent study including patients receiving modern immunosuppressive regimens demonstrated that recipients of three unmodified allogeneic red blood cell transfusions had 90% 1-year and 79% 5-year graft survivals, compared with 82% and 70% 1- and 5-year survivals, respectively, for patients who received no transfusion, which suggests continued importance.[63]

Perioperative allogeneic red blood cell transfusion may also have an adverse effect on tumor recurrence.[64–66] The data on this effect are more controversial; Blajchman[67] observed that approximately 50% of the nonrandomized studies indicate an adverse effect of transfusion on tumor recurrence. Patients with colorectal cancer who received perioperative transfusions were shown to have longer hospital stays than those who did not receive transfusion,[68] but the effect in this study was attributed to a higher incidence of postoperative infection. In surgical patients, perioperative transfusion may also predispose to bacterial infection. There appears to be a dose-response relationship between transfusion and the probability of infection; transfusion is the best predictor of infection, over such factors as extent of trauma, degree of blood loss, and presence of wound contamination,[69] although confounding factors have not been eliminated in many studies.

The mechanism for these effects may be related to the transfusion of contaminating white blood cells. The donor white blood cells could cause a downregulation of cellular immunity, mediated by secretion of T-helper 2 cytokines and inhibitors (interleukin-4, interleukin-10, and transforming growth factor β), with resultant inhibition of the T-helper 1 response.[70] The potential benefit of leukocyte reduction appears to be supported by reports that patients having colorectal surgery who received leukocyte-reduced red blood cell transfusions had fewer infections and shorter hospital stays than those who received unmodified red blood cells.[70] Animal studies also appear to support this theory. In rabbits inoculated with VX-2 tumor cells, those that received unmodified allogeneic red blood cell transfusions had significantly more pulmonary metastases than those that received 99.8% leukocyte-reduced blood.[71]

An editorial concerning TRIM stated that "prestorage WBC reduction is an intervention that is virtually risk-free and that, except for its cost, has no down side . . . the decision to implement universal prestorage WBC reduction need not be delayed until further evidence of efficacy becomes available."[72] The suggestion that leukocyte-reduced red blood cells decrease the unwanted immunosuppressive effects of transfusion may be further proof that conversion to a leukocyte-reduced blood supply enhances patients' safety.

Washed pRBCs

Washed red blood cells are prepared with isotonic saline by either manual or automated methods. Automation is more efficient, resulting in loss of fewer red blood cells with each wash cycle. Because washing takes place in an open system, the product must be used within 24 hours.

Washing red blood cells removes plasma proteins, some leukocytes, and remaining platelets. This product is indicated for patients who have suffered recurrent severe allergic transfusion reactions that are not prevented by antihistamines. Recipient IgE antibodies to donor plasma proteins mediate these reactions. Washed red blood cells are also indicated for IgA-deficient patients who have formed anti-IgA antibodies. In these patients, transfusion of blood products containing plasma with IgA can result in anaphylaxis.[73]

In patients with paroxysmal nocturnal hemoglobinuria (PNH), a rare disorder in which red blood cells are unusually sensitive to complement lysis, transfusion of washed red blood cells has been advocated to prevent hemolysis. However, a report by Brecher and Taswell[74] on 23 patients with PNH seen over 38 years appears to show that this is a needless practice.[74] A total of 431 red blood cell products (94 whole blood, 208 pRBCs, 80 leukocyte-reduced red blood cells, 38 washed red blood cells, 5 frozen red blood cells, and 6 intraoperatively salvaged units) were transfused with only one episode of hemolysis after transfusion. This single event was associated with transfusion of group O whole blood to a group AB individual. Although the need for washed red blood cells in PNH is questionable, this disorder is rare and changing established transfusion protocols may not be justified.

Irradiated pRBCs

Red blood cells are commonly irradiated using a cesium 137 source. A dose of 2500 cGy must be delivered to each unit, and quality control standards have been published to ensure that this dose is achieved with blood bank irradiators.[75] After irradiation, storage time is decreased to a maximum of 28 days[8] because of shortened red blood cell survival and increased potassium leakage.

The purpose of irradiation of cellular blood products in transfusion medicine is to inactivate immunocompetent lymphocytes. Irradiated red blood cells are indicated for the prevention of transfusion-associated graft-versus-host disease in immunocompromised patients, a frequently fatal complication. Neonates, patients with hematologic malignancies, patients with aplastic anemia, bone marrow transplant recipients, and patients with congenital immune deficiency are susceptible to transfusion-associated graft-versus-host disease; irradiated cellular blood products are indicated for these patients.[76] Graft-versus-host disease is also a potential hazard of directed donation from first-degree relatives who share

HLA haplotypes.[77] See Chapter 36 for additional information regarding this phenomenon.

REFERENCES

1. Landsteiner K: Ueber Agglutinationserscheinungen normalen menschlichen Blutes. Wein Klin Wochenschr 1901;14:1132.
2. Loutit JF, Mollison PL: Advantages of a disodium-citrate-glucose mixture as a blood preservative. Br Med J 1943;2:744.
3. Schmidt PJ: Charles Drew, a legend in our time. Transfusion 1997;37:234.
4. Goodnough L, Brecher M, Kanter M, AuBuchon J: Transfusion medicine. N Engl J Med 1999;340:438.
5. Walter C, Murphy W: A closed gravity technique for the preservation of whole blood in ACD solution utilizing plastic equipment. Surg Gynecol Obstet 1952;94:687.
6. Vengelen-Tyler V (ed): Technical Manual, 13th ed. Bethesda, Md, American Association of Blood Banks, 1999.
7. Baldini M, Costea N, Dameschek W: The viability of stored human platelets. Blood 1960;16:1969.
8. Klein HG (ed): Standards for Blood Banks and Transfusion Services, 20th ed. Bethesda, Md, American Association of Blood Banks, 2000.
9. Knutson F, Rider J, Franck V, et al: A new apheresis procedure for the preparation of high-quality red cells and plasma. Transfusion 1999;39:565.
10. Holme S, Elfath M, Whitley P: Evaluation of in vivo and in vitro quality of apheresis-collected RBC stored for 42 days. Vox Sang 1998;75:212.
11. Shi P, Ness P: Two-unit red cell apheresis and its potential advantages over traditional whole-blood donation. Transfusion 1999;39:218.
12. Lavee J, Martinowitz U, Mohr R, et al: The effect of transfusion of fresh whole blood versus platelet concentrates after cardiac operations. J Thorac Cardiovasc Surg 1989;97:204.
13. Golan M, Modan M, Lavee J, et al: Transfusion of fresh whole blood stored (4 C) for short period fails to improve platelet aggregation of extracellular matrix and clinical hemostasis after cardiopulmonary bypass. J Thorac Cardiovasc Surg 1990;99:354.
14. Schmidt P: Whole blood transfusion. Transfusion 1984;24:368.
15. Leslie SD, Toy P: Laboratory hemostatic abnormalities in massively transfused patients given red blood cells and crystalloid. Am J Clin Pathol 1991;96:770.
16. National Institute of Health Consensus Conference: Fresh frozen plasma: indications and rules. Transfus Med Rev 1987;1:201.
17. Boral L, Henry JB: Clinical Diagnosis and Management by Laboratory Methods, 19th ed. Philadelphia, WB Saunders, 1996, p 802.
18. Loutit JF, Mollison PL: Advantages of a disodium-citrate-glucose mixture as a blood preservative. Br Med J 1943;2:744.
19. Rous P, Turner JR: The preservation of living red blood cells in vitro. J Exp Med 1916;23:219.
20. Howland W, Bellville J, Zucker M, et al: Massive blood replacement: failure to observe citrate intoxication. Surg Gynecol Obstet 1957;105:529.
21. Moore GL, Peck CC, Sohmer PR, Zuck TF: Some properties of blood stored in anticoagulant CPDA-1 solution. Transfusion 1981;21:135.
22. Rapoport S: Dimensional, osmotic and clinical changes of erythrocytes in stored blood. I: Blood preserved in sodium citrate, neutral and acid citrate-glucose (ACD) mixtures. J Clin Invest 1947;26:591.
23. Nakao K, Wada T, Kamiyama T, et al: A direct relationship between adenosine triphosphate level and in vivo viability of erythrocytes. Nature 1962;194:877.
24. Hogman C: Preparation and preservation of red cells. Vox Sang 1998;74(Suppl 2):177.
25. Harken A: The surgical significance of the oxyhemoglobin dissociation curve. Surg Gynecol Obstet 1977;144:935.
26. Beutler E: What is the clinical importance of alterations of the hemoglobin oxygen affinity in preserved blood—especially as produced by variations of red cell 2,3-DPG content? Vox Sang 1978;34:113.
27. Mollison PL, Engelfriet CP, Contreras M: Blood Transfusion in Clinical Medicine, 10th ed. Boston, Blackwell Scientific Publications, 1997, p 249.
28. Hogman CF. Additive system approach in blood transfusion: birth of the SAG and Sagman systems. Vox Sang 1986;51:337.

29. Heaton A, Miripol J, Aster R, et al: Use of Adsol preservation solution for prolonged storage of low viscosity AS-1 red blood cells. Br J Haematol 1984;57:467.

30. Greenwalt TJ, McGuinness CG, Dumaswala UJ, Carter HW: Studies in red blood cell preservation. 3. A phosphate-ammonium-adenine additive solution. Vox Sang 1990;58:94.

31. Greenwalt TJ, Dumaswala UJ, Dhingra N, et al: Studies in red blood cell preservation. 7. In vivo and in vitro studies with a modified phosphate-ammonium additive solution. Vox Sang 1993;65:87.

32. Brecher ME, Zylstra-Halling VW, Pineda AA: Rejuvenation of erythrocytes preserved with AS-1 and AS-3. Am J Clin Pathol 1991;96:767.

33. Latham J, Bove J, Weirich F: Chemical and hematologic changes in stored CPDA-1 blood. Transfusion 1982;22:158.

34. Jaeger R, Rubin R: Contamination of blood stored in plastic packs. Lancet 1970;29:151.

35. Kluwe W, Haseman J, Douglas J, Huff J: The carcinogenicity of dietary di-(2-ethylhexyl)phthalate (DEHP) in Fischer 344 rats and B6C3F1 mice. J Toxicol Environ Health 1982;10:797.

36. Schulz CO, Rubin RJ, Hutchins GM: Acute lung toxicity and sudden death in rats following the intravenous administration of the plasticizer, di-(2-ethylhexyl)phthalate, solubilised with Tween surfactants. Toxicol Appl Pharmacol 1975;33:514.

37. Gray T, Butterworth K: Testicular atrophy produced by phthalate esters. Arch Toxicol Suppl 1980;4:425.

38. Bennet SH, Creelhoed GW, Aaron RK, et al: Pulmonary injury resulting from perfusion with stored bank blood in the baboon and dog. J Surg Res 1972;13:295.

39. Rubin RJ, Ness PM: What price progress? An update on vinyl plastic blood bags. Transfusion 1989;29:358.

40. Horowitz B, Stryker M, Waldman A, et al: Stabilization of red blood cells by the plasticizer, diethylhexylphthalate. Vox Sang 1985;48:150.

41. Hogman CF, Eriksson L, Ericson A, Reppucci AJ: Storage of saline-adenine-glucose-mannitol—suspended red cells in a new plastic container: polyvinylchloride plasticized with butyryl-n-trihexyl-citrate. Transfusion 1991;31:26.

42. Huggins C: Preparation and usefulness of frozen blood. Ann Rev Med 1985;36:499.

43. Meryman HT, Hornblower M: Freezing and deglycerolizing sickle-trait red blood cells. Transfusion 1976;16:627.

44. Boral L, Henry JB: Clinical Diagnosis and Management by Laboratory Methods, 19th ed. Philadelphia, WB Saunders, 1996, p 803.

45. Akerblom O, Hogman CF: Frozen blood: a method for low-glycerol, liquid nitrogen freezing allowing different postthaw deglycerolization procedures. Transfusion 1974;14:16.

46. Meryman HT, Hornblower M: A simplified procedure for deglycerolizing red blood cells frozen in a high glycerol concentration. Transfusion 1977;17:438.

47. Contreras TJ, Valeri CR: A comparison of methods to wash liquid-stored red blood cells and red blood cells frozen with high or low concentration of glycerol. Transfusion 1976;16:339.

48. Sayers M: Transfusion-transmitted viral infections other than hepatitis and human immunodeficiency virus infection: cytomegalovirus, Epstein-Barr virus, human herpes virus 6 and human parvovirus B19. Arch Pathol Lab Med 1994;118:346.

49. Valeri CR: Factors influencing the 24 hour post-transfusion survival and oxygen transport function of previously frozen red cells preserved with 40% glycerol and frozen at −80 C. Transfusion 1974;14:1.

50. Valeri CR, Zaroulis CG: Rejuvenation and freezing of outdated stored human red cells. N Engl J Med 1972;287:1307.

51. Pamphilon DH, Rider JR, Barbara JAJ, Williamson LM: Prevention of transfusion-transmitted cytomegalovirus infection. Transfus Med 1999;9:115.

52. Kreel I, Zarroff LI, Canter JW: A syndrome following total body perfusion. Surg Gynecol Obstet 1960;111:317.

53. Pamphilon DH, Foot ABM, Adeodu A, et al: Prophylaxis and prevention of CMV infection in bone marrow allograft recipients: leucodepleted platelets are equivalent to those from CMV seronegative donors. Bone Marrow Transplant 1999;23(Suppl 1):S66.

54. American Association of Blood Banks: Leukocyte Reduction for the Prevention of Transfusion-Transmitted Cytomegalovirus (AABB Association Bulletin 97-2, 10–12). Bethesda, Md, American Association of Blood Banks Press, 1997.

55. Meryman HT, Hornblower M: The preparation of red cells depleted of leukocytes. Review and evaluation. Transfusion 1986;26:101.

56. Dzik WH: Leukoreduced blood components: laboratory and clinical aspects. In Rossi EC, Simon TL, Moss GS, Gould SA (eds): Principles of Transfusion Medicine. Baltimore, Williams & Wilkins, 1995, p 353.

57. Payne R: Leukocyte agglutinins in human sera. Arch Intern Med 1957;99:587.

58. Davenport RD, Kunkel SL: Cytokine roles in hemolytic and non-hemolytic transfusion reactions. Transfus Med Rev 1994;7:157.

59. Heddle NM, Kelton JG: Febrile non-hemolytic transfusion reactions. In Popovsky MA (ed): Transfusion Reactions. Bethesda, Md, AABB Press, 1996, p 45.

60. The Trial to Reduce Alloimmunization to Platelets Study Group: leukocyte reduction and ultraviolet B irradiation of platelets to prevent alloimmunization and refractoriness to platelet transfusions. N Engl J Med 1997;337:1861.

61. Opelz G, Sengar DP, Mickey MR, et al: Effect of blood transfusions on subsequent kidney transplants. Transplant Proc 1973;5:253.

62. Blajchman MA, Singal DP: Renal transplantation: the role of red blood cell antigens, histocompatibility antigens and blood transfusions on renal allograft survival. Transfus Med Rev 1989;3:171.

63. Opelz G, Vanrentergehm Y, Kirste G, et al: Prospective evaluation of pre-transplant blood transfusion in cadaver kidney recipients. Transplantation 1997;63:964.

64. Schriemer PA, Longnecker DE, Mintz PD: The possible immunosuppressive effects of perioperative blood transfusion in cancer patients. Anesthesiology 1988;68:422.

65. Van Aken WG: Does perioperative blood transfusion promote tumor growth? Transfus Med Rev 1989;3:243.

66. Heiss MM, Jauch KW, Delanoff C, et al: Blood transfusion modulated tumor recurrence—a randomized study of autologous versus homologous blood transfusion in colorectal cancer. J Clin Oncol 1994;12:1859.

67. Blajchman MA: Immunomodulatory effects of allogeneic blood transfusions: clinical manifestations and mechanisms. Vox Sang 1998;74(Suppl 2):315.

68. Vamvakas EC, Carven JH: Allogeneic blood transfusion, hospital charges, and length of hospitalization: a study of 487 consecutive patients undergoing colorectal cancer resection. Arch Pathol Lab Med 1998;122:145.

69. Blumberg N, Heal J. Transfusion immunomodulation. In Anderson KC, Ness PM (eds): Scientific Basis of Transfusion Medicine, 2nd ed. Philadelphia, WB Saunders, 2000, p 430.

70. Blumberg N, Heal JM: Blood transfusion immunomodulation: the silent epidemic. Arch Pathol Lab Med 1998;122:117.

71. Blajchman MA, Bardossy L, Carmen R, et al: Allogeneic blood transfusion—induced enhancement of tumor growth: two animal models showing amelioration by leukocyte reduction and passive transfer using spleen cells. Blood 1993;81:1880.

72. Blajchman MA: Transfusion-associated immunomodulation and universal white cell reduction: are we putting the cart before the horse? Transfusion 1999;39:665.

73. Vyas GN, Holmdahl L, Perkins HA, Fudenberg HH: Serologic specificity of human anti-IgA and its significance in transfusion. Blood 1969;34:573.

74. Brecher ME, Taswell HF: Paroxysmal nocturnal hemoglobinuria and the transfusion of washed red cells. A myth revisited. Transfusion 1989;29:681.

75. Moroff G, Leitman SF, Luban NLC: Principles of blood irradiation, dose validation, and quality control. Transfusion 1997;37:1084.

76. Leitman SF, Holland PV: Irradiation of blood products. Indications and guidelines. Transfusion 1985;25:293.

77. Thaler M, Shamiss A, Orgad S, et al: The role of blood from HLA-homozygous donors in fatal transfusion associated graft versus host disease after open heart surgery. N Engl J Med 1989;321:25.

Chapter 14

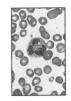

Fresh Frozen Plasma and Related Products

Silvana Z. Bucur
Christopher D. Hillyer

Component therapy has had a profound impact on the practice of transfusion medicine. The extraction of various constituents (e.g., red blood cells, platelets, granulocytes, plasma) from whole blood has led to increased efficacy and economic utilization of the blood supply. When only the component that is needed is transfused, the patient is spared untoward effects of other blood components. Plasma contains a variety of organic and inorganic elements with therapeutic value. The isolation and purification of some of these plasma constituents [e.g., cryoprecipitate, factor VIII (FVIII) concentrate, albumin, immunoglobulins] have limited the use of plasma in clinical practice. Its use is now reserved for conditions requiring therapy with multiple constituents or for which the specific component is not commercially available.

■ Physiologic Role of Plasma

Plasma is the aqueous component of blood in which cellular elements and macromolecules are transported throughout the body and other constituents are maintained in a dynamic equilibrium with the extravascular compartment. The composition of plasma is influenced by gender, age, race, diet, and other individual and environmental characteristics.[1, 2] The major component of plasma is water, which constitutes approximately 85% to 90% of the plasma volume. The solute component constitutes 0.3 mol/L, of which about 30% is made up of proteins, with colloids, crystalloids, clotting factors, hormones, vitamins, and trace elements making up the rest. Normal human plasma has a density of 1.055 to 1.063 g/mL and a pH that varies between 7.33 and 7.43 with respective temperature changes between 37 and 4°C.[3]

Although human plasma contains a multitude of substances including ionic and nonionic solutes, the practice of transfusion medicine has exploited plasma mainly for its protein content. It is estimated that human plasma contains over 700 different proteins with various physiologic characteristics and functions. Although some 120 proteins have been isolated, only a few are available for clinical use. The most abundant plasma protein is albumin, with a concentration between 3500 and 5000 mg/dL. It is responsible for maintaining colloid oncotic pressure and serves as a major transport protein for endogenous and exogenous substances. Plasma proteins with immunological functions include the immunoglobulin (Ig) family, of which IgG (5 to 14 mg/dL) is the most abundant, and the complement components, of which C3 (1.2 mg/dL) predominates quantitatively. In addition, plasma proteins include those involved in maintaining normal rheological properties of blood (e.g., coagulation and fibrinolytic proteins).[4-6]

■ Plasma Quality and Processing

Plasma can be obtained through centrifugation of whole blood, single-donor plasmapheresis, or as a by-product of cytapheresis (e.g., platelet or red blood cell). One unit of plasma is defined as the amount of plasma obtained from centrifugation of one unit of whole blood, and it usually contains 180 to 300 mL. When plasma is obtained through single-donor plasmapheresis, the amount may be two to three times greater than that obtained from whole blood processing (500 to 800 mL).

The rapidity with which plasma is collected and stored determines its quality and subsequent use.[7] Thus, several plasma products are available at various centers. Single-donor plasmapheresis can produce *source plasma* (or single-donor plasma) when it is stored at −20°C at variable times from its collection, and when stored frozen within 6 hours of its collection (at −18°C or colder) it is called *fresh frozen plasma (FFP)*. Centrifugation or sedimentation of whole blood can produce *recovered plasma*, which is obtained from a whole-blood donor; *liquid plasma*, when collected and stored refrigerated within 5 days of the expiration date of whole blood; and FFP when processed under the conditions just described. Cryo-poor plasma or cryosupernatant is the plasma product remaining after the cryoprecipitate fraction is extracted from FFP through cold precipitation.

Both source plasma and recovered plasma may be used in the manufacture of various plasma derivatives. Source plasma can also be administered as component therapy; recovered plasma, because of the less stringent conditions of collection, processing, and storage, does not meet the standards for coagulation factor concentrations and therefore is not used as component therapy. Liquid plasma is no longer used in the United States, and only FFP, source plasma, cryosupernatant, and virally inactivated plasma are approved by the U.S. Food and Drug Administration (FDA) for clinical use.

FDA-approved, virally inactivated plasma is pooled plasma subjected to a solvent-detergent process and is termed *solvent-detergent plasma* (SD plasma). This method is highly efficient in inactivating viruses using a combination of organic solvent, tri(*n*-butyl)phosphate (TNBP), and a nonionic detergent, Triton X-100. The SD method is virucidal against lipid-enveloped viruses, including human immunodeficiency virus (HIV) types 1 and 2, hepatitis viruses (HBV, HCV, HGV), human T-cell leukemia/lymphoma virus (HTLV) types I and II, vesicular stomatitis virus, Sindbis virus, and Sendai virus, but does not inactivate parvovirus or hepatitis A virus. The SD plasma is pooled from approximately 2500 donors, which results in a standard unit of 200 mL of SD plasma with a coagulation factor profile similar to that of FFP.[8–12]

■ Clinical Considerations

In clinical practice, FFP has been used as an exogenous source of proteins, specifically albumins, immunoglobulins, coagulation factors, and certain protease inhibitors. With the development of the fractionation method of Cohn and colleagues[13] and the consequent capability to administer individual plasma components, the use of FFP has been reserved for situations in which it is necessary to replace either multiple plasma constituents (e.g., multiple factor deficiency) or a plasma constituent not yet isolated (e.g., thrombotic thrombocytopenic purpura [TTP]). Indications and contraindications are listed in Table 14.1.

The Use of FFP in the Management of Coagulopathies

Patients with a known underlying coagulopathy as ascertained by an increase in the prothrombin time (PT > 16 seconds) or partial thromboplastin time (PTT > 55 seconds) exceeding 1.5 to 1.8 times the control value have an increased risk for clinically significant bleeding. In these patients, administration of FFP has decreased the risk of bleeding and reduced or stopped active bleeding. Although FFP contains all coagulation factors at normal plasma concentrations, it must be recognized that its administration in physiologically tolerable quantities results in only a 20% to 30% increase in the levels of coagulation factors.

Coagulopathy of Liver Dysfunction

The liver is essential in maintaining normal hemostasis. First, as the principal site of protein synthesis, it supplies the

Table 14.1 Fresh Frozen Plasma: Indications and Contraindications

Indications
Coagulopathies
Liver disease[25–30]
Acute hepatocellular injury
Chronic hepatic dysfunction
Hepatic surgery
Congenital factor deficiency*[31–33]
Warfarin-induced[35,38]
Dilution-induced[45–47]
Disseminated intravascular coagulopathy[48,49]
Replacement of other factor(s)
Plasma infusion or exchange[58–63] (TTP, HUS, HELLP)
C1-esterase inhibitor deficiency*[67,68]
Fluid replacement in TPE[69] (Refsum disease, frequent TPE, coagulopathy)

Contraindications
Volume expansion
Immunoglobulin replacement
Nutritional support
Reconstitution of pRBCs
Wound healing

*When factor concentrates are not available.
HELLP, hemolysis, elevated liver enzymes, and low platelets; HUS, hemolytic-uremic syndrome; pRBC, packed red blood cell; TPE, therapeutic plasma exchange; TTP, thrombotic thrombocytopenic purpura.

majority of proteins involved in the coagulation and fibrinolytic pathways and their regulators (except FVIII, von Willebrand factor [vWF], tissue plasminogen activator, and plasminogen activator inhibitor). Second, a process important in the normal function of certain coagulation proteins (e.g., prothrombin; FVII, FIX, and FX; proteins C and S), namely vitamin K–dependent γ-carboxylation of glutamic acid residues, takes place in the liver. Third, the hepatic reticulum endothelial system is also involved in the clearance of activated coagulation factors, activation complexes, and fibrin and fibrinogen degradation by-products. Therefore, the coagulopathy associated with hepatocellular injury has a complex pathogenesis including ineffective protein synthesis, consumption of coagulation factors and inhibitors, and impaired clearance of activated coagulation complexes.[14–16] In addition, end-stage liver disease is associated with a variable degree of thrombocytopenia secondary to hypersplenism[17] and a multifactorial thrombocytopathy.[18]

Impairment of hemostasis may also be encountered in hepatic surgery, including partial hepatic resection, orthotopic liver transplantation (OLT), and peritoneovenous or LeVeen shunt placement. The coagulation disorder most frequently observed in these situations is acute and chronic disseminated intravascular coagulopathy (DIC) with a predominant fibrinolytic component.[19, 20] The coagulopathy associated with OLT is usually more severe because of the underlying coagulopathy predating the transplantation, the profound hyperfibrinolysis characterizing the post-transplantation anhepatic phase, and the coagulopathy induced by massive transfusion during surgery.[21–24]

It is well recognized that patients manifesting coagulopathy associated with liver disease or hepatic surgery are at increased risk for bleeding, especially during invasive procedures (e.g., liver biopsy, paracentesis). Therefore, FFP, either alone or in conjunction with other products (e.g., platelets, prothrombin complex, or antithrombin III concentrate), has been used to control active bleeding and to decrease the risk of bleeding complications during invasive procedures.[25–28] The efficacy of FFP in these situations is assessed clinically because laboratory evidence such as normalization of PT or PTT or improvement of the thromboelastogram may be lacking with the administration of usual quantities of FFP.[25, 29, 30]

Congenital Coagulation Factor Deficiency

The introduction of specific coagulation factor concentrates has limited the use of FFP. Currently, FFP is indicated for patients with rare familial isolated factor deficiencies (e.g., FV and FXI deficiency) for which there is no commercially available factor concentrate.[31, 32] In combined FV-FVIII deficiency, FFP is the only source of FV and either FFP infusions or therapeutic plasma exchange (TPE) with FFP has been used to treat bleeding episodes. Congenital combined vitamin K–dependent factor deficiency can be treated with prothrombin complex concentrates, FFP, or occasionally high doses of vitamin K.[33] Dosages and schedules of FFP administration for congenital factor deficiencies and possible alternatives are listed in Table 14.2.

Warfarin-Induced Coagulopathy

Vitamin K is a cofactor in the γ-carboxylation of the terminal glutamic acid residues of certain coagulation (e.g., factors II, VII, IX, and X) and regulatory (e.g., protein C and S) proteins. This post-translational modification of the coagulation proteins is essential for their binding to phospholipid surfaces through calcium and the subsequent formation of activation complexes.[34] By interfering with the recovery of the active form of vitamin K, warfarin or 4-hydroxycoumarin blocks the γ-carboxylation of these coagulation proteins, rendering them inactive. Complete reversal of warfarin-induced coagulopathy occurs within 48 hours after discontinuation of the oral anticoagulant, within 12 to 18 hours after vitamin K administration, and immediately after the administration of FFP.[35] Although a single FFP infusion at a dose of 15 to 20 mL/kg

is sufficient to normalize hemostasis rapidly, it should be recognized that the incidence of spontaneous nonfatal hemorrhage in patients receiving oral anticoagulants with an International Normalized Ratio between 2.0 and 3.0 is approximately 0.7% per month.[36, 37] Therefore, FFP should be utilized in such situations involving trauma, emergent surgical procedures, or active bleeding.[38]

Dilutional Coagulopathy

The replacement of one blood volume in 24 hours with packed red blood cells (pRBCs) and crystalloid or colloid solutions is defined as massive transfusion.[39] Leslie and Toy[40] found that massively transfused patients manifest a profound hemostatic disorder as demonstrated by prolonged PT and PTT to twice control values and thrombocytopenia below $50 \times 10^6/\mu L$, which are only in part due to hemodilution.[41, 42] Although the number of units transfused, the degree of PT or PTT prolongation, and bleeding tendency are poorly correlated,[43, 44] Ciavarella and colleagues[41] reported that increases in PT or PTT greater than 1.5 to 1.8 times control values are associated with decreases in some coagulation factors (e.g., fibrinogen, FV, FVIII) to below minimum hemostatic levels. Therefore, the preceding laboratory changes, when associated with clinically significant coagulopathy, should be treated with FFP. In general, FFP should be considered when more than 50% of the blood volume has been replaced and mandatory when more than 120% to 150% of the blood volume has been replaced with pRBCs or colloid solutions, or both, within a 24-hour period. In addition, platelets should be maintained above $50 \times 10^6/\mu L$ with transfusion of platelet concentrates, and other blood products (e.g., cryoprecipitate, specific factor concentrates) may be considered for replacement of coagulation factors when the volume of FFP becomes excessive.[45–47]

Disseminated Intravascular Coagulopathy

Acute DIC is clinically characterized by a combination of diffuse microvascular hemorrhage and thrombosis. Abnormal activation of the coagulation cascade and thrombin

Table 14.2 Uses of FFP in Congenital Factor Deficiencies

Deficient Factor	Half-life (hr)	FFP Dose	Hemostatic Plasma Level	Alternative Therapy
Prothrombin (FII)	72	15–20 mL/kg, followed by 3–6 mL/kg q 12–24 hr	>30%	PE with FFP Prothrombin complex concentrates*
Factor V (FV)	36	15–20 mL/kg, followed by 3–6 mL/kg q 12–24 hr	>24%	FFP infusions or TPE with FFP
Factor VII (FVII)	3–6			Prothrombin complex concentrates* FVII concentrates[†]
Major bleed		15–20 mL/kg followed by 3–6 mL/kg q 6–12 hr	15%–25%	
Mild bleed		5–12 mL/kg q 8–12 hr	5%–10%	
Factor X (FX)	40	15–20 mL/kg, followed by 3–6 mL/kg q 24 hr	10%–15%	Prothrombin complex*
Factor XI (FXI)	80	15–20 mL/kg, followed by 3–6 mL/kg q 12 hr	30%–40%	Cryosupernatant
Factor XIII (FXIII)	9 days	3–6 mL/kg q 4–6 wk	5%	Cryoprecipitate (1 U/10–20 kg q 3–4 wk) FXIII concentrate[†]

*Prothrombin complex concentrates contain variable amounts of FII, FVII, FIX, and FX.
[†]Concentrates available only in Europe.
FFP, fresh frozen plasma; FII, factor II; TPE, therapeutic plasma exchange.

generation leads to the consumption of procoagulant factors and platelets. Hyperfibrinolysis secondary to widespread fibrin deposition further exaggerates the coagulation factor consumption. A wide variety of disorders may lead to DIC, including sepsis, liver disease, trauma, obstetrical complications, leukemia, metastatic malignancy, hypotension, and hypoperfusion.[48]

Because of the heterogeneous group of disorders that can trigger DIC, the gamut of clinical manifestations, and the lack of controlled clinical studies, the management of DIC is somewhat controversial. Therapy should be individualized and directed concomitantly at the underlying disorder and the predominant clinical manifestation (e.g., hemorrhagic versus thrombotic diathesis). Component therapy, with platelet concentrates, FFP, or cryoprecipitate, should be considered in patients with prolonged PT and PTT and active bleeding or undergoing an invasive procedure. FFP should be administered at a dose of 10 to 15 mL/kg and its effect assessed clinically and with PT-PTT measurements every 6 hours. In patients with end-stage liver disease and DIC, FFP infusions may not correct PT-PTT abnormalities and clinical responses may vary. Antifibrinolytic agents (e.g., ε-aminocaproic acid or tranexamic acid) in combination with heparin may be useful in patients with active bleeding who do not respond to coagulation factor replacement with FFP or cryoprecipitate and heparin infusions.[48, 49] In clinical situations in which the thrombotic diathesis predominates (e.g., purpura fulminans), a trial of intravenous heparin with antithrombin III (AT-III) replacement may be appropriate.[50] Initial studies have demonstrated some benefit for the use of activated protein C concentrates in patients with purpura fulminans[51] and those with DIC associated with meningococcemia,[52] although further studies are needed to confirm these results.

■ The Use of FFP as Replacement of Other Factors

Thrombotic Thrombocytopenic Purpura

Acquired or nonfamilial TTP is a clinical entity characterized by microangiopathic hemolytic anemia, thrombocytopenia, fever, and varying degrees of renal and neurological dysfunction. Although the pathogenesis of this disorder is not completely understood, there is ample evidence that endothelial cell injury is of central importance in promoting the abnormal interaction between platelets and vessel wall. In plasma of normal individuals, ultralarge von Willebrand factor (ULvWF) released by vascular endothelial cells mediates platelet aggregation under conditions of high shear stress and is modified by a specific cleaving protease, which reduces the size of the multimer. It is proposed that in patients with TTP, the damaged endothelium may release excessive amounts of ULvWF, which surpass the processing capacity of the metalloprotease, or the presence of a quantitative or qualitative abnormality or neutralizing antibodies (usually IgG) to the metalloprotease may render it ineffective.[53–57]

Thus, infusion of FFP would replace the deficient or defective metalloprotease, and TPE with FFP or cryosupernatant would remove much of the IgG metalloprotease inhibitor and simultaneously provide functional metalloprotease. Current standard therapy for TTP is TPE with FFP as replacement fluid.[58–60] Approximately 50% of patients do not respond to TPE with FFP, and in these recurrent or refractory TTP cases

the use of cryosupernatant lacking ULvWF multimers has been effective.[59–65] A few patients with TTP have responded to simple infusions of FFP.[60, 62, 63]

The standard therapy for TTP is daily exchanges with FFP or cryosupernatant replacing 1.0 to 1.5 plasma volumes. The total number of TPEs is dependent on the clinical response, and the daily schedule is continued until the serum lactic acid dehydrogenase is normal and the platelet count is above $100 \times 10^6/\mu L$ and continues to rise without the aid of TPE. A twice-daily (every 12 hours) schedule of TPE may be used in cases in which the patient's status is deteriorating despite an adequate daily regimen. The average number of TPEs necessary to achieve remission is approximately 10 procedures, and more than 90% of patients have achieved a clinical remission within 3 weeks of initiation of TPE.

C1-Esterase Inhibitor Deficiency

Deficiency of C1-esterase inhibitor, an important regulator of the complement system, is inherited in an autosomal dominant manner. Clinical manifestations of hereditary angioedema include swelling of the subcutaneous tissue and mucosa of the aerodigestive tract leading to acute respiratory distress.[66] Replacement therapy with FFP infusions has been used during acute episodes of respiratory distress and before surgical interventions. C1-esterase inhibitor concentrates are available in Europe and will eventually replace the use of FFP in this rare condition.[67, 68]

Fluid Replacement in TPE

In general, the volume of replacement fluids used in TPE is equal to the plasma volume removed, and for most situations colloid or crystalloid solutions, or both, are acceptable fluid replacement. In addition to clinical conditions in which plasma is specifically indicated (e.g., TTP, Refsum disease), there are a few situations in which the use of FFP with TPE is preferred. Plasma exchange with FFP is indicated in all patients with significant underlying coagulopathy, including DIC, liver disease, and circulating anticoagulant, as well as patients with iatrogenic coagulopathy, as observed in patients undergoing multiple TPEs within a short interval of time.[69]

Investigational Uses of FFP

Coagulation factor replacement through the use of FFP, either as simple infusions or with plasma exchange, has been explored in fulminant meningococcemia,[70, 71] in acute renal failure in the context of multiorgan failure,[72] and in the syndrome of hemolysis, elevated liver enzymes, and low platelets (HELLP).[73]

■ Authors' Approach to the Use of FFP

Although FFP is readily available for use in clinical practice, it must be recognized that its administration is not without risk. Although FFP contains albumin, coagulation proteins, immunoglobulins, and nutrients, there is no justification for its use in situations in which alternative therapy is safer and more efficacious. Therefore, crystalloid or fractionated albumin solution is preferred to FFP for volume expansion in hypovolemic shock. In conditions involving a specific coagulation factor deficiency, including hemophilia A, replacement therapy with specific coagulation factor concentrates or recombinant proteins (e.g., FVIII) is recommended. Prophylactic replacement therapy with immunoglobulin fraction and the use of approved parenteral solutions to enhance the nutritional status of debilitated patients are also currently recommended alternatives to FFP. The efficacy of FFP in other clinical situations should be determined through clinical trials.

The volume and schedule of FFP administration depend on the clinical situation for which it is intended and the patient's volume tolerance. The most common indication for the use of FFP is as a coagulation factor replacement, and the desired hemostatic level as determined by the specific coagulation factor level, PT or PTT, or clinical assessment should guide the dose, frequency, and duration of administration. It should also be noted that FFP requires 20 to 30 minutes to thaw and subsequently the labile coagulation factors (FV, FVIII) decrease gradually (adequate for 24 hours after thawing). Therapy should be coordinated with the blood bank, especially when multiple FFP infusions are anticipated (e.g, supportive therapy in massive transfusion, during OLT). FFP contains isohemagglutinins, and therefore an ABO-compatible product should be administered. AB plasma may be used in cases in which the recipient's blood group is not known at the time of administration. Compatibility testing is not routinely performed.

For the use of FFP in mild to moderate coagulopathies (e.g., liver disease, DIC), it is recommended that a usual dose of 10 to 15 mL/kg be infused as rapidly as tolerated by the patient. The calculated dose in milliliters is used to determine approximately the whole number of units of FFP, knowing that a unit of FFP is 180 to 300 mL and a unit of SD plasma is 200 mL. The frequency and duration of FFP therapy depend primarily on the clinical response.

In massive transfusion or during OLT, communication with the blood bank is essential to reserve sufficient quantities of FFP and ensure timely administration. In general, when more than 10 units of pRBCs have been transfused and abnormal hemostasis is observed, infusion of 4 units of FFP is recommended. To maintain coagulation factors above a critical hemostatic level, 4 units of FFP should be infused for every 6 units of pRBCs transfused thereafter. If the desired hemostasis is not achieved with this regimen, additional products may be considered, including cryoprecipitate, AT-III concentrate, or prothrombin concentrate.

■ Alternatives

Many factor concentrates, including FVIII, prothrombin complex concentrate, activated FIX complex, activated FVII, and AT-III, have been made available for clinical use, and a few others are at the investigational stage (e.g., C1-esterase inhibitor), Thus, the use of FFP is limited to situations in which no specific therapeutic alternative exists. FFP is no longer used for mild hemophilia A or vWD. Vitamin K should be considered for clinically stable patients with warfarin-induced coagulopathy.

■ Potential Adverse Reactions

Although FFP is considered an infrequent cause of major adverse reactions, the complexity of plasma proteins, the heterogeneity of its immunoglobulin content, and factors related to its processing and storage have the potential to

Table 14.3   Potential Adverse Reactions to FFP

Immunologically mediated
    Alloimmunization: Rh1(D), other RBC antigens
    Allergic reactions: IgA deficiency
    Transfusion-related acute lung injury (TRALI): leukoagglutinins
    Reaginic antibodies to exogenous antigens
    Alloantibodies to platelets
    Immunomodulation/immunosuppression
    Transfusion-associated graft-versus-host disease (TA-GVHD)

Related to plasma contaminants
    Donor specific: medications, infectious
    Processing/storage specific: cytokines, anaphylatoxins, plasticizers, preservatives

Related to infectious contaminants
    Bacterial contaminants
    Viral contaminants
        Leukocyte-associated: CMV, HTLV I/II
        Non–leukocyte-associated: HIV,HBV,HCV,HAV,EBV, HHV-8,prions

Related to physiochemical characteristics
    Volume overload
    Hypothermia

CMV, cytomegalovirus; EBV, Epstein-Barr virus; HAV, hepatitis A virus; HBV, hepatitis B virus; HHV, human herpes virus; HIV, human immunodeficiency virus; HTLV, human T-cell lymphotropic virus; RBC, red blood cell.

cause a wide range of reactions with various pathophysiological mechanisms (Table 14.3). Allergic reactions of variable degree, ranging from mild urticarial reactions to anaphylaxis and cardiopulmonary arrest, may be observed with FFP infusions. These reactions may be related to the immunological differences between donor and recipient or to the processing and storage of plasma.

Patients with IgA deficiency who have anti-IgA antibodies (usually IgE) are at high risk for acute and potentially fatal allergic reactions when exposed to FFP containing IgA. Patients known to be IgA deficient should receive IgA-deficient plasma available through the national registry.[74] High titers of an alloantibody in the donor plasma may induce a variety of clinical syndromes, depending on the specificity of the antibodies. When plasma contains reaginic antibodies to foreign antigens, an allergic-type reaction may ensue. Conversion to a positive direct antiglobulin test or even hemolysis can occur when plasma contains antibodies directed against red blood cells (e.g., ABO isoantibodies). Transfusion-related acute lung injury occurs when the donor plasma contains antibodies that react with recipient leukocytes (e.g., leukoagglutinins).[75–77]

Less often, febrile allergic reactions may be due to undesirable contaminants in the donor plasma. The risk of exposure to donor-specific contaminants such as infective agents and medications has been reduced considerably by careful donor screening. Febrile nonhemolytic reactions may also be related to the quality of plasma after processing, including activation of proteolytic enzymes (e.g, kinins), generation of cytokines (e.g., interleukins-1, -6, and -8 and tumor necrosis factor) and anaphylatoxins (e.g., C3a, C5a), and the presence of preservatives and plasticizers.[78–81]

■ Leukocyte-Associated Adverse Reactions

FFP has long been considered an acellular blood product with an infinitesimally small risk of leukocyte-associated complications, including transmission of cell-associated infections, alloimmunization, immunosuppression, or transfusion-associated graft-versus-host disease (TA-GVHD) in immunocompromised individuals. Several reports have documented the presence of leukocytes in FFP,[82–84] which has led to questions regarding their clinical relevance as well as the need for further processing (e.g., leukoreduction, irradiation) of FFP to reduce the risks of leukocyte-associated complications. Leukocytes have also been implicated in cytokine generation, which is responsible for febrile nonhemolytic transfusion reactions and lung injury.

Willis and colleagues[84] demonstrated that the number of leukocytes in FFP spanned a three-logarithm range depending on the method of preparation, with 43% of units obtained by the hard-spin method and 45.7% of units produced by the second-spin method containing more than 5×10^6 leukocytes. These values are higher than the American Association of Blood Banks cutoff standard ($<5 \times 10^6$ per red blood cell unit)[85] and far above the European cutoff standard ($<1 \times 10^6$ per red blood cell unit)[86] for residual donor leukocytes in the final leukoreduced product. It had been assumed that the freezing process renders FFP practically devoid of viable leukocytes.[76] Wieding[82] and Bernvil[83] and their associates demonstrated that viable lymphocytes were present, raising concern about possible adverse immunomodulation (e.g, TA-GVHD) in certain individuals at risk and the potential benefit of using irradiated FFP. Although the viability of leukocytes may be important in the pathophysiological mechanism of some adverse reactions, their destruction may release cytokines that are implicated in the pathophysiological mechanism of febrile nonhemolytic reactions.

Thus, FFP produced by certain methods may contain enough leukocytes to be categorized as a cellular blood product and justify the use of a leukoreduction filter. The use of prestorage leukodepletion filters decreases the overall leukocyte burden (viable and nonviable) in the blood component and decreases the concentration of cytokines and anaphylatoxins. Leukodepleted FFP may be indicated for certain individuals at risk for these complications, including immunosuppressed individuals and patients requiring massive transfusions.[81]

■ Infectious Potential

Although leukocytes have been shown to be present in FFP, transmission of cell-associated viruses including cytomegalovirus (CMV) and human lymphocytotropic viruses (HTLV-I and -II) has been associated with cellular blood components and not FFP. In addition to the use of donor questionnaires and serologic surrogate markers, the introduction of SD plasma, which efficiently inactivates lipid-encapsulated viruses including HBV, HCV, HGV, HTLV, and HIV, has eliminated a great majority of transfusion-transmitted pathogens. Nonetheless, nonenveloped viruses, including parvovirus B19 and hepatitis A virus, still pose concerns regarding the safety of SD plasma, especially in immunodeficient individuals, pregnant women, and patients with chronic hemolytic anemias. Although SD plasma is a pooled product and may contain parvovirus B19 and hepatitis A virus, it also contains neutralizing antibody to these viruses, which may modify the risk of infectivity or its clinical significance. Furthermore, SD plasma is screened for these viruses by

polymerase chain reaction and lots with high viral loads are eliminated.[87, 88] Another potential for transmission of infectious agents stems from the possibility of newly emerging pathogens in the donor pool, the presence of prions, or contamination during processing with agents not susceptible to inactivation by the SD process.[8–12]

REFERENCES

1. Lettellier G, Desjarlais F: Study of seasonal variations for eighteen biochemical parameters over a four-year period. Clin Biochem 1982;15:206.
2. Siest G: Human chemistry. In Siest G (ed): Reference Values in Human Chemistry: Effects, Analytical and Individual Variation, Food Intake, Drugs and Toxics—Applications in Preventive Medicine. Basel, Karger, 1973, p 134.
3. Gregersen MI, Rawson RA: Blood volume. Physiol Rev 1959;39:307.
4. Doweiko JP, Nompleggi DJ: Role of albumin in human physiology and pathophysiology. JPEN 1991;15:207.
5. Sorensen RU, Polmar SH: Immunoglobulin replacement therapy. Ann Clin Res 1987;19:293.
6. Alper CA: Inherited deficiencies of complement components in man. Immunol Lett 1987;14:175.
7. Myllyla G: Factors determining quality of plasma. Vox Sang 1998;74:507.
8. Horowitz B, Bonomo R, Prince AM, et al: Solvent/detergent-treated plasma: a virus-inactivated substitute for fresh frozen plasma. Blood 1992;79:826.
9. Prince AM, Horowitz B, Brotman B, et al: Inactivation of hepatitis B and Hutchinson strain non-A, non-B hepatitis viruses by exposing to Tween 80 and ether. Vox Sang 1984;46:36.
10. Prince AM, Horowitz B, Brotman B, et al: Sterilization of hepatitis and HTLV-III viruses by exposure to tri(n-butyl)phosphate and sodium cholate. Lancet 1986;1:706.
11. Horowitz B, Wiebe ME, Lippin A, Stryker MH: Inactivation of viruses in labile blood derivatives. Disruption of lipid-enveloped viruses by tri(n-butyl)phosphate detergent combinations. Transfusion 1985;25:516.
12. Pehta JC: Clinical studies with solvent detergent–treated products. Transfus Med Rev 1996;10:303.
13. Cohn EJ, Gurd FRN, Surgenor DM, et al: A system for the separation of the components of human blood. Qualitative procedures for the separation of protein components of human plasma. J Am Chem Soc 1950;72:465.
14. Deutsch E: Blood coagulation disorder in liver diseases. Prog Liver Dis 1965;2:69.
15. Lechner K, Nissner H, Thaler E: Coagulation abnormalities in liver disease. Semin Thromb Hemost 1977;4:40.
16. Roberts HR, Cederbaum AI: The liver and blood coagulation: physiology and pathology. Gastroenterology 1972;63:279.
17. Aster RH: Pooling of platelets in the spleen: role in the pathogenesis of "hypersplenic" thrombocytopenia. J Clin Invest 1966;45:645.
18. Laffi G, Cominelli F, Ruggiero M, et al: Altered platelet function in cirrhosis of the liver: impairment of inositol lipid and arachidonic acid metabolism in response to agonists. Hepatology 1988;8:1620.
19. Harmon DC, Demirjian Z, Ellman L, et al: Disseminated intravascular coagulation in the peritoneovenous shunt. Ann Intern Med 1979;90:774.
20. Ro JS: Hemostatic problems in liver surgery. Scand J Gastroenterol 1973;8:71.
21. Bohmig HJ: The coagulation disorder of orthotopic hepatic transplantation. Semin Thromb Hemost 1977;4:57.
22. Lewis JH, Bontempo FA, Awad SA, et al: Liver transplantation: intraoperative changes in coagulation factors in 100 first transplants. Hepatology 1989;9:710.
23. Porte RJ, Bontempo FA, Knot EA, et al: Systemic effects of tissue plasminogen activator—associated fibrinolysis and its relation to thrombin generation in orthotopic liver transplantation. Transplantation 1989;47:978.
24. Ritter DM, Owen CA Jr, Bowie EJ, et al: Evaluation of preoperative hematology-coagulation screening in liver transplantation. Mayo Clin Proc 1989;64:216.
25. McVay PA, Toy PTCY: Lack of increased bleeding after paracentesis and thoracocentesis in patients with mild coagulation abnormalities. Transfusion 1991;21:164.

26. Shanberge JN, Quattrochiocchi-Longe T: Analysis of fresh frozen plasma administration with suggestions for ways to reduce usage. Transfus Med 1992;2:189.
27. Stahl RL, Duncan A, Hooks MA, et al: A hypercoagulable state follows orthoptic liver transplantation. Hepatology 1990;12:553.
28. McNicol PL, Liu G, Harley ID, et al: Blood loss and transfusion requirements in liver transplantation: experience with the first 75 cases using thromboelastography. Anaesth Intensive Care 1994;22:666.
29. Spector I, Corn M, Ticktin HE: Effect of plasma transfusion on the prothrombin time and clotting factors in liver disease. N Engl J Med 1966;275:1032.
30. Clayton DG, Miro AM, Kramer DJ, et al: Quantification of thromboelastographic changes after blood component transfusion in patients with liver disease in the intensive care unit. Anesth Analg 1995;81:272.
31. Seeler RA: Para hemophilia. Factor V deficiency. Med Clin North Am 1972;56:119.
32. Sharland M, Palton MA, Talbot S, et al: Coagulation factor deficiencies and abnormal bleeding in Noonan's syndrome. Lancet 1992;339:19.
33. Soff GA, Levin J: Familial multiple coagulation factor deficiencies. I. Review of the literature: differentiation of single hereditary disorders associated with multiple factor deficiencies from coincidental concurrence of single factor deficiency states. Semin Thromb Hemost 1981;7:112.
34. Nakao A, Suzuki Y, Isshiki K, et al: Clinical evaluation of plasma abnormal prothrombin (des-gamma-carboxy prothrombin) in hepatobiliary malignancies and other diseases. Am J Gastroenterol 1991;86:62.
35. Shearer MJ, Barkhan P: Vitamin K1 and therapy of massive warfarin overdose. Lancet 1979;1:266.
36. Hull RD, Raskob GE, Rosenbloom D, et al: Heparin for 5 days as compared with 10 days in the initial treatment of proximal venous thrombosis. N Engl J Med 1990;322:1260.
37. Research Committee of the British Thoracic Society: Optimum duration of anticoagulation for deep-vein thrombosis and pulmonary embolism. Lancet 1992;340:873.
38. Development Task Force of the College of American Pathologists: Practice parameters for the use of fresh-frozen plasma, cryoprecipitate and platelets. JAMA 1994;271:777.
39. Sawyer PR, Harrison CR: Massive transfusion: a current review. Obstet Gynecol Surv 1991;46:289.
40. Leslie SD, Toy PT: Laboratory hemostatic abnormalities in massively transfused patients given red blood cells and crystalloid. Am J Clin Pathol 1991;96:770.
41. Ciavarella D, Reed RL, Counts RM, et al: Clotting factor levels and the risk of diffuse microvascular bleeding in the massively transfused patient. Br J Haematol 1987;67:365.
42. Hewson JR, Neame PB, Kumar N, et al: Coagulopathy related to dilution and hypotension during massive transfusion. Crit Care Med 1985;13:387.
43. Collins JA: Problems associated with the massive transfusion of stored blood. Surgery 1974;75:274.
44. Murray DJ, Olson J, Strauss R, et al: Coagulation changes during packed red cell replacement of major blood loss. Anesthesiology 1988;69:839.
45. Lundsgaard-Hansen P: Treatment of acute blood loss. Vox Sang 1992;63:241.
46. Hiippala ST, Myllyla GJ, Vahtera EM: Hemostatic factors and replacement of major blood loss with plasma-poor red cell concentrates. Anesth Analg 1995;81:360.
47. Strauss RG: Clinical perspective of platelet transfusions: defining the optimal dose. J Clin Apheresis 1995;10:124.
48. Bick RL: Disseminated intravascular coagulation. Hematol Oncol Clin North Am 1992;6:1259.
49. Rubin RN, Colman RW: Disseminated intravascular coagulation. Approach to treatment. Drugs 1992;44:963.
50. Vinazzer H: Therapeutic uses of antithrombin III in shock and disseminated intravascular coagulation. Semin Thromb Hemost 1989;15:347.
51. Dreyfus M, Masterson M, David M, et al: Replacement therapy with monoclonal antibody purified protein C concentrate in newborns with severe congenital protein C deficiency. Semin Thromb Hemost 1995;21:371.
52. Rintala E, Seppala OP, Kotilainen P, et al: Protein C in the treatment of coagulopathy of meningococcal disease [letter]. Lancet 1996;347:1767.
53. Ridolfi RL, Bell WR: Thrombotic thrombocytopenic purpura: report of 25 cases and a review of the literature. Medicine (Baltimore) 1981;60:413.
54. Moake JL, Turner NA, Stathopoulos NA, et al: Involvement of large plasma von Willebrand factor (vWF) multimers and unusually large vWF forms derived from endothelial cells in shear stress–induced platelet aggregation. J Clin Invest 1986;78:1456.
55. Furlan M, Robles R, Lammle B: Partial purification and characterization of a protease from human plasma cleaving von Willebrand factor to fragments produced by in vivo proteolysis. Blood 1996;87:4223.
56. Furlan M, Robles R, Solenthaler M, et al: Deficient activity of von Willebrand factor–cleaving protease in chronic relapsing thrombotic thrombocytopenic purpura. Blood 1996;89:3097.
57. Tsai HM, Lian ECY: Antibodies to von Willebrand factor–cleaving protease in acute thrombotic thrombocytopenic purpura. N Engl J Med 1998;339:1585.
58. Ruggenenti P, Remuzzi G: The pathophysiology and management of thrombotic thrombocytopenic purpura. Eur J Haematol 1996;56:191.
59. Kwaan HC, Soff GA: Management of thrombotic thrombocytopenic purpura and hemolytic uremic syndrome. Semin Hematol 1997;34:159.
60. Rock GA, Shumak KH, Buskard NA, et al and the Canadian Apheresis Study Group: Comparison of plasma exchange with plasma infusion in the treatment of thrombotic thrombocytopenic purpura. N Engl J Med 1991;325:393.
61. Rock GA, Shumak KH, Sutton DMC, et al and the members of the Canadian Apheresis Group: Cryosupernatant as replacement fluid for plasma exchange in thrombotic thrombocytopenic purpura. Br J Haematol 1996;94:383.
62. Moschcowitz E: An acute febrile pleiochromic anemia and hyaline thrombosis of the terminal arterioles and capillaries: an undescribed disease. Thromb & Haemost. 1978;40:4.
63. Ruggenenti P, Galbusera M, Cornejo RP, et al: Thrombotic thrombocytopenic purpura: evidence that infusion rather than removal of plasma induces remission of the disease. Am J Kidney Dis 1993;21:314.
64. Obrador GT, Ziegler ZR, Shadduck RK, et al: Effectiveness of cryosupernatant therapy in refractory and chronic relapsing thrombotic thrombocytopenic purpura. Am J Hematol 1993;42:217.
65. Onundarson PT, Rowe JM, Heal JM, et al: Response to plasma exchange and splenectomy in thrombotic thrombocytopenic purpura. Arch Intern Med 1992;152:791.
66. Agostoni A, Cicardi M: Hereditary and acquired C1-inhibitor: biological and clinical characteristics in 235 patients. Medicine (Baltimore) 1992;71:206.
67. Fritsch S, Waytes TA, Kunschak M: Recovery and half-life of C1-inhibitor in prevention and treatment of acute attacks in hereditary angioedema. Thromb Haemost 1993;69:873.
68. Laxenaire MC, Audibert G, Janot C: Use of purified C1-esterase inhibitor in patients with hereditary angioedema. Anesthesiology 1990;72:956.
69. Leitman SF, Kucera E, McLeod B, et al: Guidelines for Therapeutic Hemapheresis. Bethesda, Md, American Association of Blood Banks, 1992.
70. Churchwell KB, McManus ML, Kent P, et al: Intensive blood and plasma exchange for treatment of coagulopathy in meningococcemia. J Clin Apheresis 1995;10:171.
71. Busund R, Straume B, Revhaug A: Fatal course in severe meningococcemia: clinical predictors and effect of transfusion therapy. Crit Care Med 1993;21:1699.
72. Stegmayr BG, Jakobson S, Rydvall A, et al: Plasma exchange in patients with acute renal failure in the course of multiorgan failure. Int J Artif Organs 1995;18:45.
73. Martin JN, Files JC, Blake PG, et al: Postpartum plasma exchange for atypical preeclampsia-eclampsia as HELLP (hemolysis, elevated liver enzymes, and low platelets) syndrome. Am J Obstet Gynecol 1995;172:1107.
74. Pineda A, Taswell HF: Transfusion reactions associated with anti-IgA antibodies: report of four cases and review of the literature. Transfusion 1985;15:10.
75. Isbister JP, Fisher M: Adverse effects of plasma volume expanders. Anaesth Intensive Care 1980;8:145.
76. Isbister JP: Adverse reactions to plasma and plasma components. Anaesth Intensive Care 1993;21:31.
77. Popovsky MA, Moore SB: Mechanism of transfusion-related acute lung injury. Blood 1991;77:2299.

78. Sack G, Snyder EL: Cytokine generation in stored platelet concentrates. Transfusion 1994;34:20.
79. Sonntag J, Stiller B, Walka MM, et al: Anaphylatoxins in fresh-frozen plasma. Transfusion 1997;37:798.
80. Myhre BA: Toxicological quandary of the use of bis (2-diethylhexyl) phthalate (DEHP) as plasticizer for blood bags. Ann Clin Lab Sci 1988;18:131.
81. Nielsen HJ, Reimert C, Pedersen AN, et al: Leukocyte-derived bioactive substances in fresh frozen plasma. Br J Anaesth 1997;78:548.
82. Wieding JU, Vehmeyer K, Dittman J, et al: Contamination of fresh-frozen plasma with viable white cells and proliferative stem cells [letter]. Transfusion 1994;34:185.
83. Bernvill SS, Abdulatiff M, al-Sedairy S, et al: Fresh frozen plasma contains viable progenitor cells—should we irradiate? [Letter] Vox Sang 1994;67:405.
84. Willis JI, Lown JAG, Simpson MC, et al: White cells in fresh-frozen plasma: evaluation of a new white cell–reduction filter. Transfusion 1998;38:645.
85. Menitove JE (ed): Standards for Blood Banks and Transfusion Services, 19th ed. Bethesda, Md, American Association of Blood Banks, 1999; p 69.
86. British Committee on Standards in Haematology: Guidelines on the clinical use of leukocyte-depleted blood components. Transfus Med 1998;8:59.
87. McOmish F, Yap PL, Simonds P, et al: Detection of hepatitis A virus (HAV) in coagulation factor concentrates using the polymerase chain reaction. Thromb Haemost 1993;69:939.
88. McOmish F, Yap PL, Jorda A, et al: Detection of parvovirus B19 in donated blood: a model system for screening by polymerase chain reaction. J Clin Microbiol 1993;31:323.

Chapter 15

Cryoprecipitate and Related Products

Silvana Z. Bucur
Christopher D. Hillyer

Until the mid-1960s, hemostatic abnormalities were treated with infusions of normal human plasma in quantities sufficient to replete the deficient factors, specifically factors VIII and IX. Because these factors are contained in fresh plasma or fresh frozen plasma (FFP) at normal plasma levels and are not concentrated, the amount of plasma required to overcome some hemostatic defects was, at times, excessive. Specifically, the need for a concentrated form of factor VIII led Pool and Shannon[1] to describe a method through which factor VIII could be extracted from FFP and concentrated, now commonly known as *cryoprecipitate*, also known as cryoprecipitate antihemophilic factor. More recently, the development of purified concentrates and recombinant forms of various coagulation factors redefined the indications for use of cryoprecipitate.

Plasma Quality and Processing

To obtain a plasma derivative of acceptable quality, certain conditions must be observed: a high quality of the initial plasma (e.g., the concentration of the coagulation proteins), the rapidity of processing, and standardized conditions and duration of storage. Functional integrity of the coagulation proteins is essential to the optimal quality of cryoprecipitate. Therefore FFP, which is plasma frozen at −18°C within 6 to 8 hours of its collection, is the only acceptable plasma source. Cryoprecipitate made from FFP through the method of cold precipitation, which allows the formation of precipitate as FFP, begins to thaw at 1°C to 6°C. The cryoprecipitate thus formed is collected in individual, sterile bags, is resuspended in 5 to 10 mL (up to 20 mL in "wet cryo") of plasma, and is refrozen within 1 hour of extraction. When cryoprecipitate is stored at −18°C, the stability of the coagulation factors it contains is maintained for up to 1 year. Quality assurance

assays are performed to determine appropriate factor VIII activity (≥80 U) and fibrinogen (≥150 mg) content.[2-4]

Preparations and Mode of Administration

Cryoprecipitate is the plasma-derived product that contains the highest concentration of fibrinogen (150 to 250 mg). In addition, cryoprecipitate contains 80 to 120 U of factor VIII, 30 to 60 mg of fibronectin, and a variable percentage of the original plasma concentration of von Willebrand factor (vWF) (40% to 70%, or 80 U of vWF) and factor XIII (30% or 40 to 60 U). Before its administration, cryoprecipitate is thawed in a water bath at 30°C to 37°C for approximately 5 to 10 minutes, and several bags are pooled to a single container. Because of the need to preserve the activity of the coagulation proteins, once thawed, cryoprecipitate cannot be refrozen and may be kept at temperatures of 20°C to 24°C for no longer than 6 hours. To ensure sterility of the product, cryoprecipitate must be transfused within 4 hours if it is pooled.

Cryoprecipitate may also be used as a source of fibrinogen that can be added to a thrombin to form a *fibrin glue* or *sealant*, as in the two-component fibrin glue or sealant (Tisseel) approved by the United States Food and Drug Administration. Fibrinogen is extracted from pooled human cryoprecipitate and is reconstituted in a fibrinolysis inhibitor solution containing bovine aprotinin and plasmin. Prothrombin is prepared from pooled human plasma and is activated just before use by the addition of calcium chloride. Using a water bath (37°C), the fibrinogen concentrate/fibrinolytic inhibitor component is mixed with the thrombin solution to form a fibrin clot, the adherent sealant, at the surgical surface. Both components of Tisseel are freeze dried and are heat treated.[5]

Table 15.1 Common Uses of Cryoprecipitate

Cryoprecipitate as source of fibrinogen
Congenital hypofibrinogenemia or afibrinogenemia[6-8]
Acquired hypofibrinogenemia[6,7,9,10]
Fibrin glue-sealant[36-50]
Orthotopic liver transplant[11]
Congenital factor XIII deficiency[26-28]
von Willebrand disease (unresponsive to desmopressin)[21,22]
Hyperfibrinogenolysis (after-streptokinase therapy)
Uremic bleeding[31-34]
Hemophilia A (only in the absence of factor VIII:C concentrate)

■ Clinical Considerations

Because cryoprecipitate contains the highest concentration of fibrinogen, factor XIII, and vWF, it is most often used in the treatment of hemorrhagic disorders resulting from quantitative or qualitative deficits of these factors. As factor concentrates and recombinant factors have become more readily available and affordable, the use of cryoprecipitate has declined. Table 15.1 lists clinical indications and common uses of cryoprecipitate.

Quantitative and Qualitative Fibrinogen Deficiency

The common coagulation pathway culminates in the formation of the fibrin clot through the action of thrombin on fibrinogen. Thus, congenital abnormalities in fibrinogen synthesis, either hypofibrinogenemia/afibrinogenemia or dysfibrinogenemia, may result in spontaneous or post-traumatic hemorrhage of variable degree. Various clinical entities including hepatocellular disease, disseminated intravascular coagulopathy, and L-asparaginase therapy may be associated with clinically significant hypofibrinogenemia or dysfibrinogenemia. Although fibrinogen levels lower than 100 mg/dL result in the prolongation of the prothrombin and activated partial thromboplastin time, correction of the fibrinogen deficit is required only during episodes of active bleeding or before surgical procedures.[6-8]

In a review, Humphries[9] reported that the most common use of cryoprecipitate as fibrinogen replacement is in acquired fibrinogen deficiency. The dose and frequency of administration depend on the rate of consumption or destruction of fibrinogen, and this can be assessed by monitoring the fibrinogen level. In the absence of active bleeding, 1 U of cryoprecipitate per 10 kg body weight increases the plasma fibrinogen concentration by 40 to 50 mg/dL. In certain coagulopathies, repletion of other coagulation proteins in addition to fibrinogen may necessitate the use of FFP.[10-16]

von Willebrand Disease

The complex adhesive glycoprotein vWF is synthesized by megakaryocytes and endothelial cells and circulates in plasma as multimers of various molecular weights (500 to 10,000 kD). vWF has two important hemostatic functions: (1) it mediates platelet adhesion to the subendothelium through its interaction with platelet glycoprotein Ib, and (2) it stabilizes factor VIII by complexing with it in circulation.[17,18] Therefore, quantitative or qualitative abnormalities in vWF will result in increased bleeding tendency. Desmopressin acetate [1-deamino (8-D-arginine) vasopressin] (DDAVP) enhances the

release of vWF from the endothelial cells and augments platelet activity. DDAVP is considered effective therapy in most types of von Willebrand disease. In approximately 10% to 20% of patients with von Willebrand disease, however, DDAVP is either ineffective (type 1 and 3) or contraindicated (type 2B and 2N), or the development of tachyphylaxis prevents its prolonged use. In these circumstances, cryoprecipitate can provide adequate replacement of both vWF and factor VIII:C to shorten the bleeding time and to control clinical bleeding.[19-22]

Although precautions are taken to ensure an effective and safe plasma product (e.g., screening of blood donors) a small but definite risk of viral transmission still remains. In an effort to minimize this risk, viral inactivation procedures have been applied to various plasma products, including cryoprecipitate. Some of these procedures have been shown to affect factor recovery. Keeling and colleagues[23] demonstrated that solvent-detergent–treated cryoprecipitate does not contain high-molecular-weight vWF multimers or acceptable levels of vWF activity to maintain its efficacy in the treatment of von Willebrand disease. However, lyophilized and pasteurized plasma concentrates (e.g., intermediate-purity and high-purity factor VIII concentrates) are rich in high-molecular-weight vWF and factor VIII. The latter have largely replaced cryoprecipitate in the treatment of von Willebrand disease.[24,25]

Factor XIII Deficiency

Through the dual action of thrombin, fibrinogen is converted into fibrin, and factor XIII is activated; this process facilitates the crosslinking of polymerized fibrin and α_2-antiplasmin to fibrin clots. In the neonatal period, deficiency of this hemostatic function (factor XIII deficiency) manifests as protracted umbilical stump bleeding, whereas later in life, postsurgical bleeding and delayed or abnormal (keloid) wound healing may be observed. Factor XIII has a long biologic half-life of approximately 9 days and is effective at relatively low levels (5%). Therefore, because these patients are at increased risk of intracerebral hemorrhage, prophylactic replacement therapy with either cryoprecipitate or factor XIII (currently available only in a research setting) is feasible.[26-28]

Uremic Coagulopathy

Many patients with uremia have evidence of abnormal primary hemostasis, as documented by a prolonged bleeding time and decreased platelet aggregation, findings suggesting an abnormal interaction between platelets and vascular endothelium.[29,30] Because vWF promotes normal interaction between platelets and subendothelium, the use of cryoprecipitate in uremic bleeding has been reported in a few small studies and case reports.[31-33] Janson and associates[31] described a significant reduction in bleeding time with improvement in uremic bleeding diathesis in a group of six patients. The beneficial effect of cryoprecipitate on uremic bleeding is transient and is observed in only up to 50% of patients.[34]

Fibrin Glue or Sealant

Although the potential of a mixture of exogenous thrombin and fibrinogen to enhance local surgical hemostasis and to provide effective tissue adherence has long been explored, only in 1998 has a commercial product (Tisseel) become available and approved by the Food and Drug Administration. The elastic property, tensile strength, and tissue adhesiveness of plasma fibrin glue or sealant has made it an important

Table 15.2 Clinical Indications for Plasma Fibrin Sealant (Tisseel)

Approved indications[5]
   As adjunct to hemostasis involving cardiopulmonary bypass surgery
   As adjunct in heparinized patients undergoing coronary artery
      bypass graft
   As adjunct to conventional surgical hemostatic techniques: suture,
      ligature, cautery
   As adjunct in the closure of colostomies
   In the control of bleeding associated with splenic injury

Investigational uses
   Thoracic surgery[45]
   Cardiovascular surgery[36–40]
   Gastrointestinal surgery[37]
   Traumatology[48]
   Orthopedic surgery[40]
   Urology[52]
   Neurosurgery[46,47]
   Ophthalmology[49]
   Otorhinolaryngology[50]
   Cosmetic surgery[41–44]
   As means of delivering drugs, hormones. and cytokines to a
      target site

adjunct in microsurgical technique. In the United States, Tisseel has been approved for use as an adjunct in conventional surgical hemostasis, cardiopulmonary bypass surgery, colostomy closure, and splenic injury repair (Table 15.2).[5] Several reviews have documented a wide variety of investigational uses of plasma fibrin sealants.[35–39] Although the approved uses of Tisseel are limited, experimental uses of various fibrin tissue adhesives or sealants are numerous and are still expanding. Fibrin sealants have been used to achieve hemostatic control in patients with preexisting coagulopathy.[35, 40] In cosmetic surgery, tissue fibrin adhesives have been used in lieu of sutures to reduce scar formation and in aiding skin graft fixation in burned patients.[41–44] In various microsurgical techniques, fibrin sealants have been used not only to achieve adequate hemostasis but also to attain a fluid or air barrier, to maintain tissue adhesiveness and as adjunct in bone and cartilage repair.[45–50] As an extemporaneous fibrin glue, infusion of cryoprecipitate with thrombin into the renal pelvis facilitated the removal of small renal stones.[51]

Other Uses

As a minimum-volume fibrinogen source, cryoprecipitate has been used to decrease bleeding during orthotopic liver transplantation and after thrombolytic (streptokinase) therapy. Although cryoprecipitate is approved for use in patients with hemophilia A with factor VIII levels of 5% or greater who are unresponsive to DDAVP (tachyphylaxis), the availability of virus-safe factor VIII products has made this indication essentially obsolete. In a small, controlled study, Steinbaum and Cucinell[52] demonstrated a beneficial effect of cryoprecipitate containing fibronectin on wound healing.

■ Our Approach to the Use of Cryoprecipitate

Cryoprecipitate contains no red blood cells and only a small amount of isohemagglutinins (e.g., anti-A, anti-B). Therefore, compatibility and Rh testing are not required before its use in adults. Approximately 20 to 30 minutes must be allowed for

thawing and pooling of cryoprecipitate units before administration. The dose of cryoprecipitate is based on the desired target level of the specific factor to be repleted.

In general, the dose of cryoprecipitate necessary to replete fibrinogen deficit may be estimated using an empiric dose of 1 U of cryoprecipitate per 5 kg body weight, or alternatively, it may be calculated using the following formula:

$$\text{Desired fibrinogen increment(g/L)} = (0.2 \times \text{number of units}$$
$$\text{of cryoprecipitate)/Plasma volume(L)}$$

The frequency and duration of administration depend on the underlying condition. In acquired hypofibrinogenemia (e.g., L-asparaginase therapy, disseminated intravascular coagulation), a daily prophylactic regimen may be suitable, whereas in conditions associated with hypofibrinogenemia and active bleeding, more frequent monitoring and replacement are recommended (e.g., every 8 to 12 hours). In congenital hypofibrinogenemia, fibrinogen replacement with cryoprecipitate is indicated only during episodes of active bleeding.

The quantity, quality, and activity of vWF in cryoprecipitate are variable. Therefore, the replacement dose of vWF is estimated. The usual recommendation is daily infusions of 1 U of cryoprecipitate per 10 kg body weight. Because factor XIII has a long half-life (9 days) and levels of less than 5% are hemostatic, the recommended replacement dose and the frequency of cryoprecipitate administration in congenital factor XIII deficiency are 1 U per 10 to 20 kg body weight every 2 to 3 weeks.

■ Alternatives

The need for targeted therapy and virus-safe products led to the development of recombinant factor technology and specific factor concentrates subjected to virucidal procedures. This development, in turn, has considerably decreased the use of cryoprecipitate. Thus, virally inactivated, pooled, plasma-based, or recombinant factor VIII concentrate has entirely replaced cryoprecipitate in treatment of mild hemophilia A.[53] In certain types of von Willebrand disease in which cryoprecipitate was the treatment of choice in the past, intermediate- and high-purity factor VIII concentrates are currently preferred, because of the low risk of transmission of blood-borne viruses with the latter products.[54] As technology expands and new factors become available for clinical use, the use of cryoprecipitate may be greatly reduced.

■ Potential Adverse Reactions

Cryoprecipitate administration may be associated with nonspecific side effects related to its protein, cytokine, and isohemagglutinin content. Adverse reactions include fever, chills, and allergic reactions of variable severity. Conversion to a positive direct antiglobulin test with minimal hemolysis may occur when the isohemagglutinin titer is high in the cryoprecipitate pool.

Untoward effects of tissue fibrin adhesives (Tisseel) have been related to the source of thrombin, especially of bovine origin. These include the development of allergic-type reactions, some as severe as anaphylaxis, and factor V antibodies, which may lead to abnormal prothrombin times and postsurgical bleeding.[55]

■ Infectious Potential

As with any blood-derived product, a risk of transmission of infectious diseases, specifically viruses, is present. The concern over the long-term consequences of infection with lipid-enveloped viruses, such as human immunodeficiency virus, hepatitis B, C, and G viruses, and human T-lymphocytotropic virus (HTLV I/II), has led to the development of virucidal techniques. Treatment of plasma with an organic solvent, tri(n-butyl)phosphate, in combination with a nonionic detergent, Triton X-100 (solvent-detergent procedure), efficiently inactivates the lipid-enveloped viruses mentioned earlier and does not affect efficacy.[56, 57] Although the solvent-detergent process is efficiently virucidal, Keeling and colleagues[58] demonstrated that it interferes with recovery of high-molecular-weight multimers and activity of vWF, with little effect on the fibrinogen content. Therefore, cryoprecipitate subjected to the solvent-detergent method of viral inactivation is acceptable only for the treatment of hypofibrinogenemia.

REFERENCES

1. Pool JG, Shannon AE: Production of high potency concentrates of antihemophilic globulin in a closed bag system; assay in vitro and in vivo. N Engl J Med 273:1443, 1965.
2. Myllyla G: Factors determining quality of plasma. Vox Sang 74:507, 1998.
3. Allersma DP, Imambaks RMR, Meerhof LJ: Effect of whole blood storage on factor VIII recovery in fresh frozen plasma and cryoprecipitate. Vox Sang 71:150, 1996.
4. Hughes C, Thomas KB, Schiff P, et al: Effect of delayed blood processing on the yield of factor VIII in cryoprecipitate and factor VIII concentrate. Transfusion 28:566, 1988.
5. Tissee VH Kit: Two-component fibrin sealant, vapor-heated, kit. Fibrin sealant package insert. Manufactured by Osterreichisches Institut für Haemoderivate GES, M.B.H., Subsidiary of Immuno AG. Distributed by Baxter Healthcare Corporation, Deerfield, IL, 1998
6. Galankis DK: Fibrinogen anomalies and disease: A clinical update. Hematol Oncol Clin North Am 6:1171, 1992.
7. Mammen EF: Fibrinogen abnormalities. Semin Thromb Hemost 9:1, 1983.
8. Forbes CD, Madhok R: Genetic disorders of blood coagulation: Clinical manifestation and management. In Ratnoff OD, Forbes CD (eds): Disorders of Hemostasis. Philadelphia, WB Saunders, 1991, p 141.
9. Humphries JE: Transfusion therapy in acquired coagulopathies. Transfus Med 8:1181, 1994.
10. Ness PM, Perkins HA: Cryoprecipitate as a reliable source of fibrinogen replacement. JAMA 241:1690, 1979.
11. Nusbacher J: Blood transfusion support in liver transplantation. Transfusion 5:207, 1991.
12. Colman RW, Robboy SJ, Minna JD: Disseminated intravascular coagulation: A reappraisal. Annu Rev Med 30:359, 1979.
13. Francis JL, Armstrong DJ: Acquired dysfibrinogenemia in liver disease. J Clin Pathol 35:667, 1982.
14. Gilabert J, Estelles A, Asnar J, et al: Abruptio placentae and disseminated intravascular coagulation. Acta Obstet Gynecol Scand 64:35, 1985.
15. Sutton DM, Hauser R, Kulapongs P, et al: Intravascular coagulation in abruptio placentae. Am J Obstet Gynecol 109:604, 1971.
16. Al-Mondhiry H, Ehmann WC: Congenital afibrinogenemia. Am J Hematol 46:343–347, 1994.
17. Fischer BE, Kramer G, Mitterer A, et al: Effect of multimerization of human and recombinant von Willebrand factor on platelet aggregation, binding to collagen and binding of coagulation factor VIII. Thromb Res 84:55, 1996.
18. Sadler JE, Matsushita T, Dong Z, et al: Molecular mechanism and classification of von Willebrand disease. Thromb Haemost 74:161, 1995.
19. Rodeghiero F, Castaman G, diBona E, et al: Consistency of responses to repeated DDAVP infusions in patients with von Willebrand's disease and hemophilia A. Blood 74:1997, 1989.
20. Lusher JM: Response to 1-deamino-8-arginine vasopressin in von Willebrand disease. Haemostasis 24:276, 1994.
21. Castaman G, Rodeghiero F: Current management of von Willebrand's disease: Practical therapeutics. Drugs 602:14, 1995.
22. Mannucci PM: Biochemical characteristics of therapeutic plasma concentrates used in the treatment of von Willebrand disease. Haemostasis 24:285, 1994.
23. Keeling DM, Luddington R, Allain J-P, et al: Cryoprecipitate prepared from plasma virally inactivated by the solvent detergent method. Br J Haematol 96:194, 1997.
24. Mannucci PM, Tenconi PM, Castaman G, et al: Comparison of four virus-inactivated plasma concentrates for treatment of severe von Willebrand disease: A cross-over randomized trial. Blood 79:3130, 1992.
25. Rodeghiero F, Castaman G, Meyer D, et al: Replacement therapy with virus-inactivated plasma concentrates in von Willebrand disease. Vox Sang 62:193, 1992.
26. Stirling D, Ludlam CA: Therapeutic concentrates for the treatment of congenital deficiencies of factors VII, XI, XIII. Semin Thromb Hemost 19:48, 1993.
27. Fear JD, Miloszewski KJA, Losowsky MS: The half life of factor XIII in the management of inherited deficiency. Thromb Haemost 49:102, 1983.
28. Rodeghiero F, Castaman GC, Di Bona E, et al: Successful pregnancy in a woman with congenital factor XIII deficiency treated with substitutive therapy. Blut 55:45, 1987.
29. Remuzzi G: Bleeding disorders in uremia: Pathophysiology and treatment. Adv Nephrol 18:171, 1989.
30. Andrassy K. Ritz E: Uremia as a cause of bleeding. Am J Nephrol 5:313, 1985.
31. Janson PA, Jubelirer SJ, Weinstein MJ, et al: Treatment of the bleeding tendency in uremia with cryoprecipitate. N Engl J Med 303:1318, 1980.
32. Maierhoter W, Adams MB, Kleinman JG, et al: Treatment of the bleeding tendency in uremia with cryoprecipitate [letter]. N Engl J Med 305:645, 1981.
33. Juhl A: DDAVP, cryoprecipitate, and highly "purified" factor VIII concentrate in uremia. Nephron 43:305, 1986.
34. Triulsi DJ, Blumberg N: Variability in response to cryoprecipitate treatment for hemostatic defects in uremia. Yale J Biol Med 63:1, 1990.
35. Martinowitz U, Schulman S: Fibrin sealant in surgery of patients with a hemorrhagic diathesis. Thromb Haemost 74:486, 1995.
36. Sierra DH: Fibrin sealant adhesive systems: A review of their chemistry, material properties and clinical applications. J Biomater Appl 7:309, 1993.
37. Spotnitz WD: Fibrin sealant in the United States: Clinical use at the University of Virginia. Thromb Haemost 74:482, 1995.
38. Martinowtz U, Spotnitz WD: Fibrin tissue adhesives. Thromb Haemost 78:661, 1997.
39. Radosevich M, Goubran HA, Burnouf T: Fibrin sealant: Scientific rationale, production methods, properties, and current clinical use. Vox Sang 72:133, 1997.
40. Matinowitz U, Schulman S, Horoszowski H, et al: Role of fibrin sealants in surgical procedures on patients with hemostatic disorders. Clin Orthop 328:65, 1996.
41. Saltz R, Dimick A, Harris C, et al: Application of autologous fibrin glue in burn wounds. J Burn Care Rehabil 10:504, 1989.
42. Saltz R, Guzman G: Aesthetic reconstruction of burned hands. Plast Surg 11:23, 1992.
43. Marchac D, Pugash E, Gault D: The use of sprayed fibrin glue for face lifts. Eur J Plast Surg 10:139, 1987.
44. Vogel A, O'Grady K, Toriumi DM: Surgical tissue adhesives in facial plastic and reconstructive surgery. Fac Plast Surg 9:76, 1993.
45. Shirai T, Amano J, Takabe K: Thoracosopic diagnosis and treatment of chylothorax after pneumonectomy. Ann Thorac Surg 52:306, 1991.
46. Shaffrey CI, Spotnitz WD, Shaffrey ME, et al: Neurosurgical applications of fibrin glue: Augmentation of dural closure in 134 patients. Neurosurgery 26:207, 1990.
47. Martinowitz U, Ozer Y, Varon D, et al: Fibrin sealing in nerve repair. Thromb Haemost 69:1287, 1993.
48. Egkher E, Spangler H, Spangler HP: Indications and limits of fibrin adhesive applied to traumatological patients. In Schlag G, Redl H (eds):

Fibrin Sealant in Operative Medicine: Traumatology and Orthopaedics, vol 7. Berlin, Springer, 1986, p 144.

49. Lagoutte FM, Gauthier L, Comte PRM: A fibrin sealant for perforated and pre-perforated corneal ulcers. Br J Ophthalmol 73:757, 1989.

50. Kang DR: Fibrin tissue adhesive use in costal cartilage laryngotracheal reconstruction. Paper presented at the Cambridge Symposium on Tissue Sealants: Current Practice, Future Uses, 1996, La Jolla, CA.

51. Fischer CP, Sonda LP, Dionko AC: Further experience with cryoprecipitate coagulum in renal calculus surgery: A review of 60 cases. J Urol 126:432, 1981.

52. Steinbaum SS, Cucinell S: Effects of cryoprecipitate on the healing of chronic wounds. Mil Med 159:105, 1994.

53. Schwartz RS, Abildgaard CF, Aledort LM, et al: Human recombinant DAN-derived antihemophilic factor (factor VIII) in the treatment of hemophilia A. N Engl J Med 323:1800, 1990.

54. Lethagen S, Berntorp E, Nilsson IM: Pharmacokinetics and hemostatic effect of different factor VIII/von Willebrand factor concentrates in von Willebrand's disease type III. Ann Hematol 65:253, 1992.

55. Berguer R, Staerkel RL, Moore EE, et al: Warning: Fatal reaction to the use of fibrin glue in deep hepatic wounds. Case reports. J Trauma 126:432, 1991.

56. Hellstern P, Sachse H, Schwinn H, et al: Manufacture and in vitro characterization of a solvent/detergent-treated human plasma. Vox Sang 63:178, 1993.

57. Horowitz B, Bonomo R, Prince AM, et al: Solvent/detergent-treated plasma: a virus-inactivated substitute for fresh frozen plasma. Blood 79:826, 1992.

58. Keeling DM, Luddington R, Allain J-P, et al: Cryoprecipitate prepared from plasma virally inactivated by the solvent detergent method. Br J Haematol 96:194, 1997.

Chapter 16

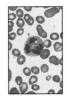

Albumin, IVIG, and Derivatives

Silvana Z. Bucur

Human plasma and its derivatives are valuable resources, and since the early 1990s, significant efforts have been made to ensure their safety, accessibility, and efficient use. Even though plasma contains several hundred proteins, only a few preparations are available using current methods of isolation, purification, and concentration. These include albumin, immunoglobulins, coagulation protein concentrates (e.g., factors VIII, IX, VII, XIII), and a few protease inhibitors (e.g., antithrombin III,C1-esterase inhibitor, α_1-proteinase inhibitor). This chapter focuses on commercially available immunoglobulin and albumin preparations and their clinical uses.

■ Plasma Quality and Processing

Regulatory organizations determine the safety and quality of plasma acceptable for the preparation of its various derivatives. Safety requirements are related to viral transmission and bacterial contamination and are the same for all plasma products. *Plasma quality* refers to the optimal conditions necessary for the functional preservation of plasma components (e.g., specific coagulation factors, immunoglobulin, albumin) such that the fractionation process will yield products of acceptable quality. The quality of plasma plays a more important role in the recuperation of coagulation factors, whereas in the preparation of immunoglobulins and albumin, less stringent requirements lead to acceptable products. Thus, plasma sources used in the manufacturing of these derivatives include plasma obtained through centrifugation of whole blood, plasmapheresis, fresh frozen plasma, and recovered plasma. The major requirements for plasma used in the production of albumin is that it be separated within 5 days of its expiration date and contain at least 60 g/L of protein. In addition, the pool of plasma used in the extraction of immunoglobulins must be obtained from a minimum of 1000 donors to ensure the presence of appropriate antibody quantities with clinically relevant specificities and acceptable anti-HAV (hepatitis A virus) titers.[1]

The commercial extraction of the various plasma components is accomplished through methods of differential protein solubility and through differential interactions of proteins with either solid or physical media. Depending on the specific plasma derivative sought, the foregoing methods may be modified and adapted for large-scale manufacture.[2] For more efficient use, plasma usually undergoes an initial cryoprecipitation step to remove coagulation factors (e.g., factor VIII–von Willebrand factor fraction) and protease inhibitors (e.g., antithrombin III). Both albumin and immunoglobulins are extracted from pooled human plasma by the method of differential protein solubility, specifically, the cold ethanol protein fractionation. This method, described by Cohn and associates[3] in 1950, employs ethanol-water mixtures of various ethanol concentration, pH, ionic strength, temperature, and protein concentrations and thus facilitates unwanted protein precipitation while maintaining the target protein in solution.

The desired protein fraction is extracted from the supernatant by filtration or centrifugation, and the ethanol is removed through methods of freeze drying or ultracentrifugation. When the target product is immunoglobulin, the process of fractionation must be specifically modified to eliminate proteolytic enzymes, because these can degrade the immunoglobulin molecule and can render it biologically ineffective. Moreover, to minimize the risk of anaphylactic reactions, immunoglobulin preparations intended for intravenous administration are rendered void of prekallikrein activator and high-molecular-weight aggregates through various physical and chemical methods.[4]

■ Albumin

Physiologic Role and Commercial Preparations

Albumin is one of the most abundant plasma proteins (4.2 g per kg body weight) and serves multiple biologic functions. It is synthesized in the liver as a symmetric molecule of approximately 66,500 D (molecular weight), possesses high negative charge and solubility, has a rapid turnover of approximately 15 g/day, and has a life span of 15 to 20 days. The distribution of albumin is predominantly extravascular, with only 35% to 40% of albumin residing intravascularly, where it is responsible for most (70% to 80%) plasma colloid oncotic pressure. The thiol group on the surface of the molecule enables albumin to function effectively as a ligand binder, a radical-scavenger, and a versatile transport protein.[5]

Albumin is extracted from pooled plasma through Cohn fractionation and is pasteurized at 60°C for 10 hours to ensure viral inactivation. Albumin preparations are sterile, nonpyrogenic protein solutions free of preservatives and coagulation factors, they are balanced to physiologic pH, and they contain approximately 145 ± 15 mEq of sodium and approximately 2 mEq/L of potassium. Commercial human albumin preparations are available in ready-to-use bottles, as 5% and 25% albumin solutions, containing either 5 or 25 g of human albumin per 100 mL of buffered diluent, respectively. Another commercially available product is plasma protein fraction, a 5% solution containing 12.5 g protein per 250 mL, of which 83% is albumin, 17% consists of α and β globulins, and less than 1% consists of γ globulins. All albumin preparations are stored at room temperature without extreme temperature fluctuations.

Clinical Considerations

Hypoalbuminemia may be associated with various conditions that affect its production, distribution, excretion, or metabolism (Table 16.1). Severe hepatic dysfunction and nutritional deficiency states result in impaired albumin synthesis. Low plasma albumin levels may be seen in hypervolemic states, or they may follow a shift from the intravascular to the extravascular compartment. Hypoalbuminemia may result from increased protein loss through the kidney, gut, or skin or

Table 16.1   Causes of Hypoalbuminemia

Decreased synthesis
  Liver disease
  Calorie-protein malnutrition
  Congenital analbuminemia
  Malignancy

Increased catabolism
  Severe burns
  Thyrotoxicosis
  Pancreatitis

Excessive extracorporeal loss
  Nephrotic syndrome
  Protein-losing enteropathy
  Exfoliative dermatitis

Redistribution
  Ascites
  Inflammatory states
  Postsurgical state

Table 16.2   Uses of Albumin

Indicated
  Following large volume paracentesis
  Nephrotic syndrome resistant to potent diuretics
  Volume/fluid replacement in plasmapheresis

Possibly indicated
  Adult respiratory distress syndrome
  Ovarian hyperstimulation syndrome
  Cardiopulmonary bypass pump priming
  Fluid resuscitation in shock/sepsis/burns
  Neonatal kernicterus
  To improve enteral feeding intolerance

Not indicated
  Correction of measured hypoalbuminemia or hypoproteinemia
  Nutritional deficiency, total parenteral nutrition
  Pre-eclampsia
  Red blood cell suspension
  Simple volume expansion (surgery, burns)
  Wound healing

Investigational
  Cadaveric renal transplantation
  Cerebral ischemia
  Stroke

Common Usages
  Serum albumin <2.0 g/dl
  Nephrotic syndrome, proteinuria and hypoalbuminemia
  Labile pulmonary, cardiovascular status
  Cardiopulmonary bypass, pump priming
  Extensive burns
  Plasma exchange
  Hypotension
  Liver disease, Hypoalbuminemia, diuresis
  Protein losing enteropathy, hypoalbuminemia
  Resuscitation
  Intraoperative fluid requirement >5–6 L in adults
  Premature infant undergoing major surgery

From Bucur SZ, Berkman EM, Hillyer CD: Transfusion of Plasma Derivatives: Fresh-Frozen Plasma, Cryoprecipitate, Albumin, and Immunoglobulins. IN Hoffman R, Benz EJ, Shattil SJ, et al: Hematology: Basic Principles and Practice, 3/e. Philadelphia, Churchill Livingstone, 2000, p 2266.

consequent to increased catabolism. Although low plasma albumin levels may be seen in many conditions, it is rarely possible or necessary to replete albumin stores. In certain conditions, however, the use of parenteral albumin therapy has been associated with a definite therapeutic benefit, although in other clinical situations, its role remains uncertain[6-9] (Table 16.2).

The concentration of the albumin solution administered is dictated by the underlying disease and by the oncotic stress of the patient. For example, 5% albumin is used as volume replacement in therapeutic plasma exchange, whereas 25% albumin is beneficial in promoting extravascular fluid mobilization in nephrotic syndromes. The volume and rate of infusion are determined by the concentration of the albumin solution and by individual tolerance and response to the product.

Paracentesis

Ascites is the accumulation of fluid in the peritoneal space that causes progressive deterioration of hemodynamic, respiratory, and renal function. This condition may be treated with paracentesis. In patients with cirrhosis, large-volume paracentesis, without plasma volume expansion, has been associated with deleterious effects including hypotension, impaired renal function, electrolyte imbalance, hepatic encephalopathy, hypoalbuminemia, and infection.[10] The use of albumin infusions after paracentesis has been evaluated, and several studies[11–15] demonstrated a beneficial effect on circulatory function and sodium balance. Ginés and associates,[16] in a large multicenter randomized trial, established that infusion of albumin after large-volume paracentesis (more than 5 L) was superior to synthetic plasma expanders (dextran 70 and polygeline) in preventing hemodynamic deterioration. Although the major and immediate effect of albumin infusion is plasma volume expansion, subsequent changes in cardiopulmonary function lead to the deactivation of the vasoconstrictor and renin-angiotensin-aldosterone systems, and this, in turn, improves electrolyte balance and renal function.[17, 18] In a randomized trial evaluating the role of albumin infusion in patients with spontaneous bacterial peritonitis, Sort and colleagues[19] demonstrated a reduction in renal impairment and mortality in patients treated with albumin and antibiotics versus antibiotics alone. This clinical benefit may be attributed to the thiol-related antioxidant effect of albumin.[20]

Nephrotic Syndrome

The hallmark of *nephrotic syndrome* is glomerular loss of albumin that results in hypoalbuminemia and decreased plasma oncotic pressure, clinically manifested as interstitial edema of variable degree.[21] Although corticosteroid and cytotoxic therapies remain the mainstays of treatment, mobilization and evacuation of peripheral edema are important in preserving patients' quality of life. Most patients have a good response to dietary sodium restriction and diuretic therapy, and only a few patients become refractory to these therapies. In an attempt to ameliorate edema and to maximize diuretic response in these treatment-refractory patients, the coadministration of albumin infusions with diuretics has been evaluated and determined by some investigators[22–24] to have a therapeutic benefit. Akcicek and associates[25] investigated the role of albumin infusion on the natriuretic effect of furosemide and could not corroborate the same beneficial results. In addition, the coadministration of albumin infusions with diuretic therapy was determined to induce response delays and frequent relapse to primary immunosuppressive therapy,[26] as well as other complications including hypertension, respiratory distress, and electrolyte abnormalities.[27] Thus, the available data suggest that coadministration of 20% to 25% albumin with diuretic therapy is a reasonable and clinically beneficial approach only in patients with nephrotic syndrome resistant to diuretic therapy.

Ovarian Hyperstimulation Syndrome

Ovarian hyperstimulation syndrome is an iatrogenic and potentially lethal complication associated with the exogenous administration of gonadotrophins within the scope of inducing ovulation in women undergoing assisted reproductive manipulations. Patients with severe ovarian hyperstimulation syndrome present with ovarian enlargement and capillary leak syndrome (ascites, pleural effusions, hypovolemia, hemoconcentration), with fluid shifts leading to electrolyte imbalance and renal failure.[28] Several vasoactive substances such as histamine, serotonin, prostaglandins, prostacyclin, angiotensin, and a prospective factor released by the hyperstimulated ovary are responsible for the increased capillary permeability.[29–32] Prophylactic administration of albumin around the time of oocyte retrieval has been shown to reduce the incidence and severity of this syndrome in high-risk patients.[33–36] It is postulated that the beneficial effect of albumin may be related to its ability to sustain plasma oncotic pressure and may thus interfere with the development of capillary leak syndrome as well as its ability to bind and possibly inactivate or enhance the clearance of various substances in plasma that may exacerbate the syndrome (e.g., hormones, vasoactive substances).[5, 37, 38] Other authors, however, did not show a beneficial effect of albumin infusion. Chen and associates[39] and Ndukwe and colleagues[40] reevaluated the efficacy of intravenous albumin in the prevention of this syndrome and found that prophylactic albumin infusions did not prevent pregnancy-associated ovarian hyperstimulation syndrome, a finding validating the need for further prospective, randomized, controlled trials.

Therapeutic Plasma Exchange

A 5% albumin solution is the replacement fluid most frequently used in *therapeutic plasma exchange*.[41, 42] Although data suggest that partial or full volume replacement with hydroxyethyl starch (HES) may be a cost-effective alternative to albumin, it is associated with more frequent untoward reactions (e.g, allergic reactions, coagulopathy),[43–46] as described in Chapter 44.

Hypovolemia and Intravascular Volume Expansion

Endogenous albumin is responsible for more than 80% of the *plasma colloid-oncotic pressure*, the force that maintains balance between the intravascular and extravascular fluids. The adverse consequences of hypoalbuminemia are primarily related to decreased plasma oncotic pressure. Thus, in extreme hypovolemic states, the therapeutic goal of fluid resuscitation is to increase plasma volume while minimizing interstitial fluid volume expansion. The type of fluid that would best accomplish this task is still being debated: crystalloid (e.g., normal saline) versus natural colloid (e.g., albumin) versus synthetic colloid solutions (e.g., HES). Although plasma oncotic pressure is raised effectively by many types of fluids, the differentiating factor is persistence of oncotic particles within the intravascular space. Although redistribution to the extravascular space occurs rapidly with crystalloid solutions, some high-molecular-weight artificial colloid solutions (e.g., HES) persist in the intravascular space for more than 48 hours, whereas exogenously administered albumin redistributes gradually; 50% will enter the extravascular compartment within 4 hours, 75% will enter the compartment within 2 days, and complete equilibration will occur within 7 to 10 days.[47–49]

The clinical benefit of volume expansion with albumin versus crystalloid solutions has been assessed in numerous trials,[50–55] which have not consistently demonstrated a superior outcome with the use of albumin. In an attempt to resolve this question, meta-analysis of preexisting trials was performed: Schierhout and Roberts[56] reviewed colloid volume replacement in critically ill patients and concluded that colloid solutions are ineffective and may even confer an increased mortality risk in this setting. The same reviewers analyzed trials involving albumin resuscitation and reported an increased mortality risk in this setting as well.[57] Conversely, the studies reviewed by Hankeln and Beez[48] surmised a clinical benefit with the use of colloid versus crystalloid solutions. The reasons for the great difficulty in interpreting data and in drawing firm conclusions from the initial trials as well as the meta-analysis reports are that the studies analyzed included small numbers of subjects and a varied patient population, they were nonrandomized trials, and they differed in types of fluids used (albumin, gelatins, and HES), resuscitation protocols, and endpoints analyzed.

Albumin supplementation in critically ill patients may result in adverse outcome through several plausible mechanisms. The administration of albumin in baboons with hemorrhagic shock resulted in rapid intravascular volume expansion and subsequent cardiac decompensation. Albumin infusion in patients with increased capillary permeability may lead to pulmonary edema and progressive hypoxemia.[58] In patients with hypovolemic shock, exogenous albumin may interfere with sodium and water excretion and may result in renal impairment[59]; it may also alter hemostasis and may lead to excessive blood loss.[60] Although most of the evidence does not favor albumin resuscitation, Quinlan and associates[20] demonstrated a potentially beneficial role of albumin infusion related to the thiol group on the surface of the albumin molecule. Repletion of plasma thiol levels by exogenous albumin may increase the antioxidative capacity in patients with sepsis, but whether this thiol-dependent antioxidant effect is translated into clinical benefit remains to be determined.

Therefore, because data to support the use (and some evidence to suggest a detrimental role) of albumin as fluid resuscitation therapy are limited, I have adopted the view of the North American consensus conference.[61] I recognize that although albumin infusion may prove beneficial in certain clinical circumstances, albumin should not be used as first-line therapy for volume expansion.

ALTERNATIVES

The two major categories of plasma volume expanders are crystalloids (e.g., 0.9% sodium chloride, Ringer's lactate) and colloids, including natural (e.g., albumin) and artificial (e.g., dextran, gelatins, and starches) substances. Both crystalloid and artificial colloid solutions have been investigated as alternatives to human albumin solutions, but none have demonstrated a definite clinical advantage over albumin. Moreover, the administration of artificial colloid solutions is associated with more frequent side effects.[68-88]

Hypoalbuminemia and Nutritional Replacement

Several randomized clinical trials have assessed the use of intravenous albumin supplementation in patients with hypoalbuminemia and have reported no effect on morbidity or mortality.[62-65] Although intravenous albumin administration does lead to a transient increase in serum albumin level, it does not translate into clinical benefit, and thus its use cannot be justified in this setting. In burned patients, crystalloid or artificial colloid solutions are used as first-line volume replacement therapy. In severe cases, albumin infusions may assist in repleting the albumin and thiol stores, although it is not clear whether this effect is clinically beneficial.[66, 67]

■ Immunoglobulins

Physiologic Role and Commercial Preparations

Immunoglobulins are produced by activated plasma cells in response to antigenic stimulation and represent a heterogeneous group of glycoproteins of variable molecular weight (150 to 1000 kD), structure, and function. All immunoglobulins consist of two sets of identical polypeptide chains—two heavy (H) and two light (L) chains—linked by disulfide bonds, and they contain a crystallizable fragment (Fc) and at least one antigen-binding fragment (Fab). Each Fab fragment contains two identical nests formed by the hypervariable (V) region of both L and H chains, which represent the antigen-binding sites and are responsible for the functional specificity and diversity of immunoglobulins. The Fc portion of immunoglobulins serves as binding site for receptors on various cells (e.g., monocyte/macrophage) and proteins (e.g., protein A, C1q). Based on physical and biologic properties, immunoglobulins may be divided into five classes or isotypes: IgG, IgA, IgM, IgD, and IgE. In plasma, IgG is the predominant isotype; it represents approximately 75% of the total plasma immunoglobulin content, and it is the only immunoglobulin class that crosses the placenta.[89-92]

Clinical Considerations

Parenteral immunoglobulins are manufactured from pooled human plasma and consist of all subclasses and allotypes of IgG, with only trace amounts of IgM and IgA. The major difference between multispecific immunoglobulin preparations for intravenous administration (IVIG) and preparations intended for intramuscular administration (immune serum globulin) is the absence in the former of immune aggregates with anticomplement activity. Hyperimmune immunoglobulin preparations are obtained from actively immunized individuals and contain high titer of disease-specific (e.g., hepatitis B virus [HBIG], varicella-zoster [VZIG], rabies [RIG]) or cell-specific (Rh immunoglobulin [RhIG]) antibodies. These preparations may be administered either intravenously or intramuscularly. In addition, various animals (e.g., bovine, equine, ovine) can be actively immunized, and the antitoxins or antisera collected may be used in clinical practice.

Parenteral immunoglobulin solutions have many clinical uses. IVIG provides active immunization when it is administered to susceptible individuals. In patients with impaired humoral immunity, IVIG augments bactericidal activity by promoting efficient opsonization, facilitates lymphocyte antigen recognition, enhances antigen elimination by the reticuloendothelial system, and induces complement activation. When administered in adequate doses, immunoglobulins can produce effective Fc receptor blockade and can thus reduce reticuloendothelial system clearance of antibody-coated cells (red blood cells, platelets). The temporary immune protection against infectious (e.g., bacteria, virus) and toxic (e.g., bacteria-associated toxins, venoms, or poisons) agents is provided either by hyperimmune immunoglobulin or IVIG preparations. The administration of antithymocyte or antilymphocyte globulin provides nonspecific immunosuppression, whereas anti-Rh(D) immunoglobulin administration provides specific immunosuppression. The specific parenteral immunoglobulin preparation and the dose, schedule, route, and rate of administration are dictated by the underlying condition and the therapeutic effect desired.[92, 93] Specific indications are described in the following sections for the use of IVIG.

Primary Immunodeficiency Syndromes

Quantitative and qualitative immunoglobulin defects predispose patients with *primary congenital immunodeficiency syndromes* to recurrent episodes of sinopulmonary infections with *Streptococcus pneumoniae* and *Haemophilus influenzae*. Prophylactic intramuscular, subcutaneous, and intravenous immunoglobulin preparations have been demonstrated to be equally effective in reducing morbidity and mortality in these patients. The intravenous route of administration offers the advantage of providing adequate and prompt delivery with minimal discomfort. The usual recommended maintenance dose is 400 mg/kg IVIG at monthly intervals to achieve a trough level between 300 and 400 mg/dL. Patients with active infections may require more frequent administrations until the infection is cleared, followed by maintenance replacement therapy.[94–102]

Secondary Immunodeficiencies

Severe *acquired immunodeficiency syndromes* may be associated with hematologic malignant diseases (e.g., chronic lymphocytic leukemia and multiple myeloma), or infection (e.g., with human immunodeficiency virus [HIV]), or they may result from immunosuppressive therapy for solid organ or bone marrow transplantation.

Hypogammaglobulinemia Associated with Malignancy. Several studies[103–110] investigated the use of prophylactic IVIG in patients with hypogammaglobulinemia associated with B-cell lymphoproliferative disorders and demonstrated a clinical benefit in those patients experiencing recurrent bacterial infections. To address the cost-effectiveness of prophylactic IVIG therapy in this setting, Chapel and associates[108] and Jurlander and colleagues[109] evaluated the efficacy of low-dose IVIG and found that a fixed low dose of IVIG (250 mg/kg every 4 weeks or 10 g every 3 weeks, respectively) was equally as effective as high-dose IVIG (400 mg/kg every 3 weeks) therapy in preventing febrile and infectious episodes.

HIV Infection. The impaired cellular and humoral immunity observed in advanced HIV infection predisposes these patients to recurrent, life-threatening infections. Studies evaluating the efficacy and cost-effectiveness of prophylactic IVIG administration in children with advanced HIV infection demonstrated a marked reduction in the frequency of severe bacterial infections, febrile episodes, and number of hospitalizations.[111, 112] In adults with advanced HIV infection, the use of prophylactic IVIG has yielded mixed results, with some studies demonstrating improved survival and decreased bacterial infections,[113, 114] whereas others have failed to detect significant clinical benefits.[115]

Neonatal Sepsis. Most of the maternal transfer of IgG occurs in the last 4 to 6 weeks of pregnancy. Therefore, preterm infants are highly susceptible to nosocomial infections with encapsulated organisms (e.g, group B streptococci, *Escherichia coli*, *H. influenzae type b*). Several preliminary studies[116–119] evaluating the use of prophylactic IVIG in premature neonates demonstrated a potential clinical benefit, although these results have not been confirmed by controlled trials. In a meta-analysis of existing trials, Lacy and Ohlsson[120] could not demonstrate decreased morbidity or mortality with routine use of IVIG in this setting. Therefore, until more convincing data become available, the routine use of prophylactic IVIG in preterm neonates cannot be recommended. The use of IVIG as adjuvant to antibiotics in the treatment of neonatal sepsis has been associated with reduced mortality and hastened recovery.[121–125]

Bone Marrow Transplantation. The preparative regimens and the anti–graft-versus-host disease immunosuppressive prophylaxis after allogeneic bone marrow transplantation delay the immune reconstitution and place patients at risk of infectious complications, especially cytomegalovirus (CMV) infection. Studies of the use of prophylactic IVIG or hyperimmune CMV-IG in preventing CMV infection after bone marrow transplantation have yielded conflicting results.[126–132] Moreover, evidence suggests that prolonged use of IVIG prophylaxis after bone marrow transplantation may delay recipient humoral responses.[128] In established CMV interstitial pneumonia, the combination of ganciclovir and IVIG is associated with decreased severity of disease and prolonged survival, and it is considered the standard therapeutic modality.[132–135] In an attempt to reduce graft-versus-host disease and transplantation-related mortality, initial studies[136, 137] demonstrated a reduction of these events in those patients receiving IVIG. Sullivan and associates,[128] however, could not confirm these results in a controlled trial evaluating IVIG after bone marrow transplantation.

Solid Organ Transplantation. Reactivation or primary infection with CMV occurs frequently after solid organ transplantation (e.g., kidney, liver) and may jeopardize allograft and patient survival. Various schedules of CMV prophylaxis that include antiviral agents (ganciclovir, acyclovir) with or without IVIG appear cost-effective in reducing the incidence of CMV primary infection and reactivation.[138–144] Some evidence suggests that IVIG prophylaxis may also be beneficial in heart and lung transplantation.[145, 146]

Disorders of the Immune System

The immunomodulatory effects of high-dose IVIG are achieved through multiple mechanisms: IVIG directly affects B lymphocytes and suppresses antibody production; it interferes with the interaction between autoantibodies and cellular targets through the anti-idiotypic antibodies it contains; high-dose IVIG can cause Fc receptor blockade; IVIG disrupts the release and action of inflammatory cytokines and impairs complement activity.[90, 147, 148] Specific uses include those described in the following sections.

Idiopathic Thrombocytopenic Purpura. Idiopathic thrombocytopenic purpura (ITP) is characterized by the production of platelet-specific autoantibodies with subsequent platelet removal by the reticuloendothelial system.[148] The use of

IVIG in both acute and chronic ITP has been shown to raise the platelet count rapidly, but transiently, within 5 days of its administration. In children with acute ITP, IVIG is as effective as corticosteroids, whereas in adults with chronic ITP unresponsive to corticosteroids or splenectomy, IVIG may be useful when platelet counts need to be acutely raised. The responses to IVIG are brief, and therapy-associated cost is high. Thus, although the efficacy of IVIG in ITP is equivalent to that of corticosteroids, its use is not recommended, except in situations requiring prompt increase in platelet counts, including the perioperative state, during acute hemorrhagic episodes, and in patients refractory to conventional therapy.[148–163] IVIG has also been demonstrated to be effective in ITP associated with pregnancy, in ITP associated with HIV infection, in postinfectious ITP, and in neonatal thrombocytopenia.[163–173]

Post-transfusion Purpura. Post-transfusion purpura is manifested by a sudden and severe decrease in platelet count 5 to 14 days after a blood transfusion. It is seen most often in women who lack the HPA-1a (Pl^{A1}) platelet antigen and who have been previously immunized through pregnancy. Occasionally, alloantibodies to other platelet antigens may be involved, including HPA-1b (Pl^{A2}), HPA-3a (Bak^a), HPA-3b (Bak^b), HPA-4a (Pen^a), HPA-5b (Br^a), and HLA-A2.[165–169] The formation and binding of immune complexes to Fc receptors, the synthesis of dually reactive autoantibody or alloantibody, and the adsorption of donor antigen to recipient's antigen-negative platelets have been postulated as possible pathophysiologic mechanisms.[174] Although post-transfusion purpura is a self-limited process with complete resolution in days to weeks, it can be associated with life-threatening bleeding complications, during which effective therapy must be instituted promptly. High-dose IVIG (400 mg/kg/day) therapy has been reported to produce rapid reversal of thrombocytopenia and has become the preferred treatment in post-transfusion purpura.[165–170, 175–178]

Disorders Resulting from Altered Immune Status. In patients with impaired immune status or those with poor bone marrow reserve (e.g., chronic hemolytic disorders), infection with parvovirus B19 can lead to pure red cell aplasia, which may be cured with high-dose IVIG.[179–181] High-dose IVIG therapy has induced either transient or permanent remissions in other immune-mediated conditions including autoimmune neutropenia,[182] autoimmune hemolytic anemia,[182, 183] hemophagocytic syndrome, and aplastic anemia.[184, 185]

Mucocutaneous Lymph Node Syndrome

Mucocutaneous lymph node syndrome, also known as Kawasaki disease, is an acute inflammatory childhood disorder manifested by fever and generalized vasculitis involving the coronary arteries. The combination of IVIG and aspirin has been demonstrated to be superior to aspirin alone in reducing and preventing coronary artery complications, as well as in shortening the febrile period of this disorder.[186–189] A single dose of IVIG, 1 to 2 g/kg, with aspirin is the current recommended regimen.

Polyneuropathies

Chronic inflammatory demyelinating polyradiculoneuropathy and *Guillain-Barré syndrome* are acquired inflammatory paralytic illnesses associated with substantial morbidity. Several double-blind, placebo-controlled studies[190–193] showed that IVIG was more effective than placebo in stabilizing symptoms and in inducing remissions in patients with chronic inflammatory demyelinating polyradiculoneuropathy. Initially, Jackson and associates[194] reported favorable preliminary results using IVIG in the treatment of Guillain-Barré syndrome. Subsequently, several other studies demonstrated the efficacy of IVIG to be superior to that of corticosteroids[195] and comparable to that of plasma exchange,[196–199] with the combined treatment modality (IVIG and plasma exchange) not demonstrating cost-effectiveness.[198, 199] In addition, IVIG has the advantage of being readily available and simple to administer, and it has less serious side effects than either plasma exchange or corticosteroids.

Other Uses of IVIG

Some clinical efficacy of IVIG has been demonstrable in women with antiphospholipid syndrome and recurrent pregnancy loss,[200–207] as well as in inflammatory myopathies including dermatomyositis, polymyositis, and inclusion-body myositis.[208–214] Cost-effective consciousness mandates that the use of IVIG in these settings be individualized. Numerous case reports and small studies have evaluated the utility of IVIG infusions in other immune-mediated disorders, including factor VIII inhibitors, rheumatoid arthritis, diabetes mellitus–associated neuropathy, and systemic vasculitides, but data remain inconclusive,[215–229] and recommendations are on a case-by-case basis. IVIG has also demonstrated some success in patients with certain childhood epileptic disorders,[230–233] multiple sclerosis,[234–237] and chronic fatigue syndrome.[238, 239]

Hyperimmune Globulins

Preparations of immunoglobulins containing high-titer, disease-specific antibodies are used as prophylactic immunization for susceptible persons. Several hyperimmune globulins are discussed in the following sections.

Rh Immune Globulin. RhIG is a high-titer IgG, anti-D immunoglobulin preparation used primarily in the prophylaxis of Rh immunization either through blood transfusions (Rh-negative recipient transfused with Rh-positive blood) or through pregnancy (antibody-negative, Rh-negative mother carrying an Rh-positive fetus). RhIG has also been demonstrated effective in Rh(D)-positive patients with ITP and intact spleens. In this setting, RhIG binds to the D-antigen on the red blood cells and enhances their destruction and elimination by the reticuloendothelial system. Thus, on the one hand, it limits exposure and prevents immunization to the D-antigen, whereas, on the other, by overwhelming the reticuloendothelial system with Rh(D)-positive red blood cells, it interferes with platelet destruction, as in ITP.[240, 241]

The necessity of suppressing Rh(D) immunization should be based on the clinical situation and the reproductive capacity of the individual patient. For the prevention of immunization of Rh(D)-negative persons exposed to Rh(D)-positive blood products (i.e., red blood cells, platelets, granulocytes), it is recommended that RhIG be administered within 72 hours of the transfusion and at a dose of 20 μg RhIG/mL red blood cells transfused. The recommendation for antepartum prophylaxis is 300 μg RhIG administered as a single intravenous or intramuscular dose at weeks 28 and 30 of gestation. A postpartum anti-D antibody titer greater than 4 represents active immunization, and, in general, no prophylaxis with RhIG is necessary. If active immunization cannot be demonstrated, postpartum prophylaxis with RhIG within 72 hours after childbirth is indicated (either 300 μg intramuscularly or 600 μg intravenously). When excessive fetomaternal hemorrhage has occurred during the delivery, an additional 300 μg RhIG per each 15 mL red blood cells should be administered irrespective of the anti-D antibody titer. Other obstetric indications include abortion, ectopic pregnancy, tubal ligation, amniocentesis, chorionic villus sampling, and other obstetric manipulations and complications.[242, 243]

In immune thrombocytopenia, RhIG is administered intravenously, and the initial dose is based on the hemoglobin content. Thus, the recommended doses are 50 μg/kg or 25 to 40 μg/kg for hemoglobin greater or less than 10 mg/dL, respectively. Additional doses of 25 to 50 μg may be administered when necessary.[163, 244, 245]

Hepatitis B Immunoglobulin. Administration of HBIG is indicated for those persons exposed to hepatitis B virus (HBV) through various routes, including sexual, oral, and perinatal or through intravenous blood product administration.[246, 247] For adults, HBIG should be administered during the first 2 weeks of the exposure, and the recommended dose is 0.06 mL/kg (up to a maximum dose of 5 mL) intramuscularly. Infants born to mothers who are carriers or who have active hepatitis B should receive 0.5 mL HBIG intramuscularly. Both adults and infants should receive HBV vaccine, 1 and 6 months thereafter.

Varicella-Zoster Immune Globulin. VZIG is indicated after exposure to herpes zoster of susceptible persons including immunocompromised children and adults, infants born to mothers with varicella infection, and pregnant women. Prophylaxis with VZIG may also be indicated to reduce the severity of disease and of complications associated with chickenpox in immunologically normal adults, in normal children to reduce the infectious risk to immunocompromised members of the household, and in health care workers. A dose of VZIG of 125 units per 10 kg body weight intramuscularly (up to a maximum of 625 units), administered within 5 days of the exposure, provides immunity for up to 3 weeks.[248]

Tetanus Immunoglobulin. Prophylactic doses of human tetanus immunoglobulin (TIG) (250 to 500 units intramuscularly) may be administered with tetanus toxoid in nonimmunized persons after a bite or injury. Treatment of tetanus with human TIG includes administration of half the total dose (500 to 3000 units) intramuscularly with the other half being infiltrated at the wound site, followed by primary immunization with tetanus toxoid. Alternatively, equine or bovine tetanus antitoxin (TAT) may be used prophylactically (3000 to 5000 units intramuscularly) and as primary treatment (50,000 to 100,000 units—20,000 units of the total dose are given by the intravenous route and the rest intramuscularly).[249, 250]

Rabies Immunoglobulin. Prophylaxis with human or equine RIG is indicated after all animal bites in which rabies cannot be excluded. Half the dose is administered at the wound site and the rest intramuscularly, and simultaneously rabies vaccine may be administered at a different site.[251]

Immunoglobulin Derivatives

Oral immunoglobulin preparations have been administered experimentally with the intent of neutralizing pathogenic microorganisms in the gastrointestinal tract. Sporadic success has been reported with the administration of oral immunoglobulin for the prevention of certain gastrointestinal illness in neonates including rotavirus infections and necrotizing enterocolitis and for the treatment of diarrhea associated with *Cryptosporidium* as well as in the period after bone marrow transplantation.[252–256] Intrathecal and aerosol administration of immunoglobulin has been attempted for the treatment of encephalitis and respiratory syncytial virus, but without proven clinical benefit.[257]

The development of various monoclonal antibodies with specificity toward cellular antigens, receptors, and cytokines led to experimentally innovative therapeutic approaches to such diseases as lymphoma (anti-CD20), leukemia (anti-CD33), and ITP (anticomplement). Antibodies (anti-CD3 and antithymocyte globulin) have also been successfully used for immunosuppression in transplantation and in certain hematologic disorders, and a sheep-derived Fab portion of IgG has been used in the treatment of digitalis toxicity. In time, antibody preparation may be engineered to provide longer half-life, enhanced complement fixation, specific cellular localization and toxicity, and better immunomodulatory capacity.

■ Potential Adverse Reactions

The manufacturing process removes all blood group isohemagglutinins from albumin products, and only trace amounts are left in immunoglobulin preparations. Thus, the process abrogates the need for ABO and Rh testing before administration of these preparations. Because of the presence of low titers of IgG anti-A and anti-B antibodies in immunoglobulin preparations, their administration may interfere with serologic testing (e.g., ABO and HLA-typing),[258] may cause a positive direct antiglobulin test, and may lead to low-grade hemolysis after high-dose IVIG therapy.[259, 260] Owing to the variable presence of IgG anti-IgA in IgA-deficient individuals, these patients are at risk of severe anaphylactic reactions after IVIG therapy with products containing IgA, and, as such, IgA-deficient products are recommended in these circumstances.[261, 262]

The incidence of adverse reactions to albumin infusions is approximately 1 in 6600 infusions, with only 1 in 30,000 infusions being life-threatening. Most side effects associated with the administration of albumin preparations may be a consequence of the biologic functions of albumin (e.g., colloid oncotic pressure and ion-binding properties), or they may be related to its physiologic properties (e.g., protein). As a protein, albumin can induce allergic-type reactions in sensitized persons. Clinical manifestations may include erythema, urticaria, and anaphylaxis. Because of its role in maintaining plasma oncotic pressure, rapid infusions of albumin may lead to circulatory overload, pulmonary edema, and hypotension in susceptible persons. Red blood cell dilution with subsequent decrease in hematocrit and hemoglobin has also been reported. Rarely, albumin may bind intravascular calcium, and this may lead to hypocalcemia and its complications.[263] The administration of plasma protein fraction has been associated with hypocoagulability resulting from platelet factor-4 and β-thromboglobulin present in the preparation, whereas in patients with renal dysfunction, metabolic acidosis may develop after administration.[264]

Immunoglobulin preparations administered intramuscularly may induce local side effects including pain at the site of injection and local irritation as well as systemic side effects. The systemic effects are allergic-type reactions related to the preservatives and stabilizer present in the solution, as well as the protein itself, and they may range from fever, headache, and flushing to urticaria and angioedema. Adverse reactions associated with intravenously administered immunoglobulin preparations are either related to infusion rate or are allergic-type reactions. Side effects related to the rate of infusion include flushing, nausea, vomiting, malaise, and anxiety, whereas allergic reactions generally manifest as pruritus, urticaria, joint pain, dyspnea, and bronchospasm. Severe anaphylactic reactions are more likely to occur in atopic persons and in those with a previous history of allergic reactions.[103, 106] Transient neutropenia,[265] acute, reversible renal failure,[266-268] and aseptic meningitis[269] have been reported as rare complications of high-dose IVIG therapy. Sensitivity testing is required before the use of all animal-derived immunoglobulin preparations (e.g., equine, bovine, ovine), because heterologous protein can induce severe allergic reactions in susceptible persons.

■ Infectious Potential

Albumin and immunoglobulin products are acellular blood byproducts obtained from pooled plasma, and preparation is thought to render these products void of cell-associated viral transmission (e.g., CMV, Epstein-Barr virus, human T-cell leukemia/lymphoma virus type I). However, a potential risk of transmission of other infectious agents (e.g., bacteria, hepatitis virus) exists. Albumin preparations undergo pasteurization (heating at 60°C for 10 hours), which is adequate for viral inactivation, but it is not efficiently bactericidal. Therefore, albumin solutions, in particular 25% albumin, remain fertile culture media for certain bacteria (e.g., *Pseudomonas* species) and require quality-control testing for pyrogenicity and bacterial contamination.[269, 270]

The process of cold ethanol fractionation successfully inactivates HIV, and although it does not inactivate hepatitis viruses, it does promote the partitioning of viruses into the different solute or precipitate fractions and results in lower viral concentration in the final product fraction. Although inactivation of hepatitis C and D viruses through pasteurization has not been specifically assessed,[271-275] there have been no reports of hepatitis transmission associated with albumin administration, with the exception of one hepatitis B outbreak thought to be related to poor manufacturing technique.[276] Unlike HIV, hepatitis viruses are generally more resistant to inactivation by the cold ethanol method. In the 1980s, four reports of transmission of non-A non-B hepatitis were published,[277-280] and it is currently estimated that more than 450 patients throughout the world have been infected with HCV through immunoglobulin preparations.[281-285] Because of these concerns, efforts have been made to reduce viral transmission by adding a viral inactivation step in the manufacturing process. This involves treatment with an organic solvent-detergent, tri-*n*-butyl phosphate octoxynol 9 and polysorbate 80, which efficiently inactivates lipid-enveloped DNA and RNA viruses, including hepatitis C virus and HIV, as demonstrated by in vitro studies.[286, 287]

REFERENCES

1. Myllylä G: Factors determining quality of plasma. Vox Sang 1998;74:507.
2. Foster PR: Fractionation, blood plasma fractionation. In Kirk-Othmer Encyclopedia of Chemical Technology, vol 11, 4th ed. London, John Wiley, 1994, p 990.
3. Cohn EJ, Gurd FRN, Surgenor DM, et al: A system for the separation of the components of human blood: Qualitative procedures for the separation of the protein components of human plasma. J Am Chem Soc 1950;72:465.
4. Vogelaar EF, deBoer-van den Berg MAG, Brummelhuis HGJ, et al: Contributions to the optimal use of human blood. IV. Quantitative analysis of the immunoglobulin isolation. Vox Sang 1974;27:193.
5. Tulis JL: Albumin 1. Background and use. JAMA 1977;237:355.
6. Kaminski MV Jr, Williams SD: Review of the rapid normalization of serum albumin with modified total parenteral nutrition solutions. Crit Care Med 1990;18:327.
7. Marik PE: The treatment of hypoalbuminemia in the critically ill patient. Heart Lung 1993;22:166.
8. Guthrie RD Jr, Hines C Jr: Use of intravenous albumin in the critically ill patient. Am J Gastroenterol 1991;86:255.
9. Rothchild MA, Ortaz M, Schreiber SS: Albumin synthesis. N Engl J Med 1972;286:748.
10. Kao HW, Rakow NE, Savage E, et al: The effect of large volume paracentesis on plasma volume: A cause of hypovolemia? Hepatology 1985;5:403.
11. Ginés P, Jiménez W, Arroyo V, et al: Atrial natriuric factor in cirrhosis with ascites: Plasma levels, cardiac release and splanchnic extraction. Hepatology 1988;8:636.
12. Tító L, Ginés P, Arroyo V, et al: Total paracentesis associated with intravenous albumin management of patients with cirrhosis an ascites. Gastroenterology 1990;98:146.
13. Ginés P, Arroyo V, Quintero E, et al: Comparison of paracentesis and diuretics in the treatment of cirrhosis with tense ascites: Results of a randomized study. Gastroenterology 1987;93:234.
14. McCormick PA, Mistry P, Kaye G, et al: Intravenous albumin infusion is an effective therapy for hyponatremia in cirrhotic patients with ascites. Gut 1990;31:204.
15. Luca A, García-Pagán JC, Bosch J, et al: Beneficial effects of intravenous albumin infusion on the hemodynamic and humoral changes after total paracentesis. Hepatology 1995;22:753.
16. Ginés A, Fernández-Esparrach G, Monescillo A, et al: Randomized trial comparing albumin, dextran 70, and polygeline in cirrhotic patients with ascites treated by paracentesis. Gastroenterology 1996;111:1002.
17. Saó J, Ginés A, Ginés P, et al: Effect of therapeutic paracentesis on plasma volume and transvascular escape rate of albumin in patients with cirrhosis. J Hepatol 1997;27:645.
18. Chang S-C, Chang H-I, Chen F-J, et al: Therapeutic effects of diuretics and paracentesis on lung function in patients with non-alcoholic cirrhosis and tense ascites. J Hepatol 1997;26:833.
19. Sort P, Navasa M, Arroyo V, et al: Effects of intravenous albumin on renal impairments and mortality in patients with cirrhosis and spontaneous bacterial peritonitis. N Engl J Med 1999;341:403.
20. Quinlan GJ, Margarson MP, Mumby S, et al: Administration of albumin to patients with sepsis syndrome: A possible beneficial role in plasma thiol repletion. Clin Sci 1998;95:459.
21. Palmer BF, Alpern RJ: Pathogenesis of edema formation in the nephrotic syndrome. Kidney Int 1997;59(Suppl):S21.
22. Davidson AM, Lambie AT, Verth AH, et al: Salt-poor human albumin in the management of nephrotic syndrome. BMJ 1974;1:481.
23. Weiss A, Schoeneman M, Griefer I: Treatment of severe nephrotic edema with albumin and furosemide. N Y State J Med 1984;84:384.
24. Fliser D, Zurbruggen I, Mutschler E, et al: Coadministration of albumin and furosemide in patients with the nephrotic syndrome. Kidney Int 1999;55:629.
25. Akcicek F, Yalniz T, Basci A, et al: Diuretic effect of furosemide in patients with nephrotic syndrome: Is it potentiated by intravenous albumin? BMJ 1995;310:162.
26. Yoshimura A, Ideura T, Iwasaki S, et al: Aggravation of minimal change nephrotic syndrome by administration of human albumin. Clin Nephrol 1992;37:109.

27. Haws RM, Baum M: Efficacy of albumin and diuretic therapy in children with nephrotic syndrome. Pediatrics 1993;91:1142.

28. Forman R, Ross C, Friedman R, et al: Severe ovarian hyperstimulation syndrome using agonist of gonadotropin-releasing hormone for in vitro fertilization: A European series and a proposal for prevention. Fertil Steril 1990;53:502.

29. Navot D, Margalioth EJ, Laufer N, et al: Direct correlation between plasma renin activity and severity of the ovarian hyperstimulation syndrome. Fertil Steril 1987;48:57.

30. Knox GE: Antihistamine blockade of the ovarian hyperstimulaton syndrome. Am J Obstet Gynecol 1974;118:992.

31. Katz Z, Lancet M, Borenstein R, et al: Absence of teratogenicity of indomethacin in ovarian hyperstimulation syndrome. Int J Fertil 1984;29:186.

32. Pollishuk W, Schenker J: Ovarian overstimulation syndrome. Fertil Steril 1969;20:443.

33. Isik AZ, Gokmen O, Zeyneloglu HB, et al: Intravenous albumin prevents moderate-severe ovarian hyperstimulation in in-vitro fertilization patients: A prospective randomized and controlled study. J Assist Reprod Genet 1995;12(Suppl):54S.

34. Shalev E, Giladi Y, Matilsky M, et al: Decreased incidence of severe ovarian hyperstimulation syndrome in high risk in-vitro fertilization patients receiving intravenous albumin: A prospective study. Hum Reprod 1995;10:1373.

35. Shoham Z, Weissman A, Barash A, et al: Intravenous albumin for the prevention of severe ovarian hyperstimulation syndrome in an in vitro fertilization program: A prospective, randomized, placebo-controlled study. Fertil Steril 1994;62:137.

36. Shaker AG, Zosmer A, Dean N, et al: Comparison of intravenous albumin and transfer of fresh embryos with cryopreservation of all embryos for subsequent transfer in prevention of ovarian hyper-stimulation syndrome. Fertil Steril 1996;65:992.

37. Asch RH, Ivery G, Goldsman M, et al: The use of intravenous albumin in patients at high risk for severe ovarian hyperstimulation syndrome. Hum Reprod 1993;8:1015.

38. Tullis JL: Albumin 2: Guidelines for clinical use. JAMA 1977;237:460.

39. Chen C-D, Wu M-Y, Yang J-H, et al: Intravenous albumin does not prevent the development of severe ovarian hyperstimulation syndrome. Fertil Steril 1997;68:287.

40. Ndukwe G, Thornton S, Fishel S, et al: Severe ovarian hyperstimulation syndrome: Is it really preventable by prophylactic intravenous albumin? Fertil Steril 1997;68:851.

41. Schumak KH, Rock GA: Therapeutic plasma exchange. N Engl J Med 1984;310:762.

42. Taft EG: Therapeutic apheresis. Hum Pathol 1983;14:235.

43. Kapiotis O, Quehenberger P, Eichler HG, et al: Effect of hydroxyethyl starch on the activity of blood coagulation and fibrinolysis in healthy volunteers. Crit Care Med 1994;22:606.

44. Brecher ME, Owen HG, Bandarenko N: Alternatives to albumin: Starch replacement for plasma exchange. J Clin Apheresis 1997;12:146.

45. Korach JM, Berger P, Giraud C, et al: Role of replacement fluids in the immediate complications of plasma exchange. Int Care Med 1998;24:452.

46. Owen HG, Brecher ME: Partial colloid replacement for therapeutic plasma exchange. J Clin Apheresis 1997;12:87.

47. Ernest D, Belzberg AS, Dodek PM: Distribution of normal saline and 5% albumin infusions in septic patients. Crit Care Med 1999;27:46.

48. Hankeln KB, Beez M: Haemodynamic and oxygen transport correlates of various volume substitutes in critically ill in-patients with various aetiologies of haemodynamic instability. Int J Intensive Care 1998;5:8.

49. Hillman K, Bishop G, Bristow P: Fluid resuscitation. Curr Anaes Crit Care 1996;7:187.

50. Lucas CE, Weaver D, Higgins RF, et al: Effects of albumin versus non-albumin resuscitation on plasma volume and renal excretory function. J Trauma 1978;18:565.

51. Lowe RJ, Moss GS, Jilek J, et al: Crystalloid vs. colloid in the aetiology of pulmonary failure after trauma: A randomized trial in man. Surgery 1977;1:676.

52. Virgilio RW, Rice CL, Smith DE, et al: Crystalloid vs. colloid resuscitation: Is one better? A randomized clinical study. Surgery 1979;85:129.

53. Zetterstrom H: Albumin treatment following major Surgery. II. Effects on postoperative lung function and circulatory adaptation. Acta Anaesthesiol Scand 1981;25:133.

54. Foely EF, Borlase BC, Dzik WH, et al: Albumin supplementation in the critically ill. Arch Surg 1990;125:739.

55. Golub R, Sorrento JJ, Cantu R, et al: Efficacy of albumin supplementation in the surgical intensive care unit: A prospective randomized study. Crit Care Med 1994;22:613.

56. Schierhout G, Roberts I: Fluid resuscitation with colloid or crystalloid solutions in critically ill patients: A systematic review of randomized trials. BMJ 1998;316:961.

57. Cochrane Injuries Group Albumin Reviewers: Human albumin administration in critically ill patients: Systematic review of randomized controlled trials. BMJ 1998;317:235.

58. Moss GS, Das Gupta TK, Brinkman R, et al: Changes in lung ultrastructure following heterologous and homologous serum albumin infusion in the treatment of hemorrhagic shock. Ann Surg 1979;189:236.

59. Moon MR, Lucas CE, Ledgerwood AM, et al: Free water clearance after supplemental albumin resuscitation for shock. Circ Shock 1989;28:1.

60. Johnson SD, Lucas CE, Gerrick SJ, et al: Altered coagulation after albumin supplements for treatment of oligemic shock. Arch Surg 1979;114:379.

61. Vermeulen LC, Ratko TA, Erstad BL, et al: A paradigm for consensus: The University Hospital Consortium guidelines for the use of albumin, non-protein colloid, and crystalloid solutions. Arch Intern Med 1995;155:373.

62. Rubin H, Carlson S, DeMeo M, et al: Randomized, double-blind study of intravenous human albumin in hypoalbuminemic patients receiving total parenteral nutrition. Crit Care Med 1997;25:249.

63. Wojtysiak SL, Brown RO, Roberson D, et al: Effect of hypoalbuminemia and parenteral nutrition on free water excretion and electrolyte-free water resorption. Crit Care Med 1992;20:164.

64. Kanarek KS, Williams PR, Blair C: Concurrent administration of albumin with total parenteral nutrition in sick newborn patients. JPEN J Parenter Enteral Nutr 1992;16:49.

65. Foley EF, Borlasse BC, Dzik WH et al: Albumin supplementation in the critically ill: A prospective, randomized trial. Arch Surg 1990;125:739.

66. Demling RH: Fluid replacement in burned patients. Surg Clin North Am 1987;67:15.

67. Sheridan RL, Prelack K, Cunningham JJ: Physiologic hypoalbuminemia is well tolerated by severely burned children. J Trauma 1997;43:448.

68. Hallowell P, Bland JHL, Dalton BC, et al: The effect of hemodilution with albumin or Ringer's lactate on water balance and blood use in open-heart surgery. Ann Thorac Surg 1979;25:22.

69. Ohqvist G, Settergren G, Bergstrom K, et al: Plasma colloid osmotic pressure during open-heart surgery using noncolloid or colloid priming solution in the extracorporeal circuit. Scand J Thorac Cardiovasc Surg 1981;15:251.

70. Marelli D, Samson R, Edgell E, et al: Does the addition of albumin to the prime solution in the cardiopulmonary bypass affect clinical outcome? J Thorac Cardiovasc Surg 1989;98:751.

71. Bodenhamer RM, Johnson RG, Randolph JD, et al: The effect of adding mannitol or albumin to a crystalloid cardioplegic solution: A prospective, randomized clinical study. Ann Thorac Surg 1985;40:374.

72. Brinson RR, Kolts BE: Hypoalbuminemia as an indicator of diarrheal incidence in critically ill patients. Crit Care Med 1987;15:506.

73. Ford EG, Jennings M, Andrassy RJ: Serum albumin (oncotic pressure) correlates with enteral feeding tolerance in the pediatric surgical patient. J Pediatr Surg 1987;22:597.

74. Stratta P, Canavese C, Dogliani M, et al: Repeated albumin infusions do not lower blood pressure in preeclampsia. Clin Nephrol 1991;36:234.

75. Brown RO, Bradley JE, Bekemeyer WB, et al: Effect of albumin supplementation during parenteral nutrition on hospital mortality. Crit Care 1988;16:1177.

76. Poppas DP, Massicotte MJ, Stewart RB, et al: Human albumin solder supplemented with TGF-b1 accelerates healing following laser welded wound closure. Lasers Surg Med 1996;19:360.

77. Massicotte JM, Stewart RB, Poppas DP: Effects of endogenous absorption in human albumin solder for acute laser wound closure. Lasers Surg Med 1998;23:18.

78. Goslinga H, Eijzenbach V, Heuvelmans JH, et al: Custom-tailored hemodilution with albumin and crystalloids in acute ischemic stroke. Stroke 1992;23:181.

79. Matsui T, Sinyama H, Asano T: Beneficial effect of prolonged administration of albumin on ischemic cerebral edema and infarction after occlusion of middle cerebral artery in rats. Neurosurgery 1993;33:293.

80. Huh PW, Belayev L, Zhao W, et al: The effect of high-dose albumin therapy on local cerebral perfusion after transient focal cerebral ischemia in rats. Brain Res 1998;804:105.

81. Gross CE, Bednar MM, Lew SM, et al: Preoperative volume expansion improves tolerance to carotid artery cross-clamping during endarterectomy. Neurosurgery 1998;43:222.

82. Belayev L, Zhao W, Pattany PM, et al: Diffusion-weighted magnetic resonance imaging confirms marked neuro-protective efficacy of albumin therapy in focal cerebral ischemia. Stroke 1998;29:2587.

83. Belayev L, Busto R, Zhao W, et al: Effect of delayed albumin hemo-dilution on infarction volume and brain edema after transient middle cerebral artery occlusion in rats. J Neurosurg 1997;87:595.

84. Dawidson IJ, Sandor ZF, Coorpender L, et al: Intraoperative albumin administration affects the outcome of cadaver renal transplantation. Transplantation 1992;53:774.

85. Roberts JS, Bratton SL: Colloid volume expanders: Problems, pitfalls and possibilities. Drugs 1998;55:621.

86. Tobias MD, Wambold D, Pilla MA, et al: Differential effects of serial hemodilution with hydroxyethyl starch, albumin and 0.9% saline on whole blood coagulation. J Clin Anesth 1998;10:366.

87. Freyburger G, Dubreuil M, Boisseau MR, et al: Rheological properties of commonly used substitutes during preoperative normovolaemic haemodilution. Br J Anaesth 1996;76:519.

88. Nearman HS, Herman ML: Toxic effects of colloids in the intensive care unit. Crit Care Clin 1991;7:713.

89. Burdette S, Schwartz RS: Current concepts: Immunology. Idiotypes and idiotypic network. N Engl J Med 1987;317:219.

90. Dwyer JM: Manipulating the immune system with immune globulin. N Engl J Med 1992;326:107.

91. Hall PD: Immunomodulation with intravenous immunoglobulin. Pharmacotherapy 1993;13:564.

92. Ballow M: Mechanisms of action of intravenous immune serum globulin therapy. Pediatr Infect Dis J 1994;13:806.

93. Seligmann M, Cunningham-Rundles C, Hanson A, et al: Appropriate uses of human immunoglobulin in clinical practice: IUIS WHO Notice 1983. Clin Exp Immunol 1983;52:417.

94. Buckley RH, Schiff RI: The use of intravenous immune globulin in immunodeficiency diseases. N Engl J Med 1991;325:110.

95. Pirofsky B: Intravenous immune globulin therapy in hypogamma-globulinemia. Am J Med 1984;76:53.

96. Litzman J, Jones A, Hann I, et al: Intravenous immunoglobulin, splenectomy, and antibiotic prophylaxis in Wiskott-Aldrich syndrome. Arch Dis Child 1996;75:436.

97. Wodzinski MA, Lilleyman JS: High-dose immunoglobulin therapy of Wiskott-Aldrich syndrome. Pediatr Hematol Oncol 1987;4:345.

98. Schwartz SA: Clinical uses of immune serum globulin as replacement therapy inpatients with primary immunodeficiency syndromes. Clin Rev Allergy 1992;10:1.

99. Nolte MT, Pirofsky B, Gerritz GA, et al: Intravenous immunoglobulin therapy for antibody deficiency. Clin Exp Immunol 1979;36:237.

100. Amman AJ, Ashman RF, Buckley RH, et al: Use of intravenous immune globulin in antibody deficiency: Results of a multicenter controlled trial. Clin Immun Immunopathol 1992;22:60.

101. Cunningham-Rundles C, Siegal FP, Smithwick EM, et al: Efficacy of intravenous immunoglobulin in primary humoral immunodeficiency disease. Ann Intern Med 1984;101:434.

102. Einstein EM, Sneller MC: Common variable immunodeficiency: Diagnosis and management. Ann Allergy 1994;73:285.

103. Cooperative Group for the Study of Immunoglobulin in Chronic Lymphocytic Leukaemia: IVIG for the prevention of infection in chronic lymphocytic leukaemia. N Engl J Med 1988;319:902.

104. Griffiths H, Brennan V, Lea J, et al: Crossover study of immunoglobulin replacement therapy in patients with low grade B cell tumors. Blood 1989;73:366.

105. Boughton BJ, Jackson N, Lim S, et al: Randomized trial of intravenous immunoglobulin prophylaxis for patients with chronic lymphocytic leukaemia and secondary hypogammaglobulinaemia. Clin Lab Haematol 1995;17:75.

106. Chapel HM, Lee M, Hargreaves R, et al: Randomized trial of intravenous immunoglobulin as prophylaxis against infection in plateau-phase multiple myeloma. Lancet 1994;343:1059.

107. Weeks JC, Tierney MR, Weinstein MC: Cost effectiveness of prophylactic intravenous immune globulin in chronic lymphocytic leukaemia. N Engl J Med 1991;325:81.

108. Chapel H, Dicato M, Gamm H, et al: Immunoglobulin replacement in patients with chronic lymphocytic leukaemia: A comparison of two dose regimes. Br J Haematol 1994;88:209.

109. Jurlander J, Hartmann Geisler C, Hansen MM: Treatment of hypogammaglobulinemia in chronic lymphocytic leukaemia by low-dose intravenous gammaglobulin. Eur J Haematol 1994;53:114.

110. Yap PL, Todd AA, Williams PE, et al: Use of intravenous immuno-globulin in acquired immune deficiency syndrome. Cancer 1991;68:1440.

111. National Institute of Child Health and Human Development Intravenous Immunoglobulin Clinical Trial Study Group: Efficacy of intravenous immunoglobulin for the prophylaxis of serious bacterial infections in symptomatic HIV-infected children. N Engl J Med 1991;325:73.

112. Moffenson LM, Moye J, Jr Korelitz J, et al: Crossover of placebo patients to intravenous immunoglobulin confirms efficacy for prophylaxis of bacterial infections and reduction of hospitalizations in human immunodeficiency virus–infected children. Pediatr Infect Dis J 1994;13:477.

113. Saint-Marc T, Touraine J-I, Berra N: Beneficial effects of intravenous immunoglobulins in AIDS. Lancet 1992;340:1347.

114. Schrappe-Bächer M, Rasokat H, Bauer P, et al: High-dose intravenous immunoglobulins in HIV-1–infected adults with AIDS-related complex and Walter-Reed 5. Vox Sang 1990;59:3.

115. Jablonowski H, Sander O, Willers R, et al: The use of intravenous immunoglobulins in symptomatic HIV infection. Clin Invest 1994;72:220.

116. Kliegman RM, Clapp DW: Rational principles for immunoglobulin prophylaxis and therapy for neonatal infections. Clin Perinatol 1991;18:303.

117. Fischer GW, Weisman LE: Therapeutic intervention of clinical sepsis with intravenous immunoglobulin, white blood cells and antibiotics. Scand J Infect Dis 1990;73:17.

118. Weisman LE, Cruess DF, Fischer GW: Current status of intravenous immunoglobulin in preventing or treating neonatal bacterial infections. Clin Rev Allergy 1992;10:13.

119. Irani SF, Wagle SU, Deshpande PG: Role of intravenous immuno-globulin in prevention and treatment of neonatal infection. Indian Pediatr 1991;28:443.

120. Lacy JB, Ohlsson A: Administration of intravenous immunoglobulins for prophylaxis or treatment of infection in preterm infants: meta-analyses. Arch Dis Child 1995;72:F151.

121. Haque KN, Remo C, Bahakim H: Comparison of two types of intravenous immunoglobulins in the treatment of neonatal sepsis. Clin Exp Immunol 1995;101:328.

122. Acunas BA, Peakman M, Liossis G, et al: Effect of fresh frozen plasma and gammaglobulin on humoral immunity in neonatal sepsis. Arch Dis Child 1994;70:F182.

123. Fischer GW, Hemming VG, Hunter KE, et al: Intravenous immuno-globulin in the treatment of neonatal sepsis: Therapeutic strategies and laboratory studies. Paediatr Infec Dis 1986;5:5171.

124. Christensen KK, Christensen P: Intravenous gammaglobulin in the treatment of neonatal sepsis with special reference to group B streptococci and pharmacokinetics. Pediatr Infect Dis J 1986; 4(Suppl):S186.

125. Haque KN, Zaidi MH, Bahakim K: IgM-enriched intravenous immunoglobulin therapy in neonatal sepsis. Am J Dis Child 1988;142:1293.

126. Wolff SN, Fay JW, Herzig RH, et al: High-dose weekly intravenous immunoglobulin to prevent infections in patients undergoing autologous bone marrow transplantation or severe myelosuppressive therapy: A study of the American Bone Marrow Transplant Group. Ann Intern Med 1993;118:937.

127. Reed E, Bowden R, Dandliker P, et al: Efficacy of cytomegalovirus immunoglobulin in marrow transplant patients with cytomegalovirus pneumonia. J Infect Dis 1987;156:641.

128. Sullivan KM, Storek J, Kopecky JK, et al: A controlled trial of long-term administration of intravenous immunoglobulin to prevent late infection and chronic graft-vs.-host disease after marrow transplantation: Clinical outcome and effect on subsequent immune recovery. Biol Blood Marrow Transplant 1996;2:44.

129. Ruutu T, Ljungman P, Brinch L, et al: No prevention of cytomegalovirus infection by anti-cytomegalovirus hyperimmune globulin in seronegative bone marrow transplant recipients. The Nordic BMT Group. Bone Marrow Transplant 1997;19:233.

130. Winston DJ, Ho WG, Bartoni K, et al: Intravenous immunoglobulin and CMV-seronegative blood products for prevention of CMV infection and disease in bone marrow transplant recipients. Bone Marrow Transplant 1993;12:283.

131. Bass EB, Powe NR, Goodman SN, et al: Efficacy of immune globulin in preventing complications of bone marrow transplantation: A meta-analysis. Bone Marrow Transplant 1993;12:273.

132. Messori A, Rampazzo R, Scroccaro G, et al: Efficacy of hyperimmune anticytomegalovirus immunoglobulins for the prevention of cytomegalovirus infection in recipients of allogeneic bone marrow transplantation: A meta-analysis. Bone Marrow Transplant 1994;13:163.

133. Verdonck LF, Degast GC, Dekker AW: Treatment of cytomegalovirus pneumonia after bone marrow transplantation with cytomegalovirus immunoglobulin combined with gancyclovir. Bone Marrow Transplant 1989;4:187.

134. Ljumgan P, Englehard D, Link H, et al: Treatment of interstitial pneumonitis due to cytomegalovirus with gancyclovir and intravenous immune globulin: Experience of European Bone Marrow Transplant Group. Clin Infect Dis 1992;14:831.

135. Emmanuel D, Cunningham I, Jules-Elysee K, et al: Cytomegalovirus pneumonia after bone marrow transplantation successfully treated with the combination of gancyclovir and high-dose intravenous immune globulin. Ann Intern Med 1988;109:777.

136. Winston DJ, Ho WG, Lin C-H, et al: Intravenous immune globulin for prevention of cytomegalovirus infection and interstitial pneumonia after bone marrow transplantation. Ann Intern Med 1987;106:12.

137. Sullivan KM, Kopecky KJ, Jocom J, et al: Immunomodulatory and antimicrobial efficacy of intravenous immunoglobulin in bone marrow transplantation. N Engl J Med 1990;323:705.

138. Snydman DR, Werner BG, Heinze-Lacey B, et al: Use of cytomegalovirus immune globulin to prevent cytomegalovirus disease in renal transplant patients. N Engl J Med 1987;317:1049.

139. Steinmueller DR, Graneto D, Swift C, et al: Use of intravenous immunoglobulin prophylaxis for primary cytomegalovirus infection post living-related-donor renal transplantation. Transplant Proc 1989;21:2069.

140. Bell R, Shei A, McDonald JA, et al: The role of CMV immune prophylaxis in patients at risk for primary CMV infection following orthotopic liver transplantation. Transplant Proc 1989;21:3781.

141. Conti DJ, Freed BM, Gruber SA, et al: Prophylaxis of primary cytomegalovirus disease in renal transplant recipients: A trial of gancyclovir vs immunoglobulin. Arch Surg 1994;129:443.

142. Dunn DL, Gillingham KJ, Kramer MA, et al: A prospective randomized study of acyclovir versus ganciclovir plus human immune globulin prophylaxis of cytomegalovirus infection after solid organ transplantation. Transplantation 1994;57:876.

143. Falagas ME, Snydman DR, Ruthazer R, et al: Cytomegalovirus immune globulin (CMVIG) prophylaxis is associated with increased survival after orthotopic liver transplantation: The Boston Center for Liver Transplantation CMVIG Study Group. Clin Transplant 1997;11:432.

144. Snydman DR, Werner BG, Dougherty NN, et al: Cytomegalovirus immune globulin prophylaxis in liver transplantation: A randomized, double-blind, placebo-controlled trial. The Boston Center for Liver Transplantation CMVIG Study Group. Ann Intern Med 1993;119:984.

145. Gould FK, Freeman R, Taylor CE, et al: Prophylaxis and management of cytomegalovirus pneumonitis after lung transplantation: A review of experience in one center. J Heart Lung Transplant 1993;12:695.

146. Smyth PL, Scott JP, Higenbottam TW, et al: Experience of cytomegalovirus infection by ganciclovir in heart-lung transplant recipients. Transplant Proc 1990;22:1820.

147. Mouthon L, Kaveri SV, Spalter SH, et al: Mechanisms of action of intravenous immune globulin in immune-mediated diseases. Clin Exp Immunol 1996;104:3.

148. Stiehm ER: Recent progress in the use if intravenous immunoglobulin. Curr Probl Pediatr 1992;22:335.

149. Hara T, Miyazaki S, Yoshida N, et al: High doses of gammaglobulin and methylprednisolone therapy for idiopathic purpura in children. Eur J Pediatr 1985;144:240.

150. Fehr J, Hofmann V, Kappeler U: Transient reversal of thrombocytopenia in idiopathic thrombocytopenic purpura by high-dose intravenous gamma globulin. N Engl J Med 1982;306:154.

151. Kerkman SA, Lee ML, Gale RP: Clinical uses of intravenous immunoglobulins. Semin Hematol 1988;25:140.

152. Bussel JB, Pham LC, Aledort L, et al: Maintenance treatment of adults with chronic refractory immune thrombocytopenic purpura using repeated intravenous infusions of gammaglobulin. Blood 1988;72:121.

153. Imholz B, Imbach P, Baumgartner C, et al: Intravenous immuno-globulin (i.v. IgG) for previously treated acute or for chronic idiopathic thrombocytopenic purpura (ITP) in childhood: A prospective multicenter study. Blut 1988;56:63.

154. Barios NJ, Humbert JR, McNeil J: Treatment of acute idiopathic thrombocytopenic purpura with high-dose methylprednisolone and immunoglobulin. Acta Haematol 1993;89:6.

155. Rosthoj S, Nielsen S, Karup F, et al: Randomized trial comparing intravenous immunoglobulin with methylprednisolone pulse therapy in acute idiopathic thrombocytopenic purpura. Acta Paediatr 1996;85:910.

156. Oxzoylu S, Sayli TR, Ozturk G: Oral megadose methylprednisolone versus intravenous immunoglobulin for acute childhood idiopathic thrombocytopenic purpura. Pediatr Hematol Oncol 1993;10:317.

157. Warrier I, Bussel JB, Valdez L, et al: Safety and efficacy of low-dose intravenous immune globulin (IVIG) treatment for infants and children with immune thrombocytopenic purpura. J Pediatr Hematol Oncol 1997;19:197.

158. Imbach P: Immune thrombocytopenic purpura and intravenous immunoglobulin. Cancer 1991;68:1422.

159. Blanchette VS, Luke B, Andrew M, et al: A prospective, randomized trial of high-dose intravenous immune globulin G therapy, oral prednisone therapy, and no therapy in childhood acute immune thrombocytopenic purpura. J Pediatr 1993;123:989.

160. Blanchette V, Imbach P, Andrew M, et al: Randomized trial of intra-venous immunoglobulin G, intravenous anti-D, and oral prednisone in childhood acute immune thrombocytopenic purpura. Lancet 1994;344:703.

161. Godeau B, Lesage S, Divine M, et al: Treatment of adult chronic autoimmune thrombocytopenic purpura with repeated high-dose intravenous immunoglobulin. Blood 1993;82:1415.

162. Scaradavou A, Woo B, Woloski BMR, et al: Intravenous anti-D treatment of immune thrombocytopenic purpura: Experience in 272 patients. Blood 1997;89:2689.

163. George JN, Woolf SH, Raskob GE, et al: Idiopathic thrombocytopenic purpura: A practical guideline developed for the American Society of Hematology. Blood 1996;88:30.

164. Boehlen F, Kaplan C, de Moerloose P: Severe neonatal alloimmune thrombocytopenia due to anti-HPA-3a. Vox Sang 1998;74:201.

165. Giers G, Hoch J, Bauer H, et al: Therapy with intravenous immunoglobulin G (ivIgG) during pregnancy for fetal alloimmune (HPA-1a(Zwa)) thrombocytopenic purpura. Prenat Diagn 1996;16:495.

166. Lucas GF, Pittman SJ, Davies S, et al: Post-transfusion purpura (PTP) associated with anti-HPA-1a, anti-HPA-2b and anti-HPA-3a antibodies. Transfus Med 1997;7:295.

167. Gonzalez J, Schwartz J, Gerstein G, et al: Case report: Post-transfusion purpura. N J Med 1996;93:101.

168. Nathan FE, Herman JH, Keashen-Schnell M, et al: Anti-Bak(a) neonatal alloimmune thrombocytopenia: Possible prevention by intravenous immunoglobulin. Pediatr Hematol Oncol 1994;11:325.

169. Nugent DJ: Alloimmunization to platelet antigens. Semin Hematol 1992;29:83.

170. Krutzberg J, Dunsmore KP: IVIG therapy in neonatal isoimmune thrombocytopenic purpura and alloimmunization thrombocytopenia. Clin Rev Allergy 1992;10:73.

171. Jahnke L, Applebaum S, Sherman LA, et al: An evaluation of intra-venous immunoglobulin in the treatment of human immunodeficiency virus–associated thrombocytopenia. Transfusion 1994;34:795.

172. Rarick MU, Montgomery T, Groshen S, et al: Intravenous immunoglobulin in the treatment of human immunodeficiency virus-related thrombocytopenia. Am J Hematol 1991;38:261.

173. Burns ER, Lee V, Rubinstein A: Treatment of septic thrombocytopenia with immune globulin. J Clin Immunol 1991;11:363.

174. Shulman NR, Reid DM: Platelet immunology. In Coleman RW, Hirsh J, Marder VJ, Salzman EW (eds): Hemostasis and Thrombosis. Philadelphia, JB Lippincott, 1994, p 414.

175. Gabriel A, Lassnigg A, Kurz M, et al: Post-transfusion purpura due to HPA-1a immunization in a male patient: Response to subsequent multiple HPA-1a–incompatible red-cell transfusions. Transfus Med 1995;5:131.

176. Berney SE, Metcalfe P, Wathen NC, et al: Post-transfusion purpura responding to high dose intravenous IgG: Further observations on pathogenesis. Br J Haematol 1986;61:627.

177. Becker T, Panzer S, Mass D, et al: High-dose intravenous immunoglobulin for post-transfusion purpura. Br J Haematol 1985;61:149.

178. Meller-Eckhardt C, Kiefel V: High-dose IgG for post-tranfusion purpura: Revisited. Blut 1988;57:163.

179. Macguire WA, Hsin Yang H, Bruno E, et al: Treatment of antibody-mediated pure red-cell aplasia with high-dose intravenous gammaglobulin. N Engl J Med 1987;137:1004.

180. Kurtzman G, Frickhofen N, Kimball J, et al: Pure red-cell aplasia of 10 years' duration due to persistent parvovirus B19 infection and its cure with immunoglobulin therapy. N Engl J Med 1989;321:519.

181. Clauvell JP, Vainchenker W, Herrera A, et al: Treatment of pure red cell aplasia by high dose intravenous immunoglobulins. Br J Haematol 1983;55:380.

182. Hilgartner MW, Bussel J: Use of intravenous gamma globulin for the treatment of autoimmune neutropenia of childhood and autoimmune hemolytic anemia. Am J Med 1987;83:25.

183. Flores G, Cunningham-Rundles C, Newland AC, et al: Efficacy of intravenous immunoglobulin in the treatment of autoimmune hemolytic anemia: Results in 73 patients. Am J Hematol 1993;44:237.

184. Kapoor N, Hvizdala E, Good RA: High dose intravenous gammaglobulin as an approach to treatment of antibody mediated pancytopenia. Br J Haematol 1988;69:98.

185. Sandowitz PD, Dobowy RL: Intravenous immunoglobulin in the treatment of aplastic anemia. Am J Pediatr Hematol Oncol 1990;12:198.

186. Fischer P, Uttenreuther-Fischer MM: Kawasaki disease: Update on diagnosis, treatment, and a still controversial etiology. Pediatr Hematol Oncol 1996;13:487.

187. Morikawa Y, Ohashi Y, Harada K, et al: A multicenter, randomized, controlled trial of intravenous gamma globulin therapy in children with acute Kawasaki disease. Acta Paediatr Jpn 1994;36:347.

188. Onouchi Z, Yanagisawa M, Hirayama T, et al: Optimal dosage and differences in therapeutic efficacy of IGIV in Kawasaki disease. Acta Paediatr Jpn 1995;37:40.

189. Durongpisitkul K, Gururaj VJ, Park JM, et al: The prevention of coronary artery aneurysm in Kawasaki disease: A meta-analysis on the efficacy of aspirin and immunoglobulin treatment. Pediatrics 1995;96:1057.

190. Hahn AF, Bolton CF, Zochodne D, et al: Intravenous immunoglobulin treatment in chronic inflammatory demyelinating polyneuropathy: A double-blind, placebo-controlled, cross-over study. Brain 1996;119:1067.

191. Thompson N, Choudhary P, Hughes RAC, et al: A novel trial design to study the effect of intravenous immunoglobulin in chronic inflammatory demyelinating polyradiculoneuropathy. J Neurol 1996;243:280.

192. Vermeulen M, van Doorn PA, Brand A, et al: Intravenous immunoglobulin treatment in patients with chronic inflammatory demyelinating polyneuropathy: A double blind, placebo controlled study. J Neurol Neurosurg Psychiatry 1993;56:36.

193. Van den Berg LH, Kerkhoff H, Oey PL, et al: Treatment of multifocal motor neuropathy with high dose intravenous immunoglobulins: A double blind, placebo controlled study. J Neurol Neurosurg Psychiatry 1995;59:248.

194. Jackson MC, Godwin-Austen RB, Whiteley AM: High-dose intravenous immunoglobulin in the treatment of Guillain-Barré syndrome: A preliminary open study. J Neurol 1993;240:51.

195. Dutch Guillain-Barré Study Group: Treatment of Guillain-Barré syndrome with high-dose immune globulins combined with methylprednisolone: A pilot study. Ann Neurol 1994;35:749.

196. Bril V, Ilse WK, Pearse R, et al: Pilot trial of immunoglobulin versus plasma exchange in patients with Guillain-Barré syndrome. Neurology 1996;46:100.

197. Gürses N, Uysal S, Çetinkaya F, et al: Intravenous immunoglobulin treatment in children with Guillain-Barré syndrome. Scand J Infect Dis 1995;27:241.

198. Haupt WF, Rosenow F, van der Ven C, et al: Sequential treatment of Guillain-Barré syndrome with extracorporeal elimination and intravenous immunoglobulin. J Neurol Sci 1996;137:145.

199. Hughes RAC, Swan AV, Cornblath DR, et al: Plasma Exchange/Sandoglobulin Guillain-Barré Syndrome Trial Group: Randomized trial of plasma exchange, intravenous immunoglobulin,

200. and combined treatments in Guillain-Barré syndrome. Lancet 1997;349:225.

201. Valensise H, Vaquero E, De Carolis C, et al: Normal fetal growth in women with antiphospholipid syndrome treated with high-dose intravenous immunoglobulin (IVIG). Prenat Diagn 1995;15:509.

201. Rehder H, Mehraein Y, Schwinger E, et al: The German RSA/IVIG Group: Intravenous immunoglobulin in the prevention of recurrent miscarriage. Br J Obstet Gynaecol 1994;101:1072.

202. Christiansen OB, Mathiesen O, Husth M, et al: Placebo-controlled trial of treatment of unexplained secondary recurrent spontaneous abortions and recurrent late spontaneous abortions with i.v. immunoglobulin. Hum Reprod 1995;10:2690.

203. Kiprov DD, Nachtigall RD, Weaver RC, et al: The use of intravenous immunoglobulin in recurrent pregnancy loss associated with combined alloimmune and autoimmune abnormalities. Am J Reprod Immunol 1996;36:228.

204. Marzusch K, Dietl J, Klein R, et al: Recurrent first trimester spontaneous abortion associated with antiphospholipid antibodies: A pilot study of treatment with intravenous immunoglobulin. Acta Obstet Gynaecol Scand 1996;75:922.

205. Spinnato JA, Clark AI, Pierangeli SS, et al: Intravenous immuno-globulin therapy for the antiphospholipid syndrome in pregnancy. Am J Obstet Gynecol 1995;172:690.

206. Coulam CB: Alternative treatment to lymphocyte immunization for treatment of recurrent spontaneous abortion. Immunotherapy with intravenous immunoglobulin for treatment of recurrent pregnancy loss: American experience. Am J Reprod Immunol 1994;32:286.

207. Mueller-Eckhardt G: Alternative treatment to lymphocyte immunization for the treatment of recurrent spontaneous abortion. Immunotherapy with intravenous immunoglobulin for prevention of recurrent pregnancy loss: European experience. Am J Reprod Immunol 1994;32:281.

208. Sansome A, Dubowitz V: Intravenous immunoglobulin in juvenile dermatomyositis: Four year review of nine cases. Arch Dis Child 1995;72:25.

209. Cherin P, Piette JC, Wechsler B, et al: Intravenous gamma globulin as first line therapy in polymyositis and dermatomyositis: An open study in 11 adult patients. J Rheumatol 1994;21:1092.

210. Basta M, Dalakas MC: High-dose intravenous immunoglobulin exerts its beneficial effect in patients with dermatomyositis by blocking endomysil deposition of activated complement fragments. J Clin Invest 1994;94:1729.

211. Dalakas MC, Sonies B, Dambrosia J, et al: Treatment of inclusion-body myositis with IVIg: A double-blind, placebo-controlled study. Neurology 1997;48:712.

212. Amato AA, Barohn RJ, Jackson CE, et al: Inclusion body myositis: Treatment with intravenous immunoglobulin. Neurology 1994;44:1516.

213. Soueidan SA, Dalakas MC: Treatment of inclusion-body myositis with high-dose intravenous immunoglobulin. Neurology 1993;43:876.

214. Sussman GL, Pruzanski W: Treatment of inflammatory myopathy with intravenous gamma globulin. Curr Opin Rheumatol 1995;7:510.

215. Lafferty TE, Smith JB, Schuster SJ, et al: Treatment of acquired factor VIII inhibitor using intravenous immunoglobulin in two patients with systemic lupus erythematosus. Arthritis Rheum 1997;40:775.

216. Sultan Y, Kazatchkine MD, Maisonneuve P, et al: Anti-idiotypic suppression of autoantibodies to factor VIII (antihemophilic factor) by high-dose intravenous immunoglobulin. Lancet 1984;2:765.

217. Sultan Y, Kazatchkine MD, Nydegger U, et al: Intravenous immunoglobulin in the treatment of spontaneously acquired factor VIII:C inhibitors. Am J Med 1991;91:35.

218. Bouvry P, Recloux P: Acquired hemophilia. Haematologica 1994;79:550.

219. Crenier L, Ducobu J, des Grottes J-M, et al: Low response to high-dose intravenous immunoglobulin in the treatment of acquired factor VIII inhibitor. Br J Haematol 1996;95:750.

220. Silverman ED, Cawkwell GD, Lovell DJ, et al: Intravenous immunoglobulin in the treatment of systemic juvenile rheumatoid arthritis: A randomized placebo controlled trial. J Rheumatol 1994;21:2353.

221. Uziel Y, Laxer RM, Schneider R, et al: Intravenous immunoglobulin therapy in systemic onset juvenile rheumatoid arthritis: A followup study. J Rheumatol 1996;23:910.

222. Kanik KS, Yarboro CH, Naparstek Y, et al: Failure of low-dose intravenous immunoglobulin therapy to suppress disease activity in

patients with treatment-refractory rheumatoid arthritis. Arthritis Rheum 1996;39:1027.

223. Krendel DA, Costigan DA, Hopkins LC: Successful treatment of neuropathies in patients with diabetes mellitus. Arch Neurol 1995;52:1053.

224. Colagiuri S, Leong GM, Thayer Z, et al: Intravenous immunoglobulin therapy for autoimmune diabetes mellitus. Clin Exp Rheumatol 1996;14(Suppl):S93.

225. Heldrich FJ, Minkin S, Gatdula CL: Intravenous immunoglobulin in Henoch-Schönlein purpura: A case study. Md Med J 1993;42:577.

226. Jayne DRW, Lockwood CM: Intravenous immunoglobulin as sole therapy for systemic vasculitis. Br J Rheumatol 1996;35:1150.

227. Richter C, Schnabel A, Csernok E, et al: Treatment of anti-neutrophilic cytoplasmic antibody (ANCA)–associated systemic vasculitis with high-dose intravenous immunoglobulin. Clin Exp Immunol 1995;101:2.

228. Richter C, Schnabel A, Csernok E, et al: Treatment of Wegener's granulomatosis with intravenous immunoglobulin. In Gross WL (ed): ANCA-Associated Vasculitides: Immunological and Clinical Aspects. New York, Plenum Press, 1993.

229. Jayne DRW, Lockwood CM: Pooled intravenous immunoglobulin in the management of systemic vasculitis. In Gross WL (ed): ANCA-Associated Vasculitides: Immunological and Clinical Aspects. New York, Plenum Press, 1993.

230. van Engelen BGM, Renier WO, Weemaes CMR, et al: Cerebrospinal fluid examination in cryptogenic West and Lennox-Gastaut syndrome before and after intravenous immunoglobulin administration. Epilepsy Res 1994;18:139.

231. Gross-Tsur V, Shalev RS, Kazir E, et al: Intravenous high-dose gammaglobulins for intractable childhood epilepsy. Acta Neurol Scand 1993;88:204.

232. van Engelen BGM, Renier WO, Weemaes CMR, et al: High-dose intravenous immunoglobulin treatment in cryptogenic West and Lennox-Gastaut syndrome: An add-on study. Eur J Paediatr 1994;153:762.

233. van Rijckevorsel-Harmant K, Delire M, Schmitz-Moorman W, et al: Treatment of refractory epilepsy with intravenous immunoglobulins: Results of the first double-blind/dose finding clinical study. Int J Clin Lab Res 1994;24:162.

234. Fazekas F, Deisenhammer F, Strasser-Fuchs S, et al. Randomized placebo-controlled trial of monthly intravenous immunoglobulin therapy in relapsing-remitting multiple sclerosis. Lancet 1997;349:589.

235. Achiron A, Rotstein Z, Noy S, et al: Intravenous immunoglobulin treatment in the prevention of childbirth-associated acute exacerbations in multiple sclerosis: A pilot study. J Neurol 1996;243:25.

236. Achiron A, Cohen IR, Lider O, et al: Intravenous immunoglobulin treatment in multiple sclerosis. Isr J Med Sci 1995;31:7.

237. Noseworthy JH, O'Brien PC, van Engelen BGM, et al: Intravenous immunoglobulin therapy in multiple sclerosis: Progress from remyelinating in the Theiler's virus model to a randomized, double-blind placebo-controlled clinical trial. J Neurol 1994;36(Suppl):S80.

238. Rowe KS: Double-blind randomized controlled trial to assess the efficacy of intravenous gammaglobulin for the management of chronic fatigue syndrome in adolescents. J Psychiatr Res 1997;31:133.

239. Vollmer-Conna U, Hickie I, Hadzi-Pavlovic D, et al: Intravenous immunoglobulin is ineffective in the treatment of patients with chronic fatigue syndrome. Am J Med 1997;103:38.

240. Contreras M, de Silva M: The prevention and management of haemolytic disease of the newborn. J R Soc Med 1994;87:256.

241. Newland AC, Macey MG: Immune thrombocytopenia and Fc receptor-mediated phagocyte function. Ann Hematol 1994;69:61.

242. Hartwell EA: Use of Rh immune globulin: ASCP practice parameter. Am J Clin Pathol 1998;110:281.

243. Peterec SM: Management of neonatal Rh Disease. Clin Perinatol 1995;22:561.

244. Rho(D) Immune Globulin Intravenous (Human): WinRho SD package insert. Winnipeg, Canada, Cangene, 1997.

245. Smith N: Intravenous anti-D immunoglobulin in the management of immune thrombocytopenic purpura. Curr Opin Hematol 1996;3:498.

246. Centers for Disease Control: Postexposure prophylaxis of hepatitis B. MMWR Morb Mortal Wkly Rep 1984;33:285.

247. Centers for Disease Control: Recommendations for protection against viral hepatitis. MMWR Morb Mortal Wkly Rep 1985;34:313.

248. Brunell PA, Gershon AA: Passive immunization against varicella-zoster infections. J Infect Dis 1973;127:415.

249. McComb JA, Dwyer RC: Passive-active immunization with tetanus immune globulin (human). N Engl J Med 1963;268:857.

250. Rubbo SD, Suri JC: Passive immunization against tetanus with human immune globulin. BMJ 1962;2:79.

251. Centers for Disease Control: Rabies prevention United States 1984: Recommendations of the Immunization Practices Advisory Committee. MMWR Morb Mortal Wkly Rep 1984;33:393.

252. Barnes GL, Doyle LW, Hewson PH, et al: A randomized trial of oral gammaglobulin in low-birth-weight infants infected with rotavirus. Lancet 1982;1:1371.

253. Losonsky GA, Johnson J, Winkelstein JA, et al: Oral administration of human serum immunoglobulin in immunodeficient patients with viral gastroenteritis: A pharmacokinetic and functional analysis. J Clin Invest 1985;76:2362.

254. Eibl MM, Wolf HM, Fumkranz H, et al: Prevention of necrotizing enterocolitis in low-birth-weight infants by IgA-IgG feeding. N Engl J Med 1988;319:1.

255. Borowitz SM, Saulsbury FT: Treatment of chronic cryptosporidial infection with orally administered human serum immune globulin. J Pediatr 1991;119:593.

256. Melamed I, Griffiths AM, Roifman CM: Benefit of oral immune globulin therapy in patients with immunodeficiency and chronic diarrhea. J Pediatr 1991;3:486.

257. Stiehm ER: Passive immunization. In Feigen RD, Cherry JD (eds): Textbook of Pediatric Infectious Diseases, 3rd ed. Philadelphia, WB Saunders, 1992, p 2261.

258. Lichtiger B, Rogge K: Spurious serologic test results in patients receiving infusions of intravenous immune gamma globulin. Arch Pathol Lab Med 1991;115:467.

259. Comenzo RL, Malachowski ME, Meissner HC, et al: Immune hemolysis disseminated intravascular coagulation and serum sickness after large doses of immunoglobulin given intravenously for Kawasaki's disease. J Paediatr Child Health 1992;120:926.

260. Nicholls MD, Cummins JC, Davies VJ, et al: Haemolysis induced by intravenously administered immunoglobulin. Med J Aust 1989;150:404.

261. Bjorkander J, Hammarstrom L, Smith CIE, et al: Immunoglobulin prophylaxis in patients with antibody deficiency syndromes an anti-IgA antibodies. J Clin Immunol 1987;7:8.

262. Burks AW, Sampson HA, Buckley RH: Anaphylactic reactions after gammaglobulin administration in patients with hypogamma-globulinemia: Detection of IgE antibodies to IgA. N Engl J Med 1986;314:560.

263. Gales BJ, Erstad BL: Adverse reactions to human serum albumin. Ann Pharmacother 1993;27:87.

264. Finlayson JS: Albumin products. Semin Thromb Haemost 1980;6:85.

265. Chetrit EB, Putterman C: Transient neutropenia induced by intravenous immune globulin [letter]. N Engl J Med 1992;326:270.

266. Cantu TG, Hoehn-Saric EW, Burgess KM, et al: Acute renal failure associated with immunoglobulin therapy. Am J Kidney Dis 1995;25:228.

267. Tan E, Hajinazarian M, Bay W, et al: Acute renal failure resulting from intravenous immunoglobulin therapy. Arch Neurol 1993;50:137.

268. Winward DB, Brophy MT: Acute renal failure after administration of intravenous immunoglobulin: Review of the literature and case report. Pharmacotherapy 1995;15:765.

269. Sekul E, Cupler E, Dalakas M: Aseptic meningitis associated with high-dose intravenous immunoglobulin therapy: Frequency and risk factors. Ann Intern Med 1994;121:259.

270. Steere AC: Adverse reactions to albumin caused by bacterial contamination. In Sgouris JT, Rene A (eds): Proceedings of the Workshop on Albumin, 1975. Publication no. (NIH) 76-925. Bethesda, MD, National Heart and Lung Institutes of Health, United States Department of Health, Education and Welfare, 1976, p 278.

271. Hochstein HD, Seligmann EB: Microbial contamination in albumin. In Sgouris JT, Rene A (eds): Proceedings of the Workshop on Albumin, 1975. Publication no. (NIH) 76-925. Bethesda, MD, National Heart and Lung Institutes of Health, United States Department of Health, Education and Welfare, 1976, p 284.

272. McClelland DB: Safety of human albumin as a constituent of biologic therapeutic products. Transfusion 1998;38:690.

273. Kempf C, Jentsch P, Poirier B, et al: Virus inactivation during production of intravenous immunoglobulin. Transfusion 1991;31:423.

274. Wells MA, Wittek AE, Epstein JS, et al: Inactivation and partition of human T-cell lymphocytotropic virus type III, during ethanol fractionation of plasma. Transfusion 1986;26:210.

275. Morgenthaler JJ, Omar A: Partitioning and inactivation of viruses during isolation of albumin and immunoglobulin by cold ethanol fractionation. In Brown F (ed): Virological Safety Aspects of Plasma Derivatives. Basel, Karger, 1993, p 185.

276. Erstad BL: Viral infectivity of albumin and plasma protein fraction. Pharmacotherapy 1996;16:996.

277. Pattison CP, Klein CA, Leger RT, et al: An outbreak of type B hepatitis associated with transfusion of plasma protein fraction. Am J Epidemiol 1976;103:399.

278. Bjorkander J, Cunningham-Rundles C, Lundin P, et al: Intravenous immunoglobulin prophylaxis causing liver damage in 16 of 77 patients with hypogammaglobulinemia or IgG subclass deficiency. Am J Med 1988;84:107.

279. Lever AML, Brown D, Webster ADB, et al: Non-A non-B hepatitis occurring in agammaglobulinemic patients after intravenous immunoglobulin. Lancet 1984;2:1062.

280. William PE, Yap PL, Gillon J, et al: Transmission of non-A non-B hepatitis by pH4 treated intravenous immunoglobulin. Vox Sang 1989;57:15.

281. Rossi G, Tucci A, Cariani E, et al: Outbreak of hepatitis C virus infection in patients with hematologic disorders treated with intra-venous immunoglobulins: Different prognosis according to the immune status. Blood 1997;90:1309.

282. Taliani G, Guerra E, Rosso R, et al: Hepatitis C virus infection in hypogammaglobulinemic patients receiving long-term replacement therapy with intravenous immunoglobulin. Transfusion 1995;35:103.

283. Bjoro K, Froland SS, Yun Z, et al: Hepatitis C infection in patients with primary hypogammaglobulinemia after treatment with contaminated immune globulin. N Engl J Med 1994;331:1607.

284. Meeks EL, Beach MJ: Outbreak of hepatitis C associated with intravenous immunoglobulin administration: United States, October 1993–June 1994. MMWR Morb Mortal Wkly Rep 1994;43:505.

285. Tong MJ, El-Farra NS, Reikes AR, et al: Clinical outcomes after transfusion-associated hepatitis C. N Engl J Med 1995;332:1463.

286. Brenner B: Clinical experience with octagam, a solvent detergent (SD) virus inactivated intravenous gammaglobulin. Clin Exp Rheumatol 1996;14(Suppl):S115.

287. Chandra S, Cavanaugh JE, Lin CM, et al: Virus reduction in the preparation of intravenous immune globulin: In vitro experiments. Transfusion 1999;39:249.

Chapter 17

Platelets and Related Products

Peter L. Perrotta
Patricia T. Pisciotto
Edward L. Snyder

Platelet transfusion therapy has dramatically improved since the 1950s, when whole blood and freshly prepared platelet-rich plasma (PRP) were the only available sources of viable platelets. Technical advances made over the past several decades have greatly facilitated the collection and storage of platelet concentrates (PCs). For example, centrifugation procedures have been optimized to allow the separation of high numbers of functionally active platelets from whole blood donation. In addition, automated cell separators are now widely used to collect even larger numbers of platelets from a single donor. Nevertheless, the shelf life of platelets was extremely limited until improved storage containers and optimization of storage conditions allowed for longer (5-day) storage. Longer-duration storage was largely prohibited before the development of gas-permeable containers, based on the adverse effects of prolonged storage on platelet structure and function—the *platelet storage defect*. Attempts to extend the shelf life of room temperature–stored PCs past 5 days were, and still are, limited by the increased risk of bacterial proliferation. These limitations have encouraged investigators to develop alternative techniques to store PCs (e.g., platelet storage solutions, cryopreservation) and platelet substitutes. The latter are either derived from donor platelets or are entirely synthetic.

Platelets are commonly transfused to bleeding patients who have low numbers of circulating platelets or functionally inactive platelets. Indeed, thrombocytopenic bleeding was a major cause of death in patients with acute leukemia until PCs became widely available.[1] Today, PCs are most commonly transfused to prevent bleeding in severely thrombocytopenic patients. These "prophylactic" platelet transfusions, which are largely provided to patients who receive intensive therapies for hematologic malignant diseases and solid tumors, are largely responsible for the dramatic increase in the number of platelet transfusions since the early 1980s.[2] Despite the widespread use of platelets in clinical practice, considerable variability in platelet transfusion practices remains.[3] Part of the difficulty in developing evidence-based guidelines for platelet transfusion therapy is that the relationship between a patient's platelet count and bleeding remains only partially understood. Furthermore, the properties of transfused platelets that best correlate with hemostatic effectiveness are not fully defined. These characteristics, which are presumably related to the efficacy of platelet transfusions, are most likely affected by the techniques used to prepare and store PCs. Thus, despite efforts to standardize platelet transfusion therapy, practices are largely determined locally. In large part, these practices are heavily influenced by the availability and cost of different platelet preparations (e.g., platelets prepared from whole blood collections or harvested by apheresis).

■ Platelet Structure and Function

Platelets play a critical role in normal hemostatic processes by preserving vascular integrity and maintaining hemostasis. They accumulate at sites of vascular injury and form hemostatic plugs. Platelets also participate in clot retraction and wound healing. The effectiveness of platelet transfusion therapy is at least partially explained by the role of endogenous platelets in normal hemostasis. The innate properties of platelets are related to their unique structure, composition, and ability to respond to a variety of stimuli. Their importance in both bleeding and thrombotic conditions has been elucidated over the past several decades. Therefore, one of the goals of transfusion practice is to prepare platelets that maintain these properties during their preparation and storage.

Alternatively, novel substances that have many of the hemostatic properties of intact human platelets are being developed as potential alternatives to standard PCs.

Platelets circulate in the blood as small, anucleate, membrane-encapsulated cell fragments (Fig. 17.1). It was recognized in the early 1900s that platelets are derived from bone marrow megakaryocytes.[4] However, the overall process of platelet production, or *thrombopoiesis*, remained poorly understood.[5] Platelets appear on Wright-stained blood smears as small, oval to round, bluish-gray bodies containing small, purple-red granules. They normally range in size from 1.0 to 2.5 μm, or less than one half the diameter of a normal red blood cell (RBC). The platelet surface is covered by a thin glycocalix that contains various membrane glycoproteins (GPs), mucopolysaccharides, glycolipids, and adsorbed plasma proteins. Sialic acid residues attached to lipids and proteins impart a net negative charge to the platelet surface that may play a role in minimizing the interaction between other platelets and negatively charged endothelial cells. The folded platelet external plasma membrane forms a surface connected canalicular or collecting system that allows plasma components to enter the platelet and internal granule contents to be released. It also greatly increases the surface area of the platelet. Sodium and calcium adenosine triphosphatase (ATPase) pumps within the plasma membrane are thought to control the platelet's ionic environment.

Platelets have a discoid shape when they are in a resting state. The discoid shape is likely maintained by a network of actin filaments near the plasma membrane and a circumferential band of microtubules composed of tubule polymers and microtubule-associated proteins.[6] On activation, platelet actin can polymerize into microfilamentous bundles that contribute to change the platelet's shape. Platelets contain both organelles found in other cells (lysosomes, peroxisomes) and platelet-specific organelles (dense bodies, α granules). Electron-dense granules (dense bodies) contain storage pool adenosine diphosphate (ADP), ATP, serotonin, and a major portion of the platelet's calcium. α Granules contain various proteins including adhesive proteins (von Willebrand factor [vWF], fibrinogen, fibronectin, thrombospondin, P-selectin), anticoagulants (platelet factor 4 [PF4], β-thromboglobulins), coagulation factors (factors V, XI, XIII, protein S), and growth factors for angiogenesis and repair (platelet-derived growth factor, transforming growth factor-β, thrombospondin).[7] Each platelet contains two to seven small mitochondria that participate in oxidative metabolic processes. α Granules are the most numerous granules seen in platelets by electron microscopy. Thus, platelets contain a large array of proteins; some are taken up into α granules from plasma, whereas others are platelet specific. The most concentrated platelet-specific proteins include PF4 and members of the β-thromboglobulin family. Both these proteins can bind heparin. PF4, in particular, binds heparin with high affinity and can neutralize heparin's anticoagulant activity.[8] Other described activities of PF4 include chemotaxis for neutrophils and monocytes,[9] inhibition of megakaryocyte maturation,[10] potentiation of platelet aggregation in vitro,[11] and widespread immunomodulatory effects.[12]

The platelet plasma membrane serves two important roles in hemostasis: (1) it provides a means for cell-to-cell or cell-to-matrix interactions and (2) it furnishes a surface that enhances the fluid phase of coagulation. Like other mammalian cells, the lipid bilayer consists of phospholipids (PLs) asymmetrically arranged between the outer and inner leaflets.[13] In a resting state, the outer leaflet is composed primarily of neutral PLs (phosphatidylcholine and sphingomyelin), whereas the inner leaflet is composed of negatively charged PLs (phosphatidylserine and phosphatidylethanolamine). An ATP-dependent amino PL translocase has been identified in platelet plasma membranes that rapidly transports phosphatidylserine and phosphatidylethanolamine from the outer to the inner leaflet. Other mechanisms also help to maintain

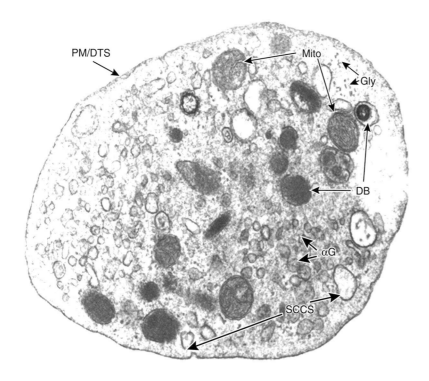

Figure 17.1 Platelets in circulation. DB, dense bodies; Gly, glycoprotein; Mito, mitochondria; PM/DTS, platelet membrane/dense tubular system; αG alpha granules; SCCS, surface connected cannulicular system.

the normal plasma membrane PL asymmetry.[14] On activation and increased intracellular calcium levels, a "flip-flop" in the normal membrane PL distribution occurs that results in an increase in phosphatidylserine and phosphatidylethanolamine exposure on the outer leaflet. This membrane alteration contributes to the procoagulant activity of platelets. Specifically, activated platelets participate in thrombin generation by providing a favorable external surface charge for the pro-thrombinase complex (X-Va) and thereby localizing fibrin generation in close proximity to the platelet plug.[15]

The most important adhesive GPs found in α granules are fibrinogen and vWF. Presumably, these substances are released after platelets accumulate at sites of vascular injury. Because megakaryocytes do not produce fibrinogen, platelets accumulate fibrinogen from plasma through processes involving the $\alpha_{IIb}\beta_3$ integrin.[16] vWF is synthesized in megakaryocytes and endothelial cells, and it is stored in platelet α granules. Platelet stores of vWF are high enough so that transfusion of platelets alone to patients with severe type 3 von Willebrand disease partially corrects their bleeding times.[17] The platelet membrane also contains certain membrane GPs, many of which function as adhesive proteins. These include the GPIb-IX-V complex, which acts as a platelet receptor for vWF in platelet adhesion and facilitates the ability of thrombin, at low concentrations, to activate platelets.[18] The $\alpha_{IIb}\beta_3$ complex, also termed GPIIb-IIIa, spans the platelet membrane and is a functional receptor for fibrinogen, vWF, fibronectin, and vitronectin.[19] The GPIa-IIa complex (GPIa-IIa, $\alpha_2\beta_1$) is the receptor for collagen,[20] and finally, GPIc-IIa (GPIc-IIa, $\alpha_5\beta_1$) is a receptor for fibronectin. The last three GPs are considered *integrins*, which are a large family of related heterodimers grouped based on their β subunit structure. P-selectin (known as CD62P, GMP-140, PADGEM) is an integral membrane protein found in α granules that becomes expressed on the surface of activated platelets after granule release.[21] Also found in Weibel-Palade bodies of endothelial cells, P-selectin is an adhesive protein that mediates the attachment of neutrophils and monocytes to activated platelets.

Platelets normally circulate in a resting state without adhering to vessel walls for approximately 7 to 10 days before they are removed, primarily in the spleen. Transfused platelets do not usually circulate for this long. Platelets rapidly respond to appropriate stimuli, such as collagen exposed on denuded endothelium, by first adhering to the subendothelial matrix. They initially undergo physical changes that include assuming a more spherical shape. Platelet membranes then form multiple extended pseudopods, an event that dramatically increases their surface area. Interaction between agonists in the microenvironment and specific receptors on the platelet surface results in the transmission of signals from the outside of the cell to the interior and generates secondary messengers that induce protein phosphorylation and the opening of ion channels.[22] The ability of platelets to aggregate on surfaces coated with type I collagen has been used in newer in vitro tests designed to measure the functional capacity of transfused platelets.[23]

Adhesion, the binding of platelets to a nonplatelet surface, is the initial event in the formation of the platelet plug. Shear forces within the vessel influence the deposition of platelets on exposed endothelium.[24] At high shear stress, as encountered within the microcirculation, the primary adhesive event is mediated by the interaction of the subendothelial-bound vWF

with the platelet GPIb receptor. vWF bound to the subendothelial matrix is believed to undergo a conformational change that exposes the binding site for the GPIb-IX-V complex.[25] The binding site for GPIb appears to reside in the A1 domain of vWF. This bond is transient, and the interaction induces a transmembrane flux of calcium ions that results in a conformational change and activation of $\alpha_{IIb}\beta_3$. Activated $\alpha_{IIb}\beta_3$ binds irreversibly to vWF to allow firm adhesion of platelets to the vessel wall. The activated $\alpha_{IIb}\beta_3$ integrin recognizes and binds to the RGD (Arg-Gly-Asp) peptide sequences of circulating vWF and fibrinogen, with resulting platelet aggregation.[26] At low shear stresses normally found in larger vessels, the role of vWF in platelet adhesion is less significant.

A critical level of ATP is required for each aspect of platelet function, including shape change, aggregation, and the release reaction. ATP is generated, in part, when glucose is metabolized by the glycolytic and oxidative pathways. As platelets are stimulated, an increase in glycolysis and Krebs cycle metabolism serves to replenish depleted ATP. Platelet adhesion does not appear to be an energy-dependent function because little ATP is consumed during primary adhesion.[27] ATP consumption mainly occurs during the early phases of platelet aggregation (e.g., shape change).[28] Adenine nucleotides present in platelets are found in two pools: ADP in the metabolic pool, which is constantly turning over, and storage pool ADP, which is found in the dense bodies and is released during platelet activation. Plasma glucose metabolism generates approximately 15% of the ATP required during normal aerobic storage, largely by glycolytic catabolism to lactate.[29] Oxidative phosphorylation, perhaps using plasma free fatty acids through β-oxidation, contributes the remaining 85%. Clearly, adequate oxygen and carbon dioxide exchange is important in maintaining aerobic capabilities of stored platelets. If deprived of oxygen, platelets increase lactate production through anaerobic glycolysis in an attempt to compensate for the loss of energy normally derived from oxidative phosphorylation. Thus, the ability to transport gases—mainly oxygen—across the platelet storage bag is critical to normal platelet metabolism and to platelet survival during storage.

■ Preparation and Storage of Platelet Concentrates

Preparation Techniques

Platelets are prepared from individual whole blood donations or are collected from a single donor by automated blood cell processors using apheresis technology.[30] Blood is drawn through wide-bore, siliconized needles to minimize platelet and clotting factor activation, and it is immediately mixed with anticoagulant. Mechanical devices are available that mix blood with anticoagulant as it is withdrawn and monitor collection volume.[31] PCs are prepared from whole blood using either the buffy coat (BC) method or the PRP method (Fig. 17.2). The BC method is favored in Europe, whereas the PRP technique is preferred in North America. In the PRP method, whole blood is first spun at a low speed (2200×g) for 3 to 4 minutes within 8 hours of collection. The resulting PRP is then spun at a higher speed (4000×g) for 5 minutes to pellet the platelets. All but about 60 mL of PRP is removed, and the pellet is left undisturbed for about 1 hour.[32] The pellet is then resuspended by gentle kneading of the bag or by

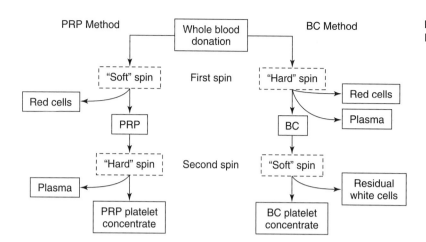

Figure 17.2 Preparation of platelet concentrates. BC, buffy coat; PRP, platelet-rich plasma.

placing the unit on a platelet agitator.[33] Generally, the platelets smoothly resuspend within several hours, after which they are stored under continuous gentle agitation. Research has shown that using a hard spin first to spin the platelets into a BC on a cushion of RBCs and then using a slow spin to isolate the platelets from the separated BC will yield a platelet product with less evidence of in vitro activation.[34] It is unclear whether differences in the properties of PCs and BC platelets affect in vivo survival and efficacy. Earlier studies suggested that 1-hour and 24-hour platelet increments were similar after transfusion of either product.[35] A more recent study comparing post-transfusion recovery and survival of radiolabeled PCs prepared by the BC and PRP methods suggested equivalent in vitro and in vivo activity.[36] After 5 days of storage, however, this preparative technique does not appear to offer better in vivo survival or functional characteristics than seen with platelets made by a soft-spin followed by a hard-spin PRP method.

Anticoagulant and Preservative Solutions

Platelets are prepared from whole blood drawn into one of several anticoagulant-preservative solutions, the most common being citrate-phosphate-dextrose solutions (CPD, CP2D) and CPD with adenine (CPDA-1). Citrate anticoagulates blood based on its ability to chelate calcium and thus inhibit the coagulation cascade. Phosphate serves as a buffer and dextrose as a source of energy. Adenine, which improves RBC survival by increasing cellular ATP levels, serves no purpose in platelet storage. Ethylene diamine tetra-acetic acid (EDTA) cannot be used because it causes platelet structural changes associated with reduced in vivo viability and is toxic to humans. Heparin is not an acceptable alternative because it activates platelets and causes them to clump. It also causes systemic anticoagulation through its effect on antithrombin. The amount of citrate in the CPD or CPDA-1 preservative does not generally produce systemic anticoagulation or hypocalcemia in blood recipients because it is quickly metabolized to bicarbonate in the liver. Apheresis-derived platelets are prepared in ACD-A (citric acid, trisodium citrate, dextrose) preservative using automated cell collectors. Citric acid is used to provide a lower pH. In some apheresis systems, platelets are collected as PRP and do not require resuspension, whereas other systems yield a concentrated platelet pellet that must be resuspended. Apheresis platelets are stored in a manner similar to that of random-donor platelets.

Although platelets stored in citrated plasma are satisfactory for clinical use, several investigators have evaluated other solutions that could extend the shelf life of PCs or improve their capacity to circulate in vivo after infusion.[37] Most alternatives studied or under development are composed of buffered salt solutions containing various additives such as acetate and gluconate.[38, 39] Glucose-free crystalloid solutions do not appear to maintain concentrate pH and are associated with reduced in vivo recovery after 5 days of storage.[40] Most studies have evaluated storage media alternatives in PRP PCs. However, synthetic storage medium has also been examined for stored BC-derived platelets.[34, 41] Other investigators have suggested placing various additives in the platelet storage bag that inhibit platelet and coagulation factor activation such as prostaglandin E₁, theophylline, aprotinin, and hirudin.[42] Although platelet shelf life can possibly be extended with these additives, the potential for harmful side effects, especially in infants and pregnant women, has slowed their commercial development. Moreover, these solutions could not be deployed to extend the shelf life of stored PCs without the availability of methods to detect or retard bacterial proliferation.

Storage Temperature

Liquid PCs were originally stored at 4°C until the late 1960s, when it was discovered that products stored at room temperature had longer in vivo survival and greater hemostatic efficacy than those stored at the colder temperature.[43–45] In fact, the shelf life of liquid platelets stored at 22°C was extended to 7 days in the 1980s, but it was later reduced to the current limit of 5 days because of concerns of bacterial proliferation and high transfusion reaction rates. The optimal platelet storage temperature appears to be 20°C to 24°C with continuous gentle agitation. Although colder storage could slow bacterial growth, platelets stored in the cold become activated and lose their normal spherical shape.[46] The mechanism for these changes may be related to the release of calcium ions from platelet dense bodies or the influx of calcium across the platelet membrane, with resulting actin filament assembly and subsequently, platelet activation.[47, 48] Membrane lipid phase transitions (liquid crystalline to gel) that occur when platelets are cooled to 4°C also negatively affect platelet membrane integrity.[49]

If changes in the platelet cytoskeleton can be prevented, long-term storage of liquid platelets could become more feasible. Platelets treated with cytochalasin B, an inhibitor of new actin filament assembly, do not develop pseudopods or undergo spreading when they are cooled to 4°C.[50] Human platelets stored for 21 days at 4°C with EGTA-AM (egtazic acid), a cytoplasmic calcium chelator, and cytochalasin B remain responsive to ADP and thrombin in the presence of exogenous calcium. Other strategies have been developed to allow preservation of platelet morphology and function during cold storage. These include trehalose, a disaccharide used during freeze-drying, and the antifreeze GPs. The latter proteins are isolated from fish that have adapted to survive in cold temperatures found in the polar regions. Antifreeze GPs have been shown to reduce platelet activation that occurs when human platelets are stored in the cold.[46] Despite these observations, the future role of cold stored platelets in clinical transfusion practice remains unclear.

Storage Containers

Plastic bags originally used to store PCs, composed of polyvinyl chloride (PVC) containing a 2-diethylhexyl phthalate (DEHP) plasticizer, did not permit storage of platelets beyond 3 days. The walls of such plastic bags did not allow adequate gas exchange and oxygen for cells to sustain aerobic metabolism. After 3 days of storage, anaerobic metabolism produced enough lactic acid that the pH of concentrates routinely fell to less than 6.0. These changes markedly reduced in vivo platelet recovery and survival.[29, 51, 52] Thus, the importance of oxygen-permeable platelet storage bags was recognized during the earliest years of platelet therapy. Entrance of oxygen into the storage bag allows platelets to maintain energy metabolism through mitochondrial oxidative phosphorylation. If oxygen supply is insufficient, platelets, like other cells, channel metabolism through anaerobic gly-colytic pathways. This pathway produces large amounts of lactic acid, which reacts with the bicarbonate buffer in the plasma. When bicarbonate is exhausted, at levels of 20 to 25 mmol/L of lactic acid, a rapid reduction in pH and a loss of platelet viability occur.

These untoward effects can be ameliorated by storing platelets in gas-permeable storage bags that permit the influx of oxygen and the efflux of carbon dioxide. It was later found that the pH of PC can be adequately maintained for 5 days by storing 50 to 65 mL of PC in more gas-permeable blood bags made of either PVC with a trimellitate, non-DEHP plasticizer such as TOTM (Fenwal PL-1240, Deerfield, Il)[53] or blow-molded polyolefin (Fenwal PL-732).[54] Other second-generation platelet storage bags were composed of thin-film PVC with a 2-DEHP plasticizer (XT-612, Terumo, Somerset, NJ) and PVC with a citrate-based non-DEHP plasticizer (butyryl-tri-hexyl citrate [BTHC], Fenwal PL-2209). The latter compound, PL-2209, allows storage of 5 to 7×10^{11} platelets per bag in 400 mL of plasma for 5 days at 20°C to 24°C with acceptable in vitro and in vivo storage characteristics.[55]

Despite the use of these containers since the 1950s, concerns remain regarding the toxicity of storage bags composed of PVC plastic with a DEHP plasticizer. Specifically, the potential adverse effects of administering quantities of DEHP plasticizer that were leached out into the blood product and were subsequently transfused were actively investigated.[56–58] These concerns, which include the potential carcinogenicity of DEHP and its mono-ethylhexyl phthalate (MEHP) metabolite, led to the development of various

alternative plasticizers used in blood storage containers.[59, 60] Animal model studies demonstrated various forms of DEHP toxicity, including reduced fertility, testicular atrophy, terato-genesis, and hepatic enlargement.[61, 62] Other investigators demonstrated immuno-globulin E antibodies specific for plastic constituents such as hexamethylene diisocyanate, methylene diphenyl diisocyanate, and toluene diisocyanate in small numbers of patients who had reactions to platelet transfusions.[63] The significance of these antibodies is unclear because they most likely would be incidentally found in some transfusion recipients.

DEHP, however, also confers a beneficial membrane-stabilizing antihemolytic effect on RBCs during storage.[64, 65] Indeed, DEHP exerts a significant RBC protective effect to reduce hemolysis by approximately 50% during a given period of storage compared with other plasticizers and with storage in glass containers. PCs prepared from units of whole blood or from plateletpheresis collections have also been stored in blood bags composed of blow-molded polyolefin plastic without a plasticizer or with a tri-2-ethylhexyl trimellitate plasticizer. Such containers are unacceptable for RBC storage because they cause significant degree of hemolysis.

Studies have suggested that transfusing platelets stored in BTHC-containing bags is safe.[66] BTHC leaches into plasma at a level 60% to 70% less than DEHP. Moreover, BTHC differs from the phthalate plasticizer in that BTHC is metabolized to physiologic compounds such as citric acid, butyric acid, and hexanol. Extensive toxicology testing has shown that BTHC has an extremely low level of toxicity, with an oral median lethal dose (LD_{50}) of more than 20 g/kg for rats and more than 48 g/kg for mice. Neither the BTHC plasticizer nor the PVC plastic polymer produces local toxic effects, as determined by dermal, ocular, and intramuscular implantation testing; extensive testing in numerous species demonstrates the lack of significant intravenous toxicity as well. The chemical compound is not mutagenic, and, unlike with DEHP, repeated oral administration does not induce peroxisome proliferation in the liver. BTHC plasticizer and its degradation products are rapidly eliminated from the body by pulmonary, fecal, and urinary routes; 70% of a single dose is excreted in 44 hours. Although gas permeability of the material is slightly less than that of PL-732 plastic, transmission of oxygen into, and carbon dioxide out of, the container is sufficient to ensure aerobic oxidative metabolism and maintenance of an acceptable pH.

Agitation

In the late 1970s, investigators found that platelets stored with gentle agitation maintained better morphology and in vitro function than platelets stored undisturbed.[67] Thus, platelets are now stored with continuous gentle agitation. Rotators are available in a face-over-face (circular) angle of rotation or in a flatbed configuration.[33] However, not all agitators are appropriate to store platelets collected in certain plastic containers. For example, platelets stored in PL-732 blow-molded polyolefin bags using 6-rpm elliptical rotators were found to show decreased post-transfusion recovery and survival.[54] These findings were thought related to platelet–plastic storage bag interactions at various shear stresses created with agitation. Platelets stored using any available storage bag–rotator combinations are associated with increasing levels of CD62P over time and progressive release of β-thromboglobulin from α granules. Agitation is also associated with discharge of cytosolic lactate dehydrogenase (LDH), a finding suggesting that some degree of platelet lysis occurs during agitation.[68]

Single-donor Platelets by Apheresis

The development of automated instruments for platelet collection was in part motivated by the need to collect large numbers of platelets from a single donor.[69] It was clear during the earliest periods of platelet transfusion therapy that some patients did not demonstrate expected increases in platelet counts after transfusion. However, these patients often had better responses when they were transfused with platelets collected from siblings with identical human leukocyte antigens (HLA antigens).[70] Later, platelets collected from unrelated donors that were HLA identical to the recipient were also found of use in unrelated platelet-refractory patients.[71] Advances in apheresis technology have resulted in improved collection efficiencies for various apheresis machines.[72, 73] These instruments are highly automated and can also be used to collect RBCs and plasma.[74] Apheresis machines routinely collect 5 to 7×10^{11} platelets from a single donor. In fact, many centers are collecting two or three individual units from a single-donor collection, each unit containing more than the 3×10^{11} platelets many standards require for a single-donor apheresis unit. The platelets are collected in larger storage containers that allow adequate transport of oxygen and maintenance of pH. Inability to provide adequate transport of oxygen into the storage bag and, to a lesser degree, adequate transport of carbon dioxide out of the bag limits the number of platelets that can be stored. Currently available citrate-based plasticizer bags can store up to 7×10^{11} platelets in a bag. Apheresis products must also be stored with continuous gentle agitation. Generally, apheresis platelets are collected in ACD-A solutions rather than the standard whole blood anticoagulant CPD, CPDA-1, or CP2D.

Apheresis platelets show in vitro characteristics comparable to those of random-donor platelets prepared from whole blood donation. Refinements in apheresis technology permit a 3- to 4-log reduction in the number of white blood cells (WBCs) contained in units of single-donor platelets. Thus, the platelets collected are collected with little WBC contamination. This form of *process leukoreduction* may provide the additional benefits of minimizing the levels of various cytokines, such as tumor necrosis factor-α, that have been implicated in febrile transfusion reactions.[75] Most transfusion specialists do not believe that it is necessary to administer these products through leukoreduction filters to reduce the number of WBCs further.

Several groups have explored the feasibility of autologous platelet donation. Platelets stored in the liquid phase at room temperature have a shelf life of only 5 days; thus, autologous collection is often not practical. However, platelets collected by apheresis and frozen preserved in dimethyl sulfoxide (DMSO) can be stored at −80°C.[76] They are then thawed, washed, and resuspended in autologous plasma or other solutions before transfusion. Platelets prepared by this technique, however, do undergo structural and metabolic changes that decreases their recovery and survival as compared with liquid-stored PCs.[77] Furthermore, most patients cannot donate enough platelets to support their needs, for instance, during a course of induction chemotherapy. It is possible, however, to store significant numbers of frozen autologous platelets for patients who are refractory to platelet transfusion, provided the blood bank is technically capable of preparing and storing these specialized products.[78]

The use of single-donor platelets prepared from a whole blood collection or by apheresis at a particular institution often depends on local issues, most importantly the availability of each product. Although platelet apheresis is well tolerated by most donors, hemodynamic instability and adverse reactions related to citrate toxicity (hypocalcemia) can occur.[79] Single-donor apheresis platelets have several potential benefits, the most often cited being decreased donor exposure. Other positive attributes include decreasing allogeneic donor antigenic stimulation with use of single-donor apheresis platelets. The transfusion community, however, is not currently able to provide all platelet products as single-donor apheresis platelets, and platelets prepared from single whole blood collections are more commonly used by most institutions.

Standards and Quality Control of Platelet Concentrates

In many respects, the standards for PCs have evolved in parallel with advances in processing and storage conditions that allow longer storage of viable platelets. *Quality assurance programs* have been developed to monitor the composition and viability of platelets.[80] These procedures are designed to minimize the variability in end products, variability that can preclude determining the efficacy of PCs. Standards for monitoring the quality of PCs vary across countries and are specific for the preparation technique. Most standards require that PC testing include platelet numbers, pH, WBC numbers for leukoreduced products, and product volume (Table 17.1).[81] In the United States, a "random-donor" platelet unit must contain a minimum of 5.5×10^{10} platelets per bag. Platelet numbers are commonly determined using automated hematology analyzers. The precision and accuracy

Table 17.1 Standards for Platelet Components

	Whole-blood–derived		Apheresis-derived	
	United States	Europe	United States	Europe
Platelets ($\times 10^{10}$)	≥5.5	>6.0	≥30	>20
pH	>6.0	>6.2	>6.0	6.5–7.4
White cells ($\times 10^6$)	<0.83	<0.2	<5.0	<1.0
Volume (mL)	To maintain pH >6.2	>50	To maintain pH >6.2	>40

of these instruments are acceptable for this purpose. Other techniques that have been developed to enumerate platelets use fluorescent dyes and monoclonal antibodies conjugated to fluorochromes.[82] These techniques, which require a flow cytometer or other instrument capable of detecting fluorescence, are not commonly used in platelet quality monitoring.

The volume of suspending plasma is not specified; however, the amount must be sufficient to maintain a pH greater than 6.0 after 5 days of storage. Single-donor platelets by apheresis must contain at least 3.0×10^{11} platelets per bag. Before release of a PC, some investigators advocate inspecting the unit for the presence of the *swirling phenomenon,* in which normal discoid platelets exposed to light and rotated display a characteristic appearance.[83] The presence of swirling, which suggests grossly normal platelet morphology, may correlate with acceptable pH values and adequate in vivo viability.[84, 85] There is no requirement, however, to check for swirling before issuing platelet components. Finally, temperature control charts should document that platelets are stored between 20°C and 24°C.

Compared with the European standard (1×10^6 WBCs/unit), the number of WBCs allowed in a leukoreduced PC is fivefold greater by United States standards (5×10^6 WBCs/unit). Automated hematology analyzers, which measure WBC numbers based on the principles of impedance or light-scattering properties, are not appropriate for determining WBC numbers in leukoreduced PCs. This is because they lack accuracy and reproducibility at the low WBC numbers found in such products. Residual WBC numbers are most commonly performed by manual chamber techniques. Larger-volume (50-μL) Nageotte-type hemacytometers are typically employed.[86, 87] The variability of chamber counts is considerable,[88] and thus alternative techniques have been developed. These include methods based on flow cytometry, microvolume fluorimetry, and quantitative polymerase chain reaction.[89–91] Most flow cytometric methods developed to count residual WBC use dyes that stain nuclear components (propidium iodide) or WBC-specific antibodies (CD45) conjugated to a fluorochrome.

Current methods of leukoreduction, when properly performed, consistently provide products that fulfill standards for WBC removal.[92] However, a proportion of products must be sampled within a quality control program to document adequate leukoreduction.[93] Only a few of the PCs produced are actually sampled because it is not currently feasible to test all products. Typically, 4 to 10 products per month, or 1% of all products collected, are tested for WBC numbers. Concerns have been expressed that such sampling numbers and sampling frequencies are not adequate.[94] Ideally, the quality control program should include a formal technique for statistical monitoring, and monitoring should be performed on a continuous basis. These steps could maximize the likelihood of detecting process failures. However, most facilities continue to perform test platelet products at weekly or monthly intervals.

Volume-reduced Platelets

Platelets prepared from whole blood collections are stored in donor plasma, which serves as a buffering agent. PCs are typically suspended in 40 to 60 mL plasma to maintain product pH.[95] Volume reducing of PCs for neonates is not usually necessary because adequate platelet increments are achieved by transfusing small volumes of platelets; a standard dose for neonates is 10 mL/kg.[96] In certain clinical situations, however,

volume-reduced platelets are considered. For example, transfusing plasma-incompatible PCs, a reasonably common adult transfusion practice, is of more potential harm to infants with smaller RBC volumes. The most dangerous situation occurs when an infant (group A) is transfused an apheresis-derived PC from a group O donor who carries high-titer anti-A.[96] For this reason, blood services that provide mainly apheresis platelets may titer group O products before they are transfused to group A recipients. If ABO compatible platelets are not available, plasma can be removed from PC by centrifugation and replaced with saline or albumin. Plasma removal is also contemplated when an antibody present in donor plasma is directed against an antigen present on a neonatal blood cell. This situation arises when an HPA-Ia mother is the only source of antigen-negative platelets for her newborn with neonatal alloimmune thrombocytopenia resulting from anti-HPA-Ia. Volume-reduced platelets may also be warranted when circulatory overload is a major concern, as part of an overall restriction of all intravenous fluids.

Investigators have shown that recentrifugation of platelets stored for up to 5 days at $1500 \times g$ for 7 minutes, $2000 \times g$ for 10 minutes, or $5000 \times g$ for 6 minutes, followed by resuspension in 10 mL of plasma after a 1-hour rest period, results in a loss of between 5% and 20% of the platelets.[97] At the latter two centrifuge speeds, in vivo survival of the platelets that tolerate centrifugation and resuspension appeared normal in healthy volunteers. Platelet loss is less than 15% after a shorter 20-minute rest period when platelets are spun at lower speeds but for longer times (e.g., $580 \times g$ for 20 minutes).[98] Platelets stored for 1 or 5 days on a flatbed or an end-over-end tumbler agitator and then volume-reduced showed no adverse effects on in vitro function, as assessed by morphology, response to hypotonic stress, aggregation, PF3 activity, pH, and discharge of LDH. Acceptable platelet increments can also be obtained in critically ill thrombocytopenic neonates transfused with volume-reduced PCs. The use of the softer spin technique to produce volume-reduced PCs has the advantage that products are available more rapidly.

Neonates usually require small-volume transfusions; therefore, blood components are often dispensed or transfused using a syringe. For platelets to maintain an acceptable pH, it is imperative that the storage container allow for sufficient gas exchange. PCs stored for up to 5 days and then maintained in gas-impermeable polypropylene syringes for 6 hours showed increases in consumption of glucose and production of lactic acid.[99] The resultant decline in pH was associated with a switch from aerobic to anaerobic metabolism. Similar results were observed when platelets were stored in syringes for 6 hours at 37°C. The pH in all these situations, however, did not fall below 6.5, which is within the accepted range for platelets stored in gas-permeable blood bags. Volume-reduced platelets produced by the soft-spin technique described earlier and stored in syringes for 6 hours at room temperature or 37°C were also evaluated.[100] Higher-temperature storage produced the greatest and most rapid decline in pH. Other in vitro parameters of platelet function, such as morphology score, response to hypotonic stress, and LDH discharge, were not adversely affected under the conditions studied. Therefore, it appears that PCs, either standard or volume-reduced, that are dispensed to neonatal nurseries in syringes for transfusion within 4 to 6 hours maintain acceptable in vitro platelet function.

■ Changes in Platelets with Storage

Platelet Storage Defect

The *platelet storage defect*, or platelet storage lesion, encompasses all untoward effects on platelet morphology, structure, and function with storage. These changes begin at the time of blood collection and component preparation and continuously progress during storage. The mechanisms responsible for the platelet storage defect are not fully understood, but they are clearly multifactorial. Development of the platelet storage lesion is in general related to collection technique, storage conditions, and postcollection manipulation.[101] For example, centrifugation can affect platelet function by exposing platelets to shear stress conditions. Shear stresses not only produce a discharge of cytosolic LDH, but also stimulate the platelet release reaction.[68] Release of β-thromboglobulin into the suspending plasma and appearance of P-selectin (CD62P, GMP-140) on the platelet membrane surface after platelet preparation are both evidence of platelet granule release.[102, 103]

During storage, the metabolic activity of platelets and residual WBCs continues to consume nutrients and to produce harmful metabolic products. Activated clotting factors, cellular debris, and proteolytic enzymes found in the suspending plasma can adversely affect platelets. Many structural changes in the platelet cytoskeleton and surface membrane antigens that occur during storage also appear related to poorer in vivo post-transfusion recovery and survival.[104] Many different in vitro tests have been used to follow changes in platelets with processing and storage (Table 17.2). In general, only platelet numbers, concentrate volumes, pH at 5 days, and WBC content are routinely measured in transfusion practice. The remaining assays, primarily relegated to research settings, correlate to varying degrees with in vivo platelet survival. Techniques used to study in vivo platelet survival—mainly radiolabeling or biotinylation of platelets before transfusion—are not commonly performed and have their own limitations.[105, 106] Many of these supplemental assays cannot be applied to large-scale platelet production. Unfortunately, no single in vitro assay can accurately predict in vivo recovery and survival of transfused platelets.

Platelet Activation during Concentrate Preparation and Storage

Various markers have been employed to examine the platelet activation that occurs during the storage of PCs. These include the following: proteins associated with the α granule, such as β-thromboglobulin, PF4, and P-selectin; dense granule proteins such as serotonin; cytosolic enzymes such as LDH; and membrane ligands including GPIb and GPIIb-IIIa.[107, 108] Little evidence suggests that the degree of platelet activation associated with routine platelet preparation and storage adversely affects the ability of transfused platelets to circulate, correct the bleeding time, produce acceptable corrected count increments, and arrest bleeding. In fact, activated platelets have been shown to continue to circulate and to function in a nonhuman primate model of platelet transfusion.[109] However, it is likely that platelet activation attributed to the preparation and storage of platelets is partially responsible for their deterioration, as assessed by certain in vivo tests of platelet function.[110]

P-selectin (CD62P, previously known as GMP-140 or PADGEM) is an important adhesive protein that is involved in platelet-WBC-endothelial interactions. Its functions are related to WBC attachment, rolling, and extravasation, as well as regulation of WBC cytokine synthesis.[111] This α granule membrane protein is sequestered on the internal membrane of the α granule in resting platelets. Platelet activation through most mechanisms results in fusion of the α granule with the platelet membrane. P-selectin then becomes expressed on the outer surface of the platelet membrane.[112] Thus, the number of platelets that have undergone α granule release can be estimated by measuring the total surface content of P-selectin.

Several investigators have used monoclonal antibodies directed against P-selectin to study platelet activation during PC preparation and storage.[113] Platelet preparation by the PRP technique can result in P-selectin expression by approximately 20% of platelets. Platelet activation is in general lower, approximately 8%, when platelets are isolated from the BC without pelleting.[114] Approximately 50% of all platelets are activated after 5 days of storage, whether they are prepared by the PRP technique or the BC method. These observations suggest that although platelet pelleting used in the PRP method causes significant α granule release, stored platelets undergo an obligatory degree of platelet activation during storage regardless of the preparative technique. In another study, it was found that the higher the platelet count in the PC, the greater the percentage of activated platelets at any given time.[115] After 5 days of storage, platelet activation averaged 15% in less concentrated stored platelets (1×10^9/mL) and 30% in more concentrated units (1.4×10^9/mL); these percentages increased to 60% and 70%, respectively, by 10 days of storage.

Table 17.2 Quantifying the Platelet Storage Defect

Routine Studies	Metabolic Activity	Platelet Lysis
Platelet number	pH, P_{O_2}, P_{CO_2}, bicarbonate changes	Supernatant lactate dehydrogenase content
Concentrate volume	Lactate production	Lysate vWF:Ag levels
pH	Glucose consumption	
Visual inspection, swirl	Intracellular calcium	Miscellaneous
Leukocyte content	ADP/ATP ratio	Cytokine levels
Morphology and shape changes	Platelet aggregation	Activated complement
Qualitative swirling	Spontaneous aggregation	Bacterial growth
Morphology score	Response to dual agonists	
Mean platelet volume		In vivo assays
Osmotic recovery	Platelet activation	Corrected count increment
Extent of shape change	CD62 P-selectin expression	Radiolabeled survival
	Annexin V binding	Biotin-labeled survival

ADP, adenosine diphosphate; ATP, adenosine triphosphate.

Investigators have suggested that activated, P-selectin–positive platelets could be preferentially removed from the circulation after transfusion. Activated platelets first bind to WBCs and are then eliminated, presumably through the mononuclear-phagocyte (reticuloendothelial) system. This hypothesis was tested by isolating platelets from normal donors, storing the platelets for 2 to 4 days under standard blood bank conditions, and then reinfusing the platelets. Pretransfusion platelet P-selectin expression was determined, and in vivo survival was estimated by indium-111 labeling.[102] Platelet recoveries at 1 hour demonstrated a modest inverse correlation with the percentage of activated platelets expressing P-selectin ($r^2 = 0.30$; $P < .05$). As in other studies of platelet survival, other factors (pH, temperature, agitation) in addition to activation may have influenced platelet recovery. The recovery of activated platelets after transfusion was also studied in thrombocytopenic patients with cancer. By quantifying the percentage of activated platelets in patients before and after transfusion and in the PCs, the observed recovery of activated platelets was compared with the predicted recovery, which was based on the increment in platelet count after transfusion. Investigators found that the observed recovery of activated platelets was always lower than predicted—averaging 38% of the predicted values—a finding implying that activated platelets may be preferentially cleared after transfusion. These data suggest that increased platelet activation, as measured by P-selectin expression, may be related to poorer in vivo survival.

Proteolysis of Platelet Cytoskeletal Proteins

The platelet cytoskeleton plays a major role in maintaining platelet shape. It also ensures the integrity of the external platelet membrane, which carries several important receptors.[116, 117] Platelet cytoskeletal proteins undergo a degree of degradation during storage. However, the contribution of this "proteolysis" in the progression of the platelet storage defect is largely unknown. Certainly, deterioration of cytoskeletal proteins could negatively affect platelet structure and function. Moreover, protein degradation may play a role in platelet microvesicle formation during platelet storage.[113, 118] Many platelet cytoskeleton proteins are known, including actin, actin-binding protein, talin, vinculin, gelsolin, tubulin, and myosin heavy chain. Of these, actin is present in greatest abundance and constitutes 15% to 20% of total platelet protein.

When PCs are stored under blood bank conditions, actin is cleaved into at least two fragments of approximately 28 kD: storage proteins 1 and 2 (SP1 and SP2).[119] Amino acid sequencing has identified that these proteins are formed when actin is cleaved at the N-terminus of residues Thr106 (SP1) and Ala114 (SP2). Actin fragments are generated when platelets are stimulated by the calcium ionophore A23187, in a reaction that can be inhibited by nonspecific protease inhibitors.[120–122] This finding suggests that actin is proteolyzed by the calcium-dependent neutral protease calpain. Degradation of other platelet cytoskeletal proteins during storage such as actin-binding protein, talin, and vinculin may also be related to calpain activation. Specifically, actin-binding protein degradation products have been seen on immunoblots of 1-day-old PCs, a finding providing further evidence that platelet activation begins during actual platelet preparation. After 6 days of platelet storage under blood bank conditions, actin-binding protein undergoes additional

degradation, as reflected by further generation of lower-molecular-weight breakdown products.

Platelets are exposed to shear stresses during their separation from blood, as well as during agitated storage. These and other physical stresses appear capable of stimulating calpain generation. Calpain activation during storage may also promote platelet microvesicle formation. Microvesicles are fragments of platelet membrane that are continuously formed during PC storage.[118] Presumably, activated calpain promotes platelet microvesicle formation by degrading actin and other cytoskeletal proteins, leading to a weakening of the actin-cytoplasmic membrane interface with resultant formation of microvesicles.[123] Despite these observations, the overall contribution of such proteases to the deterioration of platelets with storage remains unclear. Data suggest that apoptosis, possibly mediated through non–caspase-dependent mechanisms, may also play a role in platelet cytoskeletal changes during storage.[124]

Glycoprotein Ib and IIb-IIIa Expression

Changes in the expression of platelet-specific GP such as GPIb and GPIIb-IIIa occur during platelet storage. GPIb serves as the primary receptor for vWF and mediates platelet adhesion to the vasculature at high shear rates. During platelet storage, the extracellular portion of GPIb can be cleaved. Levels of the glycosylated portion of GPIb, glycocalicin, increase in the cell-free supernatant over 5 days of storage.[125] Glycocalicin is highly sensitive to enzymatic degradation and can be cleaved from the GPIb molecule by thrombin. Surface GPIb is also degraded by proteases, such as plasmin, which are clearly present in stored PCs. However, despite this increase in plasma glycocalicin, platelet surface GPIb content remains relatively constant, although a distinct subpopulation of GPIb-negative platelets does appear over time.[125] Investigators postulated that surface GPIb may be replaced through relocation of GPIb to the surface from an intracellular pool or a sequestered surface population. The observation that total platelet GPIb content is four times higher than surface amounts suggests the presence of an intraplatelet GPIb pool.

Storage conditions may play a significant role in platelet surface receptor changes. PCs stored on an elliptical rotator lose nearly 50% of their surface GPIb, whereas membrane GPIb on platelets stored on a circular tumbler rotator does not significantly decrease.[113] Therefore, comparisons of studies of stored PCs must take into account storage and preparation protocols. Postprocessing manipulation of PCs may decrease surface GPIb. For example, PCs exposed to high-dose (10,000 mJ/cm^3) ultraviolet B (UVB) irradiation have significantly reduced surface GPIb expression as compared with untreated PCs.[126] By contrast, UVB at these doses does not appear to affect GPIIb-IIIa surface density. Filtering platelets through various WBC removal filters does not appear to alter the surface expression of GPIb or GPIIb-IIIa appreciably.[127]

Seven days of storage on elliptical and tumbler rotators will cause platelet surface GPIIb-IIIa to increase slightly, as measured by iodine-125–labeled monoclonal antibodies.[113] Studies using flow cytometry and monoclonal antibodies directed against GPIIb-IIIa similarly demonstrated increasing GPIIb-IIIa expression during platelet storage.[114] After 5 days of storage, mean surface expression of GPIIb-IIIa increased 50% to 70% from baseline; expression increased by 300% or more when storage was extended to 10 days. A separate study found that preparation of platelets, especially the pelleting step, was largely responsible for the initial increase in surface GPIIb-IIIa.[115] Increased surface GPIIb-IIIa paralleled increases in β-thromboglobulin release and surface expression of P-selectin, both of which reflect α granule release. Because α granules contain a pool of GPIIb-IIIa, it seems likely that the increase in platelet surface expression of GPIIb-IIIa is the result of relocation of this protein from α granule stores to the platelet membrane. Alternatively, loss of surface GPIIb-IIIa may occur during platelet storage as a result of protease degradation or formation of microparticles from the platelet membrane.[118]

Thus, potential losses of both GPIb and GPIIb-IIIa during platelet storage can be at least partially compensated for by release of intracellular pools or from sequestration from other sources. For example, fresh plasma can restore platelet GPIb surface expression and is one possible explanation for the preservation of platelet function after transfusion.[128] Alternatively, GPIb could be relocated from platelet storage pools or sequestered at vascular surfaces. The levels of GPIb after storage, although low, are not as low as those seen on platelets collected from patients with Bernard-Soulier syndrome, which is a hereditary absence of GPIb receptors associated with a bleeding tendency. Thus, a critical level of these surface receptors may be required for platelet adhesion to the corresponding ligand.

Bacterial Contamination

Transfusion of blood products contaminated by bacteria is dangerous to a recipient and often results in the rapid development of hypotension and shock. The risk of septic transfusion reactions is higher for platelet transfusions because platelets are stored at room temperature. The actual risk is difficult to estimate; however, some deaths occurring after platelet transfusion have been attributed to bacterial contamination.[129, 130] Blood products can become contaminated by bacteria during venipuncture or when the donor is bacteremic during collection. Organisms most often implicated in septic transfusion reactions include gram-positive (Staphylococcus sp.) and gram-negative (Enterobacter, Yersinia, Pseudomonas sp.) bacteria. Contaminated units generally cannot be identified by inspection. Gram stains are relatively insensitive and are not appropriate for screening purposes, but they can be clinically useful if bacteria are identified. Commercial assays for bacteria, including polymerase chain reaction techniques, chemical tests, and tests aimed at detection of radioactive carbon dioxide, are under various stages of development.[131] Automated blood culturing systems have also been used to detect bacterially contaminated platelet units.[132] These systems are capable of identifying bacteria, often within 24 to 48 hours after sampling.[133] However, these and other systems may not always detect low-level bacterial contamination, especially if the unit is transfused shortly after preparation. Leukoreduction filters, which have been shown to remove some types of bacteria, are not sufficient to protect against septic reactions.[134]

Blood cultures should be obtained from patients who develop extremely high fevers (more than a 2°C rise) after or during platelet transfusion with or without hypotension. Other symptoms attributed to preformed endotoxin and cytokines include skin flushing, severe rigors, and rapid development of cardiovascular collapse occurring minutes to hours after

transfusion. Treatment includes fluids, cardiorespiratory support, and broad-spectrum antibiotics. The patient's blood and the suspected contaminated product should be cultured so that blood culture results can be correlated with clinical status. Culturing of blood products is associated with an approximately 3% false-positive rate. Febrile transfusion reactions can usually be distinguished from septic transfusion reactions by the self-limited nature and lack of sustained and profound hypotension in febrile reactions.

■ Postcollection Processing

Leukoreduction

Platelets, like RBCs, should be transfused through standard microaggregate filters. These filters trap larger debris including fibrin clots, but they do not remove WBCs. Filtration of platelets through microaggregate filters has been shown to result in loss of less than 5% of the platelets, a loss attributed to the filter's void volume.[135] In the 1990s, highly efficient filters were developed that were capable of removing 3 to 4 $\log_{10}$ or more of all WBCs found in a unit of RBCs or platelets.[136, 137] These filters are generally manufactured from a polyester fiber matrix to which various polymer chemicals are linked. The size of the polymer affects the degree to which WBCs are exposed to its surface and, thus, the efficiency of WBC removal. Filters that are designed to leukoreduce RBC units cannot be used to filter platelets because these filters nonspecifically adsorb both WBCs and platelets.[138] Thus, filters have been developed that are specifically designed for leukodepleting PCs.[139]

Numerous adverse effects of blood transfusion have been attributed to contaminating WBCs found in cellular blood products. The most commonly accepted complications are febrile nonhemolytic transfusion reactions (FNHTRs), alloimmunization, and cytomegalovirus transmission. In fact, many countries have instituted, or plan to institute, universal leukoreduction of all cellular blood components, including platelets. At the cellular level, lysosomal enzymes present in neutrophils are known to digest various platelet proteins. For example, elastase digests GPIb. During storage, the platelet NADPH (reduced form of nicotinamide-adenine dinucleotide phosphate) oxidase system is activated, resulting in release of platelet-activating factor.[140] Cytokines released from lymphocytes are known to produce a variety of adverse effects in vivo. Platelet-poor supernatant plasma from stored PCs is more likely to produce febrile reactions than are the platelets contained in the cellular fraction of the stored units of concentrates.[141] Other groups have shown that lymphocytes present in units of stored platelets produce cytokines such as interleukin-8 (IL-8), which may be partially responsible for febrile transfusion reactions.[142, 143] Thus, removal of WBCs before or early in storage (prestorage leukoreduction) may reduce this risk by removing the lymphocytes before they can synthesize or release various enzymes and cytokines.

Antigen-presenting cells (APCs) present in PCs appear to promote HLA alloimmunization, which is responsible for one form of platelet refractoriness. The adverse effects of neutrophilic enzyme discharge and lymphocyte cytokine release during platelet storage could be ameliorated by prestorage leukodepletion. Using a rabbit infusion model, investigators showed that supernatant plasma obtained from blood stored before filtration induces a significantly higher degree of alloimmunization than does plasma filtered before whole blood storage.[144] These results suggest that prefiltration may further decrease the incidence of HLA alloimmunization by preventing generation of soluble biologic response modifiers (BRMs), as well as by preventing the formation of platelet or RBC microparticles during storage. It is generally believed that viable donor APCs are needed to present donor HLA antigen to the recipient's T cells. Whether this mechanism would function with the infusion of plasma without donor APCs is not clear. In such cases, the recipient's APCs can also present transfused donor antigens. If so, removal of WBCs before they shed HLA antigens into the stored plasma may be beneficial. Blood bags with RBC and platelet leukoreduction filters integrally attached to provide a closed system for prestorage WBC depletion at the time of collection are available and are being used more extensively.

Gamma Irradiation

Cellular blood components are exposed to gamma irradiation, to prevent transfusion-associated graft-versus-host disease in susceptible patients. Until recently, the dose of irradiation used varied from 1500 to 5000 cGy (1 rad = 1 cGy), with most transfusion centers using doses between 1500 and 3500 cGy.[145] The United States Food and Drug Administration (FDA) recommends that a dose of 2500 cGy be delivered to the midplane of a free-standing irradiation canister, with a minimum dose of 1500 cGy delivered to any other point in the canister. Platelets stored for 1 to 5 days and subsequently irradiated with 5000 cGy have been shown to maintain normal platelet function in vitro, morphology, PF3 activity, response to hypotonic stress and synergistic aggregation, β-thromboglobulin release, and thromboxane B2 formation.[146] Irradiation with 5000 cGy causes a decrease in the initial recovery of fresh and stored platelets transfused into normal volunteers, although the platelets appear to survive normally.[147] In this study, the circulating platelets failed to neutralize the effects of aspirin on the recipient's bleeding time; however, the hemostatic effectiveness of these platelets in thrombocytopenic patients did not appear compromised. Subsequent studies have not confirmed any damaging effect of irradiation at these doses on platelets. Exposure of PCs to 3000 cGy followed by storage for 5 days[149] has been shown to have no significant effect on either in vivo platelet recovery or platelet survival.[148] Similarly, no detrimental effects on in vitro function were demonstrated in platelet units irradiated with 2000 cGy and stored for up to 5 days.[149] Evaluation of paired apheresis platelets stored for 5 days after receiving 2500 cGy on day 1 or 3 similarly showed no deleterious effects on in vivo recovery and survival or in vitro properties of platelets.[150] In contrast to the negative effects of irradiating RBCs, effects that limit their shelf life once RBCs have been irradiated, the 5-day storage period of irradiated platelets does not need to be shortened.[151] These observations are of practical importance because many transfusion services are not equipped to irradiate blood components just before transfusion. Therefore, they must maintain an inventory of irradiated platelets obtained from the collecting facility.

Ultraviolet Irradiation

Donor WBCs contained in PCs are considered to play a significant role in primary alloimmunization of recipients to class I major histocompatibility complex (MHC) antigens, which, in turn, may result in refractoriness to platelet transfusions.[152] It was originally shown, in 1971, that lymphocytes exposed to sufficient doses of UV irradiation are unable to stimulate allogeneic cells in mixed lymphocyte culture or to respond to mitogenic stimuli.[153] UVC, which has the shortest wavelength (200 to 280 nm) and the greatest biologic activity, has been found to induce the formation of pseudopods at the platelet surface and to cause a degree of platelet aggregation.[154] Medium-wavelength UVB light (280 to 320 nm) has been shown to inactivate WBCs in PCs. The UVB doses needed to damage WBCs irreversibly depends on the UV source, the type of plastic container used, and the cross-sectional depth of the PC volume.[155] PCs irradiated with 3000 J/m² UVB and then stored for 5 days experienced no adverse effects on pH, hypotonic stress, or aggregation responses.[156] In addition, transfusing healthy volunteers with autologous platelets irradiated at this dose and stored for 5 days reveals equivalent platelet recovery, half-life, and survival as compared with control nonirradiated platelets.[157] However, irradiating pooled PCs with high-dose UVB (100,000 J/m²) results in a significant decrease in morphology score and osmotic recovery after 96 hours of storage. Expression of GPIb also declines by 60% at 96 hours after irradiation at the higher dose, with no alterations in surface GPIIb-IIIa expression.[126] Therefore, long-term storage of platelets after higher-dose UVB irradiation is not recommended.

Results of one small study suggested that in vivo recovery and survival of autologous PCs irradiated with high-dose UVB (15,000 J/m²) are modestly reduced as compared with control platelets (7 versus 7.75 days; *n* = 4).[158] Differences of this magnitude would not be clinically relevant. In the Trial to Prevent Alloimmunization to Platelets, UVB irradiation at 1480 mJ/cm² was shown to be equivalent to leukofiltration for decreasing the incidence of refractoriness to platelet transfusions in patients with acute myelogenous leukemia.[159] Long-wavelength UVA (320 to 400 nm) light by itself is insufficient to inactivate WBCs. However, UVA at low doses activates 8-methoxypsoralen and transforms it into a potent DNA cross-linking agent capable of abolishing mixed lymphocyte culture activity.[160] Pretreating PCs with 8-methoxypsoralen and UVA irradiation can reduce the allogenicity of class I MHC antigen in mice without affecting platelet aggregation responses.[161]

Photochemical Treatment

The risk of transfusion-transmitted viral disease has steadily decreased with advances in donor screening and testing. Despite these improvements, a small residual risk of viral, bacterial, or protozoal transmission during platelet transfusions remains. Techniques developed to inactivate viruses in plasma, such as solvent and detergent treatment, are too harsh and cannot be applied to cellular blood components. Thus, alternative methods to inactivate infectious pathogens in cellular blood components such as platelets and RBCs are under clinical development.[162] One of the more promising systems uses a synthetic form of psoralen known as S-59, which is photoactivated by long-wavelength UVA light. In the absence of UVA light, S-59 reversibly intercalates into helical regions of DNA and RNA. On exposure to UVA light, S-59 binds to thymidine and forms nonreversible covalent mono-adducts with DNA and RNA that effectively inactivate viruses, bacteria, and WBCs. Photochemical treatment with S-59 can inactivate high concentrations (10^5 to 10^6) of cell-free human immunodeficiency virus (HIV), proviral HIV, duck hepatitis B virus (a surrogate for hepatitis B virus), bovine viral diarrhea virus (a surrogate for hepatitis C virus), cytomegalovirus, gram-positive bacteria, and gram-negative bacteria.[163, 164] This technique can also inactivate *Trypanosoma cruzi, Plasmodium malariae, Borrelia burgdorferi,* and rickettsiae in PCs.[165]

One such protocol involves first resuspending platelets in approximately 35% plasma and 65% platelet additive solution (PAS III) in a total volume of 300 mL. S-59 (150 μM) is added to the platelets through an integral closed container system and is incubated for 5 minutes. Platelets are then illuminated with shaking for 3 minutes. All procedures are performed using plastic storage bags that are transparent to UVA. After illumination, the platelets are transferred to another plastic platelet storage bag containing an S-59 reduction device (SRD) and are incubated 6 hours with shaking. After SRD, the platelets are transferred to another container and can be stored for up to 5 days. The resulting product contains extremely low levels of residual S-59 and free photoproducts. Preclinical toxicology studies performed without S-59 reduction treatment have not demonstrated clinically relevant toxicity. However, further reduction of S-59 levels may enhance the safety of this pathogen inactivation system. PCs derived from BCs have also been studied after S-59 photoinactivation.[166]

Preliminary evidence indicates that photochemical treatment with psoralen S-59 and long-wavelength UV light can prevent transfusion-associated graft-versus-host disease.[167] Using a murine transfusion model, clinical and histologic evidence of graft-versus-host disease could be prevented by either gamma irradiating or photochemically treating splenic WBCs. Other agents capable of photoinactivating viruses, such as merocyanine 540 (MC 540), a heterocyclic polymethine dye, have adverse effects on platelet structure and function. In both the presence and the absence of visible light, MC 540 has deleterious in vitro effects on platelets. This compound immediately affects the ability of platelets to aggregate, as well as hastens the fall in pH and morphology scores that occur during platelet storage.[168, 169] Thus, photoinactivation procedures must be thoroughly tested to ensure that they do not damage platelet membranes.

■ Biologic Response Modifiers

Febrile Reactions

Many of the adverse effects of platelet transfusion therapy are related to the elaboration of various biologically active molecules by the constituents of PCs or the blood recipient. These substances, often termed *biologic response modifiers* (BRMs), are clearly involved in the pathophysiology of common febrile transfusion reactions, which occur in 4% to 30% of platelet transfusions. They also play a role in more severe immune hemolytic and septic transfusion reactions. The pathogenesis of febrile reactions was originally attributed to the presence of antibodies in the transfusion recipient that react with donor WBCs.[170] After binding of these antibodies to donor WBCs, fever ensues through a cytokine-mediated inflammatory response that results in release of IL-1. Fever is then produced through IL-1–stimulated synthesis of prostaglandin E2 in the thermoregulatory center of the hypothalamus.

More recently, cytokines contained in the plasma portion of PCs have been implicated in the development of febrile reactions. After platelet preparation, whether by the PRP, BC, or apheresis method, elaboration of cytokines by viable donor WBCs continues. PCs contain not only WBCs, but also a vast array of soluble proteins that have biologic activity. It is not entirely understood what stimulates WBCs to produce cytokines during platelet storage. Platelets themselves could contribute to these reactions through the release of platelet-specific cytokines after activation or damage to platelets with component preparation and storage. The major classes of BRMs include complement fragments, ILs, chemokines, arachidonic acid metabolites, kininogens, and histamines (Table 17.3). In addition, many other biologically active and inorganic compounds are similarly capable of interacting with humoral and cellular receptors.

Direct and indirect evidence suggests a key role of BRMs in FNHTRs to platelet infusions. FNHTRs are seen in patients who are receiving their first blood transfusion and who have not been pregnant.[171] Presumably, these patients would not have developed a secondary immune response from a prior exposure to foreign blood constituents. The incidence of platelet transfusion reactions may be related to the duration of platelet storage. For example, reaction rates can be nearly double in 3- to 5-day-old platelets as compared with 1- to 2-day-old products.[141] These findings have been attributed to reactive substances contained in the plasma portion of stored PCs.

Table 17.3   Biological Response Modifiers Found in Platelet Concentrates

Class	Examples
Complement fragments	C3a, C5a
Cytokines	
Interleukins	TNF-α, IL-6, IL-10, IFN-γ, IL-10, IL-4, TGF-β
Chemokines	IL-8, MCP-1, RANTES, β-TG, NAP-2, MIP-1β
Monokines	IL-1, IL-8, TNF-α, IL-6, IL-12
Anti-inflammatory cytokines	IL-1 receptor antagonist
Kininogens	Bradykinin
Histamine	—
Other biologic response modifiers	Prostaglandins, nitric oxide, leukotrienes (LTB4), platelet-activating factor

IFN, interferon; IL, interleukin; MCP, monocyte chemoathractant protein; MIP, macrophage inflammatory protein; NAP, neutrophil activating peptide; RANTES is defined in text; TG, Thromboglobulin; TGF, transforming growth factor; TNF, tumor necrosis factor.

Specifically, supernatant levels of IL-1β and IL-6 strongly correlate with the frequency of febrile reactions. Similar relationships between storage duration and febrile reaction rates have been found after transfusion of nonfiltered pooled PCs.[172] The incidence of allergic reactions does not appear related to storage time.

Specific chemical mediators thought to play a role in FNHTRs include cytokines, complement fragments, antibodies, and cell adhesion molecules.[173] Donor WBCs can continue to produce cytokines after they are infused into a recipient—the so called *passenger leukocyte effect*. Cytokines are synthesized and elaborated by donor WBCs during storage, after which these preformed cytokines are infused during transfusion.[174] The latter mechanism, in vitro cytokine production during platelet storage, has received increasing support as the mechanism responsible for most FNHTRs.[175] Accordingly, many investigators have focused their research on modulating the effects of BRMs in platelet therapy. Most efforts are directed at limiting the formation of BRMs during platelet collection and processing, decreasing formation of BRMs during platelet storage, and removing BRMs before or during platelet transfusion. Many of these techniques involve collecting platelets with little WBC contamination (process leukoreduction) or removing WBCs from PCs shortly after their preparation.

Leukoreduction

Our understanding of the effects of BRMs in platelet therapy is largely derived from studies of leukoreduced blood components. Third-generation leukoreduction filters eliminate approximately 99.9% (less than 5×10^6 WBCs remaining per unit) of the WBCs found in a unit of blood. Generally recognized benefits of leukoreduction include reducing the incidence of febrile reactions, preventing transmission of cytomegalovirus, and decreasing alloimmunization to HLA antigens. Leukoreducing blood products, however, does not prevent allergic reactions. Prestorage leukoreduction of RBCs has been shown to reduce the likelihood of FNHTRs further, as compared with the use of bedside leukoreduction filters.[176] This study also suggested that FNHTRs are more common after infusions of single-donor apheresis platelets than of RBC transfusions, a finding that may be related to the storage of platelets at room temperature.

Several groups have shown that prestorage leukoreduction of blood components slows the accumulation of cytokines in PCs and RBCs during storage. It is now clear that prestorage leukoreduction decreases the incidence and severity of FNHTRs by minimizing the production of cytokines by residual WBCs. In particular, levels of IL-8 in PCs prepared by the PRP method and leukoreduced shortly after collection are much lower than in nonleukoreduced PCs after 5 days' storage.[142] Reductions of regulated upon activation normal T cell expressed and presumably secreted (RANTES) and C3a are also seen when PCs are filtered through third-generation filters that reliably reduce WBC numbers by $4 \times \log_{10}$ per unit filtered.[177] The filter used in the latter study (PXL-8, Pall) did not remove the proinflammatory cytokines IL-1β and IL-6.

The ability of certain platelet WBC reduction filters to remove the anaphylatoxins C3a and C5a, as well as the chemokines IL-8 and RANTES chemokines, has been studied. Levels of C3a, C5a, IL-8, and RANTES were reduced by filtration through the two bedside leukoreduction filters (PXL-8 and PXL-A, Pall Glen Cove, NY) examined, but not through a prestorage platelet filter (Sepacell PLS-5A, Ashahi, Tokyo, Japan).[178] IL-1β was not removed by any of these filters. These experiments, which used WBC free plasma, demonstrate that binding of WBCs to filters is not necessary for the trapping or degradation of most BRMs. Earlier in vitro studies showed that C5a can be removed from plasma by peripheral blood WBCs that contain high-affinity binding sites for C5a.[179] The binding of C5a to leukocyte receptors does likely represent one control mechanism that protects cells from this potent anaphylatoxin. Similar studies showed little accumulation of IL-β, IL-6, IL-8, and tumor necrosis factor-α in leukoreduced PCs.[143] More recently, investigators suggested that the frequency of reactions is significantly higher in patients receiving poststorage WBC-reduced platelets (25.8%) than plasma-depleted platelets (17.0%).[180] In this study, IL-6 levels of platelet products appeared to be associated with the risk of reaction; however, IL-6 levels were not measured in patients during or after transfusion. In addition, other cytokines that have been implicated in febrile reactions were not examined.

Hypotensive Reactions to Platelet Transfusions: Role of Bradykinin

Severe hypotensive reactions have been reported after platelet transfusion therapy.[181] The most serious reactions appear to occur in patients receiving angiotensin-converting enzyme (ACE) inhibitors who are transfused with platelets through a bedside leukoreduction filter.[182] The reactions are more common when filters bearing a net negative surface charge are used. Although the pathogenesis of this syndrome remains unclear, it appears in some cases to involve generation of plasma kallikrein by some types of biomaterials that stimulate the generation of bradykinin (BK). BK produces adverse in vivo effects such as hypotension, abdominal pain, and facial flushing, without fever or chills. In most cases, it is possible to distinguish these reactions from febrile reactions and transfusion-related acute lung injury. However, these reactions must be promptly recognized.

ACE is identical to kininase II, an enzyme that degrades BK. Accordingly, blocking kininase II prolongs the half-life of BK such that clinical symptoms can develop in susceptible patients.[183] BK levels have been directly measured in patients transfused with platelets through leukoreduction filters.[184] In this study, platelet recipient BK levels transiently increased—during the first 5 minutes—when platelets were administered through a negatively charged filter (PL-50H, Pall). BK levels were particularly high in two patients with diminished ACE inhibitor activity. Because BK has a half-life of 15 to 30 seconds, prestorage leukoreduction, as opposed to bedside leukoreduction, should eliminate reactions resulting from BK generation from contact with the filter biomaterials. Such patients could benefit from receiving blood that has been either prestorage or in-laboratory leukoreduced, as opposed to being infused through a bedside leukoreduction filter.

More recently, a metabolic abnormality that affects des-Arg⁹-BK degradation was identified in several patients with severe hypotensive transfusion reactions.[185] Des-Arg⁹-BK is an active metabolite of BK that is primarily inactivated by ACE and aminopeptidase P. With ACE inhibition, the half-life of des-Arg⁹-BK, not BK, was shown to be significantly higher in patients with pronounced hypotensive transfusion reactions when compared with control transfusion recipients. These findings suggest that failure to metabolize active vasodilatory peptides could contribute to transfusion reactions. However, the findings do not imply that bedside leukoreduction of blood components is absolutely contraindicated in patients receiving ACE inhibitors.

■ Platelet Transfusion Therapy

Early in the 20th century, freshly drawn whole blood was the only source of viable platelets.[186] Although whole blood was neither a convenient nor an optimal source of platelets, such transfusions reportedly reduced bleeding times and halted hemorrhage in thrombocytopenic patients. PCs became widely available only after the development of plastic collection and storage containers in the late 1960s and early 1970s, which allowed the separation of platelets from whole blood. These products contained large numbers of viable platelets in a relatively small volume. Oncology patients use most of the PCs produced, and increasing numbers of PCs used since the 1980s were transfused to patients being supported during chemotherapy. Significant numbers of PCs are also provided to trauma and surgical patients and to solid-organ transplant recipients.

Platelet transfusion therapy is mainly used to treat or prevent bleeding in patients with thrombocytopenia. In fact, most PCs are transfused to nonbleeding thrombocytopenic patients as a prophylactic measure.[187] The thrombocytopenia can result from marrow suppression (e.g., drugs, radiation, infiltration), massive transfusion (dilutional thrombocytopenia), or immune destruction (e.g., neonatal alloimmune thrombocytopenia, immune thrombocytopenic purpura). Patients with congenital or acquired platelet disorders may benefit from platelet transfusion. These patients often have normal numbers of poorly functioning platelets. Platelet transfusions are also considered in disseminated intravascular coagulation and during or after cardiopulmonary bypass, as well as to support patients undergoing extracorporeal membrane oxygenation.

Despite vast clinical experience, few trials have demonstrated the effectiveness of platelet transfusion therapy in controlling and preventing thrombocytopenic bleeding.[188] Thus, practices followed for platelet therapy often vary among and within medical facilities. This situation has resulted in clinical controversies that have not been entirely resolved (Table 17.4). For example, it is unclear at what

Table 17.4 Clinical Controversies in Platelet Transfusion Therapy

Prophylactic platelet transfusions
    Higher versus lower platelet transfusion triggers

Platelet dosing
    Larger versus smaller platelet doses

Platelet preparation and product selection
    ABO-matched versus unmatched platelet concentrates
    Fresh versus stored platelet concentrates
    Single donor platelets by apheresis versus pooled donor platelet concentrates
        Decreased exposure to infectious agents in single donor units

Platelet-refractory patients
    Crossmatched versus HLA-selected platelets

platelet count a nonbleeding patient should receive prophylactic platelet transfusions. Additionally, the optimal dose of platelets for an individual patient has not been clearly defined. Some practitioners advocate larger doses of platelets than those routinely provided (e.g., 10 random-donor PCs [RDPs] instead of 4 to 6 RDPs). Various separation techniques have been developed to prepare PCs. Each of these has certain advantages and disadvantages; however, platelets isolated by each of the commonly used methods have been successfully used in the clinical arena. Finally, numerous strategies have been used to manage platelet-refractory patients. These patients are often difficult to manage, and they can consume large quantities of platelets.

Prophylactic Platelet Transfusion

Decisions to transfuse platelets, as well as any blood product, are no longer made based solely on transfusion thresholds. Patient factors should be considered when deciding when an individual patient should receive a transfusion. These factors may include the patient's disease, concurrent medications, and overall coagulation status.[189] Until recently, physicians typically transfused platelets to maintain a patient's platelet count at more than 20,000/μL. This level was believed necessary to prevent spontaneous bleeding.[190] However, serious spontaneous bleeding is unusual unless platelet counts fall to less than 5000/μL in the absence of other irregularities (e.g., aspirin use, decreased clotting factors) of the hemostatic system.[191] In fact, the earliest studies of the effectiveness of prophylactic platelet transfusions were limited by the widespread use of aspirin as an antipyretic agent before the antiplatelet effects of this drug were recognized.

Other difficulties have hindered efforts to determine an optimal prophylactic platelet transfusion "trigger." First, serious thrombocytopenic hemorrhage is unusual, even at extremely low platelet counts. This fact was recognized early in the history of platelet transfusion therapy. Results of an early small clinical trial suggested that RBC usage and major bleeding were no different in patients who received prophylactic platelet transfusions at the 20,000/μL threshold as compared with those transfused only when bleeding from sites other than the skin or mucous membranes.[192] Second, it is difficult to quantify minor clinical bleeding. Investigators have estimated stool RBC loss by chromium-51 RBC labeling as an indicator of spontaneous bleeding. One study that used such a technique found that patients with aplastic anemia did not have significantly elevated stool blood loss until platelet levels dropped to less than 5000/μL.[193] Finally, platelet counts, as determined by automated counters or manual methods, are less reliable in severely thrombocytopenic patients.

In the 1990s, studies were performed that were designed to define platelet transfusion thresholds more clearly. In one of the earlier studies, Gmur and associates prospectively followed 102 consecutive patients with acute leukemia.[194] Patients with platelet levels lower than 6000/μL received prophylactic platelet transfusions, whereas those with levels higher than 20,000/μL received transfusions only when major bleeding developed or before invasive procedures. Intermediate thresholds included 6000 to 11,000/μL for patients with minor bleeding or fever and 11,000 to 20,000/μL for patients with coagulation disorders and before minor procedures. Overall, 31 episodes of major bleeding occurred on 1.9% of total study days when platelet counts were less than or equal to 10,000/μL and on 0.07% of study days when counts were between 10,000 and 20,000/μL. The investigators suggested that prophylactic levels of 5000/μL were safe in the absence of fever or bleeding. However, several serious hemorrhages occurred in patients in the 6000 to 10,000/μL groups who did not receive prophylactic transfusions.

Several prospective trials compared the bleeding risks and platelet transfusion needs of thrombocytopenic patients. Most of these trials grouped patients using 10,000/μL (10K) and 20,000/μL (20K) thresholds. In a nonrandomized trial, Gil-Fernandez and colleagues found no difference in bleeding using the 10K or 20K threshold in 190 bone marrow transplant recipients.[195] Heckman and associates randomized 78 patients with acute leukemia to the 10K or 20K threshold and could demonstrate no difference in bleeding between these two levels.[196] Similarly, Wandt and colleagues were unable to demonstrate a difference in bleeding risk when they prospectively compared transfusion thresholds in 105 patients with acute myeloid leukemia.[197] Finally, in a large randomized multi-institution study of 255 patients with newly diagnosed acute myeloid leukemia, Rebulla and associates found no difference in major bleeding or in RBC transfusions when patients received transfusions at the 10K or 20K threshold.[198] Although most of these studies were limited to patients with acute leukemia, similar studies performed in other patient groups, such as those with severe aplastic anemia, have shown that platelet thresholds can be safely lowered.[199]

These studies suggest no clear differences in serious hemorrhage or hemorrhagic death when the platelet transfusion trigger is set at less than 20,000/μL. When lower prophylactic platelet transfusion thresholds are used, recipients are exposed to less donor blood and the potential complications of such a transfusion. Despite the results of these studies, no clear consensus on the clinical indications for prophylactic platelet transfusion remains. Accordingly, the thresholds selected for prophylactic platelet transfusions vary widely.[200] For most patients, the lower 10,000/μL threshold is likely as safe as higher levels. Patients with other risk factors for bleeding such as fever and sepsis are probably best transfused at higher thresholds, although specific triggers for these groups of patients have not been defined. In addition, profound anemia can alter hemostatic capabilities and, accordingly, should be avoided in severely thrombocytopenic patients.[201] Platelet counts higher than 20,000/μL are indicated before invasive procedures. Typically, platelet counts are increased to more than 50,000/μL before lumbar puncture, indwelling catheter insertion, thoracentesis, liver biopsy, or transbronchial biopsy.[202] However, children with acute lymphoblastic leukemia may tolerate lumbar puncture without serious complication when platelet levels are lower than 10,000/μL.[203] Platelet transfusions are usually not necessary before bone marrow aspiration or biopsy if adequate surface pressure can be applied to the site after the procedure.

Platelet Dosing

Doses of platelets, as determined by the number of platelets in single or pooled PCs, have not been standardized. In general, a single dose of transfused platelets contains approximately 3×10^{11} platelets, corresponding to one single-donor apheresis product or five to six pooled RDPs. The optimal adult dose of platelets has not been clearly established, and doses are

often determined based on factors unrelated to efficacy, such as cost and availability.[204] For example, an adult's body weight is not usually considered when determining the number of platelets to administer. In general, the higher a patient's post-transfusion platelet increment, the longer the interval will be before the next platelet transfusion is required. Endogenously produced platelets normally survive approximately 9 to 10 days in the absence of diseases that decrease platelet survival. Transfused platelets do not circulate this long in thrombocytopenic patients because they are more rapidly consumed, for instance, to maintain vascular integrity. For this reason, patients undergoing chemotherapy for various malignant diseases often require platelet transfusions at least every 3 days.[205] During periods of severe bone marrow hypoplasia, daily platelet transfusions are often required.

Several transfusion specialists advocate transfusing doses of platelets larger than the standard six-RDP pool, albeit at longer intervals between transfusions (e.g., 10 to 12 RDPs every 2 to 3 days). The rationale for this practice is largely based on decreasing the number of individual transfusion episodes. This is more convenient for many patients transfused in outpatient settings. As expected, it is possible to obtain higher post-transfusion platelet increments by transfusing higher platelet numbers.[206, 207] However, it is unclear whether this practice is more effective than the use of standard platelet doses in reducing the risk of spontaneous bleeding. Alternatively, smaller doses of platelets transfused at shorter intervals (e.g., three to four RDPs per transfusion) may reduce the total number of platelets required during a patient's thrombocytopenic period.[208] This strategy could decrease the overall number of platelets needed for a large patient population and could decrease the number of exposures for an individual patient. Thus, smaller platelet doses may be more economical, but this practice has been criticized for possibly increasing the number of individual transfusions and thereby increasing overall costs.[209] Therefore, an "optimal" dose of platelets has not been clearly defined, and transfusion practices will likely remain largely based on local preferences. These preferences are often heavily influenced by costs and supply.

Platelet Preparation and Product Selection

Platelets express ABH, Lewis, P, and I blood group antigens. They also carry class I HLA-A, HLA-B, and HLA-C, as well as platelet-specific antigens (human platelet antigens [HPA antigens]). Those that are most relevant to allogeneic platelet survival are the ABH, class I HLA, and HPA antigens. The presence of recipient antibodies directed against these antigens does not imply that all platelets carrying these antigens will be rapidly destroyed. Platelet survival is clearly decreased when recipients with higher-titer anti-A or anti-B immunoglobulin G antibodies in their plasma are transfused with platelets carrying one of these antigens. This incompatibility can be avoided by using ABO-identical platelets and should be considered as a first step in patients who are not responding appropriately to platelet transfusions.[210] Unfortunately, ABO-identical platelets are often unavailable during blood shortages. Transfusing ABO-incompatible apheresis-derived platelets does not usually produce measurable hemolysis in adults, although significant hemolysis has occurred, especially in patients with small plasma volumes.[211, 212]

There appears to be little difference in the efficacy of platelet transfusions whether the concentrates are prepared from PRP or BCs or are collected by apheresis. The decision to use any of these products—or a mixture of such products—is often based largely on cost and availability. Advocates of BC-prepared platelets, the technique widely practiced in Europe, note that cytokine production is lower in such concentrates.[213] BC platelets have also been reported as less activated immediately after preparation. However, this difference is not appreciable after storage for 48 hours, and transfusion of such products does not infer improved 5-day post-transfusion platelet recovery.[36, 115] Thus, although various in vitro measurements of PCs compared by any technique may differ, these differences are not usually associated with decreased platelet survival in vivo. Human transfusion studies are difficult to perform and to compare for several reasons, one being that thrombocytopenic patients often have extremely variable responses to platelet transfusion.[214]

Many blood centers provide only platelets collected from apheresis donors based on several potential benefits. Apheresis transfusions do decrease donor exposures, and this theoretically could reduce the risk of transfusion-associated infection. Donor testing has improved to such a point that the most important human viruses are detected in potentially infectious blood donors. Nucleic acid testing for viruses will likely reduce this risk further and will make the advantage of apheresis platelets more difficult to justify. It has been difficult to demonstrate that platelet alloimmunization rates are lower in patients who receive only apheresis-derived platelets.[159] This may be because these patients often receive an extremely large number of platelet transfusions during treatment. Platelets prepared by apheresis are usually more expensive than those prepared from single whole blood donations because of equipment and personnel costs for such a collection. Moreover, the apheresis platelet donors themselves have risks inherent to this collection technique.[215]

Platelet-Refractory Patients

Investigators have long recognized that some patients who receive long-term platelet support may begin to destroy transfused platelets rapidly.[216] This apparent *platelet-refractory state* can occur in clinical conditions that hasten platelet removal from the circulation. These conditions are often classified as immune mediated or nonimmune mediated, based on the presumed mechanism of platelet destruction (Table 17.5).[214, 217] Overall, nonimmune platelet destruction caused by splenomegaly (platelet sequestration), antibiotic treatment, and infection is more common than immune-mediated removal.[218, 219] From a practical standpoint, the effects of amphotericin B on platelet survival can be minimized by transfusing platelets 2 hours after completing amphotericin

infusion.[220] Antibody-related platelet destruction is often related to the development of HLA-specific antibodies in response to foreign donor HLA antigens.[70] Presumably, these antibodies coat donor platelets that carry antigens these immunoglobulins are capable of recognizing.[221] The antibody-coated platelets are then removed by the reticuloendothelial system or through mechanisms involving platelet activation and deposition on endothelial surfaces.[222] Less commonly, patients develop platelet-specific antibodies.

Strategies used to manage platelet-refractory patients vary across institutions and are often developed based on the availability of specialized testing and platelet products.[223] It may be possible to withhold platelet transfusion in nonbleeding patients with uncomplicated cases. If transfusion is absolutely necessary, such as if bleeding develops or before an invasive procedure, several strategies have been proposed. First, the dose of platelets can be simply increased by transfusing more platelets (e.g., 6 to 12 RDPs per pool or 2 single-donor platelets by apheresis). Other options include HLA-selected platelets and crossmatch-compatible platelets. Ideally, anti-HLA antibodies should be present in the patient before HLA-specific platelets are used because of the difficulties encountered in obtaining such products. The HLA system is extremely polymorphic, and thus a large pool of HLA-typed donors is needed to maximize the likelihood of an ideal platelet match.[224] These products are usually collected by apheresis and are selected based on the HLA-A and HLA-B types of the donor and recipient. HLA-C antigens are only weakly expressed by platelets, and mismatch of this antigen does not appear to influence platelet survival.[225] The use of HLA-selected platelets in patients who are not alloimmunized for the purpose of preventing HLA alloimmunization does not appear useful.[226, 227]

An alternative to HLA-selected platelets is crossmatch-compatible platelets. Platelet crossmatching is performed by reacting recipient serum or plasma with donor platelets that are fixed to a solid support. Compatibility is based on the presence or absence of reactivity. An incompatible platelet crossmatch predicts a poor response (platelet increment) in more than 90% of transfusions. Conversely, a compatible crossmatch does not guarantee good survival—a compatible crossmatch is predictive of a successful transfusion only 50% of the time.[228] For this reason, large collection facilities may combine the two approaches. Platelet units are selected for crossmatch based on the class I HLA types of the recipient and potential donor. This approach is also of potential use in the unusual patient who has developed both HLA and platelet-specific antibodies. Other approaches that have been proposed to transfuse heavily alloimmunized patients include techniques to reduce class I HLA antigen expression on platelets.[229] These methods, which are largely based on eluting HLA antigens, are not available for routine clinical practice.

Table 17.5 Conditions Associated with the Rapid Destruction of Transfused Platelets

Immune-Mediated	Non–immune-Mediated
HLA class I alloantibodies	Splenomegaly
Platelet-specific alloantibody formation	Drugs (amphotericin B, other antibiotics)
Platelet-specific autoantibodies	Sepsis and fever
Circulating immune complexes	Disseminated intravascular coagulation
	Graft-versus-host disease

■ Platelet Substitutes

Numerous products have been explored as alternatives to liquid PCs stored at 22°C. These *platelet substitutes,* in general, are either derived from platelets themselves or are synthetic. Platelet substitutes are designed to mimic the normal hemostatic properties of intact human platelets. Other advantageous properties of platelet substitutes include (1) an ability to retain efficacy when sterilized to prevent bacterial or viral infection, (2) a long biologically active shelf life, (3) few specialized storage requirements, and (4) ease of preparation and administration. Substitutes should be hemostatically effective in vivo without causing dangerous thromboses, and, in addition, they should be nonimmunogenic. Novel products derived from human platelets include platelet-derived microparticles (PMPs), lyophilized platelets, and cryopreserved (frozen) platelets. Synthetic platelet substitutes include RBCs carrying surface-bound fibrinogen or surface-bound RGD peptides, fibrinogen-coated microspheres, and liposome-based agents.

Platelet-derived Microparticles

PMPs are platelet membrane microvesicles that are formed during platelet storage. They are also found in fresh frozen plasma and cryoprecipitate. PMPs are strongly procoagulant and retain many of the biologic properties of intact platelets. Specifically, they can both adhere to vascular endothelium and enhance platelet adhesion.[230] PMPs range in size from 0.1 to 1.0 μm in diameter and are identified based on their expression of surface receptors for platelet-endothelial interactions including GPIIb-IIIa, Ib-IX, and P-selectin.[111] Early studies using infusions of platelets disrupted by sonication were discouraging.[231] This product had no apparent hemostatic effect in thrombocytopenic dogs, and it produced significant tachycardia and hypotension in recipients. More recently, human "infusible platelet membranes" were developed and tested in animal models.[232] This material is prepared from outdated platelets that are lysed by freeze-thawing, virally heat inactivated for 20 hours at 60°C, and, finally, sonicated. The fragments are then formulated with a preservative solution, lyophilized, and stored at 4°C; the product is reported stable for 3 years. The resulting spherical vesicles measure less than 1 μm in diameter and express detectable GPIb but not GPIIb-IIIa. This preparation has a PL content similar to that of natural platelets, retains so-called PF3 activity, and may have reduced class I HLA expression.[233] Studies have demonstrated shortening of the bleeding time in thrombocytopenic rabbits.[232] Preliminary evidence indicates that platelet membrane fragments prepared in this fashion are tolerated by human recipients and possess hemostatic effectiveness.[234]

This product has not been licensed by the FDA because of the difficulties in demonstrating efficacy. Measurement of postinfusion platelet count increments is not possible because they consist of platelet fragments that are not routinely measured. In addition, it is difficult to quantify the effects of any platelet substitute in thrombocytopenic patients who typically have other conditions associated with a bleeding tendency.

Lyophilized Platelets

The process of *lyophilization*—rapidly freezing a substance at an extremely low temperature and then dehydrating in a high vacuum—has been investigated as a means of long-term platelet storage. In fact, studies of rehydrated lyophilized platelets were originally performed in the 1950s. Unfortunately, these studies failed to demonstrate hemostatic efficacy in animal models of thrombocytopenia.[235] A more recently developed lyophilization procedure appears to allow better preservation of platelet structure.[236] This technique involves fixing washed platelets in 1.8% paraformaldehyde, followed by freezing in 5% albumin and lyophilization at −20°C to −40°C. The resulting fixed and lyophilized platelets retained important hemostatic properties after rehydration in studies of thrombocytopenic rats and canine models of von Willebrand disease. Their ultrastucture by electron microscopy is similar to that of fresh platelets, and they also express the GP surface receptors Ib and IIb-IIIa, albeit at decreased concentration. Reconstituted, lyophilized platelets appear capable of supporting thrombin generation and of facilitating fibrin deposition of exposed vascular endothelium in a vascular perfusion model.[237] Despite encouraging animal studies, concerns remain regarding the toxicity, in vivo survival (short in vivo life span), thrombogenicity, and reticuloendothelial blockade of such preparations; results of clinical trials using rehydrated lyophilized platelets are not available.

Platelet Cryopreservation

Cryopreservation has been used to store RBC units since the 1960s. However, similar techniques evaluated for preserving platelets at low temperatures have been less successful. Platelets that are frozen or stored for prolonged periods at 4°C demonstrate abnormalities in aggregation, hypotonic stress response, clot retraction, and, most important, in vivo survival. These changes are related to irreversible cytoskeletal and membrane alterations.[49] Adverse effects of freezing platelets could be minimized by using high concentrations of a cryoprotectant; however, cryoprotectants can themselves harm platelets. These effects can result from direct chemical damage and osmotic changes that develop as the cryoprotectant crosses the cell membrane.

Numerous compounds have been evaluated as potential platelet cryoprotective agents including glucose, DMSO, propylene glycol, polyvinylpyrrolidone, hydroxyethyl starch, polyethylene glycol, ethylene glycol, and others.[238] Propane-1,2-diol (propylene glycol), which is an effective agent for other hematopoietic elements, has a higher permeability rate than glycerol and is an ineffective platelet cryoprotectant.[239] Glycerol, used extensively for RBC cryopreservation, has little direct toxic chemical effects on platelets at the concentrations needed for effective protection. However, this compound enters the cell relatively slowly and results in severe osmotic damage. Use of a 5% glycerol–4% glucose solution may minimize freeze-thaw platelet loss and, in initial studies, preserved platelet function.[240] Despite these precautions, adverse effects of freezing on in vitro platelet function have been demonstrated. This damage consists of platelet morphologic and ultrastructural changes, decreased ATP levels, an inability to undergo the release reaction or aggregation, decreased recovery from hypotonic stress, and decreased in vivo recovery.[241, 242] Modifications of the original procedure, including optimizing the platelet count before freezing and use of a nonplasma diluent, did improve in vitro function.[243] Thus, platelet cryopreservation using glucose-glycerol solutions has not been successfully adapted for use in clinical transfusion practice.[244]

DMSO rapidly penetrates the platelet membrane and has less of an osmotic effect than glucose-glycerol. In addition, both in vitro and in vivo studies suggest that DMSO is a more effective cryoprotective agent than glycerol.[245] Long-term studies showed that DMSO-preserved platelets remain functional when they are stored for 3 years at $-80^\circ C$.[246] However, cryopreservation with 5% to 6% DMSO does result in a clear loss of platelet structure and function in terms of platelet morphology, aggregation responses, and platelet recovery after transfusion.[247] The average post-transfusion recovery of cryopreserved platelets is approximately 50% to 70% that of fresh platelets; those platelets that do survive the freeze-thaw cycle appear to circulate normally.[234] The nearly 50% of platelets that are damaged during cryopreservation become unresponsive to various platelet agonists. In addition, the content of secretory granules decreases, and the metabolic activity typically seen after platelet activation is almost completely absent. Investigators postulated that these findings reflect a defect in the stimulus-response coupling mechanisms that follow plasma membrane damage. Although these effects generally appear equally distributed among subpopulations of platelets, larger platelets may be most capable of retaining normal aggregatory responses.[248] Platelets stored frozen in liquid nitrogen with DMSO as a cryoprotectant have also been shown to have lower adhesive capacity in vitro as compared with fresh platelets from the same platelet unit.[249]

PCs cryopreserved using DMSO are used clinically as an alternative to liquid-stored platelets. However, the use of this technique is limited because it is reasonably time-consuming, laborious, and quite costly.[238] In addition, the platelets must be washed before transfusion to remove DMSO, which can produce clinical side effects such as nausea, vomiting, and local vasospasm. Frozen platelets have generally been reserved to store autologous platelets for patients with acute leukemia who have become heavily alloimmunized and hence refractory to allogeneic platelet products. The efficacy of cryopreserved and liquid-preserved platelets was compared in cardiopulmonary bypass surgery.[250] Cryopreserved platelets appeared effective in minimizing blood loss and the need to transfuse blood products. However, these authors suggested that procoagulant activity, not common in in vitro measures of platelet quality (e.g., aggregation, hypotonic stress), more accurately reflects the ability of cryopreserved platelets to maintain hemostasis. Solutions containing platelet-stabilizing agents (e.g., ThromboSol [Life Cell, The Woodlands, Tex.] containing amiloride, adenosine, and nitroprusside) have been developed that allow reducing the DMSO concentration while preserving recovery and survival on transfusion.[251, 252] These solutions allow using only 2% DMSO while better maintaining platelet viability and both in vitro and in vivo function.

Synthetic Platelet Alternatives

Several synthetic products are produced without the use of platelets or platelet fragments, yet they display hemostatic properties similar to those of intact platelets. Peptides containing Arg-Gly-Asp (RGD) sequences have been covalently coupled to RBCs.[253] Platelet GPIIb-IIIa receptors recognize RGD sequences on fibrinogen. Fibrinogen is primarily responsible for cross-linking activated platelets and forming platelet aggregates at sites of injury. These peptides are designed to bind only activated GPIIb-IIIa molecules, and this limits their reactivity to platelets activated at sites of vascular injury. Other platelet substitutes being studied include inert polyacrylonitrile beads coated with fibrinogen, RBCs with fibrinogen covalently bound to the membrane, and liposome-based agents.[233] For example, recombinant fragments of the platelet GPIbα have been incorporated into liposomes.[254] In vitro tests showed that these GPIbα liposomes can mediate vWF accumulation on subendothelial tissues and can enhance platelet function. Intravenous infusions of procoagulant liposomes in conjunction with activated factor X were studied in dogs with hemophilia; however, such a strategy had unacceptable toxic effects.[234] Fibrinogen-coated albumin microcapsules (Synthocytes Quadrant Healthcare, Nottingham, UK) were shown to facilitate platelet adhesion to the endothelial cell matrix and to reduce bleeding from surgical wounds in a rabbit model of severe thrombocytopenia.[255] Although many of these products face long research and development times, problems with current platelet preparations and antigenicity of certain formulations of thrombopoietic cytokines are encouraging many companies to pursue these products further.

■ Thrombopoietic Growth Factors

Hematopoietic growth factors used in clinical medicine are designed to limit the exposure of patients to allogeneic blood components. The isolation, characterization, and subsequent synthesis of erythropoietin by recombinant technology have reduced the need for RBC transfusions in certain patient populations. A product that would similarly reduce the need for platelet transfusions has not been developed. However, the limitations and risks of platelet transfusion therapy continue to drive the development of agents that stimulate platelet production.[256] Thrombopoietic growth factors have the potential to stimulate platelet apheresis donors, to increase stem cell harvest yields, and to expand progenitor cells ex vivo.[257] Rapid developments in the use of growth factors include FLT-3 ligand, c-MPL ligand (thrombopoietin [TPO]), and various combinations of growth factors. IL-11, a 199-amino acid protein coded for on chromosome 19q, directly stimulates the proliferation of hematopoietic stem cells and megakaryocyte progenitors, and it induces increased megakaryocyte maturation. A commercial form of IL-11 was approved by the FDA in 1997 for preventing severe thrombocytopenia in patients receiving myelosuppressive chemotherapy. However, IL-11 effects on platelet production are modest, and IL-11 is not recommended for patients with myeloid leukemias.[258]

TPO, a key regulator of platelet production, is a 38-kD protein that is synthesized in the liver and kidney.[259] It undergoes post-translational glycosylation to form a 90-kD protein. Its effects are mediated by binding to the TPO receptor. In vitro effects of TPO include increasing the number, size, and ploidy of megakaryocytes in culture. TPO does not appear to be involved in the release of platelets from mature megakaryocytes. Its receptor, c-MPL, was discovered during study of a viral oncogene v-MPL in the myeloproliferative (mpl) leukemia virus. Once this receptor was identified, the ligand (TPO) was directly isolated. TPO isolated from humans is a two-domain structure with an N-terminus that is partially (50%) homologous with erythropoietin. The "erythropoietin-like" domain appears to confer its biologic activity. Two recombinant forms of TPO have undergone clinical testing: a glycosylated recombinant human TPO (rHuTPO) identical in amino acid sequence to endogenous TPO, and pegylated recombinant megakaryocyte growth and development factor (polyethylene glycol [PEG]-rHuMGDF). The latter is a nonglycosylated, truncated form of TPO that contains the first 163 amino acids of endogenous TPO. The molecule is covalently linked to PEG to extend the half-life of the molecule to more than 20 hours. Using a baboon model, research showed that PEG-MGDF does not increase platelet secretory granule membrane protein P-selectin expression, nor does it increase the binding of annexin V to platelet membranes.[260] In addition, direct exposure of platelets to various concentrations of PEG-rHuMGDF does not appear to hasten or retard development of platelet storage defect, as defined by a battery of in vitro tests of platelet structure and function.[261]

Both rHuTPO and PEG-rHuMGDF are potent stimulators of platelet production in humans. They have been shown to stimulate the production of platelets in thrombocytopenic oncology patients after chemotherapy and may reduce the need for platelet transfusion.[262–264] Moreover, PEG-rHuMGDF has been effective in increasing platelet counts in chimpanzees with HIV-related thrombocytopenia.[260] The platelets produced in response to these growth factors demonstrate the expected responses to platelet agonists and ATP release in vivo, and their function is abrogated by aspirin.[265] PEG-rHuMGDF was administered to normal donors; single 2 μg/kg doses produced a doubling of the platelet count 9 to 14 days after administration. A single 3 μg/kg dose reliably produced a platelet count of $600 \times 10^9/L$. Single intravenous doses of PEG-rHuMGDF produced higher platelet elevations on day 5 after administration, whereas daily administration for 5 days produced more prolonged thrombocytosis. Thus, PEG-rHuMGDF was evaluated to increase the yield of platelets from volunteer platelet apheresis donors.[266] Apheresis platelets collected from such donors were stored and, when transfused, improved the platelet corrected count increment in the recipient. The development of neutralizing antibodies against endogenous TPO has plagued clinical testing of thrombopoietic growth factors, in particular, PEG-rHuMGDF. These antibodies have caused severe thrombocytopenia in healthy volunteers and in oncology patients undergoing intensive chemotherapy.[267]

Thrombopoietic growth factors have also been used in combination with other growth factors to produce megakaryocytic progenitors ex vivo that can then be administered to autologous donors.[268] Other cytokines under development are designed to mimic the effects of TPO. A peptide agonist has been described that is a 14-amino acid peptide with a high affinity for the TPO receptor.[269] This molecule was shown to be equipotent to the 332-amino acid natural cytokines in cell-based assays. These small molecules, which can activate receptors and can replace the need for large peptide ligands, may open the way for production of new types of hematopoietic stem cell growth factors.

■ Conclusions

For at least the near future, clinicians will continue to rely on PC transfusions for bleeding or thrombocytopenic patients. Efforts to employ methods that safely extend the shelf life of currently available platelet products and to develop platelet alternatives that provide similar hemostatic effects are ongoing. Unfortunately, it is difficult to determine which in vitro platelet functions are essential for in vivo hemostasis

after platelet transfusion. For example, should these alternatives demonstrate aggregation responses or procoagulant properties that parallel those of freshly drawn platelets? Numerous functions have been attributed to platelets, yet it has not been determined which of these properties are most critical to controlling or preventing bleeding. Clearly, more basic research is required to delineate these mechanisms further. Similarly, a generally poor correlation exists between in vitro tests and in vivo animal or human models of platelet function and survival. Thus, more innovative and useful in vitro assays are needed that more reliably predict in vivo platelet recovery, survival, and function. Pathogen inactivation systems that further decrease the risk of known—and possibly unknown—threats to the blood supply are being actively pursued. These processes must inactivate pathogens without adversely affecting platelets. The role of TPOs in transfusion medicine remains unclear, but novel molecules are under development that can stimulate platelet production, molecules that are less antigenic than some of the TPO forms evaluated thus far.[270, 271]

REFERENCES

1. Hersh EM, Bodey GP, Boyd AN, Freireich EJ: Causes of death in acute leukaemia: A ten year study of 414 patients from 1954–1963. JAMA 1965;193:99–103.
2. Wallace EL, Churchill WH Surgenor DM, et al: Collection and transfusion of blood and blood components in the United States, 1994. Transfusion 1998;38:625–636.
3. Schiffer CA, Anderson KC, Bennett CL, et al: Platelet transfusion for patients with cancer: Clinical practice guidelines of the American Society of Clinical Oncology. J Clin Oncol 2001;19:1519–1538.
4. Wright JH: The histogenesis of blood platelets. J Morphol 1910;21:263.
5. Bruno E, Hoffman R: Human megakaryocyte progenitor cells. Semin Hematol 1988;35:183–191.
6. Fox JE: The platelet cytoskeleton. Thromb Haemost 1993;70:884–893.
7. Holt JC, Niewiarowski S: Biochemistry of alpha granule proteins. Semin Hematol 1985;22:151–163.
8. Rucinski B, Niewiarowski S, Strzyzewski M, et al: Human platelet factor 4 and its C-terminal peptides: Heparin binding and clearance from the circulation [published erratum appears in Thromb Haemost 1991;66:269]. Thromb Haemost 1991;63:493–498.
9. Deuel TF, Senior RM, Chang D, et al: Platelet factor 4 is chemotactic for neutrophils and monocytes. Proc Natl Acad Sci U S A 1981;78:4584–4587.
10. Gewirtz AM, Calabretta B, Rucinski B, et al: Inhibition of human megakaryocytopoiesis in vitro by platelet factor 4 (PF4) and a synthetic COOH-terminal PF4 peptide. J Clin Invest 1989;83:1477–1486.
11. Capitanio AM, Niewiarowski S, Rucinski B, et al: Interaction of platelet factor 4 with human platelets. Biochim Biophys Acta 1985;839:161–173.
12. Zucker MB, Katz IR, Thorbecke GJ, et al: Immunoregulatory activity of peptides related to platelet factor 4. Proc Natl Acad Sci U S A 1989;86:7571–7574.
13. Bevers EM, Comfurius P, Dekkers DW, et al: Transmembrane phospholipid distribution in blood cells: Control mechanisms and pathophysiological significance. Biol Chem 1998;379:973–986.
14. Comfurius P, Senden JM, Tilly RH, et al: Loss of membrane phospholipid asymmetry in platelets and red cells may be associated with calcium-induced shedding of plasma membrane and inhibition of aminophospholipid translocase. Biochim Biophys Acta 1990;1026:153–160.
15. Rosing J, van Rijn JL, Bevers EM, et al: The role of activated human platelets in prothrombin and factor X activation. Blood 1985;65:319–332.
16. Harrison P, Wilbourn B, Cramer E, et al: The influence of therapeutic blocking of Gp IIb/IIIa on platelet alpha-granular fibrinogen. Br J Haematol 1992;82:721–728.
17. Castillo R, Escolar G, Monteagudo J, et al: Hemostasis in patients with severe von Willebrand disease improves after normal platelet transfusion and normalizes with further correction of the plasma defect. Transfusion 1997;37:785–790.

18. Kieffer N, Phillips DR: Platelet membrane glycoproteins: functions in cellular interactions. Annu Rev Cell Biol 1990;6:329–357.

19. Nachman RL, Leung LL: Complex formation of platelet membrane glycoproteins IIb and IIIa with fibrinogen. J Clin Invest 1982;69:263–269.

20. Nieuwenhuis HK, Akkerman JW, Houdijk WP, et al: Human blood platelets showing no response to collagen fail to express surface glycoprotein Ia. Nature 1985;318:470–472.

21. Berman CL, Yce EL, Wencel-Drake JD, et al: A platelet alpha granule membrane protein that is associated with the plasma membrane after activation: Characterization and subcellular localization of platelet activation-dependent granule-external membrane protein. J Clin Invest 1986;78:130–137.

22. Clemetson KJ: Platelet activation: Signal transduction via membrane receptors. Thromb Haemost 1995;74:111–116.

23. Eriksson L, Kristensen J, Olsson K, et al: Evaluation of platelet function using the in vitro bleeding time and corrected count increment of transfused platelets: Comparison between platelet concentrates derived from pooled buffy coats and apheresis. Vox Sang 1996;70:69–75.

24. Weiss HJ: Flow-related platelet deposition on subendothelium. Thromb Haemost 1995;74:117–122.

25. Perutelli P, Biglino P, Mori PG: von Willebrand factor: Biological function and molecular defects. Pediatr Hematol Oncol 1997;14:499–512.

26. Ruggeri ZM: Mechanisms initiating platelet thrombus formation [published erratum appears in Thromb Haemost 1997;78:1304]. Thromb Haemost 1997;78:611–616.

27. Lyman B, Rosenberg L, Karpatkin S: Biochemical and biophysical aspects of human platelet adhesion to collagen fibers. J Clin Invest 1971;50:1854–1863.

28. Homsen H, Setkowsky CA, Day HJ: Effects of antimycin and 2-deoxyglucose on adenine nucleotides in human platelets:Role of metabolic adenosine triphosphate in primary aggregation, secondary aggregation and shape change of platetets. Biochem J 1974;144:385–396.

29. Kilkson H, Holme S, Murphy S: Platelet metabolism during storage of platelet concentrates at 22 degrees C. Blood 1984;64:406–414.

30. Moroff G, Holme S:Concepts about current conditions for the preparation and storage of platelets. Transfus Med Rev 1991;5:48–59.

31. Murphy S, Heaton WA, Rebulla P: Platelet production in the Old World—and the New. Transfusion 1996;36:751–754.

32. Mourad N: A simple method for obtaining platelet concentrates free of aggregates. Transfusion 1968;8:48.

33. Snyder EL, Pope C, Ferri PM, et al: The effect of mode of agitation and type of plastic bag on storage characteristics and in vivo kinetics of platelet concentrates. Transfusion 1986;26:125–130.

34. Fijnheer R, Veldman HA, van den Eertwegh AJ, et al: In vitro evaluation of buffy-coat-derived platelet concentrates stored in a synthetic medium. Vox Sang 1991;60:16–22.

35. Bishop D, Tandy N, Anderson N, et al: A clinical and laboratory study of platelet concentrates produced by pooled buffy coat and single donor apheresis technologies. Transfus Sci 1995;16:187–188.

36. Keegan T, Heaton A, Holme S, et al: Paired comparison of platelet concentrates prepared from platelet-rich plasma and buffy coats using a new technique with ^{111}In and [51]Cr. Transfusion 1992;32:113–120.

37. Murphy S: The efficacy of synthetic media in the storage of human platelets for transfusion. Transfus Med Rev 1999;13:153–163.

38. Rock G, White J, Labow R: Storage of platelets in balanced salt solutions: A simple platelet storage medium. Transfusion 1991;31:21–25.

39. Gulliksson H, Eriksson L, Hogman CF, et al: Buffy-coat-derived platelet concentrates prepared from half-strength citrate CPD and CPD whole-blood units: Comparison between three additive solutions: in vitro studies. Vox Sang 1995;68:152–159.

40 Murphy S, Kagen L, Holme S, et al: Platelet storage in synthetic media lacking glucose and bicarbonate. Transfusion 1991;31:16–20.

41.. Bertolini F, Rebulla P, Riccardi D, et al: Evaluation of platelet concentrates prepared from buffy coats and stored in a glucose-free crystalloid medium. Transfusion 1989;29:605–609.

42. Bode AP, Holme S, Heaton WA, et al: Extended storage of platelets in an artificial medium with the platelet activation inhibitors prostaglandin E1 and theophylline. Vox Sang 1991;60:105–112.

43. Murphy S, Gardner FH: Effect of storage temperature on maintenance of platelet viability: Deleterious effect of refrigerated storage. N Engl J Med 1969;280:1094–1098.

44. Slichter SJ, Harker LA: Preparation and storage of platelet concentrates. II. Storage variables influencing platelet viability and function. Br J Haematol 1976;34:403–419.

45. Filip DJ, Aster RH: Relative hemostatic effectiveness of human platelets stored at 4 degrees and 22 degrees C. J Lab Clin Med 1978;91:618–624.

46. Vostal JG, Mondoro TH: Liquid cold storage of platelets: A revitalized possible alternative for limiting bacterial contamination of platelet products. Transfus Med Rev 1997;11:286–295.

47. Hartwig JH: Mechanisms of actin rearrangements mediating platelet activation. J Cell Biol 1992;118:1421–1442.

48. Hoffmeister KM, Falet H, Toker A, et al: Mechanisms of cold-induced platelet actin assembly. J Biol Chem 2001;27:27.

49. Reid TJ, LaRussa VF, Esteban G, et al: Cooling and freezing damage platelet membrane integrity. Cryobiology 1999;38:209–224.

50. Winokur R, Hartwig JH: Mechanism of shape change in chilled human platelets. Blood 1995;85:1796–1804.

51. Murphy S, Gardner FH: Platelet storage at 22 degrees C: Role of gas transport across plastic containers in maintenance of viability. Blood 1975;46:209–218.

52. Moroff G, Friedman A, Robkin-Kline L: Factors influencing changes in pH during storage of platelet concentrates at 20–24 degrees C. Vox Sang 1982;42:33–45.

53. Snyder EL, Ezekowitz M, Aster R, et al. Extended storage of platelets in a new plastic container. II. In vivo response to infusion of platelets stored for 5 days. Transfusion 1985;25:209–214.

54. Murphy S, Kahn RA, Holme S, et al: Improved storage of platelets for transfusion in a new container. Blood 1982;60:194–200.

55. Snyder EL, Aster RH, Heaton A, et al: Five-day storage of platelets in a non-diethylhexyl phthalate-plasticized container. Transfusion 1992;32:736–741.

56. Jaeger RJ, Rubin RJ: Migration of a phthalate ester plasticizer from polyvinyl chloride blood bags into stored human blood and its localization in human tissues. N Engl J Med 1972;287:1114–1118.

57. Jaeger RJ, Rubin RJ: Di-2-ethylhexyl phthalate, a plasticizer contaminant of platelet concentrates. Transfusion 1973;13:107–111.

58. Sasakawa S, Mitomi Y: Di-2-ethylhexylphthalate (DEHP) content of blood or blood components stored in plastic bags. Vox Sang 1978;34:81–86.

59. Rock G, Secours VE, Franklin CA, et al: The accumulation of mono-2-ethylhexylphthalate (MEHP) during storage of whole blood and plasma. Transfusion 1978;18:553–558.

60. Peck CC, Odom DG, Friedman HI, et al: Di-2-ethylhexyl phthalate (DEHP) and mono-2-ethylhexyl phthalate (MEHP) accumulation in whole blood and red cell concentrates. Transfusion 1979;19:137–146.

61. Conway JG, Tomaszewski KE, Olson MJ, et al: Relationship of oxidative damage to the hepatocarcinogenicity of the peroxisome proliferators di(2-ethylhexyl)phthalate and Wy-14,643. Carcinogenesis 1989;10:513–519.

62. Albro PW, Chapin RE, Corbett JT, et al: Mono-2-ethylhexyl phthalate, a metabolite of di-(2-ethylhexyl) phthalate, causally linked to testicular atrophy in rats. Toxicol Appl Pharmacol 1989;100:193–200.

63. Salkie ML, Hannon JL: Anti-plasticizer specific IgE is present in the serum of transfused patients. Clin Invest Med 1995;18:419–423.

64. Horowitz B, Stryker MH, Waldman AA, et al: Stabilization of red blood cells by the plasticizer, diethylhexylphthalate. Vox Sang 1985;48:150–155.

65. AuBuchon JP, Estep TN, Davey RJ: The effect of the plasticizer di-2-ethylhexyl phthalate on the survival of stored RBCs. Blood 1988;71:448–452.

66. Gulliksson H, Shanwell A, Wikman A, et al: Storage of platelets in a new plastic container: Polyvinyl chloride plasticized with butyryl-n-trihexyl citrate. Vox Sang 1991;61:165–170.

67. Holme S, Vaidja K, Murphy S: Platelet storage at 22 degrees C: effect of type of agitation on morphology, viability, and function in vitro. Blood 1978;52:425–435.

68. Snyder EL, Hezzey A, Katz AJ, Bock J: Occurrence of the release reaction during preparation and storage of platelet concentrates. Vox Sang 1981;41:172–177.

69. Graw RG Jr, Herzig GP, Eisel RJ, Perry S: Leukocyte and platelet collection from normal donors with the continuous flow blood cell separator. Transfusion 1971;11:94–101.

70. Yankee RA, Grumet FC, Rogentine GN: Platelet transfusion: The selection of compatible platelet donors for refractory patients by lymphocyte HLA typing. N Engl J Med 1969;281:1208–1212.

71. Thorsby E, Helgesen A, Gjemdal T: Repeated platelet transfusions from HLA-compatible unrelated and sibling donors. Tissue Antigens 1972;2:397–404.

72. Burgstaler EA, Pineda AA, Wollan P: Plateletapheresis: comparison of processing times, platelet yields, and white blood cell content with several commonly used systems. J Clin Apheresis 1991;12:170–178.

73. Yockey C, Murphy S, Eggers L, et al: Evaluation of the Amicus Separator in the collection of apheresis platelets. Transfusion 1998;38:848–854.

74. Elfath MD, Whitley P, Jacobson MS, et al: Evaluation of an automated system for the collection of packed RBCs, platelets, and plasma. Transfusion 2000;40:1214–1222.

75. Chalandon Y, Mermillod B, Beris P, et al: Benefit of prestorage leukocyte depletion of single-donor platelet concentrates. Vox Sang 1999;76:27–37.

76. Bock M, Schleuning M, Heim MU, Mempel W: Cryopreservation of human platelets with dimethyl sulfoxide: Changes in biochemistry and cell function. Transfusion 1995;35:921–924.

77. Funke I, Wiesneth M, Koerner K, et al: Autologous platelet transfusion in alloimmunized patients with acute leukemia. Ann Hematol 1995;71:169–173.

78. Torretta L, Perotti C, Pedrazzoli P, et al: Autologous platelet collection and storage to support thrombocytopenia in patients undergoing high-dose chemotherapy and circulating progenitor cell transplantation for high-risk breast cancer. Vox Sang 1998;75:224–229.

79. McLeod BC, Price TH, Owen H, et al: Frequency of immediate adverse effects associated with apheresis donation. Transfusion 1998;38:938–943.

80. Sweeney J: Quality assurance and standards for red cells and platelets. Vox Sang 1998;74:201–205.

81. Menitove J (ed): Standards for Blood Banks and Transfusion Services, 19th ed. Bethesda, MD, American Association of Blood Banks, 1999.

82. Dickerhoff R, Von Ruecker A: Enumeration of platelets by multiparameter flow cytometry using platelet-specific antibodies and fluorescent reference particles. Clin Lab Haematol 1995;17:163–172.

83. Bertolini F, Murphy S: A multicenter inspection of the swirling phenomenon in platelet concentrates prepared in routine practice: Biomedical Excellence for Safer Transfusion (BEST) Working Party of the International Society of Blood Transfusion. Transfusion 1996;36:128–132.

84. Bertolini F, Murphy S: A multicenter evaluation of reproducibility of swirling in platelet concentrates: Biomedical Excellence for Safer Transfusion (BEST) Working Party of the International Society of Blood Transfusion. Transfusion 1994;34:796–801.

85. Bertolini F, Agazzi A, Peccatori F, et al: The absence of swirling in platelet concentrates is highly predictive of poor posttransfusion platelet count increments and increased risk of a transfusion reaction. Transfusion 2000;40:121–122.

86. Lutz P, Dzik WH: Large-volume hemocytometer chamber for accurate counting of white cells (WBCs) in WBC-reduced platelets: Validation and application for quality control of WBC-reduced platelets prepared by apheresis and filtration. Transfusion 1993;33:409–412.

87. Moroff G, Eich J, Dabay M: Validation of use of the Nageotte hemocytometer to count low levels of white cells in white cell-reduced platelet components. Transfusion 1994;34:35–38.

88. Finch SJ, Chen JB, Chen CH, et al: Process control procedures to augment quality control of leukocyte-reduced red cell blood products. Stat Med 1999;18:1279–1289.

89. Dzik WH Ragosta A, Cusack WF: Flow-cytometric method for counting very low numbers of leukocytes in platelet products. Vox Sang 1990;59:153–159.

90. Adams MR, Johnson DK, Busch MP, et al: Automatic volumetric capillary cytometry for counting white cells in white cell-reduced plateletpheresis components. Transfusion 1997;37:29–37.

91. Dzik S, Moroff G, Dumont L: A multicenter study evaluating three methods for counting residual WBCs in WBC-reduced blood components: Nageotte hemocytometry, flow cytometry, and microfluorometry. Transfusion 2000;40:513–520.

92. Sirchia G, Rebulla P, Sabbioneda L, et al: Optimal conditions for white cell reduction in red cells by filtration at the patient's bedside. Transfusion 1996;36:322–327.

93. Seghatchian J, Krailadsiri P: Current methods for the preparation of platelet concentrates: Laboratory and clinical aspects. Transfus Sci 1997;18:27–32.

94. Dumont LJ, Dzik WH Rebulla P, Brandwein H: Practical guidelines for process validation and process control of white cell-reduced blood components: Report of the Biomedical Excellence for Safer Transfusion (BEST) Working Party of the International Society of Blood Transfusion (ISBT). Transfusion 1996;36:11–20.

95. Holme S, Heaton WA, Moroff G: Evaluation of platelet concentrates stored for 5 days with reduced plasma volume. Transfusion 1994;34:39–43.

96. Blanchette VS, Kuhne T, Hume H, Hellmann J: Platelet transfusion therapy in newborn infants. Transfus Med Rev 1995;9:215–230.

97. Simon TL, Sierra ER:. Concentration of platelet units into small volumes. Transfusion 1984;24:173–175.

98. Moroff G, Friedman A, Robkin-Kline L, et al: Reduction of the volume of stored platelet concentrates for use in neonatal patients. Transfusion 1984;24:144–146.

99. Pisciotto PT, Snyder EL, Napychank PA, Hopfer SM: In vitro characteristics of volume-reduced platelet concentrate stored in syringes. Transfusion 1991;31:404–408.

100. Pisciotto PT, Snyder EL, Snyder JA, et al: In vitro characteristics of white cell-reduced single-unit platelet concentrates stored in syringes. Transfusion 1994;34:407–411.

101. Seghatchian J, Krailadsiri P: The platelet storage lesion. Transfus Mod Rev 1997;11:130–144.

102. Rinder HM, Murphy M, Mitchell JG, et al: Progressive platelet activation with storage: evidence for shortened survival of activated platelets after transfusion. Transfusion 1991;31:409–414.

103. Triulzi DJ, Kickler TS, Braine HG: Detection and significance of alpha granule membrane protein 140 expression on platelets collected by apheresis. Transfusion 1992;32:529–533.

104. Chernoff A, Snyder EL: The cellular and molecular basis of the platelet storage lesion: A symposium summary. Transfusion 1992;32:386–390.

105. Snyder EL, Moroff G, Simon T, Heaton A: Recommended methods for conducting radiolabeled platelet survival studies. Transfusion 1986;26:37–42.

106. Heilmann E, Friese P, Anderson S, et al: Biotinylated platelets: A new approach to the measurement of platelet life span. Br J Haematol 1993;85:729–735.

107. Rinder HM, Bonan JL, Rinder CS, et al: Dynamics of leukocyte-platelet adhesion in whole blood. Blood 1991;78:1730–1737.

108. Murphy S, Rebulla P, Bertolini F, et al: In vitro assessment of the quality of stored platelet concentrates: The BEST (Biomedical Excellence for Safer Transfusion) Task Force of the International Society of Blood Transfusion. Transfus Med Rev 1994;8:29–36.

109. Michelson AD, Barnard MR, Hechtman HB, et al: In vivo tracking of platelets: Circulating degranulated platelets rapidly lose surface P-selectin but continue to circulate and function. Proc Natl Acad Sci U S A 1996;93:11877–11882.

110. Metcalfe P, Williamson LM, Reutelingsperger CP, et al: Activation during preparation of therapeutic platelets affects deterioration during storage: A comparative flow cytometric study of different production methods. Br J Haematol 1997;98:86–95.

111. Dumont LJ, VandenBroeke T, Ault KA: Platelet surface P-selectin measurements in platelet preparations: An international collaborative study. Biomedical Excellence for Safer Transfusion (BEST) Working Party of the International Society of Blood Transfusion (ISBT). Transfus Med Rev 1999;13:31–42.

112. McEver RP: GMP-140: A receptor for neutrophils and monocytes on activated platelets and endothelium. J Cell Biochem 1991;45:156–161.

113. George JN, Pickett EB, Heinz R: Platelet membrane glycoprotein changes during the preparation and storage of platelet concentrates. Transfusion 1988;28:123–126.

114. Fijnheer R, Modderman PW, Veldman H, et al: Detection of platelet activation with monoclonal antibodies and flow cytometry: Changes during platelet storage. Transfusion 1990;30:20–25.

115. Fijnheer R, Pietersz RN, de Korte D, et al: Platelet activation during preparation of platelet concentrates: A comparison of the platelet-rich plasma and the buffy coat methods. Transfusion 1990;30:634–638.

116. Fox JE, Reynolds CC, Morrow JS, et al: Spectrin is associated with membrane-bound actin filaments in platelets and is hydrolyzed by the Ca2+-dependent protease during platelet activation. Blood 1987;69:537–545.

117. Pollard TD, Cooper JA: Actin and actin-binding proteins: A critical evaluation of mechanisms and functions. Annu Rev Biochem 1986;55:987–1035.

118. Bode AP, Orton SM, Frye MJ, Udis BJ: Vesiculation of platelets during in vitro aging. Blood 1991, 77:887–895.

119. Snyder EL, Horne WC, Napychank P, et al: Calcium-dependent proteolysis of actin during storage of platelet concentrates. Blood 1989;73:1380–1385.

120. Robey FA, Freitag CM, Jamieson GA: Disappearance of actin binding protein from human blood platelets during storage. FEBS Lett 1979;102:257–260.

121. Tsujinaka T, Sakon M, Kambayashi J, Kosaki G: Cleavage of cytoskeletal proteins by two forms of Ca2+ activated neutral proteases in human platelets. Thromb Res 1982;28:149–156.

122. Fox JE, Goll DE, Reynolds CC, Phillips DR: Identification of two proteins (actin-binding protein and P235) that are hydrolyzed by endogenous Ca2+-dependent protease during platelet aggregation. J Biol Chem 1985;260:1060–1066.

123. Wiedmer T, Shattil SJ, Cunningham M, Sims PJ: Role of calcium and calpain in complement-induced vesiculation of the platelet plasma membrane and in the exposure of the platelet factor Va receptor. Biochemistry 1990;29:623–632.

124. Brown SB, Clarke MC, Magowan L, et al: Constitutive death of platelets leading to scavenger receptor-mediated phagocytosis: A caspase-independent cell clearance program. J Biol Chem 2000;275:5987–5996.

125. Michelson AD, Adelman B, Barnard MR, et al: Platelet storage results in a redistribution of glycoprotein Ib molecules: Evidence for a large intraplatelet pool of glycoprotein Ib. J Clin Invest 1988;81:1734–1740.

126. Snyder EL, Beardsley DS, Smith BR, et al: Storage of platelet concentrates after high-dose ultraviolet B irradiation. Transfusion 1991;31:491–496.

127. Bertolini F, Rebulla P, Porretti L, Sirchia G: Comparison of platelet activation and membrane glycoprotein Ib and IIb-IIIa expression after filtration through three different leukocyte removal filters. Vox Sang 1990;59:201–204.

128. Michelson AD, Barnard MR: Plasmin-induced redistribution of platelet glycoprotein Ib. Blood 1990;76:2005–2010.

129. Goldman M, Blajchman MA: Blood product-associated bacterial sepsis. Transfus Med Rev 1991;5:73–83.

130. Morrow JF, Braine HG, Kickler TS, et al: Septic reactions to platelet transfusions: A persistent problem. JAMA 1991;266:555–558.

131. Mitchell KM, Brecher ME: Approaches to the detection of bacterial contamination in cellular blood products. Transfus Med Rev 1999;13:132–144.

132. Liu HW, Yuen KY, Cheng TS, et al: Reduction of platelet transfusion-associated sepsis by short-term bacterial culture. Vox Sang 1999;77:1–5.

133. Brecher ME, Means N, Jere CS, et al: Evaluation of an automated culture system for detecting bacterial contamination of platelets: An analysis with 15 contaminating organisms. Transfusion 2001;41:477–482.

134. Buchholz DH, AuBuchon JP, Snyder EL, et al: Effects of white cell reduction on the resistance of blood components to bacterial multiplication. Transfusion 1994;34:852–857.

135. Snyder EL, Mosher DF, Hezzey A, Golenwsky G: Effect of blood transfusion on in vivo levels of plasma fibronectin. J Lab Clin Med 1981;98:336–341.

136. Kickler TS, Bell W, Drew H, Pall D: Depletion of white cells from platelet concentrates with a new adsorption filter. Transfusion 1989;29:411–414.

137. Sirchia G, Wenz B, Rebulla P, et al: Removal of white cells from red cells by transfusion through a new filter. Transfusion 1990;30:30–33.

138. Kao KJ, Mickel M, Braine HG, et al: White cell reduction in platelet concentrates and packed red cells by filtration: A multicenter clinical trial. The Trap Study Group. Transfusion 1995;35:13–19.

139. Snyder EL, DePalma L, Napychank P: Use of polyester filters for the preparation of leukocyte-poor platelet concentrates. Vox Sang 1988;54:21–23.

140. Silliman CC, Dickey WO, Paterson AJ, et al: Analysis of the priming activity of lipids generated during routine storage of platelet concentrates. Transfusion 1996;36:133–139.

141. Heddle NM, Klama L, Singer J, et al: The role of the plasma from platelet concentrates in transfusion reactions. N Engl J Med 1994;331:625–628.

142. Stack G, Snyder EL: Cytokine generation in stored platelet concentrates. Transfusion 1994;34:20–25.

143. Aye MT, Palmer DS, Giulivi A, Hashemi S: Effect of filtration of platelet concentrates on the accumulation of cytokines and platelet release factors during storage. Transfusion 1995;35:117–124.

144. Blajchman MA, Bardossy L, Carmen RA, et al: An animal model of allogeneic donor platelet refractoriness: The effect of the time of leukodepletion. Blood 1992;79:1371–1375.

145. Anderson KC, Goodnough LT, Sayers M, et al: Variation in blood component irradiation practice: Implications for prevention of transfusion-associated graft-versus-host disease. Blood 1991;77:2096–2102.

146. Moroff G, George VM, et al: The influence of irradiation on stored platelets. Transfusion 1986;26:453–456.

147. Button LN, DeWolf WC, Newburger PE, et al: The effects of irradiation on blood components. Transfusion 1981;21:419–426.

148. Read EJ, Kodis C, Carter CS, Leitman SF: Viability of platelets following storage in the irradiated state: A pair-controlled study. Transfusion 1988;28:446–450.

149. Rock G, Adams GA, Labow RS: The effects of irradiation on platelet function. Transfusion 1988;28:451–455.

150. Sweeney JD, Holme S, Moroff G: Storage of apheresis platelets after gamma radiation. Transfusion 1994;34:779–783.

151. Moroff G, Luban NL: The irradiation of blood and blood components to prevent graft-versus-host disease: Technical issues and guidelines. Transfus Med Rev 1997;11:15–26.

152. Pamphilon DH: The rationale and use of platelet concentrates irradiated with ultraviolet-B light. Transfus Med Rev 1999;13:323–333.

153. Lindahl-Kiessling K, Safwenberg J: Inability of UV-irradiated lymphocytes to stimulate allogeneic cells in mixed lymphocyte culture. Int Arch Allergy Appl Immunol 1971;41:670–678.

154. Doery JC, Dickson RC, Hirsh J: Induction of aggregation of human blood platelets by ultraviolet light: Action spectrum and structural changes. Blood 1973;42:551–555.

155. Kahn RA, Duffy BF, Rodey GG: Ultraviolet irradiation of platelet concentrate abrogates lymphocyte activation without affecting platelet fiunction in vitro. Transfusion 1985;25:547–550.

156. Pamphilon DH, Corbin SA, Saunders J, Tandy NP: Applications of ultraviolet light in the preparation of platelet concentrates. Transfusion 1989;29:379–383.

157. Pamphilon DH, Potter M, Cutts M, et al: Platelet concentrates irradiated with ultraviolet light retain satisfactory in vitro storage characteristics and in vivo survival. Br J Haematol 1990;75:240–244.

158. Andreu G, Boccaccio C, Lecrubier C, et al: Ultraviolet irradiation of platelet concentrates: Feasibility in transfusion practice. Transfusion 1990;30:401–406.

159. Trial to Reduce Alloimmunization to Platelets Study Group: Leukocyte reduction and ultraviolet B irradiation of platelets to prevent alloimmunization and refractoriness to platelet transfusions. N Engl J Med 1997;337:1861–1869.

160. Kraemer KH, Levis WR, Cason JC, Tarone RE: Inhibition of mixed leukocyte culture reaction by 8-methoxypsoralen and long-wavelength ultraviolet radiation. J Invest Dermatol 1981;77:235–239.

161. Grana NH, Kao KJ: Use of 8-methoxypsoralen and ultraviolet-A pretreated platelet concentrates to prevent alloimmunization against class I major histocompatibility antigens. Blood 1991;77:2530–2537.

162. Corash L: Inactivation of viruses, bacteria, protozoa, and leukocytes in platelet concentrates: Current research perspectives. Transfus Med Rev 1999;13:18–30.

163. Lin L, Londe H, Janda JM, et al: Photochemical inactivation of pathogenic bacteria in human platelet concentrates. Blood 1994;83:2698–2706.

164. Lin L, Cook DN, Wiesehahn GP, et al: Photochemical inactivation of viruses and bacteria in platelet concentrates by use of a novel psoralen and long-wavelength ultraviolet light. Transfusion 1997;37:423–435.

165. Corash L: Inactivation of viruses, bacteria, protozoa, and leukocytes in platelet concentrates. Vox Sang 1998;74:173–176.

166. van Rhenen DJ, Vermeij J, Mayaudon V, et al: Functional characteristics of S-59 photochemically treated platelet concentrates derived from buffy coats. Vox Sang 2000;79:206–214.

167. Grass JA, Wafa T, Reames A, et al: Prevention of transfusion-associated graft-versus-host disease by photochemical treatment. Blood 1999;93:3140–3147.

168. Produoz KN, Lytle CD, Keville EA, et al: Inhibition by albumin of merocyanine 540-mediated photosensitization of platelets and viruses. Transfusion 1991;31:415–422.

169. Dodd RY, Moroff G, Wagner S, et al: Inactivation of viruses in platelet suspensions that retain their in vitro characteristics: Comparison of

psoralen-ultraviolet A and merocyanine 540-visible light methods. Transfusion 1991;31:483–490.

170. Payne R: The association of febrile transfusion reactions with leukoagglutinins. Vox Sang 1957;2:233.

171. Chambers LA, Kruskall MS, Pacini DG, Donovan LM: Febrile reactions after platelet transfusion: The effect of single versus multiple donors. Transfusion 1990;30:219–221.

172. Sarkodee-Adoo CB, Kendall JM, Sridhara R, et al: The relationship between the duration of platelet storage and the development of transfusion reactions. Transfusion 1998;38:229–235.

173. Snyder EL: The role of cytokines and adhesive molecules in febrile non-hemolytic transfusion reactions. Immunol Invest 1995;24:333–339.

174. Ferrara JL: The febrile platelet transfusion reaction: a cytokine shower [editorial]. Transfusion 1995;35:89–90.

175. Heddle NM, Klama LN, Griffith L, et al: A prospective study to identify the risk factors associated with acute reactions to platelet and red cell transfusions. Transfusion 1993;33:794–797.

176. Federowicz I, Barrett BB, Andersen JW, et al: Characterization of reactions after transfusion of cellular blood components that are white cell reduced before storage. Transfusion 1996;36:21–28.

177. Snyder EL, Mechanic S, Baril L, Davenport R: Removal of soluble biologic response modifiers (complement and chemokines) by a bedside white cell-reduction filter. Transfusion 1996;36:707–713.

178. Geiger TL, Perrotta PL, Davenport R, et al: Removal of anaphylatoxins C3a and C5a and chemokines interleukin 8 and RANTES by polyester white cell-reduction and plasma filters. Transfusion 1997;37:1156–1162.

179. Oppermann M, Gotze O: Plasma clearance of the human C5a anaphylatoxin by binding to leucocyte C5a receptors. Immunology 1994;82:516–521.

180. Heddle NM, Klama L, Meyer R, et al: A randomized controlled trial comparing plasma removal with white cell reduction to prevent reactions to platelets. Transfusion 1999;39:231–238.

181. Hume HA, Popovsky MA, Benson K, et al: Hypotensive reactions: A previously uncharacterized complication of platelet transfusion? Transfusion 1996;36:904–909.

182. Hild M, Soderstrom T, Egberg N, Lundahl J: Kinetics of bradykinin levels during and after leucocyte filtration of platelet concentrates. Vox Sang 1998;75:18–25.

183. Mair B, Leparc GF: Hypotensive reactions associated with platelet transfusions and angiotensin converting enzyme inhibitors. Vox Sang 1998;74:27–30.

184. Shiba M, Tadokoro K, Sawanobori M, et al: Activation of the contact system by filtration of platelet concentrates with a negatively charged white cell-removal filter and measurement of venous blood bradykinin level in patients who received filtered platelets. Transfusion 1997;37:457–462.

185. Cyr M, Hume HA, Champagne M, et al: Anomaly of the des-Arg9-bradykinin metabolism associated with severe hypotensive reactions during blood transfusions: A preliminary study. Transfusion 1999;39:1084–1088.

186. Duke WW: The relation of blood platelets to hemorrhagic disease: Description of a method for determining the bleeding time and coagulation time and report of 3 cases of hemorrhagic disease relieved by transfusion. JAMA 1910;55:1185–1192.

187. Pisciotto PT, Benson K, Hume H, et al: Prophylactic versus therapeutic platelet transfusion practices in hematology and/or oncology patients. Transfusion 1995, 35:498–502.

188. Hunt BJ: Indications for therapeutic platelet transfusions. Blood Rev 1998;12:227–233.

189. Ancliff PJ, Machin SJ: Trigger factors for prophylactic platelet transfusion. Blood Rev 1998;12:234–238.

190. Gaydos LA, Freireich EJ, Mantel N: The quantitative relation between platelet count and hemorrhage in patients with acute leukemia. N Engl J Med 1962;13:283–290.

191. Beutler E: Platelet transfusions: The 20,000/microL trigger. Blood 1993;81:1411–1413.

192. Solomon J, Bofenkamp T, Fahey JL, et al: Platelet prophylaxis in acute non-lymphoblastic leukaemia. Lancet 1978;1:267.

193. Slichter SJ, Harker LA: Thrombocytopenia: mechanisms and management of defects in platelet production. Clin Haematol 1978;7:523–539.

194. Gmur J, Burger J, Schanz U, et al: Safety of stringent prophylactic platelet transfusion policy for patients with acute leukaemia. Lancet 1991;338:1223–1226.

195. Gil-Fernandez JJ, Alegre A, Fernandez-Villalta MJ, et al: Clinical results of a stringent policy on prophylactic platelet transfusion: Non-randomized comparative analysis in 190 bone marrow transplant patients from a single institution. Bone Marrow Transplant 1996;18:931–935.

196. Heckman KD, Weiner GJ, Davis CS, et al: Randomized study of prophylactic platelet transfusion threshold during induction therapy for adult acute leukemia: 10,000/microL versus 20,000/microL. J Clin Oncol 1997;15:1143–1149.

197. Wandt H, Frank M, Ehninger G, et al: Safety and cost effectiveness of a 10×10^9/L trigger for prophylactic platelet transfusions compared with the traditional 20×10^9/L trigger: A prospective comparative trial in 105 patients with acute myeloid leukemia. Blood 1998;91:3601–3606.

198. Rebulla P, Finazzi G, Marangoni F, et al: The threshold for prophylactic platelet transfusions in adults with acute myeloid leukemia: Gruppo Italiano Malattie Ematologiche Maligne dell'Adulto. N Engl J Med 1997;337:1870–1875.

199. Sagmeister M, Oec L, Gmur J: A restrictive platelet transfusion policy allowing long-term support of outpatients with severe aplastic anemia. Blood 1999;93:3124–3126.

200. Murphy MF, Murphy W, Wheatley K, Goldstone AH: Survey of the use of platelet transfusions in centres participating in MRC leukaemia trials. Br J Haematol 1998;102:875–876.

201. Ho CH: The hemostatic effect of packed red cell transfusion in patients with anemia. Transfusion 1998;38:1011–1014.

202. Murphy MF, Brozovic B, Murphy W, et al: Guidelines for platelet transfusions: British Committee for Standards in Haematology, Working Party of the Blood Transfusion Task Force. Transfus Med 1992;2:311–318.

203. Howard SC, Gajjar A, Ribeiro RC, et al: Safety of lumbar puncture for children with acute lymphoblastic leukemia and thrombocytopenia. JAMA 2000;284:2222–2224.

204. Rinder HM, Arbini AA, Snyder EL: Optimal dosing and triggers for prophylactic use of platelet transfusions. Curr Opin Hematol 1999;6:437–441.

205. Hanson SR, Slichter SJ: Platelet kinetics in patients with bone marrow hypoplasia: Evidence for a fixed platelet requirement. Blood 1985;66:1105–1109.

206. Klumpp TR, Herman JH, Innis S, et al: Factors associated with response to platelet transfusion following hematopoietic stem cell transplantation. Bone Marrow Transplant 1996;17:1035–1041.

207. Norol F, Bierling P, Roudot-Thoraval F, et al: Platelet transfusion: A dose-response study. Blood 1998;92:1448–1453.

208. Hersh JK, Hom EG, Brecher ME: Mathematical modeling of platelet survival with implications for optimal transfusion practice in the chronically platelet transfusion-dependent patient. Transfusion 1998;38:637–644.

209. Ackerman SJ, Klumpp TR, Guzman GI, et al: Economic consequences of alterations in platelet transfusion dose: analysis of a prospective, randomized, double-blind trial. Transfusion 2000;40:1457–1462.

210. Lee EJ, Schiffer CA: ABO compatibility can influence the results of platelet transfusion: Results of a randomized trial. Transfusion 1989;29:384–389.

211. McManigal S, Sims KL: Intravascular hemolysis secondary to ABO incompatible platelet products: An underrecognized transfusion reaction. Am J Clin Pathol 1999;111:202–206.

212. Larsson LG, Welsh VJ, Ladd DJ: Acute intravascular hemolysis secondary to out-of-group platelet transfusion. Transfusion 2000;40:902–906.

213. Flegel WA, Wiesneth M, Stampe D, Koerner K: Low cytokine contamination in buffy coat-derived platelet concentrates without filtration. Transfusion 1995;35:917–920.

214. Ishida A, Handa M, Wakui M, et al: Clinical factors influencing posttransfusion platelet increment in patients undergoing hematopoietic progenitor cell transplantation: A prospective analysis. Transfusion 1998;38:839–847.

215. Despotis GJ, Goodnough LT, Dynis M, et al: Adverse events in platelet apheresis donors: A multivariate analysis in a hospital-based program. Vox Sang 1999;77:24–32.

216. Howard JE, Perkins HA: The natural history of alloimmunization to platelets. Transfusion 1978;18:496–503.

217. Bishop JF, McGrath K, Wolf MM, et al: Clinical factors influencing the efficacy of pooled platelet transfusions. Blood 1988;71:383–387.

218. Doughty HA, Murphy MF, Metcalfe P, et al: Relative importance of immune and non-immune causes of platelet refractoriness. Vox Sang 1994;66:200–205.

219. Bock M, Muggenthaler KH, Schmidt U, Heim MU: Influence of antibiotics on posttransfusion platelet increment. Transfusion 1996;36:952–954.

220. Hussein MA, Fletcher R, Long TJ, et al: Transfusing platelets 2 h after the completion of amphotericin-B decreases its detrimental effect on transfused platelet recovery and survival. Transfus Med 1998;8:43–47.

221. Green D, Tiro A, Basiliere J, Mittal KK: Cytotoxic antibody complicating platelet support in acute leukemia: Response to chemotherapy. JAMA 1976;236:1044–1046.

222. Brandt JT, Julius CJ, Osborne JM, Anderson CL: The mechanism of platelet aggregation induced by HLA-related antibodies. Thromb Haemost 1996;76:774–779.

223. McFarland JG: Alloimmunization and platelet transfusion. Semin Hematol 1996;33:315–328.

224. Bolgiano DC, Larson EB, Slichter SJ: A model to determine required pool size for HLA-typed community donor apheresis programs. Transfusion 1989;29:306–310.

225. Mueller-Eckhardt G, Hauck M, Kayser W, Mueller-Eckhardt C: HLA-C antigens on platelets. Tissue Antigens 1980;16:91–94.

226. Messerschmidt GL, Makuch R, Appelbaum F, et al: A prospective randomized trial of HLA-matched versus mismatched single-donor platelet transfusions in cancer patients. Cancer 1988;62:795–801.

227. Schonewille H, Haak HL, van Zijl AM: Alloimmunization after blood transfusion in patients with hematologic and oncologic diseases. Transfusion 1999;39:763–771.

228. Friedberg RC, Donnelly SF, Mintz PD: Independent roles for platelet crossmatching and HLA in the selection of platelets for alloimmunized patients. Transfusion 1994;34:215–220.

229. Novotny VM, Doxiadis II, Brand A: The reduction of HLA class I expression on platelets: A potential approach in the management of HLA-alloimmunized refractory patients. Transfus Med Rev 1999;13:95–105.

230. Owens MR, Holme S, Cardinali S: Platelet microvesicles adhere to subendothelium and promote adhesion of platelets. Thromb Res 1992;66:247–258.

231. Hjort PF, Perman V, Cronkite EP: Fresh, disintegrated platelets in radiation thrombocytopenia: Correction of prothrombin consumption without correction of bleeding. Proc Soc Exp Biol Med 1959;102:31–35.

232. Chao FC, Kim BK, Houranieh AM, et al: Infusible platelet membrane microvesicles: A potential transfusion substitute for platelets. Transfusion 1996;36:536–542.

233. Lee DH, Blajchman MA: Novel platelet products and substitutes. Transfus Med Rev 1998;12:175–187.

234. Alving BM, Reid TJ, Fratantoni JC, Finlayson JS: Frozen platelets and platelet substitutes in transfusion medicine. Transfusion 1997;37:866–876.

235. Fliedner TM, Sorensen DK, Bond VP: Comparative effectiveness of fresh and lyophilized platelets in controlling irradiation hemorrhage in the rat. Proc Soc Exp Biol Med 1958;99:731–733.

236. Read MS, Reddick RL, Bode AP, et al: Preservation of hemostatic and structural properties of rehydrated lyophilized platelets: Potential for long-term storage of dried platelets for transfusion. Proc Natl Acad Sci U S A 1995;92:397–401.

237. Bode AP, Read MS, Reddick RL: Activation and adherence of lyophilized human platelets on canine vessel strips in the Baumgartner perfusion chamber. J Lab Clin Med 1999;133:200–211.

238. Gao DY, Neff K, Xiao HY, et al: Development of optimal techniques for cryopreservation of human platelets. I. Platelet activation during cold storage (at 22 and 8 degrees C) and cryopreservation. Cryobiology 1999;38:225–235.

239. Arnaud FG, Pegg DE: Cryopreservation of human platelets with propane-1,2-diol. Cryobiology 1990;27:130–136.

240. Dayian G, Pert JH: A simplified method for freezing human blood platelets in glycerol-glucose using a statically controlled cooling rate device. Transfusion 1979;19:255–260.

241. Kotelba-Witkowska B, Schiffer CA: Cryopreservation of platelet concentrates using glycerol-glucose. Transfusion 1982;22:121–124.

242. Redmond JD, Bolin RB, Cheney BA: Glycerol-glucose cryopreservation of platelets: In vivo and in vitro observations. Transfusion 1983;23:213–214.

243. Dayian G, Harris HL, Vlahides GD, Pert JH: Improved procedure for platelet freezing. Vox Sang 1986;51:292–298.

244. Arnaud FG, Pegg DE: Cryopreservation of human platelets with 1.4 m glycerol at −75 degrees C in PVC blood packs. Thromb Res 1990;57:919–924.

245. Taylor MA: Cryopreservation of platelets: An in-vitro comparison of four methods. J Clin Pathol 1981;34:71–75.

246. Daly PA, Schiffer CA, Aisner J, Wiernik PH: Successful transfusion of platelets cryopreserved for more than 3 years. Blood 1979;54:1023–1027.

247. van Prooijen HC, van Heugten JG, Mommersteeg ME, Akkerman JW: Acquired secretion defect in platelets after cryopreservation in dimethyl sulfoxide. Transfusion 1986;26:358–363.

248. van Prooijen HC, van Heugten JG, Riemens MI, Akkerman JW: Differences in the susceptibility of platelets to freezing damage in relation to size. Transfusion 1989;29:539–543.

249. Owens M, Cimino C, Donnelly J: Cryopreserved platelets have decreased adhesive capacity. Transfusion 1991;31:160–163.

250. Khuri SF, Healey N, MacGregor H, et al: Comparison of the effects of transfusions of cryopreserved and liquid-preserved platelets on hemostasis and blood loss after cardiopulmonary bypass. J Thorac Cardiovasc Surg 1999;117:172–183.

251. Currie LM, Livesey SA, Harker JR, Connor J: Cryopreservation of single-donor platelets with a reduced dimethyl sulfoxide concentration by the addition of second-messenger effectors: Enhanced retention of in vitro functional activity. Transfusion 1998;38:160–167.

252. Currie LM, Lichtiger B, Livesey SA, et al: Enhanced circulatory parameters of human platelets cryopreserved with second-messenger effectors: an in vivo study of 16 volunteer platelet donors. Br J Haematol 1999;105:826–831.

253. Coller BS, Springer KT, Beer JH, et al: Thromboerythrocytes: In vitro studies of a potential autologous, semi-artificial alternative to platelet transfusions. J Clin Invest 1992;89:546–555.

254. Kitaguchi T, Murata M, Iijima K, et al: Characterization of liposomes carrying von Willebrand factor-binding domain of platelet glycoprotein Ibalpha: A potential substitute for platelet transfusion. Biochem Biophys Res Commun 1999;261:784–789.

255. Levi M, Friederich PW, Middleton S, et al: Fibrinogen-coated albumin microcapsules reduce bleeding in severely thrombocytopenic rabbits. Nat Med 1999;5:107–111.

256. Webb IJ, Anderson KC: Risks, costs, and alternatives to platelet transfusions. Leuk Lymphoma 1999;34:71–84.

257. Kuter DJ: Thrombopoietins and thrombopoiesis: A clinical perspective. Vox Sang 1998;74:75–85.

258. Tepler I, Elias L, Smith JW 2nd, et al: A randomized placebo-controlled trial of recombinant human interleukin-II in cancer patients with severe thrombocytopenia due to chemotherapy. Blood 1996;87:3607–3614.

259. Kaushansky K: Thrombopoietin. N Engl J Med 1998;339:746–754.

260. Harker LA, Marzec UM, Novembre F, et al: Treatment of thrombocytopenia in chimpanzees infected with human immunodeficiency virus by pegylated recombinant human megakaryocyte growth and development factor. Blood 1998;91:4427–4433.

261. Snyder E, Perrotta P, Rinder H, et al: Effect of recombinant human megakaryocyte growth and development factor coupled with polyethylene glycol on the platelet storage lesion. Transfusion 1999;39:258–264.

262. Basser RL, Rasko JE, Clarke K, et al: Thrombopoietic effects of pegylated recombinant human megakaryocyte growth and development factor (PEG-rHuMGDF) in patients with advanced cancer. Lancet 1996;348:1279–1281.

263. Fanucchi M, Glaspy J, Crawford J, et al: Effects of polyethylene glycol-conjugated recombinant human megakaryocyte growth and development factor on platelet counts after chemotherapy for lung cancer. N Engl J Med 1997;336:404–409.

264. Vadhan-Raj S, Verschraegen CF, Bueso-Ramos C, et al: Recombinant human thrombopoietin attenuates carboplatin-induced severe thrombocytopenia and the need for platelet transfusions in patients with gynecologic cancer. Ann Intern Med 2000;132:364–368.

265. O'Malley CJ, Rasko JE, Basser RL, et al: Administration of pegylated recombinant human megakaryocyte growth and development factor to humans stimulates the production of functional platelets that show no evidence of in vivo activation. Blood 1996;88:3288–3298.

266. Kuter DJ, Goodnough LT, Romo J, et al: Thrombopoietin therapy increases platelet yields in healthy platelet donors. Blood 2001;98:1339–1345.
267. Kuter DJ: Future directions with platelet growth factors. Semin Hematol 2000;37:41–49.
268. Bertolini F, Battaglia M, Pedrazzoli P, et al: Megakaryocytic progenitors can be generated ex vivo and safely administered to autologous peripheral blood progenitor cell transplant recipients. Blood 1997;89:2679–2688.
269. Cwirla SE, Balasubramanian P, Duffy DJ, et al: Peptide agonist of the thrombopoietin receptor as potent as the natural cytokine. Science 1997;276:1696–1699.
270. Reid TJ, Snider R, Hartman K, et al: A method for the quantitative assessment of platelet-induced clot retraction and clot strength in fresh and stored platelets. Vox Sang 1998;75:270–277.
271. Krishnamurti C, Maglasang P, Rothwell SW: Reduction of blood loss by infusion of human platelets in a rabbit kidney injury model. Transfusion 1999;39:967–974.

Chapter 18

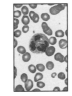

Granulocytes

Thomas H. Price

Infection associated with severe neutropenia continues to be a major limiting factor in the application of aggressive chemotherapeutic regimens and bone marrow transplantation to patients with malignant disease.[1-3] In the Trial to Reduce Alloimmunization to Platelets, 7% of patients undergoing induction therapy for acute myelocytic leukemia died of infection.[4] The spectrum of these therapy-related infections has shifted since the 1980s. Improved antibiotic regimens have reduced the incidence of refractory bacterial infection, and fungal infections have emerged as the principal infectious cause of mortality and morbidity. Fungal infection is now responsible for approximately 40% of fatalities in acute leukemia and bone marrow transplantation.[5] Prophylactic use of fluconazole has reduced the incidence of disseminated *Candida* infection, and the leading cause of mortality has become infection with invasive molds such as *Aspergillus* and *Fusarium*.[6, 7] The incidence of invasive *Aspergillus* infection in patients undergoing bone marrow transplantation is approximately 5%, with a mortality rate of 65% to 85%.[8-10] *Fusarium* infection in these patients is associated with a 70% mortality rate.[7]

The provision of normally functioning neutrophils is a logical approach to the problem of infection in the setting of severe neutropenia or neutrophil dysfunction. The first reports of modern neutrophil transfusion therapy occurred in the mid-1960s, with large numbers of neutrophils obtained from donors with chronic myelocytic leukemia. The development of apheresis equipment shortly thereafter allowed the collection of transfusion doses of neutrophils from hematologically normal donors, and favorable clinical reports ushered in an era of enthusiasm for this therapeutic approach. A series of controlled trials followed that, on aggregate, indicated efficacy in terms of a survival advantage for patients given transfusions. In spite of these results, granulocyte transfusion therapy all but disappeared from clinical use from about 1985 to 1995. This change in attitude occurred for several reasons. Improvement in antibiotic and general supportive care rendered refractory bacterial infection a less common clinical problem. Reports also surfaced of adverse effects of granulocyte transfusion, particularly adverse pulmonary reactions. Finally, and probably most important, the clinical results in most patients were, at best, marginal.

This unimpressive clinical efficacy had two probable causes. First, the dose of neutrophils supplied to patients with the best standard collection techniques, even in the mid-1990s (20 to 30×10^9), was probably inadequate. Normal neutrophil production in an average-sized adult is approximately 60×10^9 cells per day in the uninfected state.[11] Although reliable quantitative information is lacking, the normal bone marrow is probably capable of increasing production severalfold in the presence of severe infection. Thus, the number of neutrophils routinely provided to patients undergoing neutrophil transfusion therapy was likely only about one tenth of the normal need. The second problem is that neutrophils rapidly undergo apoptosis after collection, a phenomenon that may be responsible for both the failure of the transfused cells to circulate and the short shelf life of these components.

Since the mid-1990s interest in granulocyte support therapy has been rekindled with the availability of granulocyte colony-stimulating factor (G-CSF), a cytokine that may be administered to granulocyte donors to increase the number of cells that can be collected.[3, 12] G-CSF also inhibits neutrophil apoptosis, and this feature raises the possibility that in vitro and in vivo survival of these cells may be enhanced.

The features of traditional granulocyte transfusion are discussed first, including issues such as collection, storage, indications, evidence of efficacy, and adverse effects. This is followed by a discussion of the more recent experience using G-CSF to stimulate donors to obtain greatly increased numbers of cells for transfusion.

■ Traditional Granulocyte Transfusion Therapy

Procurement of Granulocytes

Granulocyte donors are selected from pools of community apheresis donors, or, perhaps more commonly, they are family members or friends of the patient. The ABO blood group is not important for granulocyte compatibility,[13] but donors should be ABO compatible with the patient because of the relatively large number of red blood cells contained in a typical granulocyte concentrate. Donors should be generally healthy and must meet the American Association of Blood Banks (AABB) and the United States Food and Drug Administration standards for blood donation. There should be no contraindication to their receiving the institution's stimulation regimen (e.g., corticosteroids) for increasing the donor's blood neutrophil count. Infectious disease screening and testing must be the same as with any blood product, but modifications are often made in the timing of this testing to accommodate the need to transfuse the granulocytes as soon as possible after collection. In some centers, blood for infectious disease testing is drawn up to 24 hours before leukapheresis so that release of the cells will not be delayed.

If the patient is cytomegalovirus seronegative, consideration should be given to requiring that the donor also be cytomegalovirus seronegative, particularly because most granulocyte recipients are in a patient population that normally requires cytomegalovirus-safe components. The incidence of cytomegalovirus transmission appears to be higher with granulocyte concentrates than with other cellular blood products because the latent virus resides in the leukocytes,[14, 15] and the risk of transmission can be eliminated by selecting seronegative donors. Needless to say, leukocyte reduction (leukoreduction), a technique available to render other blood components cytomegalovirus-safe, is not appropriate for granulocyte concentrates.

If the patient is not alloimmunized, it is not necessary to select granulocyte donors on the basis of HLA or granulocyte typing or to perform leukocyte compatibility testing.[16] However, convincing evidence indicates that alloimmunized recipients who are transfused with incompatible leukocytes are more likely to experience adverse pulmonary reactions or febrile transfusion reactions.[17–21] In addition, the infused granulocytes will be rapidly cleared from the circulation and will be ineffective.[16, 17, 20, 22–25] The difficulty is in knowing which patients are alloimmunized. Leukocyte antibodies detected in the laboratory do not necessarily correlate well with clinical evidence of alloimmunization, such as the ability of the transfused cells to circulate or to accumulate at sites of inflammation. In addition, reliable detection of clinically significant antibodies requires that a panel of sophisticated tests be performed,[18, 23] tests that are not available in most institutions. In the absence of such results, a common approach is to attempt to gauge the likelihood of alloimmunization on the basis of information such as the patient's history of febrile transfusion reactions, the response to random donor platelet transfusions, and the results of a lymphocytotoxic antibody screen. If these results are normal,

it is not likely that the patient is alloimmunized. Significant abnormalities in these parameters do not necessarily mean that the patient will have difficulty with granulocyte transfusions, but they do suggest that one proceed gingerly, and further clinical or laboratory evaluation should be considered.

Granulocytes are collected from donors by a leukapheresis procedure. Historically, two methods have been used: filtration and centrifugation. In the former, the donor's blood was passed over nylon wool filters to which the neutrophils adhered; the cells were subsequently eluted from the columns. Although large numbers of granulocytes could be collected by this technique, subsequent studies showed that the cells were functionally impaired.[26–28] In addition, the process itself activated complement and was associated with transfusion reactions in recipients and with occasional and sometimes serious adverse effects in donors.[29, 30] This technique is no longer in use. For centrifugal leukapheresis, the cells are separated from other components by centrifugation. Numerous acceptable cell separators are on the market for this purpose. Usually, one processes 7 to 10 L of the donor's blood in a procedure that takes approximately 3 hours.

It is necessary to add a red blood cell sedimenting agent to the donor's blood to effect an adequate separation of the granulocytes from the red blood cells. Hydroxyethyl starch has traditionally been used for this purpose, and in modern cell separating machines, this allows for 30% to 50% efficiency in granulocyte collection. Two preparations of hydroxyethyl starch are available for this purpose. Hetastarch, a high-molecular-weight compound, was the substance used originally, but it was shown to persist in the circulation for months. This persistence led to a concern for its safety, although long-term effects were not actually observed. The lower-molecular-weight version, Pentastarch, was shown to have a much more rapid elimination time and appeared to function equivalently for the purposes of granulocyte collection.[31] Many collection centers switched to Pentastarch as a result of these findings. More recent controlled studies showed, however, that collection efficiency is much greater when the high-molecular-weight preparation of hydroxyethyl starch is used.[32]

In an effort to increase the number of granulocytes collected, donors are routinely stimulated with corticosteroids to mobilize cells from the marrow storage pool and to increase the circulating granulocyte count, thereby increasing the number of granulocytes that can be collected. Numerous stimulation regimens have been proposed over the years, the most successful using up to 60 mg prednisone or 8 mg dexamethasone and raising the donor's neutrophil count two- to threefold from baseline values.[33, 34] Short-term administration of such doses of corticosteroids are well tolerated by most donors; persons with medical conditions in whom such stimulation may be considered contraindicated, such as active peptic ulcer disease or diabetes, should not be donors. Even higher donor granulocyte counts can be obtained by stimulation with G-CSF, a strategy discussed later in this chapter.

Granulocyte concentrates are not licensed by the Food and Drug Administration and therefore have no defined regulatory specifications. AABB standards require that at least 75% of concentrates contain at least 10×10^9 granulocytes,[35] a value intended to serve as a benchmark for adequate collection technique, not to imply that 10×10^9 granulocytes is an adequate clinical dose. With the techniques discussed earlier, including adequate corticosteroid stimulation of the donor, one typically achieves mean yields of 20 to 30 × 10⁹ granulocytes. Depending on the particular cell separator used, the granulocytes are suspended in 200 to 400 mL plasma and contain 10 to 30 mL red blood cells and 1 to 6 × 10¹¹ platelets.

The functional capabilities of granulocytes obtained by these techniques have been the subject of many reports. In vitro and in vivo studies have shown repeatedly that cells collected by centrifugal apheresis are normal or near normal functionally, and these capabilities are not compromised by the use of hydroxyethyl starch or by stimulation of normal donors with corticosteroids.[26, 36, 37]

Storage of Neutrophils

After collection, granulocytes rapidly undergo apoptosis,[3, 38, 39] and this process greatly limits one's ability to store the cells before transfusion. Although the hardier cell functions persist after a few days of liquid storage, the more sensitive ones, such as the ability to migrate, deteriorate much more quickly.[40, 41] In vivo studies have shown that blood recovery and survival are adversely affected by as little as 24 hours of storage, and the ability of the transfused cells to localize to areas of inflammation is decreased as much as 75% after 8 to 24 hours of storage.[26, 42] As a result of these observations, granulocytes should be administered as soon as possible after collection. In the event that this is not possible, the cells should be stored without agitation for no more than 24 hours.[35, 43] The preponderance of evidence to date indicates that the cells should be maintained at room temperature for any period of storage.[40, 44]

Transfusion of Granulocytes

Once the decision is made to initiate granulocyte support, one should strive to provide daily transfusions until the patient's infection clears or until the patient's neutrophil count has returned to at least 500/µL. Data are insufficient to determine whether higher neutrophil counts are more appropriate as stopping points for certain clinical conditions. Outside these parameters, it is generally not appropriate to stop and start transfusion support on the basis of the patient's daily clinical status.

Granulocyte concentrates usually contain 10 to 30 mL red blood cells, enough to cause a hemolytic transfusion reaction if the donor and patient are incompatible. Therefore, AABB standards require that a red blood cell crossmatch be performed before transfusion.[35]

Granulocyte preparations contain viable lymphocytes, and graft-versus-host disease has been reported after granulocyte transfusion.[45] Although this complication can easily be prevented by gamma irradiation of the component, the decision to irradiate granulocyte concentrates routinely is controversial. Those who oppose routine irradiation note that graft-versus-host disease is an extremely rare complication, express concern that irradiation may compromise the integrity of the cells, and argue that, as with any other blood product, the decision to irradiate the cells should be based on a clinical evaluation of the patient.[46] However, most studies have suggested that standard irradiation does not impair neutrophil function,[47–50] a finding that makes it more reasonable to irradiate these cells routinely.

Granulocytes should be administered through a standard blood administration set filter (170 µm) and infused over 1 to 2 hours. Premedication with antipyretics or corticosteroids is not recommended routinely, but it should be reserved for those patients who experience symptoms such as chills and fever.

Clinical Efficacy of Neutrophil Transfusion Therapy

Neutropenia

The first reports of treating infected neutropenic patients with granulocyte transfusions occurred in the 1960s. In these studies, granulocytes were harvested from donors with chronic myelocytic leukemia by a manual leukapheresis technique whereby leukocyte-rich plasma was prepared from individual units of donor blood by sedimenting the red blood cells. Schwarzenberg and associates[51] treated 33 patients with various malignant diseases and reported that approximately half showed a favorable response. In several of the patients, the postinfusion rise in the patient's neutrophil count persisted, and the Philadelphia chromosome could be demonstrated in the patient's marrow cells, findings suggesting that a temporary graft had occurred. Morse and associates[52] used a similar technique and transfused 40 patients with leukopenia, most of whom had acute leukemia. Of 81 transfusions given to patients who were febrile before the transfusion, more than half of them were afebrile by 36 hours after the transfusion. Lowenthal and colleagues[53] collected granulocytes from normal donors and those with chronic myelocytic leukemia by continuous-flow centrifugation and treated 41 febrile patients with acute leukemia or aplastic anemia. Two thirds of the patients responded by defervescence. Response was more likely in those patients with proven or probable bacterial or fungal infection than it was in those with fever of unknown origin.

With the development of the automated cell separator, it became possible to collect large numbers of granulocytes from normal donors, and the use of donors with chronic myelocytic leukemia fell into disuse. A flurry of reports of granulocyte transfusion therapy in patients with neutropenia then followed. The aggregate experience was reviewed by Strauss[54] and is summarized in Table 18.1. In this review, patients were categorized by the infection for which the transfusions were begun and were counted only once. All patients with documented fungal infection were categorized as such, whether or not they fit into other categories. After excluding these patients, all patients with sepsis were listed only in the sepsis section. The number of patients indicated in Table 18.1 represents the number of patients who could actually be evaluated for treatment efficacy, sometimes a much smaller number than actually treated. Therapy was considered

Table 18.1 Treatment of Neutropenic Patients with Granulocyte Transfusions

Infection	N	Success (%)
Bacterial sepsis	206	62
Sepsis, organism unspecified	39	46
Pneumonia, organism unspecified	11	64
Invasive fungal infection	77	36
Localized infection	47	83
Nonspecific fever	85	75

Adapted from strauss RG: Granulocyte transfusion. In McLeod BC, Price TH, Drew MJ (eds): Apheresis: Principles & Practice, Bethesda, MD, AABB Press, 1997, pp 195–209.

successful if so indicated by the authors of the study. Although these results indicate the general experience with granulocyte transfusion therapy, one must be cautious in overinterpreting the data. The number of patients was often small, and the studies represented were heterogeneous, with very different inclusion criteria, granulocyte preparations, and criteria for success.

Included in the foregoing aggregate experience were seven controlled trials, reported between 1972 and 1982, and designed to assess the efficacy of therapeutic granulocyte transfusion in adults.[55–61] In each of these studies, neutropenic patients with clinical evidence of infection who treated with granulocyte transfusions were compared with a group of similar patients who received only conventional antibiotic therapy. All but two of the studies were randomized trials; in those that were not,[55, 57] patients were assigned to the control group if no suitable granulocyte donor could be identified. When patient survival was compared, three of the studies showed a clear beneficial effect of transfusion. Higby and associates[56] treated patients with clinically evident infection with 4 daily transfusions and found that 15 of 17 treated patients and 5 of 19 control patients survived until day 20. Vogler and Winton[58] studied 30 patients with documented infection who had failed to respond to at least 72 hours of appropriate antibiotic therapy; survival to 22 days was 59% in the transfused group and 31% in the control group. Herzig and associates[60] treated 27 patients with documented gram-negative septicemia; 75% (12 of 16) of the treated group survived compared with 36% (5 of 14) of the control group. When these results were further analyzed, the survival advantage was entirely in the subset of patients who did not recover bone marrow function. Two of the controlled trials showed no statistically significant overall beneficial effect of transfusion, but subset analysis suggested efficacy in certain groups.

In the study of Graw and colleagues[55] of patients with documented gram-negative septicemia, overall survival was not improved in the treatment group, but survival was improved for those who received at least four transfusions. In the other study with partial benefit, that of Alavi and associates,[59] no advantage of granulocyte transfusion was apparent for the overall patient population; however, in the subgroup with persistent bone marrow failure, 75% of the transfused patients survived compared with 20% of the controls. In two of the controlled studies, no benefit to transfusion was identified. Fortuny and associates[57] treated 58 febrile episodes in 39 patients with acute nonlymphocytic leukemia. Survival of the episode was 78% in the transfused group versus 80% in the control group. Winston and colleagues[61] studied 95 neutropenic patients with documented infections; 63% (30 of 48) of the transfused patients and 72% (34 of 47) of the controls survived the infection.

In trying to understand the somewhat disparate results of these controlled trials, it is useful to keep in mind that the number of patients involved in many of the studies was relatively small, and the study designs and evaluation parameters were different. Whether efficacy was demonstrated or not may have been primarily influenced by the survival of the control group. In those trials in which the control group did well, it would be difficult to demonstrate that additional benefit was provided by transfusion therapy, even if the therapy itself was generally useful. As discussed later, subsequent analysis of these studies also suggested that the positive studies generally were those in which larger numbers of functional neutrophils were provided, as well as those in which some attempt was made to take leukocyte compatibility into account.[62, 63] Moreover, by modern standards, only one of the controlled studies[58] provided adequate numbers of functional neutrophils as a transfusion dose. In four of the studies, cells were collected by filtration leukapheresis, a technique now known to produce damaged cells.

Despite the foregoing caveats, the aggregate message from the controlled therapeutic trials is that, in the proper clinical circumstances, granulocyte transfusion therapy is likely beneficial, a conclusion that is bolstered by meta-analysis.[63] Based on the information from these trials, it seems reasonable to consider transfusion therapy in severely neutropenic patients with documented serious bacterial infection who have failed to respond to appropriate antibiotic therapy after 48 to 72 hours.

No systematic studies have been conducted to evaluate the role of granulocyte transfusion therapy in the treatment of fungal infection. Experimental studies in dogs suggested that transfused neutrophils may be effective. Ruthe and associates[64] used a dog *Candida* sepsis model to show that the extent of infection could be reduced by granulocyte transfusions. Chow and colleagues[65] developed a *Candida* meningitis model in dogs and showed that transfused neutrophils were capable of migrating into the cerebrospinal space and increasing survival. Reports of granulocyte transfusions in patients with fungal infection have mostly consisted of case reports.[66, 67] Bhatia and associates[68] conducted a retrospective study of granulocyte transfusion therapy in 87 patients who were undergoing bone marrow transplantation and who had various systemic fungal infections. No beneficial effect of transfusion was seen. It is difficult to draw conclusive answers from this study for several reasons: it was a retrospective study in which patient entry was controlled only by the patient's physician; the control group and the treatment group were not comparable; the dose of granulocytes delivered was largely unknown and was probably not adequate because the granulocyte donors were not stimulated with corticosteroids; and the collection parameters were not optimal. Clinical trials are obviously needed to address the issue of efficacy in fungal infection. In the meantime, it is probably reasonable to provide granulocytes to patients with a serious systemic fungal infection that is refractory to conventional therapy.

If granulocytes are effective in treating an established infection, it would seem logical that they could even be more effective in preventing infection in neutropenic patients. Numerous controlled trials of prophylactic granulocyte support were reported from 1977 to 1984 and were summarized by Strauss.[69] As with the trials of therapeutic transfusion, positive effects were limited to those in which larger doses of granulocytes were provided. The effects were modest, however, and some studies reported a high rate of adverse effects.[19, 70] Cost-effectiveness analysis contemporary to these studies showed that provision of prophylactic support was also very expensive.[71] As a result of these findings, prophylactic transfusion cannot be recommended.

Neonatal Sepsis

Bacterial sepsis occurs in 1 to 10 per 1000 neonates and is associated with an average mortality of approximately 20%, approaching 100% in premature neonates with group B streptococcal sepsis.[69] A contributing factor to this high mortality is relative dysfunction of neonatal neutrophils, cells that have been shown to exhibit quantitative abnormalities in chemotaxis, adhesion, and oxidative metabolism.[69] As a result, neonates with sepsis whose blood neutrophil counts are less than 3000/µL and who have diminished marrow neutrophil stores have been shown to have a high mortality in spite of antibiotic treatment.[72] The efficacy of granulocyte transfusion therapy in the setting of neonatal sepsis was evaluated in six controlled trials[73–78] and reviewed by Strauss.[69] In four of the six studies, a survival benefit was identified in patients who received granulocyte transfusions, although subsequent meta-analysis concluded that the studies were so heterogeneous that no definite conclusion could be reached about efficacy.[63]

In the study of Laurenti and associates,[73] which was controlled but not randomized, 20 neonates with sepsis received 2 to 15 granulocyte transfusions, and these patients were compared with 18 similar patients who did not receive transfusions. Survival was 90% in the transfused group and 28% in the control group. The granulocytes were collected by filtration leukapheresis and, for half of the transfused patients, were stored for up to 2 days before transfusion; these features would suggest that the cells were probably nonfunctional. Christensen and colleagues[74] randomized 16 neonates with bacterial infection and depleted marrow neutrophil storage pools. All the transfused patients (7 of 7) and 11% (1 of 9) of the controls survived. Cairo and associates[75] randomized 23 newborns with clinical sepsis; those who received transfusions were transfused every 12 hours for a total of 5 transfusions. Survival of the transfused group (13 of 13) was significantly higher than that of the control group (6 of 10). When analysis was limited to those patients with positive blood cultures, there was still a survival advantage to those who received transfusions (100% versus 57%), but the difference was no longer statistically significant.

In a subsequent randomized study, Cairo and associates compared granulocyte transfusion therapy with intravenous immune globulin treatment in the same clinical population.[76] Again, all the neonates who recaeived transfusions (21 of 21) survived, whereas only 64% (9 of 14) of those treated with immune globulin survived. In the remaining two studies,[77, 78] no survival advantage was seen with transfusion, but in both studies the granulocytes were prepared from units of whole blood, rather than by leukapheresis, and this makes the viability of the cells suspect.

In summary, the role of granulocyte transfusion therapy in neonatal sepsis is not clear. As a practical approach, it is probably reasonable to recommend that in institutions experiencing high mortality in this clinical situation, granulocyte support be considered in neonates with sepsis who have blood neutrophil counts less than 3000/µL with evidence that the marrow storage pool is depleted.

Granulocyte Function Disorders

Patients with severe neutrophil dysfunction, who may have normal or even elevated blood neutrophil counts, may also benefit from granulocyte transfusion therapy. Some investigators have reported, usually as single case studies, apparent clinical success in treatment of antibiotic-resistant bacterial or fungal infection in patients with disorders such as chronic granulomatous disease and leukocyte adhesion deficiency.[79–83] Although few patients have these disorders and controlled trials have not been performed, efficacy of such therapy can be very convincing with an individual patient who has recurring infections. At the Puget Sound Blood Center in Seattle, we treated a patient with leukocyte adhesion deficiency (originally described by Bowen and associates[83]) over the course of 15 to 20 years. He was repeatedly unable to clear bacterial infections until he received a course of granulocyte transfusion therapy. The indications for transfusion in patients with neutrophil function disorders are not firmly established. One should probably be conservative, however, because these patients ordinarily have normal immune systems, and alloimmunization can be a significant problem.[18]

Adverse Effects

Fever and chills are fairly commonly seen after the administration of granulocytes. Precise figures are not available, but the incidence depends on the likelihood of alloimmunization.[18] As an approximation, nonimmunized patients can expect to experience mild to moderate fever or chills with about 10% of transfusions. Routine premedication is not necessary, but for those patients experiencing reactions, premedication with acetaminophen or corticosteroids will often prevent recurrences. Moderate to severe pulmonary reactions can occur in these patients, but true transfusion reactions are often difficult to distinguish from other conditions such as fluid overload or underlying pulmonary disease.[84] Wright and associates[85] reported a high incidence of severe pulmonary reactions in patients receiving both granulocyte transfusions and amphotericin B, a finding that several investigators have failed to confirm.[21, 84, 86, 87] Nevertheless, it remains common practice to space the administration of amphotericin from that of granulocytes by several hours.

In addition to being a factor complicating the ability to provide effective granulocyte support, alloimmunization may be a complication of such support. The incidence likely depends on the integrity of the patient's immune system as well as the tests used to detect antibody. Stroncek and colleagues[18] reported that approximately 75% of patients with chronic granulomatous disease who receive repeated courses of granulocyte support will develop clinically significant antibodies. Other studies have detected leukocyte antibodies after granulocyte transfusion in 40% to 80% of patients with acute leukemia or various marrow failure states.[88, 89]

As previously discussed, graft-versus-host disease, a highly fatal but unusual complication of granulocyte transfusion therapy, can be prevented by gamma irradiation (2500 rads) of the concentrate.

■ Use of Granulocyte Colony-Stimulating Factor to Stimulate Donors

An important reason for the unimpressive efficacy of traditional granulocyte transfusion therapy is the inadequacy of the cell dose usually provided. Evidence of the importance of dose comes from several quarters. First, in the early uncontrolled trails of granulocyte transfusion therapy, in which large doses of cells could be obtained from donors with marked leukocytosis, clinical responses were reported to be associated with the dose delivered. Morse and associates[52] observed that the increase in the patient's neutrophil count was directly related to the dose of cells provided and was detectable only if the dose exceeded $10^{10}/m^2$. The clinical response, as defined by defervescence, was also proportional to the dose, the fraction of patients responding ranging from 30% to 100% with mean doses of $2.6 \times 10^{10}/m^2$ and $15.6 \times 10^{10}/m^2$, respectively. Lowenthal and colleagues[53] reported that patients with clinical responses received, on average, four times as many cells as patients without responses. Second, retrospective analysis of the controlled trials of therapeutic granulocyte transfusion therapy suggested that higher doses of cells were provided in the studies that showed efficacy.[62, 63] Third, the experience with the provision of granulocytes to neonates, in whom the relative dose is much higher because of the size of these patients, suggests that efficacy is determined by dose. Finally, studies in animals indicated the importance of dose. Appelbaum and associates[90] examined the clinical effect of granulocyte support in dogs with *Pseudomonas* sepsis and showed that dogs receiving 10^8 cells/kg did not survive the infection, whereas 100% (five of five) survived when they were given 2×10^8 cells/kg. Epstein and Chow[91] provided granulocytes to dogs with *Candida albicans* meningitis and showed a direct relationship among the dose of cells administered, the blood granulocyte increments, and the number of granulocytes migrating to the cerebrospinal fluid.

With the availability of recombinant G-CSF, the possibility of greatly increasing the number of granulocytes for transfusion raised the hope that the efficacy of granulocyte transfusion therapy could be improved.[3, 12] When administered to normal subjects, G-CSF causes a rapid dose-dependent increase in the neutrophil count, beginning within 2 hours and peaking at approximately 12 hours.[92] This phenomenon is the result of the rapid release of neutrophils from the marrow storage pool into the blood. When given daily, G-CSF also stimulates the proliferation of granulocyte precursors and accelerates the transit time of the developing cells through the maturation pool into the blood.[93] G-CSF also affects neutrophil function. It increases phagocytosis as well as bactericidal and fungicidal activity.[38, 94, 95] It primes neutrophils and enhances their metabolic responses to second agonists.[38] It affects the expression of cell surface proteins such as CD64, CD35, CD14, and CD11/18,[38, 96, 97] proteins that are important in cell adhesion processes. G-CSF also inhibits neutrophil apoptosis,[38, 98] a finding that may explain, in part, the prolonged blood survival of neutrophils from subjects given the drug.[93]

The use of G-CSF to stimulate normal granulocyte donors has been reported by numerous investigators (Table 18.2). In most of these studies, G-CSF was administered repeatedly to donors who were family members or friends of the patient who received the transfusions, although in the study of Price and associates,[99] the donors were community apheresis donors who were fairly easily recruited to donate for patients whom they did not know. The dose of G-CSF in these studies ranged from 5 to 10 µg/kg, and it resulted in granulocyte concentrates containing an average of 40 to 60×10^9 cells. Leitman and associates[100] and Price and colleagues[99] achieved substantially higher average yields (80×10^9 cells) by administering both G-CSF and dexamethasone (8 mg) to normal subjects. Liles and associates[101] determined that the addition of corticosteroids resulted in higher donor blood neutrophil counts, irrespective of the dose of G-CSF, and the maximum neutrophil counts occurred approximately 12 hours after stimulation. Administration of G-CSF, with or without corticosteroids, is well tolerated by donors.[102, 103] Most donors experience mild to moderate bone aching, headache, or insomnia. In one study, 98% of donors were willing to undergo future G-CSF stimulation.[99]

Because G-CSF has been shown to inhibit neutrophil apoptosis,[38, 98] this cytokine may be useful in lengthening the acceptable storage time for neutrophils and thereby improving the logistics of granulocyte therapy programs. Whether this will turn out to be true must await further studies.

In marked contrast to the situation in traditional granulocyte transfusion therapy, the postinfusion neutrophil increments seen in patients receiving these large doses of cells are quite large. Hester and associates[104] reported a mean post-transfusion neutrophil increment of $0.6 \times 10^3/\mu L$ after infusion of 40×10^9 granulocytes, and the value remained higher than the baseline value for 24 hours. In the study of Adkins and colleagues,[105] patients received a mean granulocyte dose of 51×10^9 and exhibited a post-transfusion neutrophil increment of $1 \times 10^3/\mu L$, a value that was maintained for 1 to 1.5 days. With even higher cell doses (78×10^9), as reported by Bowden and associates,[106] post-transfusion

Table 18.2   Granulocyte Colony-Stimulating Factor (G-CSF)–Stimulated Granulocyte Collections

	N	G-CSF	Donor PMN ($10^3/\mu L$)	PMN Yield (10^9)
Caspar et al.[116]	22	300 µg	20	44
Hester et al.[104]	124	5 µg/kg/d	24–36	41
Bensinger et al.[117]	58	5 µg/kg/d	15–40	42
Jendiroba et al.[118]	221	5 µg/kg/d	—	42
	179	5 µg/kg/qod	—	46
Adkins et al.[105]	29	5 µg/kg/d	20–30	51
Grigg et al.[114]	55	10 µg/kg/d	—	59
Leitman et al.[100]	7	5 µg/kg Dexa 8 mg	28	78
Price et al.[99]	175	600 µg Dexa 8 mg	31	82

PMN, polymorphonuclear leukocytes; Dexa, dexamethasone.

neutrophil increments were $2 \times 10^3/\mu L$, with an average next morning count of $1.6 \times 10^3/\mu L$. It thus appears that donors stimulated with G-CSF and corticosteroids are able to provide enough granulocytes to sustain a normal or near-normal blood neutrophil count in a severely neutropenic patient. Strong evidence indicates that these granulocytes are also capable of migrating to extravascular sites. Dale and associates[107] showed that neutrophils collected from G-CSF–stimulated normal donors were able to accumulate in skin chambers. Adkins and colleagues[108] reported that indium-111–labeled granulocytes obtained from G-CSF–stimulated donors were able to localize to areas of infection in neutropenic recipients. Bowden and associates[106] measured buccal neutrophil accumulation in neutropenic granulocyte recipients and demonstrated the ability of the transfused cells to migrate to the extravascular compartment.

The evidence that providing large numbers of granulocytes from G-CSF–stimulated donors is clinically efficacious is limited to that derived from case reports[109–113] and from small uncontrolled series.[104, 106, 114, 115] Hester and associates[104] transfused 15 patients with fungal infection and reported that 60% responded. Eighty-three percent of patients (15 of 18) with established bacterial or fungal infection recovered in the series reported by Taylor and associates.[115] Results were more discouraging in the study of Grigg and associates,[114] in which 3 of 3 patients with bacterial infection survived, but 5 of 5 with fungal infection died. Bowden and associates[106] treated 11 bone marrow transplant recipients with a variety of bacterial and fungal infections. Infection cleared in 3 patients, and 5 patients survived until engraftment.

Transfusion of granulocytes obtained from G-CSF–stimulated donors has generally been well tolerated by recipients. In the study of Adkins and associates,[105] 29 HLA-matched transfusions were administered to 10 patients. After one of the transfusions, the patient experienced dyspnea, cough, and the sensation of a large tongue, all of which disappeared after treatment with antihistamines. No febrile or other respiratory reactions were seen. Hester and associates[104] reported adverse pulmonary reactions in approximately 5% of transfusions, reactions characterized by varying degrees of dyspnea, hypoxia, and changes on the chest radiograph. In the study of Bowden and associates,[106] chills and fever were seen in only about 10% of patients. These reactions were mild to moderate and were preventable in subsequent transfusions by treatment with antipyretics or corticosteroids. No changes were seen in blood oxygen saturation measured before and after the transfusions. Although this experience is encouraging, the likelihood of alloimmunization is low in the groups of patients studied to date. Similar results may not occur with transfusion of multitransfused patients with intact immune systems, such as those with neutrophil function disorders.

Thus, the administration of G-CSF, particularly in addition to corticosteroids, causes marked neutrophilia in donors and permits the collection of large numbers of granulocytes. These cells circulate in patients and, on average, increase the patient's neutrophil count to a normal or near-normal level. The cells are capable of migrating from the vasculature to tissue sites of inflammation. Although the preliminary results are encouraging and suggest that one may now be able to provide meaningful neutrophil support for infected neutropenic patients, large-scale clinical trials are needed to determine efficacy.

REFERENCES

1. Pizzo PA: Management of fever in patients with cancer and treatment-induced neutropenia. N Engl J Med 328:1323–1332, 1993.
2. Hughes WT, Armstrong D, Bodey GP, et al: 1997 Guidelines for the use of antimicrobial agents in neutropenic patients with unexplained fever. Clin Infect Dis 25:551–573, 1997.
3. Dale DC, Liles WC, Price TH: Renewed interest in granulocyte transfusion therapy. Br J Haematol 98:497–501, 1997.
4. Trial to Reduce Alloimmunization to Platelets Study Group: Leukocyte reduction and ultraviolet B irradiation of platelets to prevent alloimmunization and refractoriness to platelet transfusions. N Engl J Med 337:1861–1869, 1997.
5. Bodey G, Bueltmann B, Duguid W, et al: Fungal infections in cancer patients: An international autopsy survey. Eur J Clin Microbiol Infect Dis 11:99–109, 1992.
6. Wingard JR: Fungal infections after bone marrow transplant. Biol Blood Marrow Transplant 5:55–68, 1999.
7. Boutati EI, Anaissie EJ: *Fusarium*, a significant emerging pathogen in patients with hematologic malignancy: Ten years' experience at a cancer center and implications for management. Blood 90:999–1008, 1997.
8. Pannuti C, Gingrich R, Pfaller MA, et al: Nosocomial pneumonia in patients having bone marrow transplant: Attributable mortality and risk factors. Cancer 69:2653–2662, 1992.
9. Iwen PC, Reed EC, Armitage JO, et al: Nosocomial invasive aspergillosis in lymphoma patients treated with bone marrow or peripheral stem cell transplants. Infect Control Hosp Epidemiol 14:131–139, 1993.
10. Saugier-Veber P, Devergie A, Sulahian A, et al: Epidemiology and diagnosis of invasive pulmonary aspergillosis in bone marrow transplant patients: Results of a 5 year retrospective study. Bone Marrow Transplant 12:121–124, 1993.
11. Dancey JT, Deubelbeiss KA, Harker LA, et al: Neutrophil kinetics in man. J Clin Invest 58:705–715, 1976.
12. Strauss RG: Neutrophil (granulocyte) transfusions in the new millennium. Transfusion 38:710–712, 1998.
13. McCullough J, Clay M, Loken M, et al: Effect of ABO incompatibility on the fate in vivo of [111]indium granulocytes. Transfusion 28:358–361, 1988.
14. Winston DJ, Ho WG, Howell CL, et al: Cytomegalovirus infections associated with leukocyte transfusions. Ann Intern Med 93:671–675, 1980.
15. Hersman J, Meyers JD, Thomas ED, et al: The effect of granulocyte transfusions on the incidence of cytomegalovirus infection after allogeneic marrow transplantation. Ann Intern Med 96:149–152, 1982.
16. Dutcher JP, Schiffer CA, Johnston GS, et al: Alloimmunization prevents the migration of transfused indium-111–labeled granulocytes to sites of infection. Blood 62:354–360, 1983.
17. Dutcher JP, Riggs JR, Fox JJ, et al: Effect of histocompatibility factors on pulmonary retention of indium-111–labeled granulocytes. Am J Hematol 33:238–243, 1990.
18. Stroncek DF, Leonard K, Eiber G, et al: Alloimmunization after granulocyte transfusions. Transfusion 36:1009–1015, 1996.
19. Schiffer CA, Aisner J, Daly PA, et al: Alloimmunization following prophylactic granulocyte transfusion. Blood 54:766–774, 1979.
20. Goldstein IM, Eyre HJ, Terasaki PI, et al: Leukocyte transfusions: Role of leukocyte alloantibodies in determining transfusion response. Transfusion 11:19–24, 1971.
21. Dutcher JP, Kendall J, Norris D, et al: Granulocyte transfusion therapy and amphotericin B: Adverse reactions? Am J Hematol 31:102–108, 1989.
22. Westrick MA, Debelak-Fehir KM, Epstein RB: The effect of prior whole blood transfusion on subsequent granulocyte support in leukopenic dogs. Transfusion 17:611–614, 1977.
23. McCullough J, Clay M, Hurd D, et al: Effect of leukocyte antibodies and HLA matching on the intravascular recovery, survival, and tissue localization of 111-indium granulocytes. Blood 67:522–528, 1986.
24. McCullough J, Weiblen BJ, Clay ME, et al: Effect of leukocyte antibodies on the fate of in vivo of indium-111–labeled granulocytes. Blood 58:164–170, 1981.
25. Appelbaum FR, Trapani RJ, Graw JR: Consequences of prior alloimmunization during granulocyte transfusion. Transfusion 17:460–464, 1977.
26. Price TH, Dale DC: Blood kinetics and in vivo chemotaxis of transfused neutrophils: Effect of collection method, donor corticosteroid treatment, and short-term storage. Blood 54:977–986, 1979.

27. Wright DG, Kauffmann JC, Chusid MJ, et al: Functional abnormalities of human neutrophils collected by continuous flow filtration leukopheresis. Blood 45:901–911, 1975.

28. McCullough J, Weiblen BJ, Deinard AR, et al: In vitro function and post-transfusion survival of granulocytes collected by continous-flow centrifugation and by filtration leukapheresis. Blood 48:315–326, 1976.

29. Nusbacher J, Rosenfeld SI, MacPherson JL, et al: Nylon fiber leukapheresis: Associated complement component changes and granulocytopenia. Blood 51:359–365, 1978.

30. Wiltbank TB, Nusbacher J, Higby DJ, et al: Abdominal pain in donors during filtration leukapheresis. Transfusion 17:159–162, 1977.

31. Strauss RG, Hester JP, Vogler WR, et al: A multicenter trial to document the efficacy and safety of a rapidly excreted analog of hydroxyethyl starch for leukapheresis with a note on steroid stimulation of granulocyte donors. Transfusion 26:258–264, 1986.

32. Lee J-H, Leitman SF, Klein HG: A controlled comparison of the efficacy of hetastarch and pentastarch in granulocyte collections by centrifugal leukapheresis. Blood 86:4662–4666, 1995.

33. Hinckley ME, Huestis DW: Premedication for optimal granulocyte collection. Plasma Ther 2:149–152, 1981.

34. Winton EF, Vogler WR: Development of a practical oral dexamethasone premedication schedule leading to improved granulocyte yields with the continuous-flow centrifugal blood cell separator. Blood 52:249–253, 1978.

35. Standards Committee of the American Association of Blood Banks (Menitove JE [ed]): Standards for Blood Banks and Transfusion Services, 19th ed. Bethesda, MD, American Association of Blood Banks, 1999.

36. Glasser L, Huestis DW, Jones JF: Functional capabilities of steroid-recruited neutrophils harvested for clinical transfusion. N Eng J Med 297:1033–1036, 1977.

37. Price TH: Neutrophil transfusion. In vivo function of neutrophils collected using cell separators. Transfusion 23:504–507, 1983.

38. Dale DC, Liles WC, Summer WR, et al: Granulocyte colony-stimulating factor: Role and relationships in infectious diseases. J Infect Dis 172:1061–1075, 1995.

39. Colotta F, Re F, Mantovani A: Granulocyte transfusions from granulocyte colony-stimulating factor-treated donors: Also a question of cell survival? Blood 82:2258, 1993.

40. Lane TA, Windle B: Granulocyte concentrate function during preservation: Effect of temperature. Blood 54:216–225, 1979.

41. McCullough J, Carter SJ, Quie PG: Effects of anticoagulants and storage on granulocyte function in bank blood. Blood 43:207–217, 1974.

42. McCullough J, Weiblen BJ, Fine D: Effects of storage of granulocytes on their fate in vivo. Transfusion 23:20–24, 1983.

43. Glasser L, Lane TA, McCullough J, et al: Panel VII: Neutrophil concentrates—functional considerations, storage, and quality control. J Clin Apheresis 1:179–184, 1983.

44. McCullough J, Weiblen BJ, Peterson PK, et al: Effects of temperature on granulocyte preservation. Blood 52:301–310, 1978.

45. Anderson KC, Weinstein HJ: Transfusion-associated graft-versus-host disease. N Engl J Med 323:315–321, 1990.

46. McCullough J: Granulocyte transfusion. In Petz LD, Swisher SN, Kleinman S, et al (eds): Clinical Practice of Transfusion Medicine, 3rd ed. New York, Churchill Livingstone, 1996, pp 413–432.

47. Valerius NH, Johansen KS, Nielsen OS, et al: Effect of in vitro x-irradiation on lymphocyte and granulocyte function. Scand J Haematol 27:9–18, 1981.

48. Eastlund DT, Charbonneau TT: Superoxide generation and cytotactic response of irradiated neutrophils. Transfusion 28:368–370, 1988.

49. Wolber RA, Duque RE, Robinson JP, et al: Oxidative product formation in irradiated neutrophils: A flow cytometric analysis. Transfusion 27:167–170, 1987.

50. Button LN, DeWolf WC, Newburger PE, et al: The effects of irradiation on blood components. Transfusion 21:419–426, 1981.

51. Schwarzenberg L, Mathé G, de Grouchy J, et al: White blood cell transfusions. Isr J Med Sci 1:925–956, 1965.

52. Morse EE, Freireich EJ, Carbone PP, et al: The transfusion of leukocytes from donors with chronic myelocytic leukemia to patients with leukopenia. Transfusion 6:183–192, 1966.

53. Lowenthal RM, Grossman L, Goldman JM, et al: Granulocyte transfusions in treatment of infections in patients with acute leukaemia and aplastic anaemia. Lancet 1:353–358, 1975.

54. Strauss RG: Granulocyte transfusion. In McLeod BC, Price TH, Drew MJ (eds): Apheresis: Principles and Practice. Bethesda, MD, AABB Press, 1997, pp 195–209.

55. Graw RG, Herzig GH, Perry S, et al: Normal granulocyte transfusion therapy: Treatment of septicemia due to gram-negative bacteria. N Engl J Med 287:367–371, 1972.

56. Higby DJ, Yates JW, Henderson ES, et al: Filtration leukapheresis for granulocyte transfusion therapy: Clinical and laboratory studies. N Engl J Med 292:761–766, 1975.

57. Fortuny IE, Bloomfield CD, Hadlock DC, et al: Granulocyte transfusion: A controlled study in patients with acute nonlymphocytic leukemia. Transfusion 15:548–557, 1975.

58. Vogler WR, Winton EF: A controlled study of the efficacy of granulocyte transfusions in patients with neutropenia. Am J Med 63:548–555, 1977.

59. Alavi JB, Root RK, Djerassi I, et al: A randomized clinical trial of granulocyte transfusions for infection in acute leukemia. N Engl J Med 296:706–711, 1977.

60. Herzig RH, Herzig GP, Graw RG, et al: Successful granulocyte transfusion therapy for gram-negative septicemia: A prospectively randomized controlled study. N Engl J Med 296:701–705, 1977.

61. Winston DJ, Ho WG, Gale RP: Therapeutic granulocyte transfusions for documented infections: A controlled trial in ninety-five infectious granulocytopenic episodes. Ann Intern Med 97:509–515, 1982.

62. Strauss RG: Therapeutic granulocyte transfusions in 1993. Blood 81:1675–1678, 1993.

63. Vamvakas EC, Pineda AA: Meta-analysis of clinical studies of the efficacy of granulocyte transfusions in the treatment of bacterial sepsis. J Clin Apheresis 11:1–9, 1996.

64. Ruthe RC, Andersen BR, Cunningham BL, et al: Efficacy of granulocyte transfusions in the control of systemic candidiasis in the leukopenic host. Blood 52:493–497, 1978.

65. Chow HS, Sarpel SC, Epstein RB: Pathophysiology of *Candida albicans* meningitis in normal, neutropenic, and granulocyte transfused dogs. Blood 55:546–551, 1980.

66. Spielberger RT, Falleroni MJ, Coene AJ, et al: Concomitant amphotericin B therapy, granulocyte transfusions, and GM-CSF administration for disseminated infection with *Fusarium* in a granulocytopenic patient. Clin Infect Dis 16:528–530, 1993.

67. Swerdlow B, Deresinski S: Development of *Aspergillus* sinusitis in a patient receiving amphotericin B treatment with granulocyte transfusions. Am J Med 76:162–166, 1984.

68. Bhatia S, McCullough J, Perry EH, et al: Granulocyte transfusions: Efficacy in treating fungal infections in neutropenic patients following bone marrow transplantation. Transfusion 34:226–232, 1994.

69. Strauss RG: Granulocyte transfusions. In Rossi EC, Simon TL, Moss GS, et al (eds): Principles of Transfusion Medicine, 2nd ed. Baltimore, Williams & Wilkins, 1996, pp 321–328.

70. Strauss RG, Connett JE, Gale RP, et al: A controlled trial of prophylactic granulocyte transfusions during initial induction chemotherapy for acute myelogenous leukemia. N Engl J Med 305:597–603, 1981.

71. Rosenshein MS, Farewell VT, Price TH, et al: The cost effectiveness of therapeutic and prophylactic leukocyte transfusion. N Engl J Med 302:1058–1062, 1980.

72. Christensen RD, Anstall HB, Rothstein G: Deficiencies in the neutrophil system of newborn infants, and the use of leukocyte transfusions in the treatment of neonatal sepsis. J Clin Apheresis 1:33–41, 1982.

73. Laurenti F, Ferro R, Isacchi G, et al: Polymorphonuclear leukocyte transfusion for the treatment of sepsis in the newborn infant. J Pediatr 98:118–123, 1981.

74. Christensen RD, Rothstein G, Anstall HB, et al: Granulocyte transfusions in neonates with bacterial infections, neutropenia, and depletion of mature marrow neutrophils. Pediatrics 70:1–6, 1982.

75. Cairo MS, Rucker R, Bennetts GA, et al: Improved survival of newborns receiving leukocyte transfusions for sepsis. Pediatrics 74:887–892, 1984.

76. Cairo MS, Worcester C, Rucker RW, et al: Randomized trial of granulocyte transfusions versus intravenous immune globulin therapy for neonatal neutropenia and sepsis. J Pediatr 120:281–285, 1992.

77. Baley JE, Stork EK, Warkentin PI, et al: Buffy coat transfusions in neutropenic neonates with presumed sepsis: A prospective, randomized trial. Pediatrics 80:712–720, 1987.

78. Wheeler JG, Chauvenet AR, Johnson CA, et al: Buffy coat transfusions in neonates with sepsis and neutrophil storage pool depletion [abstract]. Pediatrics 79:422–425, 1987.

79. Pflieger H, Arnold R, Bhaduri S, et al: Beneficial effect of granulocyte transfusions in patients with defects in granulocyte function and severe infections. Scand J Haematol 22:33–41, 1979.

80. Buescher ES, Gallin JI: Leukocyte tranfusions in chronic granulomatous disease: Persistence of transfused leukocytes in sputum. N Engl J Med 307:800–803, 1982.

81. Yomtovian R, Abramson J, Quie P, et al: Granulocyte transfusion therapy in chronic granulomatous disease: Report of a patient and review of the literature. Transfusion 21:739–743, 1981.

82. Dougherty SH, Peterson PK, Simmons RL: Granulocyte transfusion as adjunctive therapy for qualitative granulocytopenia: Multiple liver abscesses in a patient with chronic granulomatous disease. Arch Surg 118:873–874, 1983.

83. Bowen TJ, Ochs HD, Altman LC, et al: Severe recurrent bacterial infections associated with defective adherence and chemotaxis in two patients with neutrophils deficient in a cell-associated glycoprotein. J Pediatr 101:932–940, 1982.

84. Dana BW, Durie BG, White RF, et al: Concomitant administration of granulocyte transfusions and amphotericin B in neutropenic patients: absence of significant pulmonary toxicity. Blood 57:90–94, 1981.

85. Wright DG, Robichaud KJ, Pizzo PA, et al: Lethal pulmonary reactions associated with the combined use of amphotericin B and leukocyte transfusions. N Engl J Med 304:1185–1189, 1981.

86. Bow EJ, Schroeder ML, Louie TJ: Pulmonary complications in patients receiving granulocyte transfusions and amphotericin B. Can Med Assoc J 130:593–597, 1984.

87. Karp DD, Ervin TJ, Tuttle S, et al: Pulmonary complications during granulocyte transfusions: Incidence and clinical features. Vox Sang 42:57–61, 1982.

88. Pegels JG, Bruynes ECE, Engelriet CP, et al: Serological studies in patients on platelet- and granulocyte-substitution therapy. Br J Haematol 52:59–68, 1982.

89. Arnold R, Goldmann SF, Pflieger H: Lymphocytotoxic antibodies in patients receiving granulocyte transfusion. Vox Sang 38:250–258, 1980.

90. Appelbaum FR, Bowles CA, Makuch RW, et al: Granulocyte transfusion therapy of experimental *Pseudomonas* septicemia: Study of cell dose and collection technique. Blood 52:323–331, 1978.

91. Epstein RB, Chow HS: An analysis of quantitative relationships of granulocyte transfusion therapy in canines. Transfusion 21:360–362, 1981.

92. Chatta GS, Price TH, Allen RC, et al: Effects of in vivo recombinant methionyl human granulocyte colony-stimulating factor on the neutrophil response and peripheral blood colony-forming cells in healthy young and elderly adult volunteers. Blood 84:2923–2929, 1994.

93. Price TH, Chatta GS, Dale DC: Effect of recombinant granulocyte colony-stimulating factor on neutrophil kinetics in normal young and elderly humans. Blood 88:335–340, 1996.

94. Liles WC, Huang JE, van Burik JH, et al: Granulocyte colony-stimulating factor administered in vivo augments neutrophil-mediated activity against opportunistic fungal pathogens. J Infect Dis 175:1012–1015, 1997.

95. Gaviria JM, van Burik J-A, Dale DC, et al: Comparison of interferon-gamma, granulocyte colony-stimulating factor, and granulocyte-macrophage colony-stimulating factor for priming leukocyte-mediated hyphal damage of opportunistic fungal pathogens. J Infect Dis 179:1038–1041, 1999.

96. Liles WC, Rodger ER, Dale DC: Differential regulation of human neutrophil surface expression of CD14, CD11b, CD18, and L-selection following the administration of G-CSF in vivo and in vitro [abstract]. Clin Res 42:304A, 1994.

97. Stroncek DF, Jaszcz W, Herr GP, et al: Expression of neutrophil antigens after 10 days of granulocyte-colony-stimulating factor. Transfusion 38:663–668, 1998.

98. Liles WC: Regulation of apoptosis in neutrophils: Fast track to death? J Immunol 155:3289–3291, 1995.

99. Price TH, Bowden RA, Boeckh M, et al: Neutrophil collection from community apheresis donors after granulocyte colony-stimulating factor and dexamethasone stimulation: feasibility and efficacy [abstract]. Blood 90(Suppl 1):137B, 1997.

100. Leitman SF, Yu M, Lekstrom J: Pair-controlled study of granulocyte colony stimulating factor (G-CSF) plus dexamethasone (DEXA) for granulocytapheresis donors [abstract]. Transfusion 35:53S, 1995.

101. Liles WC, Huang JE, Llewellyn C, et al: A comparative trial of granulocyte-colony-stimulating factor and dexamethasone, separately and in combination, for the mobilization of neutrophils in the peripheral blood of normal volunteers. Transfusion 37:182–187, 1997.

102. Stroncek DF, Clay ME, Petzoldt ML, et al: Treatment of normal individuals with granulocyte-colony-stimulating factor: Donor experiences and the effects on peripheral blood CD34$^+$ cell counts and on the collection of peripheral blood stem cells. Transfusion 36:601–610, 1996.

103. Anderlini P, Przepiorka D, Seong D, et al: Clinical toxicity and laboratory effects of granulocyte-colony-stimulating factor (filgrastim) mobilization and blood stem cell apheresis from normal donors, and analysis of charges for the procedures. Transfusion 36:590–595, 1996.

104. Hester JP, Dignani MC, Anaissie EJ, et al: Collection and transfusion of granulocyte concentrates from donors primed with granulocyte stimulating factor and response of myelosuppressed patients with established infection. J Clin Apheresis 10:188–193, 1995.

105. Adkins D, Spitzer G, Johnston M, et al: Transfusions of granulocyte-colony-stimulating factor–mobilized granulocyte components to allogeneic transplant recipients: Analysis of kinetics and factors determining posttransfusion neutrophil and platelet counts. Transfusion 37:737–748, 1997.

106. Bowden R, Price T, Boeckh M, et al: Phase I/II study of granulocyte transfusions from G-CSF–stimulated unrelated donors for treatment infections in neutropenic blood and marrow transplant (BMT) patients [abstract]. Blood 90(Suppl 1):435A, 1997.

107. Dale DC, Liles WC, Llewellyn C, et al: Neutrophil transfusions: Kinetics and functions of neutrophils mobilized with granulocyte colony-stimulating factor (G-CSF) and dexamethasone. Transfusion 38:713–721, 1998.

108. Adkins D, Goodgold H, Hendershott L, et al: Indium-labeled white blood cells apheresed from donors receiving G-CSF localize to sites of inflammation when infused into allogeneic bone marrow transplant recipients. Bone Marrow Transplant 19:809–812, 1997.

109. Leitman SF, Oblitas JM, Emmons R, et al: Clinical efficacy of daily G-CSF-recruited granulocyte transfusions in patients with severe neutropenia and life-threatening infections [abstract]. Blood 88(Suppl 1):331A, 1996.

110. Clarke K, Szer J, Shelton M, et al: Multiple granulocyte transfusions facilitating successful unrelated bone marrow transplantation in a patient with very severe aplastic anemia complicated by suspected fungal infection. Bone Marrow Transplant 16:723–726, 1995.

111. Di Mario A, Sica S, Salutari P, et al: Granulocyte colony-stimulating factor–primed leukocyte transfusions in *Candida tropicalis* fungemia in neutropenic patients. Haematologica 82:362–363, 1997.

112. von Planta M, Ozsahin H, Schroten H, et al: Greater omentum flaps and granulocyte transfusions as combined therapy of liver abscess in chronic granulomatous disease. Eur J Pediatr Surg 7:234–236, 1997.

113. Catalano L, Fontana R, Scarpato N, et al: Combined treatment with amphotericin-B and granulocyte transfusion from G-CSF–stimulated donors in an aplastic patient with invasive aspergillosis undergoing bone marrow transplantation. Haematologica 82:71–72, 1997.

114. Grigg A, Vecchi L, Bardy P, et al: G-CSF–stimulated donor granulocyte collections for prophylaxis and therapy of neutropenic sepsis. Aust N Z J Med 26:813–818, 1996.

115. Taylor K, Moore D, Kelly C, et al: Safety and logistical use of filgrastim (FG) mobilised granulocytes (FMG) in early management of severe neutropenic sepsis (SNS) in acute leukemia (AL)/autograft [abstract]. Blood 88(Suppl 1):349A, 1996.

116. Caspar CB, Seger RA, Burger J, et al: Effective stimulation of donors for granulocyte transfusions with recombinant methionyl granulocyte colony-stimulating factor. Blood 81:2866–2871, 1993.

117. Bensinger WI, Price TH, Dale DC, et al: The effects of daily recombinant human granulocyte colony-stimulating factor administration on normal granulocyte donors undergoing leukapheresis. Blood 81:1883–1888, 1993.

118. Jendiroba DB, Lichtiger B, Anaissie E, et al: Evaluation and comparison of three mobilization methods for the collection of granulocytes. Transfusion 38:722–728, 1998.

PART III

Transfusion Medicine

Chapter 19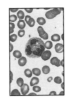

Leukocyte Reduced Products

Walter H. Dzik

Zbigniew M. Szczepiorkowski

Recipient exposure to allogeneic donor leukocytes results in several complications of blood transfusion. To reduce the likelihood of these complications, leukoreduction of red blood cells (RBCs) and platelets is widely practiced. This chapter addresses the basis for the adverse effects of recipient exposure to donor leukocytes and presents the evidence supporting the scientific foundation for leukoreduction of cellular blood products. In particular, we address the biophysical mechanisms involved in the preparation of leukoreduced RBCs and platelets and the biologic mechanisms accounting for febrile nonhemolytic reactions, primary human leukocyte antigen (HLA) alloimmunization, transmission and reactivation of cytomegalovirus (CMV), transfusion-associated immunosuppression, and adverse effects from transfusion of leukoreduced blood. The reader is referred to other sources for a discussion of additional aspects of leukoreduction, including clinical outcomes studies, device evaluations, quality control, cost-effectiveness, and operational issues.[1-3]

Standards defining leukoreduced blood exist in both the United States and Europe. In the United States, a leukoreduced RBC or apheresis platelet contains less than 5×10^6 leukocytes (WBCs) per unit. Leukoreduced RBCs should retain more than 85% of the original erythrocytes. For platelet concentrates derived from whole blood, the standard requires that each unit contain no more than 0.83 WBCs/unit, so that a pool of six such units would contain no more than 5×10^6 WBCs. In Europe, a leukoreduced RBC or platelet should contain no more than 1×10^6 WBCs. These standards are used in the evaluation of new technologies for leukoreduction and in quality control validation.

No standards address the relative proportion of residual leukocyte subpopulations in leukoreduced blood. As described later, some complications of donor leukocytes depend on exposure to particular subsets of leukocytes, such as mononuclear cells for transmission of CMV or HLA class II–bearing cells for direct alloimmunization. One study demonstrated that the leukocyte subsets found in process-reduced apheresis platelets differed significantly from the subsets found in filtered platelets, the latter product containing a lower relative concentration of mononuclear cells.[4] The significance of this finding was challenged in a subsequent study comparing leukocyte subsets in products obtained from different apheresis instruments.[5] A study of prestorage leukoreduced RBCs using Sepacell filters (Asahi Medical Corporation, Baxter Healthcare, Round Lake, IL) and flow cytometry demonstrated greater removal of monocytes and lymphocytes compared with neutrophils. The study also noted progressive loss of all leukocyte subsets during refrigerated storage after leukoreduction.[6] However, no major clinical study has examined outcomes among patients supported with leukofiltered whole blood platelets compared with processed leukoreduced apheresis platelets, and so the clinical impact of differences in leukocyte subpopulations cannot be determined at this time. Currently, all methods of leukoreduction that meet the threshold standard for total number of residual donor leukocytes are considered equivalent.

The issue of whether all cellular blood components should be leukoreduced has generated interest in many nations. Several countries announced plans to convert to a universally leukoreduced blood supply during the latter half of the 1990s. The rationale was different in different nations and was linked to a program of hemovigilance in France, to concern over the potential for spread of transmissible spongiform encephalopathies by donor leukocytes in the United Kingdom, and to a general reorganization of blood services in Canada. In the United States, the Blood Product Advisory Committee of the Food and Drug Administration (FDA) voted in 1998 in favor of universal leukoreduction in the absence

---

Box 19.1   Indications for Leukoreduced Blood Components

Reduce rate of recurrent febrile nonhemolytic transfusion reactions (FNHTRs)

Reduce rate of HLA alloimmunization among hematology-oncology patients

Reduce rate of cytomegalovirus transmission to susceptible recipients

---

of any consideration of cost to the health care system and sponsored a conference in 1999 that was geared toward implementation of universal leukoreduction. However, studies estimated that universal leukoreduction would cost more than $500 million per year in the United States. Moreover, most studies of cost-effectiveness have demonstrated an unfavorable cost-benefit ratio for universal leukoreduction (Box 19.1).

Technologies for the Preparation of Leukoreduced Blood

To achieve a 10,000-fold reduction in the leukocyte content of blood requires specialized technologies of leukofiltration or apheresis collection. Numerous factors affect the performance of leukoreduction, including the temperature of filtration, the speed of blood flow through the filter, the number of leukocytes presented to the filter, the protein content of the suspending medium, the platelet content of blood, the use of a rinse step after filtration, the storage age of blood, and the presence of the hemoglobin S in the RBCs to be filtered.

Leukofilter Device Design

Removal of leukocytes from whole blood, packed RBCs, or platelets depends on a combination of barrier filtration and cell adsorption to the filter material. Certain principles of design are common to leukofiltration devices.[7] A large surface area of filter medium is required to allow sufficient opportunity for contact of blood leukocytes with the medium. This requirement for surface area can be met through the use of filter media composed of fibers with a very small diameter (microfibers) or open-cell media with a geometry like "Swiss cheese."

Three different approaches to manufacturing such nonwoven media have been commercially viable. The first is a dry formation process in which a polymer (typically a polyester) is melted and extruded through very fine nozzles into a turbulent gas stream at high velocity. The melted polyester is simultaneously stretched and cooled to form thin strands of fibers in a process akin to the making of cotton candy. These fibers are then collected, matted, and hot compressed to a controlled density. Some variation of this basic technique is used in products from Pall Corporation, Asahi Medical Company, and Fresenius AG, among others.

An alternative approach to making nonwoven media is wet formation. This process is similar to papermaking. Fibrous ingredients are first dispersed in water to form a suspension. The suspension is deposited on a fine-mesh screen, and the water is allowed to drain. As water is removed, the fibers settle into a soft mat. The spaces created within the interlocking scaffold are determined by key properties such as length and thickness of the fine fibers. The mat is then heated and dried to stabilize the structure into a fibrous sheet. This manufacturing process is used in products made by Hemasure, Inc.

A third approach has been to prepare superfine glass fiber membranes.[8] Foam-like structures with open-cell geometry contain interconnecting voids that allow a circuitous flow passage. Manufacture of such media derives from principles used in the manufacture of sponges. For example, filters from Terumo Corporation are made with the use of a porous polycarbonate medium that exhibits an open-cell architecture.

Because they offer an effective pore size that is extremely small, filter media must be designed to have a hydrophilic surface. Otherwise, the material will fail to "wet" as blood encounters the medium, owing to the inherent surface tension of blood. The synthetic materials used in leukoreduction filters—polyester microfibers, porous polycarbonate, and glass microfibers—are all naturally hydrophobic. Manufacturers modify the surface chemistry of these materials to increase their ability to "wet." Failure to wet would prevent blood from passing through the filter under gravity conditions. Although prefiltration rinsing with a more hydrophilic liquid (e.g., saline rinse) can wet the filter medium, prerinsing introduces an inconvenience that manufacturers of filters generally wish to avoid.

The volume of blood left inside the filter after filtration is referred to as the "hold-up volume." Filters that have a hard external housing often include a venting step at the end of filtration, which allows sterile air to enter the filter and displace blood that would otherwise have been held up in the device. One manufacturer (MacoPharma, Tourcoing, France) packages the filter medium in a flexible plastic housing that collapses under atmospheric pressure as blood drains out of the filter. U.S. FDA guidelines require that the filtration process result in loss of no more than 15% of the original amount of therapeutic blood elements.[9]

The filtration medium is packaged in an external housing. It is essential that the medium completely fill the housing, allowing no opportunity for the path of blood to flow around (bypass) the filter and thereby circumvent the leukodepletion medium. To appreciate the stringency required, consider that the leukocyte content of an entire unit of leukoreduced RBC is equal to the leukocyte content of only one drop (100 μL) of nonleukoreduced blood. Therefore, even a trivial amount of filter bypass would foil the leukoreduction process.

Mechanisms of Leukoreduction

Barrier Filtration

Simple barrier filtration, in which the effective pore size of the filter medium is smaller than the size of the leukocyte, is a major mechanism used by leukoreduction filters. Modern leukoreduction filters have an effective pore size on the order of 4 μm. This space is sufficient for passage of platelets and deformable erythrocytes but is able to retain leukocytes. Because effective leukoreduction by barrier-based filtration is tightly linked to the deformability of blood cells, factors affecting cell deformability have an impact on filter performance. Increased leukocyte deformability at higher temperatures probably accounts for the poorer performance of leukofiltration when it is applied to room-temperature RBCs, compared with refrigerated RBCs (see later discussion).

Cell Adhesion

Contact-mediated adhesion between leukocytes and the filter medium also contributes to the performance of leukofiltration devices. For contact to occur, there must be a sufficient dwell time of the blood with the medium. In order that the cells do not detach from the medium, shear forces of the flowing blood must not be too strong. High flow rates can result in insufficient contact and excess detachment of leukocytes from the medium. Because cell adhesion to filter media involves a complex surface chemistry that is not fully understood, filter media development has been largely determined by experimentation. The nature of the fluid in which cells are suspended, including the plasma protein content and the platelet content, affects the adhesion of leukocytes to synthetic media. Steneker[10] demonstrated that during leukofiltration of fresh RBCs the presence of viable platelets improves the performance of leukofiltration. This has been attributed to sticking of platelets to protein-coated fibers in the filter medium, with subsequent binding of leukocytes to these activated platelets. Ledent and Berlin[11] demonstrated that replacement of plasma with crystalloid can decrease the performance of leukofiltration, presumably by decreasing the concentration of adhesive plasma proteins that participate in leukocyte adhesion to the medium.

Leukofiltration of platelet concentrates presents the added complexity that platelets are naturally adhesive under shear conditions in a plasma environment, as a result of von Willebrand factor–mediated platelet adhesion. Therefore, manufacturers of leukoreduction filters designed for platelets have further modified the surface chemistry of the filter media to decrease binding of platelets to the filter. For example, Nishimura and colleagues[12] documented that by adjusting the molar ratio of positively charged diethyl-amino ethyl methacrylate to negatively charged hydroxy ethyl methacrylate, the net surface charge on the filter medium could be adjusted to optimize leukocyte adhesion but minimize platelet adhesion to the medium.

Biophysical Reasons for Reduced Performance of Leukofiltration

The reduced efficiency of leukofiltration applied to warmed RBCs compared with cold RBCs has repeatedly been demonstrated. For example, Beaujean and coworkers[13] split RBCs (storage age, 2 to 10 days) into two equal aliquots, which were then filtered at either at 4° or 37°C. The mean postfiltration leukocyte content was 10-fold higher for units filtered at 37°C. Ledent and associates[11] found leukocyte content to be 100-fold higher among units filtered at 37° compared with 4°C. Sirchia and colleagues[14] studied filtration under conditions designed to mimic bedside use. They found that cold RBCs warmed to room temperature within 90 minutes after removal of the units from the refrigerator. They also documented that as the blood warmed, filtration performance declined, so that the majority of units filtered slowly (and allowed to warm) failed to meet minimum requirements for leukoreduced blood. The performance of newer versions of leukoreduction filters may be less sensitive to temperature. van der Meer and colleagues[15] demonstrated enhanced performance at 4°C, but the difference between the results at 4° and at 22°C was less than that seen in earlier studies.[15] In a small study of 10 units examined only at day 14 of storage,

Smith and Leitman[16] were unable to demonstrate enhanced filtration performance at 4° compared with 22°C.

The importance of the temperature of RBC leukofiltration has had a direct bearing on the timing of leukoreduction. Laboratory-based leukofiltration (either before or after storage) can be done under refrigerated conditions. In contrast, because bedside filtration is done more slowly, blood warms to room temperature and filtration performance may decline. The reduced performance of bedside filtration, especially with earlier versions of leukofilters, is very important in the interpretation of major clinical trials of leukoreduction technology. For example, both the CMV prevention trial of Bowden and associates[17] and the HLA alloimmunization trial of Williamson and coworkers[18] used bedside filtration with filters subsequently determined to have reduced performance under warm conditions.

Several other factors may reduce the effectiveness of leukofiltration. Excess shear force and resulting cell detachment from the filter medium may be an important consideration when bedside leukofiltration is combined with mechanical blood delivery systems that may "pull" blood through the filter at excessive rates. Postfiltration rinsing of filters may also occur during bedside transfusion and has been documented to result in leukocyte detachment. Filtration of excessive volumes of blood or of blood containing excessive numbers of leukocytes can overwhelm the capacity of the filter medium, leading to ineffective leukoreduction.

Leukofiltration of RBCs has been shown to be less effective if the blood carries the hemoglobin S mutation.[19, 20] This occurs with hemoglobin AS blood (sickle cell trait). The exact mechanism for poor leukofiltration of hemoglobin AS blood is not known. It is possible that under conditions of reduced pH and oxygen, such as occur in blood storage bags, RBC deformability of hemoglobin AS erythrocytes is reduced. This would result in "filling" of the filter with RBCs (rather than leukocytes), leading to a decrease in the effective area of medium available for retention of leukocytes. Because sickle trait is relatively common, the frequency of failure of leukoreduction by filtration may be higher than expected.

Leukoreduced Apheresis Platelets

Modern apheresis devices are able to collect platelets that are leukoreduced during collection; this is referred to as "process leukoreduction." The Spectra LR (COBE BCT, Lakewood, CO) apheresis device is widely used for the preparation of leukoreduced apheresis platelets. Three design principles of this device enhance its ability to separate platelets from leukocytes during donor collection. Centrifugation in the rotating chamber of the machine establishes an initial gradient in which the less dense plasma and platelets "float" on top of the more dense leukocytes and RBCs. In order to leave the spinning chamber, the more dense RBCs and leukocytes must flow in a direction opposite to that of plasma and platelets. This establishes a flow pattern in which the less dense cells "slip" in the opposite direction to the more dense cells and represents a first-order separation of leukocytes from platelets. Second, platelets must flow over a "dam," which serves to further separate the less dense platelets from the more dense leukocytes. Finally, the platelet-rich plasma enters a conically shaped chamber that further separates platelets from leukocytes based on the principle of particle-bed separation. Platelets and leukocytes enter the small end of the conical chamber.

As when a rapidly flowing narrow river empties into a large bay, the linear flow rate of the cells slows as the chamber widens. This slowing causes the leukocytes, with a larger mass, to become unable to traverse the chamber against the centrifugal force of the spinning chamber. As a result, the leukocytes accumulate in the chamber during the collection. In contrast, the smaller platelets are able to exit the chamber and continue in the flow path to the collection bag. The final product is rich in platelets and highly depleted in leukocytes. Further leukoreduction by filtration usually is not required.

The Amicus apheresis system (Baxter Healthcare, Round Lake, IL) is a second widely used apheresis system for the preparation of leukoreduced platelets. The device incorporates three design features to achieve leukoreduction—active interface control, autoelutriation, and fluid flow dynamics. An optical interface detector is positioned within the separation chamber to monitor changes in the platelet interface. The system recirculates some of the donor plasma into the interface in order to separate platelets from leukocytes by elutriation. Just as a wind blows lightweight leaves but not heavy objects across a street, plasma pumped through the interface dislodges the platelets but not the leukocytes into the collection path. The collection path for platelet collection is in the opposite direction to the flow path for the return of RBCs and plasma to the donor, promoting further separation between donor platelets and donor leukocytes.

Process control monitoring of apheresis platelet collections documents that these are reliable systems for the collection of leukoreduced platelets.[21] However, as with leukoreduction filters, the apheresis process can fail. Sudden changes in the rate of blood entering the machine or pauses in blood flow during collection will disturb the centrifugal separation of blood in the chambers and may interrupt the controlled flow paths upon which the cells travel during separation. These interruptions can lead to "spillover" of leukocytes into the platelet collection stream. Manufacturers have attempted to engineer alarms into the software that will alert operators to conditions that might result in the failure to collect a leukoreduced product. The leukocyte content of these collections can then be tested to determine whether the product is leukoreduced.

Studies of leukoreduction "failure" have documented problems with both leukofiltration and apheresis technologies. For example, Kao and colleagues[22] reported quality control data from the Trial to Reduce Alloimmunization to Platelets (TRAP). Using a propidium iodide stain and microscopic chamber counting, they found that 7% of apheresis platelets and 5% of pooled platelets contained more than 5×10^6 residual donor leukocytes. Depending on the kind of leukodepletion filter used, the frequency of units with greater than 5×10^6 residual WBCs ranged from 0.3% to 2.7%. In addition, they reported substantial losses of platelets and

RBCs as a result of the process of leukofiltration. Although refinements in filter design and apheresis technology have improved on these results,[23] the findings demonstrate the need for continuous quality monitoring of blood component preparation and modification (Box 19.2).

■ Prevention of Febrile Nonhemolytic Transfusion Reactions by Leukoreduction

One of the first indications for the use of leukocyte filters was prevention of febrile nonhemolytic transfusion reactions (FNHTRs). Original studies suggested that the frequency of FNHTRs to packed RBCs is reduced when the residual leukocyte content is less than 5×10^8 WBCs/unit.[24–28] Although FNHTRs are one of the most common transfusion reactions experienced by recipients of blood components, they are also relatively easy to manage. Many, but not all FNHTRs, can be prevented by leukoreduction of blood components (Box 19.3).

Fever is a hallmark and part of the clinical definition of FNHTR. In addition to fever, patients may experience chills, rigors, cold, a sense of discomfort, headache, and nausea. Because the pathophysiology of fever involves a rigor/chill response before the temperature rises, the initial signs of an FNHTR may document only rigors without temperature elevation. Therefore, the presence of fever should not be required to diagnose an FNHTR.[29, 30] FNHTRs tend to develop toward the end of a transfusion and in 10% to 20% of cases reactions are noted after the transfusion has been discontinued. Such clinical observations underlie the fact that reactions are dose-related and require time to develop.

Box 19.3   Pros and Cons of Universal Leukoreduction

Pro: Patients with selected indications to receive LR blood will be more likely to receive LR units

Improves "purity" of blood

Inventory management is streamlined

May have favorable effect on viral reactivation

May have favorable effect on cancer recurrence and survival in colorectal cancer

May have favorable effect on other aspects of immune modulation

Con: Removes physician choice from product selection

Adds > $500 million each year to health care costs

May adversely affect availability of an adequate supply of blood in setting of recalls of LR devices; may interfere with supply of blood donors with African ancestry (sickle trait blood)

Large randomized study suggests no benefit of LR for viral reactivation*

Large randomized study suggests no benefit of LR for recurrence in colorectal cancer†

Studies fail to demonstrate clear benefit of LR on immunomodulation

*Collier AC, Kalish LA, Busch MP, et al. *JAMA* 2001;285:1592–1601.
†van de Watering LMG, Brand A, Houbiers JGA, et al. *Br J Surg* 2001;88:267–272.

Box 19.2   Methods for Quality Control of Leukoreduced Products

Large-volume hemocytometer (e.g., Nageotte chamber)
Flow cytometer
Volumetric cytometer

The Pathophysiology of Fever

Fever is one the oldest signs and symptoms recognized in medicine. Fever results from cytokine generation by activated monocytes, macrophages, and Kupffer cells. The involved cytokines, including interleukin-1β (IL-1β), IL-6, interferon-β (IFN-β), IFN-γ, and tumor necrosis factor-α (TNF-α), are polypeptides that act on the organum vasculosum of lamina terminalis (OVLT).[31] The OVLT interacts with the preoptic area of the hypothalamus. In the case of TNF-α, the induction of cyclooxygenase-2 in brain blood vessels leads to increased production of prostaglandins (mainly prostaglandin E_2)[32] and subsequently to fever.[33] Engel and associates[34] reported the peripheral blood levels of cytokines measured in patients with fever and neutropenia. The median peak concentration for IL-6 was 400 pg/mL (range, 100 to 41,000 pg/mL); for IL-8, it was 1025 pg/mL (range, 600 to 26,000 pg/mL); for TNF-α, less than 10 pg/mL; and for IL-1β, 17 pg/mL (range, <10 to 36 pg/mL).

Incidence and Mechanisms of FNHTR

The reported incidence of FNHTR depends on the transfused component. Transfusions of nonleukoreduced RBCs are associated with 0.5% to 6.0% risk, whereas transfusions of platelet concentrates carry a risk as high as 20% to 30%.[35–37] This significant difference between RBCs and platelet concentrates can be attributed to different mechanisms involved in development of febrile reactions.

Three mechanisms may account for FNHTRs (Fig. 19.1). The original (classic) mechanism implicated the presence of recipient antibodies against donor leukocytes. Anti-leukocyte antibodies reacting with transfused donor leukocytes result in the release of "endogenous pyrogens" (now known to be cytokines) from leukocytes. This explanation failed to account for the fact that FNHTRs were more common among recipients of platelets compared with packed RBCs, and it failed to explain the observation that FNHTRs may occur among men with no history of prior transfusions. A second mechanism (passive cytokine infusion) acknowledges the accumulation during storage of fever-producing cytokines in platelet concentrates. This mechanism may account for the majority of FNHTRs to nonleukoreduced platelets, but it fails to explain reactions to leukoreduced platelets and packed RBCs. A third (immune complex) mechanism for FNHTRs is based on the formation of immune complexes that trigger activation of recipient macrophages to release inflammatory cytokines. In practice, FNHTRs may depend on all three of these mechanisms.

FNHTR Caused by Destruction of Transfused Donor Leukocytes

First proposed in the 1960s, the classic mechanism suggests that donor leukocytes react with recipient anti-leukocyte antibodies, causing the donor cells to release endogenous pyrogens (cytokines). This mechanism is consistent with the prevention of FNHTRs by leukoreduction of donor blood, and it is supported by studies of DeRie and colleagues,[38] Decary and colleagues,[39] Perkins and colleagues,[40] Brubaker,[41] and others[42] that documented the high prevalence of anti-lymphocyte or anti-granulocyte antibodies in the sera of patients who

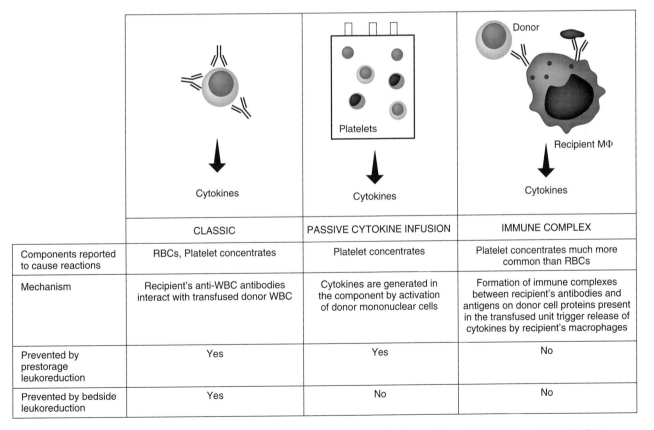

	CLASSIC	PASSIVE CYTOKINE INFUSION	IMMUNE COMPLEX
Components reported to cause reactions	RBCs, Platelet concentrates	Platelet concentrates	Platelet concentrates much more common than RBCs
Mechanism	Recipient's anti-WBC antibodies interact with transfused donor WBC	Cytokines are generated in the component by activation of donor mononuclear cells	Formation of immune complexes between recipient's antibodies and antigens on donor cell proteins present in the transfused unit trigger release of cytokines by recipient's macrophages
Prevented by prestorage leukoreduction	Yes	Yes	No
Prevented by bedside leukoreduction	Yes	No	No

Figure 19.1 Mechanisms underlying febrile nonhemolytic transfusion reactions. (Adapted from Klein HG, Dzik WH, Slichter SJ, et al: Leukocyte-Reduced Blood Components: Current Status. Educational Program, American Society of Hematology, 1998, pp 154–177.)

experienced FNHTRs. The mechanism can be challenged, however, because leukocytes are not known to store IL-1 and TNF,[43] and because patients with anti-HLA antibodies have febrile reactions when transfused with leukocyte-reduced platelet concentrates.

FNHTRs Caused by Passive Transfer of Cytokines

In a series of simple and well-designed experiments, Heddle and associates[44] focused attention on the plasma constituent of stored platelet concentrates, rather than the platelets themselves, as the source of febrile reactions after transfusion of platelet concentrates.[44] The authors selected 4- and 5-day-old platelet concentrates. Using centrifugation, the platelet-poor plasma was separated from the platelet pellet, which was resuspended in fresh plasma. Patients were then transfused with both components in random sequence, with a 2-hour washout period between transfusions. Signs and symptoms suggestive of FNHTR were assessed. Transfusions of the platelet-poor plasma obtained from stored platelet concentrates were associated with a significantly higher rate of FNHTR, compared with the resuspended platelet pellets. The authors concluded that soluble substances that had accumulated in the plasma during platelet storage were primarily responsible for febrile reactions in the older platelet concentrates. Increased levels of two cytokines, IL-1β and IL-6, were present in stored platelets and correlated with the frequency of observed reactions.

MECHANISM OF CYTOKINE ACCUMULATION IN PLATELET CONCENTRATES

Cytokines include a large family of molecules involved in innate immunity and cell signaling. After release by mononuclear phagocytes, T lymphocytes, and several other cell types, cytokines bind to specific receptors on target cells. Cytokine receptor chains cluster, and their intracellular portions are phosphorylated by Janus kinases (Jaks). The phosphorylation step is required for the Src homology-2 (SH-2) portion of the Jak to bind to the receptor. SH-2 facilitates binding of a signal transducer and activator of transcription (STAT) protein. After phosphorylation, these STAT proteins form homodimers, which migrate to the nucleus and bind to nuclear factors such as nuclear factor-κB (NF-κB) or activation protein-1 (AP-1) transcription factors. The transcription factors then activate genes involved in innate immunity.[45]

A number of reports showed increased accumulation of cytokines, especially IL-1β, IL-6, IL-8, TNF-α, and RANTES (regulated on activation, normal T expressed and secreted), with prolonged storage of platelet concentrates.[46–48] Increased cytokine levels were observed especially on the fourth and fifth day of storage. Stack and Snyder[47] assayed 2-, 3-, 4- and 5-day-old platelet concentrates for IL-1β, IL-6, IL-8, and TNF-α. Although IL-8 was the cytokine most frequently detected, IL-8 is not regarded as a fever-producing cytokine. Increased IL-1β was observed in the units with elevated IL-8. In general, the highest levels of IL-8 were found in the units with the longest storage times and highest leukocyte counts. Only 8% and 10% of tested units showed detectable levels of IL-6 and TNF-α, respectively. Leukoreduction before storage prevented the accumulation of IL-8 and IL-1β to day 5 of storage. This study underscored the importance of storage time and initial number of leukocytes before storage in the generation of cytokines.

Palmer and coworkers[49, 50] combined results of their two studies and showed that cytokine accumulation during storage of platelet concentrate correlated with the number of leukocytes present before storage. Units with a leukocyte concentration greater than 100/μL resulted in detectable levels of IL-8 and IL-1β. Although prestorage leukoreduction prevented cytokine accumulation, leukoreduction had no beneficial effect on markers of platelet activation such as P-selectin, transforming growth factor-β1 (TGF-β1), platelet-derived growth factor AB (PDGF-AB), von Willebrand factor, and serotonin. These results were confirmed in a study by Fujihara and colleagues,[51] who showed that accumulation of platelet-derived RANTES and TGF-β1 was independent of leukocyte concentration but correlated with platelet concentration.

MONOCYTE ACTIVATION

Monocytes are a major constituent of the leukocyte population in platelet concentrates. They are also capable of secreting cytokines, namely IL-1β, IL-6, and TNF-α. Several authors have investigated monocyte activation in platelet concentrates as a potential explanation for cytokine accumulation. Muller-Steinhardt and associates[52] studied the influence of storage time, temperature, and type of anticoagulant on the capability of mononuclear cells to secrete cytokines. Mononuclear cells were harvested on days 1, 3, and 5 from platelet concentrates stored under routine conditions, and the response to mitogenic stimulants, such as lipopolysaccharide (LPS), phytohemagglutinin, and staphylococcal enterotoxin B, was evaluated by measuring secretion of IL-1α, IL-2, IL-6, and IFN-γ. The ability of monocytes to secrete cytokines did not change significantly during the first 3 days of storage and decreased to 25% to 50% of original levels by day 5 of storage. Mitogenic response of mononuclear cells was significantly higher at 37°C than at 22°C. These findings showed that under normal storage conditions mononuclear cells in platelet concentrates preserve the ability to synthesize and secrete cytokines for at least 5 days. Heddle and coworkers[53] demonstrated that cytokine accumulation during storage is temperature-dependent. Platelet concentrates were split into two identical portions, one of which was stored for 5 days at 22°C and the other at 4°C. Cytokines failed to accumulate in the aliquots stored at 4°C.

Grey and associates[54] reported in vivo activation of monocytes in platelet concentrates. They analyzed platelet concentrates for leukocyte and monocyte total count, CD14 and CD16 monocyte-associated antigen expression, and IL-1β and IL-6 concentrations on days 1, 2, 3, 4, and 5. The analyzed monocytes expressed increased levels of CD14 (LPS receptor) and CD16 (FcγRIII), which are both markers of activation, starting on the first day of storage. On day 3, more than 50% of platelet concentrates had an increased IL-6 concentration. The elevation of IL-6 and IL-1β correlated with the number of monocytes in the unit on day 1. However, increased IL-6 levels occurred earlier during storage. Several hypotheses have sought to explain the delay between monocyte activation and detectable elevation of interleukins. TNF-α and IL-1 are known to induce IL-1 synthesis and together with PDGF can stimulate IL-6 synthesis.[55] Both IL-1α and IL-1β were found in the cytoplasm of resting and thrombin-activated platelets.[56] It is possible that the cumulative effect of PDGF and IL-1 derived from platelets reaches a threshold concentration necessary to trigger monocytes to generate additional cytokines such as IL-8 and IL-6. This hypothesis is supported by the findings by Aye and colleagues[57] indicating that, despite uniform release of PDGF from platelets during preparation and storage, only components with high leukocyte content had a detectable level of cytokines.

Mononuclear cells in stored platelet concentrates may be activated by other mechanisms. Activation of monocytes by the plastic used in storage bags was studied by El-Kattan and coworkers.[58] Whole blood–derived platelets were stored in plastic bags made of polyolefin (POF), and apheresis platelets were stored in the bags made of polyvinyl chloride (PVC). Mononuclear cells showed preferential adherence to POF compared with PVC. This adherence was associated with increased mean cytokine levels (IL-1β, TNF, IL-6) that were 11- to 48-fold higher in POF bags compared with PVC bags.

FNHTRs Caused by Cytokine Production by Recipient Macrophages

A third mechanism for FNHTRs depends on cytokine release by the recipients' own macrophages. It has been proposed that recipient antibody bound to donor-cell antigen may form an immune complex that serves to activate recipient macrophages to release inflammatory cytokines.[59] This mechanism does not depend on release of preformed stored cytokines contained within donor leukocytes but acknowledges that immune complexes are a known stimulus for macrophage activation. Indirect support for this hypothesis comes from a number of observations, including the development of fever among alloimmunized recipients of prestorage leukoreduced platelets; fever after transfusion of platelets to patients with immune thrombocytopenia or drug-induced thrombocytopenia; fever among recipients of incompatible RBC transfusions; and the fever reactions to the cellular portion of platelet concentrates seen in the study by Heddle and associates[44] cited earlier.

Cytokine Concentrations In Vivo and In Vitro

Sacher[60] attempted to establish the causality between cytokines and FNHTR. IL-6 levels were measured in vivo before and after transfusion in a group of 42 patients. Acute transfusion reactions occurred in 26 patients. The mean post-transfusion IL-6 level was 3.7-fold higher than in pretransfusion specimens. Patients without acute reactions had insignificant increases in IL-6 levels. Unfortunately, the concentration of IL-6 in the transfused components was not measured, leaving uncertainty as to the origin of the cytokine elevation (i.e., a blood component or the recipient).

In the absence of conclusive clinical trials, one may question whether the level of cytokines found in platelet concentrates is high enough to cause FNHTRs. The amount of TNF-α known to cause fever and chills is approximately 5 to 10 μg/m^2, or 8500 to 17,000 ng of TNF-α for a 70-kg person.[61, 62] In order to achieve such an amount after transfusion of a blood component, the amount of TNF-α present should be approximately 28,000 to 56,000 ng/L in a 300-mL unit, or 170,000 to 340,000 ng/L in a 50-mL unit. However, the measured levels of TNF-α in platelet concentrates were far below this level, with the highest reported concentration being 1890 ng/L and the median concentration in the range of 42 to 571 ng/L.[47–49] The data suggest that passive transfer of

TNF-α cannot be solely responsible for symptoms observed in patients with FNHTR.

The situation is slightly different with the other endogenous pyrogen, IL-1. This cytokine can cause clinical symptoms at concentrations as low as 10 to 100 ng/kg, corresponding to 700 to 7000 ng in a 70-kg recipient.[63–65] The maximum measured levels of accumulated IL-1 in platelet concentrates vary from 143 to 26,000 ng/L, with medians ranging from 14 to 5250 ng/L.[47–49] These median values correspond to 0.7 to 260 ng in a 50-mL unit or 4.2 to 1560 ng in a 300-mL unit. Passive transfer of such quantities of IL-1 might be able to cause fever in a 70-kg person.

Clinical Evaluation of FNHTRs

Studies[26, 27] in chronically transfused patients with thalassemia have documented that leukoreduction is a highly effective means to prevent FNHTRs to RBCs. Current methods of leukoreduction—whether done before storage, just before blood issue, or at the bedside—are capable of reducing the residual donor leukocyte concentration to levels well below those that result in FNHTRs. Moreover, owing to refrigerated blood storage (and in contrast to platelet concentrates), RBCs do not accumulate clinically important levels of cytokines during storage. Indeed, fever reactions to properly leukoreduced RBCs are sufficiently rare that patients who receive leukoreduced RBCs and experience fever should be evaluated for the presence of hemolytic reactions due to RBC blood group incompatibility and for the presence of bacterial contamination of the transfused product. In contrast to RBCs and as described earlier, FNHTRs to platelet concentrates are much more common and are not completely eliminated by leukoreduction. Patients experiencing FNHTRs to platelet concentrates should be evaluated for platelet increments, for evidence of alloimmunization, for drug-induced platelet refractoriness, for bacterial contamination of platelets, and for passive transfer of antibodies to ABO antigens from donor to recipient.

■ Prevention of HLA Alloimmunization

Alloimmunization to HLA donor antigens is a well-recognized complication of blood transfusion. Clinical consequences of HLA alloimmunization include FNHTRs, renal allograft rejection, and platelet refractoriness. There are many nonimmune causes of platelet refractoriness, including fever, use of amphotericin B, drug-related anti-platelet antibodies, hypersplenism, consumptive coagulopathy, and idiopathic thrombocytopenic purpura. Because these conditions contribute to platelet refractoriness, no studies have documented that prevention of alloimmunization by leukoreduction prevents *bleeding complications* due to platelet refractoriness. Nevertheless, prevention of HLA alloimmunization is generally regarded as an important benefit of leukoreduction (see Box 19.3).

After the demonstration in rodents by Claas and colleagues that leukocytes and not platelets are responsible for primary alloimmunization,[66] leukoreduction of blood components was the subject of numerous clinical trials assessing alloimmunization to donor HLA antigens. The reported rate of anti-HLA alloimmunization due to unmodified components in randomized controlled trials varied from 20% to 50% in the control arm, with median incidence of 42%.[67] Meta-analysis of eight controlled, randomized trials demonstrated a 70% reduction in the incidence of HLA alloimmunization in the group of patients who received leukoreduced blood components.[67–75] The same report identified a corresponding reduction in platelet refractoriness. The currently recommended level of leukoreduction to prevent allosensitization is less than 5×10^6 WBCs/unit (3 to 17 WBCs/μL).[76, 77]

Immune recognition of foreign donor cells requires at least three fundamental elements: binding of the antigen to the antigen receptor, binding of costimulatory molecules mediating cell–cell contact, and local elaboration of cytokines and appropriate cytokine receptors. In whole blood, the majority (70%) of class I HLA antigen is found on the surface of platelets, which express 50,000 to 100,000 copies at their surface.[78, 79] The rest of the HLA molecules are distributed among RBCs (3%), granulocytes (2%), lymphocytes (2%), and plasma (23%). Platelet concentrates contain approximately 3.4 mg of HLA molecules, of which 3.2 mg (94%) is associated with platelets, 0.2 mg is in plasma, and 17 μg is present on leukocytes.[78] Therefore, most of the HLA antigens in nonleukoreduced platelet concentrates are found on the platelets themselves. For this reason, it may seem counterintuitive that leukoreduction decreases the risk of alloimmunization.

The recipient of platelet concentrates is exposed to different forms of HLA antigens: soluble class I/II antigens in the plasma, class I/II antigens on cell fragments shed from leukocytes and platelets during processing and storage, class I antigens present on intact platelets, and class I/II antigens expressed on leukocytes. The route by which the antigen presentation occurs influences the likelihood of alloimmunization. Indeed, an important feature of transfusion-induced alloimmunization is the availability of two different sets of antigen-presenting cells (APCs), those of donor origin and those of recipient origin. Stimulation of recipient T or B cells by donor APCs has been called "direct" alloimmunization. In contrast, stimulation by recipient APCs, presenting peptides of donor origin, has been called "indirect" alloimmunization. The data derived from clinical trials of leukoreduction and from basic research suggest that the direct alloimmunization pathway plays a more important role in transfusion-induced alloimmunization.[78]

Direct Alloimmunization Pathway

Direct alloimmunization refers to the process by which recipient immune cells respond directly to donor HLA antigens without the processing of donor antigens by recipient APCs. The mixed lymphocyte reaction is an in vitro example of direct T-cell recognition. Direct sensitization to donor class I antigens results when the recipient is exposed to donor cells bearing class II structures. The route by which donor peptides derived from class I antigens are directly presented has not been precisely delineated. Class II–positive donor cells might carry within the peptide-binding groove oligopeptides representing the cell's own HLA class I antigen. It is known, for example, that a proportion of the endogenous peptides eluted from major histocompatability class (MHC) molecules are from degraded self-MHC molecules.[80, 81] In addition, donor CD4+ T cells were shown in a rodent transfusion model to serve as direct APCs to recipient CD8+ cells.[82]

Kao and Del Rosario[83] provided additional direct experimental evidence for the importance of HLA class II cells in

transfusion-induced alloimmunization to class I MHC antigens.[83] Using a rodent transfusion system, they compared alloantigen response to transfusion of unmodified donor mononuclear cells versus transfusion of mononuclear cells that were first depleted of cells bearing class II MHC antigens. Alloantibodies against class I MHC antigens were generated in 100% of mice infused with unmodified mononuclear cells, whereas only 25% of mice transfused with the modified components became alloimmunized. This study confirmed the validity of direct immunization mediated by donor APCs and also showed variability in response among different strains.

Clinical studies of transfusion-induced HLA alloimmunization suggest that donor class I peptides presented by class II cells are more immunogenic than intact class I molecules found on donor platelets. The failure of platelets to directly provoke immunization presumably reflects the absence of critical costimulatory molecules on platelets. For example, Gouttefangeas and coworkers[84] showed that HLA class I molecules from platelets cannot directly induce allogeneic CD8+ cytotoxic T-cell response in vitro. Moreover, pure platelet suspensions are unable to stimulate cells in a mixed lymphocyte reaction. Because leukoreduction depletes blood of cells bearing the combination of HLA antigens and costimulatory molecules, and because neither RBCs nor platelets display the combination of class I antigen, costimulatory molecule, and relevant cytokine, leukoreduction of RBCs or platelets prevents direct HLA alloimmunization.

Indirect Allorecognition Pathway

Indirect allorecognition refers to the process by which recipient APCs first engulf donor cells and then process donor antigen for redisplay to the recipient immune system. Donor cells, cell fragments, and soluble donor antigens undergo endocytosis by phagocytosis, macropinocytosis, or a clathrin mediated process.[85] The proteins are degraded to small peptides within a specialized lysosomal compartment termed the MHC class II compartment of the recipient APCs. The peptides are then loaded onto class II molecules as follows. The MHC invariant chain (Ii), a chaperone molecule that guides α and β chains of class II molecules from the endoplasmic reticulum, is digested proteolytically. A fragment of Ii, the class II–associated Ii peptide (CLIP), remains associated with $\alpha\beta$ dimers and occupies the peptide-binding groove. In addition, HLA-DM stabilizes the $\alpha\beta$ complex and facilitates binding of the peptides to the peptide-binding groove. The allogeneic peptides are then loaded into the MHC class II groove, replacing CLIP or HLA-DM.[86] Empty class II molecules—those that contain neither peptide, invariant chain, nor HLA-DM—are unstable and are degraded in the low pH compartment of the lysosomes. Because HLA-DM is found at a fivefold lower concentration than HLA class II in the late endosomal compartments, excess self-HLA class II molecules are presumably degraded and their peptide fragments recycled.

Because transfusion typically results in alloimmunization to class I HLA antigens, trafficking of class I molecules in donor APCs is of special interest to transfusion science. Although no evidence currently documents that class I peptides are concentrated in the MHC class II compartment, current technical limitations make it hard to determine the proportion of peptides bound to class II that originated from class II compared with class I molecules.[87] However, Turley and colleagues[88] reported that class I HLA molecules can accompany class II HLA molecules from the endoplasmic reticulum, where the class I molecules may be potentially degraded and their peptides loaded onto class II structures ultimately expressed on the surface of the cell.

Expression of costimulatory molecules by APCs is presumably required for transfusion alloimmunization. Both CD80 and CD86 can bind to CD28 found on T-helper lymphocytes, thereby promoting T-cell activation. Activated helper T cells in turn increase their expression of CD40 ligand (CD40L) and the IL-2 receptor. CD40L interacts with CD40 present on B cells to induce activation of B cells and expression of B7-2, and later B7-1, on the surface. Resting B cells do not express CD80/CD86 on their membrane, but on activation, either by cytokines or by activated T lymphocytes, B cells are able to fully interact with T cells and follicular dendritic cells in germinal centers. In addition, a profile of cytokines secreted by T cells is needed for B-cell activation and antibody synthesis. A Th1 response is associated with increased secretion of IL-2 and IFN-γ, whereas a Th2 response is characterized by secretion of IL-4, -5, -10, and -13. The cytokines generated by T cells allow for B-cell proliferation, maturation, and antibody production.

Investigators have attempted to dissect the pathway of antigen processing by recipient APCs in response to transfusion. Bang and colleagues[89] developed a system in which allogeneic platelets were incubated with the recipient's APCs in the presence of various compounds that potentially affect intracellular peptide processing, such as IFN-γ, aminoguanidine, L-arginine, colchicine, ammonium chloride, chloroquine, brefeldin A, and a cytosolic proteasome inhibitor (MG115). The pulsed APCs (enriched spleen macrophages) were then injected into recipients, and anti-donor IgG production was evaluated. Forty-five percent of recipients developed alloantibodies after two infusions, and all recipients were alloimmunized by the sixth transfusion. Two patterns of response were observed. The first was consistent with the classic endosomal-dependent processing of exogenous antigen and resulted in production of IgG$_1$ antibodies. The second pattern was insensitive to both chloroquine and pH suggesting a nonendosomal pathway and led to an IgG$_{2\alpha}$ alloimmune response.

Clinical Studies of Leukoreduced Blood Components for the Prevention of Alloimmunization

There have been eight prospective, randomized clinical trials of filter-leukoreduced blood components to prevent platelet alloimmunization. The populations studied were patients with chronic thrombocytopenia and, in most of the investigations, acute myelogenous leukemia. As reviewed by Heddle[90] and by Vamvakas,[67] these trials varied greatly in experimental design. For example, they differed in such fundamental issues as exclusion criteria, definition of alloimmunization and platelet refractoriness, methods of leukoreduction, consistency of leukoreduction, and numbers and types of patients enrolled. The majority of studies showed that fewer patients in the study arm receiving leukoreduced components developed lymphocytotoxic antibodies (Table 19.1). However, this difference between groups was less pronounced when the researchers looked at clinically significant platelet refractoriness. Not surprisingly, these studies documented that alloimmunization to platelet-specific antigens was not affected by leukoreduction.

The largest and the most authoritative prospective randomized trial was the TRAP study, which enrolled 268 patients with acute myelogenous leukemia.[75] The results demonstrated conclusively that leukoreduction of blood components reduces the rate of alloimmunization among patients with leukemia. The study also demonstrated that leukoreduced, pooled, whole blood–derived platelets are as effective as apheresis platelets for the prevention of alloimmunization. Although the rate of HLA alloimmunization was higher among patients with a history of prior pregnancy, compared with never-pregnant patients, the alloimmunization rate among previously pregnant patients was lower in the leukoreduced arms than in the control arm. The finding that patients who were previously pregnant might benefit from leukoreduction differed from the results of other studies that showed lack of efficacy of leukoreduction for such patients.[74] Despite the size of the TRAP trial, the measured rate of platelet refractoriness was low: 16% in the control arm and 7% in the study

Table 19.1 Prospective Randomized Controlled Trials in Hematology-Oncology Patients using Leukocyte Reduction (LR) to Prevent Primary Alloimmunization

Author	Year	No. of Patients	% of Patients with Lymphocytotoxic Antibodies		% of Patients with Platelet Antibodies		% of Patients with Platelet Refractoriness	
			Control	LR	Control	LR	Control	LR
Elghouzzi et al	1981	160	28	15	NT	NT	NA	NA
Schiffer et al	1983	56	42	20	NT	NT	19	16
Murphy et al	1986	50	48	16	10	11	23	5
Sniecinski et al	1988	40	50	15	35	15	50	15
Andreu et al	1988	69	31	12	NT	NT	47	21
Oksanen et al	1991	31	26	13	33	31	26	13
Van Marwijk Kooy et al	1991	53	42	7	NT	NT	46	11
Lane et al	1994	46	35	11	NT	NT	NA	NA
Williamson et al	1994	123	38	22	NT	NT	30	26
TRAP Trial	1997	268	45	18	11	6	16	7

Adapted from Klein HG, Dzik WH, Slichter S, et al: Leukocyte-Reduced Blood Components: Current Status. Educational Program, American Society of Hematology, 1998, pp 154–177.

arm (P = .03). Platelet refractoriness was strictly defined as corrected count increments of less than 5000/µL on two sequential transfusions. The study defined the primary outcome as concurrent development of both antibodies and platelet refractoriness. Platelet refractoriness (defined as described) that was present within 2 weeks after the development of antibodies constituted alloimmune platelet refractoriness. By these criteria, 13% of patients in the control arm and 3% of those in the treatment arm had alloimmune platelet refractoriness (P = .004).

The collective results from existing clinical trials support the use of leukoreduced components to prevent primary alloimmunization in patients with acute myelogenous leukemia who are receiving induction chemotherapy. However, there have been few studies of leukoreduction and alloimmunization in other patient groups. Because treatment of leukemia is itself immunosuppressive, the impact of leukoreduction may be different in other patient groups, and the efficacy of leukoreduction for prevention of HLA alloimmunization among nonleukemic patients has not been formally demonstrated. Moreover, even among patients with hematologic malignancies, there are no studies documenting that leukoreduction has a significant impact on bleeding complications secondary to platelet refractoriness.

◼ Cytomegalovirus: Transmission and Reactivation

CMV is a member of the herpes family of DNA viruses and is a significant pathogen for immunocompromised individuals. Approximately 2 decades of clinical and basic research provide evidence that CMV can be transmitted by donor leukocytes and that transmission can be reduced by leukoreduction (see Box 19.3). Clinical trials documenting the effectiveness of leukoreduction as a means to reduce the risk of transmission of CMV have been reviewed elsewhere.[91, 92] Testing of donors for evidence of antibodies to CMV is another widely practiced method for reducing the risk of CMV transmission by blood components. Comparative trials of leukoreduction versus serotesting have not shown a clear benefit of one method over the other.[17] In addition to primary transmission of CMV by blood transfusion, there is broad interest in understanding whether transfusion leads to reactivation of latent host CMV infection in the blood recipient. The scientific basis for prevention of CMV transmission or of reactivation by leukoreduction is discussed in the following sections.

CMV Is Present in Blood Donors as a Latent Infection in Mononuclear Cells

Almost all studies of the epidemiology of CMV infection identify that the virus is common in healthy individuals and that the prevalence of serologic markers for prior infection increases with age. Although carriers of CMV may intermittently shed virus in their saliva, they do not have continuous viremia. Rather, CMV is present in latent form—viral genome is present, but gene expression is limited and infectious virus is not produced. Blood cells, endothelial cells, tissue macrophages, stromal cells, and neural cells are all sites of CMV latency.

Leukoreduction as a method of prevention of transmission of CMV is based on the finding that the virus is tropic for leukocytes and is not found in erythrocytes, platelets, or plasma of healthy blood donors. Multiple lines of evidence document that CMV is tropic for leukocytes and that CMV DNA can be recovered from leukocyte DNA of healthy carriers. The particular subset of leukocytes that harbors CMV has been investigated. Whereas CMV is found in polymorphonuclear leukocytes of patients with *active* infection, viral DNA is found in mononuclear cells of healthy donors.[93, 94] Use of polymerase chain reaction (PCR) techniques to detect CMV DNA has demonstrated that blood monocytes and macrophages (rather than T and B cells) are the principal sites of latent CMV infection. More detailed evidence that monocytes are an important reservoir of latent CMV infection was presented by Bolovan-Fritts and associates,[95] who provided evidence that viral DNA could be recovered from cells expressing the monocyte marker CD14. CMV DNA in these cells migrated on agarose gels as a circular plasmid. Neither linear, complex, nor integrated proviral configurations were identified.

Cells susceptible to viral latency are different from those that are permissive for viral replication and lytic infection. Differentiation of monocytes to macrophages increases the likelihood of successful in vitro infection of the cell by CMV or reactivation of latent CMV. Experimental evidence suggests that less differentiated cells are less permissive to active CMV replication. In vitro studies have demonstrated that undifferentiated cell lines express transcriptional regulators that suppress CMV intermediate-early gene expression.[96] Although the full range of transcriptional regulators has not been resolved, data from Sinclair and Sissons[97] suggest that the so-called YY1 factor binds to the immediate-early gene promotor region and downregulates its expression. Binding of YY1 may act by preventing binding of the general transcription factor TFIIB to the preinitiation complex directly upstream from the immediate-early gene.

Using reverse transcriptase–PCR, Taylor-Wiedeman and colleagues[98] demonstrated that monocytes from latently infected, healthy, seropositive individuals failed to transcribe CMV genes. However, when the cells were cultured in vitro after exposure either to granulocyte-monocyte colony-stimulating factor plus hydrocortisone or to phorbol 12–myristate 13–acetate plus hydrocortisone, they differentiated into macrophages and expressed messenger RNA for the CMV early-intermediate gene. However, late CMV gene transcripts were not produced, and the cells failed to shed complete virus, suggesting an arrest in productive viral transcription at the early gene phase. Recently, Crapnell and Zanjani[99] provided in vitro evidence that CMV can infect megakaryocytes and that latently infected progenitor cells become permissive for CMV replication as they differentiate into megakaryocytes.

Hematopoietic progenitors may also serve as an important reservoir for latent CMV infection. In an interesting study Zhuravskaya and associates[100] deliberately infected highly purified CD34+ progenitor cells and allowed them to undergo differentiation in culture. As in the studies already described, these researchers found that undifferentiated cells failed to express CMV transcripts but that both CMV intermediate-early and late gene products (both mRNA and protein) were detected as cells differentiated into terminal macrophages. Because progenitor cells are self-renewing, their infection with CMV may be one mechanism for the long-term persistence of latent infection with this virus.

Few Mononuclear Cells in Healthy Donors Harbor CMV

Among healthy blood donors, the proportion of mononuclear cells infected with CMV bears directly on the ability of 3- to 4-logarithm leukoreduction to prevent CMV transmission by transfusion. Earlier studies reported that CMV immediate-early gene transcripts were present in 0.03% to 2% of peripheral blood mononuclear cells from healthy seropositive individuals.[94, 101] More recently, Slobedman and Mocarski[102] analyzed the proportion of infected cells by PCR and in situ hybridization and by quantitative competitive PCR. Using normal donors undergoing granulocyte colony-stimulating factor mobilization of hematopoietic progenitors, they found that 0.004% to 0.01% of mononuclear cells contained viral genomes at a copy number of 2 to 13 genomes per infected cell. Among healthy blood donors who are not undergoing growth factor–mediated mobilization, the proportion of infected cells presumably would be lower. These findings generate a plausible explanation for the ability of leukoreduction to reduce the transmission of CMV. If a unit of blood contains approximately 10^7 monocytes and if 1 in 10,000 to 1 in 100,000 monocytes are infected, then the unit contains 10^3 to 10^2 latently infected cells. Therefore, a 3- to 4-log leukoreduction may be expected to render the unit noninfectious. Moreover, it is unlikely that clinical infections in humans can be established by exposure to a single latently infected cell, even though the threshold level required to acquire infection is not known. Quantitative studies of the level of viremia in patients after liver transplantation have documented that levels greater than 10^4 genomes per milliliter are required for infections to become symptomatic.[103] In addition, earlier clinical transfusion trials documented that less efficient leukoreduction processes, such as cell washing, resulted in a significant decrease in transmission of CMV, suggesting that transmission requires far more than one virion.

Seronegative Healthy Subjects Frequently Test Positive for CMV DNA

Although serologic testing has proved of great practical value for reducing the transmission of CMV to immunocompromised recipients, PCR-based testing has documented that a substantial minority of healthy individuals who are considered to be CMV-negative by serologic testing may be positive for CMV DNA (Table 19.2).

CMV-seronegative, PCR-positive blood donors may account for the finding that patients supported with CMV-seronegative units experience a 1% to 4% rate of CMV transmission, as measured by CMV seroconversion, viremia, or viruria.[104] Moreover, the frequent observation that seronegative, healthy donors carry CMV viral DNA has called into question the reliability of serologic screening methods for CMV risk reduction. As a consequence, efforts to prevent transmission of CMV by blood transfusion should concentrate not only on CMV-seropositive donors but also on CMV-seronegative donors.

Infection with More Than One Strain of CMV

Molecular typing methods have demonstrated that some patients are infected with more than one strain of CMV. Using restriction enzyme analysis, Chou[105] compared the patterns of isolates among 36 pairs of recipients of CMV-seropositive renal allografts. Although donor material was not analyzed, two patients were found whose CMV strain was different from that present in the recipient before organ transplantation. One of these two virus strains was simultaneously present after transplantation. Follow-up studies confirmed that solid organ transplants were capable of infecting recipients with a second strain of CMV.[106] Multiple-strain infection has also been documented in community-acquired cases of CMV. Chandler and colleagues[107] reported molecular evidence for multiple-strain infection among four of eight women attending a clinic for sexually transmitted diseases. Spector and associates[108] reported multiple-strain infection in two persons with serologic evidence of infection with the human immunodeficiency virus (HIV) who were diagnosed with acquired immunodeficiency syndrome. However, the interpretation of studies of second-strain infection has been confounded by the fact that strain mutations develop under the selective pressure of antiviral therapy.[109] These mutations lead to a different pattern of restriction digest, which can be misinterpreted as a second independent strain.

Recognition of second-strain infection via organ transplantation or multiple sexual contacts raises the possibility of transfusion-transmitted second-strain infection and the question of whether CMV-seropositive transfusion recipients should receive CMV–reduced-risk blood components. The risk of second-strain infection by transfusion remains only theoretical to date, because no such cases have been reported. Using restriction endonuclease analysis, Winston and coworkers[110] observed no second-strain infections in a study

Table 19.2 Studies Documenting Cytomegalovirus (CMV) Positivity by Assays using Nucleic Acid Testing (NAT) in CMV-Seronegative Blood Donors

Author (Ref. No.)	CMV Seronegative, NAT Negative	CMV Seronegative, NAT Positive	% CMV Seronegative, NAT Positive	Comment
Cassol et al[183]	281	4	1.4	PCR, one primer pair; IE gene
Stanier et al[184]	20	5	20	PCR, one primer pair; IE gene
Bevan et al [185]	312	108	25.6	PCR, three primer pairs
Taylor-Wiedeman et al[94]	6	3	33	Nested PCR; IE gene
Zhang et al[186]	110	86	44	RNA hybridization assay
Larsson et al[187]	29	16	55	PCR on adherent cell fraction
Larsson et al[187]	129	19	13	PCR on peripheral blood mononuclear cells

PCR, polymerase chain reaction.

of 18 allogeneic bone marrow transplant recipients who developed CMV during the course of their treatment.

Reactivation of Latent CMV by Transfusion of Allogeneic Donor Leukocytes

It is not known whether recipient exposure to allogeneic donor leukocytes results in reactivation of latent CMV infection in recipients. Furthermore, it is not known whether the use of leukoreduced blood components would prevent recipient CMV reactivation or prevent clinical disease from reactivation infection. Demonstration of clinical reactivation infection resulting from donor leukocytes would provide a rationale for widespread leukoreduction.

Decades ago, the hypothesis was put forward that allogeneic transfusion would result in an in vivo mixed lymphocyte reaction and that this immunologic stimulus might result in reactivation of latent CMV infection.[111] The hypothesis was addressed in several experimental studies that attempted to induce viral reactivation in vitro. For example, Olding and colleagues[112] documented reactivation of murine CMV in response to an in vitro allogeneic challenge with mouse embryo cells. Reactivation did not occur after exposure to syngeneic embryo cells. In a detailed study using human blood cells, Soderberg-Naucler and associates[113] reported evidence that prolonged in vitro allogeneic stimulation was able to induce CMV reactivation. They incubated equal numbers of peripheral blood mononuclear cells from healthy individuals for 48 hours, removed nonadherent cells, washed the cultures, and then continued incubation for up to 90 days, periodically sampling the cultures for evidence of CMV reactivation. Their culture conditions were established to promote the differentiation of monocytes into macrophages and thereby render the cells more permissive for CMV gene expression and viral assembly. By day 17, they found evidence for CMV immediate-early gene and late gene expression. Between days 17 and 60, they found expression of immediate-early protein in the culture supernatants. Sonicated cultures applied to fibroblast targets were able to induce CMV infection in vitro between days 26 and 60, documenting whole-virus production from the originally latently infected cells. The restriction endonuclease pattern of the isolates from the infected fibroblasts matched that of the original, latently infected cells. The cells that reactivated CMV were found to express markers of macrophages (CD14 and CD64) and dendritic cells (CD1a and CD83). Control cultures of either CMV-negative allogeneic cells or CMV-positive cells that were stimulated only with conconavalin failed to induce viral reactivation in vitro. Although this study documented that reactivation is possible in vitro, the experimental conditions may not be relevant to clinical blood transfusion.

Experimental attempts to induce CMV reactivation in vivo with transfusions have been contradictory. Chueng and Lang[114] studied viral reactivation in a mouse model using C3H and BALB/c allogeneic strains. When they gave intraperitoneal injections of cells from uninfected BALB/c donors to latently infected CH3 recipients, virus was recoverable in the recipient's salivary gland 3 weeks after inoculation. However, virus was also recovered after syngeneic inoculation of CH3 donor cells. Bruggerman[115] studied CMV reactivation in a rat model. He was not able to induce reactivation by transfusion of 10^7 thoracic duct lymphocytes or spleen cells from uninfected LEW rats to immunocompetent, allogeneic, latently infected BN strain recipients. However, CMV infection could be induced by transfusion if the recipients were first exposed to 500 cGy of total-body irradiation.

Clinical studies of CMV reactivation by transfusion have provided evidence that donor leukocytes do not result in CMV reactivation. Initial studies documented that increases in CMV antibody titers occurred more frequently among transfused patients compared with nontransfused patients.[116] Whether this finding resulted from a stimulus posed by transfusion or from the fact that transfusion is a correlate of more intensively treated patients cannot be resolved from the data. A major clinical trial in the United States, the Viral Activation Transfusion Study (VATS), was initiated to investigate whether the use of leukoreduced blood would result in a lower incidence of CMV reactivation and disease in a cohort of HIV-positive transfusion recipients.[117] The study was a randomized, double-blind trial comparing the effects of allogeneic blood with and without leukoreduction on the outcomes of 531 patients infected with HIV-1 and CMV. The investigators found no evidence for viral reactivation as measured by HIV viral load or CMV replication assays in either the group transfused with unmodified allogeneic blood or the group transfused with leukoreduced blood. Moreover, the use of leukoreduced blood had no effect on disease progression or duration of survival. This clinical trial provides the strongest evidence to date that viral reactivation does not result from exposure of the recipient to allogeneic donor leukocytes.

Based on the evidence, CMV reactivation in patients may depend more on factors unrelated to blood transfusion. Increased understanding of the regulation of CMV gene expression should ultimately lead to a full understanding of the mechanism of viral reactivation. Studies of the regulation of the CMV immediate-early gene have identified a strong promoter site consisting of at least four repetitive sequence elements, termed 17-bp, 18-bp, 19-bp, and 21-bp repeats, each of which is present in multiple copies within the CMV promoter region.[118] The 18-bp repeat contains a consensus sequence for binding NF-κB that leads to enhanced transcription of the immediate-early gene.[119] In contrast, the 21-bp region binds to a negative regulatory factor that appears to be specific for undifferentiated cells and represses CMV gene transcription. This latter site may account for the nonpermissiveness to CMV replication of undifferentiated cells. Activation of the immediate-early gene has also been demonstrated for other transcription factors, including cyclic AMP response element binding activation transcription factor (CREB/ATF) and AP-1.[120, 121] The immediate-early gene promoter may also contain elements responsive to cyclic adenosine monophosphate and prostaglandin E_2.[118]

Activation of CMV gene expression by nuclear factors such as NF-κB may account for the clinical observation that CMV reactivation accompanies organ allograft rejection, graft-versus-host disease, and bacterial or viral infection. The immune response to these comorbid events may lead to local production of cytokines such as TNF-α, IL-1, or IL-6, which in turn increase levels of NF-κB and activate the CMV promoter site. Organs rich in immune cells capable of releasing these cytokines may generate high local concentrations of such cytokines in response to inflammatory stimuli. Indeed, Loser and colleagues[119] demonstrated in a mouse model that reactivation of the immediate-early gene in the liver occurred in response to partial hepatectomy (without transfusion) and correlated with increased NF-κB expression. Therefore, local inflammatory signals may prove to be more important than blood transfusion as a signal for CMV reactivation. Currently, the evidence does not support the use of leukoreduced blood components for the prevention of CMV reactivation.

■ Donor Leukocytes and Immunomodulation

Allogeneic blood transfusion is purported to cause, in some individuals, a mild state of immunosuppression. The original suggestion for this effect arose from the observation in 1973 by Opelz and associates[122] that allogeneic transfusions given before renal transplantation resulted in improved allograft survival. Although this finding was confirmed by numerous subsequent reports, including studies conducted in the era of modern antirejection therapy,[123] the exact mechanism has never been conclusively explained. In 1981 Gantt[124] questioned whether transfusions might also downregulate host antitumor immunity, thereby resulting in either an increased rate of tumor relapse or a shorter interval from primary tumor resection to time of relapse. Subsequently, the topic of transfusion-associated immunosuppression was extended to include concern that transfusion might result in an increased frequency of postoperative bacterial infections. A detailed account of the possible immunomodulatory effects of transfusion was published by Vamvakas and Blajchman.[2]

Whether blood transfusions result in a clinically measurable increase in tumor recurrence or postoperative bacterial infection has never been adequately resolved. The issue is difficult to address experimentally in human subjects. A large number of observational studies have documented that patients who receive transfusions are more likely than their untransfused counterparts to develop tumor recurrence or bacterial infection. This observation, however, represents a correlation and does not imply that the transfusions resulted in these adverse effects. Indeed, blood transfusion is generally viewed as an identifier of patients with more severe or advanced disease. Moreover, the finding that transfusion correlates with tumor recurrence or bacterial infection does not imply that leukoreduction would have a beneficial effect on the frequency of these complications. The clinical question of the effect of leukoreduction is best addressed by randomized, prospective, blinded clinical trials in which patients are assigned to receive either leukoreduced or nonleukoreduced blood components. Few such trials have been conducted, and their results speak both for and against an immunosuppressive effect of blood transfusion (Table 19.3). Interested readers will find an authoritative review of this controversy by Vamvakas and Blajchman.[2]

Blood Transfusion and the Immune Response

The human immune system has been divided into the innate immune response and the adaptive immune response. The *innate immune response* represents a first line of defense against foreign intrusion into the host and may account not only for an early response against microbial invasion but also for early tumor surveillance. Components of the innate immune response include plasma proteins such as complement, antibacterial proteins, polymorphonuclear leukocytes, and immune cells such as natural killer (NK) cells. Given the strong clinical suspicion that transfusion has an immunosuppressive effect resulting in decreased tumor surveillance or decreased resistance to postoperative bacterial infection, it is perhaps striking that so little research on the transfusion effect has focused on studies of the innate immune response.

In contrast to the innate immune response, the *adaptive immune response* consists of both humoral and cellular reactions specifically directed against antigen. Response to antigen depends on antigen presentation by mature dendritic cells (and other APCs) and expansion of populations of both B cells and T cells whose receptors are specific for that antigen. Examples of the adaptive immune response include alloimmunization, transplant rejection, T-cell clones cytotoxic for virally infected tissues, and response to vaccination. In contrast to the innate immune response, a large body of literature has sought to uncover a link between transfusion and suppression of the adaptive immune response. Much of this literature addresses the development of tolerance to organ transplantation—an experimental system that serves as a model for the study of adaptive immune recognition.

Common Themes in Studies of Transfusion-Associated Immunosuppression

Four themes regularly appear in experimental studies of the induction of tolerance by pretransplantation blood

Table 19.3   Randomized Controlled Clinical Trials Concerning Transfusion and Risk of Cancer Recurrence or Postoperative Infection

Study	End Point	Sample Size	RBCs Used in Test Group*	Relative Risk (95% Confidence Interval)	Probability Value	Percentage with Complication
Busch	Cancer	423	Buffy coat RBC	0.66–1.59	0.18	25
Houbiers	Cancer	697	Buffy coat RBC	0.69–1.37	0.93	25
Heiss	Cancer	100	Buffy coat RBC	0.77–5.33	0.16	23
Jensen (1993)	Infection	197	Whole blood	1.62–33.12	0.0033	8
Heiss	Infection	120	Buffy coat RBC	1.05–7.24	0.042	20
Busch	Infection	470	Buffy coat RBC	0.59–1.34	0.60	26
Houbiers	Infection	697	Buffy coat RBC	0.64–1.19	0.42	33
Jensen (1996)	Infection	589	Buffy coat RBC	2.16–5.20	0.001	17
Van de Watering	Infection	909	Buffy coat RBC	1.00–1.99	0.05	19
Tartter	Infection	221	Allogeneic RBC	0.89–3.85	0.11	16

*Buffy coat RBCs are packed red blood cells from which the buffy coat has been removed by centrifugation.
Adapted from Vamvakas EC, Blajchman MA (eds): Immunomodulatory Effects of Blood Transfusion. Bethesda, MD: American Association of Blood Banks Press, 1999.

transfusion: recipient conditioning, the histocompatibility relationship between donor and recipient, the presentation of antigen, and the persistence of donor antigen. First, experimental tolerance induction appears to require proper *"conditioning" of the recipient.* Conditioning regimens usually consist of mild immunosuppression with anti–T-cell globulins, chemotherapy, or steroids. One may speculate that these agents weaken the immune response in such a way as to prevent the transfused cells or proteins from resulting in direct alloimmunization and to allow the transfused cells or proteins to persist within the recipient long enough to induce tolerance.

Second, antigen-specific tolerance induction appears to depend on the proper *relationship between the MHC antigens of the donor and those of the recipient.* Transfusions from donors who are highly mismatched at MHC loci appear more likely to provoke alloimmunization than immunosuppression. Immune tolerance may depend on partial histocompatibility matching of donor and recipient. However, the details of the MHC relationship required for the induction of tolerance are poorly defined and appear to vary among species and with the experimental conditions. In human studies, HLA class II antigen matching appears to be particularly relevant. For example, van Twuyver and associates[125] studied 23 untransfused first-time renal allograft recipients, each of whom was deliberately transfused before transplantation with donor fresh blood containing approximately 7×10^8 leukocytes. After transfusion, cytotoxic T-cell precursors directed against donor antigen targets were measured. Ten patients demonstrated a significant decline in the level of anti–donor T cell response at 1 month after transfusion. Nine of them were found to share one HLA haplotype (HLA-B and HLA-DR match) with their donor. In contrast, those patients transfused with mismatched blood maintained strong anti–T cell responsiveness after transfusion. In a similar way, Leivestad and Thorsby[126] studied in vitro cocultures of donor and recipient lymphocytes after deliberate transfusion of fresh blood containing donor leukocytes. They demonstrated suppression of the in vitro mixed lymphocyte response after transfusion if the donor and the recipient shared one HLA haplotype. However, other studies have been unable to demonstrate a conclusive effect of transfusions matched for one haplotype on the recipient immune system.

Third, the *dose and molecular presentation of transfused antigens* may affect whether the recipient response is directed toward alloimmunization or tolerance. Evidence for the induction of tolerance by infusion of large intravenous doses of antigen (high-zone tolerance) has existed for years in experimental immunology. In the case of blood transfusion, it may be that a sufficiently large dose of donor blood is required to induce an immunosuppressive effect. For example, Van de Watering and colleagues[127] randomly assigned more than 900 patients undergoing cardiac surgery to receive transfusion support with either leukoreduced blood or blood that was depleted of buffy coat but not extensively leukoreduced. Among patients receiving fewer than 4 units of blood, there was no difference in 60-day mortality. However, among those receiving more than 4 units, there was a higher observed mortality among patients who received buffy coat–depleted blood, compared with those who received blood that was leukoreduced by filtration. The inability to detect any immunosuppressive effect after the transfusion of smaller

doses of blood may account for some of the discrepant findings in published studies on this topic.

The molecular presentation of donor antigen may also play a critical role in the immune response of the transfusion recipient. Transfusions expose the recipient not only to whole cells displaying cell-surface antigens but also to soluble antigens, including soluble HLA peptides of the donor type. There is evidence supporting a role for both cells and soluble antigens in the induction of experimental tolerance. Hypotheses attributing immune suppression to whole cells form the basis for the conjecture that leukoreduction at the time of transfusion prevents transfusion-associated immunosuppression.

However, large intravenous doses of soluble antigen may be central to recipient immune downregulation. Experimental work from several laboratories has demonstrated that soluble HLA antigens can downregulate in vitro immune responses by several different mechanisms.[128] For example, peptides from the nonpolymorphic 3 region of the class I HLA molecule were able to inhibit the differentiation of cytotoxic T cells in response to an alloantigen stimulus.[129] Of even greater interest, soluble HLA peptides may be directly inhibitory to NK cells. As members of the innate immune system, NK cells are likely to play an important role in tumor surveillance. Infusion of soluble HLA peptides has been introduced into clinical trials of organ transplantation. In one study, patients who received infusions of soluble HLA peptides demonstrated a significant reduction in NK cell cytotoxicity lasting 2 months beyond the end of treatment.[130]

If soluble HLA antigen accounts for the immunosuppressive effect of transfusion, then one hypothesis for the prevention of transfusion-associated immunomodulation is based on prestorage leukoreduction as a method to prevent release of leukocyte antigens into plasma during blood storage. Whether leukocytes actually do release soluble antigens during storage is unresolved. Dzik and colleagues[131] measured soluble HLA antigens in units of RBCs that were stored either with or without prestorage leukoreduction and found no difference between them and no increase in soluble HLA substance during storage. In contrast, Ghio and associates[132] measured increased concentrations of soluble class I HLA antigens and soluble Fas ligand in units of RBCs and platelets during storage. They found that concentrations of soluble antigens and Fas ligand were proportionate to the number of residual donor leukocytes in the blood components.

If leukocytes do in fact release soluble antigens during blood storage, and if the infusion of large doses of these antigens is relevant for immune downregulation as a result of transfusion, then *prestorage* leukoreduction would be the most effective method for preventing transfusion-associated immunosuppression. This approach would be consistent with the experimental findings of Blajchman and coworkers,[150] whose results in a mouse tumor model demonstrated that the immunosuppressive effect of transfusion was ameliorated by prestorage but not by poststorage leukoreduction. In contrast, the large, prospective, randomized clinical trial of Van de Watering and associates[127] found no difference in rate of postoperative infection among recipients of blood that had undergone prestorage leukoreduction compared with blood that was leukoreduced after storage. However, all units in the latter study were first buffy coat–depleted, so those units that were leukoreduced after storage may not have contained sufficient leukocytes during storage to develop high concentrations of soluble HLA antigen.

Fourth, the *persistence of donor antigen* in the recipient is a common finding in experimental models for the induction of tolerance.[133] During the last decade a large body of literature has developed on the topic of microchimerism—specifically, the persistence of low levels of donor cells in the recipient. There appears to be little doubt that microchimerism accompanies tolerance. However, it is uncertain whether the persistence of donor cells contributes to the induction of tolerance or is merely a consequence of tolerance. Microchimerism after clinical solid organ transplantation is unquestionably present and has been verified by numerous assays. Donor cells infiltrate and coexist with recipient cells in lymphoid organs and in skin for years after solid organ transplantation, suggesting that either long-lived lymphocytes or stem cells with self-renewing capacity (or both) survive immune clearance by the recipient. Microchimerism with fetal cells may also exist in women after normal pregnancy and delivery. One provocative study identified the presence of male DNA in the circulation of women who had given birth to male children years before the blood sampling.[134]

Whether microchimerism develops after blood transfusion is controversial. Adams and coworkers[135] used PCR techniques to study the persistence of donor DNA material in recipients after transfusion of routine blood components but were able to identify donor signal for only 5 days after transfusion.[135] However, the study investigated routine donor units that had undergone refrigerated storage. In contrast, Lee and colleagues[136] reported evidence for extended microchimerism after blood transfusion. Using a PCR assay directed against donor-type HLA genes, they detected donor signal in one recipient for up to 1.5 years after transfusion. Of note, the transfusions occurred in the setting of trauma and included infusions of fresh blood, which might have contained more viable donor cells than the blood used in the study by Adams' group. Also of interest, in one of the recipients who demonstrated prolonged persistence of donor material, the recipient and donor shared (by chance) two HLA antigens. Clinically, patients with microchimerism demonstrated neither obvious signs of immune downregulation nor evidence for graft-versus-host disease.

Mechanisms of Transfusion-Associated Immunosuppression

Three major immunologic mechanisms account for the majority of experimental findings in transfusion-induced immunosuppression: clonal deletion, anergy, and immune suppression. Research supporting each of these mechanisms in transfusion-associated immunosuppression is considered in the following sections. Clonal deletion refers to immune suppression resulting from the removal of responding cells. Clones may be deleted either in the thymus gland (so-called central clonal deletion) or in lymph nodes, spleen, gut, or other tissues (peripheral clonal deletion). Anergy refers to immune nonresponsiveness; the term implies that the immune cells are still present but have been rendered unable to respond. Immune suppression implies that the responding cells are present and capable of response but are prevented from doing responding by a suppressive signal, such as a suppressive cytokine.

Clonal Deletion

The thymus gland plays a key role in the development of the immune system and in the recognition of "self." During normal T-cell development, T cells come into contact with specialized APCs within the thymus, which display self-antigens. Those developing T cells that are highly reactive with "self" are deleted. In this way the organism protects itself from autoreactive cells. This physiology has been demonstrated in studies in which foreign antigen was directly placed into thymic tissue, where the antigen is displayed as if it were "self." When antigen is directly placed in the thymus, developing T cells that are directed against the foreign antigen and would normally have survived passage through the thymus are deleted. As a result, the manipulated recipient becomes tolerant to the foreign antigen through a process of thymic clonal deletion.

Induction of tolerance by direct inoculation of donor antigen into the recipient's thymus has been successfully accomplished in a number of experimental systems. For example, Campos and coworkers[137] used a rat liver transplant model among inbred but MHC-disparate rats. Use of pretransplantation antilymphocyte globulin alone resulted in graft survival of 29 days. However, if 5×10^7 donor marrow cells were inoculated into the recipient thymus gland of animals treated with antilymphocyte globulin, then the liver transplant was tolerated indefinitely without any posttransplantation immunosuppression. Among animals given the marrow cells by intravenous infusion (rather than intrathymic inoculation), tolerance induction was far less successful. Nevertheless, the transplant allografts survived 44 days, which was significantly longer than the survival time observed in control animals. Numerous other experimental studies have documented tolerance induction by the direct inoculation of donor cells into the recipient thymus.[124]

Central thymic tolerance has also been induced by the inoculation of MHC peptide into the recipient thymus. These peptides are presumably taken up by recipient APCs and displayed as if they were self-antigens. For example, Chowdhury and colleagues[138] were able to induce prolonged cardiac allograft acceptance in a rat model by intrathymic injection of synthetic class I allopeptides. Whether central tolerance is relevant for blood transfusion is unknown. It is conceivable that donor HLA peptide present in blood becomes localized in the recipient thymus gland. Because the thymus involutes with age, the role of central thymic tolerance may be more relevant for pediatric transfusions than for those given to adults.

T-cell clones may also undergo deletion outside the environment of the thymus gland. Activation-induced apoptosis occurs when T cells respond to antigen via their T-cell receptor but are not sustained by costimulatory molecules or by proper cytokine support. Normally, for any given environmental antigen, only approximately 1 in 10^5 to 1 in 10^6 T cells have a matching T-cell receptor and are able to respond to the antigen. However, in the setting of an allogeneic HLA stimulus, such as occurs with organ transplantation or blood transfusion, approximately 1% to 10% of T cells are able to respond. This remarkable finding is the basis of the strong blastogenic response of the routine mixed lymphocyte culture. It is possible that this large activation signal leads to considerable activation-induced apoptosis of recipient cells and subsequent peripheral clonal deletion.

Development of Cellular Anergy

Multiple lines of experimental evidence demonstrate that immune activation of T cells depends on the cell's receiving not only a primary signal (the antigen signal) but also a secondary signal known as a costimulatory signal. Mature dendritic cells and other APCs deliver costimulatory signals through cell-surface molecules, including CD40, CD80/CD86, LFA-3, and ICAM-1. T cells that interact with dendritic cells have corresponding receptors for each of the costimulatory molecules. Initial studies suggested that when a T cell binds to antigen in the absence of the secondary costimulatory signal, T cells are induced to undergo an anergic response rather than an activation response.[139] Subsequent research has suggested that certain costimulatory molecules send an activation signal, whereas others send an anergy signal. The CD40 and the CD80/CD86 molecules on APCs and their respective ligands on T cells (CD40-L and CD28) represent an important costimulatory system for activation of T cells. In contrast, the CTLA-4 receptor on T cells (also called CD152) appears to be critical to the induction of T-cell anergy. CTLA-4 knockout mice succumb to massive T-cell overgrowth, suggesting that CTLA-4 plays a physiologic role in downregulation of T cells. Therefore, tolerance may be induced either by blocking activation costimulatory molecules or by activating anergy-inducing receptors on T cells. For example, Larsen and associates[140] induced long-term acceptance of skin and cardiac allografts in mice by the combination of transfusion of donor cells and blockade of CD40 and CD28 pathways. More recently, Kirk and colleagues[141] demonstrated that blockade of CD40L on T cells resulted in induction of tolerance to fully mismatched kidney allografts in primates.

One hypothesis concerning the immunomodulatory effect of blood transfusion suggests that during refrigerated blood storage donor leukocytes undergo alterations that interfere with their ability to express costimulatory molecules. When the recipient immune system encounters these altered cells after transfusion, anergy is induced. There is little direct experimental evidence to support this contention, although Minchef and coworkers[142] reported that refrigerated storage resulted in a mixture of both necrosis and apoptosis of donor leukocytes. In a rodent model, they demonstrated that transfusion of necrotic mononuclear cells led to suppression of delayed-type hypersensitivity in the recipients. Other experimental evidence has also suggested that apoptotic cells are directly immunosuppressive.[143]

The infusion of large doses of soluble HLA antigen might also result in T-cell anergy.[128, 144] Soluble HLA peptides would be expected to bind directly to the T-cell antigen receptor without providing a costimulatory signal. Experimental work suggests that soluble HLA molecules are internalized and bind to an intracellular protein that belongs to the heat shock 70 protein family. This binding is accompanied by inhibition of the NF-AT transcription factor, which is required for T-cell activation. As a result, T-cell nonresponsiveness occurs.[145] Other anergic signals may also result from blockade of costimulatory receptors.[146]

Development of Suppressor Cells

The explosive growth in understanding of cytokine signals between immune cells has provided a foundation for the molecular understanding of immune suppression. T cells are now functionally divided into subsets based on the pattern of cytokines that they release. Th1 cells are characterized by strong expression of IFN-γ and IL-2. Th2 cells release IL-4 -5, -6, and -10. Th3 cells release TGF. Each of these subsets derives from a more primitive Th0 cell. Certain clinical immune reactions appear to be characterized by polarization of the immune response toward one of these subsets. One important hypothesis for the immunosuppressive effect of blood transfusion suggests that transfusion may drive the recipient toward a Th2 or Th3 response.

In a series of experiments in mice, Chen and associates[147] showed evidence for tolerance induced by a suppressor T cell found in the spleen. BALB/c mice (H-2d) were donors of cardiac allografts to MHC-disparate CBA/Ca (H-2k) recipients. In the absence of any conditioning, the recipients promptly rejected the cardiac allografts. Transplant tolerance was induced by pretransplantation blood transfusion from the donor after conditioning with nonlytic antilymphocyte globulin. Under these conditions, the animals retained the cardiac allografts for more than 100 days. Splenic lymphocytes taken from these tolerant animals were then transferred to naive CBA/Ca animals, which were then tolerant of BALB/c heart allografts in the absence of any immunosuppression. In fact, tolerance could be transferred successfully through nine passages of splenic lymphocytes into new animals. The suppressor cell was localized to the CD4+ subset of T cells. Studies, such as this one, that demonstrate adoptive transfer of tolerance argue strongly in favor of a suppressor cell mechanism. Similar findings were reported by Yang and colleagues,[148] who suggested than the CD45RC+ subset of CD4+ T cells accounted for the immune suppression.

More direct evidence that allogeneic blood transfusion can induce suppressor T cells in recipients comes from the studies of Blajchman and colleagues,[149, 150] who examined the potential of transfusions to promote tumor growth in animals. In one series of experiments, animals were first transfused with either unmodified allogeneic blood, leukoreduced allogeneic blood, or syngeneic blood (as a control). After the transfusions, the animals were challenged with an injection of tumor cells. After a waiting period, the animals were sacrificed and the number of pulmonary metastases were counted. The investigators found that transfusion with unmodified blood promoted increased numbers of pulmonary metastases, compared with leukoreduced or syngeneic blood. Moreover, spleen cells transferred to naive animals from animals that had received unmodified allogeneic blood transfusions promoted greater numbers of pulmonary metastases than did spleen cells transferred from animals that had not been transfused or had received transfusion of leukoreduced blood. These findings argue for the induction of suppressor spleen cells in the animals who had received unmodified donor blood.

Further evidence for splenic suppressor cells induced by blood transfusion was presented by Kao.[151] He was able to induce humoral immune nonresponsiveness in CBA mice (H-2k) using transfusions of ultraviolet B–irradiated leukocytes from BALB/c (H-2d) donor mice. Ultraviolet B irradiation is known to interfere with the expression of costimulatory molecules (see earlier discussion). When spleen cells from the tolerant animals were transferred to naive CBA recipients, the recipients also became tolerant to BALB/c donor antigens. Presumably, the transferred cells suppressed the ability of CBA recipients to form a humoral immune response.

In humans, direct evidence for the induction of Th2-type suppressor cells by blood transfusion is lacking. However, Kirkley and associates[152] reported in vitro cytokine release in 43 patients transfused with either allogeneic or autologous blood at the time of hip surgery. Mean levels of IL-10 and IL-4 released in vitro were slightly higher among recipients of allogeneic blood, suggesting polarization by allogeneic transfusion toward a Th2 phenotype. However, other studies of transfused patients have not found statistically significant differences in cytokine profiles as a result of transfusion.[153, 154]

Transfusion-Associated Immunosuppression and CMV Infection

Although the VATS study[117] found no evidence for transfusion-induced reactivation of CMV, it is possible that preexisting CMV infection might contribute to a state of mild generalized immunosuppression of the innate immune system, especially of NK cells. The enormous prevalence of CMV in the human population is testimony to the success of viral mechanisms in escaping host immune surveillance. The virus uses two complementary strategies to avoid host immune clearance. First, viral transcripts of the US2, US3, US6, and US11 genes interfere with host cell class I HLA transport and antigen presentation. These gene products interfere with the association of class I heavy chains with β_2 microglobulin, interfere with transport of HLA proteins out of the endoplasmic reticulum, and facilitate the premature destruction of HLA class I proteins before reaching the cell surface. In this way, host cells fail to display viral peptides that would be recognized by the recipient adaptive immune system. However, because NK cells recognize and respond to the presence of a reduction in the surface expression of class I HLA molecules, the virus has evolved a second strategy to avoid NK cell recognition. CMV produces a NK cell decoy protein using the viral UL18 gene. This protein is homologous to the human class I HLA molecule and binds to CD94, the inhibitory receptor of NK cells. Although there is no direct experimental evidence for CMV as the mediator of transfusion-associated immune suppression, it is conceivable that downregulation of NK cell activity mediated by the CMV decoy protein could contribute to the impairment of host innate immunity.

Future Research in Transfusion-Associated Immunosuppression

Despite an enormous experimental effort stretching over decades and the explosion in understanding of the molecular nature of immune stimulation and suppression, we remain uncertain as to whether routine clinical blood transfusions in humans are immunosuppressive and the mechanism by which they might result in immunosuppression. Although much evidence implicates recipient exposure to allogeneic donor leukocytes, other possible mediators include the infusion of large amounts of soluble HLA antigens present in blood. Three organ systems may play an important role in the adaptive immune response to transfusion. The thymus gland is the site for central immune tolerance mediated by deletion of self-reacting clones of T cells. The collective lymphoid organ represented by lymph nodes, lymphatic tissue of the gut, and immune cells of the lungs may represent important sites of cell–cell interaction resulting in T-cell anergy or activation-induced apoptosis. Experimental evidence suggests that the spleen may be critical for suppressor T-cell activity in response to the intravenous administration of antigen. Nevertheless, clinical studies of blood transfusion recipients suggest that transfusion may have immunosuppressive effects related more to functions of the innate immune system. Future work in the area of transfusion-associated immunomodulation is likely to include investigation into elements of the innate immune response—the details of which are just beginning to emerge in research laboratories around the world.

■ Hypotensive Reactions to Bedside Leukoreduction

Leukoreduction of blood components is generally safe with few adverse effects. However, there have been several case reports of severe hypotension, occasionally accompanied by skin flushing and loss of consciousness, developing in patients who received bedside filtered blood components.[155–162] Although the reported incidence of these reactions is relatively low, some reactions have been severe. Four clinical features intersect to result in these reactions: transfusion of plasma-containing blood components; use of a bedside leukoreduction filter; use of a filter whose medium carries a net negative charge; and, most importantly, the concurrent administration of angiotensin-converting enzyme (ACE) inhibitors to the recipient. The sudden elaboration of bradykinin was a prime suspect as the cause of these reactions, because bradykinin had previously been implicated in anaphylactic reactions observed among patients receiving ACE inhibitors and undergoing low-density lipoprotein apheresis or hemodialysis.[163–165]

Kinins and Activation of the Contact Pathway Are Implicated in the Pathogenesis of Hypotensive Reactions

Two related vasodilator peptides—the nonapeptide bradykinin and the decapeptide lysyl-bradykinin (kallidin)—exert strong hypotensive effects in humans. Both peptides are metabolized by kininase I, a carboxypeptidase that removes one amino acid (arginine) from the carboxyl-terminal end. Kininase II, also known as ACE, removes two amino acids (phenylalanine and arginine) from the carboxyl-terminal end, rendering the peptides inactive. Bradykinin and lysyl-bradykinin are formed from two precursor proteins, high-molecular-weight kininogen or HMWK (approximately 110,000 D) and low-molecular-weight kininogen or LMWK (approximately 68,000 D). The physiologic function of both kinins is exerted through their action on two receptors, B1 and B2. These receptors were cloned and identified as serpentine receptors coupled to G proteins. Because bradykinin and lysyl-bradykinin are primarily tissue hormones, their concentration in the circulation is usually low. Reported physiologic levels vary from less than 3 to 55 pg/mL.[166, 167] Both peptides are responsible for contraction of visceral smooth muscles, but they relax vascular smooth muscles through the action of nitric oxide. In addition to the effect on smooth muscle cells, the kinins cause increased capillary permeability, accumulation of leukocytes, and pain after injection under the skin. Bradykinin acting on the B2 receptor triggers nitric oxide formation, which activates guanylate cyclase in smooth muscle cells, leading to increased concentrations of cyclic guanosine monophosphate (cGMP) and smooth muscle relaxation.[168] Previous studies have shown that bradykinin also activates phospholipase A_2, phospholipase C, protein kinases, and prostaglandins, thereby resulting in the accumulation of cGMP and cyclic adenosine monophosphate in cells.[169] Although bradykinin can activate tissue mast cells, leading to release of histamine,[170] histamine release does not account for the full vasodilatory effects of bradykinin. Dachman and colleagues[171] demonstrated a residual vasodilatory effect even in the presence of a histamine$_1$ receptor antagonist (brompheniramine) and a histamine$_2$ receptor antagonist (cimetidine).[171]

In healthy individuals, approximately 95% of injected bradykinin is metabolized during the first passage through the lungs. Pulmonary kininases rapidly degrade bradykinin, thereby preventing its effect on the arterial circulation. Indeed, these pulmonary kininases may normally provide transfusion recipients with protection against bradykinin-induced vasodilation. However, pulmonary breakdown of bradykinin is significantly diminished among patients with genetically low activity of pulmonary kininases and patients receiving ACE-inhibitor medications. In addition, patients undergoing cardiopulmonary bypass are at increased risk for bradykinin-mediated hypotensive reactions, because during the bypass venous blood flow is diverted around the pulmonary circulation. The largest series of severe hypotensive reactions accompanying bedside leukoreduction filtration was reported among patients undergoing cardiopulmonary bypass.[157]

The vasodilatory effect of bradykinin was studied in several experimental settings. Forearm blood flow increased after doses of 10 and 100 ng/min.[172, 173] Icatibant, a B2-kinin receptor antagonist, was used to demonstrate dose-dependent vasodilation in response to bradykinin. With increased dosage of icatibant, blood flow diminished significantly. L-NG-Monomethyl-arginine, a specific inhibitor of nitric oxide synthase, was used to demonstrate that bradykinin-induced vasodilation is mediated in part by nitric oxide.[172]

Bonner and colleagues[174] reported on the hemodynamic effects of bradykinin on the systemic and pulmonary circulation in normotensive and hypertensive subjects. Bradykinin was injected intravenously and intra-arterially at doses ranging from 42.4 to 6413 ng/kg. Bradykinin lowered blood pressure by decreasing systemic vascular resistance. ACE inhibitors potentiated this effect by approximately 20- to 50-fold. Systolic blood pressure declined by more than 20 mm Hg when the arterial bradykinin concentration reached at least 100 pg/mL. The study demonstrated that the physiologic effect of bradykinin is very rapid, with a hypotensive effect demonstrable within seconds after administration.

The Contact System Is Activated During Passage of Blood through Leukoreduction Filters

Because bradykinin elaboration would occur if the contact system were activated, investigators have examined whether leukofiltration could induce contact activation of blood. Studies have measured either an increase in bradykinin or its stable metabolite 1,5-bradykinin or a decrease in the substrates HMWK or LMWK.

Although direct measurement of bradykinin is more appealing, bradykinin is technically difficult to assay owing to ex vivo activation of the contact system. Shiba and coworkers[175]

measured bradykinin during leukofiltration of platelet concentrates, using a negatively charged filter and a positively charged filter. After filtration through the negatively charged filter, decreased levels of prekallikrein and increased levels of bradykinin were observed. The bradykinin level was inversely related to the activity of ACE in the platelet concentrates.

The same group studied the effects of storage time, plasma dilution, and filtration on contact-system activation in packed RBCs preserved in mannitol–adenine phosphate solution.[176] The authors noted an increase in the bradykinin level, up to 500 pg/mL on the 10th day of storage. The level decreased to 200 pg/mL during the subsequent 5 days and remained at this low level until the end of the storage time. A significantly decreased level of ACE activity was noted in the packed RBCs stored in solutions containing mannitol. Filtration using two different negatively charged filters generated bradykinin levels up to 6000 pg/mL. The authors concluded that mannitol may act as an ACE inhibitor, slowing down catabolism of bradykinin and leading to its accumulation in stored RBCs.

Hild and colleagues[177] studied generation of bradykinin during leukofiltration of platelets using three different filters—negatively charged, positively charged, and neutral. Only the negatively charged filter contributed significantly to bradykinin production. The levels of bradykinin detected in the eluate varied from less than 200 pg/mL to as much as 10,000 pg/mL in samples collected after processing of 50 and 100 mL of platelet concentrates. The final concentration in units ranged from 200 to 2500 pg/mL. Interestingly, bradykinin present after filtration was rapidly metabolized; after 60 minutes of storage, the bradykinin level was below the limit of detection. However, when an ACE inhibitor was added to the storage bag, bradykinin levels remained elevated for as long as 90 minutes.[177] Significant differences in bradykinin production were observed among the donors, so that some components generated measurable levels of bradykinin but others did not. The highest bradykinin levels (>20,000 pg/mL) were observed after leukofiltration of apheresis platelets.

Scott and associates[178] investigated bradykinin generation by negatively charged filters by measuring substrates of the contact system during leukoreduction of apheresis platelets. The number of WBCs before leukoreduction varied from 0.5 to 1000 cells/µL. Two different leukocyte filters were used. Measurements of the cleavage products of HMWK and LMWK were used as markers of contact-phase activation and the potential for bradykinin production. Although no significant changes were detected in kininogen cleavage products, the assay could not exclude conversion of small amounts (<5%) of kininogen to kinin. The authors concluded that clinically significant activation of the contact system did not occur as a result of leukofiltration. However, they did observe a temporary decrease in kininogen levels with one of the studied filters. The interpretation of this study is difficult because, on a molar basis, kininogen is a very abundant molecule. Therefore, conversion of a minor fraction of kininogen could result in very significant levels of bradykinin.

Why is it that not all patients react uniformly when given bedside transfusions while receiving ACE inhibitors? Cyr and colleagues[179] studied the influence of ACE-inhibitor medication on the in vitro generation of bradykinin and its active metabolite des-Arg^9-bradykinin. The in vitro half-life of bradykinin and of des-Arg^9-bradykinin was measured in the presence of an ACE inhibitor in serum from four patients who had experienced hypotensive reactions during blood transfusions of leukoreduced products. Although the half-life of bradykinin did not differ between the patients and controls, the degradation of des-Arg^9-bradykinin was significantly slower in the patient samples (1549 versus 661 seconds). The authors proposed the hypothesis that an anomalous metabolism of des-Arg^9-bradykinin might contribute to selection of patients who experience clinical reactions to bedside leukodepletion.

Based on the published studies, bradykinin produced during bedside filtration of platelets seems to be responsible for reactions during bedside leukofiltration in patients taking ACE-inhibitor medications. Reactions to RBC components may be less likely, because cold storage of RBCs inhibits contact activation enzymes and because RBCs contain less plasma and kininogens. Concern regarding hypotensive reactions among patients receiving blood components filtered at the bedside prompted the FDA to issue a letter to physicians in May 1999. The FDA recommended use of blood products leukoreduced at the time of collection or during laboratory storage whenever available.

REFERENCES

1. Dzik S, Aubuchon J, Jeffries L, et al: Leukocyte reduction of blood components: public policy and new technology. Transfus Med Rev 2000;14:34–52.
2. Vamvakas EC, Blajchman MA (eds): Immunomodulatory Effects of Blood Transfusion. Bethesda, MD: American Association of Blood Banks Press, 1999.
3. Miller JP, Aubuchon JP: Leukocyte-reduced and cytomegalovirus-reduced risk blood components. In Mintz PD (ed): Practice Guidelines for Transfusion Therapy. Bethesda, MD: American Association of Blood Banks Press, 1998, pp 163–189.
4. Sowemimo-Coker SO, Kim A, Tribble E, et al: White cell subsets in apheresis and filtered platelet concentrates. Transfusion 1998;38:650–657.
5. Triulzi DJ, Meyer EM, Donnenberg AD: WBC subset analysis of WBC-reduced platelet components. Transfusion 2000;40:771–780.
6. Ruback JD, Bray RA, Hillyer CD: Longitudinal monitoring of WBC subsets in packed RBC units after filtration: Implications for transfusion transmission of infections. Transfusion 2000;40:500–506.
7. Dzik S: Leukodepletion blood filters: Filter design and mechanisms of leukocyte removal. Transfus Med Rev 1993;7:65–77.
8. Yuanguo Z, Qijun S, Aihua L, et al: Efficiency of leukocyte removal by filters made of superfine glass fiber membranes. Vox Sang 1999;76:22–26.
9. www.fda.gov/cber/gdlns/preleuk.htm
10. Steneker I: Leukocyte depletion from fresh red cell concentrates by fiber filtration: Filtration mechanisms. Amsterdam: VU University Press, 1992, pp 1–149.
11. Ledent E, Berlin G: Factors influencing white cell removal from red cell concentrates by filtration. Transfusion 1996;36:714–718.
12. Nishimura T, Kuroda T, Mizoguchi Y, et al: Advanced methods for leukocyte removal by blood filtration. In Brozovic B (ed): The Role of Leukocyte Depletion in Blood Transfusion Practice: Proceedings of the International Workshop. Oxford: Blackwell Scientific, 1989, pp 35–40.
13. Beaujean F, Segier JM, le Forestier C, Duedari N: Leucocyte depletion of red cell concentrates by filtration: Influence of blood product temperature [letter]. Vox Sang 1992;62:242.
14. Sirchia G, Rebulla P, Sabbioneda L, et al: Optimal conditions for white cell reduction in red cells by filtration at the patient's bedside. Transfusion 1996;36:322–327.
15. van der Meer PF, Pietersz RN, Nelis JT, et al: Six filters for the removal of white cells from red cell concentrates, evaluated at 4 degrees C and/or at room temperature. Transfusion 1999;39:265–270.
16. Smith JD, Leitman SF: Filtration of RBC units: Effect of storage time and temperature on filter performance. Transfusion 2000;40:521–526.
17. Bowden RA, Slichter SJ, Sayers M, et al: A comparison of filtered leukocyte-reduced and cytomegalovirus (CMV) seronegative blood products for the prevention of transfusion-associated CMV infection after marrow transplant. Blood 1995;86:3599–3603.
18. Williamson LM, Wimperis JZ, Williamson P, et al: Bedside filtration of blood products in the prevention of HLA alloimmunization: A prospective randomized trial. Blood 1994;83:3028–3035.
19. Mijovic V, Kruse A: Filtration of blood from donors with HbAS: An unexpected problem. In Brozovic B (ed): The Role of Leukocyte Depletion in Blood Transfusion Practice. Oxford: Blackwell Scientific, 1989, pp 48–50.
20. Gotlin JB, Adams CL, Stefan MM, et al: Variable leukoreduction on units from donors with sickle cell trait: a time-temperature donor reproducibility study [abstract]. Transfusion 2000;40(Suppl 1):55s.
21. Burgstaler EA: Current instrumentation for apheresis. In McLeod BC, Price TH, Drew MI (eds): Apheresis: Principles and Practice. Bethesda, MD: American Association of Blood Banks Press, 1997, pp 85–112.
22. Kao KJ, Mickel M, Braine HG, et al: White cell reduction in platelet concentrates and packed red cells by filtration: A multicenter clinical trial. Transfusion 1995;35:13–19.
23. Popovsky MA: Quality of blood components filtered before storage and at the bedside: implications for transfusion practice. Transfusion 1996;36:470–474.
24. Mintz PD: Febrile reactions to platelet transfusions. Am J Clin Pathol 1991;95:609–612.
25. Dzieczkowski JS, Barrett BB, Nester D, et al: Characterization of reactions after exclusive transfusion of white cell-reduced cellular blood components. Transfusion 1995;35:20–25.
26. Sirchia G, Rebulla P, Parravicine A, et al: Leukocyte depletion of red cell units at the bedside by transfusion through a new filter. Transfusion 1987;27:402–405.
27. Sirchia G, Wenz B, Rebulla P, et al: Removal of white cells from red cells by transfusion through a new filter. Transfusion 1990;30:30–33.
28. Wenz B: Microaggregate blood filtration and the febrile transfusion reaction: A comparative study. Transfusion 1983;23:95–98.
29. Heddle NM, Kelton JG: Febrile nonhemolytic transfusion reactions in transfusion reactions. In Popovsky MA (ed). Transfusion Reactions. Bethesda, MD: American Association of Blood Banks Press, 1996, pp 45–80.
30. Vengelen-Tyler V (ed): Technical Manual, 13th ed. Bethesda, MD: American Association of Blood Banks Press, 1999, p 577.
31. Luheshi GN: Cytokines and fever: Mechanisms and sites of action. Ann N Y Acad Sci 1998;856:83–89.
32. Cao C, Matsumura K, Yamagata K, Watanabe Y: Cyclooxygenase-2 is induced in brain blood vessels during fever evoked by peripheral or central administration of tumor necrosis factor. Brain Res Mol Brain Res 1998;56:45–56.
33. Ganong WF: Central regulation of visceral function. In Review of Medical Physiology, 19th ed. Stamford, CT: Appleton & Lange, 1999, p 242.
34. Engel A, Kern WV, Murdter G, Kern P: Kinetics and correlation with body temperature of circulating interleukin-6, interleukin-8, tumor necrosis factor alpha and interleukin-1 beta in patients with fever and neutropenia. Infection 1994;22:160–164.
35. Menitove JE, McElligott MD, Aster RH: Febrile transfusion reaction: What component should be given next? Vox Sang 1982;42:318–321.
36. Chambers LA, Donovan LM, Pacini DG, Kruskall MS: Febrile reactions after platelet transfusion: The effect of single versus multiple donors. Transfusion 1990;30:219–221.
37. Heddle NM, Klama LN, Griffith L, et al: A prospective study to identify the risk factors associated with acute reactions to platelet and red cell transfusions. Transfusion 1993;33:794–797.
38. DeRie M, van der Plas-van Daken CM, Engelfriet CP, von dem Borne AEG: The serology of febrile transfusion reactions. Vox Sang 1985;49:126–134.
39. Decary F, Ferner P, Giavedoni L, et al: An investigation of nonhemolytic transfusion reactions. Vox Sang 1984;46:277–285.
40. Perkins HA, Payne R, Ferguson J, Wood M: Nonhemolytic febrile transfusion reactions: Quantitative effects of blood components with emphasis on isoantigenic incompatibility of leukocytes. Vox Sang 1966;11:578–600.
41. Brubaker DB: Clinical significance of white cell antibodies in febrile nonhemolytic transfusion reactions. Transfusion 1990;30:733–737.

42. Thulstrup H: The influence of leukocyte and thrombocyte incompatibility on non-hemolytic transfusion reactions. I: A retrospective study. Vox Sang 1971;21:233–250, 434–442.

43. Arend WP, Joslin FG, Massoni J: Effects of immune complexes on production by human monocytes of interleukin 1 or an interleukin 1 inhibitor. J Immunol 1985;134:3868–3875.

44. Heddle NM, Klama L, Singer J, et al: The role of the plasma from platelet concentrates in transfusion reactions. N Engl J Med 1994;331:625–628.

45. Abbas AK, Lichtman AN, Pober JS: Cytokines in Cellular and Molecular Immunology, 3rd ed. Philadelphia: WB Saunders, 1997, pp 249–277.

46. Muylle L, Joos M, Wouters E, et al: Increased tumour necrosis factor α (TNFα), interleukin 1, and interleukin 6 (IL-6) levels in the plasma of stored platelet concentrates: Relationship between TNFα and IL-6 levels and febrile transfusion reactions. Transfusion 1993;33:195–199.

47. Stack G, Snyder EL: Cytokine generation in stored platelet concentrates. Transfusion 1994;34:20–25.

48. Muylle L: Ex Vivo Cytokine Production in Blood Components: Relevant and Irrelevant. In Smit-Sibinga CTh (ed): Proceedings of the 21st International Symposium on Blood Transfusion, Groningen, 1996. Dordrecht, the Netherlands, Kluwer Academic Press, 1996, pp 63–70.

49. Aye MT, Palmer DS, Giulivi A, et al: Effect of filtration of platelet concentrates on the accumulation of cytokines and platelet release factors during storage. Transfusion 1995;35:117–124.

50. Palmer DS, Aye MT, Dumont L, et al: Prevention of cytokine accumulation in platelets obtained with the Cobe Spectra apheresis system. Vox Sang 1998;75:115–123.

51. Fujihara M, Ikebuchi K, Wakamoto S, et al: Effects of filtration and gamma irradiation on the accumulation of RANTES and transforming growth factor-beta1 in apheresis platelet concentrates during storage. Transfusion 1999;39:495–505.

52. Muller-Steinhardt M, Kirchner H, Kluter H: Impact of storage at 22°C and citrate anticoagulation on the cytokine secretion of mononuclear leukocytes. Vox Sang 1998;75:12–17.

53. Heddle NM, Tan M, Klama L, Shroeder J: Factors affecting cytokine production in platelet concentrates [abstract]. Transfusion 1994;34(Suppl):67S.

54. Grey D, Erber WN, Saunders KM, Lown JAG: Monocyte activation in platelet concentrates. Vox Sang 1998;75:110–114.

55. Molloy RG, Mannick JA, Rodrick ML: Cytokines, sepsis, and immunomodulation. Br J Surg 1993;82:3170–3176.

56. Hawrylowicz CM, Howells GL, Feldman M: Platelet-derived interleukin 1 induces human endothelial adhesion molecule expression and cytokine production. J Exp Med 1991;174:785–790.

57. Aye MT, Palmer DS, Giulivi A, Hashemi S: Effect of filtration of platelet concentrates on the accumulation of cytokines and platelet release factors during storage. Transfusion 1995;35:117–124.

58. El-Kattan I, Anderson J, Yun JK, et al: Mononuclear cell (MC) adhesion to platelet storage bag plastic polymers correlates with cytokine levels. Transfusion 1995;35(Suppl):44S.

59. Dzik WH: Is the febrile response to transfusion due to donor or recipient cytokine? Transfusion 1992;32:594.

60. Sacher RA: High circulating interleukin 6 levels associated with acute transfusion reaction: Cause or effect? [letter]. Transfusion 1993;33:962.

61. Schiller JH, Storer BE, Witt PL, et al: Biological and clinical effects of intravenous tumor necrosis factor-alpha administered three times weekly. Cancer Res 1991;51:1651–1658.

62. Agosti JM, Coombs RW, Collier AC, et al: A randomized, double-blind, phase I/II trial of tumor necrosis factor and interferon-gamma for treatment of AIDS-related complex (Protocol 025 from the AIDS Clinical Trials Group). AIDS Res Hum Retroviruses 1992;8:581–587.

63. Tewari A, Buhles WC, Starnes HF: Preliminary report: Effects of interleukin-1 on platelet counts. Lancet 1990;336:712–714.

64. Crown J, Jakubowski A, Kemeny N, et al: A phase I trial of recombinant human interleukin-1 beta alone and in combination with myelosuppressive doses of 5-fluorouracil in patients with gastrointestinal cancer. Blood 1991;78:1420–1427.

65. Dinarello CA: Interleukin-1 and interleukin-1 antagonism. Blood 1991;77:1627–1652.

66. Claas FHJ, Smeenk RJT, Schmidt R, et al: Alloimmunization against the MHC antigens after platelet transfusions is due to contaminating leukocytes in the platelet suspension. Exp Hematol 1981;9:84–89.

67. Vamvakas EC: Meta-analysis of randomized controlled trials of the efficacy of white cell reduction in preventing HLA-alloimmunization and refractoriness to random-donor platelet transfusions. Transfus Med Rev 1998;12:258–270.

68. Schiffer CA, Dutcher JP, Aisner J, et al: A randomized trial of leukocyte-depleted platelet transfusion to modify alloimmunization in patients with leukemia. Blood 1983:62;815–820.

69. Sniecinski I, O'Donnell MR, Nowicki B: Prevention of refractoriness and HLA-alloimmunization using filtered blood products. Blood 1988;71;1402–1407.

70. Andreu G, Dewailly J, Leberre C, et al: Prevention of HLA immunization with leukocyte-poor packed red cells and platelet concentrates obtained by filtration. Blood 1988;72;964–969.

71. Van Marwijk Kooy M, Van Prooijen HC, Moes M, et al: Use of leukocyte-depleted platelet concentrates for the prevention of refractoriness and primary HLA alloimmunization: A prospective, randomized trial. Blood 1991;77;201–205.

72. Oksanen K, Kekomaki R, Runtu T, et al: Prevention of alloimmunization in patients with acute leukemia by the use of white cell reduced blood components: A randomized trial. Transfusion 1991;31;588–594.

73. Willamson LM, Wimperis JZ, Williamson P, et al: Bedside filtration of blood products in the prevention of HLA alloimmunization: A prospective randomized study. Blood 1994;83;3028–3035.

74. Sintnicolaas K, Van Marwijk Kooy M, Van Prooijen HC, et al: Leukocyte depletion of random single-donor platelet transfusions does not prevent secondary human leukocyte antigen-alloimmunization and refractoriness: A randomized prospective study. Blood 1995;85;824–828.

75. The Trial to Reduce Alloimmunization to Platelets Study Group: Leukocyte reduction and ultraviolet B irradiation of platelets to prevent alloimmunization and refractoriness to platelet transfusions. N Engl J Med 1997:337;1861–1869.

76. Fisher M, Chapman JR, Ting A, Morris PJ: Alloimmunization to HLA antigens following transfusion with leukocyte-poor and purified platelet suspensions. Vox Sang 1985;49:331.

77. Petranyi GG, Padanyi A, Horuzsko A, et al: Mixed lymphocyte culture: Evidence that pretransplant transfusion with platelets induces FcR and blocking antibody production similar to that induced by leukocyte transfusion. Transplantation 1988;45:823.

78. Kao KJ, Luz de Rosario M: Platelet alloimmunization. In Anderson K, Ness P (eds): Scientific Basis of Transfusion Medicine: Implications for Clinical Practice. Philadelphia: WB Saunders, 2000, pp 409–419.

79. Kao KJ, Cook DJ, Scornik JC: Quantitative analysis of platelet surface HLA by W6/32 anti-HLA monoclonal antibody. Blood 1986;68:627–632.

80. Rudensky AY, Preston-Hurlburt P, Hong SC, et al: Truncation variants of peptides isolated from MHC class II molecules suggest sequence motifs. Nature 1991;353:622–627.

81. Chicz RM, Urban RG, Gorga JC, et al: Specificity and promiscuity among naturally processed peptides bound to HLA-DR alleles. J Exp Med 1993;178:27–47.

82. Fast L: Recipient elimination of allogeneic lymphoid cells: Donor CD4+ cells are effective alloantigen-presenting cells. Blood 2000;96:1144–1149.

83. Kao KJ, Del Rosario MLU: Role of class II major histocompatibility complex (MHC)-antigen-positive donor leukocytes in transfusion-induced alloimmunization to donor class I MHC antigens. Blood 1998;92;690–694.

84. Gouttefangeas C, Diehl M, Keilholz W, et al: Thrombocyte HLA molecules retain nonrenewable endogenous peptides of megakaryocyte lineage and do not stimulate direct allocytotoxicity in vitro. Blood 2000 May 15;95:3168–3175.

85. Mellman R, Turley SJ, Steinman RM: Antigen processing for amateurs and professionals. Trends Cell Biol 1998;8:233–237.

86. Vogt AB, Kropshofer H: HLA-DM: An endosomal and lysosomal chaperone for the immune system. Trends Biochem Sci 1999;24:150–154.

87. Gould DS, Auchincloss H: Direct and indirect recognition: The role of MHC antigens in graft rejection. Immunol Today 1999;20:77–82.

88. Turley SJ, Inaba K, Garrett WS, et al: Transport of peptide-MHC class II complexes in developing dendritic cells. Science 2000;288:522–527.

89. Bang KWA, Speck ER, Blanchette VS, et al: Unique processing pathway within recipient antigen-presenting cells determines IgG immunity against donor platelet MHC antigens. Blood 2000;95:1735–1742.

90. Heddle NM: The efficacy of leukodepletion to improve platelet transfusion response: A critical appraisal of clinical studies. Transfus Med Rev 1994;8:15.

91. Hillyer CD, Emmens RK, Zago-Novaretti M, et al: Methods for the reduction of transfusion-transmitted cytomegalovirus infection: Filtration versus the use of seronegative donor units. Transfusion 1994;34:929–934.

92. Smith DM, Shoos-Lipton K: Leukocyte-reduction for the prevention of transfusion-transmitted cytomegalovirus. American Association of Blood Banks Bulletin 97-2. Bethesda, MD: American Association of Blood Banks Press, 1997.

93. Taylor-Wiedeman J, Hayhurst GP, Sissons JGP, Sinclair JH: Polymorphonuclear cells are not sites of persistence of human cytomegalovirus in healthy individuals. J Gen Virol 1993;74:265–268.

94. Taylor-Wiedeman J, Sissons JGP, Borysiewicz LK, Sinclair JH: Monocytes are a major site of persistence of human cytomegalovirus in peripheral blood mononuclear cells. J Gen Virol 1991;72:2059–2064.

95. Bolovan-Fritts CA, Mocarski ES, Wiedeman JA: Peripheral blood CD14+ cells from healthy subjects carry a circular conformation of latent cytomegalovirus genome. Blood 1999;93:394–398.

96. Sinclair JH, Baillie J, Bryant LA, et al: Repression of human cytomegalovirus major immediate early gene expression in a monocytic cell line. J Gen Virol 1992;73:433–435.

97. Sinclair JH, Sissons P: Latent and persistent infections of monocytes and macrophages. Intervirology 1996;39:293–301.

98. Taylor-Wiedeman J, Sissons P, Sinclair J: Induction of endogenous human cytomegalovirus gene expression after differentiation of monocytes from healthy carriers. J Virol 1994;68:1597–1604.

99. Crapnell K, Zanjani ED, Chaudhuri A, et al: In vitro infection of megakaryocytes and their precursors by human cytomegalovirus. Blood 2000;95:487–493.

100. Zhuravskaya T, Maciejewski JP, Netski DM, et al: Spread of human cytomegalovirus (HCMV) after infection of human hematopoietic progenitor cells: Model of HCMV latency. Blood 1997;90:2482–2491.

101. Stanier P, Taylor DL, Kitchen AD, et al: Persistence of cytomegalovirus in mononuclear cells in peripheral blood from blood donors. Br Med J 1989;299:897–898.

102. Slobedman B, Mocarski ES: Quantitative analysis of latent human cytomegalovirus. J Virol 1999;73:4806–4812.

103. Cope AV, Sabin C, Burroughs A, et al: Interrelationships among quality of human cytomegalovirus (HCMV) DNA in blood, donor-recipient serostatus, and administration of methylprednisolone as risk factors for HCMV disease following liver transplantation. J Infect Dis 1997;176:1484–1490.

104. Miller WJ, McCullough J, Balfour HH, et al: Prevention of cytomegalovirus-infection following bone marrow transplantation: A randomized trial of blood product screening. Bone Marrow Transplant 1991;7:227–234.

105. Chou S: Acquisition of donor strain of cytomegalovirus by renal transplant recipients. N Engl J Med 1986;314:1418–1423.

106. Chou S: Reactivation and recombination of multiple cytomegalovirus strains from individual organ donors. J Infect Dis 1989;160:11–15.

107. Chandler SH, Handsfield HH, McDougall JK: Isolation of multiple strains of cytomegalovirus from women attending a clinic for sexually transmitted diseases. J Infect Dis 1987;155:655–660.

108. Spector SA, Kirata KK, Newman TR: Identification of multiple cytomegalovirus strains in homosexual men with acquired immunodeficiency syndrome. J Infect Dis 1984;150:953–956.

109. Baldanti F, Simoncini L, Sarasini A, et al: Ganciclovir resistance as a result of oral ganciclovir in a heart transplant recipient with multiple human cytomegalovirus strains in blood. Transplantation 1998;66:324–329.

110. Winston DJ, Huang ES, Miller MJ, et al: Molecular epidemiology of cytomegalovirus infections associated with bone marrow transplantation. Ann Intern Med 1985;102:16–20.

111. Lang DJ: Cytomegalovirus infection in organ transplantation and post-transfusion: A hypothesis. Arch Ges Virusforsch 1972;37:365–370.

112. Olding LB, Jensen FC, Oldstone MB: Pathogenesis of cytomegalovirus infection. I: Activation of virus from bone marrow derived lymphocytes by in vitro allogeneic reaction. J Exp Med 1975;141:561–572.

113. Soderberg-Naucler C, Fish KN, Nelson JA: Reactivation of latent human cytomegalovirus by allogeneic stimulation of blood cells from healthy donors. Cell 1997;91:119–126.

114. Cheung KS, Lang DJ: Transmission and activation of cytomegalovirus with blood transfusion: A mouse model. J Infect Dis 1977;135:841–845.

115. Bruggerman CA: Reactivation of latent CMV in the rat. Transplant Proc 1991;23(Suppl 3):22–24.

116. Adler SP, Baggett J, McVoy M: Transfusion-associated cytomegalovirus infections in seropositive cardiac surgery patients. Lancet 1985;1:743–746.

117. Collier AC, Kalish LA, Busch MP, et al: Leukocyte-reduced red blood cell transfusions in patients with anemia and human immunodeficiency virus infection: the Viral Activation Transfusion Study: a randomized controlled trial. JAMA 2001;285:1592–1601.

118. Sweet C: The pathogenicity of cytomegalovirus. FEMS Microbiol Rev 1999;23:457–482.

119. Loser P, Jennings GS, Strauss M, Sandig V: Reactivation of the previously silenced cytomegalovirus major immediate-early promoter in the mouse liver: Involvement of NFκB. J Virol 1998;72:180–190.

120. Rodems SM, Clark CL, Spector DH: Separate DNA elements containing ATF/CREB and IE86 binding sites differentially regulate the human cytomegalovirus UL112-113 promoter at early and late times in the infection. J Virol 1998;72:2697–2707.

121. Chau NH, Vanson CD, Kerry JA: Transcriptional regulation of the human cytomegalovirus US11 early gene. J Virol 1999;73:863–870.

122. Opelz G, Sengar DPS, Mickey MR, et al: Effect of blood transfusions on subsequent kidney transplants. Transplant Proc 1973;5:253–259.

123. Opelz G, Vanrenterghem Y, Kirste G, et al: Prospective evaluation of pretransplant blood transfusions in cadaver kidney recipients. Transplantation 1997;63:964–967.

124. Gantt CL: Red blood cells for cancer patients. Lancet 1981;ii:363.

125. Van Twuyver E, Mooijaart RJD, ten Berge IJM, et al: Pretransplantation blood transfusion revisited. N Engl J Med 1991;325:1210–1213.

126. Leivestad T, Thorsby E: Effects of HLA-haploidentical blood transfusion on donor specific immune responsiveness. Transplantation 1984;37:175–181.

127. Van de Watering LMG, Hermans J, Houbiers JGA, et al: Beneficial effects of leukocyte depletion of transfused blood on postoperative complications in patients undergoing cardiac surgery: A randomized clinical trial. Circulation 1998;97:562–568.

128. Murphy B, Krensky AM: HLA-derived peptides as novel immunomodulatory therapeutics. J Am Soc Nephrol 1999;10:1346–1355.

129. Clayberger C, Lyu SC, DeKruyff R, et al: Peptides corresponding to the CD8 and CD4 binding domain of HLA molecules block T lymphocyte immune responses in vitro. J Immunol 1994;153:946–951.

130. Giral M, Cuturi MC, Nguyen JM, et al: Decreased cytotoxic activity of natural killer cells in kidney allograft recipients treated with human HLA-derived peptide. Transplantation 1997;63:1004–1011.

131. Dzik WH, Szuflad P, Eaves S: HLA antigens on leukocyte fragments and plasma proteins: Prestorage leukoreduction by filtration. Vox Sang 1994;66:104–111.

132. Ghio M, Contini P, Mazzei C, et al: Soluble HLA class I, HLA class II, and Fas ligand in blood components: A possible key to explain the immunomodulatory effects of allogeneic blood transfusions. Blood 1999;93:1770–1777.

133. Starzl TE, Zinkernagel RM: Antigen localization and migration in immunity and tolerance. N Engl J Med 1998;339:1905–1913.

134. Bianchi DW, Zickwolf GK, Weil GJ, et al: Male fetal progenitor cells persist in maternal blood for as long as 27 years postpartum. Proc Natl Acad Sci U S A 1996;93:705–708.

135. Adams PT, Davenport RD, Reardon DA, Roth MS: Detection of circulating donor white blood cells in patients receiving multiple blood transfusion. Blood 1992;80:551–555.

136. Lee TH, Paglieroni T, Ohto H, et al: Survival of donor leukocyte subpopulations in immunocompetent transfusion recipients: Frequent long-term microchimerism in severe trauma patients. Blood 1999;93:3127–3139.

137. Campos L, Alfrey EJ, Posselt AM, et al: Prolonged survival of rat orthotopic liver allografts after intrathymic inoculation of donor-strain cells. Transplantation 193;55:86–70.

138. Chowdhury NC, Murphy B, Sayegh MH, et al: Acquired systemic tolerance to rat cardiac allografts induced by intrathymic inoculation of synthetic polymorphic MHC class I allopeptides. Transplantation 1996;62:1878–1882.

139. Harding FA, McArthur JG, Gross JA, et al: CD28-mediated signalling co-stimulates murine T cells and prevents induction of anergy in T-cell clones. Nature 1992;356:607–609.

140. Larsen CP, Elwood ET, Alexander DZ, et al: Long-term acceptance of skin and cardiac allografts after blocking CD40 and CD28 pathways. Nature 1996;381:434–438.

141. Kirk AD, Burkly LC, Batty DS, et al: Treatment with humanized monoclonal antibody against CD154 prevents acute renal allograft rejection in nonhuman primates. Nat Med 1999;5:686–693.

142. Minchef MS, Getsov SI, Meryman HT: Mechanisms of alloimmunization and immunosuppression by blood transfusion in an inbred rodent model. Transplantation 1995;60:815–821.

143. Voll RE, Herrmann M, Roth EA, et al: Immunosuppressive effects of apoptotic cells. Nature 1997;390:350–351.

144. Magee CC, Sayegh MH: Peptide-mediated immunosuppression. Curr Opin Immunol 1997;9:669–675.

145. Nossner E, Goldberg JE, Naftzger C, et al: HLA-derived peptides which inhibit T cell function to members of the heat-shock protein 70 family. J Exp Med 1996;183:339–348.

146. Gudmundsdottir H, Turka LA: T cell costimulatory blockade: New therapies for transplant rejection. J Am Soc Nephrol 1999;10:1356–1365.

147. Chen ZK, Cobbold SP, Waldmann H, Metcalfe S: Amplification of natural regulatory immune mechanisms for transplantation tolerance. Transplantation 1996;62:1200–1206.

148. Yang CP, McDonaugh M, Bell EB: CD45RC + CD4 T cell subsets are maintained in an unresponsive state by the persistence of transfusion-derived alloantigen. Transplantation 1995;60:192–199.

149. Blajchman MA, Bardossy L, Carmen R, et al: Allogeneic blood transfusion induced enhancement of tumor growth: Two animal models showing amelioration of leukodepletion and passive transfer using spleen cells. Blood 1993;81:1880–1882.

150. Bordin JO, Bardossy L, Blajchman MA: Growth enhancement of established tumors by allogeneic blood transfusion in experimental animals and its amelioration by leukodepletion: The importance of timing of the leukodepletion. Blood 1994;84:344–348.

151. Kao KJ: Induction of humor immune tolerance to major histocompatibility complex antigens by transfusions of UV-B irradiated leukocytes. Blood 1996;88:4375–4382.

152. Kirkley SA, Cowles J, Pellegrini VD, et al: Cytokine secretion after allogeneic or autologous blood transfusion [letter]. Lancet 1995;345:527.

153. Quintilliani L, Iudicone P, DeGirolamo M, et al: Immunoresponsiveness of cancer patients: Effect of blood transfusion and immune reactivity of tumor infiltrating lymphocytes. Cancer Detect Prev 1995;19:518–526.

154. Tietze M, Kluter H, Troch M, Kirchner H: Immune responsiveness in orthopedic surgery patients after transfusion of autologous or allogeneic blood. Transfusion 1995;35:378–383.

155. Sano H, Koga Y, Hamasaki K, et al: Anaphylaxis associated with white-cell reduction filter [letter]. Lancet 1996;347:1053.

156. Fried MR, Eastlund T, Christie R, et al: Hypotensive reactions to white cell-reduced plasma in a patient undergoing angiotensin-converting enzyme inhibitor therapy. Transfusion 1996;36:900.

157. Mair B, Leparc GF: Hypotensive reactions associated with platelet transfusions and angiotensin-converting enzyme inhibitor therapy. Vox Sang 1998;74:27–30.

158. Yenicesu I, Tezcan I, Tuncer AM: Hypotensive reactions during platelet transfusions [letter]. Transfusion 1998;38:410.

159. Sweeney JD, Dupuis M, Mega AJ: Hypotensive reactions to red cells filtered at the bedside, but not to those filtered before storage, in patients taking ACE inhibitors [letter]. Transfusion 1998;38:410.

160. Abe H, Ikebuchi K, Shimbo M, Sekiguchi S: Hypotensive reactions with a white cell reduction filter: Activation of kallikrein-kinin cascade in a patient [letter]. Transfusion 1998;38:411.

161. Belloni M, Alghisi A, Bettini C, et al: Hypotensive reactions associated with white cell reduced apheresis platelet concentrates in patients not receiving ACE inhibitors [letter]. Transfusion 1998;38:412.

162. Myers T, Uhl L, Kruskall MS: Association between angiotensin-converting enzyme (ACE) inhibitors and hypotensive transfusion reactions [abstract]. Transfusion 1996;36:60S.

163. Verresen L, Waer M, Venrenterghem Y, Michielsen P: Angiotensin-converting enzyme inhibitors and anaphylactoid reactions to high flux membrane dialysis. Lancet 1990;336:1360–1362.

164. Olbricht CJ, Schaumann D, Fisher D: Anaphylactoid reactions, LDL apheresis with dextran sulphate and ACE inhibitors. Lancet 1992;340:908–909.

165. Davidson DC, Pearl I, Turner S, Sangster M: Prevention with icatibant of anaphylactoid reactions to ACE inhibitor during LDL apheresis. Lancet 1994;343:1575.

166. Nielsen F, Damkjar Nielsen M, et al: Bradykinin in blood and plasma: Facts and fallacies. Acta Med Scand Suppl 1983;677:54–59.

167. Scicli AG, Mindroiu T, Scicli G, Carretero OA: Blood kinins, their concentration in normal subjects and in patients with congenital deficiency in plasma prekallikrein and kininogen. J Lab Clin Med 1982;100:81–93.

168. Berridge MJ: Inositol trisphosphate and diacylglycerol: Two interacting second messengers. Ann Rev Biochem 1987;56:159–193.

169. Sung CP, Arleth AJ, Shikano K, Berkowitz BA: Characterization and function of bradykinin receptors in vascular endothelial cells. J Pharmacol Exp Ther 1988;247:8–13.

170. Mousli M, Bueb JL, Bronner C, et al: G protein activation: A receptor-independent mode of action for cationic amphiphilic neuropeptides and venom peptides. Trends in Pharmacol Sci 1990;11:358–362.

171. Dachman WD, Ford GA, Blaschke TF, Hoffman BB: Mechanism of bradykinin-induced venodilation in humans. J Cardiovasc Pharmacol 1993;21:241–248.

172. O'Kane KP, Webb DJ, Collier JG, Vallance PJ: Local L-NG-monomethyl-arginine attenuates the vasodilator action of bradykinin in the human forearm. Br J Clin Pharmacol 1994;38:311–315.

173. Cockroft JR, Chowienczyk PJ, Brett SE, et al: Inhibition of bradykinin-induced vasodilation in human forearm vasculature by icatibant. Br J Clin Pharmacol 1994;38:317–321.

174. Bonner G, Preis S, Schunk U, et al: Hemodynamic effects of bradykinin on systemic and pulmonary circulation in healthy and hypertensive humans. J Cardiovasc Pharmacol 1990;15(Suppl 6):S46–56.

175. Shiba M, Tadokoro K, Sawanobori M, et al: Activation of the contact system by filtration of platelet concentrates with negatively charged white cell-removal filter and measurement of venous blood bradykinin level in patients who received filtered platelets. Transfusion 1997;37:457–462.

176. Shiba M, Tadokoro K, Nakajima K, Juji T: Bradykinin generation in RC-MAP during storage at 4 degrees C and leukocyte removal filtration. Thromb Res 1997;87:511–520.

177. Hild M, Soderstrom T: Kinetics of bradykinin levels during and after leukocyte filtration of platelet concentrates. Vox Sang 1998;75:18–25.

178. Scott CF, Brandwein H, Whitbread J, Colman RW: Lack of clinically significant contact system activation during platelet concentrate filtration by leukocyte removal filters. Blood 1998;92:616–622.

179. Cyr M, Hume HA, Champagne M, et al: Anomaly of the des-Arg9-bradykinin metabolism associated with severe hypotensive reactions during blood transfusions: A preliminary study. Transfusion 1999;39:1084–1088.

180. Klein HG, Dzik WH, Slichter SJ, et al: Leukocyte-Reduced Blood Components: Current Status. Educational Program, American Society of Hematology, 1998, pp 154–177.

181. Elghouzzi MH, Vedreen JB, Jullien AM, et al: Etude technique immunologique et clinique des performances de filtration du sang a la l'aide de l'apparell Erypur. Rev Fr Transfus Immunohematol 1981;24:579–595.

182. Lane TA, Myllyla G: Leukocyte-depleted blood products. Curr Stud Hematol Blood Transfus 1994;60:1–145.

183. Cassol SA, Poon MC, Pal R, et al: Primer-mediated enzymatic amplification of cytomegalovirus (CMV) DNA: Application to the early diagnosis of CMV infection in marrow transplant recipients. J Clin Invest 1989;83:1109–1115.

184. Stanier P, Kitchen AD, Taylor DL, et al: Detection of human cytomegalovirus in peripheral mononuclear cells and urine samples using PCR. Mol Cell Probes. 1992 Feb;6(1):51–58

185. Bevan IS, Daw RA, Day PJ, et al: Polymerase chain reaction for detection of human cytomegalovirus infection in a blood donor population. Br J Haematol 1991;78:94–99.

186. Zhang LJ, Hanff P, Rutherford C, et al: Detection of human cytomegalovirus DNA, RNA, and antibody in normal donor blood. J Infect Dis 1995;171:1002–1006.

187. Larsson S, Soderberg-Naucler C, Wang FZ, Moller E: Cytomegalovirus DNA can be detected in peripheral blood mononuclear cells from all seropositive and most seronegative healthy blood donors over time. Transfusion 1998;38:271–278.

Chapter 20

Virus "Safe" Products/Pathogen Reduction

Laurence Corash

Despite the increased safety of blood achieved through continued improvements in donor screening and testing, concern remains about the safety of blood components. Transfusion of blood components has been implicated in transmission of viral, bacterial, and protozoan diseases.[1] While it is commonly recognized that hepatitis B virus (HBV), hepatitis C virus (HCV), cytomegalovirus (CMV), and the retroviruses, such as human immunodeficiency virus (HIV) and the human lymphotrophic viruses (HTLV), can be transmitted through cellular components, other pathogens are emerging as potentially significant transfusion-associated infectious agents.[2] For example, transmission of protozoan infections due to trypanosomes[3–5] and babesia have been documented.[6] Although protozoan agents have typically been thought of as unimportant pathogens in transfusion-associated infection, recent experience with babesia suggests seroprevalence rates among blood donors as high as 4%.[7] Bacterial contamination of platelet and red blood cell (RBC) concentrates continues to be reported[8–10] and may be an underreported transfusion complication.[11] More importantly, new infectious agents may periodically enter the donor population before they can be definitively identified and tested for to maintain consistent safety of the blood supply.[12] The paradigm for this possibility is the HIV pandemic that erupted in 1979. During the past decade a number of methods to inactivate infectious pathogens in blood components have been investigated as a strategy to improve the safety of blood component therapy. Two methods for the inactivation of pathogens during the preparation of fresh frozen plasma (FFP) are in clinical practice. Methods for the inactivation of pathogens in platelet and RBC concentrates have now reached the clinical trial phase in the United States and Europe.

Currently, prevention of transfusion-associated viral disease depends on predonation evaluation of potential donors followed by serologic testing for infectious pathogens, including HIV-1, HIV-2, HTLV-I, HBV, and HCV. CMV screening is usually performed after blood collection, when CMV seronegative products are required. In addition to these agents, blood is tested for the syphilis pathogen (*Treponema pallidum*). Testing is not routinely done for parvovirus B19, hepatitis A virus (HAV), hepatitis G virus (HGV), hepatitis E virus (HEV), bacteria, or protozoa. Although continued improvements in testing have greatly reduced the transmission of viral disease by blood components, viruses may still contaminate the blood supply because diagnostic tests may be insensitive during the "window period," before serologic conversion of an infected donor. Even direct tests for a virus, such as the hepatitis B surface antigen test, have a sensitivity limitation, below which contaminated components escape detection. Current estimates of the frequency of viral transmission from blood components are 1 in 100,000 donors for HCV, 1 in 63,000 for HBV, and 1 in 680,000 for HIV.[13] The aggregate risk of receiving a blood component contaminated with one of the viruses for which sensitive tests are in place has been estimated to be 1 in 34,000 blood donors.[14] A recent U.S. government report estimated that the average transfusion episode results in exposure to five blood donors.[15] Therefore, per transfusion episode, the risk of receiving a component contaminated with virus may be as high as 1 in 6800. Clearly, the impending implementation of nucleic acid testing for HIV and HCV may have a further impact on these risk assessments. However, failure to detect an infectious blood donor has already been reported for nucleic acid testing.[16]

Bacterial contamination of platelet concentrates is a persistent problem owing to storage at room temperature (20° to 24°C) for up to 5 days before use. Bacterial contamination may come directly from the donor or from an external source. A small number of contaminating bacteria can replicate to more than 10^7 organisms per milliliter after 5 days of storage. A wide variety of bacteria have been cultured from patients with transfusion-transmitted septicemia.[9, 17, 18] Although the number of reported cases of serious transfusion-transmitted sepsis is small, there are no routine laboratory tests to detect bacterial contamination of platelet units. Estimates of the frequency of bacterial contamination range up to 0.4% per unit of platelet concentrate.[19] A 1991 survey by Morrow and coworkers[18] identified bacterial contamination culminating in a septic response from 6 of 10,219 transfusions of pooled random donor platelets, a frequency of approximately 1 in 1700. A prospective study of 3584 platelet transfusions in 161 bone marrow transplantation patients demonstrated the risk of symptomatic bacteremia to be 1 per 16 patients, 1 per 350 transfusions, and 1 per 2100 platelet units.[20] These frequencies are significant considering that more than 8 million units of platelet concentrates are transfused annually in the United States alone.[21]

Although better methods of donor selection and testing have yielded substantial improvements in blood safety, the risk of infectious disease transmission persists. The logistics and costs of continued expansion of testing processes (e.g., nucleic acid testing) have been questioned.[13] Despite these efforts, testing remains a reactive strategy to ensure blood component safety, because new pathogens may enter the donor population before adequate tests can be implemented. A complementary approach to improving the safety of blood component transfusion is inactivation of infectious pathogens in blood components. Treatment of plasma fractions with the solvent detergent (SD) process has demonstrated the benefits of this approach.[22] A robust inactivation technology that is compatible with current blood component processing procedures offers the potential for improving transfusion safety. To be highly effective, a successful technology must inactivate pathogens in extracellular, intracellular, and nuclear compartments (Fig. 20.1). In the last case, inactivation also must be effective against pathogen nucleic acid sequences integrated into donor leukocytes. Furthermore, a technology capable of inactivating residual leukocytes may confer additional benefits, by inhibition of critical leukocyte functions including cytokine synthesis, lymphocyte proliferation, and antigen presentation. Donor leukocytes may be associated with a variety of adverse immune events, ranging in severity from febrile transfusion reactions to alloimmunization and graft-versus-host disease.[23, 24] Although a number of measures have been implemented to reduce the likelihood of these adverse immune reactions, a robust nucleic acid–targeted pathogen inactivation process offers the potential to inactivate leukocytes as well as infectious pathogens. Over the past decade, a number of laboratories have reported investigations of methods to inactivate pathogens in platelet and RBC concentrates, as well as in plasma used for preparation of FFP.

■ Potential Systems for Inactivation of Pathogens in Platelet Concentrates

Considerable effort has been devoted to developing methods for pathogen inactivation in platelet concentrates (Tables 20.1 and 20.2). The potential processes can be divided into two basic groups: nucleic acid–targeted and photodynamic methods. The nucleic acid–targeted methodology has been focused on the use of psoralens. The photodynamic methods generally do not provide sufficient pathogen inactivation and are associated with unacceptable levels of platelet injury.[25] The psoralen methods have been more extensively investigated, and more progress has been made with psoralens than with other systems.

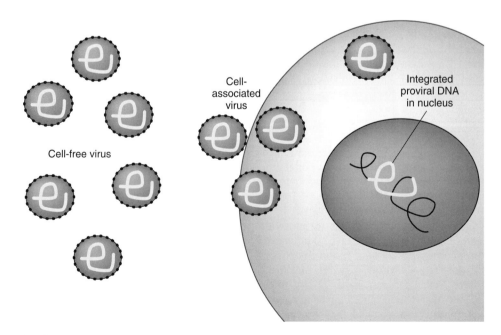

Figure 20.1 Infectious pathogens such as viruses may be present in the plasma as cell-free virus, associated with cell membranes, in the cell cytoplasm, or in the nucleus. Some viruses, such as retroviruses, may integrate nucleic acid sequences into host genomic nucleic acid.

Table 20.1 Psoralen Methods Used to Inactivate Infectious Pathogens and Leukocytes in Platelet Concentrates

Photoreactive Agent	Target	Ref. No.
8-MOP	fd, R17, FeLV, *E. coli* S. aureus	26
8-MOP	MCMV,FeRTV	70
8-MOP	HIV	71
8-MOP	DHBV	72
8-MOP	12 pathogenic bacteria	73
AMT	VSV	30
AMT	HIV	31,74
AMT	VSV, Sindbis	75
PSR-Br	Bacteriophage	76,77
S-59	Pathogenic bacteria	34
S-59	Leukocytes	35
S-59	HIV, DHBV, BVDV CMV, bacteria	34

fd, bacteriophage; R17, bacteriophage; MCMV, murine cytomegalovirus; FeRTV, feline rhinotracheitis virus; HIV, human immunodeficiency virus; HSV, herpes simplex virus; CMV, cytomegalovirus; VSV, vesicular stomatitis virus; FeLV, feline leukemia virus; Sindbis, Sindbis virus; 8-MOP, 8-methoxysoralen; AMT, aminomethyltrimethylpsoralen; PSR-Br, brominated psoralens.

Table 20.2 Photodynamic Methods Used to Inactivate Infectious Pathogens in Platelet Concentrates

Photoreactive Agent	Target	Ref. No.
UVB	Poliovirus	78
Merocyanine 540	VSV	79
Merocyanine 540	HSV, MS2, F6	30
Methylene blue	Unspecified	80
Phthalocyanines	VSV	81

VSV, vesicular stomatitis virus; MS2, bacteriophage; F6, bacteriophage; HSV, herpes simplex virus; HIV, human immunodeficiency virus; UVB, ultraviolet B light (280–320 nm).

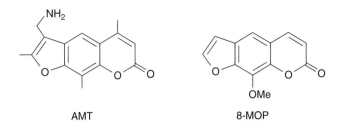

Figure 20.2 Psoralen structures. The structures of aminomethyltrimethyl psoralen (AMT) and 8-methoxypsoralen (8-MOP).

Psoralen-mediated processes generally are based on the formation of nucleic acid–specific adducts, whereas the photodynamic processes tend to use the production of active oxygen species as the primary effector mechanism for pathogen inactivation. Psoralens are low-molecular-weight, planar furocoumarins (Fig. 20.2). In the absence of ultraviolet light (UVA), psoralens reversibly intercalate into helical regions of DNA and RNA, under equilibrium kinetics. On illumination with UVA, psoralens react with pyrimidine bases to form covalent monoadducts and cross-links with nucleic acids (Fig. 20.3). Bacteria, viruses, and nucleated cells with genomes that have been modified by psoralens are unable to replicate.

Early investigations with psoralen-mediated pathogen inactivation were conducted with 8-methoxypsoralen (8-MOP),[26] based on its prior use in humans to treat psoriasis and cutaneous T-cell lymphoma.[27, 28] The initial studies by Lin and coworkers[26, 29] established the principle of psoralen-mediated pathogen inactivation, but 8-MOP photochemical treatment was not a sufficiently rapid process for treatment of platelet concentrates in clinical use.

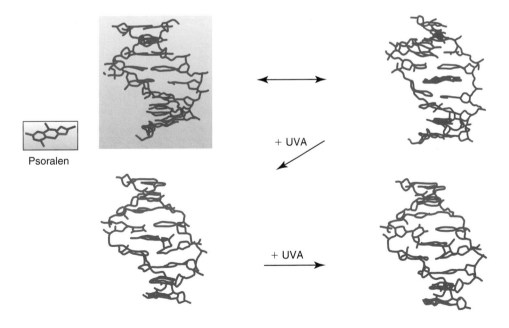

Figure 20.3 The mechanism of psoralen binding to nucleic acid. In the dark, psoralens intercalate into helical regions of nucleic acid, either DNA or RNA *(upper images)*. This phase is a reversible equilibrium process without covalent addition to nucleic acid. During illumination with long-wavelength ultraviolet light (UVA), monoadducts and diadducts between psoralen and pyrimidine form *(lower images)*. Both types of adducts inhibit the function of polymerases and block nucleic acid replication.

Two laboratories have investigated the use of amino-methyltrimethyl psoralen (AMT), a synthetic psoralen with enhanced nucleic acid binding efficiency.[30, 31] Although AMT has increased nucleic acid binding affinity compared to 8-MOP, it exhibits mutagenicity in the absence of light and therefore has an unfavorable toxicology profile.

Several classes of new psoralens have been synthesized that offer potential advantages over AMT and 8-MOP. The halogenated psoralens do not appear to be sufficiently effective for viral inactivation, and in preliminary studies they demonstrated adverse effects on platelet viability.[32, 33] A new class of amino psoralens has been synthesized and shown to be highly effective for inactivation of pathogenic viruses, bacteria, and leukocytes in platelet concentrates, with preservation of in vitro platelet function properties (Table 20.3).[34, 35] Lin and coworkers[34] reported that human platelet concentrates (300 mL) contaminated with high titers of HCV ($10^{4.5}$) and HBV ($10^{5.5}$), when treated with the aminopsoralen S-59, did not transmit hepatitis after transfusion into naive chimpanzees. Other studies demonstrated that these novel psoralens inactivate high levels of T cells, inhibit leukocyte cytokine synthesis during platelet storage, and inhibit nucleic acid amplification.[35] More importantly, treatment of T cells with the S-59 process prevented transfusion-associated graft-versus-host disease in both immune-competent and immunocompromised murine bone marrow transplantation models.[35]

One of these novel amino psoralens, S-59, has entered human clinical trials.[36] The prototype S-59 system is a closed system with a series of plastic containers that are carried through a sequence of processing steps (Fig. 20.4). A pooled buffy-coat or single-donor platelet concentrate, suspended in approximately 35% plasma and 65% platelet additive solution, is connected to a container of S-59. The platelet concentrate is passed through the S-59 container into a PL 2410 Plastic container (Baxter Healthcare Corporation, Round Lake, IL). The platelet concentrate containing S-59 (150 µM) is illuminated with long-wavelength UVA for 3 minutes (3 J/cm^2 treatment), with reciprocal shaking at 20° to 24°C in a microprocessor-controlled light source. After illumination, the platelets are transferred to an S-59 reduction device (SRD) in order to passively reduce the residual S-59 and free S-59 photoproducts to low levels (<0.5 µM). The SRD consists of resin beads integrated into the PL 2410 Plastic container. After SRD exposure, the platelets are transferred to a final PL 2410

Table 20.3 Summary of S-59 Pathogen Inactivation in Platelet Concentrates

Pathogen	Strain	Inactivation Achieved
HIV-1	IIIB, cell-free	>$10^{6.2}$ pfu/mL
	IIIB, cell-associated	>$10^{6.1}$ pfu/mL
	Integrated provirus*	No p24 expression using 0.1 µM S-59 + 1 J/cm^2
	Clinical isolate Z84, cell-free†	>$10^{3.4}$ TCID$_{50}$/mL
HIV-2	Clinical isolate CBL20, cell-free†	>$10^{2.5}$ TCID$_{50}$/mL
HBV	MS-2‡	>$10^{5.5}$ CID$_{50}$/mL
	DHBV as a model	>$10^{6.2}$ ID$_{50}$/mL
HCV	Hutchinson‡	>$10^{4.5}$ CID$_{50}$/mL
	BVDV as a model	>$10^{6.0}$ pfu/mL
HCMV	AD169, cell-associated	>$10^{5.9}$ pfu/mL
	AD169, cell-associated*	Below limit of detection using 1.5 µM S59 + 1.4 J/cm^2
	MCMV as a model, Smith strain, cell-associated*	>$10^{3.3}$–$10^{5.1}$ ID$_{50}$/mL
Bacteria	*Staphylococcus epidermidis*	>$10^{6.6}$ cfu per unit
	Listeria monocytogenes	>$10^{6.3}$ cfu per unit
	Corynebacterium minutissimum	>$10^{6.3}$ cfu/mL
	Streptococcus pyogenes	>$10^{6.8}$ cfu per unit
	Staphylococcus aureus	$10^{6.6}$ cfu per unit
	Escherichia coli	>$10^{6.4}$ cfu per unit
	Yersinia enterocoliticus	>$10^{5.9}$ cfu/mL
	Serratia marcescens	>$10^{6.7}$ cfu per unit
	Salmonella choleraesuis	>$10^{6.2}$ cfu/mL
	Enterobacter cloacae	$10^{5.9}$ cfu/mL
	Klebsiella pneumoniae	>$10^{5.6}$ cfu per unit
	Pseudomonas aeruginosa	$10^{4.5}$ cfu/mL
	Bacillus cereus	>$10^{3.6}$, ≤$10^{3.9}$ cfu per unit

HIV, human immunodeficiency virus; HBV, hepatitis B virus; HCV, hepatitis C virus; HCMV, human cytomegalovirus; DHBV, duck hepatitis B virus; BVDV, bovine viral diarrhea virus; MCMV, murine cytomegalovirus; pfu/mL, plaque-forming units per mL; ID$_{50}$/mL, infectious dose per mL measured from an endpoint dilution that causes infection in 50% of inoculated animals; cfu/mL, colony-forming units per mL; TCID$_{50}$/mL, tissue culture infectious dose per mL measured from an endpoint dilution that causes infection in 50% of inoculated samples; CID$_{50}$/mL, chimpanzee infectious dose per mL measured from an endpoint dilution that causes infection in 50% of inoculated chimpanzees.
*Three studies are indicated: the HIV-1 provirus inactivation was performed in cell culture medium, and the other two studies were performed with platelet sample size less than 300 mL.
†Highest titers possible.
‡The infectivity of the MS-2 strain of HBV and the Hutchinson strain of HCV was measured in susceptible chimpanzees.

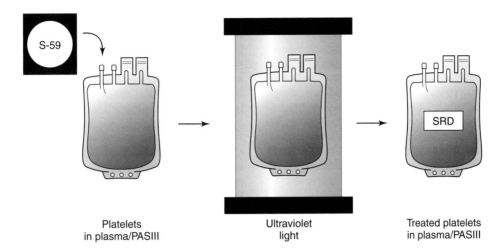

Figure 20.4 The prototype psoralen S-59 process for treatment of platelet concentrates. In a series of connected containers, S-59 is added to the platelet concentrate suspended in approximately 300 mL of 35% plasma and 65% of a platelet additive solution (PAS III). The platelet concentrate is illuminated with 3 J/cm^2 ultraviolet light treatment for approximately 3 minutes. After illumination, the platelet concentrate is transferred to another plastic container containing the S-59 reduction device (SRD). Platelets are incubated with shaking in the SRD for 6 hours to lower the levels of residual S-59 and free S-59 photoproducts. This is followed by transfer to a final plastic container for up to 5 days of storage at 20° to 24°C. The final transfused dose of residual S-59 ranges from 25 to 50 μg per 300 mL of platelet concentrate.

Plastic container for storage. The treated platelet concentrates can be stored for up to 5 days with standard platelet storage conditions and reciprocal shaking at 20° to 24°C.

Phase I and II studies with S-59-treated, 5-day-old platelets transfused to healthy subjects have shown adequate viability.[36] The average post-transfusion recovery of 5-day-old S-59-treated platelets was 42.5%, with an average lifespan of 4.8 days. Interestingly, the rate of radiolabel elution from S-59 platelets was greater than that from control platelets (3.3% versus 2.1%). In these studies, S-59-treated platelets were well tolerated during and after transfusion of full therapeutic doses (300 mL, 3.0×10^{11} platelets) into healthy subjects. This study also provided information regarding the peak plasma S-59 concentrations after transfusion and the kinetics of S-59 clearance, including the area under the curve and terminal half-life. The median peak S-59 plasma level was less than 1 ng/mL and rapidly fell to concentrations below the limits of quantitative measurement.

An additional clinical trial was conducted to evaluate the hemostatic, therapeutic efficacy of S-59-treated platelet concentrates and to expand the safety experience in a spectrum of patients requiring platelet transfusion support.[37] In this randomized, double-blinded, crossover trial, patients received double-dose transfusions ($>6.0 \times 10^{11}$ platelets) of S-59-treated platelets and standard platelets in random order. Platelet transfusions were ordered based on the daily platelet count by physicians blinded to the type of platelet product. Platelet counts and cutaneous template bleeding times were performed before each platelet transfusion and at 1 and 24 hours after each study platelet transfusion. Secondary endpoints included the following: clinical hemostasis before and after transfusion, frequency of transfusion reactions, corrected count increments (CCIs), and adverse events. Before platelet transfusion, the average platelet count was less than 13×10^9/L and the median bleeding time was greater than 30 minutes. After transfusion of S-59-treated platelets,

the average platelet count increased to 53.2×10^9/L and the median bleeding time decreased to 15 minutes. Control platelet transfusions demonstrated an average post-transfusion platelet count of 63.3×10^9/L and a median bleeding time of 12 minutes. The improvements in bleeding times persisted for up to 24 hours after platelet transfusion: 17 minutes for S-59 platelets and 19 minutes for standard platelets. The S-59-treated platelets were well tolerated.

In 1998, a large, randomized, controlled, double-blinded clinical trial[38] was initiated using pooled random-donor buffy-coat platelets prepared with S-59 treatment or by standard methods. This study enrolled 103 patients at four European centers. The S-59 platelet concentrates were pooled, treated with S-59, and then stored for up to 5 days before transfusion. Patients were randomly assigned to receive all platelet transfusions of the assigned type for up to 8 weeks of transfusion support. The primary endpoint of this trial was the CCI 1 hour after platelet transfusion. Secondary endpoints included the CCI 24 hours after transfusion, clinical hemostasis, frequency of platelet transfusion, frequency of acute transfusion reactions, frequency of refractoriness to platelet transfusion, frequency of platelet-associated bacteremia, and overall safety. A second, large clinical trial[39] of S-59-treated platelets commenced enrollment in the United States in July 1999. This is a randomized, controlled, double-blinded trial designed to enroll 600 patients at 12 clinical centers. It is being conducted with single-donor platelets collected on the Amicus (Baxter Healthcare Corporation, Round Lake, IL) cell separator system. Platelet concentrates are prepared at each study center. Patients are randomly divided into two treatment groups: those receiving S-59-treated platelets and those receiving standard platelets. Patients receive all platelet transfusion support of the assigned type for up to 4 weeks. Patients who require additional platelet transfusion support after the initial 4-week period will be invited to enroll into a second transfusion 4-week cycle. The primary endpoint of this trial is the frequency of clinical bleeding among the two treatment groups. Secondary endpoints include 1- and 24-hour platelet CCIs, interval between platelet transfusions, frequency of acute transfusion reactions, frequency of platelet-associated bacterial sepsis, rate of refractoriness to platelet transfusion, and safety. The study was completed and demonstrated that transfusions of photochemically treated platelets were equivalent to conventional platelets for the prevention and treatment of bleeding during periods of prolonged thrombocytopenia.[39]

Potential Systems for Inactivation of Pathogens in RBC Concentrates

A number of laboratories have investigated the application of pathogen inactivation to RBC concentrates (Table 20.4). RBCs present a difficult environment for pathogen inactivation owing to the light absorbance by hemoglobin and the viscosity of packed RBCs. To date, most research efforts have explored the use of photodynamic methods, but more recently several groups have developed nucleic acid–targeted processes that do not require light activation. The latter approach offers the potential to minimize nonspecific damage by active oxygen species to RBCs and plasma proteins. Photodynamic-associated damage may be further increased during prolonged RBC storage. Moreover, significant defects of the photodynamic systems have included incomplete inactivation of pathogens, damage to RBCs resulting in hemolysis and potassium leakage, increased binding of immunoglobulins, long treatment times, and the necessity to work at a reduced hematocrit or in thin-layer configurations to facilitate light activation. Cellular damage due to active oxygen species can be ameliorated by the inclusion of scavengers or quenchers of active oxygen species,[40, 41] but this modification further complicates the treatment process.

The initial RBC studies were conducted with porphyrin-based compounds and dyes such as merocyanine 540, methylene blue (MB), and phthalocyanine (see Table 20.4). Each of these methodologies had limited viral inactivation capacity and induced various levels of RBC injury. Subsequently, Wagner and colleagues[42] described the use of a new phenothiazine compound, dimethylene blue, which exhibited an improved inactivation spectrum compared to MB and demonstrated less hemolysis and less immunoglobulin binding during storage after treatment.

More recently, two groups reported studies using nucleic acid–targeted compounds that do not require photoactivation for nucleic acid inactivation. Inactine, a nucleic acid–targeted compound, was reported to inactivate a series of model viruses in RBC suspensions.[43] No data have been reported with respect to inactivation of bacteria. This compound does not require light for activation. Although limited information has been presented, the inactines appear to be stable monoalkylators that are immediately active on addition to blood or RBC concentrates. The inactine compound PEN 110 has been used to evaluate the effect of treatment on the viability of chimpanzee RBCs.[44] RBCs treated with PEN 110 were stored for 28 days, radiolabeled, and then transfused into chimpanzees. Post-transfusion RBC recovery and lifespan were reported to be similar to those of untreated RBCs. PEN 110 is currently under study in a phase I trial of 16 healthy subjects to evaluate the effect of treatment on post-transfusion RBC recovery and lifespan. This trial was designed as a crossover study and uses autologous RBCs stored for 28 days before transfusion. After treatment, the concentration of residual PEN 110 is reduced in the RBC concentrate by cell washing, and levels as low as 30 ng/mL have been achieved.[45]

Cook and associates[46] developed a class of compounds known as anchor linker effectors (ALE) and frangible anchor

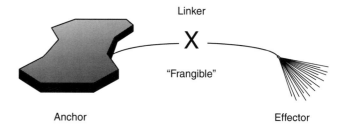

Figure 20.5 The generic structure of the frangible anchor linker effector (FRALE) compounds, for example S-303. The molecule consists of three parts: an anchor for nucleic acid intercalation, an effector region for covalent addition to nucleic acid, and a labile "frangible" linker to facilitate S-303 degradation.

Table 20.4 Methods Used to Inactivate Infectious Pathogens in Red Blood Cell Concentrates

Reactive Agent	Target	Ref. No.
Dihematoporphyrin	HIV, HSV, CMV, SIV, *T. cruzi*	82
Benzoporphyrin A	VSV, FeLV	83
Merocyanine 540	Friend LV	84
Merocyanine 540	HSV-1	85
Merocyanine 540	*P. falciparum*	86
Methylene blue	VSV	87
Methylene blue	VSV, Φ6, Sindbis, M13	88
Phthalocyanines	VSV	89
Phthalocyanines	VSV, Sindbis	81
PSR-Br	Φ6	90
Hypericin	HIV	91
Dimethylene blue	VSV, PRV, BVDV, Φ6, R17, EMC	40
Inactine	Porcine parvovirus, BVDV, HIV-1, VSV	41
S-303	HIV, DHBV, BVDV, bacteria	44

HIV, human immunodeficiency virus; HSV, herpes simplex virus; CMV, cytomegalovirus; SIV, simian immunodeficiency virus; *T. cruzi*, *Trypanosoma cruzi*; VSV, vesicular stomatitis virus; FeLV, feline leukemia virus; Friend LV, Friend erythroleukemia virus; Sindbis, Sindbis virus; Φ6, bacteriophage; PSR-Br, brominated psoralen; PRV, pseudorabies virus; BVDV, bovine viral diarrhea virus; EMC, encephalo-myocarditis virus; R17, bacteriophage.

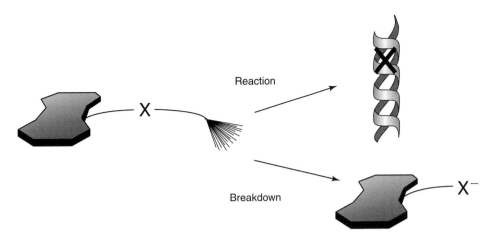

Figure 20.6 The mechanism of action for FRALE compounds. After addition to red blood cells, S-303 rapidly adds to nucleic acid, and then degrades to S-300, a negatively charged compound that does not bind to nucleic acid.

linker effectors (FRALE) for inactivation of pathogens in RBC concentrates. The FRALE compounds comprise three moieties (Fig. 20.5): consisting of a nucleic acid–targeted intercalator group, an effector group for covalent addition to nucleic acid, and a central frangible bond that facilitates compound degradation. The FRALEs are stable at low pH and are activated by a pH shift on addition to packed RBCs suspended in residual plasma and an RBC additive solution at neutral pH. The FRALE compounds rapidly degrade to a negatively charged, inactive species after reaction, preventing further binding to DNA and RNA (Fig. 20.6). On addition to packed RBCs (60% hematocrit), the lead compound, S-303 (100 mg/mL) inactivated high titers of cell-free and cell-associated HIV, duck HBV (DHBV), vesicular stomatitis virus, herpes simplex virus, bovine viral diarrhea virus (BVDV), and both gram-negative and gram-positive bacteria.[47] During the treatment process, S-303 degraded to the negatively charged compound S-300.

S-303-treated RBCs exhibited post-transfusion recovery and lifespan comparable to those of untreated RBCs in a murine transfusion model,[46] and similar results were found in a second series of studies using S-303-treated dog RBCs.[47] Dogs transfused multiple times with allogeneic-treated S-303 RBCs failed to develop antibodies to S-303-treated autologous RBCs, but some dogs did develop alloantibodies to untreated donor cells, indicating an intact alloimmune response not directed against S-303-treated RBCs. Other dogs transfused with S-303-treated RBCs (10 mL/kg) 12 times over a 1-month period had no evidence of clinical or histopathologic toxicity. In addition, replacement of 80% of the blood volume of dogs with S-303-treated RBCs using treatment concentrations up to 500 μg/mL resulted in no toxicity.[47]

A prototype S-303 system was designed to inactivate infectious pathogens in plastic containers (Fig. 20.7). With the use of a closed system with a series of connected containers,

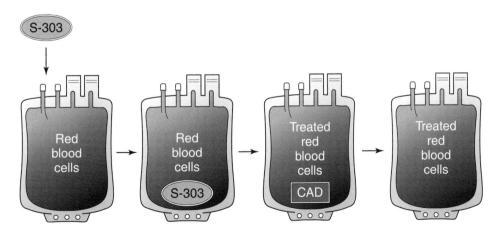

Figure 20.7 The prototype FRALE, S-303 process for treatment of red blood cell (RBC) concentrates. The treatment is conducted in a closed system. S-303 is maintained at low pH and is activated by addition to RBC concentrates at neutral pH. The inactivation process is conducted in full-sized units ranging in hematocrit from 60% to 80%. After addition of S-303 to the RBCs, the plastic container is incubated at room temperature for 6 to 8 hours to complete pathogen inactivation. Then, the RBCs are transferred to a plastic container with a compound absorption device (CAD) to reduce the levels of S-300. The RBCs remain in contact with the CAD for up to 35 days of storage at 4°C.

S-303 is added to RBC concentrates (200 to 250 mL). The RBCs are incubated at room temperature for 8 hours, during which time pathogen inactivation is completed and S-303 degrades to the inert compound S-300. After incubation, the treated RBCs are transferred to a plastic storage container with an integral compound absorption device (CAD) for storage up to 42 days at 4°C. Evaluation of in vitro RBC properties after 42 days of storage compared with untreated RBC demonstrated no differences in the following parameters: RBC levels of adenosine triphosphate, extracellular potassium, hemolysis, and glucose consumption.[46] S-303-treated RBCs advanced through preclinical safety studies and entered the clinical phase in 1998.[48–50]

Two phase I clinical trials with S-303-treated RBCs have been completed in healthy subjects. The first study was a controlled, two-arm, randomized trial in which the post-transfusion viability of S-303-treated, autologous RBCs stored for 35 days after treatment was compared with that of untreated RBCs stored for 35 days.[51] Twenty-one subjects were enrolled into the S-303 treatment group and 22 into the control group. The average post-transfusion recovery of 35-day-old S-303 RBCs was 77.7%, and the average recovery of control RBCs was 82.6%; both types exceeded 75%, the generally accepted threshold for viability of stored RBCs. No adverse events were observed after transfusion of S-303 RBCs.

A second phase I study evaluated the viability and potential immune response to multiple exposures of S-303-treated RBCs.[52] Subjects from the first study, from either treatment group, were invited to participate in this second study. The second study was initiated approximately 6 months after completion of the first study; thus, there was an interval of 6 to 9 months before the next transfusion exposure. In the second study, each subject donated a unit of blood that was processed into packed RBCs. All of the units were treated with S-303, and the units were stored for 35 days. At four times during the 35-day storage period, subjects were transfused with an aliquot of autologous S-303-treated RBCs. The final aliquot on day 35 was radiolabeled with chromium 51 to measure post-transfusion viability. The RBC recovery 24 hours after transfusion of S-303-treated RBCs was compared with each subject's RBC recovery in the first study. Twelve subjects received control RBCs in the first study and S-303 RBCs in the second study; the average RBC recovery in the first study with control cells was 82.6%, and the average recovery in the second study was 84.3% with S-303-treated cells. Sixteen subjects received S-303 RBCs in the first study, with an average recovery of 77.7%; after transfusion in the second study, these subjects demonstrated an average recovery of 78.1%. After exposure to either four or five aliquots of S-303-treated RBCs, no subjects developed antibodies directed against S-303 RBCs.[52]

■ Potential Systems for Inactivation of Pathogens in Preparation of Fresh Frozen Plasma

The SD process for inactivation of enveloped viruses in plasma for use as FFP has entered clinical practice.[53] The SD process is generally effective against enveloped viruses, although evidence has been reported recently to suggest that some enveloped viruses, such as vaccinia, may be resistant to SD treatment.[54] Moreover, because SD treatment is not

effective against nonenveloped viruses, concern has been expressed regarding the potential for transmission of these pathogens due to pooling with failure to inactivate resistant viruses.[55] Despite these issues, SD-FFP has demonstrated therapeutic efficacy for replacement of congenital[56] and acquired coagulation factor deficiencies[57] and for plasma exchange therapy of thrombotic thrombocytopenic purpura (TTP).[56] Of note, SD-FFP does not contain high-molecular-weight multimers of von Willebrand factor (vWF) and has been advocated for use in the treatment of TTP.[56] Transfusion of SD-FFP has been well tolerated, with a low incidence of transfusion reactions and adverse events.[58]

Other studies with SD-FFP have documented mild to marked decreased levels of antithrombotic proteins: protein C, protein S, and plasmin inhibitor.[59] Mast and associates[60] confirmed that SD-FFP has markedly reduced levels of the antithrombotic proteins antiplasmin and antitrypsin, and that these reduced levels are the result of conformational changes induced by the detergent treatment process. The clinical significance of these observations remains unclear at present but may be important for patients treated with FFP in clinical settings in which the coagulation cascade has been activated, such as disseminated intravascular coagulation.

The SD process uses pooled plasma from 2500 donors and is not amenable to a single-unit viral inactivation process. In Europe, a single-unit treatment process using the phenothiazine dye MB and long-wavelength visible light was developed and has been used in clinical practice for preparation of fresh frozen plasma (MB-FFP).[61] Although MB does demonstrate limited binding affinity for nucleic acid, the predominant mechanism of action is photodynamic, via production of active oxygen species. More importantly, MB is not effective against intracellular viruses due to conversion into the leukomethylene blue species. Certain coagulation proteins, primarily factor VIII and fibrinogen, are sensitive to MB treatment and undergo a decrease in functional activity during treatment, ranging from 30% to 40% of the levels in untreated plasma.[62] However, MB-FFP did provide adequate levels of fibrinogen, factor VIII, factor XIII, and vWF in cryoprecipitate,[63] and the corresponding cryosupernatant fraction was depleted of the high-molecular-weight vWF multimers.[63] The MB process requires long treatment times, and recent concerns about the preclinical safety profile have led to decreased use of this technique in Europe. MB-FFP has been well tolerated when transfused into healthy subjects.[64]

A photochemical treatment device using the psoralen S-59 and UVA has been developed to inactivate viruses in plasma prepared as single-donor FFP. After 3 J/cm^2 of UVA delivered in 3 minutes, the average log reductions of virus were 6.4 ± 0.2 for cell-associated HIV, more than 5.9 (95% confidence interval) for cell-free HIV, 5.4 ± 0.4 for DHBV; a reduction of 6.7 ± 0.4 was achieved for BVDV after only 0.5 J/cm^2. Because the S-59 process is nucleic acid–targeted, it has demonstrated inactivation of several nonenveloped viruses (e.g., rotavirus, calicivirus, blue tongue virus). After photochemical treatment, FFP units were treated for 1 hour with an SRD to reduce residual S-59 concentration, followed by freezing (−20°C). Coagulation activity of thawed S-59 FFP units (N = 7) was compared with that of matched control FFP units that had been exposed to no photochemical treatment or SRD. Factor activities (percentage of control ± SD) were as follows: clottable fibrinogen, $87 \pm 3\%$; factor V, $98 \pm 2\%$; factor VII, $86 \pm 2\%$; factor VIII, $73 \pm 4\%$; factor IX, $95 \pm 4\%$; factor X, $98 \pm 4\%$; and factor XI, $91 \pm 5\%$.[65] A single-blind, crossover, stepwise, ascending-dose clinical trial (100 to 1000 mL) was conducted in 15 healthy subjects; there were no adverse events attributed to transfusion of S-59 FFP at any dose and no clinically significant changes in post-transfusion coagulation, chemistry, or hematology profiles.[66]

There are no published pharmacokinetic analyses of coagulation factors in response to FFP transfusion. In a second study using a novel design, Wages and colleagues[67] compared the pharmacokinetics of factor VII and the post-transfusion recovery of factors II, VII, IX, and X in 27 healthy subjects treated with a 4-day regimen (7.5 mg/day) of warfarin. Healthy subjects donated 2 L of FFP by apheresis collection. One liter of plasma was treated with S-59 and frozen at -18°C; the other liter was prepared as standard FFP and stored at -18°C. Subjects were given 4 days of warfarin therapy followed by transfusion of 1 L of S-59-treated or untreated FFP. Warfarin therapy resulted in reduction of factor VII levels to approximately 30% of normal. Each subject received both types of FFP in random order. No statistical differences (Wilcoxon signed-rank test) were observed between S-59-treated and control FFP in clearance, recovery, half-life, or mean residence time for factor VII.[67] No differences in recoveries of other factors (II, IX, and X) were observed. Transfusion of single-unit S-59 FFP provided acceptable coagulation factor preservation without adverse effects. The anticoagulant challenge crossover trial demonstrated that transfusion of S-59-treated FFP yielded therapeutic coagulation factor increments similar to those of standard FFP.

A phase II, randomized, controlled, pilot study of S-59-treated FFP was completed in 13 patients with acquired coagulopathy to evaluate the response of prolonged prothrombin (PT) and partial thromboplastin times (PTT) to transfusion after S-59 treatment.[68] Patients with a diagnosis of acquired coagulopathy were randomly assigned to transfusion with either S-59-treated or standard FFP. The average PT and PTT were prolonged before FFP transfusion and responded similarly to transfusion with either S-59-treated or standard FFP. The response lasted 8 to 12 hours, and S-59-treated FFP demonstrated acceptable control of bleeding in patients undergoing invasive procedures (e.g., liver biopsy).

A phase III trial program for S-59-treated FFP has been initiated in the United States (personal communication). The first protocol will evaluate the post-transfusion recovery and clearance of specific coagulation factors in 20 patients with congenital coagulopathies requiring FFP transfusion. This open-label, single-arm study has enrolled patients with deficiencies of factors I, II, V, VII, X, and XI. Enrolled patients receive at least one transfusion of S-59-treated FFP (15 mL/kg) to measure the recovery and clearance of the specified deficient clotting factor. Patients are then eligible to receive additional transfusions of S-59-treated FFP as required to manage active bleeding or for prophylaxis during surgical procedures. A second controlled, double-blinded, randomized study of 120 patients with acquired coagulopathy has been completed. Patients are randomly assigned to receive either standard FFP or S-59-treated FFP for up to 7 days of support. The primary endpoint of this study is the response of the PT and PTT to FFP transfusion. A third controlled,

double-blinded randomized study of 30 patients with TTP is open for enrollment (personal communication). In this study, patients are randomly assigned to receive up to 30 days of therapeutic plasma exchange (TPE) with either standard FFP or S-59-treated FFP. The primary endpoint is the proportion of patients in remission in each treatment group after 30 days of TPE. Patients who fail to reach remission after 30 days of TPE are eligible to continue TPE for an additional 30 days.

■ Conclusions

Robust pathogen inactivation systems for the treatment of each blood component have been developed and are in various stages of clinical trials in the United States and Europe. In addition, two systems for treatment of plasma, SD and MB, are in clinical use. Beyond inactivation of infectious pathogens, these treatments offer additional opportunities for improving transfusion safety, such as leukocyte inactivation. The availability of pathogen inactivation systems for all blood components may permit modification of current testing strategies to take advantage of a stratified, integrated approach to transfusion safety by using pathogen inactivation and a modified testing strategy to improve blood component transfusion safety. As new pathogens of clinical importance are identified in the donor population, both pathogen inactivation and testing strategies will require further modification to meet new challenges.

REFERENCES

1. Dodd RY: Will blood products be free of infectious agents? In Nance SJ (ed): Transfusion Medicine in the 1990s. Arlington, VA: American Association of Blood Banks, 1990, pp 223–251.
2. McQuiston JH, Childs JE, Chamberland ME, Tabor E: Transmission of tick-borne agents of disease by blood transfusion: a review of known and potential risks in the United States. Transfusion 2000;40:274–284.
3. Schmunis GA: *Trypanosoma cruzi*, the etiologic agent of Chagas' disease: Status in the blood supply in endemic and nonendemic countries. Transfusion 1991;31:547–557.
4. Grant IH, Gold JMW, Wittner M, et al: Transfusion-associated acute Chagas disease acquired in the United States. Ann Intern Med 1989;111:849–851.
5. Nickerson P, Orr P, Schroeder ML, et al: Transfusion-associated *Trypanosoma cruzi* infection in a non-endemic area. Ann Intern Med 1989;111:851–853.
6. Mintz ED, Anderson JF, Cable RG, Hadler JL: Transfusion-transmitted babesiosis: A case report from a new endemic area. Transfusion 1991;31:365–368.
7. Linden JV, Wong SJ, Chu FK, et al: Transfusion-associated transmission of babesiosis in New York state. Transfusion 2000;40:285–289.
8. McDonald CP, Hartley S, Orchard K, et al: Fatal *Clostridium perfringens* sepsis from a pooled platelet transfusion. Transfusion Med 1998;8:19–22.
9. Goldman M, Blajchman MA: Blood product–associated bacterial sepsis. Transfus Med Rev 1991;5:73–83.
10. Blajchman MA, Ali AM: Bacteria in the blood supply: An overlooked issue in transfusion medicine. In Nance SJ (ed): Blood Safety: Current Challenges. Bethesda, MD: American Association of Blood Banks, 1992, pp 213–228.
11. Sazama K: Reports of 355 transfusion-associated deaths: 1976 through 1985. Transfusion 1990;30:583–590.
12. Handa A, Dickstein B, Young NS, Brown KE: Prevalence of the newly described circovirus, TTV, in United States blood donors. Transfusion 2000;40:245–251.
13. AuBuchon JP, Birkmeyer JD, Busch MP: Safety of the blood supply in the United States: Opportunities and controversies. Ann Intern Med 1997;127:905–909.

14. Schreiber GB, Busch MP, Kleinman SH, Korelitz JJ: The risk of transfusion-transmitted viral infections. N Engl J Med 1996;334:1685–1690.

15. Chan K: Blood supply: FDA oversight and remaining issues of safety. In U.S. General Accounting Office, 1997.

16. Schuttler GC, Caspari C, Jursch CA, et al: Hepatitis C virus transmission by a blood donation negative in nucleic acid amplification tests for viral RNA. Lancet 2000;355:41–42.

17. Zaza S, Tokars JI, Yomtovian R, et al: Bacterial contamination of platelets at a university hospital: Increased identification due to intensified surveillance. Infect Control Hosp Epidemiol 1994;15:82–87.

18. Morrow JF, Braine HG, Kickler TS, et al: Septic reactions to platelet transfusions: A persistent problem. JAMA 1991;266:555–558.

19. Blajchman MA, Ali A, Lyn P, et al: Bacterial surveillance of platelet concentrates: quantitation of bacterial load. Transfusion 1997;37(Suppl):74s.

20. Chiu EKW, Yuen KY, Lie AKW, et al: A prospective study of symptomatic bacteremia following platelet transfusion and of its management. Transfusion 1994;34:950–954.

21. Wallace EL, Churchill WH, Surgenor DM: Collection and transfusion of blood components in the United States, 1992. Transfusion 1992;35:802–812.

22. Horowitz B, Wiebe ME, Lippin A, Stryker MH: Inactivation of viruses in labile blood derivatives: I. Disruption of lipid-enveloped viruses by tri(n-butyl)phosphate detergent combinations. Transfusion 1985;25:516–522.

23. Heddle NM, Kalma L, Singer J, et al: The role of plasma from platelet concentrates in transfusion reactions. N Engl J Med 1994;331:625–628.

24. Ohto H, Anderson KC: Survey of transfusion-associated graft-versus-host disease in immunocompetent recipients. Transfus Med Rev 1996;10:31–43.

25. Corash L: Photochemical decontamination of cellular blood components. Anaesth Pharmacol Rev 1995;3:138–149.

26. Lin L, Wiesehahn GP, Morel PA, Corash L: Use of 8-methoxypsoralen and long wavelength ultraviolet radiation for decontamination of platelet concentrates. Blood 1989;74:517–525.

27. Edelson R, Berger C, Gasparro F, et al: Treatment of cutaneous T-cell lymphoma by extracorporeal photochemotherapy. N Engl J Med 1987;316:297–303.

28. McEvoy MT, Stern RS: Psoralens and related compounds in the treatment of psoriasis. Pharmacol Ther 1987;34:75–97.

29. Alter HJ, Morel PA, Dorman BP, et al: Photochemical decontamination of blood components containing hepatitis B and non-A, non-B virus. Lancet 1988;2:1446–1450.

30. Dodd RY, Moroff G, Wagner S, et al: Inactivation of viruses in platelet suspensions that retain their in vitro characteristics: Comparison of psoralen-ultraviolet A and merocyanine 540-visible light methods. Transfusion 1991;31:483–490.

31. Margolis-Nunno H, Bardossy L, Robinson R, et al: Psoralen-mediated photochemical decontamination of platelet concentrates: Inactivation of cell-free and cell-associated forms of human immunodeficiency virus and assessment of platelet function in vivo. Transfusion 1997;37:889–895.

32. Goodrich RP, Yerram NR, Tay GB, et al: Selective inactivation of viruses in the presence of human platelets: UV sensitization with psoralen derivatives. Proc Natl Acad Sci U S A 1994;91:5552–5556.

33. Goodrich RP, Yerram NR, Crandall SL, Sowemimo-Coker SO: In vivo survival of platelets subjected to virus inactivation protocols using psoralen and coumarin photosensitizers. Blood 1995;86(Suppl 1):354a.

34. Lin L, Corten L, Murthy KK, et al: Photochemical inactivation of hepatitis B (HBV) and hepatitis C (HCV) virus in human platelet concentrates as assessed by a chimpanzee infectivity model. Blood 92 (Suppl 1):502a, 1998.

35. Grass JA, Hei DJ, Metchette K, et al: Inactivation of leukocytes in platelet concentrates by psoralen plus UVA. Blood 1998;91:2180–2188.

36. Corash L, Behrman B, Rheinschmidt M, et al: Post-transfusion viability and tolerability of photochemically treated platelet concentrates (PC). Blood 1997;90(Suppl 1):267a.

37. Slichter SJ, Corash L, Grabowski M, et al: Viability and hemostatic function of photochemically treated (PCT) platelets in thrombocytopenic patients. Blood 1999;94(Suppl 1):376a.

38. vanRhenen D, Gulliksson H, Pamphilon D, et al: S-59 Helinx photochemically treated platelets (plt) are safe and effective for support of thrombocytopenia: results of the EUROSPRITE Phase 3 trial. Blood 96:819a, 2000.

39. McCullough J, Vesole D, Benjamin RJ, et al: Pathogen inactivated platelets (plt) using Helinx technology (INTERCEPT plt) are hemostatically effective in thrombocytopenic patients (tcp pts): the SPRINT trial. Blood 98 (Suppl 1):450a, 2001.

40. Rywkin S, Ben-Hur E, Reid ME, et al: Selective protection against IgG binding to red cells treated with phthalocyanines and red light for virus inactivation. Transfusion 1995;35:414–420.

41. Ben-Hur E, Rywkin S, Rosenthal I, et al: Virus inactivation in red cell concentrates by photosensitization with phthalocyanine: Protection of red cells but not of vesicular stomatitis virus with a water-soluble analogue of vitamin E. Transfusion 1995;35:401–406.

42. Wagner SJ, Skirpchenko A, Robinette D, et al: Preservation of red cell properties after virucidal phototreatment with dimethylene blue. Transfusion 1998;38:729–737.

43. Zhang QX, Edson C, Budowsky E, Purmal A: Inactine: A method for viral inactivation in red blood cell concentrate. Transfusion 1998;38(10S):75S.

44. Edson CM, Purmal A, Brown F, et al: Viral inactivation of red blood cell concentrates by Inactine: Mechanism of action and lack of effect on red cell physiology. Transfusion 1999;39(Suppl 1):108s.

45. AuBuchon JP, Pickard CA, Herschel LH, et al: In vivo recovery of red cells of virally inactivated by INACTINE and stored for 28 days. Blood 96(Suppl 1):819a, 2000.

46. Cook D, Stassinopoulos A, Merritt J, et al: Inactivation of pathogens in packed red blood cell (PRBC) concentrates using S-303. Blood 1997;90(Suppl 1):409a.

47. Cook D, Stassinopoulos A, Wollowitz S, et al: In vivo analysis of packed red blood cells treated with S-303 to inactivate pathogens. Blood 1998;92(Suppl 1):503a.

48. Rios JA, Viele M, Greenwalt TJ, et al: Helinx treated RBC transfusions are well tolerated and show comparable recovery and survival to control RBCs. Transfusion 41 (Suppl 1):38S, 2001.

49. Greenwalt TJ, Hambleton J, Wages D, et al: Viability of red blood cells treated with a novel pathogen inactivation system. Transfusion 39(Suppl 1):109s, 1999.

50. Hambleton J, Greenwalt T, Viele M, et al: Post transfusion recovery after multiple exposures to red blood cell concentrates (RBCS) treated with a novel pathogen inactivation (P.I.) process. Blood 94(suppl 1): 376a, 1999.

51. Greenwalt TJ, Hambleton J, Wages D, et al: Viability of red blood cells treated with a novel pathogen inactivation system. Transfusion 1999;39(Suppl 1):109s.

52. Hambleton J, Greenwalt T, Viele M, et al: Post transfusion recovery after multiple exposures to red blood cell concentrates (RBCs) treated with a novel pathogen inactivation (P.I.) process. Blood 1999;94 (Suppl 1):376a.

53. Horowitz B, Bonomo R, Prince AM, et al: Solvent/detergent treated plasma: A virus-inactivated substitute for fresh frozen plasma. Blood 1992;79:826–831.

54. Roberts P: Resistance of vaccinia virus to inactivation by solvent/ detergent treatment of blood products. Biologicals 2000;28:29–32.

55. Luban NLC: Human parvovirus: Implications for transfusion medicine. Transfusion 1994;34:821–827.

56. Horowitz MS, Pehta JC: SD plasma in TTP and coagulation factor deficiencies for which no concentrates are available. Vox Sang 1998;74(Suppl 1):231–235.

57. Williamson LM, Llewelyn CA, Fisher NC, et al: A randomized trial of solvent/detergent-treated and standard fresh-frozen plasma in the coagulopathy of liver disease and liver transplantation. Transfusion 1999;39:1227–1234.

58. Baudoux E, Margraff U, Coenen A, et al: Hemovigilance: Clinical tolerance of solvent-detergent treated plasma. Vox Sang 1998;74 (Suppl 1):237–239.

59. Beeck H, Hellstern P: In vitro characterization of solvent/detergent-treated human plasma and of quarantine fresh frozen plasma. Vox Sang 1998;74(Suppl 1):219–223.

60. Mast AE, Stadanlick JE, Lockett JM, Dietzen DJ: Solvent/detergent-treated plasma has decreased antitrypsin activity and absent antiplasmin activity. Blood 1999;94:3922–3927.

61. Mohr H, Lambrecht B, Knueyer-Hopf J: Virus inactivated single-donor fresh plasma preparations. Infusionstherapie 1992;19:79–83.

62. Aznar JA, Molina R, Montoro JM: Factor VIII/von Willebrand factor complex in methylene blue-treated fresh plasma. Transfusion 1999;39:748–750.

63. Aznar JA, Montoro JM, Bonnad S, et al: Clotting factors in cryoprecipitate and cryosupernatant prepared from MB-treated fresh plasma. Transfusion 2000;40:493.
64. Simonsen AC, Sorensen H: Clinical tolerance of methylene blue virus-inactivated plasma: A randomized crossover trial in 12 healthy volunteers. Vox Sang 1999;77:210.
65. Alfonso R, Lin C, Dupuis K, et al: Inactivation of viruses with preservation of coagulation function in fresh frozen plasma. Blood 1996;88(Suppl 1):526a.
66. Wages D, Smith D, Walsh J, et al: Transfusion of therapeutic doses of virally inactivated fresh frozen plasma in healthy subjects. Blood 1997;90(Suppl 1):409a.
67. Wages D, Radu-Radurescu L, Adams M, et al: Quantitative analysis of coagulation factors in response to transfusion of S-59 photochemically treated fresh frozen plasma (S-59 FFP) and standard FFP. Blood 1998;92(Suppl 1):503a.
68. Wages D, Bass N, Keefe E, et al: Treatment of acquired coagulopathy by transfusion of fresh frozen plasma (FFP) prepared using a novel, single unit photochemical. Blood 1999;94(Suppl 1):247a.
69. Mintz P, Steadman R, Blackall D, et al: Pathogen inactivated fresh frozen plasma prepared using Helinx™ technology is efficacious and well tolerated in treatment of end-stage liver disease patients—the STEP AC trial. Blood 98(Suppl 1):709a, 2001.
70. Londe H, Damonte P, Corash L, Lin L: Inactivation of human cytomegalovirus with psoralen and UVA in human platelet concentrates. Blood 1995;86(Suppl 1):544a.
71. Lin L, Londe H, Hanson CV, et al: Photochemical inactivation of cell-associated human immunodeficiency virus in platelet concentrates. Blood 1993;82:292–297.
72. Eble BE, Corash L: Photochemical inactivation of duck hepatitis B virus in human platelet concentrates: A model of surrogate human hepatitis B virus infectivity. Transfusion 1996;36:406–418.
73. Lin L, Londe H, Janda M, et al: Photochemical inactivation of pathogenic bacteria in human platelet concentrates. Blood 1994;83:2698–2706.
74. Benade LE, Shumaker J, Xu Y, Dodd R: Inactivation of free and cell-associated HIV in platelet suspensions by aminomethyltrimethyl (AMT) psoralen and ultraviolet light. Transfusion 1992;32S:33S.
75. Margolis-Nunno M, Williams B, Rywkin S, Horowitz B: Photochemical virus sterilization in platelet concentrates with psoralen derivatives [abstract]. Thromb Haemost 1991;65:1162.
76. Rai S, Kasturi C, Grayzar J, et al: Dramatic improvements in viral inactivation with brominated psoralens, napthalenes and anthracenes. Photochem Photobiol 1993;58:59–65.
77. Yerram N, Forster P, Goodrich T, et al: Comparison of virucidal properties of brominated psoralen with 8-methoxy psoralen (8-MOP) and aminomethyl trimethyl psoralen (AMT) in platelet concentrates. Blood 1993;82(Suppl 1):402a.
78. Prodouz KN, Fratantoni JC, Boone EJ, Bonner RF: Use of laser-UV for inactivation of virus in blood products. Blood 1987;70:589–592.
79. Prodouz KN, Lytle CD, Keville EA, et al: Inhibition by albumin of merocyanine 540-mediated photosensitization of platelets and viruses. Transfusion 1991;31:415–422.
80. Klein-Struckmeier A, Mohr H: Virus inactivation by methylene blue/light in thrombocyte concentrates. Vox Sang 1994;67 (Suppl 2):36.
81. Horowitz B, Rywkin S, Margolis-Nunno H, et al: Inactivation of viruses in red cell and platelet concentrates with aluminum phthalocyanine (AlPc) sulfonates. Blood Cells 1992;18:141–150.
82. Matthews JL, Sogandares-Bernal F, Judy M, et al: Inactivation of viruses with photoactive compounds. Blood Cells 1992;18:75–89.
83. North J, Neyndorff H, King D, Levy JG: Viral inactivation in blood and red cell concentrates with benzoporphyrin derivative. Blood Cells 1992;18:129–140.
84. Sieber F, Krueger GJ, O'Brien JM, et al: Inactivation of Friend erythroleukemia virus and friend virus-transformed cells by merocyanine 540-mediated photosensitization. Blood 1989;73: 345–350.
85. O'Brien JM, Gaffney DK, Wang TP, Sieber F: Merocyanine 540-sensitized photoinactivation of enveloped viruses in blood products: site and mechanism of phototoxicity. Blood 1992;80:277–285.
86. Smith OM, Dolan SA, Dvorak JA, et al: Merocyanine 540-sensitized photoinactivation of human erythrocytes parasitized by *Plasmodium falciparum*. Blood 1992;80:21–24.
87. Wagner SJ, Storry JR, Mallory DA, et al: Red cell alterations associated with virucidal methylene blue phototreatment. Transfusion 1993;33:30–36.
88. Wagner SJ, Abe H, Benade L: Differential sensitivity to methylene blue (MB) photosensitization. Photochem Photobiol 1993;57(Suppl):67S.
89. Horowitz B, Williams B, Rywkin S, et al: Inactivation of viruses in blood with aluminum phthalocyanine derivatives. Transfusion 1991;31:102–108.
90. Yerram N, Platz MS, Forster P, et al: Selective viral inactivation in RBC, platelets, and plasma using a novel psoralen derivative plus ultraviolet A (UVA) light. Transfusion 1993;33(Suppl 9S):50S.
91. Lavie G, Mazur Y, Lavie D, et al: Hypericin as an inactivator of infectious viruses in blood components. Transfusion 1995;35:392–400.

Chapter 21

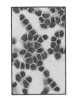

Irradiated Products and Washed/Volume Reduced Products

Naomi L. C. Luban
Edward C. C. Wong

Transfusion-associated graft-versus-host disease (TA-GVHD), an often fatal immunological complication, was first reported in the 1960s in individuals with hematologic malignancies and infants with congenital immunodeficiencies who received blood and then developed what was called runting disease.[1]

Since these early reports, the spectrum of individuals at risk has expanded, the pathogenesis has been more fully explained, and preventive strategies have been established.[2–4] Despite these advances, there are still many unanswered questions. There are no adequate estimates of prevalence, as most at-risk patients receive irradiated products. No registries or systems are in place to collect data on incidences in the United States. In Japan, a Japanese Red Cross GVHD Study Group and a registry exist. On the basis of the homozygosity for one-way human leukocyte antigen (HLA) haplotype sharing in Japan, the use of familial donors, and the use of fresh rather than stored red blood cells (RBCs), an estimated 40 cases per year are expected in Japan.[5] No estimates are available in the United States.

The clinical manifestations of TA-GVHD differ from those of GVHD in the setting of hematopoietic stem cell transplantation, but why this is the case is unknown. There is no well-established animal model, forcing investigators to utilize the classic parent-to-F1 hybrid mouse model of GVHD, which may or may not provide the correct tool for TA-GVHD investigations.[6] Lastly, as the indications for universal leukodepletion of blood and blood products have expanded, there has been less interest in mechanistic studies of TA-GVHD because of difficulties in performing such studies with blood products that would simulate the product to be used by patients at risk. Indeed, despite no studies to confirm that leukodepleted blood and blood products might obviate the need to attenuate lymphocyte reactivity (see later), some blood filter manufacturers imply such an advantage.

■ Pathogenesis

Three prerequisites for the development of GVHD have been proposed in the transplant setting: (1) differences in histocompatibility between recipient and donor, (2) presence of immunocompetent cells in the graft, and (3) inability of the host to reject the immunocompetent cells. In TA-GVHD, a similar set of circumstances can occur. Most immunocompetent recipients destroy the donor-derived T cells through lymphocytolysis. However, transfusion from an HLA homozygous donor into an HLA heterozygous recipient who shares one HLA haplotype may result in failure of recognition of the donor cells as foreign, and engraftment ensues.[7, 8] In both cases, the foreign major histocompatibility complex (MHC) antigens or minor histocompatibility antigens of the host, or both, stimulate clonal T-cell expansion and the induction of an inflammatory response with cytokine release that is ultimately responsible for the induction of the process and clinical manifestations of the disorder.

Ferrara and colleagues[6] have described the paradigm of the T-helper subsets Th1 and Th2, which delineates the cellular origins and differential biological functions of T-cell–derived cytokines on the basis of murine CD4 differentiation. Th1 CD4 T cells secrete interleukin-2 (IL-2) as their allostimulator. Th2 CD4 T cells produce IL-4, IL-5, IL-6, IL-10, IL-13, and lesser amounts of tumor necrosis factor-α (TNF-α), and Th1 and Th2 both produce IL-3 and granulocyte-macrophage colony-stimulating factor. The type 1 cell is proinflammatory and induces cell-mediated immunity, whereas the type 2 cell is considered anti-inflammatory. Differentiation toward type 1 or type 2 is a complicated process that involves early exposure to IL-4 or IL-12, the type of antigen-presenting cells, costimulating molecules, and the presence of macrophages and their unique cytokines.

On the basis of their work in mice, Ferrera and colleagues proposed a three-step process for the development of acute GVHD in the transplant setting. In this model (Fig. 21.1), host tissue damaged through irradiation or chemotherapy secretes TNF-α and IL-1, which enhance recognition of host MHC or minor histocompatibility antigens, or both, by donor T cells. Donor T-cell activation results in proliferation of Th1 T cells and secretion of IL-2 and TNF-α, which in turn activate T cells further and induce cytotoxic T lymphocyte (CTL) and natural killer (NK) responses. Whether there is direct comparability to TA-GVHD remains a question.

Additional donor and residual host phagocytes are stimulated to produce IL-1 and TNF-α; stimulated macrophages release the free radical nitric oxide (NO), which has further deleterious effects on host tissues. In addition, NO upregulates alloreactivity and mediates the cytotoxic function of macrophages.[9] A secondary triggering signal initiates step 3, wherein

lipopolysaccharide (LPS) stimulates gut-associated macrophages and lymphocytes, stimulates keratocytes and dermal fibroblasts, and further promotes the inflammatory response and end-organ damage that are classic hallmarks of the disorder.

The importance of CD4 and CD8 cells in the pathogenesis of TA-GVHD has been studied by Fast and coworkers[10] in a mouse model and by Nishimura and associates[11] in a patient with TA-GVHD and is further supported by clinical correlation with human immunodeficiency virus (HIV) and acquired immunodeficiency syndrome (AIDS).[12] In the mouse, depletion of CD4+ cells increased the number of donor cells needed to induce TA-GVHD, and depletion of CD8+ or NK cells, or both, decreased the number of donor cells needed to induce the disorder. In HIV and AIDS, there has been only one report of TA-GVHD[13] despite widespread use of supportive transfusion and profound immunosuppression. Early depletion of

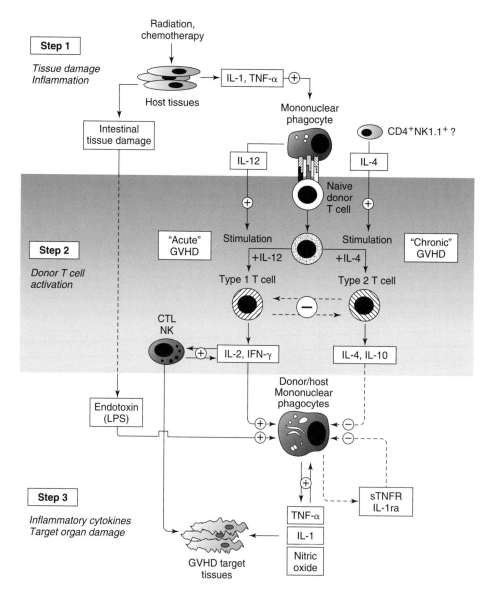

Figure 21.1   Proposed interactions between T-cell cytokines and mononuclear phagocyte–derived cytokines during graft-versus-host disease (GVHD). IFN, interferon; IL-1, interleukin-1; LPS, lipopolysaccharide; sTNFR, soluble tumor necrosis factor receptor; TNF-α, tumor necrosis factor-α.

CD4 may well protect against establishment of GVHD. Alternatively, activation of CD8+ lymphocytes against HIV-infected CD4 T cells may limit the development of the GVHD process.[12]

Clinical Manifestations

Fever, anorexia, nausea, vomiting, and diarrhea are seen. Skin manifestations are variably severe and begin as an erythematous maculopapular eruption that may proceed to erythroderma with bullae and frank desquamation. Gastrointestinal bleeding is commonly seen, usually as bloody diarrhea. Hepatic dysfunction with hyperbilirubinemia, with a progressively increasing direct fraction, is also seen. TA-GVHD differs from acute GVHD in the setting of allogeneic transplantation in that the pancytopenia seen is severe and often results in the death of the patient. The diagnosis is often made at postmortem examination and is based on pathognomonic histopathological findings of lymphocyte infiltration in skin, lymph nodes, liver, and the gastrointestinal tract.[14]

Diagnosis of TA-GVHD

Clinical suspicion may warrant a skin biopsy. Skin biopsy often reveals vacuolization of the epidermal basal cell layer, dermal-epithelial layer separation, and formation of bullae; other findings include mononuclear cell migration into the epidermis, hyperkeratosis, and dyskeratosis. Liver biopsies may reveal eosinophilic infiltration and degeneration of small bile ducts, peripheral inflammation, and lymphocyte infiltration. The bone marrow findings are those classically associated with "empty marrow," with pancytopenia, fibrosis, and some lymphocytic infiltration.

Definitive confirmation is more complicated. Several methods have been utilized to identify lymphocytes of foreign origin in the patient's circulation or in affected tissue. Serological HLA typing, DNA-based HLA class II typing, karyotype analysis, restriction fragment length polymorphism analysis using probes from both HLA and non-HLA regions, and genetic fingerprinting have all been used.[15–19] Fibroblast and buccal mucosal cells of the recipient are often needed as the lymphocytolysis accompanying the disorder prohibits standardized serological HLA typing. Parental or familial specimens may be necessary to deduce a recipient's HLA type.[20] Donor lymphocytes obtained from suspected blood products present in attached remaining blood bag segments often require polymerase chain reaction (PCR) amplification and sequence-specific oligonucleotide probe methodologies to provide confirmation of donor cell origin.[21]

In 1996, Busch and Lee and their colleagues[22] demonstrated a thousandfold expansion of donor lymphocytes in the circulation of otherwise healthy recipients 3 to 5 days after transfusion for elective orthopedic procedures; within 2 weeks, the allogeneic cells were cleared. In another study of adult trauma victims who received large numbers (4 to 18 units) of fresh packed RBCs, 8 of 10 had confirmed microchimerism (MC). Two of the eight had persistence of MC when studied as long as 1.5 years after transfusion.[23] Wang-Rodriquez and associates[24] studied post-transfusion immune modulation in 14 premature infants. Through collaboration with Busch and Lee, they identified two of six female infants, transfused with nonleukodepleted RBCs, who experienced transient MC detected by Y chromosome PCR amplification; in both, these cells were cleared by 2 weeks after transfusion. An additional three infants who received leukodepleted RBCs also had transient MC.

Vietor and coworkers[25] studied 9 surviving recipients of intrauterine transfusion whose donors were still available for testing. Using fluorescence in situ hybridization, PCR of Y chromosome–specific sequences, and assays for the frequencies of CTL and T-helper lymphocyte precursors, they detected true MC in 6 of 7 young adults studied 20 years after transfusion. Reed and colleagues[26] have developed sequence-specific amplification of DRB1, which permitted identification of minor chimeric populations at the 0.01% level. The establishment of stable MC and identification of its biological consequences are critical for pediatric patients who are expected to live to adulthood and may well be stable transfusion-induced chimeras, an intriguing and at the same time worrying concept. The persistence of MC may predispose to autoimmune disease,[27–29] chronic GVHD, and recurrent abortion[30] and may serve as an allogeneic stimulus of latent viral reactivation in the recipient.

Groups at Risk

Among methodologies (e.g., photoinactivation, pegylation, ultraviolet [UV] light, and irradiation) that can be used to prevent TA-GVHD, only irradiation of whole blood and cellular components is currently accepted by the Food and Drug Administration (FDA). Patients in whom TA-GVHD may develop have been described in a number of reviews,[2–4, 7, 8, 31, 32] and there has been growing concern about the types of patients who may be affected. For example, on the basis of two reports of TA-GVHD in older infants with severe combined immunodeficiency,[13, 21] it has been recommended that the age range of irradiation be extended well past the neonatal age group.[33, 34] Because of the lack of adequate animal models and laboratory tests to identify individual TA-GVHD risk, many reports stratify the need for irradiation using such terms as "clearly indicated" or "probably indicated."[3, 31, 32] In reality, the spectrum of individuals at risk is likely to grow as intensive immunomodulatory therapies expand beyond oncological disease and transplantation (Table 21.1).

The Irradiation Process

Irradiation of cellular components with ionizing radiation results in the inactivation of T lymphocytes by damaging nuclear DNA either directly or by generating ions and free radicals that have damaging biological actions. The irradiation prevents post-transfusion donor T-cell proliferation in response to host antigen-presenting cells, which, in turn, abrogates GVHD.[35–37] Two types of ionizing radiation, gamma rays and x-rays, are equivalent in inactivating T lymphocytes in blood components at a given absorbed dose. Gamma rays originate from the radioactive decay process within the atomic nucleus of cesium 137 (^{137}Cs) or cobalt 60 (^{60}Co). Freestanding blood bank gamma irradiators, which are the predominant instruments for blood component irradiation, use either of these two isotopes as an irradiation source. In contrast, x-rays are generated from the interaction of a beam of electrons with a metallic surface.

Table 21.1   Clinical Indications for Irradiated Products

Fetus/Infant

Intrauterine transfusion

Premature infants

Congenital immunodeficiency

Those undergoing exchange transfusion for erythroblastosis

Child/Adult

Congenital immunodeficiency

Hematologic malignancy or solid tumor (neuroblastoma, sarcoma, Hodgkin disease receiving ablative chemotherapy or radiotherapy)

Recipient of peripheral blood stem cell or marrow transplant

Recipient of familial blood donation

Recipient of human leukocyte antigen–matched products

Lupus or any other condition requiring fludarabine

Potential Indications

Term infant

Recipient and donor pair from a genetically homogeneous population

Other patients with hematologic malignancy or solid tumor receiving immunosuppressive agents

Linear accelerators that generate x-rays for patients' therapy (teletherapy) may serve as an irradiation source for blood and blood components. The FDA has also approved the use of a freestanding x-ray machine (Rad-Source RS3000, Coral Springs, FL) for irradiation of blood components.

■ Instrumentation for Irradiation

The basic operating principles and configurations of a freestanding irradiator with either a cesium (^{137}Cs) source or a linear accelerator are shown schematically in Figure 21.2. With a freestanding ^{137}Cs irradiator, blood components are contained within a metal canister that is positioned on a rotating turntable. Continuous rotation allows the gamma rays, originating from one to four closely positioned pencil sources, to penetrate all portions of the blood component. The number of sources and their placement depend on the instrument and model. The speed of rotation of the turntable also depends on the make or model of the instrument. A lead shield encloses the irradiation chamber. Freestanding irradiators employing ^{60}Co as the source of gamma rays are comparable except that the canister containing the blood component does not rotate during the irradiation process; rather, tubes of ^{60}Co are placed in a circular array around the entire canister within the lead chamber. When freestanding irradiators are used, the gamma rays are attenuated as they pass through air and blood but at different rates.[37] The magnitude of attenuation is greater with ^{137}Cs than with ^{60}Co sources.

Linear accelerators generate a beam of x-rays over a field of given dimensions. Routinely, the field is projected on a tabletop structure. The blood component is placed (flat) between two sheets of biocompatible plastic several centimeters thick. The plastic on the top of the blood component (i.e., nearer to the radiation source) generates electronic equilibrium of the secondary electrons at the point where they pass through the component container. The plastic sheet on the bottom of the blood component provides radiation backscattering that helps to ensure homogeneous delivery of the x-rays. The blood component is usually left stationary when the entire x-ray dose is being delivered. Alternatively, it may be flipped over when half of the dose has been delivered; this process involves turning off and restarting the linear accelerator during the irradiation procedure. Although the practice of flipping seems not to be required, further data are needed.

A   FREE-STANDING IRRADIATOR

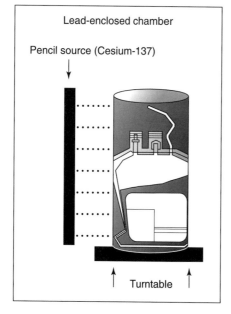

Lead-enclosed chamber

Pencil source (Cesium-137)

Turntable

· · · · · · Gamma irradiation

B   LINEAR ACCELERATOR

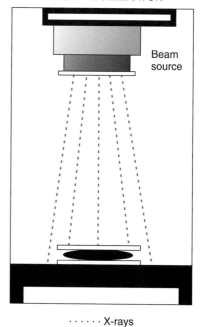

Beam source

· · · · · · X-rays

Figure 21.2   Diagrammatic views of two common types of instrumentation used for blood irradiation. *A*, Configuration of a freestanding irradiator using a cesium 137 source. *B*, Configuration of a linear accelerator.

In June 1999, the FDA licensed the first x-ray irradiator based on principles utilized in standard x-ray machines. This irradiator does not require federal or nuclear regulatory licensing or reporting, a shielded room for operation, or special floor reinforcement.

Components to Be Irradiated

The single most important characteristic of a blood component's ability to induce TA-GVHD is its white blood cell content, specifically its lymphocyte content. On the basis of animal models and estimates from the bone marrow transplant literature, 5×10^4 to 1×10^5 T cells per kilogram in an ablated host induce GVHD,[38] and a greater number is probably needed in a nonablated host. The content of lymphocytes in each blood component differs depending on the donor's initial lymphocyte count, the method of collection, and any postcollection manipulation and processing; there are probably enough lymphocytes in almost all blood products to induce TA-GVHD in a susceptible recipient. (Table 21.2). During storage, fewer lymphocytes can be isolated from both RBC and platelet concentrates. The detailed nature of lymphocyte subsets in different blood products has not been well studied, making assessment of the risk for a specific class of product and a subcategory of at-risk patients impossible. Further, there could be a cumulative or synergistic effect of viable T cells present in the multiple transfusions received by a given patient whose own immunological status fluctuates with time from treatment and infectious disease state.

For patients at risk for GVHD, all components that might contain viable T lymphocytes should be irradiated. These include units of whole blood and cellular components (RBCs, platelets, granulocytes), whether prepared from whole blood or by apheresis (Table 21.3). All types of RBCs should be irradiated, whether they are suspended in citrated plasma or in an additive solution. There are data supporting the retention of the quality of irradiated RBCs after freezing and thawing.[39, 40] If frozen/thawed units are intended for GVHD-susceptible

Table 21.2   White Blood Cell (WBC) Content of Different Blood Components

Component	Volume (mL)	Average WBC Content
Whole blood	450	1–2×10^9
Red blood cells	250	2–5×10^9
Washed red blood cells	Variable	$< 5 \times 10^8$
Deglycerolized red blood cells	250	$\sim 10^7$
Platelet concentrate	50–75	4×10^7
Plateletpheresis unit	200–500	$3 \times 10^{8*}$
Cryoprecipitate	25	0
Fresh frozen plasma	125	0
Pediatric frozen plasma	Variable	0
Liquid plasma	125	1.5×10^5
Single-donor plasma	125	0
Granulocyte concentrate	200–500	1×10^{10}

*Less with new modified chambers.
Adapted from Luban NLC: Basics of transfusion medicine. In Fuhrman BP, Zimmerman JJ (eds): Pediatric Critical Care. St. Louis, Mosby–Year Book, 1992, pp. 829–840.

Table 21.3   Blood Components Requiring Irradiation for Patients at Risk of Graft-versus-Host Disease

Products <u>known</u> to contain viable T-cells
  Whole blood
  Packed red blood cells (pRBC)
  Frozen/deglycerolized RBC
  Leukoreduced pRBC
  Platelet concentrates, pooled
  Platelets, pheresis
  Granulocytes
  Non-frozen plasma (fresh plasma)
Products that <u>may</u> contain viable T-cells
  Fresh frozen plasma
  Frozen plasma (e.g. F24)
Products <u>unlikely</u> to contain viable T-cells
  Cryoprecipitate
  SD-Plasma
  "Pathogen-reduced" products (in development)

individuals and have not been previously irradiated, they should be irradiated because it is known that such components contain viable T lymphocytes.[41]

Filtered RBC products should also be irradiated. Extensive leukoreduction through filtration may decrease the potential for GVHD and serve as an alternative to irradiation in the future when questions about the minimum level of viable T lymphocytes that can lead to GVHD are resolved. There are reports of TA-GVHD in patients who received leukodepleted (filtered) RBCs; however, the extent of leukoreduction of the components was not uniformly quantified in such reports.[42–45]

In addition, the number and specific subtype of T lymphocytes present in a product that induce TA-GVHD may depend on the patient's immunocompetence at the time of transfusion. It is likely that the greater the degree of immunosuppression, the fewer viable T lymphocytes are required to produce GVHD in susceptible patients. It was suggested that CTLs or IL-2–secreting precursors of helper T lymphocytes may be more predictive of GVHD than the number of proliferating T cells alone. Accordingly, until further data are available to confirm adequate removal of these T-cell subtypes by leukoreduction, irradiation should be used for blood products destined for patients at risk for GVHD.[45]

Irradiated RBCs undergo enhanced efflux of potassium during storage at 1 to 6°C.[46, 47] Comparable levels of potassium leakage occur with or without prestorage leukoreduction.[48] Washing of units of RBCs before transfusion to reduce the supernatant potassium load does not seem to be warranted for most RBC transfusions because post-transfusion dilution prevents increases in plasma potassium.[49] On the other hand, when irradiated RBCs are used for neonatal exchange transfusion or the equivalent of a whole blood exchange is anticipated, RBC washing should be considered to prevent the possible adverse cardiotoxicity caused by hyperkalemia associated with irradiation and storage.[50]

Blood components containing lymphocytes that are homozygous for an HLA haplotype that is shared with the recipient, whether immunocompromised or immunocompetent, pose a specific risk for TA-GVHD. This circumstance occurs when first- and second-degree relatives serve as directed donors[7, 8, 32, 34] and when HLA-matched platelet components donated by related or unrelated individuals are transfused.[51, 52]

Irradiation of blood components must be performed in these situations.

Platelet components that have low levels of leukocytes because of their collection through the apheresis process or leukofiltration, or both, should also be irradiated if intended for transfusion to susceptible patients because the minimum number of T lymphocytes that induces TA-GVHD has not yet been delineated.

In contrast, there is controversy about fresh frozen plasma. It is generally accepted that the freezing and thawing processes destroy the T lymphocytes that are present in such plasma. However, two brief articles have suggested that immunocompetent progenitor cells may be present in frozen/thawed plasma, and the authors recommended that frozen/thawed plasma be irradiated.[53, 54] Further studies are needed to validate these findings and to assess whether the number of immunocompetent cells that may be present in thawed fresh frozen plasma is sufficient to induce GVHD. In the rare instances in which nonfrozen plasma (termed *fresh plasma)* is transfused, it should be irradiated because of the presence of a sizable number of viable lymphocytes, approximately 1×10^7 cells, in a component prepared from a unit of whole blood.

■ Storage of Red Blood Cells and Platelets after Irradiation

Red Blood Cells

Irradiation of RBCs is not a benign process. The viability in vivo of irradiated RBCs, evaluated as the 24-hour recovery, is reduced during storage compared with that of nonirradiated RBCs.[55–59] This reduced viability has raised questions concerning the maximum storage time for RBCs after irradiation. Davey and colleagues[55] found that the 24-hour recovery for RBCs preserved in a solution containing adenine, sodium chloride, dextrose, and mannitol (Adsol) and treated with 300 cGy on day 0 was $68.5 \pm 8.1\%$ (mean ± standard deviation [SD]) after 42 days of storage compared with $78.4 \pm 7.1\%$ for control, nontreated RBCs. Subsequent studies employed total storage periods of 21 to 35 days after irradiation on day 0 or day 1. After storage for 35 days, the mean (± SD) 24-hour recovery for irradiated (3000 cGy) and control Adsol-preserved RBCs was $78.0 \pm 6.8\%$ and $81.8 \pm 4.4\%$, respectively. In studies with a 28-day storage period, the values for irradiated (2500 cGy) and control Adsol-preserved RBCs were $78.6 \pm 5.9\%$ and $84.2 \pm 5.1\%$, respectively.[57] With Nutricel-preserved RBCs treated with 2000 cGy on day 1, mean 24-hour recoveries for control and irradiated RBCs were 90.4% and 82.7% after 21 days of storage and 85.0% and 80.7% after 28 days of storage.[58]

Moroff and colleagues[59] evaluated the effect of irradiation on Adsol-preserved RBCs stored from day 1 to 28 (irradiated day 1, protocol 1), day 14 to 28 (irradiated day 14, protocol 2), day 14 to 42 (irradiated day 14, protocol 3), and day 26 to 28 (irradiated day 26, protocol 4). In comparison with previous investigations, this study was unique because RBCs were studied after being irradiated for various times in storage and then studied after further storage. For protocol 1 the mean ± SD recovery was $84.2 \pm 5.1\%$ for control RBCs and $78.6 \pm 5.9\%$ for irradiated RBCs ($n = 16$; $p < .01$). With protocol 3, the recoveries were $76.3 \pm 7.0\%$ for control RBCs and $69.5 \pm 8.6\%$ for irradiated RBCs ($n = 16$; $p < .01$). Protocols 2 and 4 demonstrated comparable 24-hour recoveries for control and irradiated RBCs. Long-term survival was comparable for control and irradiated RBCs in all protocols, confirming previous data showing that the long-term survival of RBCs is minimally influenced by irradiation. On the basis of multiple linear regression analysis, only the length of storage after irradiation had a significant effect on the 24-hour recovery. No effect was observed with day of irradiation or total storage time.

In another study by Moroff and colleagues,[59] in vitro RBC properties such as adenosine triphosphate (ATP) levels and the amount of hemolysis were altered to only a small extent compared with control values with extended storage after irradiation, but potassium leakage from the RBCs during storage was substantially enhanced by irradiation.[36, 40, 46, 47] Despite elevated potassium levels, the irradiation-induced changes in RBC viability and potassium leakage were not complementary. On the basis of analysis of these studies, the FDA guidelines call for a 28-day maximum storage period for RBCs after irradiation, irrespective of the day of storage on which the treatment was performed, with the provison that the total storage time cannot exceed that for nonirradiated RBCs.

Platelets

In contrast to RBCs, platelets appear to be unaffected by irradiation. The storage period at 20 to 24°C for irradiated platelet components does not need to be modified. Both in vitro and in vivo platelet properties are not influenced to any extent by irradiation. Many studies have confirmed that platelet properties are retained immediately after conventional levels of irradiation and at the conclusion of a 5-day storage period, whether irradiation is performed before storage or in the middle of storage.[60–67] One report indicated some differences in selected in vitro parameters between irradiated and control platelets after storage.[66]

■ Selection of Radiation Dose

In the past, there were no standards pertaining to the dose of radiation that should be used. A survey in 1989 indicated that a range of irradiation dose levels between 1500 and 5000 cGy (1 rad = 1 cGy) were being used, with the majority of facilities employing 1500 cGy.[68] These reported irradiation doses were for the most part estimates and retrospective calculations because most facilities were not performing any type of dosimetry measurement. Furthermore, such values may be different from current values determined through dose mapping because there was no standardized way of calculating or reporting irradiation dose. The selection of 1500 cGy as the target irradiation dose was based on studies in the 1970s that showed that 500 cGy abrogated the mixed lymphocyte response of isolated lymphocytes.[69–71]

Later studies from our laboratory with a more sensitive limiting dilution assay (LDA) indicated that 2500 cGy (measured at the internal midplane of a component) is the most appropriate dose.[72, 73] In these experiments, RBC and platelet components were irradiated in their original plastic containers (blood bags) with increasing doses of radiation. Our laboratory selected LDA as a tool to study the effect of gamma irradiation for several reasons. LDA measures the clonogenic potential of both CD4+ and CD8+ T cells in a functional assay. It provides a quantification at low T-cell numbers. It has been used to determine residual, functional T cells in bone marrows purged of T cells, thus providing a clinical correlate of prevention of GVHD.[74] Assays of T-cell proliferation using mixed lymphocyte culture (MLC) or mitogens or detection of T cells by flow cytometry can detect up to a two logarithm (log) reduction. PCR techniques are capable of detecting up to a six log reduction but cannot distinguish between viable and nonviable cells and hence are not informative if cells are inactivated. The LDA assay may fail to detect an as yet undescribed human T-cell subset that contributes to GVHD, but despite this limitation we believe our work has contributed significantly to the selection of irradiation doses for plateletpheresis and RBC components to abrogate TA-GVHD.

In our studies, after each irradiation dose, the LDA samples were removed and the clonogenic proliferation of T lymphocytes was measured. With RBC units, 500 cGy had a minimal influence, whereas 1500 cGy inactivated T-lymphocyte proliferation by approximately four logs; however, some growth was still observed in each experiment. Increasing the dose to 2000 cGy resulted in no T-lymphocyte proliferation in all but one experiment. No growth was observed after 2500 cGy.[72] In a subsequent study using plateletpheresis components with sufficient T lymphocytes to perform the LDA, the influence of 1500 and 2500 cGy was evaluated.[73] With 1500 cGy, substantial inactivation was measured; however, some growth was still observed in all experiments. As noted with the RBC experiments, 2500 cGy resulted in complete abrogation of clonogenic T-lymphocyte proliferation. Another laboratory used more traditional assay methods to assess T-lymphocyte inactivation and recommended an irradiation dose of 2800 to 3000 cGy.[75] The FDA has recommended that the irradiation process should deliver 2500 cGy to the internal midplane of a freestanding irradiation instrument canister, with a minimum of 1500 cGy at any other point within the canister.[75]

◼ Quality Assurance Measures

One must document that the instrument being used for irradiation is operating appropriately and confirm that blood components have been irradiated. To ensure that the irradiation process is being conducted correctly, specific procedures are recommended for free-standing irradiators and linear accelerators, which are summarized in Table 21.4 and discussed in detail in a review article.[76]

Dose mapping measures the delivery of radiation within a simulated blood component or over an area in which a blood component is placed. This applies to an irradiation field when a linear accelerator is used or to the canister of a freestanding irradiator. Dose mapping is the primary means of ensuring that the irradiation process is being conducted correctly. It documents that the intended dose of irradiation is being delivered at a specific location (such as the central midplane of a canister), and it describes the variation of the delivered irradiation dose within a simulated component or over a given area. This allows conclusions to be drawn about the maximum and minimum doses being delivered. Dose mapping should be performed with sensitive dosimetry techniques. A number of commercially available systems have been developed.

Other quality assurance measures include the routine confirmation that the turntable is operating correctly

Table 21.4   Quality Assurance Guidelines for Irradiating Blood Components

Dose
  2500 cGy to the central midplane of a canister (freestanding irradiator) or to the center of an irradiation field (linear accelerator) with a minimum of 1500 cGy

Dose mapping (freestanding irradiators)
  Routinely, once a year (^{137}Cs) or twice a year (^{60}Co) and after major repairs; using a fully filled canister (water/plastic) with a dosimetry system to map the distribution of the absorbed dose

Dose mapping (linear accelerators)
  Recommend yearly dose mapping with an ionization chamber and a water phantom; more frequent evaluation of instrument conditions to ensure consistency of x-rays.

Correction for radioisotopic decay
  With ^{137}Cs as the source, annually
  With ^{60}Co as the source, quarterly

Turntable rotation (freestanding ^{137}Cs irradiators)
  Daily verification

Storage time for red blood cells after irradiation
  For up to 28 days; total storage time cannot exceed maximum storage time for unirradiated red blood cells

Storage time for platelets after irradiation
  No change related to irradiation procedure

Adapted from Moroff G, Luban NLC: The irradiation of blood and blood components to prevent graft-versus-host disease: technical issues and guidelines. Transfus Med Rev 1997;11:15–26.

(for ^{137}Cs irradiators), measurements to ensure that the timing device is accurate, and periodic lengthening of the irradiation time to correct for source decay. With linear accelerators, it is necessary to measure the characteristics of the x-ray beam to ensure consistency of delivery. Confirming that a blood component has, in actuality, been irradiated is also an important part of a quality assurance program. Several firms have developed indicator labels for this purpose.

◼ Dose Mapping with Freestanding Irradiators

For freestanding irradiators, a dose-mapping procedure measures the dose delivered throughout the circular canister in which the blood component is placed. To establish a two-dimensional map, a dosimetry system is placed in a canister that is completely filled with a blood/tissue-compatible phantom composed of water or an appropriate plastic such as polystyrene.[77, 78] The dosimetry material is placed within the phantom in a predetermined way. This approach provides data showing the minimum levels of radiation that would be absorbed by a blood component placed in the canister and recognizes that maximum attenuation occurs when the canister is completely filled with a blood-compatible material. The absorbed dose at the central midplane of a canister (i.e., at the center point) may be decreased by 25% (from 3100 to 2500 cGy) in a [137]CS irradiator (JL Shepherd and Associates, San Francisco, CA) when the loading of the canister is changed from 0% (air) to 100% (with blood components).[79] An irradiation-sensitive film dosimetry system (International Specialty Products) was used in this study.

Other studies have shown that the variability in the dose delivered to the interior of simulated blood units (water or saline in plastic blood storage containers) depended on the model of the ^{137}Cs freestanding irradiator.[80, 81] An immobilized grid of thermoluminescent dosimeters in a plastic sheet was placed within the simulated blood units to measure dose delivery. A spacer in the bottom of the canister increased the minimum level of radiation within the simulated blood units, as expected from the results of full-canister dose mapping involving a phantom.[81] The variability with ^{137}Cs irradiation is influenced by a number of factors, including the blood-compatible environment. Cumulatively, these studies underscore the need for consistency in loading the canister.

When an irradiator is purchased, the distributor provides a central dose level that is determined in a blood-compatible environment. In the 1970s and 1980s, manufacturers provided a central dose that was determined in air, resulting in the use of timer settings that provided a dose level somewhat less than was expected. Since the issuing of the FDA guidelines in July 1993[75] and the use of dose mapping, it has been necessary to readjust irradiation times with some instruments because the attenuation effect had not been considered previously.

The dose map can also be used to assess whether the turntable of a ^{137}Cs irradiator is rotating in an appropriate manner. The occurrence of comparable readings at the two edges of the two-dimensional map, as depicted in the theoretical dose map, indicates that the canister is rotating evenly in front of the ^{137}Cs source. If the turntable were not rotating, the dose levels at the edge of the map closest to the source would be much higher than those on the opposite edge, that is, the side farthest from the source.

■ Dosimetry Systems in Use

The radiation dose delivered can be measured by a variety of dosimetry systems. Several commercial systems have been introduced to the market; each system consists of a phantom that fills the canister and a sensitive dosimeter. These dosimeters are referred to as routine dosimeters. They are calibrated against standard systems, usually at national reference laboratories such as the National Institute of Standards and Technology in the United States. The routine dosimeter measurement systems were initially developed for use with irradiators because this is the predominant irradiation source for blood. Subsequently, they were also developed for use with ^{60}Co irradiators.

Thermoluminescent dosimeters (TLD chips) are one type of routine dosimeter. TLD chips are small plastic chips with millimeter dimensions having a crystal lattice that absorbs ionizing radiation. Specialized equipment is used to release and measure the energy absorbed by the TLD chip at the time of the test irradiation. In one commercially available system, chips are placed at nine different locations within a polystyrene phantom that fits into the canister for the IBL 437C irradiator (CIS US, Inc, Bedford, MA). The timer setting used routinely for an instrument is used in the test procedure.

There are two systems that use radiochromic film. On exposure to irradiation, the film darkens, resulting in an increase in optical density. The optical density, determined at various locations on the film, is linearly proportional to the absorbed radiation dose. Standard films that are irradiated at a given dose level with a calibrated source at a national reference laboratory provide the means to assess the absolute level of absorbed irradiation. This type of dosimeter is basically an x-ray film comparable with that used in clinical practice. With this device, the map that is developed identifies the absorbed radiation dose that is measured at a large number of locations.

In one system, a film contained in a thin watertight casement is placed into the canister (International Specialty Products, Wayne, NJ). This approach is being used with a variety of irradiators. The canister is filled completely with water before the irradiation procedure. This system provides a direct readout of the dose that is delivered throughout the canister. The timer setting used routinely is employed for the test procedure. In a second system, a film having different radiation-sensitive characteristics is embedded between two halves of a circular-fitting polystyrene plastic phantom (Nordion International, Kanata, Ontario, Canada). Irradiation of specialized films is performed with a number of timer settings, each larger than that used routinely. The map produced is normalized for a central midplane dose of 2500 cGy. The time to produce the 2500 cGy is predetermined with a different dosimeter system, the Fricke system, in which absorbed radiation causes a change in the state of an iron salt that can be assessed spectrophotometrically.

Another approach to irradiation dose mapping employs a solid-state electronic dosimeter that is technically referred to as a metal oxide semiconductor field effect transistor (MOSFET). A board contains a number of small transistors in an arrangement that provides data for a dose map. The board is placed between two halves of a circular polystyrene phantom that fits into the canister. This dosimeter absorbs and stores the radiation dose imparted to it electronically. The radiation causes the formation of holes in the metal oxide layer that become trapped within the transistor. The magnitude of the holes is evaluated by measuring the voltage across the transistor with a voltmeter. The voltages measured are converted to absorbed dose.

With each dosimetry system, measurements are used to express the absorbed radiation dose of grays (or centigrays). All dosimetry measurements are associated with a degree of uncertainty or possible error. The magnitude of the uncertainty depends on the kind of dosimeter used. For most dosimeters, the level is ±5% of the measured value. For a central absorbed dose level of 2560 cGy (see theoretical dose map in Fig. 21.3), the value could be as high as 2788 cGy or as low as 2432 cGy. Correspondingly, a measured value of 2400 cGy could be as high as 2520 cGy or as low as 2380 cGy. Because the measured value could in actuality meet the 2500 cGy standard, it is appropriate to accept a value of 2400 cGy as meeting the current standard. The same approach should be used when evaluating the minimum value on a dose map. Albeit arbitrary and cautious, the actual minimum on an irradiation dose map should not be below 1500 cGy.

■ Other Measures with Freestanding Irradiators

Correction for Isotopic Decay

It is important to lengthen the time of irradiation periodically to correct for decay of the isotopic source that emits the gamma irradiation. Previously, this was the only major quality assurance measure that was performed routinely. With the half-life of ^{137}Cs of 30 years, annual lengthening of the timer setting is appropriate. On the other hand, with the half-life of ^{60}Co of only 5 years, the time of irradiation should be increased on a quarterly basis. The additional seconds of irradiation that are needed can be calculated using formulas that

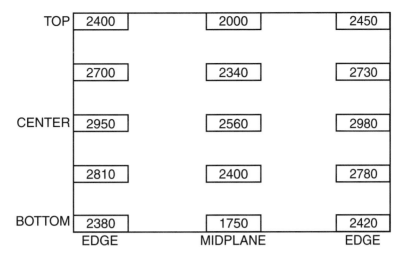

Figure 21.3   Two-dimensional dose map showing the irradiation dose distribution through a fully filled canister of a freestanding cesium 137 irradiator.

can be found in a physics textbook. Alternatively, distributors of irradiators provide a chart that specifies the appropriate setting as a function of calendar time.

Turntable Rotation

For ^{137}Cs irradiators, it is essential that the turntable operates at a constant speed in a circular pattern to ensure that all parts of a blood component are exposed equally to the source. Daily verification of turntable rotation is an appropriate quality assurance measure. With some free-standing irradiator models, rotation of the turntable can be observed before the door of the compartment in which the canister is positioned is closed. In other models, it can be observed only indirectly by ensuring that an indicator light is operating appropriately. With some older models, there have been occasional reports that the turntable failed to rotate because of mechanical problems. Such problems should not be encountered with the newer models because of changes in the turntable mechanisms.

Assessing Radioactivity Leakage

Irradiators are constructed so that the isotopic sources are contained in a chamber heavily lined with a protective lead shield to prevent leakage of radioactivity. Accordingly, gamma irradiators are considered to be very safe instruments. Although there have been no reports of source leakage of radioactivity, periodic measurements are warranted. Attaching a film badge to the outside of the irradiator, using a Geiger counter periodically, and performing a wipe test of the inside of the chamber where the canister is positioned at least semiannually are measures that are being used.

■ Dose Mapping with Linear Accelerators

Linear accelerators that are used to provide radiation therapy are carefully monitored to ensure appropriateness of dose to an irradiation field. When blood components are treated with x-rays, the instrument settings are different from those used to treat oncology patients. Hence, additional periodic quality control measures, primarily to assess the dose delivered to blood components, are needed to ensure that linear accelerators are being operated appropriately when used for blood irradiation.

Currently, there are no commercially available systems for assessing the dose delivered throughout the area of an irradiation field in which blood components are placed for treatment with x-rays. An ideal dosimeter for this purpose would be made of a tissue-compatible plastic phantom containing appropriate dosimeter material and a covering that could be placed at the appropriate distance from the source. An alternative approach might involve use of a blood bag filled with water (simulating a blood unit) containing TLD chips, as described earlier. In comparative studies using such simulated blood units, it was determined that radiation delivery was more uniform with linear accelerators than with ^{137}Cs freestanding irradiators.[80] This uniformity reflects the relative homogeneity of x-ray beams.

In the absence of an available system modified for the irradiation of blood bags, the dose delivered throughout an irradiation field should be mapped with the dosimetric measuring system known as an ionization chamber. The ionization chamber is used to calibrate linear accelerators for use with patients. In addition, on a yearly basis, dose mapping should be performed using a tissue-compatible phantom. In view of the widely divergent conditions that are used during the operation of linear accelerators, other parameters pertaining to the x-ray beam should be evaluated on at least a quarterly basis to provide assurance that the instrument is being used appropriately for the irradiation of blood components. The goal is to ensure that the instrument is being set in a consistent fashion.

When setting a linear accelerator for blood component irradiation, the following should be measured: (1) the distance between the x-ray source and the position where the blood components are to be placed, (2) consistency of the strength of the x-ray beam, and (3) the intensity of the x-ray beam. The distance between the source and position on the table where blood components will be placed (referred to as the target) can be evaluated easily with a calibrated measuring device. This is a simple task that can be performed routinely. The consistency of beam output can be evaluated by measuring the beam current. Beam intensity can be evaluated by measuring the ionization current in a monitoring ionization chamber array, which can be expressed in terms of the number of photons delivered per square centimeter. These parameters should be assessed routinely as part of quality control programs used by radiation physicists. A code of blood practice was published in 1994 by the Radiation Therapy Committee of the American Association of Physicists in Medicine for the quality control of radiotherapy accelerators.[82, 83]

Confirming That Irradiation Occurred

It is important to have positive confirmation that the irradiation process has taken place. The process would not take place if an operator failed to initiate the electronically controlled irradiation process or there was an instrumentation malfunction. A radiation-sensitive indicator label has been developed specifically for this purpose (International Specialty Products, Wayne, NJ). The label containing a radiation-sensitive film strip is placed on the external surface of the blood component. Irradiation causes distinct visually observable changes. The appearance changes from clear red to opaque with obliteration of the word "NOT." When the label is placed on a blood component, there is a visual record that the irradiation process took place. The reliability of this type of indicator has been documented in a multisite study.[84]

Two versions of the indicator label have been manufactured. They differ the range of radiation needed to cause a change in the radiation-sensitive film. The ratings for these indicators are 1500 and 2500 cGy. The ratings serve as an approximate guideline for the amount of absorbed radiation needed to change the window completely from reddish to opaque with complete obliteration of the word NOT. Because the indicator labels are designed and used to confirm that the irradiation process has occurred, our laboratory utilizes the 1500 cGy label as the most appropriate tool to perform this quality control measure. This is based on the routinely observed pattern of dose distribution to a blood component in a canister of a freestanding irradiator. Despite a targeted central dose of 2500 cGy, there are spots at which the dose is less. If the theoretical dose map presented in Figure 21.3 is used as an example, there is a spot that receives only 1800 cGy. If the label rated 2500 cGy was located on the external surface of a component, there might be minimal changes in the appearance of the radiation-sensitive film window. This would result in a judgment that the blood component was not irradiated when in actuality it was treated satisfactorily.

New Methods

Photochemical treatment (PCT) using psoralens and long-wavelength UV irradiation (UVA) have been developed to reduce the risks of bacterial and viral contaminants of platelet transfusions. Psoralens bind reversibly to nucleic acids by intercalation and, after UVA illumination, form covalent monoadducts and cross-links with RNA and DNA. The process modifies bacterial and viral genomes sufficiently to permit replication. Among a broad group of compounds, the psoralen S-59 has been shown to be particularly effective in inactivating bacteria and viruses without adversely affecting platelet function in vitro and in vivo.[85] Clinical trials are under way to confirm adequate in vivo survival and lack of adverse effects and equivalence (L. Corash, personal communication).

The use of S-59 and PCT has been studied for possible inactivation of leukocytes in platelet concentrates.[86, 87] PCT inactivation of T cells was evaluated with four assay systems. These included T-cell quantitation, inhibition of cytokine synthesis, modification of leukocyte genomic DNA by quantification of psoralen-DNA adducts, and inhibition of replication of T cells using PCR amplification of genomic DNA sequences. This work built on previous studies in which IL-8, a marker of cytokine generation in platelet concentrates, was significantly reduced in pools treated with PCT compared with those treated with irradiation.[86]

A more detailed study by Grass and coworkers[87] compared PCT with irradiation at 2500 cGy; cytokine synthesis was not inhibited and induction of DNA strand breaking was inhibited less than with S-59 and PCT. LDA was used to confirm inactivation of T cells in the platelet concentrates. The efficacy of S-59 and PCT was further supported by a study of transfusion-induced GVHD in a murine F1 hybrid model.[88] No GVHD was noted in mice receiving splenocytes treated with either 2500 cGy or S-59 at 150 μmol/L and UVA at 2.1 J/cm. Another set of experiments was performed to study the use of PCT to prevent GVHD in an immunocompromised mouse model.[89] Taken together, these studies suggest that PCT may well be an alternative to irradiation and may provide a mechanism to prevent an increase in cytokine concentration in platelet concentrates. The limitation of PCT methodology is the need for UVA penetration, which is not currently possible with RBC products.

REFERENCES

1. von Fliedner V, Higby DJ, Kim U: Graft-versus-host reaction following blood product transfusion. Am J Med 1972;72:951–961.
2. Anderson KC, Weinstein HJ: Transfusion-associated graft-versus-host disease. N Engl J Med 1990;323:315–321.
3. Webb IJ, Anderson KC: Transfusion-associated graft-versus-host disease. In Anderson KC, Ness PM (eds): Scientific Basis of Transfusion Medicine. Philadelphia, WB Saunders, 2000, pp 420–425.
4. Linden JV, Pisciotto PT: Transfusion-associated graft-versus-host disease and blood irradiation. Transfus Med Rev 1992;6:116–123.
5. Ohto H, Anderson KC: Survey of transfusion-associated graft-versus-host disease in immunocompetent recipients. Transfus Med Rev 1996;10:31–43.
6. Ferrera JM, Krenger W: Graft-versus-host disease. The influence of type 1 and type 2 T cell cytokines. Transfus Med Rev 1998;12:1–17.
7. McMilan KD, Johnson RL: HLA-homozygosity and the risk of related-donor transfusion-associated graft-versus-host disease. Transfus Med Rev 1993;7:37–41.
8. Petz LD, Calhoun L, Yam P, et al: Transfusion-associated graft-versus-host disease in immunocompetent patients: report of a fatal case associated with transfusion of blood from a second-degree relative, and a survey of predisposing factors. Transfusion 1993;33:742–750.
9. Worrall NK, Lazenby WD, Misko TP, et al: Modulation of in vivo alloreactivity by inhibition of inducible nitric oxide synthetase. J Exp Med 1995;181:63–70.
10. Fast LD, Valeri CR, Crowley JP: Immune responses to major histocompatibility complex homozygous lymphoid cells in murine F1 hybrid recipients: implications for transfusion-associated graft-versus-host disease. Blood 1995;86:3090–3096.
11. Nishimura M, Uchida S, Mitsunaga S, et al: Characterization of T-cell clones derived from peripheral blood lymphocytes of a patient with transfusion-associated graft-versus-host disease: FAS-mediated killing by CD4+ and CD8+ cytotoxic T-cell clones and tumor necrosis factor beta production by CD4+ T-cell clones. Blood 1997;89:1440–1445.
12. Ammann AJ: Hypothesis: absence of graft-versus-host disease in AIDS is a consequence of HIV-1 infection of CD4+ T cells. J Acquir Immune Defic Syndr 1993;6:1224–1227.
13. Klein C, Fraitag S, Foulon E, et al: Moderate and transient transfusion-associated cutaneous graft versus host disease in a child infected by human immunodeficiency virus. Am J Med 1996;101:445–446.

14. Brubaker DB: Immunopathogenic mechanisms of post-transfusion graft versus host disease. Proc Soc Exp Biol Med 1993;202:122–147.
15. Blundell EL, Pamphilon DH, Anderson NA, et al: Transfusion-associated graft-versus-host disease, monoclonal gammopathy and PCR. Br J Haematol 1992;82:622–623.
16. Capon SM, DePond WD, Tyan DB, et al: Transfusion associated graft-versus-host disease in an immunocompetent patient. Ann Intern Med 1991;114:1025–1026.
17. Drobyski W, Thibodeau S, Truitt RL, et al: Third-party–mediated graft rejection and graft-versus-host disease after T-cell–depleted bone marrow transplantation, as demonstrated by hypervariable DNA probes and HLA-DR polymorphism. Blood 1989;74:2285–2294.
18. Kunstmann E, Bocker T, Roewer L, et al: Diagnosis of transfusion-associated graft versus-host disease by genetic fingerprinting and polymerase chain reaction. Transfusion 1992;32:766–770.
19. Depalma L, Bahrami KR, Kapur S, et al: Amplified fragment length polymorphism analysis in the evaluation of post-transfusion graft versus host disease. J Thorac Cardiovasc Surg 1994;108:182–184.
20. Wang L, Juji T, Tokunaga K, et al: Polymorphic microsatellite markers for the diagnosis of graft-versus-host disease. N Engl J Med 1994;330:398–401.
21. Friedman DF, Kwittken P, Cizman B, et al: DNA-based HLA typing of nonhematopoietic tissue used to select the marrow transplant donor for successful treatment of transfusion-associated graft-versus-host disease. Clin Diagn Lab Immunol 1994;1:590–596.
22. Lee TH, Donegan E, Slichter S, Busch MP: Transient increase in circulating donor leukocytes after allogeneic transfusions in immunocompetent recipients compatible with donor cell proliferation. Blood 1996;85:1207–1214.
23. Lee TH, Paglieroni T, Ohto H, et al: Survival of donor leukocyte subpopulations in immunocompetent transfusion recipients: frequent long term microchimerism in severe trauma patients. Blood 1999;93:3127–3139.
24. Wang-Rodriguez J, Fry E, Fiebig E, et al: Immune response to blood transfusion in very-low-birthweight infants. Transfusion 2000;40:25–34.
25. Vietor HE, Hallensleben E, van Bree SP, et al: Survival of donor cells 25 years after intrauterine transfusion. Blood 2000;95:2709–2714.
26. Reed WF, Lee TH, Trachlenberg E, et al: Detection of microchimerism by PCR as a function of amplification strategy. Transfusion 2001;41:39–44.
27. Nelson J, Furst D, Maloney S, et al: Microchimerism and HLA compatible relationships of pregnancy in scleroderma. Lancet 1998;351:559–562.
28. Arlett CM, Smith JB, Jimenez SA: Identification of fetal DNA and cells in skin lesions from women with systemic sclerosis. N Engl J Med 1998;333:1186–1191.
29. Evans PC, Lambert N, Maloney S, et al: Long-term fetal microchimerism in peripheral blood mononuclear cell subsets in healthy women and women with scleroderma. Blood 1999;93:2033–2037.
30. Daya S, Gunby J, Clark DA: Intravenous immunoglobulin therapy for recurrent spontaneous abortion: a meta-analysis. Am J Reprod Immunol 1998;39:69–76.
31. Williamson LM, Warwick RM: Transfusion-associated graft-versus-host disease and its prevention. Blood Rev 1995;9:251–261.
32. Kanter MH: Transfusion-associated graft-versus-host disease: do transfusions from second-degree relatives pose a greater risk than those from first-degree relatives? Transfusion 1992;32:323–327.
33. Luban NL, DePalma L: Transfusion-associated graft-versus-host disease in the neonate--expanding the spectrum of disease [editorial]. Transfusion 1996;36:101–103.
34. Ohto H, Anderson KC: Post-transfusion graft-versus-host disease in Japanese newborns. Transfusion 1996;36:117–123.
35. Shlomchik WD, Couzens MS, Tang CB, et al: Prevention of graft versus host disease by inactivation of host antigen-presenting cells. Science 1999;285:412–415.
36. Davey RJ: The effect of irradiation on blood components. In Baldwin ML, Jefferies LC (eds): Irradiation of Blood Components. Bethesda, Md, American Association of Blood Banks, 1992, pp 51–62.
37. Fearon TC, Luban NLC: Practical dosimetric aspects of blood and blood product irradiation. Transfusion 1986;26:457–459.
38. Korngold R: Biology of graft-versus-host disease. Am J Pediatr Hematol Oncol 1993;15:18–37.
39. Suda BA, Leitman SF, Davey RJ: Characteristics of red cells irradiated and subsequently frozen for long term storage. Transfusion 1993;33:389–392.
40. Miraglia CC, Anderson G, Mintz PD: Effect of freezing on the in vivo recovery of irradiated red cells. Transfusion 1994;34:775–778.
41. Crowley JP, Skrabut EM, Valeri CR: Immunocompetent lymphocytes in previously frozen washed red cells. Vox Sang 1974;26:513–517.
42. Akahoshi M, Takanashi M, Masuda M, et al: A case of transfusion-associated graft-versus-host disease not prevented by white cell-reduction filters. Transfusion 1992;32:169–172.
43. Heim MU, Munker R, Sauer H, et al: Graft-versus-host Krankheit (GVH mit letalem ausgang nach der gabe von gefilterten erythrozytenkonzentraten). Infusionstherapie 1991;18:8–9.
44. Hayashi H, Nishiuchi T, Tamura H, et al: Transfusion associated graft-versus-host disease caused by leukocyte filtered stored blood. Anesthesiology 1993;79:1419–1421.
45. Anderson KC: Leukodepleted cellular blood components for prevention of transfusion-associated graft-versus-host disease. Transfus Sci 1995;16:265–268.
46. Ramirez AM, Woodfield DG, Scott R, et al: High potassium levels in stored irradiated blood. Transfusion 1987;27:444–445.
47. Rivet C, Baxter A, Rock G: Potassium levels in irradiated blood. Transfusion 1989;29:185.
48. Swann ID, Williamson LM: Potassium loss from leukodepleted red cells following γ–irradiation. Vox Sang 1996;70:117–118.
49. Strauss RG: Routine washing of irradiated red cells before transfusion seems unwarranted. Transfusion 1990;30:675–677.
50. Luban NLC, Strauss RG, Hume HA: Commentary on the safety of red cells preserved in extended-storage media for neonatal transfusion. Transfusion 1991;31:229–235.
51. Benson K, Marks AR, Marshall MJ, et al: Fatal graft-versus-host disease associated with transfusions of HLA-matched, HLA-homozygous platelets from unrelated donors. Transfusion 1994;34:432–437.
52. Grishaber JE, Birney SM, Strauss RG: Potential for host transfusion-associated graft-versus-host disease due to apheresis platelets matched for HLA class I antigens. Transfusion 1993;33:910–914.
53. Wielding JU, Vehmeyer K, Dittman J, et al: Contamination of fresh-frozen plasma with viable white cells and proliferable stem cells [letter]. Transfusion 1994;34:185–186.
54. Bernvill SS, Abdulatiff M, Al-Sedairy S, et al: Fresh frozen plasma contains viable progenitor cells--should we irradiate [letter]? Vox Sang 1994;67:405.
55. Davey RJ, McCoy NC, Yu M, et al: The effect of pre-storage irradiation on post-transfusion red cell survival. Transfusion 1992;32:525–528.
56. Mintz PD, Anderson G: Effect of gamma irradiation on the in vivo recovery of stored red blood cells. Ann Clin Lab Sci 1993;23:216–220.
57. Moroff G, Holme S, Heaton A, et al: Effect of gamma irradiation on viability of AS-1 red cells [abstract]. Transfusion 1992;32(Suppl):70S.
58. Friedman KD, McDonough WC, Cimino DF: The effect of pre-storage gamma irradiation on post-transfusion red blood cell recovery [abstract]. Transfusion 1991;31:50S.
59. Moroff G, Holme S, AuBuchon JP, et al: Viability and in vitro properties of AS-1 red cells after gamma irradiation. Transfusion 1999;39:128–134.
60. Moroff G, George VM, Siegl AM, et al: The influence of irradiation on stored platelets. Transfusion 1986;26:453–456.
61. Espersen GT, Ernst E, Christiansen OB, et al: Irradiated blood platelet concentrates stored for five days--evaluation by in vitro tests. Vox Sang 1988;55:218–221.
62. Duguid JK, Carr R, Jenkins JA, et al: Clinical evaluation of the effects of storage time and irradiation on transfused platelets. Vox Sang 1991;60:151–154.
63. Read EJ, Kodis C, Carter CS, et al: Viability of platelets following storage in the irradiated state. A paired-controlled study. Transfusion 1988;28:446–450.
64. Rock G, Adams GA, Labow RS: The effects of irradiation on platelet function. Transfusion 1988;28:451–455.
65. Sweeney JD, Holme S, Moroff G: Storage of apheresis platelets after gamma irradiation. Transfusion 1994;34:779–783.
66. Seghatchian MJ, Stivala JFA: Effect of 25 Gy gamma irradiation on storage stability of three types of platelet concentrates: a comparative analysis with paired controls and random preparation. Transfus Sci 1995;16:121–129.
67. Bessos H, Atkinson A, Murphy WG, et al: A comparison of in vitro storage markers between gamma-irradiated and non-irradiated apheresis platelet concentrates. Transfus Sci 1995;16:131–134.
68. Anderson KC, Goodnough LT, Sayers M, et al: Variation in blood component irradiation practice: implications for prevention of

transfusion-associated graft-versus-host disease. Blood 1991;77:2096–2102.

69. Sprent J, Anderson RE, Miller JF: Radiosensitivity of T and B lymphocytes. II. Effect of irradiation on response of T cells to alloantigens. Eur J Immunol 1974;4:204–210.

70. Valerius NH, Johansen KS, Nielsen OS, et al: Effect of in vitro x-irradiation on lymphocyte and granulocyte function. Scand J Hematol 1981;27:9–18.

71. Rosen NR, Weidner JG, Bold HD, et al: Prevention of transfusion-associated graft-versus-host disease: selection of an adequate dose of gamma irradiation. Transfusion 1993;33:125–127.

72. Pelszynski MM, Moroff G, Luban NLC, et al: Effect of γ-irradiation of red blood cell units on T-cell inactivation as assessed by limiting dilution analysis: implications for preventing transfusion-associated graft-versus-host disease. Blood 1994;83:1683–1689.

73. Luban NLC, Drothler D, Moroff G, et al: Irradiation of platelet components: inhibition of lymphocyte proliferation assessed by limiting dilution analysis. Transfusion 2000;40:348–352.

74. Quinones RR, Gutierrez RH, Dinndorf PA, et al: Extended cycle elutriation to adjust T-cell content in HLA-disparate bone marrow transplantation. Blood 1993;82:307–317.

75. Center for Biologics Evaluation and Research, Food and Drug Administration: Recommendations Regarding License Amendments and Procedures for Gamma Irradiation of Blood Products. Bethesda, Md, Department of Health and Human Services, July 22, 1993.

76. Moroff G, Luban NL: The irradiation of blood and blood components to prevent graft-versus-host disease: technical issues and guidelines. Transfus Med Rev 1997;11:15–26.

77. Masterson ME, Febo R: Pre-transfusion blood irradiation: clinical rationale and dosimetric considerations. Med Phys 1992;19:649–657.

78. Leitman SF: Dose, dosimetry and quality improvements of irradiated blood components [editorial]. Transfusion 1993;33:447–449.

79. Perkins JT, Papoulias SA: The effect of loading conditions on dose distribution within a blood irradiator [abstract]. Transfusion 1994;34:75S.

80. Moroff G, Luban NLC, Wolf L, et al: Dosimetry measurements after gamma irradiation with cesium-137 and linear acceleration sources [abstract]. Transfusion 1993;33:52S.

81. Luban NLC, Fearon T, Leitman SF, et al: Absorption of gamma irradiation in simulated blood components using cesium irradiators [abstract]. Transfusion 1995;35:63S.

82. Kutcher GJ, Coia L, Gillin M, et al: Comprehensive QA for radiation oncology: report of AAPM Radiation Therapy Committee Task Group 40. Med Phys 1994;21:581–618.

83. Nath R, Biggs PJ, Bova FJ, et al: AAPM code of practice for radiotherapy accelerators: report of AAPM Radiation Therapy Task Group No. 45. Med Phys 1994;21:1093–1121.

84. Leitman SF, Silberstein L, Fairman RM, et al: Use of a radiation-sensitive film label in the quality control of irradiated blood components [abstract]. Transfusion 1992;32:4S.

85. Lin L, Cook DN, Wiesehahn GP, et al: Photochemical inactivation of viruses and bacteria in human platelet concentrates using a novel psoralen and long wavelength UV light. Transfusion 1997;37:423–435.

86. Hei DJ, Grass J, Lin L, et al: Elimination of cytokine production in stored platelet concentrate aliquots by photochemical treatment with psoralen plus ultraviolet A light. Transfusion 1999;39:239–248.

87. Grass JA, Hei DJ, Metchette K, et al: Inactivation of leukocytes in platelet concentrates by psoralen plus UVA. Blood 1998;91:2180–2188.

88. Grass JA, Wafa T, Reames A, et al: Prevention of transfusion-associated graft-versus-host disease by photochemical treatment. Blood 1999;93:3140–3147.

89. Grass J, Delmonte J, Wages D, et al: Prevention of transfusion-associated graft vs. host disease (TA-GVHD) in immunocompromised mice by photochemical treatment (PCT) of donor T cells. Blood 1997;90(Suppl 1):207a.

Chapter 22

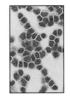

Blood Substitutes

Robert M. Winslow

Replacement of blood after acute loss has two main goals: restitution of blood volume and delivery of oxygen to tissues. In contrast, administration of red blood cells in chronic anemia or hypoxia is aimed only at restitution of oxygen delivery to tissues. Non–oxygen-carrying solutions such as saline, Ringer's lactate, albumin, dextran, and the starches are widely used to replace lost blood volume in surgery and trauma, and they can be used satisfactorily to expand blood volume. The term *red blood cell substitutes* usually refers to oxygen-carrying solutions that can both expand the blood volume and oxygenate tissues. These solutions contain a delivery system for oxygen, commonly modified hemoglobin or perfluorocarbon emulsions, and they are intended to carry out the primary function of red blood cells: transport of oxygen to tissues.

Development of a red blood cell substitute has been an elusive goal: for centuries, an alternative to allogeneic blood for transfusion has been sought by scientists, by the military, and by industry. Early attempts included the use of milk, wine, gum, and red blood cell hemolysates.[1] In the modern era (since about 1965), three general types of products have been under development: modified hemoglobin solutions, perfluorocarbon emulsions, and lipid vesicle-encapsulated hemoglobin. None is as yet approved for clinical use.

The current forces driving the development of red blood cell substitutes are the perceived danger of transfusion of allogeneic blood (Table 22.1), as well as the diminishing numbers of donors of allogeneic blood. In fact, blood is safer now than it ever has been. However, the aggregate risks listed in Table 22.1 are frightening to many patients, their families, and their doctors, and the demand for a safe and efficacious alternative is increasing. Beyond the risks listed in Table 22.1, in regions of the world where the frequency of human immunodeficiency virus infection is high, development of these solutions would

be particularly important. Furthermore, the risks listed in Table 22.1 are for the United States; in other parts of the world, additional risks include contamination of blood with parasites, prions, other retroviruses, tick-borne illnesses, and malaria. Bacterial infections represent a growing risk as the length of time blood can be stored is increased, because the risk of contamination is proportional to storage time.

Because of the risks of allogeneic blood transfusion, and because of the large markets that could be generated for red blood cell substitutes, considerable efforts are now being expended by industry to develop safe products. It is likely that red blood cell substitutes will find their way into clinical practice within the next decade.

■ Principles

Several major issues must be addressed to develop a successful red blood cell substitute.

Table 22.1 Pre-NAT Risks of Allogeneic Blood in the United States

Event	Risk
Human immunodeficiency virus infection	1/676,000
Human T-cell leukemia lymphoma virus I and II infection	1/641,000
Hepatitis B	1/66,000
Hepatitis C	1/125,000
Fever, chills	1/100
Hemolytic transfusion reaction	1/6,000
Fatal hemolytic transfusion reaction	1/100,000

Data from Klein HG: Oxygen carriers and transfusion medicine. Artif Cells Blood Substit Immobil Biotechnol 22:123–135, 1994; and Schreiber GB, Busch MP, Kleinman SH, Korelitz JJ: The risk of transfusion-transmitted viral infections. N Engl J Med 334:1685–1690, 1996.

1. *Oxygen transport.* Must a red blood cell substitute transport oxygen in the same way as red blood cells do? Oxygen affinity and cooperativity of cell-free or encapsulated hemoglobin may be very different from that of red blood cells. Perfluorocarbons carry oxygen physically dissolved, rather than chemically bound, and therefore the dissociation curve is linear. Whether these factors are important, physiologically or clinically, is still not known, and extensive clinical experience will be required for definite conclusions to be drawn.

2. *Plasma retention.* The normal red blood cell life span is about 120 days. However, the plasma half-life of cell-free hemoglobin may be only 12 hours, and that of encapsulated or surface-modified hemoglobin and perfluorocarbon emulsions may be 24 to 48 hours. Are these times clinically useful? If the effect of a red blood cell substitute is so short that a transfusion with allogeneic blood is only delayed, not eliminated, then the usefulness of the product becomes questionable.

3. *Efficacy.* It will be necessary to demonstrate efficacy for any red blood cell substitute to be used clinically. At present, it is taken as a matter of faith that a solution carrying oxygen will be more useful than one with no oxygen carrier, if it is without side effects. However, conclusive demonstrations will be necessary because no red blood cell substitute currently being developed is without side effects. For example, if a particular substitute increases systemic pressure and vascular resistance (as many hemoglobin-based solutions do), this property could counteract any increase in oxygen transported. At present, the United States Food and Drug Administration has accepted reduced use of allogeneic blood as a valid end-point for clinical testing and licensure, but whether this is sufficient for widespread clinical use by physicians will not be known until products are actually on the market.

4. *Toxicity.* No candidate product developed to date is without toxicity. Cell-free hemoglobin has vasoconstrictor properties that could limit its use in shock and trauma. Lipid vesicles and perfluorocarbon emulsions stimulate macrophages to elaborate cytokines that can produce diverse effects, including fever, flu-like symptoms, and thrombocytopenia.

5. *Commercial viability.* To be successful, a red blood cell substitute must be competitive with allogeneic red blood cells in effect, toxicity, and cost. The cost of providing human red blood cells for transfusion is complex and very difficult to determine with any accuracy, but it is probably in the range of $250 to $500 per unit. The technology required for the production of red blood cell substitutes is complex and possibly expensive, but the final cost of a product, whose safety and efficacy is equivalent to banked blood, will need to be in the same range.

■ Clinical Applications

Products

Hemoglobin-Based Products

The red blood cell substitute products that have gained the most attention are based on hemoglobin, an extraordinarily complex molecule consisting of four polypeptide chains, each one made up of about 140 amino acids. Normally packaged in the red blood cell, when it is free in solution it is fragile: it tends to oxidize, is unstable and toxic, and is excreted by the kidneys as the subunits dissociate. Over the years, the strategy for making a hemoglobin-based red blood cell substitute has been based on crosslinking hemoglobin to correct these problems.[1]

Hemoglobin has the desirable properties of high capacities to bind oxygen and to release it cooperatively. However, hemoglobin, free in solution, has several unique properties: (1) its oxygen affinity is high because outside the red blood cell the allosteric effectors, 2,3-diphosphoglycerate and adenosine triphosphate, for example, are not present; (2) its effectiveness as an oxygen carrier is limited because it dissociates into half-molecules (dimers) (haptoglobin is rapidly saturated, and excess dimers are quickly removed from the circulation by the kidney after filtration in the glomerulus); (3) once it is filtered, a high concentration of protein in the renal tubules can cause tubular obstruction and consequent renal failure; (4) cell-free hemoglobin binds nitric oxide, an endothelium-derived relaxing factor that may contribute to vasoconstriction; (5) iron, when released from hemoglobin, can promote the formation of toxic oxygen radicals and bacterial growth.

Thus, to be an effective oxygen carrier in the cell-free state, hemoglobin must be chemically modified to avoid these problems. Whether all these must be solved completely for a product to be useful is a matter of intense debate. All the reactions currently considered useful in the production of hemoglobin-based red cell substitutes use chemical modification at one or more sites on the surface of the protein.[1]

Table 22.2 Classes of Hemoglobin-Based Red Blood Cell Substitutes

Class	Examples (see Table 22.3)	Molecular Radius (nm)	Intravascular Persistence (hr)	Oncotic Pressure	Viscosity	Vasoactivity
Crosslinked tetramers	Diaspirin crosslinked hemoglobin (DCLHb) αα-Hemoglobin	2.7	~12	Low	Low	Marked
Polymerized tetramers	HemoPure Hemolink PolyHeme	4.9	~12–24	Low	Low	Moderate
Surface-modified tetramers	Pyridoxalated hemoglobin polyoxyethylene Polyethylene glycol-hemoglobin	14.1	~24–48	Moderate-high	Moderate-high	Mild

Data from Vandegriff K, McCarthy M, Rohlfs R, Winslow R: Colloid osmotic properties of modified hemoglobins: Chemically cross-linked versus polyethylene glycol surface-conjugated. Biophys Chem 69:23–30, 1997.

The dimensions and reactivity of the crosslinking reagents determine differences in the reactions. Because the function of hemoglobin in binding and releasing oxygen is intricately connected to a structural transition, it is not surprising that the oxygen half-saturation pressure and yield are highly variable. Even small differences among structures of the reagents can yield products with quite different properties. In addition, the conditions of the reaction are important, in regard to not only the state of ligation (i.e., oxygen saturation), but also the presence of agents or molecules that lack or compete for certain reactive sites.

A further complication of these reactions is that many nonhemoglobin proteins, copurified with hemoglobin, contain reactive groups and may also be modified to produce new, potentially toxic, contaminants. It is understandable that it has been difficult to produce "pure" modified hemoglobin for toxicity studies when most processes start with relatively crude "stroma-free" hemoglobin.[2] One classification of the various types of modified hemoglobins is given in Table 22.2.

An example of a crosslinked hemoglobin is a product studied intensively by the United States Army and numerous academic laboratories. Crosslinking of hemoglobin isolated from outdated human blood was carried out with bis-(3,5-dibromosalicyl)fumarate (DBBF),[3] and it was called $\alpha\alpha$-hemoglobin by the Army and DCL Hb by Baxter Healthcare, which produced it in commercial quantities. The reaction results in a four-carbon covalent link between adjacent α chains at position 99 (Lys$\alpha_1$99-Lys$\alpha_2$99) (Fig. 22.1). This covalently crosslinked hemoglobin cannot break down into subunits in the circulation and therefore cannot be excreted as filtered globin chains.

The production process is complex.[4] Stroma-free hemoglobin is separated from red blood cell membranes and is deoxygenated to achieve the proper molecular conformation for crosslinking, and the 2,3-diphosphoglycerate pocket is blocked reversibly with an allosteric effector. It is then crosslinked, heated to pasteurize it and also to remove unreacted hemoglobin, and passed through a series of cross-flow filters. It is finally sterilized by filtration through a 0.2-μm filter.

The product has an oxygen equilibrium curve with an oxygen half-saturation pressure under physiologic conditions of 28 mm Hg. The degree of cooperativity (the slope of the dissociation curve) is similar to that of blood (Hill coefficient 2.62 for blood, 2.31 for crosslinked hemoglobin), and the Bohr[5] and carbon dioxide[6] effects are nearly intact.

Based on its oxygen equilibrium curve, this product should have in vivo oxygen transport properties similar to those of whole blood; its oxygen equilibrium curve is closer to that of red blood cells than that of other types of red blood cell substitutes (Fig. 22.2). The intravascular persistence is markedly extended in the rat: uncrosslinked hemoglobin has a half-life of about 1.2 hours, and crosslinked hemoglobin has a half-life of about 4.3 hours. In the rabbit, the persistence is longer, approximately 16 hours for crosslinked hemoglobin, for monkey about 14 hours, and for pig about 7 hours.[7] No doubt exists that cell-free hemoglobin transports oxygen. Many studies in the literature have demonstrated the ability of hemoglobin solutions to resuscitate animals in lethal hemorrhagic shock.[1]

The commercial version of $\alpha\alpha$-hemoglobin, called DCL Hb and HemAssist by Baxter Healthcare, was studied extensively in clinical trials. However, the product was found to be severely vasoactive; it raised blood pressure and increased systemic and pulmonary vascular resistance.[8,9] Phase III clinical trials were carried out in numerous clinical applications and led to disappointing results. In fact, trials in trauma[10] and in stroke[11] both showed reduced survival in patients who received the product.

Closely related to $\alpha\alpha$-hemoglobin is a recombinant product (RHb1.1) produced in *Escherichia coli*.[12] Starting material for hemoglobin modification can also be produced in transgenic animals.[13] Hemoglobin also can be polymerized using various polyfunctional reagents to yield molecules with markedly increased molecular weights. One example is

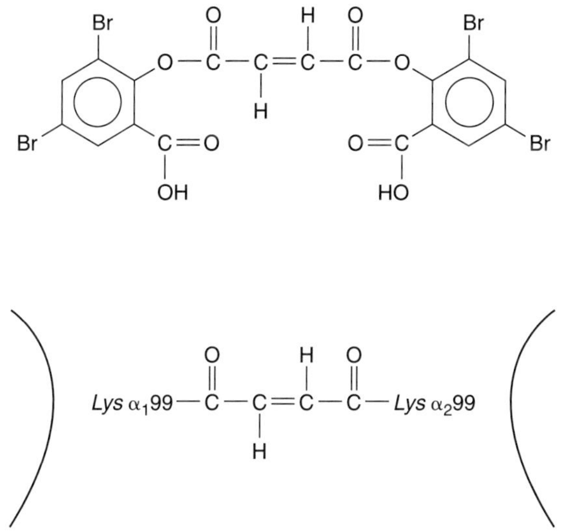

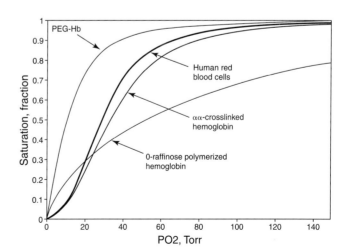

Figure 22.1 Structure of the crosslinker, bis-(2,3-dibromosalicyl) fumarate (DBBF, *top*) and crosslinked hemoglobin (*bottom*). The brominated acetyl groups of the DBBF are leaving groups in the reaction, which results in a four-carbon bridge between the two α-chain polypeptide subunits of hemoglobin.

Figure 22.2 Oxygen equilibrium curves for some respresentative red blood cell substitutes. Note the large difference between the curves for polyethylene glycol hemoglobin (PEG-Hb), o-raffinose polymerized hemoglobin, and red blood cells.

human hemoglobin, reacted first with pyridoxal-5' phosphate and then polymerized with glutaraldehyde.[14] This product has a reduced colloidal osmotic (oncotic) pressure and longer intravascular persistence compared with smaller molecules, but the polymerization reaction is notoriously difficult to control.[15, 16]

Another promising approach is to couple hemoglobin to polyethylene glycol[17] or a similar molecule, such as polyoxyethylene[18] or dextran.[19] These conjugated hemoglobins may also have prolonged plasma retention times and may have reduced interactions with the reticuloendothelial systems.

Liposome-Encapsulated Hemoglobin

Because hemoglobin is normally packaged inside a membrane, it seems intuitively correct that encapsulated hemoglobin would be the ultimate solution of the red blood cell substitute problem. In 1957, Thomas Chang reported the use of microencapsulated hemoglobin as artificial red blood cells.[20] Since that time, dramatic results have been reported in the complete exchange transfusion of laboratory animals,[21, 22] but progress toward development of an artificial red blood cell for human use has been slow because of problems of reticuloendothelial and other macrophage stimulation.[23] Other problems include maintaining sterility and large-scale production.

In the years that have followed Chang's initial descriptions of encapsulated hemoglobin, much work with lipid vesicles (liposomes) has been done. Liposomes have served as models for understanding natural cell membranes. They also have been used investigationally as vehicles for gene transfer, as targeted carriers, for pharmacological agents, and even as lubricants for degenerated joint surfaces. The most extensively studied liposomes used to encapsulate hemoglobin are composed of phospholipid in combination with cholesterol and other lipids that confer flexibility and stability, such as ganglioside GM_1 or cholesterol.[24] When injected into animals, such liposomes are rapidly coated with immunoglobulin G, albumin, and other opsonins.[25] Newer formulations include the use of surface components such as polyethylene glycol or dextran, which can stabilize the liposomes in the circulation.[26]

The limitations to the development of liposome-encapsulated hemoglobin as a red blood cell substitute are difficulties in stabilizing the final product and the massive scale that would be required to produce a commercial product. The size of most liposome particles is approximately 0.2 to 1.0 μm, too large to be filter sterilized. In addition, neither the liposome nor its hemoglobin contents can withstand pasteurization temperature. Other potential approaches to the solution of these problems could include polymerizable phospholipids[27] and other polymers.[28]

Perfluorocarbon-Based Products

A resurgence has occurred in the development of perfluorocarbons for two reasons. First, Fluosol-DA (Fluosol, Green Cross Corp., Osaka, Japan) was approved for marketing by the Food and Drug Administration for use in coronary angioplasty in 1990 (manufacture was discontinued in 1995). Second, new perfluorocarbon emulsions now being developed by industry carry much more oxygen than previous products.[29] Still, a fundamental difference exists between perfluorocarbon- and hemoglobin-based red blood cell substitutes: oxygen is transported by perfluorocarbons as dissolved gas, whereas hemoglobin carries oxygen chemically bound to the protein itself. The oxygen dissociation curve for hemoglobin is sigmoid, whereas oxygen dissociation from perfluorocarbons is linear. One product, Oxygent (Alliance Pharmaceutical Corp.) is an emulsion of perflubron and egg yolk phospholipid, which contains about five times more fluorocarbon than Fluosol and therefore five times more dissolved oxygen.

Initially, it would appear that it is better to have a sigmoid oxygen dissociation curve because (1) it is natural and (2) maximum oxygen carriage in blood is achieved at an alveolar partial oxygen pressure (PO_2) of about 100 mm Hg, whereas only about 20% of the perfluorocarbon carries oxygen at the same PO_2. To carry as much oxygen in this fluorocarbon as 7 g/dL hemoglobin, an arterial PO_2 of about 450 mm Hg is needed. Therefore, it seems that the utility of fluorocarbon red blood cell substitutes will depend on a high inspired PO_2. In many elective surgical procedures, arterial PO_2 much higher than 300 mm Hg can be achieved, but in trauma, emergencies, and pulmonary patients, these levels of PO_2 may not be possible.

In practice, a margin of safety could be achieved with relatively low doses of perfluorocarbon emulsions, which could have a significant impact; increased tolerance to a reduced hematocrit would further reduce the "transfusion trigger." In a theoretical analysis of transfusion, mixed venous PO_2 is nearly constant from a hematocrit of 25% to 45% because as oxygen is added in the form of transfused red blood cells, cardiac output decreases.[30] If the hematocrit is kept low but oxygen is added in the form of perfluorocarbon, a significant increase in mixed venous PO_2 occurs because the cardiac output remains high. Cell-free hemoglobin solutions would not offer this advantage if their use does not result in increased cardiac output.

Safety

Demonstration of safety of red blood cell substitutes is a critical issue, because the risks of transfusion of allogeneic blood are well known (see Table 22.1). To be used, a substitute should be at least as safe as red blood cells, unless a decisive therapeutic advantage can be demonstrated.

In a review of almost a century of clinical trials with red blood cell substitutes, reported side effects involved renal dysfunction and systemic symptoms (fever, chills, nausea, headache, flushing, vomiting, allergic reactions, tachycardia, bradycardia, hypertension, rigors, low back pain, chest pain, abdominal pain, decreased platelets, and increased partial thromboplastin time).[1] Many of these effects could be explained by the depletion of nitric oxide, in the case of hemoglobin-based products, or by stimulation of macrophages, in the case of liposomes or perfluorocarbon emulsions. Many are smooth muscle effects, and some involve macrophages and platelets. Clinical trials with hemoglobin-based products have not been extensively reported in the literature. However, preclinical animal studies clearly have not been completely successful in predicting human reactions to the products.[31]

Cell-free hemoglobin is widely distributed in the tissues after administration. Studies of the distribution of crosslinked hemoglobin in the intact animal show that significant amounts of hemoglobin are retained in the kidney, spleen, liver, adrenal gland, lung, heart, brain, and muscle well after any hemoglobin is detected in the plasma.[32–34] Thus, cell-free hemoglobin is distributed in almost every tissue of the body, and therefore we may expect toxic effects that could be unpredictable or unknown. Extensive histologic studies were carried out in animals after exchange transfusion and were summarized.[1]

Perhaps the effect of cell-free hemoglobin of most concern is its known ability to cause vasoconstriction and hypertension. This vasoconstriction can be mediated in part by the reaction of hemoglobin with nitric oxide, an endothelium-derived relaxing factor.[35] Nitric oxide is synthesized from arginine in endothelial cells (as well as in other cells) by an enzyme, nitric oxide synthase, which produces nitric oxide and citrulline. It binds to a heme group in guanylate cyclase that activates cyclic guanosine monophosphate. Nitric oxide diffuses rapidly out of endothelial cells into the vessel lumen, the interstitial space, and smooth muscle cells, where it binds to a heme group in guanylate cyclase, activating cyclic guanosine monophosphate and moving calcium from the unbound to bound state. The result is smooth muscle relaxation. Nitric oxide also stimulates platelets and polymorphonuclear leukocytes and macrophages. Hemoglobin binds nitric oxide very tightly, more tightly, in fact, than it binds oxygen, whether hemoglobin is in the red blood cell or is free in solution.[36] The reaction is virtually irreversible. Whether this interaction of hemoglobin with nitric oxide will limit clinical usefulness of hemoglobin-based red blood cell substitutes remains to be determined.

In addition to its effect as a scavenger of nitric oxide, cell-free hemoglobin may also induce vasoconstriction by disrupting normal autoregulation of vascular tone. In other words, it may make oxygen so readily available to regulatory arterioles that reflexive vasoconstriction could occur that paradoxically limits blood flow.[37, 38] This concept is suggested by the direct observation in the microcirculation[39] and may lead to potentially new design strategies for cell-free red blood cell substitutes.

Perfluorocarbon emulsions have the most extensive history of use in humans. Fluosol was approved by the Food and Drug Administration for use in coronary angioplasty and therefore was been given to many human patients. In addition, similar formulations have been used on the battlefield in China and Afghanistan, although data are generally not available. Perfluorocarbon emulsions have also been tested in humans as imaging agents. The principal toxicity of perfluorocarbon emulsions appears to be in their stimulation of macrophages.[40, 41] This can result in pulmonary hypertension and elaboration of thromboxane in swine and could lead to nonspecific symptoms such as fever, chills, and flu-like symptoms in humans.

Biocompatibility studies with liposome-encapsulated hemoglobin have been generally favorable,[22] but such products tend to be removed from the circulation by the phagocytic cells of the reticuloendothelial system.[42] This situation leads to significant enlargement of the liver and spleen. Current research is aimed at prolongation of the intravascular persistence to minimize this problem.[43]

Efficacy

It seems intuitively obvious that a plasma expander that carries oxygen would be superior to one that does not, and experimental proof of this concept should be relatively straightforward. However, the problem of efficacy can be appreciated by considering the difficulties in showing efficacy for red blood cell transfusions. The problem is a lack of clear endpoints: no single measure of oxygen transport is accurate and easily obtainable. It may be possible to show improved clinical outcome after transfusion of red blood cells to patients with extremely low hematocrits, but the bulk of allogeneic blood is given intraoperatively in response to blood loss, not severe anemia.

Most demonstrations of efficacy have been either by exchange transfusions with test material or by resuscitation from shock. Resuscitation from shock is exceedingly complex, however, and the most urgent requirement is for volume replacement.[44] Clinical trials involving trauma patients are particularly difficult to design because of the problems of controls and informed consent. Future clinical trials will most likely be aimed at, for example, reduced use of allogeneic blood, rather than at specific oxygen transport parameters, which may be controversial, at best. For example, one trial with Fluosol during surgical procedures showed that its use did not reduce the need for allogeneic blood transfusions in the postoperative period.[45]

Clinical Trials

Early trials with various cell-free hemoglobin solutions were reviewed and showed an array of side effects that involve every organ of the body.[1] However, most of these are mild or reversible, and only 1 death in more than 211 patients was reported in the early literature; this patient was terminally ill and would likely have died even without the administration of hemoglobin.[46]

Certain red blood cell substitute products are in various stages of advanced clinical trials (Table 22.3). The greatest

Table 22.3 Red Blood Cell Substitutes in Clinical Trials

Product (Manufacturer)	Composition	Indication	Clinical Testing Stage
Hemopure (BioPure)	Glutaraldehyde-polymerized bovine hemoglobin	Hemodilution, trauma	III
Hemolink (Hemosol)	o-raffinose–polymerized human hemoglobin	Hemodilution, trauma	III
PolyHeme (Northfield)	Glutaraldehyde-polymerized human hemoglobin	Trauma	III
Oxygent (Alliance)	Emulsified perflubron	Hemodilution, bypass	III

Table 22.4 Potential Clinical Applications for Red Blood Cell Substitutes

Hemodilution, elective surgery
Trauma
Chronic anemia
Ischemic disease (angioplasty, stroke)
Red cell incompatibility (rare blood types)
Extracorporeal circulation (bypass)
Cell culture media
High blood-use surgery
Cardioplegia
Tumor oxygenation
Organ transplantation
Bone marrow transplant support
Sickle cell anemia
Research on oxygen delivery and circulation

concern for hemoglobin-based products is that the known vasoactivity of the solutions could lead to hypertension or underperfusion of ischemic tissue. Perfluorocarbon emulsions are also being tested in humans, and a major concern appears to be thrombocytopenia.[47] No liposome-based product has yet been approved for use in human trials.

Advanced clinical trials have been reported for one polymerized hemoglobin product, Northfield's Polyheme.[48] This report, although preliminary, is highly optimistic. In contrast, the published reports of clinical trials with HemAssist have been disappointing.[10, 11]

■ Implications and Future Applications

Potential Clinical Applications

The need for red blood cell substitutes to replace all use of allogeneic blood is both unnecessary and naive. The red blood cell substitute candidates now being developed will probably be used initially in surgical hemodilution to provide a margin of safety and perhaps to reduce the need for the 2 or 3 units of blood used in most surgical procedures.

Many clinical applications in addition to hemodilution for the products now being developed will be targeted by industry (Table 22.4). Applications for perfluorocarbon emulsions other than as red blood cell substitutes could surpass their use in trauma, surgery, and shock. For example, emulsions have been shown to increase the radiosensitivity of solid tumors,[49] to be excellent nuclear magnetic resonance and ultrasound imaging agents,[50] to be capable of removing gaseous microemboli during cardiopulmonary bypass,[51] and to measure tissue P_{O_2}.[52]

Availability in the Future

It seems unlikely that cell-free hemoglobin as a red blood cell substitute with vasoactive effects will be accepted broadly by clinicians. Indeed, vasoconstriction is a hallmark of the shock state. Perfluorocarbon emulsions may well be the first red blood cell substitutes to reach the clinic. However, they may not find wide application as such. More likely, they will be used as imaging enhancers, liquid-breathing agents, or adjuncts to radiotherapy of solid tumors. In addition, the low cost and simplicity of production of perfluorocarbon emulsions are favorable qualities for commercialization.

Liposome-encapsulated hemoglobin may well be the ultimate solution to the red blood cell substitute problem.

To be successful, however, an inexpensive and simple process will need to be developed, and any problems of reticuloendothelial blockade and engorgement of organs such as liver and spleen will have to be thoroughly studied and understood.

The present commercial climate is such that few, if any, of these products are being used in scientific studies that can be evaluated in the peer-reviewed literature until they are approved for use by the Food and Drug Administration. This unfortunate situation has retarded development in the past and is likely to do so in the future.[31]

REFERENCES

1. Winslow R: Hemoglobin-based Red Cell Substitutes. Baltimore, Johns Hopkins University Press, 1992.
2. Christensen S, Medina F, Winslow R, et al: Preparation of human hemoglobin Ao for possible use as a blood substitute. J Biochem Biophys Methods 17:143–154, 1988.
3. Walder J, Chatterjee R, Arnone A: Electrostatic effects within the central cavity of the hemoglobin tetramer [abstract 2228]. Fed Proc 41:651, 1982.
4. Winslow R, Chapman K: Pilot-scale preparation of hemoglobin solutions. In: Everse J, Vandegriff K, Winslow R (eds): Hemoglobin Part B: Biochemical and Analytical Methods. San Diego, Academic Press, 1994, pp 3–16.
5. Vandegriff K, Medina F, Marini M, Winslow R: Equilibrium oxygen binding to human hemoglobin cross-linked between the alpha chains by bis-(3,5-dibromosalicyl)fumarate. J Biol Chem 264:17824–17833, 1989.
6. Vandegriff K, Benazzi L, Ripamonti M, et al: Carbon dioxide binding to human hemoglobin cross-linked between the alpha chains. J Biol Chem 266:2697–2700, 1991.
7. Hess J, Fadare S, Tolentino L, et al: The intravascular persistence of crosslinked human hemoglobin. In: Brewer G (ed): The Red Cell Seventh Ann Arbor Conference. New York, Alan R. Liss, 1989, pp 351–360.
8. Hess J, Macdonald V, Brinkley W: Systemic and pulmonary hypertension after resuscitation with cell-free hemoglobin. J Appl Physiol 74:1769–1778, 1993.
9. Winslow RM, Gonzales A, Gonzales M, et al: Vascular resistance and the efficacy of red cell substitutes. J Appl Physiol 85:993–1003, 1998.
10. Sloan EP, Koenigsberg M, Gens D, et al: Diaspirin cross-linked hemoglobin (DCLHb) in the treatment of severe traumatic hemorrhagic shock: A randomized controlled efficacy trial. JAMA 282:1857–1864, 1999.
11. Saxena R, Wijnhoud AD, Carton H, et al: Controlled safety study of a hemoglobin-based oxygen carrier, DCLHb, in acute ischemic stroke. Stroke 30:993–996, 1999.
12. Hoffman S, Looker D, Roehrich J, et al: Expression of fully functional tetrameric human hemoglobin in *Escherichia coli*. Proc Natl Acad Sci U S A 87:8521–8525, 1990.
13. Sharma A, Martin MJ, Okabe JF, et al: An isologous porcine promoter permits high level expression of human hemoglobin in transgenic swine. Biotechnology 12:55–59, 1994.
14. Gould S, Sehgal L, Sehgal H, Moss G: Artificial blood: Current status of hemoglobin solutions. Crit Care Clin 8:293–309, 1992.
15. Marini M, Moore G, Fishman R, et al: Reexamination of the polymerization of pyridoxylated hemoglobin with glutaraldehyde. Biopolymers 29:871–882, 1990.
16. Marini M, Moore G, Fishman R, et al: A critical examination of the reaction of pyridoxal 5-phosphate with human hemoglobin Ao. Biopolymers 28:2071–2083, 1989.
17. Nho K, Glower D, Bredehoeft S, et al: PEG-bovine hemoglobin: Safety in a canine dehydrated hypovolemic-hemorrhagic shock model. Artif Cells Blood Substit Immobil Biotechnol 20:511–524, 1992.
18. Malchesky P, Takahashi T, Iwasaki K, et al: Conjugated human hemoglobin as a physiological oxygen carrier—pyridoxalated hemoglobin polyoxyethylene conjugate (PHP). Int J Artif Organs 13:442–450, 1990.
19. Wong J: Rightshifted dextran-hemoglobin as blood substitute. Artif Cells Blood Substit Immobil Biotechnol 16:237–245, 1988.

20. Chang T: Red blood cell substitutes: Microencapsulated hemoglobin and cross-linked hemoglobin including pyridoxylated polyhemoglobin conjugated hemoglobin. Artif Cells Blood Substit Immobil Biotechnol 16:11–29, 1988.

21. Djordjevich L, Mayoral J, Ivankovich A: Synthetic erythrocytes: Cardiorespiratory changes during exchange transfusions [abstract]. Anesthesiology 63:109, 1985.

22. Hunt C, Burnette R, MacGregor R, et al: Synthesis and evaluation of a prototypal artificial red cell. Science 230:1165–1168, 1985.

23. Rudolph A: Encapsulated hemoglobin: Current issues and future goals. Artif Cells Blood Substit Immobil Biotechnol 22:347–360, 1994.

24. Farmer M, Gaber B: Liposome-encapsulated hemoglobin as an artificial oxygen-carrying system. Methods Enzymol 149:184–200, 1987.

25. MacGregor R, Hunt C: Artificial red cells: A link between the membrane skeleton and RES detectability? Artif Cells Blood Substit Immobil Biotechnol 18:329–343, 1990.

26. Allen T, Hansen C, Martin F, et al: Liposomes containing synthetic lipid derivatives of poly(ethylene glycol) show prolonged circulation half-times in vivo. Biochim Biophys Acta 1066:29–36, 1991.

27. Nakachi O, Tokuyama S, Satoh T, Tsuchida E: Characteristics of polylipid/Hb vesicles (ARC) (in vitro and in vivo test). Artif Cells Blood Substit Immobil Biotechnol 20:635–640, 1992.

28. Yu WP, Chang TM: Submicron polymer membrane hemoglobin nanocapsules as potential blood substitutes: Preparation and characterization. Artif Cells Blood Substit Immobil Biotechnol 24:169–183, 1996.

29. Long C, Long D, Riess J, et al: Preparation and application of highly concentrated perfluorooctylbromide fluorocarbon emulsions. Artif Cells Blood Substit Immobil Biotechnol 16:441–442, 1988.

30. Winslow R: A model for red cell O_2 uptake. Int J Clin Monit Comput 2:81–93, 1985.

31. Naval Research Advisory Committee: Delivery of Artificial Blood to the Military. Washington, DC: United States Navy, 1992.

32. Keipert P, Verosky M, Triner L: Plasma retention and metabolic fate of hemoglobin modified with an interdimeric covalent cross link. Trans Am Soc Artif Intern Organs 35:153–159, 1989.

33. Keipert PE, Gomez CL, Gonzales A, et al: Diaspirin cross-linked hemoglobin: Tissue distribution and long-term excretion after exchange transfusion. J Lab Clin Med 123:701–711, 1994.

34. Hsia J, Song D, Er S, et al: Pharmacokinetic studies in the rat on an O-raffinose polymerized human hemoglobin. Artif Cells Blood Substit Immobil Biotechnol 20:587–595, 1992.

35. Palmer R, Ferrige A, Moncada S: Nitric oxide release accounts for the biological activity of endothelium-derived relaxing factor. Nature 327:524–526, 1987.

36. Gibson QH, Roughton FJW: The kinetics and equilibria of the reactions of nitric oxide with sheep hemoglobin. J Appl Physiol 136:123–134, 1956.

37. Vandegriff K, Winslow R: A theoretical analysis of oxygen transport: A new strategy for the design of hemoglobin-based red cell substitutes. In Winslow R, Vandegriff K, Intaglietta M (eds): Blood Substitutes: Physiological Basis of Efficacy. Boston, Birkhäuser, 1995.

38. Winslow RM, Vandegriff KD: Hemoglobin oxygen affinity and the design of red cell substitutes. In Winslow R, Vandegriff K, Intaglietta M (eds): Advances in Blood Substitutes: Industrial Opportunities and Medical Challenges. Boston, Birkhäuser, 1997, pp 167–188.

39. Intaglietta M, Johnson P, Winslow R: Microvascular and tissue oxygen distribution. Cardiovasc Res 32:632–643, 1996.

40. Ingram D, Forman M, Murray J: Phagocytic activation of human neutrophils by the detergent component of Fluosol. Am J Pathol 140:1081–1087, 1992.

41. Bucala R, Kawakami M, Cerami A: Cytotoxicity of a perfluorocarbon blood substitute to macrophages in vitro. Science 220:965–967, 1983.

42. Beach M, Morley J, Spiryda L, Weinstock S: Effects of liposome encapsulated hemoglobin on the reticuloendothelial system. Artif Cells Blood Substit Immobil Biotechnol 20:771–776, 1992.

43. Flaim S: Perflubron-based emulsion: Efficacy as temporary oxygen carrier. In Winslow R, Vandegriff K, Intaglietta M (eds): Advances in Blood Substitutes: Industrial Opportunities and Medical Challenges. Boston, Birkhäuser, 1997.

44. Pope A, French G, Longnecker DE (eds): Fluid Resuscitation: State of the Science for Treating Combat Casualties and Civilian Injuries. Washington, DC, National Academy Press, 1999.

45. Gould S, Rosen A, Sehgal L, et al: Fluosol-DA as a red-cell substitute in acute anemia. N Engl J Med 314:1653–1656, 1986.

46. Amberson W, Jennings J, Rhodes C: Clinical experience with hemoglobin-saline solutions. J Appl Physiol 1:469–489, 1949.

47. Kaufman R: Clinical development of perfluorocarbon-based red cell substitutes. In Winslow R, Vandegriff K, Intaglietta M (eds): Blood Substitutes: Physiological Basis of Efficacy. Boston, Birkhäuser, 1995.

48. Gould SA, Moore EE, Hoyt DB, et al: The first randomized trial of human polymerized hemoglobin as a blood substitute in acute trauma and emergent surgery. J Am Coll Surg 187:113–120, 1998.

49. Teicher B, Herman T, Menon K: Enhancement of fractionated radiation therapy by an experimental concentrated perflubron emulsion (Oxygent) in the Lewis lung carcinoma. Artif Cells Blood Substit Immobil Biotechnol 20:899–902, 1992.

50. Mattrey R: Perfluorooctylbromide: A new contrast agent for CT, sonography, an MR imaging. AJR Am J Roentgenol 152:247–252, 1988.

51. Blauth C, Smith P, Newman S, et al: Retinal microembolism and neuropsychological deficit following clinical cardiopulmonary bypass: Comparison of a membrane and bubble oxygenator. A preliminary communication. Eur J Cardiothorac Surg 3:135–138, 1989.

52. Mason R, Shukla H, Antich P: Oxygent: A novel probe of tissue oxygen tension. Artif Cells Blood Substit Immobil Biotechnol 20:929–932, 1992.

53. Klein HG: Oxygen carriers and transfusion medicine. Artif Cells Blood Substit Immobil Biotechnol 22:123–135, 1994.

54. Schreiber GB, Busch MP, Kleinman SH, Korelitz JJ: The risk of transfusion-transmitted viral infections. N Engl J Med 334:1685–1690. 1996.

55. Vandegriff K, McCarthy M, Rohlfs R, Winslow R: Colloid osmotic properties of modified hemoglobins: Chemically cross-linked versus polyethylene glycol surface-conjugated. Biophys Chem 69:23–30, 1997.

Chapter 23

Autologous Blood and Related Alternatives to Allogeneic Transfusion

Margot S. Kruskall

Autologous blood can be collected from a patient in advance of anticipated blood loss (preoperative donation) or at the start of the procedure (acute normovolemic hemodilution); in addition, shed blood can be salvaged for reinfusion both during surgery and in the postoperative period (perioperative salvage) (Table 23.1). In the 19th century allogeneic transfusions were fraught with immunologic risks; the concept of using a patient's own blood as a source of transfusable red blood cells (RBCs) was born of necessity. Early authors proposed the recovery of blood shed during childbirth, ectopic pregnancy, and splenectomy.[1, 2] With the discovery of the ABO blood group system, the development of approaches for storage of blood and preparation of components, and the need during two world wars for a large and immediately available blood supply, interest in autologous blood waned. The appearance in the early 1980s of the human immuno-deficiency virus (HIV) as a transfusion-transmissible complication of allogeneic transfusion fostered a recurrence of interest in autologous blood techniques. Blood collection statistics bear this trend out: donations of blood for autologous use increased from 28,000 units in 1982 to 1,117,000 units 10 years later.[3, 4]

■ Advantages and Disadvantages of Autologous Blood Transfusion

Advantages

A number of advantages have been associated with the use of autologous blood. Originally, autologous techniques were viewed as options for obtaining blood to augment short allogeneic supplies. More relevant in current times is the use of autologous blood to eliminate the risk of transfusion-transmitted microorganisms, in particular HIV and hepatitis viruses. The institution of increasingly sensitive tests for such infections, including nucleic acid testing, has softened the impact of this argument; however, the risk of future incursions into the blood supply by new infectious agents remains a threat. Immunologic complications such as antibody-mediated hemolysis and leukocyte-associated febrile reactions are eliminated with the use of autologous blood. Supported by recent human and animal data, some authors also believe that allogeneic transfusions induce immunosuppression in the recipient, and that autologous blood might not.[5] Other advantages include the stimulation of erythropoiesis in the repeatedly bled autologous donor, which could speed recovery from postoperative anemia.[6] Intraoperatively salvaged RBCs are typically transfused back to the patient within a few hours after collection, thus precluding the acquired membrane defects and enzyme deficiencies (2,3-diphosphoglycerate and adenosine triphosphate) that develop during refrigeration (the "storage lesion").[7]

Disadvantages

Autologous techniques are not without drawbacks. Although an ideal preoperative donation schedule should allow sufficient time for compensatory erythropoiesis to occur, some individuals develop donation-induced anemia at the time of admission for surgery. Concerns regarding complications of donation in patients with underlying cardiac disease have been raised,[8] although it can be difficult in such settings to distinguish between an untoward effect of blood letting and the natural history of the baseline condition. Clerical errors, including release of the wrong unit of blood, may still occur.[9] Finally, although it is rare, autologous blood may itself pose infectious risks. *Yersinia enterocolitica*, a common cause of community-acquired diarrhea, persists in the blood stream for many weeks after infection and can grow at refrigerator temperatures; an individual who donates blood during this

Table 23.1 Indications for Autologous Blood Techniques

Surgical Procedure	Preoperative Donation	Perioperative Salvage	Acute Normovolemic Hemodilution
Vascular surgery (intra-abdominal procedures)	Yes	Yes	Yes
Open heart surgery	Yes	Yes	Yes
Total hip surgery	Yes	No*	No*
Total knee surgery	Yes	Yes†	No*
Scoliosis surgery	Yes	Yes	Yes
Radical prostatectomy	Yes	Yes‡	Yes
Liver resection/ transplantation	Yes	Yes	Yes
Placenta previa	Yes	No§	No*
Multiple gestations	Yes	No§	No*

*Need not conclusively established.
†Intraoperative salvage is unnecessary when a tourniquet is used; postoperative salvage may be of value in cementless procedures.
‡Hypothetical risk of cancer spread after transfusion of intraoperatively salvaged blood.
§The safety of blood containing amniotic fluid has not been conclusively established.

time period can be made severely ill by later transfusion of the component.[10]

Costs of Autologous Blood Techniques

As the allogeneic blood supply has become safer, more attention has been focused on the costs associated with autologous transfusion techniques. Costs come from unused autologous collections (for example, when a patient has donated enough blood to match the mean number of components used by others undergoing the procedure but requires less). This problem is magnified by overcollection and unnecessary utilization (e.g., in plastic surgery) and by the extra work involved in deviation from routine large-scale allogeneic collection practices.[11] In one hypothetical cost-utility analysis of patients undergoing primary elective hip replacement, the cost-effectiveness of autologous transfusion per quality-adjusted life year (QALY) was estimated at an extremely high $3,400,000. However, if allogeneic transfusions were assumed to increase the risk of postoperative bacterial infection, a possibility suggested by some workers,[12–14] the cost of using autologous blood fell to less than $50,000 per QALY, and the procedure became dominant (cheaper to use than allogeneic blood) as the infection risk rose.[15] Some authors have suggested that autologous blood could be kept cost-effective by streamlining collection and processing, including forgoing infectious disease testing of autologous donors.[16, 17] As of the fall of 1999, however, the U.S. Food and Drug Administration is considering a requirement for such testing as a means of reducing the risks associated with misdirected autologous units. Reducing costs through the intentional use of autologous blood by a recipient other than the donor ("crossover") is not recommended. Only 30% of collections are typically eligible for allogeneic use, and the costs, complexity, and risk of error of the transition all serve to negate the value.[18]

▪ Preoperative Autologous Transfusion

Indications for Autologous Whole Blood Collection

The decision to use preoperative autologous blood donations should be predicated on the type of surgery, the amount of time available for donation and hematopoietic reconstitution, the patient's hematocrit, and the predicted vigor of the erythropoietic response to donation. Patients planning to undergo elective orthopedic surgery are ideal candidates for autologous transfusion, because they require moderate amounts of blood during and immediately after surgery, and they typically have sufficient time in advance of surgery to make multiple donations.[19–21] Open heart surgery and vascular surgery are other areas in which autologous blood collections have led to reduction or elimination of allogeneic blood use.[6] The use of preoperative autologous blood donation has also been reported for a variety of other surgical procedures, including radical prostatectomies, hysterectomies and other gynecologic procedures, gastrointestinal surgery, and neurosurgery.[22, 23] Donors of bone marrow for transplantation undergo multiple iliac crest aspirations and may develop a moderate anemia; advance donation of autologous blood forestalls the need for allogeneic transfusions.[24] As surgical techniques change, the need for blood transfusions may be affected, and in such instances the role of autologous blood should be re-examined. Radical prostatectomy is a case in point: Ten years ago many hospitals encouraged patients undergoing the procedure to donate autologous blood,[25, 26] but today in some hands fewer than 2% of patients require blood, and autologous blood donations may be superfluous.[27, 28] Blood transfusion is also rarely necessary in plastic surgical procedures, and the collection of autologous blood in such cases is often frivolous.[29]

Autologous blood can be collected from a pregnant woman for use during childbirth. The expanded maternal blood volume contributes a substantial safety cushion, and the donation process appears safe for both mother and fetus.[30, 31] However, the use of blood transfusions in uncomplicated pregnancies is exceedingly low (<2.5%).[32] A role for autologous collections may exist for patients with multiple gestations or placenta previa, situations in which the likelihood of transfusion may exceed 25% and the condition is often identified with sufficient time for advance blood donations.[33] In addition, autologous blood has been collected from patients with unusual antibodies discovered during the pregnancy.[34]

Long-term frozen storage of autologous RBCs in the absence of an anticipated transfusion episode is both ineffective and expensive. An exception is the storage of blood by individuals with high-frequency or complex alloantibodies, for whom stockpiling of rare autologous units may be beneficial. Even here, however, the likelihood that such blood would be helpful is slim. To be of value, sufficient autologous blood would have to be available to meet the needs of an unexpected emergency; furthermore, delays in sending the blood expeditiously to the hospital where it is needed and in preparing units (thawed and washed free of the glycerol cryoprotectant) would make its use unwieldy.

Indications for Other Autologous Components

Although autologous plasma is easily prepared from whole blood, little need exists for plasma in most elective surgery.[35] Autologous fibrin glue can be prepared from the cryoprecipitated portion of autologous plasma; after thawing, this material is mixed with bovine thrombin immediately before application to the surgical field site. This tissue adhesive has been employed in a variety of surgical procedures, including the control of bleeding in cardiovascular and cardiothoracic surgery,[36] adhesion in middle ear surgery,[37] repair of the dura mater in neurosurgical procedures,[38] application of skin grafts,[39] and closure of gastrointestinal fistulas.[40] Fibrin glue has also been used in pancreatic and hepatic resection and trauma.[41, 42] In the latter settings, occasional reports of severe hypotension have been noted, possibly caused by allergic or other reactions to systemically absorbed bovine thrombin.[43] Another rare complication is the development of an acquired factor V inhibitor, associated with life-threatening bleeding. This results from recipient immunization to bovine factor V, present in the bovine thrombin; the bovine antibodies recognize cross-reactive epitopes on human factor V.[44–46] An alternative to autologous fibrin glue is a commercial tissue sealant that uses pooled (virally inactivated) human plasma as a source of both fibrinogen and thrombin (plus bovine aprotinin to inhibit fibrinolysis).[47]

Autologous platelet-rich plasma can be prepared at the start of open heart surgery, using apheresis equipment before bypass, to be returned to the patient after heparin reversal.[48] Because thrombocytopenia or an acquired platelet defect can occur after blood passes through the membrane oxygenator,[49] the theoretical advantages of transfusing platelet-rich plasma should include an improvement in hemostasis and reduced transfusion requirements. Although initial studies of this approach provided supportive data,[48, 50–52] later prospective, blinded protocols were not able to demonstrate a reduction in blood use in either primary heart surgery or reoperations.[53, 54] In addition, the harvesting of platelet-rich plasma has been followed by intraoperative heparin resistance, possibly owing to release of platelet factor 3 and other procoagulants from platelets damaged during the collection.[55] A recent meta-analysis of 17 trials that used platelet-rich plasma in cardiac surgery noted that most studies had serious methodologic problems, so no conclusion regarding efficacy could be made.[56]

Collecting Autologous Blood

Autologous blood donations are well tolerated by a variety of ostensibly high-risk donors, including the elderly,[22, 57] children,[58] pregnant women,[30, 31] and patients with atherosclerotic coronary artery disease.[59] One group reported an increased frequency of serious reactions among autologous donors at blood collection facilities, although this may reflect an intentionally conservative approach to patients (compared with the normal volunteers that donor centers are accustomed to).[60] A weekly phlebotomy schedule fosters some degree of RBC regeneration before surgery (in one study, a mean of 522 mL of RBCs donated over 3 weeks resulted in a mean RBC production of 351 mL).[61] However, the most important medical problem associated with autologous donation is anemia developing during the collection interval. When this occurs, it is typically as a result of marginal iron stores and insufficient erythropoietic response (with little or no increase in serum erythropoietin levels), probably because the hematocrit of most donors is not allowed to fall below 30%.[62] This situation may be improved by the administration of recombinant human erythropoietin.[63] Many variables affect the response of blood donors to this drug, including route of administration, adequacy of iron stores, and method of iron supplementation (oral versus parenteral).[64, 65] Especially in the United States, the expense of recombinant human erythropoietin has limited its use to situations in which autologous blood donation might otherwise be difficult or impossible (e.g., in a patient who is already anemic).[66, 67] An alternative approach employs RBC apheresis—collection of two units of RBCs (without plasma)—because each collection enhances the rate of compensatory erythropoiesis.[68]

Provided that the donor has satisfactory iron stores and that bone marrow erythropoiesis can occur in a timely fashion, blood may be comfortably collected from an autologous donor on a weekly schedule. Oral ferrous sulfate is commonly prescribed (325 mg three times daily), although the amount absorbed may not be sufficient to counter the iron lost with the donations.[69, 70] The shelf life of refrigerated whole blood is limited to 42 days with current formulations of anticoagulant-preservative solutions, and a schedule for multiple donations is usually fit into this 6-week window. Alternatively, some or all of the units can be frozen at −65°C, using glycerol as a cryopreservative, for up to 10 years. Although frozen units allow collections to occur over a longer period, the flexibility of utility at the time of surgery is affected: thawing and deglycerolizing takes a few hours, and the thawed units have an outdate of 24 hours.

■ Intraoperative Autologous Transfusion: Blood Salvage

A number of techniques has been developed for the salvage and reinfusion of blood lost during an operative procedure. Interest in intraoperative salvage has been spurred by the introduction of pumps, separation chambers for washing RBCs, and increasing automation of the collection process.[71, 72] The simplest approach, direct reinfusion without washing, involves collection of blood under low vacuum pressure into a plastic bag seated within a hard outer cannister. An anticoagulant, usually citrate, is added. As soon as the bag is full, or within 4 hours after the start of the collection (to prevent bacterial growth), the contents of the bag are reinfused through a standard blood filter to the patient (Fig. 23.1). RBCs shed into a surgical field, already potentially damaged by their travail, are accompanied by activated coagulation factors and platelets, cellular debris and soluble factors

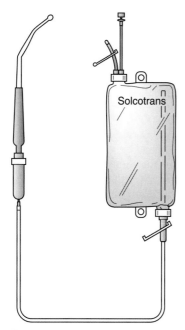

Figure 23.1 Equipment for the direct reinfusion of perioperatively salvaged blood without washing. A 600-mL plastic bag is seated within the rigid plastic outer shell. A suction aspirator wand and filter are connected to the bottom port; vacuum suction is connected to the top left port. The top right port is connected to a blood filter for transfusion to the autologous recipient. (From Solco Basle, Rockland, MA, and Williams and Wilkins, with permission.)

released from injured tissue cells, pharmaceuticals applied to the field, and irrigant solutions. Despite this scenario, salvaged blood has been reinfused directly into patients with few untoward consequences.

Alternatively, the contents in the bag can be washed with saline. Devices that include a reservoir for collecting the salvaged blood and a centrifuge for washing are now available (Fig. 23.2) to collect and process large volumes (e.g., 225 mL of RBCs with a final hematocrit of 50% in less than 3 minutes).[73] With these techniques, intraoperative blood salvage has become practical in situations in which blood loss may be extremely rapid, such as trauma or liver transplantation. Approximately one half of the blood lost during a surgical procedure can be recovered; the rest is irretrievably absorbed in drapes and sponges or damaged during collection.[74]

Complications of intraoperative salvage are surprisingly infrequent. The hematocrit of salvaged unprocessed blood is typically low because of a combination of dilution from irrigation fluids and some degree of mechanical hemolysis.[75] Free hemoglobin levels may exceed 1000 mg/dL, and in the recipient this can result in hemoglobinemia and hemoglobinuria (Table 23.2). Nevertheless, renal sequelae are uncommon.[76] The survival of chromium 51–labeled salvaged cells is normal in most patients, presumably because damaged cells are cleared with processing.[77, 78]

Coagulation abnormalities are often observed in recipients of large volumes of salvaged blood and include hypofibrinogenemia, elevated fibrin degradation products, thrombocytopenia, and prolonged prothrombin and partial thromboplastin times.[79, 80] In general, this clinical picture is related to a combination of the characteristics of the salvaged blood and hemodilution in the recipient. After exposure to serosal surfaces in the operative field, blood becomes depleted of coagulation factors and platelets; in the case of unwashed autologous blood, fibrin degradation products accumulate.[81] Although the clinical picture can resemble that of disseminated intravascular coagulation, which in theory might be initiated by phospholipids and other materials released from damaged blood cells, no evidence exists to support a cause-and-effect relationship.

Other substances in salvaged blood include fat, fibrin, and microaggregates. Infusion of unprocessed blood has not been shown to be harmful in either animals or humans, possibly because of the removal of most particulate matter by standard blood filters.[82, 83] Pharmaceutical contaminants, such as heparin, topical antibiotics, hemostatic agents, and biologic substances such as tissue enzymes and hormones, can be removed, but usually not completely, by washing.[84, 85]

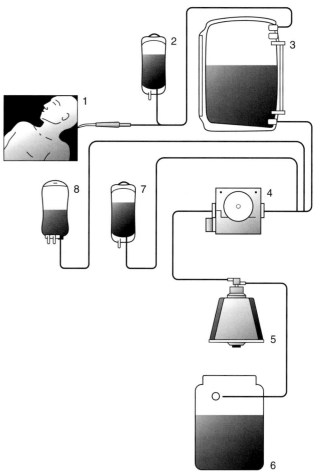

Figure 23.2 Schematics of an instrument used for collection and washing of perioperatively salvaged blood. Shed blood is suctioned from the operative field (1), an anticoagulant is added (2), and the blood moves past a mesh filter into a reservoir (3). A pump (4) forces the blood into a spinning plastic centrifuge bowl (5). With separation, plasma flows into a waste bag (6); saline (7) is continuously pumped into the bowl to wash the packed red blood cells. At the completion of washing, the red blood cells are moved into a reinfusion bag (8) for return to the patient. (From Haemonetics, Braintree, MA, and Williams and Wilkins, with permission.)

Table 23.2   Characteristics of Perioperatively Salvaged Blood Compared with Banked Blood and Normal Patient Values.*

Component	Hematocrit	Free Hemoglobin (mg/dL)	Platelet Count (/mm³)	Coagulation Factors	Fibrin Degradation Products
Salvaged blood, unwashed	Low (25%)	Very high (≥200)	Low (100,000)	Low (35%–75%)	High (300 mg/dL)
Salvaged blood, washed	High (60%)	Low (<50)	Very low (<10,000)	Absent	Absent
Allogeneic blood (packed red blood cells)	High (60%)	Variable with age of component	Low and dysfunctional (100,000)	Low	Increased
Normal patient	Normal (40%)	<5	300,000	100%	<10 mg/dL

*Typical results of laboratory tests are given. The transfusion of large volumes of salvaged blood could result in similar alterations in the recipient. From Noon GP: Intraoperative autotransfusion. Surgery 1978; 84:719–721, and Silva R, Moore EE, Bar-Or D, et al: The risk:benefit ratio of autotransfusion: Comparison to banked blood in a canine model. J. Trauma 1984;24:557–564, with permission.

Bacterial contamination during the collection and processing of autologous blood is also inevitable due to environmental organisms such as coagulase-positive and -negative staphylococci, propionibacteria, and *Corynebacterium* species. Administration of antibiotics to the patient reduces the microorganisms but does not eliminate them,[86] and complete removal of bacteria after collection also is not possible, even when the washing solution includes antibiotics.[87] There is no apparent clinical significance to such low levels of contamination. Larger bacterial counts are of more concern. Collection of blood from a contaminated site, such as that associated with spilled intestinal contents, is probably contraindicated, although some authors have argued that, if no other blood is available, such transfusions may be life-saving and worth the risk.[88, 89] Tumor cells have also been found in salvaged blood during cancer surgery; their malignant potential is unknown, and many consider cancer another contraindication.[90, 91]

Finally, although it is uncommon, the collection process can be associated with fatal air embolism; such events were originally reported in association with a device that allowed reservoir contents to be pumped directly into a venous catheter, without an air detection system.[92] Although instruments with this design are no longer marketed, rare fatalities are still reported. A 1997 report cautioned that external pressure devices magnify the risk of air embolism and should never be used with perioperatively salvaged blood except if absolutely necessary and under close supervision.[93]

The collection and transfusion of intraoperatively salvaged blood has been associated with substantial reductions in allogeneic transfusions (>50%), particularly in spine surgery,[94, 95] in hip replacement,[96] and in vascular procedures such as aortic reconstruction.[97] During cardiac surgery, the largest volume of blood that can be processed for return to the patient comes from the membrane oxygenator. Although this blood is not technically shed, in that it is removed from the extracorporeal circuit at the end of surgery, the processing is helpful in concentrating the RBCs and removing cardioplegia solution.[98, 99] In liver transplantation volumes as large as 25 units have been salvaged,[100–102] and salvage during trauma is also feasible.[87, 103, 104] The collection of autologous blood during cesarean section carries theoretical risks associated with transfusing amniotic fluid; however, an analysis of 139 women who received processed salvaged blood identified no increased incidence of obstetric complications.[105] Blood has also been recovered from the hemoperitoneum in association with ectopic pregnancy,[106] during radical prostatectomy,[107] and during splenectomy.[108] Intraoperatively salvaged blood has been a useful adjunct in the treatment of some Jehovah's Witnesses, whose literal acceptance of the Bible includes abstention from routine allogeneic blood transfusions. In this situation, an uninterrupted circuit between the salvaged blood processor and the patient facilitates acceptance.[109]

■ Postoperative Autologous Transfusion: Blood Salvage

Both cannister systems and RBC processors can be used to collect postoperative blood drainage, such as that from the mediastinum after heart surgery,[110] from the peritoneal cavity after hepatic injury,[111] or from the knee or hip site after orthopedic procedures.[112] Blood salvaged from a serosal cavity has little residual fibrinogen or platelets, and clotting is usually not a problem; therefore the addition of anticoagulants to the collection is usually not necessary.[113] Despite the substantial levels of free hemoglobin in the salvaged blood, RBCs survive normally, as documented by studies involving radiolabeled markers.[114]

In addition to free hemoglobin, the salvaged blood may be contaminated with tissue exudate, bone, bone marrow, and other biologic and surgical materials; nevertheless, most patients tolerate the infusions well. Bioactive substances measured in the unwashed drainage include histamine, interleukin-6 and other cytokines, prostaglandins, and activated complement components; however, these levels have not been associated with transfusion reactions, and measurements in patients after infusion are not significantly affected.[115–117] Similarly, methyl methacrylate (used as a cement in orthopedic surgery) and its breakdown product, methanol, can be measured in blood salvaged postoperatively from the surgical site; however, these materials have not been detected in recipients after transfusion.[118] Occasional complications do occur, however, including respiratory distress,[119] hypotension with anaphylaxis,[120] and fever,[121] the last more likely to occur when the product is collected over a long time interval (6 to 12 hours). The pathophysiology of these events remains unclear.

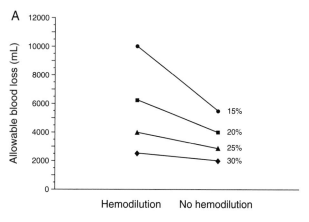
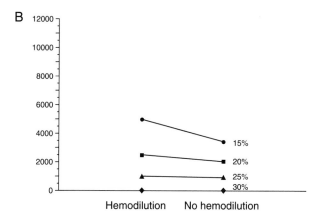

Figure 23.3   The volume of surgical blood loss (Y-axis) that could occur before transfusion of allogeneic blood is needed, in a patient of either 45% (graph A) or 30% (graph B) with a starting hematocrit and a blood volume of 5 L who either has or has not undergone isovolemic hemodilution. Each curve represents a different target hematocrit (the hemodilution endpoint, which is then maintained during surgery with autologous blood). (From Weiskopf RB: Mathematical analysis of isovolemic hemodilution indicates that it can decrease the need for allogeneic blood transfusion. Transfusion 1995;35:37–41. With permission).

After open heart surgery, mediastinal blood may contain very high levels of cardiac muscle enzymes, especially creatine phosphokinase, as well as lactate dehydrogenase from hemolyzed RBCs.[81, 122] The reinfusion of shed mediastinal blood can result in increased levels of these enzymes and can confound the diagnosis of myocardial infarction in the postoperative period.[123, 124]

The volume of RBCs actually salvaged is often small, and the effect on reducing transfusions debatable. Infusion of shed mediastinal blood after cardiac operations appears to have the potential to reduce the volume of allogeneic blood required (by 1.4 units in one study).[125] In other situations, the benefit is less clear. Although the volume of postoperative drainage is often substantial in orthopedic procedures,[126, 127] much of the collection is plasma and other serosanguineous fluids, rather than RBCs. One study reported a mean total collection of only 55 ± 29 mL of RBCs in drains after hip surgery.[128] Arthroplasty procedures performed without cement are associated with larger perioperative blood losses, and postoperative salvage may be more effectively used in such cases.[129]

■ Acute Normovolemic Hemodilution

The collection of autologous blood at the start of a surgery, for return to the patient at the end of the procedure, had its origins in open heart surgery. The original goal was prevention of postoperative coagulopathies through ex vivo maintenance of a supply of platelets undamaged by exposure to the membrane oxygenator.[130, 131] However, additional advantages to the intentionally created anemia were also identified. Hemodilution can contribute to a reduction in RBC loss. In simplest terms, a patient with a hematocrit of 45% and a 2-L blood loss during surgery loses roughly 900 mL of RBCs, whereas a similar patient with a hematocrit of 20% loses only 400 mL of RBCs. More elaborate mathematical modeling studies have been published that take into account the dynamic nature of the patient's RBC mass as it is affected by blood loss, fluid replacement, and blood transfusions (Fig. 23.3).[132, 133] Hemodilution is probably less expensive to accomplish than preoperative autologous blood donation, and

it may be the only option available when surgery is performed in other than elective settings.[134]

The technique involves removal of blood into standard collection bags with the citrate anticoagulation (unless the patient is already heparinized) and replacement of lost volume with either crystalloids or colloids. Close monitoring of the patient's cardiovascular status is necessary during the hemodilution process. Units are stored in the operating room during surgery and reinfused as needed, in reverse order of collection, reserving the bags with the highest concentration of RBCs for the end of the procedure, after blood loss has been controlled.

In orthopedic and cardiovascular surgery, reductions in allogeneic blood use have been reported after extreme hemodilution (reduction of the patient's RBC mass by as much as 50%).[133, 135] More modest hemodilution (e.g., removal of 2 units of blood at the beginning of surgery) may also be beneficial, according to some workers,[136, 137] but this is not accepted by others.[132, 138, 139] The severity of the anemia could affect oxygen transport, although the concomitant drop in blood viscosity, and compensatory cardiac output increases, could restore oxygen delivery. However, one group has provided evidence that hemodilution may jeopardize patients at risk for myocardial infarction.[140] Further clinical studies appear necessary to resolve the continued controversy over the value of hemodilution in contemporary transfusion practice.[141, 142]

REFERENCES

1. Highmore W: Practical remarks on an overlooked source of blood supply for transfusion in postpartum hemorrhage, suggested by a recent fatal case. Lancet 1874;1:89.
2. Theis HJ: Zur Behandlung der Estrauteringraviditar. Zentralbl Gynakol 1914;38:1191–1193.
3. Surgenor DM, Wallace EL, Hao SL, Chapman RH: Collection and transfusion of blood in the United States, 1982–1988. N Engl J Med 1990;322:1646–1651.
4. Wallace EL, Churchill WH, Surgenor DM, et al: Collection and transfusion of blood and blood components in the United States, 1992. Transfusion 1995;35:802–812.
5. Blajchman MA: Transfusion-associated immunomodulation and universal white cell reduction: Are we putting the cart before the horse? Transfusion 1999;39:665–670.

6. Owings DV, Kruskall MS, Thurer RL, Donovan LM: Autologous blood donations prior to elective cardiac surgery: Safety and effect on subsequent blood use. JAMA 1989;262:1963–1968.
7. Wolfe LC, Byrne AM, Lux SE: Molecular defects in the membrane skeleton of blood bank-stored red cells: Abnormal spectrin-protein 4.1-actin complex formation. J Clin Invest 1986;78:1681–1686.
8. Spiess BD, Sassetti RJ, McCarthy RJ, et al: Autologous blood donation: Hemodynamics in a high-risk patient population. Transfusion 1992;32:17–22.
9. Linden JV: Autologous blood errors and incidents [Abstract]. Transfusion 1994;34:28S.
10. Haditsch M, Binder L, Garbriel C, et al: *Yersinia enterocolitica* septicemia in autologous blood transfusion. Transfusion 1994;34:907–909.
11. Etchason J, Petz L, Keeler E, et al: The cost-effectiveness of preoperative autologous blood donations. N Engl J Med 1995;332:719–724.
12. Heiss MM, Mempel W, Jauch KW, et al: Beneficial effect of autologous blood transfusion on infectious complications after colorectal cancer surgery. Lancet 1993;342:1328–1333.
13. Busch OR, Hop WC, van Papendrecht MAH, et al: Blood transfusion and prognosis in colorectal cancer. N Engl J Med 1993;328:1372–1376.
14. Jensen LS, Kissmeyer-Nielsen P, Wolff B, Qvist N: Randomised comparison of leucocyte-depleted versus buffy-coat-poor blood transfusion and complications after colorectal surgery. Lancet 1996;348:841–845.
15. Sonnenberg FA, Gregory P, Yomtovian R, et al: The cost-effectiveness of autologous transfusion revisited: Implications of an increased risk of bacterial infection with allogeneic transfusion. Transfusion 1999;39:808–817.
16. Kruskall MS, Yomtovian R, Dzik WH, et al: On improving the cost-effectiveness of autologous blood transfusion practices. Transfusion 1994;34:259–264.
17. Kruskall MS: Cost effectiveness of autologous blood donation. N Engl J Med 1995;333:461–462.
18. Blum LN, Allen JR, Genel M, Howe JPI: Crossover use of donated blood for autologous transfusion: Report of the Council on Scientific Affairs, American Medical Association. Transfusion 1998;38:891–895.
19. Haugen RK, Hill GE: A large-scale autologous blood program in a community hospital: A contribution to the community's blood supply. JAMA 1987;257:1211–1214.
20. Woolson ST, Marsh JS, Tanner JB: Transfusion of previously deposited autologous blood for patients undergoing hip-replacement surgery. J Bone Joint Surg Am 1987;69:325–328.
21. Woolson ST, Pottorff G: Use of preoperatively deposited autologous blood for total knee replacement. Orthopedics 1993;16:137–141.
22. Kruskall MS, Glazer EE, Leonard SS, et al: Utilization and effectiveness of a hospital autologous preoperative blood donor program. Transfusion 1986;26:335–340.
23. Toy PTCY, Strauss RG, Stehling LC, et al: Predeposited autologous blood for elective surgery. N Engl J Med 1987;316:517–520.
24. Thompson HW, McCullough J: Use of blood components containing red cells by donors of allogeneic bone marrow. Transfusion 1986;26:98–100.
25. Peters CA, Walsh PC: Blood transfusion and anesthetic practices in radical retropubic prostatectomy. J Urol 1985;134:81–83.
26. Toy PTCY, Menozzi D, Strauss RG, et al: Efficacy of preoperative donation of blood for autologous use in radical prostatectomy. Transfusion 1993;33:721–724.
27. Koch MO, Smith JA Jr: Blood loss during radical retropubic prostatectomy: Is preoperative autologous blood donation indicated? J Urol 1996;156:1077–1080.
28. Goh M, Kleer CG, Kielczewski P, et al: Autologous blood donation prior to anatomical radical retropubic prostatectomy: Is it necessary? Urology 1996;49:569–574.
29. Kruskall MS: Autologous blood transfusions and plastic surgery [Editorial]. Plast Reconstr Surg 1989;84:662–664.
30. Kruskall MS, Leonard S, Klapholz H: Autologous blood donation during pregnancy: Analysis of safety and blood utilization. Obstet Gynecol 1987;70:938–941.
31. McVay PA, Hoag RW, Hoag MS, Toy PT: Safety and use of autologous blood donation during the third trimester of pregnancy. Am J Obstet Gynecol 1989;160:1479–1486.
32. Kamani AA, McMorland GH, Wadsworth LD: Utilization of red blood cell transfusion in an obstetric setting. Am J Obstet Gynecol 1988;159:1177–1181.
33. Klapholz H: Blood transfusion in contemporary obstetric practice. Obstet Gynecol 1990;75:940–943.
34. Katz AR, Ali V, Ross PJ, Gammon E: Management of a rare blood type: Oh "Bombay" in pregnancy. Obstet Gynecol 1981;57:16S–17S.
35. Consensus conference: Fresh-frozen plasma—Indications and risks. JAMA 1985;253:551–553.
36. Matthew TL, Spotnitz WD, Kron IL, et al: Four years' experience with fibrin sealant in thoracic and cardiovascular surgery. Ann Thorac Surg 1990;50:40–44.
37. Silberstein LE, Williams LJ, Hughlett MA, et al: An autologous fibrinogen-based adhesive for use in otologic surgery. Transfusion 1988;28:319–321.
38. Stechison MT: Rapid polymerizing fibrin glue from autologous or single-donor blood: Preparation and indications. J Neurosurg 1993;76:626–628.
39. Dahlstrom KK, Weis-Fogh US, Medgyesi S, et al: The use of autologous fibrin adhesive in skin transplantation. Plast Reconstr Surg 1992;89:968–972.
40. Abel ME, Chui YS, Russell TR, Volpe PA: Autologous fibrin glue in the treatment of rectovaginal and complex fistulas. Dis Colon Rectum 1993;36:447–449.
41. Kram HB, Clark SR, Ocampo HP, et al: Fibrin glue sealing of pancreatic injuries, resections, and anastomoses. Am J Surg 1991;161:479–481.
42. Dulchavsky SA, Geller ER, Maurer J, et al: Autologous fibrin gel: Bactericidal properties in contaminated hepatic injury. J Trauma 1991;31:991–994.
43. Berguer R, Staerkel RL, Moore EE, et al: Warning: Fatal reaction to the use of fibrin glue in deep hepatic wounds. Case reports. J Trauma 1991;31:408–411.
44. Rapaport SI, Zivelin A, Minow RA, et al: Clinical significance of antibodies to bovine and human thrombin and factor V after surgical use of bovine thrombin. Am J Clin Pathol 1992;97:84–91.
45. Ortel TL, Quinn-Allen MA, Charles LA, et al: Characterization of an acquired inhibitor to coagulation factor V: Antibody binding to the second C-type domain of factor V inhibits the binding of factor V to phosphatidylserine and neutralizes procoagulant activity. J Clin Invest 1992;90:2340–2347.
46. Berruyer M, Amiral J, French P, et al: Immunization by bovine thrombin used with fibrin glue during cardiovascular operations. J Thorac Cardiovasc Surg 1993;105:892–897.
47. Radosevich M, Goubran HA, Bumouf T: Fibrin sealant: Scientific rationale, production methods, properties, and current clinical use. Vox Sang 1997;72:133–143.
48. Giordano GF, Rivers SL, Chung GK, et al: Autologous platelet-rich plasma in cardiac surgery: Effect on intraoperative and postoperative transfusion requirements. Ann Thorac Surg 1988;46:416–419.
49. Harker LA, Malpass TW, Branson HE, et al: Mechanism of abnormal bleeding in patients undergoing cardiopulmonary bypass: Acquired transient platelet dysfunction associated with selective alpha-granule release. Blood 1980;56:824–834.
50. Boldt J, von Bormann B, Kling D, et al: Preoperative plasmapheresis in patients undergoing cardiac surgery procedures. Anesthesiology 1990;72:282–288.
51. Davies GG, Wells DG, Mabee TM, et al: Platelet-leukocyte plasmapheresis attenuates the deleterious effects of cardiopulmonary bypass. Ann Thorac Surg 1992;53:274–277.
52. DelRossi AJ, Cernaianu AC, Venrees RA, et al: Platelet-rich plasma reduces postoperative blood loss after cardiopulmonary bypass. J Thorac Cardiovasc Surg 1990;100:281–286.
53. Tobe CE, Vocelka C, Sepulvada R, et al: Infusion of autologous platelet rich plasma does not reduce blood loss and product use after coronary artery bypass. J Thorac Cardiovasc Surg 1993;105:1007–1014.
54. Ereth MH, Oliver WC, Beynen FMK, et al: Autologous platelet-rich plasma does not reduce transfusion of homologous blood products in patients undergoing repeat valvular surgery. Anesthesiology 1993;79:540–547.
55. Wickey GS, Keifer JC, Larach DR, et al: Heparin resistance after intraoperative platelet-rich plasma harvesting. J Thorac Cardiovasc Surg 1992;103:1172–1176.
56. Rubens FD, Fergusson D, Wells PS, et al: Platelet-rich plasmapheresis in cardiac surgery: A meta-analysis of the effect on transfusion requirements. J Thorac Cardiovasc Surg 1998;116:641–647.

57. Greenwalt TJ: Autologous and aged blood donors. JAMA 1987;257:1220–1221.

58. Silvergleid AJ: Safety and effectiveness of predeposit autologous transfusions in preteen and adolescent children. JAMA 1987;257:3403–3404.

59. Goldfinger D, Capon S, Czer L, et al: Safety and efficacy of preoperative donation of blood for autologous use by patients with end-stage heart or lung disease who are awaiting organ transplantation. Transfusion 1993;33:336–340.

60. Popovsky MA, Whitaker B, Arnold NL: Severe outcomes of allogeneic and autologous blood donation: Frequency and characterization. Transfusion 1995;35:734–737.

61. Kasper SM, Gerlich W, Buzello W: Preoperative red cell production in patients undergoing weekly autologous blood donation. Transfusion 1997;37:1058–1062.

62. Kickler TS, Spivak JL: Effect of repeated whole blood donations on serum immunoreactive erythropoietin levels in autologous donors. JAMA 1988;260:65–67.

63. Goodnough LT, Price TH, Rudnick S, Soegiarso RW: Preoperative red cell production in patients undergoing aggressive autologous blood phlebotomy with and without erythropoietin therapy. Transfusion 1992;32:441–445.

64. Brugnara C, Chambers LA, Malynn E, et al: Red blood cell regeneration induced by subcutaneous recombinant erythropoietin: Iron-deficient erythropoiesis in iron-replete subjects. Blood 1993;81:956–964.

65. Rutherford CJ, Schneider TJ, Dempsey H, et al: Efficacy of different dosing regimens for recombinant human erythropoietin in a simulated perisurgical setting: The importance of iron availability in optimizing response. Am J Med 1994;96:139–145.

66. Mercuriali F, Zanella A, Barosi G, et al: Use of erythropoietin to increase the volume of autologous blood donated by orthopedic patients. Transfusion 1993;33:55–60.

67. Price TH, Goodnough LT, Vogler WR, et al: Improving the efficacy of preoperative autologous blood donation in patients with low hematocrit: A randomized, double-blind, controlled trial of recombinant human erythropoietin. Am J Med 1996;101:22S–27S.

68. Smith KJ, James DS, Hunt WC: A randomized, double-blind comparison of donor tolerance of 400 mL, 200 mL, and sham red cell donation. Transfusion 1996;36:674–680.

69. Monsen ER, Critchlow CW, Finch CA, Donohue DM: Iron balance in super donors. Transfusion 1983;23:221–225.

70. Lieden G, Hoglund S, Ehn L: Iron supplement to blood donors: II. Effect of continuous iron supply. Acta Med Scand 1975;197:37–41.

71. Wilson JD, Utz DC, Taswell HF: Auto transfusion during transurethral resection of the prostate: Technique and preliminary clinical evaluation. Mayo Clin Proc 1969;44:374–386.

72. Long GW, Glover JL, Bendick PJ, et al: Cell washing versus immediate reinfusion of intraoperatively shed blood during abdominal aortic aneurysm repair. Am J Surg 1993;166:97–102.

73. Williamson KR, Taswell HF: Intraoperative blood salvage: A review. Transfusion 1991;31:662–675.

74. O'Hara PJ, Hertzer NR, Santilli PH, Beven EG: Intraoperative autotransfusion during abdominal aortic reconstruction. Am J Surg 1983;145:215–220.

75. Aaron RK, Beazley RM, Riggle GC: Hematologic integrity after intraoperative allotransfusion: Comparison with bank blood. Arch Surg 1974;108:831–837.

76. Brener BJ, Raines JK, Darling RC: Intraoperative autotransfusion in abdominal aortic resections. Arch Surg 1973;107:78–84.

77. Ansell J, Parrilla N, King M, et al: Survival of autotransfused red blood cells recovered from the surgical field during cardiovascular operations. J Thorac Cardiovasc Surg 1982;84:387–391.

78. Buth J, Raines JK, Kolodny GM, Darling RC: Effect of intraoperative autotransfusion on red cell mass and red cell survival. Surg Forum 1975;26:276–278.

79. Stillman RM, Wrezlewicz WW, Stanczewski BS, et al: The haematological hazards of auto transfusion. Br J Surg 1976;63:651–654.

80. Moore EE, Dunn EL, Breslich DJ, Galloway WB: Platelet abnormalities associated with massive autotransfusion. J Trauma 1980;20:1052–1056.

81. Griffith LD, Billman GF, Daily PO, Lane TA: Apparent coagulopathy caused by infusion of shed mediastinal blood and its prevention by washing of the infusate. Ann Thorac Surg 1989;47:400–406.

82. Dorang LA, Klebanoff G, Kemmerer WT: Autotransfusion in long-segment spinal fusion: An experimental model to demonstrate the efficacy of salvaging blood contaminated with bone fragments and marrow. Am J Surg 1972;123:686–688.

83. Bennett SH, Geelhoed GW, Terrill RE, Hoye RC: Pulmonary effects of autotransfused blood: A comparison of fresh autologous and stored blood with blood retrieved from the pleural cavity in an in situ lung perfusion mode. Am J Surg 1973;125:696–702.

84. Umlas J, O'Neill TP: Heparin removal in an autotransfusor device. Transfusion 1981;21:70–73.

85. Paravicini D, Thys J, Hein H: Use of neomycin-bacitracin irrigating solution with intraoperative autotransfusions during orthopedic operations. Arzneimittelforschung 1983;33:997–999.

86. Wollinsky KH, Oethinger M, Buchele M, et al: Autotransfusion—Bacterial contamination during hip arthroplasty and efficacy of cefuroxime prophylaxis: A randomized controlled study of 40 patients. Acta Orthop Scand 1997;68:225–230.

87. Rumisek JD, Weddle RL: Autotransfusion in penetrating abdominal trauma. In Hauer JM, Thurer RL, Dawson RB (eds). Auto Transfusion. New York: Elsevier/North Holland, 1981, pp 105–113.

88. Timberlake GA, McSwain NE: Autotransfusion of blood contaminated by enteric contents: A potentially life-saving measure in the massively hemorrhaging trauma patient? J Trauma 1988;28:855–857.

89. Ozmen V, McSwain NE Jr, Nichols RL, et al: Autotransfusion of potentially culture-positive blood (CPB) in abdominal trauma: Preliminary data from a prospective study. J Trauma 1992;32:36–39.

90. Yaw PB, Sentany M, Link WJ, et al: Tumor cells carried through auto transfusion: Contraindication to intraoperative blood recovery? JAMA 1975;231:490–491.

91. Lane TA: The effect of storage on the metastatic potential of tumor cells collected in autologous blood: An animal model. Transfusion 1989;29:418–420.

92. Duncan SE, Klebanoff G, Rogers W: A clinical experience with intraoperative auto transfusion. Ann Surg 1974;180:296–304.

93. Linden JV, Kaplan HS, Murphy MT: Fatal air embolism due to perioperative blood recovery. Anesth Analg 1997;84:422–426.

94. Lennon RL, Hosking MP, Gray JR, et al: The effects of intraoperative blood salvage and induced hypotension on transfusion requirements during spinal surgical procedures. Mayo Clin Proc 1987;62:1090–1094.

95. Kruger LM, Colbert JM: Intraoperative autologous transfusion in children undergoing spinal surgery. J Pediatr Orthop 1985;5:330–332.

96. Bovill DF, Moulton CW, Jackson WST, et al: The efficacy of intraoperative autologous transfusion in major orthopedic surgery: A regression analysis. Orthopedics 1986;9:1403–1407.

97. Hallett JW Jr, Popovsky M, Ilstrup D: Minimizing blood transfusions during abdominal aortic surgery: Recent advances in rapid auto transfusion. J Vasc Surg 1987;5:601–606.

98. Keeling MM, Gray LA, Brink MA, et al: Intraoperative autotransfusion: Experience in 725 consecutive cases. Ann Surg 1983;197:536–541.

99. McCarthy PM, Popovsky MA, Schaff HV, et al: Effect of blood conservation efforts in cardiac operations at the Mayo Clinic. Mayo Clin Proc 1988;63:225–229.

100. Dzik WH, Jenkins R: Use of intraoperative blood salvage during orthotopic liver transplantation. Arch Surg 1985;120:946–948.

101. Van Voorst SJ, Peters TG, Williams JW, et al: Autotransfusion in hepatic transplantation. Am J Surg 1985;51:623–626.

102. Williamson KR, Taswell HF, Rettke SR, Krom RAF: Intraoperative autologous transfusion: Its role in orthotopic liver transplantation. Mayo Clin Proc 1989;64:340–345.

103. Reul GJ Jr, Solis RT, Greenberg SD, et al: Experience with autotransfusion in the surgical management of trauma. Surgery 1974;76:546–555.

104. Smith RS, Meister RK, Tsoi EKM, Bohman HR: Laparoscopically guided blood salvage and autotransfusion in splenic trauma: A case report. J Trauma 1993;34:313–314.

105. Rebarber A, Lonser R, Jackson S, et al: The safety of intraoperative autologous blood collection and autotransfusion during cesarean section. Am J Obstet Gynecol 1998;179:715–720.

106. Merrill BS, Mitts DL, Rogers W, Weinberg PC: Auto transfusion: Intraoperative use in ruptured ectopic pregnancy. J Reprod Med 1980;24:14–16.

107. Klimberg I, Sirois R, Wajsman Z, Baker J: Intraoperative autotransfusion in urologic oncology. Arch Surg 1986;121:1326–1329.

108. Witte CL, Esser MJ, Rappaport WD: Updating the management of salvageable splenic injury. Ann Surg 1992;215:261–265.

109. Spence RK, Alexander JB, DelRossi AJ, et al: Transfusion guidelines for cardiovascular surgery: Lessons learned from operations in Jehovah's Witnesses. J Vasc Surg 1992,16:825–831.

110. Johnson RG, Rosenkrantz KR, Preston RA, et al: The efficacy of postoperative autotransfusion in patients undergoing cardiac operations. Ann Thorac Surg 1983;36:173–179.

111. Semkiw LB, Schurman DJ, Goodman SB, Woolson ST: Postoperative blood salvage using the Cell Saver after total joint arthroplasty. J Bone Joint Surg Am 1989;71:823–827.
112. Reiner DS, Tortolani AJ: Postoperative peritoneal blood salvage with autotransfusion after hepatic trauma. Surg Gynecol Obstet 1991;173:501–504.
113. Glover JL, Broadie TA: Intraoperative auto transfusion. World J Surg 1987;11:60–64.
114. Schmidt H, Lund JO, Nielsen SL: Autotransfused shed mediastinal blood has normal erythrocyte survival. Ann Thorac Surg 1996;62:105–108.
115. Jensen CM, Pilegaard R, Hviid K, et al: Quality of reinfused drainage blood after total knee arthroplasty. J Arthroplasty 1999;14:312–318.
116. Schmidt H, Bendtzen K, Mortensen PE: The inflammatory cytokine response after autotransfusion of shed mediastinal blood. Acta Anaesthesiol Scand 1998;42:558–564.
117. Mottl-Link S, Russlies M, Klinger M, et al: Erythrocytes and proinflammatory mediators in wound drainage. Vox Sang 1998;75:205–211.
118. Hand GCR, Henderson M, Mace P, et al: Methyl methacrylate levels in unwashed salvage blood following unilateral total knee arthroplasty. J Arthroplasty 1998;13:576–579.
119. Woda R, Tetzlaff JE: Upper airway oedema following autologous blood transfusion from a wound drainage system. Can J Anaesth 1992;390:290–292.
120. Dich-Nielsen JO, Rajan RM, Jensen J-J: An anaphylactoid reaction following infusion of salvaged unwashed drain blood. Can J Anaesth 1998;45:189.
121. Faris PM, Ritter MA, Keating EM, Valeri CR: Unwashed filtered shed blood collected after knee and hip arthroplasties: A source of autologous red blood cells. J Bone Joint Surg Am 1991;73:1169–1178.
122. Klebanoff G: Early clinical experience with a disposable unit for the intraoperative salvage and reinfusion of blood loss (intraoperative autotransfusion). Am J Surg 1970;120:718–722.
123. Schmidt H, Mortensen PE, Folsgaard SL, Jensen EA: Cardiac enzymes and autotransfusion of shed mediastinal blood after myocardial revascularization. Ann Thorac Surg 1997;63:1288–1292.
124. Nguyen DM, Gilfix BM, Dennis F, et al: Impact of transfusion of mediastinal shed blood on serum levels of cardiac enzymes. Ann Thorac Surg 1996;62:109–114.
125. Kilgore ML, Pacifico AD: Shed mediastinal blood transfusion after cardiac operations: A cost-effectiveness analysis. Ann Thorac Surg 1998;65:1248–1254.
126. Gannon DM, Lombardi AV, Mallory TH, et al: An evaluation of the efficacy of postoperative blood salvage after total joint arthroplasty. J Arthroplasty 1991;1:109–114.
127. Majkowski RS, Currie IC, Newman JH: Postoperative collection and reinfusion of autologous blood in total knee arthroplasty. Ann R Coll Surg Engl 1991;73:381–384.
128. Umlas J, Foster RR, Dalal SA, et al: Red cell loss following orthopedic surgery: The case against postoperative blood salvage. Transfusion 1994;34:402–406.
129. Martin JW, Whiteside LA, Milliano MT, Reedy ME: Postoperative blood retrieval and transfusion in cementless total knee arthroplasty. J Arthroplasty 1992;7:205–210.
130. Cooley DA, Beall AC Jr, Grondin P: Open-heart operations with disposable oxygenators, 5 per cent dextrose prime, and normothermia. Surgery 1962;52:713–719.
131. Petry AF, Jost T, Sievers H: Reduction of homologous blood requirements by blood-pooling at the onset of cardiopulmonary bypass. J Thorac Cardiovasc Surg 1994;107:1210–1214.
132. Brecher ME, Rosenfeld M: Mathematical and computer modeling of acute normovolemic hemodilution. Transfusion 1994;34:176–179.
133. Weiskopf RB: Mathematical analysis of isovolemic hemodilution indicates that it can decrease the need for allogeneic blood transfusion. Transfusion 1995;35:37–41.
134. Monk TG, Goodnough LT, Brecher ME, et al: Acute normovolemic hemodilution can replace preoperative autologous blood donation as a standard of care for autologous blood procurement in radical prostatectomy. Anesth Analg 1997;85:953–958.
135. Milam JD, Austin SF, Nihill MR, et al: Use of sufficient hemodilution to prevent coagulopathies following surgical correction of cyanotic heart disease. J Thorac Cardiovasc Surg 1985;89:623–629.
136. Ness PM, Bourke DL, Walsh PC: A randomized trial of perioperative hemodilution versus transfusion of preoperatively deposited autologous blood in elective surgery. Transfusion 1992;32:226–230.
137. Johnson LB, Plotkin JS, Kuo PC: Reduced transfusion requirements during major hepatic resection with use of intraoperative isovolemic hemodilution. Am J Surg 1998;176:608–611.
138. Pliam MB, McGoon DC, Tarhan S: Failure of transfusion of autologous whole blood to reduce banked-blood requirements in open-heart surgical patients. J Thorac Cardiovasc Surg 1975;70:338–343.
139. Sherman MM, Dobnik DB, Dennis RC, Berger RL: Autologous blood transfusion during cardiopulmonary bypass. Chest 1976;70:592–595.
140. Weisel RD, Charlesworth DC, Mickleborough LL, et al: Limitations of blood conservation. J Thorac Cardiovasc Surg 1984;88:26–38.
141. Goodnough LT, Monk TG, Brecher ME: Acute normovolemic hemodilution should replace the preoperative donation of autologous blood as a method of autologous-blood procurement. Transfusion 1998;38:473–476.
142. Rottman G, Ness PM: Acute normovolemic hemodilution is a legitimate alternative to allogeneic blood transfusion. Transfusion 1999;38:477–480.
143. Noon GP: Intraoperative autotransfusion. Surgery 1978;84:719–721.
144. Silva R, Moore EE, Bar-Or D, et al: The risk:benefit ratio of autotransfusion: Comparison to banked blood in a canine model. J Trauma 1984;24:557–564.

i. Approach to the Anemic Patient

Chapter 24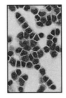

Red Blood Cell Transfusion and the Transfusion Trigger, Including the Surgical Setting

Pearl Toy

In the United States, approximately 13 million units of blood are collected per year.[1] An estimated two thirds of red blood cell transfusions are given in the perioperative period to treat acute blood loss.[2] At 15 hospitals in the University Health Consortium Clinical Database in 1994 to 1995, the top 10 procedures and conditions for which transfusion was given were as follows, in order of descending frequency: vaginal delivery, coronary artery bypass graft, hip replacement, back and neck procedures, craniotomy except for trauma, major cardiovascular procedures, cardiac valve procedures, percutaneous coronary angiography, gastrointestinal hemorrhage, and other vascular procedures.[3] This chapter discusses red blood cell transfusion in the perioperative period.

■ Physiology of Oxygen Transport

Tissues have no storage system for oxygen and rely on a continuous supply delivered by blood. Oxygen transport from air to mitochondria occurs in several steps[4] (Fig. 24.1). Inspired oxygen is taken up by the lungs and is transported by the heart into the arterial circulation. The arterial oxygen tension (Pa_{O_2}) is determined by the inspired oxygen concentration and barometric pressure, alveolar ventilation, diffusion of oxygen from alveoli to pulmonary capillaries, and distribution and matching of ventilation and perfusion. Oxygen is carried in the blood mostly on hemoglobin, with only a small amount (normally less than 2%) dissolved in the plasma. Oxygen content of blood is the product of hemoglobin content, arterial oxygen saturation, and a constant. Oxygen delivery (D_{O_2}) from lung to tissue is a product of cardiac output and oxygen content. Oxygen is off-loaded from hemoglobin in the red blood cells to interstitial fluid and then into intracellular mitochondria. As oxygen is off-loaded from hemoglobin, nitric oxide bound to hemoglobin and attached to the anion exchange protein AE1 is also exported.[5] The nitric oxide exported from red blood cells causes local vasodilation and an increase in local blood flow. Normally, oxygen delivery is adequate to meet oxygen consumption (V_{O_2}). Oxygen consumption can be measured directly or calculated as the product of cardiac output and the difference between arterial

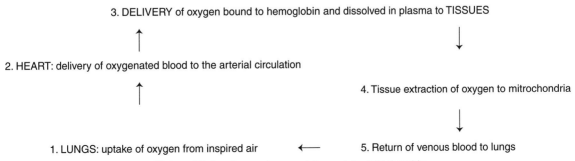

Figure 24.1 Oxygen transport from air to mitochondria.

and mixed venous oxygen content. The amount of oxygen consumed (Vo_2) divided by oxygen delivery (Do_2) is the oxygen extraction ratio (Vo_2/Do_2). In a normal adult with normal activity, the extraction ratio is 25%. The oxygen not extracted by the tissues returns to the lungs. Once the extraction ratio exceeds 60% to 70% for most tissues, consumption exceeds supply, and hypoxia occurs. Hypoxia can be the result of inadequate hemoglobin concentration, inadequate oxygen uptake by the lungs, or inadequate cardiac output.

■ Preoperative Correction of Anemia

Minimum Acceptable Hemoglobin Concentration

The National Institutes of Health Perioperative Consensus Conference concluded that "otherwise healthy patients with hemoglobin values of 10 g/dL or greater rarely require perioperative transfusion, whereas those with acute anemia with resulting hemoglobin values of less than 7 g/dL will frequently require red cell transfusions."[2] Whether patients with hemoglobin values between 7 and 10 g/dL should receive transfusions depends on the patient's clinical status. Since the conference, many specialty groups have issued similar guidelines on red cell transfusion.[6–14]

The minimum acceptable level of hemoglobin varies for patients because individual persons vary in their ability to tolerate and compensate for anemia. For example, at rest, normovolemic young healthy persons with normal cardiorespiratory function tolerate, at least briefly, a hemoglobin concentration of 5 g/dL. Serum lactate and oxygen consumption do not increase,[15] and mild cognitive impairment is reversible.[16] However, this low level of hemoglobin may not be benign to elderly patients with cardiopulmonary disease. Many questions remain regarding when we should transfuse red cells for acute anemia.[17]

Anemia from Nutritional Deficiencies: Iron, Vitamin B$_{12}$, and Folate Deficiency

If a preoperative patient is anemic, the cause should be found and, ideally, corrected preoperatively. Anemia resulting from nutritional deficiencies is easily correctable, but treatment takes weeks to months. If surgical procedures are required sooner and red blood cell transfusions must be given, transfusion should be given slowly to elderly patients to avoid circulatory overload. If surgical treatment is not urgent, nutritional replacement will correct the anemia and may obviate the need for red cell transfusion.

Iron is required for the synthesis of hemoglobin. Iron deficiency anemia can occur with blood loss or decreased iron intake or absorption. Blood loss can result from menses, gastrointestinal bleeding, hookworm infestation, or phlebotomy. Decreased iron absorption occurs after gastrectomy and in sprue or regional enteritis. Iron requirements increase in infancy, adolescence, and pregnancy. The laboratory findings are decreased serum iron and serum ferritin and increased iron binding capacity. If anemia is severe, the red blood cells are microcytic and hypochromic. Therapy with oral iron (e.g., ferrous sulfate 325 mg PO three times daily) improves the anemia slowly over months, and iron supplementation should be continued for 6 months after correction of the anemia to replenish iron stores.

Vitamin B$_{12}$ is required for DNA synthesis, and high-turnover tissues such as the marrow are sensitive to deficiency.

Vitamin B$_{12}$ deficiency can occur uncommonly with decreased intake, as in the strictest vegetarians, or more commonly with decreased absorption resulting from gastrointestinal disease. Causes include pernicious anemia, gastrectomy, pancreatic insufficiency, intestinal bacterial overgrowth, ileitis or ileal resection, and intestinal parasites. Serum vitamin B$_{12}$ is low, and the red blood cells are macrocytic. Therapy with intramuscular cyanocobalamin is effective, and the hemoglobin will rise in 6 to 8 weeks.

Folate is also required for DNA synthesis and is found in many foods, especially leafy green vegetables. Folate deficiency is commonly seen in patients with poor diets and gastrointestinal disease, and it is especially common in patients with alcoholism because of their poor diet and the interference of folate metabolism by alcohol. Other causes of folate deficiency include malabsorption, increased folate use (hemolytic anemia and pregnancy), and drugs that interfere with folate metabolism (e.g., anticonvulsants, oral contraceptives). Red blood cell folate levels are low, and the red blood cells are macrocytic in folate deficiency. Therapy consists of oral folate 1 mg PO three times daily.

Anemia from Preoperative Blood Donation

Patients who donate autologous blood preoperatively often do not regenerate all the red blood cells they donated. As a result, their hemoglobin concentration is lower at the time of the operation than at baseline before blood donation. Donors who have a lower preoperative hemoglobin concentration and who have operative blood loss will be more likely to reach the transfusion threshold and thus are more likely to receive a red blood cell transfusion. To prevent this increased likelihood of transfusion as a result of autologous donation, several preventive measures can be taken. First, unnecessary autologous donations should not be made by patients who are unlikely to need a transfusion for the surgical procedure. Second, donations should be made early, to allow time for red blood cell regeneration. Red blood cells donated a few days preoperatively will not be regenerated. Oral iron supplements are usually given to autologous donors.

Use of Recombinant Erythropoietin

Recombinant erythropoietin given subcutaneously to presurgical patients with or without autologous donation can increase preoperative hemoglobin concentration and the amount of autologous red blood cells collected and can reduce the need for allogeneic transfusion in patients undergoing orthopedic[18–21] and cardiac surgical procedures.[22–24] However, its administration is not believed to be cost-effective.[25, 26] Even the least expensive schedules in randomized trials that showed reduction in allogeneic transfusion cost an estimated $1000 per unit of red blood cells[26]: For orthopedic surgery, the least expensive effective subcutaneous erythropoietin dose was 100 units/kg per day for 15 doses without autologous donation.[21] For cardiac surgery, the least expensive effective subcutaneous dose was 400 units/kg weekly for 4 weeks.[23]

As the risks of transfusion decrease, the cost-effectiveness of autologous blood donation and erythropoietin therapy also decrease. Criteria that predict that patients will benefit from autologous donation and erythropoietin therapy would be helpful. To determine clinical predictive criteria for autologous donation and erythropoietin, the Mayo Clinic group in Rochester, Minnesota performed a retrospective analysis of patients undergoing primary total hip replacement.[27] Their data suggest that for primary total hip replacement, a patient with a predonation hemoglobin level higher than 14.7 g/dL does not need preoperative autologous donation. Preoperative donation would be effective for men with hemoglobin concentrations of 14.7 g/dL or less and for women with hemoglobin concentrations of 13.2 to 14.7 g/dL. Women with hemoglobin levels less than 13.2 g/dL may benefit from erythropoietin therapy together with autologous donation. Further similar studies for other surgical procedures are needed to identify cost-effective strategies for the use of autologous donation and erythropoietin therapy. Currently, erythropoietin is used for some Jehovah's Witness patients before surgical procedures that are expected to incur large blood losses.

■ Procedures that Usually Do Versus Do Not Require Transfusion

Surgical procedures that usually require transfusion include coronary artery bypass graft, major vascular surgery, hip replacement, major spine surgery with instrumentation, hepatic resections, radical prostatectomy, and selected neurologic procedures such as resection of arteriovenous malformation. Surgical procedures that usually do not require transfusion include cervical spine fusion, intervertebral discectomy, mastectomy, hysterectomy, reduction mammoplasty, cholecystectomy, tonsillectomy, transurethral resection of the prostate, and vaginal and cesarean deliveries.[28]

■ Preoperative Red Blood Cell Orders

Maximum surgical blood order schedules (MSBOSs) recommend amounts of red blood cells to be crossmatched, based on historical red blood cell use for operative procedures. Although the concept is not new, hospitals that only recently introduced an MSBOS continue to reduce cost and blood outdate by preventing overordering and unnecessary crossmatching.[29] Use of the immediate-spin crossmatch when the patient has no red blood cell antibodies allows crossmatched blood to be quickly available. Adoption of the immediate-spin crossmatch (instead of the 45-minute full crossmatch) has reduced clinician concern regarding reduced amounts of blood crossmatched preoperatively. The electronic crossmatch can also facilitate rapid blood availability for eligible patients. Despite the benefits, MSBOSs are not ideal for accurate preoperative blood ordering. Historically, at a time when the abbreviated crossmatch was not used, the amount of blood recommended was designed to cover the transfusion needs of 90% of patients who underwent the procedure and resulted in a crossmatch-to-transfusion ratio of 2:1. Thus, even with the MSBOS, half of the units crossmatched are not used. Ideally, the surgeon determines the transfusion need for a patient by determining the patient's preoperative hemoglobin level, estimating the amount of blood loss for the procedure, and deciding on the patient's minimal allowable hemoglobin level. In the future, schedules that incorporate specific patient variables for surgical patients, like that developed for total hip replacement,[30] may further reduce the crossmatch-to-transfusion ratio.

Although red blood cells are appropriate for most patients undergoing elective surgical procedures, whole blood is preferable for patients having operations in which massive transfusion (one or more blood volume blood loss) may occur, such as complex spine surgery. To reduce wastage of unused whole blood, the whole blood units can be separated into red blood cells with plasma attached. Whole blood can be reconstituted by anesthesiologists on transfusion. If unused, the units can be returned to the blood bank and detached into red blood cell and plasma units for future transfusion without additional processing.

■ Special Problems with Autologous and Directed Donor Blood

Special problems associated with autologous and directed donor blood may lead to unavailability of the units when needed by the patient. For example, unless unused autologous and directed donor blood is promptly returned from the operating suites to the blood bank refrigerator and computer inventory, such blood may be unavailable for the patient postoperatively, and random volunteer-donated blood may be issued. Unless blood bank personnel and anesthesiologists are alert and informed about the appropriate sequence of transfusion (autologous, then directed, then random volunteer-donated blood), random volunteer-donated blood may be transfused before autologous and directed donor blood. Unless the patient is registered in the hospital system preoperatively, the intended recipient will be unknown to the blood bank, and autologous and directed donor blood that arrives before the surgical procedure may not be set aside for the intended recipient, or special units collected for the patient may not arrive at the hospital in time. Unless communication is clearly maintained between the blood bank and clinicians, autologous and directed donor blood could be prematurely discarded postoperatively and be unavailable when the patient requires it. Usually, a special donations coordinator, clear policies, education, and good communication among hospital personnel are required for a successful autologous and directed donor program.

■ Special Problems with Same-Day Surgery

Even for major surgical procedures, patients are now frequently admitted on the day of the operation. This practice may give rise to situations in which blood is not available to the patient on the day of surgery because the blood bank has not received a patient specimen or has received the specimen too late to complete compatibility testing. To prevent this situation, a patient sample should be obtained within 3 days of the surgical procedure, if the patient has been pregnant or has had a transfusion in the preceding 3 months, or if the history is uncertain. If the patient is known not to have been pregnant or to have received a transfusion in the preceding 3 months, a sample can be obtained more than 3 days before the operation. In the, one hopes, rare situation in which the patient arrives on the day of the surgical procedure with no or incomplete compatibility testing, and blood is required for the operation, procedures for emergency blood (described later) may have to be used, or the procedure may have to be postponed.

■ Delivery of Blood to the Operating Room

Blood can be delivered to the operating room and stored in the operating room refrigerator, or blood can be delivered in patient-specific coolers to the operating rooms of individual patients. If it is stored in the operating room refrigerator, blood bank personnel must ensure the refrigerator is monitored by blood bank standards. If coolers are used, these also must be subjected to quality control standards to ensure maintenance of proper storage temperatures for a specified number of hours. Despite the additional work involved in packing coolers, some blood banks favor such a system because the patient's blood is stored in the patient's room; this system ensures availability of the blood when needed and enhances the likelihood of return of unused units back to the blood bank when the operation is completed. Timely return of unused autologous and directed units back into the blood bank computer inventory is especially essential, to prevent premature issue of random units when autologous or directed units are actually available (Table 24.1).

Emergency Requirement for Red Blood Cells

Red blood cells may be urgently needed for the surgical patient because of unexpected rapid or large blood loss. In, one hopes, rare cases, red blood cells may be urgently needed because the patient is already in the operating room ready for the surgical procedure and blood has not been set up for use. Reasons for such cases include failure to obtain a patient specimen preoperatively or insufficient time to complete antibody identification preoperatively. Such cases may be more frequent with same-day surgery, especially if the patient was not evaluated at the institution several days preoperatively.

In these cases, blood can be made quickly available in several ways, depending on the situation. If there is no patient specimen for ABO Rh grouping, group O negative red blood cells can be issued. If there is a patient specimen and ABO Rh grouping can be performed, ABO and Rh type-specific red blood cells can be issued. Even for emergency transfusion, patients prefer to receive directed donor before volunteer blood, and type-specific directed donor red blood cells should be transfused first. If the patient specimen shows a positive antibody screen but the antibody has not yet been identified, transfusion medicine specialists should evaluate available information and should issue red blood cells most likely to be compatible, such as antigen-matched or crossmatch-compatible red blood cells. Transfusion medicine specialists should

consult with the surgeons and anesthesiologists to weigh the risks of an emergency transfusion versus a delayed transfusion after further compatibility testing is completed.

Reduction of Intraoperative Red Blood Cell Loss

Several methods for reduction of intraoperative red blood cell loss are available in addition to meticulous surgical hemostasis. Intraoperative and postoperative salvage procedures are commonly used to limit transfusion requirements. Induced, controlled hypotension is another method anesthesiologists can use to reduce blood loss. Acute, normovolemic hemodilution is another strategy, but it must be performed by anesthesiologists trained in the procedure.

Blood-Loss Reduction Drugs During Surgery

Desmopressin

Desmopressin (DDAVP) releases von Willebrand factor and factor VIII coagulant activity from endothelial cells and thus increases their circulating levels. The increased factor VIII coagulant activity allows patients with mild hemophilia A to undergo minor surgical procedures. The increase in von Willebrand factor level can control mild bleeding in some patients with von Willebrand disease, such as with tooth extractions or minor surgical procedures. Desmopressin may also improve the bleeding tendency in uremia, liver disease, and use of some antiplatelet drugs. Its efficacy is less certain in surgical patients without hemophilia A or von Willebrand disease. In double-blind, randomized trials, desmopressin did not significantly decrease blood loss in complex spine surgery[31, 32] or in aortic surgery.[33] Desmopressin decreased blood loss but not transfusion requirements in bilateral osteotomy[34] and in complex cardiac surgery.[35]

Antifibrinolytic Agents

Tranexamic acid, ε-aminocaproic acid, and aprotinin are antifibrinolytic agents that are used to decrease surgical bleeding. Tranexamic acid is the least expensive. In a randomized study comparing the three agents in patients undergoing cardiac surgical procedures, tranexamic acid was as effective as aprotinin in decreasing bleeding and transfusion requirements, whereas ε-aminocaproic acid showed higher postoperative bleeding.[36] Tranexamic acid also reduced blood

Table 24.1 Management: Blood Delivery to Operating Room Beginning with Perceived Need

Elective Cases	Emergency Cases
Consider autologous and directed donor blood.	Consider whether uncrossmatched blood is indicated
Request blood bank to coordinate autologous, directed, and random blood needed. Draw blood specimen from patient for blood bank, before the day of surgery, if possible.	Request to blood bank with patient's blood specimen and indicate urgency.
Transport blood to operating room on the day of surgery.	Facilitate transport logistics if urgent, e.g., send person to blood bank to pick up blood.
Check blood units and patient identity by two persons before transfusion.	Check blood units and patient identity by two persons before transfusion.
Transfuse autologous before directed and directed before random units. Monitor for adverse reactions.	Monitor for adverse reactions.
Return unused units to blood bank inventory.	Return unused units to blood blank inventory.

loss in orthotopic liver transplantation, transurethral prostatic surgery, menstrual bleeding, and urgent operations in patients with upper gastrointestinal bleeding.[37]

Local Fibrin Glue

Fibrin glue or sealant is a source of concentrated fibrinogen. After activation by thrombin, the mixture is applied to surgical wound surfaces to form fibrin, which decreases local bleeding in thoracic and cardiovascular surgery,[38] in general surgery and endoscopy,[39] and in vascular surgery.[40] Current research investigates fibrin sealant's ability to incorporate drugs and cytokines into the fibrin matrix for slow release as a drug delivery system, for example, as an antibiotic coating or as an agent for endothelialization of grafts.[40] Although mixtures of cryoprecipitate and bovine thrombin were popular before the availability of commercial sources of fibrin sealant in the United States, the commercial materials are virally inactivated and avoid the problems of antibodies to coagulation factors induced by bovine thrombin.

■ Intraoperative Monitoring of Tissue Oxygen

Approach and Rationale

The goal of red blood cell transfusion is to prevent inadequate oxygenation, which causes tissue ischemia and damage. Hypovolemia and hypoxemia can also cause tissue ischemia and damage. Prolonged inadequate oxygenation that causes enough tissue damage can result in disseminated intravascular coagulation and a bleeding diathesis intraoperatively. The anesthesiologist must monitor and distinguish among inadequate blood volume, inadequate arterial oxygen content, and inadequate oxygen-carrying capacity. These factors can occur together or separately. Therapy must be directed appropriately to increase blood volume with fluids, arterial oxygen content by inspired oxygen, or hemoglobin concentration by red blood cell transfusion.

Monitoring of Systemic Tissue Oxygenation

Anesthesiologists cannot monitor the adequacy of systemic, whole-body tissue oxygenation by measuring hemoglobin concentration alone. Hemoglobin concentration is merely a measure of oxygen-carrying capacity. The primary method for assessing adequacy of oxygenation is oxygen consumption, which is not routinely clinically measured. A surrogate measure of total-body tissue oxygenation is base excess and is measured by arterial blood gas. Serum lactate is useful, but the results are usually not available for short-term patient management. Mixed venous partial pressure of oxygen and saturation are useful, but they require the placement of a central arterial line.

Using the acute isovolemic hemodilution model, there is no evidence of inadequate systemic tissue oxygenation for a brief period at hemoglobin concentration of 5 g/dL in healthy awake humans.[15] At a hemoglobin concentration of 5 g/dL, further reduction of oxygen delivery to 7.3 mL oxygen/kg/min by reducing the patient's heart rate does not result in inadequate systemic tissue oxygenation.[41] These results were found in awake, healthy, young adults and may not apply to older, less healthy patients.

Monitoring of Local Tissue Oxygenation

When no evidence suggests inadequate total-body tissue oxygenation, local tissue may still be compromised. Anesthesiologists monitor the adequacy of local tissue oxygenation in limited ways. ST segments are monitored to detect cardiac ischemia. In patients with cardiac disease, myocardial wall motion may be monitored by transesophageal echocardiography. In the nervous system, evoked potentials are measured intraoperatively to detect ischemia to the spinal cord and brain resulting from hypovolemia. Gastric tissue pH has not been found to be useful.[42] Using the acute isovolemic hemodilution model, young healthy subjects were found to have mild, reversible impairment in cognitive function and memory at hemoglobin concentrations of 5 g/dL. The impairment was reversible with red blood cell transfusion.[16]

Monitoring of Factors that Affect Tissue Oxygenation

In the absence of adequate methods to measure oxygen in all local tissues, anesthesiologists monitor the three variables that affect tissue oxygen: blood volume, arterial oxygen content, and hemoglobin concentration. First, anesthesiologists monitor blood volume during surgical procedures by measuring blood pressure, pulse, and urine output and by monitoring peripheral perfusion. In patients undergoing operations during which large blood loss is expected, a central venous line is needed to monitor central venous pressure. In patients undergoing surgical procedures in which large blood loss is expected and volume control is critical, an arterial line may be inserted into the left atrium to monitor pulmonary artery wedge pressure.

Second, anesthesiologists monitor arterial oxygen content by measuring arterial blood gases. If the arterial partial pressure of oxygen is low, the fraction of inspired oxygen is increased, and the cause of the hypoxemia is determined to facilitate specific treatment.

Third, anesthesiologists monitor oxygen-carrying capacity by measuring hemoglobin concentration. In hypovolemic patients, the hemoglobin concentration is falsely high and decreases when fluid is restored and blood volume equilibrates.

Controversy: Old Versus Fresh Blood

On storage, 2,3-diphosphoglycerate levels decrease in red blood cells, and the result is hemoglobin with higher oxygen affinity. After transfusion, 2,3-diphosphoglycerate levels recover by about 50% in 6 hours.[43] Whether the increased oxygen affinity in stored red blood cells impairs tissue oxygenation has been a matter of controversy. Two studies suggest that stored red blood cells, when transfused, may not improve tissue oxygenation immediately. Red blood cell transfusion failed to increase oxygen consumption despite an increase in oxygen content, in patients after trauma.[44] The authors concluded that red blood cell transfusion may not improve tissue oxygenation in a rapid manner. In a study of septic, critically ill patients undergoing mechanical ventilation, 3 units of packed red blood cells did not increase systemic oxygen uptake measured by indirect calorimetry for up to 6 hours after transfusion.[45] Another retrospective study suggested an adverse effect of length of storage of transfused red blood cells on postoperative pneumonia in coronary artery

Table 24.2   Clinical Controversies

Fresh red blood cells or whole blood
    PRO: Less potassium in plasma of these stored products
        Lower oxygen affinity of hemoglobin and increased delivery
            to tissues
    CON: Clinical significance of potassium in stored products
            unclear
        Clinical significance of higher hemoglobin oxygen affinity
            unclear
        Difficulty in procurement and management of fresh products

Use of erythropoietin
    PRO: Increases endogenous red cell production
    CON: Expensive and unnecessary in most patients

Value of autologous blood
    PRO: No risk of viral transmission
        Peace of mind for the patient
    CON: Not cost-effective

Value of directed donor blood
    PRO: Peace of mind for the patient and family
    CON: Not safer

bypass graft surgery.[46] At our institution, red blood cells that are less than 5 days old are provided for infants with severe pulmonary or cardiac disease, such as those undergoing extracorporeal membrane oxygenation or complex cardiac operations for congenital heart disease. More studies are needed to define the indication, if any, for fresh red blood cells (Table 24.2).

Intraoperative Indications for Red Blood Cell Transfusion

The Anesthesiologists Task Force[8] recommended the following: (1) transfusion is rarely indicated when the hemoglobin concentration is greater than 10 g/dL and is almost always indicated when it is less than 6 g/dL, especially when the anemia is acute; (2) the determination of whether intermediate hemoglobin concentrations (6 to 10 g/dL) justify or require red blood cell transfusion should be based on the patient's risk of complications of inadequate oxygenation; (3) the use of a single hemoglobin "trigger" for all patients and other approaches that fail to consider all important physiologic and surgical factors affecting oxygenation are not recommended; (4) when appropriate, preoperative autologous blood donation, intraoperative and postoperative blood salvage, acute normovolemic hemodilution, and measures to decrease blood loss (deliberate hypotension and pharmacologic agents) may be beneficial; and (5) the indications for transfusion of autologous red blood cells may be more liberal than for allogeneic red blood cells because of the lower (but still significant) risks associated with autologous blood.

The foregoing guidelines were based on the best evidence and expert opinion available at the time. More studies are needed. For example, whether hemoglobin concentration is a significant variable in the morbidity and mortality of surgical patients is unclear. Hemoglobin concentration in the range of 5.8 to 7.2 g/dL was not a significant variable affecting myocardial lactate flux (as an index of ischemia) in patients undergoing coronary artery bypass grafting who had an ejection fraction greater than 50%.[47] Similarly, in a retrospective multicenter study of patients with hip fractures who were

60 years old or older, perioperative transfusion in patients with lowest hemoglobin levels of 8 g/dL or higher did not influence the risk of 30- or 90-day mortality.[48] In contrast, in a retrospective study of elderly men undergoing radical prostatectomy, intraoperative or postoperative myocardial ischemia was more likely to occur in patients with hematocrit levels lower than 28%, particularly in the presence of tachycardia.[49] Oxygen delivery may be the more important factor. Oxygen delivery was an important predictor of outcome in patients with ruptured abdominal aortic aneurysms.[50] More studies are needed.

Postoperative Indications for Red Blood Cell Transfusion

Current guidelines do not distinguish between indications for red blood cell transfusion in the postoperative period and those during other perioperative periods. Furthermore, guidelines do not distinguish between uncomplicated postoperative patients and those who are critically ill.

In uncomplicated postoperative patients, those undergoing cardiac and hip operations have been studied. In a randomized study of autologous donors undergoing elective myocardial revascularization, those transfused to a hematocrit of 31% had improved exercise endurance compared with those transfused to a hematocrit of 28%. However, there was no difference in duration or degree of exercise between the two groups.[51] In a randomized pilot study of postoperative patients with hip fractures, patients transfused based on symptoms received transfusion of fewer units than those transfused for a threshold lower than 8 g/dL. However, it is unknown whether these two strategies have comparable mortality, morbidity, or functional status.[52]

In critically ill postoperative patients, a retrospective study showed that mortality rates were lowest with hematocrit values between 27% and 33%.[53] Similarly, in a prospective, case-control study of high-risk patients undergoing infrainguinal arterial bypass procedures, a hematocrit of 28% was found to be the best threshold hematocrit value below which morbid cardiac events were most likely to occur.[54] In contrast to these studies, a randomized trial suggests that transfusion to such hematocrit levels may be harmful to some critically ill patients. A randomized trial of acutely anemic, nonbleeding, intensive care patients found that a restrictive strategy of red blood cell transfusion (average daily hemoglobin, 8.5 g/dL) was at least as effective as and possibly superior to a liberal transfusion strategy (average daily hemoglobin, 10.7 g/dL) in the subgroups of patients less than 55 years of age and patients with APACHE (Acute Physiology and Chronic Health Evaluation) II scores of less than 20.[55] The exception was patients with acute myocardial infarction and unstable angina in whom there was no difference between the two strategies. Among the restrictive-strategy group, 39% were postoperative patients; among the liberal-strategy group, 34% were postoperative patients. These data suggest that harm may be caused by liberal use of transfusion in younger, less severely ill patients in the intensive care unit. The mechanisms for these observations are not understood.[56] Thus, further studies are clearly needed to clarify these conflicting data relevant to postoperative transfusion.

REFERENCES

1. Wallace EL, Churchill WH, Surgenor DM, et al: Collection and transfusion of blood and blood components in the United States. Transfusion 38:625–635, 1998.
2. Consensus conference: Perioperative red blood cell transfusion. JAMA 260:2700–2703, 1988.
3. Cummings JP: Technology Assessment: Red Blood Cell Transfusion Guidelines 1997. Oak Brook, IL, UHC Clinical Practice Advancement Center, 1997.
4. Treacher DF, Leach RM: ABC of oxygen: Oxygen transport. I. Basic principles. BMJ 317:1302–1306, 1998.
5. Pawloski JR, Hess DT, Stamler JS: Export by red blood cells of nitric oxide bioactivity. Nature 409:622–626, 2001.
6. American College of Obstetricians and Gynecologists: ACOG technical bulletin: Blood component therapy. Int J Gynecol Obstet 48:233–238, 1995.
7. American College of Physicians: Practice strategies for elective red blood cell transfusion. Ann Intern Med 116:403–406, 1992.
8. American Society of Anesthesiologists Task Force on Blood Component Therapy: Practice guidelines for blood component therapy. Anesthesiology 84:732–747, 1996.
9. Blanchette VS, Hume HA, Levy GJ, et al: Guidelines for auditing pediatric blood transfusion practices. Am J Dis Child 145:787–796, 1991.
10. Blood Management Practice Guidelines Conference: Surgical red blood cell transfusion practice policies. Am J Surg 170(Suppl 6A): 3S–15S, 1995.
11. Royal College of Physicians of Edinburgh: Consensus statement on red cell transfusion. Transfus Med 4:177–178, 1994.
12. Simon TL, Alverson DC, AuBuchon J, et al: Practice parameter for the use of red blood cell transfusions: Developed by the Red Blood Cell Administration Practice Guideline Development Task Force of the College of American Pathologists. Arch Pathol Lab Med 122:130–138, 1998.
13. Stehling L, Luban NLC, Anderson KC, et al: Guidelines for blood utilization review. Transfusion 34:438–448, 1994.
14. Wedgewood JJ, Thomas JG, for the Royal College of Anesthetists. Peri-operative haemoglobin: An overview of current opinion regarding the acceptable level of haemoglobin in the peri-operative period. Eur J Anesthesiol 13:316–324, 1996.
15. Weiskopf RB, Viele MK, Feiner J, et al: Human cardiovascular and metabolic response to acute, severe, isovolemic anemia. JAMA 279:217–221, 1998.
16. Weiskopf RB, Kramer J, Viele M, et al: Acute severe isovolemic anemia impairs cognitive function and memory in humans. Anesthesiology 92:1646–1652, 2000.
17. Weiskopf RB: Do we know when to transfuse red cells to treat acute anemia[editorial]? Transfusion 38:517–521, 1998.
18. Canadian Orthopedic Perioperative Erythropoietin Study Group: Effectiveness of perioperative recombinant human erythropoietin in elective hip replacement. Lancet 341:1227–1232, 1993.
19. Biesma DH, Karraijenhagen RJ, Dalmulder, et al: Recombinant human erythropoietin in autologous blood donors: A dose-finding study. Br J Haematol 86:30–35, 1994.
20. Biesma DH, Van de Wiel A, Beguin Y, et al: Erythropoietic activity and iron metabolism in autologous blood donors during recombinant human erythropoietin therapy. Eur J Clin Invest 24:426–432, 1994.
21. Faris PM, Ritter MA, Abels RI: The effects of recombinant human erythropoietin on perioperative transfusion requirements in patients having a major orthopaedic operation: The American Erythropoietin Study Group. J Bone Joint Surg Am 78:62–72, 1996.
22. Watanabe Y, Fuse K, Naruse Y, et al: Subcutaneous use of erythropoietin in heart surgery. Ann Thorac Surg 54:479–484, 1992.
23. Kulier AH, Gombotz H, Fuchs G, et al: Subcutaneous recombinant human erythropoietin and autologous blood donation before coronary bypass surgery. Anesth Analg 76:102–106, 1993.
24. Hayashi J, Kumon K, Takanashi S, et al: Subcutaneous administration of recombinant human erythropoietin before cardiac surgery: A double-blind, multicenter trial in Japan. Transfusion 34:142–146, 1994.
25. Etchason J, Petz L, Keeler E, et al: The cost effectiveness of preoperative autologous blood donations. N Engl J Med 332:719–724, 1995.
26. Jafari-Fesharaki M, Toy P: Effect and cost of subcutaneous recombinant human erythropoietin in preoperative patients. Orthopedics 20:1159–1165, 1997.
27. Nuttall GA, Santrach PJ, Oliver WC Jr, et al: A prospective randomized trial of the surgical blood order equation for ordering red cells for total hip arthroplasty patients. Transfusion 38:828–833, 1998.
28. NIH Expert Panel on Autologous Blood: Transfusion alert: Use of autologous blood. Transfusion 335:703–713, 1995.
29. Richardson NG, Bradley WN, Donaldson DR, O'Shaughnessy DF: Maximum surgical blood ordering schedule in a district general hospital saves money and resources. Ann R Coll Surg Engl 80:262–265, 1998.
30. Nuttall GA, Santrach PJ, Oliver WC Jr, et al: Possible guidelines for autologous red blood cell donations before total hip arthroplasty based on the surgical blood order equation. Mayo Clin Proc 75:10–17, 2000.
31. Theroux MC, Cordry DH, Tietz AE, et al: A study of desmopressin and blood loss during spinal fusion for neuromuscular scoliosis: A randomized, controlled, double-blinded study. Anesthesiology 87:260–267, 1997.
32. Letts M, Pang E, D'Astous J, et al: The influence of desmopressin on blood loss during spinal fusion surgery in neuromuscular patients. Spine 23:475–478, 1998.
33. Clagett GP, Valentine RJ, Myers SI, et al: Does desmopressin improve hemostasis and reduce blood loss from aortic surgery? A randomized, double-blind study. J Vasc Surg 22:223–230, 1995.
34. Guyuron B, Vaughan C, Schlecter B: The role of DDAVP (desmopressin) in orthopathic surgery. Ann Plast Surg 37:516–519, 1996.
35. Cattaneo M, Harris AS, Stromberg U, Mannucci PM: The effect of desmopressin on reducing blood loss in cardiac surgery: A meta-analysis of double-blind, placebo-controlled trials. Thromb Haemost 74:1064–1070, 1995.
36. Casati V, Guzzon D, Oppizzi M, et al: Hemostatic effects of approtinin, tranexamic acid and epsilon-aminocaproic acid in primary cardiac surgery. Ann Thorac Surg 68:2252–2257, 1999.
37. Dunn CJ, Goa KL: Tranexamic acid: A review of its use in surgery and other indications. Drugs 57:1005–1032, 1999.
38. Spotnitz WD: As originally published in 1990: Four years' experience with fibrin sealant in thoracic and cardiovascular surgery. Updated in 1998. Ann Thorac Surg 65:592–593, 1998.
39. Dunn CJ, Goa KL: Fibrin sealant: A review of its use in surgery and endoscopy. Drugs 58:863–886, 1999.
40. Shireman PK, Greisler HP: Fibrin sealant in vascular surgery: A review. J Long Term Eff Med Implants 8:117–132, 1998.
41. Lieberman JA, Weiskopf RB, Kelley SD, et al: Critical oxygen delivery in conscious humans is less than 7.3 mL $O_2.kg.^{-1}min.^{-1}$ Anesthesiology 92:407–413, 2000.
42. Knudson MM, Bermudex KM, Doyle CA, et al: Use of tissue oxygen tension measurements during resuscitation from hemorrhagic shock. J Trauma 42:608–616, 1997.
43. Beutler E, Wood L: The in vivo regeneration of red cell 2,3-diphosphoglyceric acid (DPG) after transfusion of stored blood. J Lab Clin Med 74:300–304, 1969.
44. Shah DM, Gottlieb ME, Rahm RL, et al: Failure of red blood cell transfusion to increase oxygen transport or mixed venous Po_2 in injured patients. J Trauma 22:741–746, 1982.
45. Marik PE, Sibbald WJ: Effect of stored-blood transfusion on oxygen delivery in patients with sepsis. JAMA 269:3024–3029, 1993.
46. Vamvakas EC, Carven JH: Transfusion and postoperative pneumonia in coronary artery bypass graft surgery: Effect of the length of storage of transfused red cells. Transfusion 39:701–709, 1999.
47. Doak GJ, Hall RI: Does hemoglobin concentration affect perioperative myocardial lactate flux in patients undergoing coronary artery bypass surgery? Anesth Analg 80:910–916, 1995.
48. Carson JL, Duff A, Berlin JA, et al: Perioperative blood transfusion and postoperative mortality. JAMA 279:199–205, 1998.
49. Hogue CW Jr, Goodnough LT, Monk TG: Perioperative myocardial ischemic episodes are related to hematocrit level in patients undergoing radical prostatectomy. Transfusion 38:924–931, 1998.
50. Peerless JR, Alexander JJ, Pinchak AC, et al: Oxygen delivery is an important predictor of outcome in patients with ruptured abdominal aortic aneurysms. Ann Surg 227:726–734, 1998.
51. Johnson RG, Thurer RL, Kruskall MS, et al: Comparison of two transfusion strategies after elective operations for myocardial revascularization. J Thorac Cardiovasc Surg 104:307–314, 1992.

52. Carson JL, Terrin ML, Barton FB, et al: A pilot randomized trial comparing symptomatic vs. hemoglobin-level-driven red blood cell transfusion following hip fracture. Transfusion 38:522–529, 1998.

53. Czer LS, Shoemaker WC: Optimal hematocrit value in critically ill postoperative patients. Surg Gynecol Obstet 147:363–368, 1978.

54. Nelson AH, Fleisher LA, Rosenbaum SH: Relationship between postoperative anemia and cardiac morbidity in high-risk vascular patients in the intensive care unit. Crit Care Med 21:860–866, 1993.

55. Hebert PC, Wells G, Blajchman MA, et al: A multicenter, randomized, controlled clinical trial of transfusion requirements in critical care. N Engl J Med 340:409–417, 1999.

56. Ely EW, Bernard GR: Transfusions in critically ill patients [editorial]. N Engl J Med 340:467–468, 1999.

Chapter **25**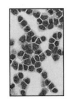

Transfusion of the Patient with Congenital Coagulation Defects

Suzanne Shusterman
Catherine S. Manno

Tremendous progress has been made since the 1980s in the diagnosis and management of congenital bleeding disorders. DNA diagnostic testing that permits accurate prenatal diagnosis is widely available for most cases of severe hemophilia. Recombinant factor concentrates for factor VIII (FVIII) and factor IX (FIX) deficiencies have been licensed and are now commonly used in the management of bleeding episodes or, in prophylaxis regimens, for the prevention of bleeding episodes. This chapter reviews the clinical and laboratory features of hemophilia A and B, von Willebrand disease (vWD), and less well-known congenital bleeding disorders. Treatment options for bleeding episodes and for prevention of bleeding are presented. Although certain clinical challenges such as the management of high-titer inhibitor patients still exist, the outlook for children born today with hemophilia and other congenital bleeding disorders is brighter than ever before.

■ Hemophilia A and Hemophilia B

Hemophilia A and *hemophilia B* are serious congenital clotting disorders caused by a deficiency in FVIII and FIX, respectively. Both diseases have an X-linked recessive pattern of inheritance. The incidence of hemophilia A (classic hemophilia) is 1 in 5000 to 10,000 male births, and the incidence of hemophilia B (Christmas disease) is approximately 1 in 30,000 to 50,000 male births.[1, 2]

Hemophilia is a clinically heterogeneous disorder with severity and symptoms dependent on an individual person's factor activity level. FVIII and FIX activity levels are measured in units (U/mL), with 1 U/mL corresponding to 100% of the factor found in 1 mL of normal plasma. Normal FVIII and FIX activity levels range from 0.5 to 1.5 U/mL (50% to 150%), with measurements lower than this range defining

three levels of clinical severity of hemophilia. Patients with *mild hemophilia* have factor activity levels of approximately 0.05 to 0.30 U/mL (5% to 30%) and tend to have bleeding difficulties only after severe trauma or surgical procedures. *Moderate hemophilia* is defined by factor activity levels between 0.01 and 0.05 U/mL (1% to 5%) and is characterized by bleeding with moderate trauma. Persons with factor activity levels of less than 0.01 U/mL (less than 1%) are designated as having *severe hemophilia* and bleed spontaneously into joints and soft tissues.[1] Affected boys and men tend to have the same factor levels and clinical manifestations of disease as other family members.[3]

Although most patients with hemophilia A have a positive family history, 20% to 30% of affected persons have no previous family history of disease.[1] Hemophilia should be suspected in any male patient with a history of spontaneous bleeding into joints or muscles or excessive bleeding with trauma. Children may have excessive bruising. A common presentation in the absence of a positive family history is excessive bleeding after circumcision. The diagnosis of hemophilia is made by direct assay of FVIII or FIX levels in plasma, and this test can be performed on umbilical cord blood. The cloning of the genes for FVIII and IX on the X chromosome has made prenatal diagnosis of hemophilia possible in some families. Forty to 50% of patients with severe hemophilia A have an inversion in the FVIII gene at intron 22, and carriers can be detected using direct gene mutation analysis for this inversion.[4, 5] If this mutation is not present, carriers can be identified for both hemophilia A and B by linkage analysis, if affected and unaffected family members are available. Direct gene mutation and linkage analysis can also be done on the fetus in the prenatal period by chorionic villus sampling at 10 to 12 weeks of gestation or amniocentesis at 15 weeks of gestation.[4] If genetic analysis is not possible, fetal blood sampling, when available, can be used to assay plasma FVIII levels.[6] FIX plasma assays are less reliable in making the definitive diagnosis before or at birth because of normally low levels of vitamin K–dependent factors in the prenatal and postnatal periods.[7]

Therapeutic Options for Factor Replacement in Hemophilia

Historical Perspective

Before the availability of products to replace specific clotting factor deficiencies, patients with hemophilia were treated with whole blood or fresh frozen plasma. Many patients died of hemorrhage or were incapacitated with progressive joint disease because products were either unavailable or contained inadequate amount of factor. In the 1960s, fractionation of large pools of plasma allowed crude separation of FVIII and FIX from other plasma proteins. Cryoprecipitate, that portion of a unit of fresh frozen plasma that precipitates during thawing at 4°C to 6°C, contains FVIII, von Willebrand factor (vWF), FXIII, and fibrinogen and was the first concentrate available for more specific factor replacement for hemophilia A.[8, 9]

Prothrombin complex concentrates (PCCs), containing FII, FVII, FIX, and FX, were developed for treatment of hemophilia B in 1967.[10] In the 1970s, development of clotting factors was aimed at improving solubility, yield (units of clotting factor recovered from plasma), and purity. Lyophilized specific FVIII and FIX concentrates became commercially available, and their ease of storage and reconstitution made home infusion for early signs of hemorrhage possible, thus markedly improving the quality of life of patients with hemophilia.[1, 9, 11] These concentrates, however, were prepared from pooled plasma obtained from 2000 to 200,000 largely paid donors,[9] and by 1980, the transmission of hepatitis from these concentrates was recognized.[1] In 1982, the first case of acquired immunodeficiency syndrome in a patient with hemophilia was reported; by 1988, the prevalence of seropositivity for human immunodeficiency virus (HIV) was 77% in patients with severe hemophilia A and 42% in patients with hemophilia B.[3, 12–14] As a result of the tragic transmission of HIV and hepatitis to so many patients with hemophilia, by the mid-1980s, the major goal of factor concentrate development was further improvement of product purity and elimination of viral transmission.[15]

Purification Methods

The purity of factor concentrates is classified according to *specific activity* (SA), the ratio of clotting protein to total protein contained in a factor concentrate.[16] Improved separation techniques have resulted in the availability of increasingly pure products. Cryoprecipitate is a low-purity concentrate.[1] The first specific factor concentrates made in the 1970s were intermediate-purity products with SA levels between 1 and 10 IU/mg total protein.[9] High-purity concentrates with an SA ranging from 50 to 150 IU/mg total protein were later produced using ion exchange, affinity, or gel filtration chromatography to improve removal of contaminating proteins.[15] The use of monoclonal antibodies to FVIII or FIX in combination with immunoaffinity chromatography produces very high-purity products (SA 200 to 2000 IU/mg total protein).[15] In addition to enhancing the separation of clotting from nonclotting proteins, purification processes separate the clotting proteins from transfusion-transmitted viruses.[11, 15]

Virus-Inactivation Methods

Purification techniques alone are not sufficient to eliminate the risk of viral contamination from plasma-derived factor concentrates. Since the mid-1980s, all concentrates made in the United States have undergone some form of viral inactivation, either physical or chemical.[3] HIV is exquisitely heat labile, and effective eradication can be accomplished with heat or a combination of heat and pressure.[3, 17] Hepatitis viruses are more resistant to heat inactivation than HIV, although the degree of eradication improves with increased temperature, moisture, and length of heating.[15] One problem, however, with heat treatment of factor concentrates is a reduction in factor yield. HIV and hepatitis B and C viruses are lipid-coated viruses and are readily inactivated with a combination of solvent and detergent treatments. FVIII concentrates treated with a combination of solvent and detergent were first licensed in 1985, and the combination of the solvent tri-*n*-butyl phosphate and the detergent polysorbate-80 is now widely used.[15] No transmission of lipid-coated viruses has been seen in clinical trials using solvent–detergent combinations,[18] and product yield is high using this method.[17] Hepatitis A and parvovirus B19, however, are not lipid-coated; as such, they elude inactivation with solvent and detergent and therefore remain potential contaminants in concentrates.[3, 11, 19]

Factor VIII Concentrates

Many different specific FVIII concentrates are licensed in the United States (Table 25.1). All products have undergone viral attenuation since the mid-1980s.[3] Products of intermediate, high and very high purity (the latter including immunoaffinity purified and recombinant products) are available today.[1] Certain high- and intermediate-purity FVIII products contain vWF and fibrinogen in addition to FVIII,[3] and these are used for treatment of vWD (see later). In 1984, two biotechnology companies (Genentech, San Francisco, and Genetics Institute, Boston) cloned and expressed the FVIII gene and made the production of recombinant FVIII (rFVIII) possible.[20, 21] After this, four first-generation rFVIII products were developed and were licensed by the United States Food and Drug Administration for use in patients with FVIII deficiency in the United States. Two of these products, Recombinate (Baxter Hyland Immuno, Glendale, CA) and Bioclate (Aventis Behring, Kankakee, IL) are made through co-expression of FVIII and vWF cDNA in Chinese hamster ovary cells, with purification of rFVIII from cell culture by immunoaffinity chromatography with antihuman mouse FVIII antibody.[11] The other products, Kogenate (Bayer Corp., Berkeley, CA) and Helixate (Aventis Behring) are derived from the medium of hamster kidney cell cultures transfected with FVIII cDNA alone.[11, 22] All four products contain trace amounts of hamster proteins and mouse immunoglobulin G.[11] However, no cases of development of antibodies against rodent protein or transmission of animal viruses to recipients of these products have been reported.[16] Their biochemical profiles are similar to those of plasma-derived FVIII.

After preclinical safety evaluations, clinical studies were done, initially in previously treated patients. In 1989, White and associates[23] reported on efficacy in two previously treated

Table 25.1   Factor VIII Concentrates Available in the United States in 2000

A. Recombinant Factor VIII Concentrates

Product	Manufacturer	Method of Viral Inactivation or Depletion	Stabilizer	Specific Activity of Final Product[*]
Recombinate	Baxter Hyland Immuno	IAC	Human albumin	1.65–19
Bioclate	Baxter Hyland Immuno[†]	IAC	Human albumin	1.65–19
Kogenate	Bayer	IAC	Human albumin	8–30
Helixate	Bayer[†]	IAC	Human albumin	8–30
Kogenate SF	Bayer	IAC	Sucrose	4,000
Helixate SF	Bayer[†]	IAC	Sucrose	4,000
ReFacto	Pharmacia Upjohn AB[‡]	IAC, SD1	Sucrose	11,200–15,5000

B. Very High-Purity (Immunoaffinity-Purified) Plasma-Derived Factor VIII Concentrates

Product	Manufacturer	Method of Viral Inactivation or Depletion	Specific Activity of Final Product[*]
Hemphil M	Baxter Hyland Immuno	IAC, SD1	2–15
Monarc M	Baxter Hyland Immuno[§]	IAC, SD1	2–15
Monoclate P	Aventis Behring	IAC, P	5–10

C. High- and Intermediate-Purity Plasma-Derived Factor VIII Concentrates[||]

Product	Manufacturer	Method of Viral Inactivation or Depletion	Specific Activity of Final Product[*]
Alphanate SD	Alpha Therapeutics	IAC, SD2	8–30
Humate P	Aventis Behring	P	1–2
Koate-DVI	Bayer	SD2, DH	9–22

D. Porcine Factor VIII Products[¶]

Product	Manufacturer	Method of Viral Inactivation or Depletion	Specific Activity of Final Product[*]
Hyate:C	Ipsen, Inc.	P	>50

IAC, immunoaffinity chromatography, SD1, solvent–detergent (TNBP and Triniton X-100); P, pasteurization (60°C, 10 hr); DH, dry heat (72°C, 72 hr); SD2 (TNBP and polysorbate-80).

[*]IU factor VIII/mg total protein, including stabilizer.
[†]Distributed by Aventis Behring.
[‡]Distributed by Genetics Institute.
[§]Manufactured from American Red Cross–collected plasma, distributed by American Red Cross.
[||]Contain von Willebrand factor.
[¶]For use in patients with inhibitors to factor VIII.

patients with severe hemophilia and HIV seropositivity treated with Recombinate for 12 months. In patients, clinical effectiveness and factor recovery were comparable to those observed with plasma-derived products; neither patient developed alloantibodies after exposure to the product. Larger studies were then done concurrently with previously untreated patients (PUPs) to assess efficacy, safety, and inhibitor formation after treatment with the recombinant products. In 1993, Lusher and associates[24] reported on 95 PUPs who were treated with Kogenate exclusively for a median of 1.5 years. All patients responded well when they were treated for spontaneous or traumatic hemorrhages or invasive procedures. Three minor local reactions were noted, with no detection of antibody to hamster or murine protein. Of some concern, early inhibitor formation was detected; 28.6% of patients with severe disease developed an inhibitor after a median of 9 days

of factor exposure. Most patients, however, had low-titer inhibitor levels.

In 1994, Bray and colleagues[25] reported on 71 PUPs with severe hemophilia who were treated with Recombinate. Ninety-two percent of bleeding episodes responded well to Recombinate infusion, and only 0.1% of these infusions were associated with a minor local reaction. Again, an unanticipated high rate of early inhibitor formation was observed. Seventeen patients (23.9%) developed inhibitors after a median of 9 days of factor exposure, and 12 of these patients had a low-titer inhibitor and continued good clinical response to Recombinate.

As these reports show, both rFVIII products were found to have clinical efficacy equal to intermediate- or high-purity plasma-derived products and were well tolerated. Both PUP studies showed a higher incidence of inhibitor formation than previously described; however, prior estimates were collected retrospectively and included patients with mild hemophilia as well as extensively pretreated patients, all of which likely contribute to previous underestimation of the risk of inhibitor formation.[24, 25] In addition, longitudinal follow-up of PUPs in both rFVIII trials demonstrated that the inhibitors were transient in more than 50% of those in whom they developed.[26]

Although recombinant products are not derived from human plasma and are ultrapure, they require the addition of a stabilizer such as human albumin to prevent such highly concentrated clotting protein from adhering to the surface of the container.[27] Recombinate and Bioclate have an SA greater than 3000 IU/mg protein and Kogenate and Helixate have an SA greater than 4500 IU/mg protein before the addition of human albumen.[28] Many investigators have raised safety concerns about the addition of albumin, a human plasma protein, although none of these recombinant products have been associated with either hepatitis or HIV transmission. New rFVIII product development is focused on decreasing or eliminating human albumin. Second-generation FVIII products use only a small amount of human albumin in the production process and use sugar as a stabilizer.[3] These products include Kogenate SF (sucrose formulated) and Helixate FS (Bayer Corp.)[29] as well as ReFacto (Genetics Institute), which is a B-domain–deleted rFVIII product.[30, 31]

Factor IX Concentrates

Three types of factor concentrates are available for treatment of patients with FIX deficiency. These are PCCs, coagulation FIX concentrates, and recombinant FIX (rFIX) (Table 25.2).

PCCs, also known as FIX complex concentrates, first became available in the late 1960s and contain FIX as well as prothrombin, FVII and FX, some of which become activated during preparation.[16] PCCs are low-purity products with an SA less than 50 IU/mg total protein.[1] When PCCs are used at frequent intervals or for prolonged periods, they have been associated with paradoxic thrombotic complications such as myocardial infarction, venous thromboembolism, and disseminated intravascular coagulation.[15, 32] These problems are caused either by the presence of activated factors that serve to trigger coagulation or by accumulation of high levels of the factors.[15] High-purity FIX concentrates, also known as coagulation FIX concentrates, were first licensed in 1992.[15] They are purified by immunoaffinity or gel chromatography, contain only FIX, and have little or no thrombotic potential.[15, 16] High-purity concentrates are preferred over PCCs for treatment, particularly when frequent replacement is required,

Table 25.2   Factor IX Concentrates Available in the United States in 2000

A. Recombinant Factor IX Concentrates				
Product	Manufacturer	Method of Viral Inactivation or Depletion	Stabilizer	Specific Activity of Final Product*
BeneFix	Genetics Institute	IAC, UF	Sucrose	>200

B. Coagulation Factor IX Concentrates (Human Plasma Derived)			
Product	Manufacturer	Method of Viral Inactivation or Depletion	Specific Activity of Final Product*
Alphanine SD	Alpha	DAC, SD, NF	230
Mononine	Aventis Behring	IAC, ST, UF	>160

C. Factor IX Complex Concentrates (Prothrombin Complex Concentrates), Human Plasma Derived			
Product	Manufacturer	Method of Viral Inactivation or Depletion	Specific Activity of Final Product*
Bebulin VH	Baxter Hyland Immuno	VH	2
Konyne 80	Bayer	DH	1.25
Profilnine SD	Alpha	SD	4.5
Proplex-T	Baxter Hyland Immuno	DH	3.9

D. Activated Factor IX Complex Concentrates (Activated Prothrombin Complex Concentrates), Human Plasma Derived			
Product	Manufacturer	Method of Viral Inactivation or Depletion	Specific Activity of Final Product*
Autoplex T	Baxter Hyland Immuno[†]	DH	5
FEIBA VH	Baxter Hyland Immuno	VH	0.8

*IU factor VIII/mg total protein, including stabilizer.
[†]Distributed by Nabi.
DAC, dual-affinity chromatography; DH; dry heat (72°C, 72 hr); IAC, immunoaffinity chromatography; NF, nanofiltration; SD, solvent-detergent (TNBP and polysorbate-80); ST, sodium thiocyanate; UF, ultrafiltration; VH, vapor heat (10 hr, 60°C, 1190 mbar pressure plus 1 hr, 80°C, 1375 mbar).

such as in surgical patients or in clinical situations associated with an increased risk of thrombosis, as in patients with advanced liver disease.[11] FIX concentrates currently available in the United States include Alphanine SD (Alpha Therapeutic Corp., Los Angeles) and Mononine (Aventis Behring).[15, 33, 34]

The gene for FIX was cloned in 1982 and was successfully transfected into Chinese hamster ovarian cells, a process leading to rFIX production in 1985 by Genetics Institute.[35–38] Initially, rFIX was tested in a canine model and in previously treated patients and was shown to have clinical efficacy comparable to that of plasma-derived products, with a low thrombogenic potential even at high doses.[36, 39] Inhibitor formation was also low; only 1 of 44 previously treated patients developed a low-titer inhibitor that was detectable for 11 months.[40]

In October of 1995, a trial of rFIX in PUPs was initiated. Although the final results of this trial are not yet published, preliminary reports show good clinical efficacy with no adverse effects, including no viral transmission. The only difference detected between plasma-derived and rFIX in these initial studies was that recovery of rFIX is approximately 20% less than in the plasma-derived products. Poorer than anticipated recovery has been attributed to minor differences in post-translational modifications between rFIX and plasma-derived products.[39] One rFIX concentrate, BeneFix (Genetics Institute), is currently available in the United States. The SA of BeneFix is greater than 200 IU/mg protein, and the final preparation does not contain human albumin.[28]

Nonconcentrate Therapeutic Options for Hemophilia

Desmopressin

Desmopressin (DDAVP or 1-deamino, 8-D-arginine vasopressin) is a synthetic analogue of vasopressin that stimulates endothelial cell release of FVIII, vWF, and plasminogen activator. If a patient with mild hemophilia has previously been shown to have a therapeutic elevation of factor levels after drug administration, DDAVP is given at a dose of 0.3 μg/kg, is diluted in 30 to 50 mL of saline, and is administered intravenously over 15 to 30 minutes.[41, 42] The side effects are mostly minor and include facial flushing, mild headaches, nausea, or lightheadedness.[3] DDAVP can rarely cause inappropriate water retention and subsequent hyponatremia that can be avoided with fluid restriction after treatment.[1, 3] A concentrated nasal spray (Stimate, Aventis Behring) is also available that is given at a dose of 300 μg (one spray in each nostril) for patients weighing 50 kg or more and 150 μg (one spray in one nostril) for patients weighing less than 50 kg.[16, 41]

Antifibrinolytic Therapy

Antifibrinolytic therapy inhibits clot lysis and stabilizes clot formation by saturating the fibrin binding sites on plasminogen and preventing its attachment to a developing clot.[43] Antifibrinolytic therapy is particularly helpful in the treatment of oral hemorrhage because saliva contains a high concentration of fibrinolytic proteins, so clot formation is rendered more difficult. Two antifibrinolytic agents— ε-aminocaproic acid (Amicar, Immunex Corp., Seattle) and tranexamic acid (Cyklokapron, Pharmacia-Upjohn, Bridgewater, NJ)—are available for clinical use. Amicar is recommended at a dose of 100 mg/kg every 6 hours either orally or intravenously and is available both as a syrup and as a tablet.[1] The recommended dose of Cyklokapron is 25 mg/kg orally (as a tablet only) or 10 mg/kg intravenously every 8 hours.[1] These drugs are contraindicated in patients who have received PCCs or activated PCCs within 12 hours because of the possibility for enhanced thrombosis.[3]

Therapeutic Contraindications

Patients with hemophilia and other congenital coagulopathies should avoid the use of drugs that interfere with platelet function. These drugs include, but are not limited to, aspirin and other nonsteroidal anti-inflammatory agents.[16]

Clinical Management

General Principles

The goal of hemophilia care is to prevent morbidity caused by both acute blood loss and chronic, repeated bleeding episodes. Treatment or prevention of acute hemorrhage requires intravenous replacement of FVIII or FIX to hemostatic plasma levels. Factor concentrate infusions can be given to induce and to maintain hemostasis at the time of a bleeding episode, an approach known as *on-demand therapy*, or at prescribed intervals to prevent hemorrhage, an approach known as *prophylactic therapy.* Traditionally in the United States, factor replacement has been given on demand; however, increasing evidence demonstrating the benefits of prophylactic therapy is causing this practice to change.

Factor Dosing

The dose of concentrate required for factor replacement is calculated on the basis of the volume of distribution and the half-life of the specific concentrate, the patient's type and severity of hemophilia, and the severity of the particular bleeding episode.[1, 3] Factor concentrates are administered in international units (IU) per kg body weight, with 1 IU of FVIII or FIX concentrate equal to the amount of factor present in 1 mL of normal pooled plasma.[1]

Based on the severity of a specific bleeding episode, the minimum plasma factor level required to sustain hemostasis is determined. Potentially severe bleeding episodes that are life-threatening or limb-threatening require factor replacement to maintain a plasma factor level of 50% to 100% of normal. As discussed later, depending on the specific situation, these levels may need to be maintained for several days. Less severe bleeding episodes require factor replacement to reach a plasma factor level of 30% to 50% of normal. Under these circumstances, usually only a few doses of factor are required to control bleeding.[3]

The dose of concentrate required to reach these plasma factor goals is calculated using the volume of distribution of the specific factor concentrate. In general, 1 IU of plasma-derived FVIII concentrate per kilogram raises the plasma factor level by 1% in children, whereas 1 IU of plasma-derived factor concentrate per kilogram raises the plasma factor level by 2% in adults.[44] Using rFVIII, 1 IU of factor concentrate raises the plasma factor level by 2% in both children and adults.[45] For FIX products, 1 IU of plasma-derived FIX concentrate per kilogram raises the plasma factor level by 1%,[16] and 1 IU of rFIX concentrate per kilogram raises the patient's plasma level by approximately 0.6%.[39] The volume of distribution of rFIX is variable among patients, and therefore a recovery study should be done for each patient to determine the optimal dosing regimen.[1]

Subsequent dosing of factor concentrate is based on the half-life of the specific concentrate. Both factors have an initial short half-life secondary to diffusion that becomes longer with repeat dosing. The initial half-life of FVIII is 6 to 8 hours, and the subsequent half-life is 8 to 12 hours. The initial half-life of FIX is 4 to 6 hours, and the subsequent half-life is 18 to 24 hours.

Treatment of Acute Bleeding Episodes (On-Demand Therapy)

Early treatment of bleeding episodes is essential to limit the amount of blood loss and the subsequent tissue damage caused by chronic blood exposure. Replacement factor recommendations for a specific bleeding episode depend on its location and the potential for complications secondary to blood loss. Laboratory measurements of the partial thromboplastin time and FVIII or FIX levels are important guides to successful therapy and should be ordered when managing a serious bleeding episode such as intracranial hemorrhage. Management of common bleeding problems in hemophilia is discussed later, and factor replacement guidelines for specific hemorrhages are listed in Table 25.3.

INTRACRANIAL HEMORRHAGE

Intracranial hemorrhage is a major cause of morbidity and mortality in patients with hemophilia. Patients with severe factor deficiency are at higher risk of central nervous system bleeding than are patients with higher baseline factor levels. Before the wide availability of prophylaxis, about half of all cases of intracranial hemorrhage were not preceded by head trauma. Given the consequence of delayed or absent treatment, all patients with moderate or severe hemophilia with any type of head injury or a significant headache should be treated immediately with a factor replacement of 100%. Patients with a history of significant trauma should then be evaluated with a computed tomography scan. If the scan shows no sign of hemorrhage, the patient should be admitted to an inpatient setting for observation and should receive one to two subsequent 50% corrections to protect against possible delayed or slow bleeding.[41] Patients with mild hemophilia generally need factor replacement only after severe trauma. Management of actual intracranial bleeding requires prolonged maintenance of 100% of normal factor levels and includes the same life-support measures and indications for surgery used in children without coagulation disorders.

JOINT BLEEDING

Hemarthroses are a common cause of significant morbidity in hemophilia and often occur in the absence of known trauma in patients with severe disease. The joints most commonly involved are the knees, elbows, and ankles.[1] To limit long-term joint damage, initial replacement therapy should be instituted as early as possible to raise the plasma factor level to 50% to 70%. For minor or early joint bleeding, an additional factor replacement should be given to maintain a plasma factor level of 30% for approximately 24 hours. For late or significant joint hemorrhage or bleeding in a joint that has been the site of recurrent hemorrhages (target joint), a factor level of 30% should be maintained for 36 to 48 hours. In addition, for all hemarthroses, the joint should be immobilized with a splint for 48 to 72 hours. These recommendations apply to all hemarthroses, regardless of the severity of an individual patient's disease.

MUSCLE BLEEDING

Most muscle hemorrhages are superficial and are easily controlled with a single dose of replacement therapy to 30% correction, if correction is necessary at all. However, substantial blood loss can occur with internal muscle bleeding in large cavities such as with thigh and iliopsoas hemorrhages. These hemorrhages should be treated with an initial 70% correction, and plasma factor levels should be maintained at more than 30% for several days while healing occurs. These severe muscle hemorrhages are best treated with hospital admission and bed rest. The patient's hemoglobin level should be checked initially and later, as clinically indicated, because significant blood loss can occur with minimal swelling, particularly with thigh hemorrhages.

MOUTH BLEEDING

Oral bleeding is particularly common in young children with hemophilia and may occur with primary tooth eruption or in association with loose deciduous teeth. In addition, bleeding can occur after trauma leads to a laceration of the tongue or frenulum. Antifibrinolytic therapy or local measures such as topical thrombin, pressure, or ice may be sufficient to control bleeding. However, if these measures are not adequate,

Table 25.3   Factor Replacement Guidelines for Common Bleeding Problems in Hemophilia

Type of Bleeding	Target Factor Level (IU/dL)	Duration of Factor Replacement	Comments
Intracranial	0.8–1.0	10–14 days	Secondary prophylaxis to prevent recurrent bleeding
Head trauma, no intracranial hemorrhage	1.0 initially, then 0.5–1.0 if significant trauma	24–36 hours	Computed tomography scan even if normal exam for significant trauma
Joints	0.5–0.7 initially, then 0.3–0.5	24–48 hours	Immobilize for 48–72 hours
Deep muscle	0.7–1.0 initially, then 0.3–0.5	5–7 days	Hospitalize, bed rest, monitor for blood loss
Superficial muscle	0.3	12–24 hours	Immobilize for 24–48 hours
Oral mucosa	0.3	12–24 hours	Antifibrinolytics or topical therapy may be sufficient
Persistent hematuria	0.3–0.5	Until hematuria clears	Bed rest, adequate hydration, no antifibrinolytics, consider renal ultrasound
Trauma or surgery	1.0 initially, then 0.5–0.7	7–14 days	Shorter duration for minor procedure; recovery study preoperatively

factor concentrate replacement should be given to obtain a 30% correction. If bleeding persists or recurs, additional replacement doses may be required.

HEMATURIA

Painless, atraumatic hematuria can occur in patients with severe hemophilia. Bed rest and increased fluid intake is sufficient initial treatment. If symptoms persist for more than 24 hours, bed rest should be continued and the plasma factor level should be corrected to 30% until the bleeding clears. If the patient has a history of trauma, bleeding is persistent, or bleeding occurs in a patient with mild or moderate hemophilia, an ultrasound scan should be performed to look for an intracapsular or intrarenal hemorrhage so that appropriate factor replacement can be given.

SOFT TISSUE BLEEDING

Soft tissue hemorrhages do not require factor replacement unless they lead to compression of critical organs. For example, a soft tissue hemorrhage in the neck could lead to airway compression. In this situation, 100% correction should be given immediately, and appropriate measures should be taken to ensure airway patency.

Prophylactic Therapy

The major long-term morbidity of hemophilia is joint disease caused by repeated exposure of the synovium to blood. Blood acts as an irritant in a joint and leads to synovial membrane proliferation, which, in turn, makes the joint more susceptible to repeated injury and bleeding. Recurrent bleeding then causes chronic synovitis, damage to the underlying cartilage, and finally erosion of the bone.[46] Before the availability of specific factor concentrates, people with severe hemophilia had an average of 30 to 35 joint hemorrhages per year, and 90% developed subsequent degenerative joint disease.[47, 48] The introduction of specific factor concentrates, which allowed earlier and more complete treatment of hemarthrosis, markedly decreased the incidence of hemophiliac arthropathy, but it did not eliminate it entirely, thus necessitating an alternate treatment strategy.

Dr. Nilsson and colleagues in Malmo, Sweden first developed the concept of prophylaxis in 1958.[46] Based on the observation that people with moderate and mild hemophilia rarely developed joint disease, these investigators hypothesized that by giving regular factor infusions with the goal of maintaining a factor level of at least 1% in patients with severe hemophilia, they could in a sense convert severe disease to mild or moderate disease and could prevent frequent hemorrhage and subsequent arthropathy.[49, 50] These investigators published several case series demonstrating the benefits of their theory, and their data have been confirmed by others around the world.[46, 51, 52] A longitudinal, uncontrolled outcome study from 21 centers in the United States, Europe, and Japan published in 1994 reported that patients with severe hemophilia, who were treated with adequate prophylaxis, experienced a reduced number of hemorrhages and a reduced rate of joint degeneration, whereas patients receiving on-demand treatment had signs of progressive joint deterioration.[53]

Two prophylactic treatment strategies have been developed that vary according to the timing of initiation of regular infusions relative to joint status. *Primary prophylaxis* is defined as the initiation of regular factor concentrate infusions before the development of recurrent joint bleeding and clinical or radiologic abnormalities.[54] *Secondary prophylaxis* indicates the initiation of regular factor concentrate infusions after the development of chronic clinical or radiologic abnormalities in a particular joint, considered a "target" joint.[55] Until recently, secondary prophylaxis was the treatment strategy most commonly used in the United States. It has been shown to be beneficial in preventing frequent rebleeding in a target joint and to improve orthopedic examination and quality of life.[51, 56, 57] However, eventual joint deterioration, as evidenced by radiologic evaluation, is not stopped in most cases by secondary prophylaxis.[53] In contrast, primary prophylaxis has been shown to prevent permanent, chronic joint damage. An update of the Swedish prophylaxis experience demonstrates that boys who began primary prophylaxis at a mean age of 1.2 years had no clinical or radiologic evidence of joint damage when they were evaluated 3 to 12 years after the initiation of therapy.[50, 52]

In 1994, the National Hemophilia Foundation's Medical and Scientific Advisory Counsel recommended that primary prophylaxis be the treatment of choice for severe hemophilia.[1] However, this recommendation has met several obstacles. An important obstacle to prophylaxis is its expense. Smith and colleagues[58] compared 27 boys receiving prophylactic factor concentrate infusions with 70 boys receiving episodic infusions over a 2-year interval and showed that the median cost of prophylaxis is at least three times the cost of on-demand therapy. One way to decrease the cost of prophylaxis, as suggested by Carlsson and colleagues,[59] is to give prophylactic factor infusions more frequently; therefore, smaller doses are required to maintain a factor trough level higher than the baseline value. This may become possible when home continuous factor infusion becomes available.

Another major obstacle to prophylaxis is venous access. Placement of central venous access devices is often necessary to provide consistent venous access in young children receiving prophylaxis and is associated with an increased risk of infection compared with intermittent intravenous access.[60, 61] The incidence of central line infections in a survey of 81 hemophilia treatment centers from 33 states was 28% in patients receiving prophylaxis.[62] A third concern preventing the widespread adoption of prophylaxis is that frequent exposure to large quantities of factor may exacerbate inhibitor formation. Fortunately, this has not been shown to occur, and, in fact, regular factor infusion may prevent inhibitor formation because it may mimic immune tolerance, which is discussed in detail later.[28, 50]

A final obstacle to widespread adoption of prophylaxis is the lack of prospective randomized trials directly comparing prophylaxis with on-demand therapy. In 1996, a multicenter randomized control study comparing joint and psychosocial outcomes in young children using either a prophylactic regimen or an aggressive on-demand regimen was begun and will likely address this issue.[28]

When prophylaxis is implemented, factor should be administered at a dose to maintain a trough factor activity of more than 1%, and recombinant factor should be given to minimize the risk of infection.[46, 59] In general, this requires doses of rFVIII every other day or three times a week and twice-weekly dosing of rFIX.

Surgical Procedures

The goal of hemophilia care for elective surgery is to maintain factor levels of 50% to 70% throughout the surgical procedure and the postoperative period.[41] A factor recovery study should be done preoperatively to ensure that the patient has the expected response to therapy and to predict the half-life of the concentrate accurately. Regular factor infusion should continue 2 to 7 days postoperatively and then can be tapered.[41]

Treatment of Newborns

The newborn with unsuspected hemophilia born to a woman with no family history may pass through the newborn period with no clinical evidence of disease.[63] The likelihood of excess bleeding at circumcision is 50%[64]; bleeding from circumcision often prompts a diagnostic workup and definitive diagnosis. Male children born to obligate carrier mothers or those infants diagnosed prenatally with hemophilia present a perplexing question of management. Some practitioners recommend prophylactic infusion of factor concentrate in either case, to prevent neonatal intracranial hemorrhage that could result from a vaginal delivery. Others recommend immediate measurement of neonatal factor levels and concomitant head ultrasounds to rule out intracranial hemorrhage.[65, 66]

Treatment for Patients with Inhibitors

One of the greatest challenges in the treatment of hemophilia is the development of inhibitors, high-affinity neutralizing immunoglobulin G antibodies directed against FVIII or FIX.[1] Based on both prospective and retrospective studies, inhibitor development occurs in 21% to 33% of patients with severe hemophilia A[28] and in 1% to 4% of patients with hemophilia B.[26] Most inhibitors form in young children who have had less than 20 treatment days and occur more often in black patients than in white patients.[26] There is also an increased incidence of inhibitors in brothers of boys who have already developed an inhibitor, a finding suggesting a genetic predisposition.[67] Patients with severe hemophilia are more likely to develop inhibitors than those with milder forms of disease. This may be because the low levels of factor produced in patients with mild and moderate hemophilia induce immune tolerance, whereas in severely affected patients, the endogenous factor level is so low that infused factor is regarded as a foreign protein and more easily provokes an immune response.[68] Among patients with severe hemophilia, there is a higher rate of inhibitor development among persons with large gene mutations that lead to undetectable factor levels. The rate of inhibitor development is lower in patients with severe hemophilia with missense mutations and small deletions in whom circulating, but abnormal, factor is present.[69, 70]

The development of an inhibitor is suspected when the patient has decreased clinical response to factor replacement, or it can be found in an asymptomatic person during routine laboratory screening.[68] The presence of an inhibitor is confirmed using the Bethesda assay that measures the titer of neutralizing antibody and is reported in Bethesda Units (BU). One BU is defined as the amount of inhibitor needed to inactivate 50% of the FVIII or FIX in a mixture of inhibitor-containing plasma and normal plasma.[71] Inhibitor patients are classified as *high responders* or *low responders*, depending on the extent of amnestic response on repeat exposure to the factor against which the inhibitor has formed.[28] Patients with high-responder inhibitors develop an increased antibody level within a few days of repeat exposure to FVIII or FIX, whereas low-responder inhibitors only minimally increase after repeat exposure to factor. High-responder inhibitors have antibody titers greater than 10 BU and are also called *high-titer inhibitors*, whereas low responders have titers lower than 10 BU and are referred to as *low-titer inhibitors*.[26] The inhibitor titer level is a useful guide for determining the optimal replacement therapy. Specific treatment recommendations for patients with hemophilia A with inhibitors are outlined in Table 25.4.

Patients with low-titer inhibitors can be treated for acute hemorrhage with higher doses of their specific replacement therapy.[1] Patients often require doses two to three times higher than the normal replacement dose to effect hemostasis. FVIII or FIX levels should be monitored before and after treatment

Table 25.4 Treatment of Hemorrhage in Patients with Hemophilia with Inhibitors

Type of Patient	Titer at Time of Hemorrhage	Minor Hemorrhage		Major Hemorrhage	
		Agent	Dosage	Agent/Method	Dosage
High responder	<10 BU	PCC	75 IU/kg q12h	Human FVIII	100–200 IU/kg, q12h*
		aPCC	75 IU/kg q12h	Porcine FVIII	50–200 IU/kg*†
				aPCC	75–100 IU/kg q12h
				rFVIIa	90–120 µg/kg q2h
	>10BU	PCC	75 IU/kg q12h	Porcine FVIII	50–200 IU/kg*†
		aPCC	75 IU/kg q12h	aPCC	75–100 IU/kg q12h
				rFVIIa	90–120 µg/kg q 2h
				Plasmapheresis and high-dose human FVIII	100–200 IU/kg q12h
Low responder	<5 BU	Human FVIII	50–75 IU/kg q 8–12 h	Human FVIII	100–200 IU/kg*
	<10 BU	PCC	75 IU/kg q12h	Human FVIII	100–200 IU/kg q12h*
		aPCC	75 IU/kg q12h	Porcine FVIII	20–50 IU/kg*†
				aPCC	50–100 IU/kg q12h
				rFVIIa	60–120 µg/kg q2h

*Monitor FVIII levels.
†Use porcine FVIII only if porcine FVIII inhibitor level < 20 BU.
aPCC, activated prothrombin complex concentrates; BU, Bethesda units; FVIII, factor VIII; PCC, prothrombin complex concentrates; rFVIII, recombinant factor VIII.
From Manno, CS: Treatment options for bleeding episodes in patients undergoing immune tolerance therapy. Haemophilia 5:33–41, 1999.

to help assess, along with clinical measurements, the treatment's usefulness. Adjuvant measures including restriction of limb motion and bed rest should also be used to preserve fragile clots.

First-line treatment of hemorrhage in patients with high-titer inhibitors is aimed at bypassing the factor against which the inhibitor is directed. The most commonly used treatments for patients with hemophilia A and hemophilia B with high-titer inhibitors are PCCs and activated PCCs (aPCCs), which contain FII, FVII, FIX, and FX, as previously described. These products are effective in stopping bleeding in approximately half of the inhibitor patients treated, with some studies suggesting increased efficacy of aPCCs compared with PCCs.[72] PCCs and aPCCs should be infused at doses of 50 to 100 IU/kg every 12 to 24 hours with the maximum dose not to exceed 200 IU/kg in 24 hours.[26] As described previously, these bypass agents can be associated with thrombotic complications with repeated dosing. In addition, patients with hemophilia B occasionally develop an increased inhibitor titer or a severe allergic response when they are treated with these products containing FIX and therefore must be monitored closely.[73] One licensed alternative treatment for bleeding episodes in patients with high-titer FVIII or FIX inhibitors is recombinant activated FVIIa (rFVIIa), (NovoSeven, Novo-Nordisk, Copenhagen, Denmark), which bypasses FVIII and FIX by activating the extrinsic pathway of the clotting cascade. rFVIIa is thought to initiate hemostasis only at the site of tissue injury and therefore should not be thrombogenic.[74] In addition, rFVIIa is not plasma derived and is not associated with an anamnestic response. A drawback to using rFVIIa is its short half-life, which requires dosing every 2 to 3 hours, a feature that makes treatment cumbersome and costly.[75] Laboratory coagulation parameters have not been shown to correlate directly with the establishment of hemostasis when one uses bypassing agents. Dosing is therefore empiric, based largely on clinical response.

Porcine FVIII (Hyate:C, Ipsen, Inc., Wales, UK) is an alternative for high-responding inhibitor patients with hemophilia A, particularly for treatment of a major hemorrhage. It has an efficacy of more than 75% and has been shown to be most useful when the human FVIII antibody is less than 50 BU and porcine FVIII antibody is less than 15 BU.[26, 68] Hyate:C has 30% homology with human FVIII, so that it can participate in the coagulation cascade while having potentially limited cross-reactivity with inhibitor antibodies.[16, 26] However, cross-reactivity is often seen, and patients should be assessed for this before administration of the product. Potential side effects of porcine FVIII include severe allergic reactions and thrombocytopenia, and anamnesis to both human and porcine factor frequently occurs.[73] In cases of serious bleeding, plasmapheresis followed by high-dose factor replacement is another treatment option. However, traditional plasmapheresis results in inhibitor reduction of only 40%, and this may not lead to adequate hemostasis in patients with titers higher than 40 BU. Use of a protein A sepharose column has been shown to improve the efficacy of plasma exchange by more than twofold.[68]

None of the transfusion options for patients with high-titer inhibitors are as reliable as specific factor replacement, and therefore elimination of inhibitors with immune tolerance therapy (ITT) is a major emphasis of management. ITT involves the regular exposure to high doses of FVIII or FIX for weeks to years with or without concurrent immunosuppressive therapy. Several available ITT regimens are available, with an overall success rate of 60% to 80%, but these regimens often require central venous access and can be time intensive and costly.[1] Data from the North American ITT registry shows a higher efficacy and shorter interval to inhibitor elimination when ITT is initiated when the inhibitor titer is low.[76] Other data show improved outcomes when the interval between inhibitor detection and starting ITT is short.[76] It is therefore important to start ITT as soon as a patient's high-titer, high-response status is confirmed. Once immune tolerance has been achieved, management of bleeding episodes can be the same as before inhibitor development.

Comprehensive Hemophilia Care

Patients with hemophilia have lifelong disease punctuated by hospitalization and the need for expensive intravenous medication. The management of such complicated patients is best supervised by a multidisciplinary expert team that includes a hematologist, a hemophilia nurse specialist, a physical therapist, a social worker, an orthopedist, and a dentist. Regular clinic visits for evaluation by these health care providers give the patient with hemophilia a solid foundation for managing the long-term medical and psychosocial issues associated with chronic disease.

Gene Therapy

Hemophilia is a good model for a gene therapy approach for several reasons.[77] First, small increases in circulating levels of FVIII or FIX through transgene expression would likely result in significant reduction of bleeding episodes. Second, tight regulation of transgene expression is not necessary because normal levels of FVIII and FIX extend to 150%. Gene therapy trials are under way using numerous different viral and nonviral approaches to transfer the recombinant gene to human cells, including liver and muscle cells.[77, 78] Whether a gene therapy approach will be safe or effective has yet to be determined, but preliminary results are encouraging.[79]

■ Von Willebrand Disease

vWD is the most common congenital coagulation disorder, occurring in approximately 1% to 2% of the population.[80, 81] It is actually a collection of disorders caused by either quantitative or qualitative abnormalities of vWF, a glycoprotein that is important in both primary and secondary hemostasis.[82] In contrast to hemophilia, mucosal bleeding, especially epistaxis and menorrhagia, and easy bruising are the most frequent clinical signs, although more significant bleeding can occur with trauma or surgery. Bleeding symptoms are often most severe in children and adolescents.[83] vWD occurs at the same rate in male and female patients and is generally inherited as an autosomal trait with variable penetrance.[84] In contrast to hemophilia, bleeding symptoms may vary among members of affected families.[83]

Structure and Function of von Willebrand Factor

The gene for vWF is located on chromosome 12 and is 178 kb in length with 52 exons.[85] There is also a pseudogene on chromosome 22 with 97% homology.[86] vWF is initially transcribed as a large, single-chain protein with 2813 amino acids (pre-pro VFW) that undergoes a series of changes to become the mature multimeric vWF.[83] First, a small signal peptide is removed to form pro-vWF. Next, the remaining peptide undergoes glycosylation, sulfation, and dimer formation leading to the formation of vWF multimers of various sizes ranging in molecular weight from 500 to 20,000 kD.[87] vWF is the largest soluble protein in humans. Its plasma concentration and functional activity are generally expressed either as a percentage of normal or as units per milliliter related to a normal plasma pool calibrated against an international plasma standard for vWF.[87]

vWF is synthesized in endothelial cells and megakaryocytes. vWF from the endothelial cells is stored in Weibel-Palade bodies and is secreted into the plasma or subendothelial matrix, and it consists of predominantly high-molecular-weight multimers.[88] Platelet vWF, consisting of mostly low-molecular-weight multimers, is synthesized in the megakaryocyte and is stored in platelet α granules.[87] vWF multimers with the highest molecular weight are most effective in hemostasis because they have a large surface area with a high concentration of binding sites for various ligands and receptors.[87]

vWF is important in both primary and secondary hemostasis. It is a cofactor in platelet adhesion and a participant in platelet aggregation. In response to vascular injury, a conformational change occurs in plasma vWF that allows it to bind to platelet glycoprotein Ib.[83, 88] Platelets then adhere to the site of endothelial damage and become activated after interactions with subendothelial components such as collagen. Platelet activation causes release of stored platelet components, including vWF from α granules, and expression of activated glycoprotein IIb/IIIa, the receptor that is involved in platelet aggregation.[88] Platelet vWF can bind to glycoprotein IIb/IIIa to facilitate aggregation, although fibrinogen is the main cofactor in this reaction.[83] vWF multimers with the highest molecular weight are most effective in hemostasis because they have a large surface area with a high concentration of binding sites for various ligands and receptors. vWF also plays an important role in the coagulation cascade, by acting as a carrier protein for FVIII so that it is protected from proteolytic cleavage in the plasma.[88] Deficiency of vWF causes FVIII to have a reduced half-life and leads to a deficiency in plasma FVIII. In addition, vWF plays a role in stimulating FVIII release into plasma. This is shown in vitro, where cells transfected with the FVIII gene express rFVIII more efficiently when vWF is present in the media or is co-transfected along with FVIII. In addition, in vivo, when plasma from FVIII-deficient patients is infused into patients with vWD, an increase in FVIII in the patients with vWD is seen.[83]

Classification

As is evident from the previous discussion, vWF plays several critical roles in platelet function and thrombus formation. For vWF to function normally, several requirements must be met, including the presence of high-molecular-weight multimer forms, the appropriate release of activated vWF, and the presence of binding sites for platelet glycoproteins, FVIII, and constituents of the subendothelial cell matrix. Abnormalities of any of these components can lead to vWD, with particular deficiencies leading to different clinical phenotypes. In addition, because the vWF locus is autosomal and the protein is polymeric, the phenotype of a particular patient with vWD is the result of interactions between two different alleles and protein products that lead to the further clinical heterogeneity of this disorder.[89] More than 20 subtypes of vWD have been identified so far.[90] The current classification system for vWD, approved by the Subcommittee on vWF at the 39th Annual Meeting of the Scientific and Standardization Committee of the International Society of Thrombosis and Haemostasis in 1993, attempts to simplify this clinical heterogeneity by classifying patients based on pathophysiology, clinical behavior, and genetic abnormalities.[89] This classification scheme is based on the principle that all vWD is the result of mutations of the vWF locus. In the scheme are three major categories of vWD: type 1 disease, a partial quantitative deficiency of vWF; type 2 vWD, a qualitative deficiency of vWF; and type 3 disease, a complete quantitative deficiency of vWF. The clinical course and genetic implications can be predicted by type. Mixed phenotypes can exist, resulting from compound heterozygosity.[89]

Type 1

Type 1 disease is most common and accounts for 70% to 80% of patients diagnosed with vWD.[87, 91] Patients with type 1 disease have a mild to moderate decrease in plasma levels of vWF with a normal vWF multimer pattern. Type 1 disease is usually inherited in an autosomal dominant pattern. Clinically, patients with type 1 disease usually have only mild symptoms and are often identified during routine preoperative screening tests.[83, 87]

Type 2 (2A, 2B, 2M, and 2N)

Type 2 vWD disease is diagnosed in 15% to 20% of affected patients and is characterized by a qualitative defect in vWF caused by missense mutations and small inframe deletions or insertions.[82, 87] Typically, patients have more significant bleeding symptoms than are seen in type 1 disease. Family history is often positive with this diagnosis, with both autosomal dominant and recessive patterns of inheritance seen.[87] Type 2 disease can be further classified into four variants according to the particular vWF abnormality.

Type 2A vWD is the most frequent subtype and is characterized by decreased vWF platelet-dependent function and an absence of high- and intermediate-molecular-weight vWF multimers.[82, 89] This multimer abnormality can result from either abnormal synthesis of vWF or increased breakdown of circulating vWF. Type 2A vWD is usually inherited as a dominant trait.[88, 89]

Type 2B is a rarer form of vWD in which an abnormal vWF has excessive affinity for platelet glycoprotein Ib. This causes excessive platelet activation and removal from the circulation and leads to variable thrombocytopenia as well as decreased plasma concentrations of vWF.[82, 84] Thrombocytopenia may be intermittent and is often exacerbated by stress such as infection.[84] Type 2B is inherited as a dominant trait and is associated with absence of high-molecular-weight multimers.[82, 91]

Type 2M disease describes patients with decreased platelet-dependent function that is similar to type 2A disease, except high-molecular-weight multimers are not absent. Decreased platelet function is instead caused by structural or functional defects in binding regions of the vWF protein. Like type 2A and 2B disease, this type is usually inherited as a dominant trait.[82, 91]

Type 2N vWD (also known as vWD Normandy) refers to patients with vWF variants with decreased binding affinity for FVIII. This leads to decreased survival of FVIII in the circulation and a moderate to severe reduction of FVIII plasma levels with normal vWF levels. Affected persons therefore have a mild hemophilia phenotype. This type usually has an autosomal recessive inheritance.[82–84]

Type 3

Type 3 vWD is characterized by near-complete deficiency of vWF (less than 10%) as well as a secondary deficiency of FVIII, resulting in a severe bleeding disorder with abnormalities in both primary and secondary hemostasis.[91] This type of vWD is very rare, with a prevalence of 1 to 3 cases per 1,000,000, and is inherited as an autosomal recessive disorder.[92]

Diagnosis

vWD should be suspected in patients with a history of increased bruising, prolonged bleeding after minor trauma, or mucosal bleeding, particularly epistaxis and menorrhagia, and is supported by a family history of abnormal bleeding. Initial screening tests include prothrombin time, partial thromboplastin time, platelet count, and bleeding time. The prothrombin time is usually normal, whereas the partial thromboplastin time may be prolonged by a decrease in FVIII.[91] The platelet count is also usually normal, although, as described earlier, thrombocytopenia can be present in patients with type 2B disease.[84] The bleeding time is usually prolonged secondary to abnormal platelet function, but it may be normal in patients with type 1 disease and normal platelet vWF content.[91] All these screening tests may be normal in persons with vWD, so further testing may be needed when suspicion of disease is significant.[93]

Specific tests used to evaluate patients for vWD include vWF antigen, FVIII assay, ristocetin cofactor activity, and vWF multimer analysis. Because normal physiologic variation can occur in plasma levels of vWF, FVIII, and ristocetin cofactor, repeated plasma measurements over time may be necessary to establish a diagnosis of disease.[84, 93] Results of these tests vary according to type of vWD.

vWF antigen is decreased in type 1 disease, decreased or normal in type 2, and undetectable in type 3 disease.[91] vWF is an acute-phase reactant, and factors such as pregnancy, exercise, infection, and cigarette smoking as well as medications including corticosteroids, birth control pills, and DDAVP can increase plasma concentrations of vWF and need to be taken into consideration when one evaluates test results.[84] In addition, vWF antigen varies with ABO blood types and therefore should be interpreted in reference to values specific for the patient's blood type; persons with blood group O have the lowest mean vWF antigen level.[94] FVIII levels are normal or mildly decreased in patients with types 1 and 2 vWD.[91] In contrast, patients with type 2N and type 3 vWD can have an extremely low FVIII level.[84] The ristocetin cofactor activity assay measures the vWF function, specifically the interaction of vWF with platelet glycoprotein Ib. Patients with type 1 and type 3 vWD tend to have a decrease in ristocetin cofactor activity that is proportional to their decrease in vWF antigen, whereas those with type 2 disease have a more substantial decrease in ristocetin cofactor activity than vWF antigen.[84, 91] Studies have shown that measurement of ristocetin cofactor activity is the most sensitive test for diagnosing type 1 vWD.[80, 93] Finally, the vWF can be separated by agarose gel electrophoresis into high-, intermediate-, and low-molecular-weight multimers. All the multimers are present in type 1 disease and are absent in type 3 disease. In type 2 vWD, gel electrophoresis can vary with disease type, but generally it shows a reduction in high- and intermediate-weight multimer.[84] Table 25.5 summarizes the laboratory findings according to vWD type.

Therapeutic Products

Superficial bleeding, particularly in type 1 vWD, can usually be managed by applying local pressure, ice, or a local hemostatic agent such as topical thrombin. Systemic therapy is generally reserved for bleeding at sites not controllable by local measure or as prophylaxis before and after surgical treatment. The two main approaches to systemic therapy of vWD are: (1) increasing the release of endogenous vWF and (2) exogenous replacement of vWF. Selecting the appropriate therapy for an individual patient depends on the specific type of vWD and clinical treatment goal.[43]

Desmopressin

As previously discussed, DDAVP, a synthetic analogue of vasopressin, causes immediate endothelial cell release of vWF, FVIII, and plasminogen activator.[42] It is effective in patients with vWD who have adequate stores of functional vWF. Therefore, it is useful in type 1 disease but ineffective in type 3 disease. DDAVP can be used in some patients with type 2A vWD, but it is not recommended in patients with type 2B disease because it can exacerbate thrombocytopenia.[88, 95]

Table 25.5 Laboratory Findings in von Willebrand Disease According to Subtype

Study	Type 1	Type 2A	Type 2B	Type 2M	Type 2N	Type 3
von Willebrand factor antigen	↓	↓	+/–↓	↓	↓	Absent
Ristocetin cofactor activity	↓	↓↓↓	+/–↓	↓↓↓	↓	Absent
Factor VIII	↓	Normal	Normal	Normal	↓↓	Absent
Ristocetin-induced platelet aggregation	+/–↓	↓↓	Normal	↓	Normal	Absent
Multimers	Normal	Absent Intermediate- and high-molecular weight multimers	Absent high-molecular-weight multimers	Normal	Normal	Absent

Adapted from Montgomery RR, Gill JC, Scott JP: Hemophilia and von Willebrand Disease. In Nathan DH, Orkin SH (eds): Naton and OSKI's Hematology of Infancy and Childhood, vol 2, 5th ed, Philadelphia, WB Sandeps. 1998, p 1646.

Patients with type 2N disease generally have high FVIII levels in response to DDAVP, but the released FVIII has a shorter than normal half-life that limits its therapeutic utility in major bleeding episodes.[95] DDAVP is given at the same dose used in mild FVIII deficiency, both intravenously and as a concentrated nasal spray (Stimate). Infusion of 0.3 µg/kg body weight results in an average three to fivefold increase in vWF and FVIII; nasal dosing is slightly less effective.[42, 88] Before therapeutic use, patients should have a trial to measure individual response to DDAVP.[96] Response to DDAVP is generally consistent over time, and family members usually have similar responses.[97] DDAVP is used preferentially over plasma-derived products in patients who have an adequate response, because of viral safety. In addition, DDAVP is substantially less expensive than exogenous vWF replacement.[42]

DDAVP may not be useful when prolonged hemostasis is required. When administered more often than once every 24 to 48 hours, decreased effectiveness may be observed because of depletion of storage pools (tachyphylaxis).[97] Therefore, when DDAVP is used for several days, coagulation parameters should be followed closely (vWF, FVIII, and ristocetin cofactor) to monitor the need for alternate replacement therapy.

Exogenous von Willebrand Factor Replacement

Exogenous replacement of vWF is used in patients in whom DDAVP is not effective. This includes most patients with type 2B, type 2M, and type 3 vWD, as well as those with type 1 and 2A disease who do not show adequate response in a DDAVP trial. Fresh frozen plasma contains both FVIII and vWF; however, the large volumes required to achieve hemostasis limit its clinical use.[96] Cryoprecipitate, containing vWF, FVIII, and fibrinogen, was the treatment of choice for patients with vWD from the early 1960s until the early 1980s.[43, 98] The development of products with higher purity that are more convenient to store and have decreased volumes of infusion subsumed the need for cryoprecipitate. However, if other alternatives are not available, transfusion of cryoprecipitate will produce hemostasis.[88] Each bag of cryoprecipitate contains 80 to 100 IU of vWF, and the usual starting dose is 1 bag/10 kg body weight every 12 to 24 hours.[88, 96] Cryoprecipitate from a single donor who has been pretreated with DDAVP contains supraphysiologic amounts of vWF and is another treatment option.[83]

The early plasma-derived FVIII concentrates were not effective in treating vWD because the vWF multimers were partially proteolyzed; this resulted in a loss of functional high-molecular-weight multimers.[43] In addition, the newer high-purity (monoclonal antibody-derived) FVIII and rFVIII also cannot be used to treat vWD because they do not contain appreciable amounts of vWF.[88] A few plasma-derived, virus-inactivated intermediate- and high-purity products contain sufficient amounts of functional vWF in addition to FVIII. One product is currently licensed in the United States, Humate-P, and two others also contain high-molecular-weight multimers; Alphanate (Alpha Therapeutic Corp.) and Koate-DVI (Bayer Corp.).[88, 98, 99] These latter products are not yet licensed by the Food and Drug Administration for use in vWD. In general, dosing for vWD is in units of ristocetin cofactor. In addition a recombinant vWF concentrate is currently under development.[92]

Adjunctive Treatment

As previously described for hemophilia treatment, antifibrinolytic therapy, which inhibits lysis of newly formed clots, is also useful in the treatment of vWD. ε-Aminocaproic acid and tranexamic acid are the agents most commonly used and are given at the same doses used in hemophilia. Both agents may be useful alone in mild type 1 disease or as adjuncts in the treatment of oral hemorrhage, epistaxis, gastrointestinal bleeding, and menorrhagia. As previously described, these agents may increase the risk of thrombosis and are contraindicated in patients with a known preexisting prothrombotic state and in the treatment of genitourinary bleeding.[88, 96]

Estrogen causes an increase in plasma vWF. This effect is variable and is not dose related and therefore is not widely clinically applicable. However, estrogen therapy, particularly in the form of oral contraceptives, is useful in reducing the severity of menorrhagia, a common problem in women with vWD.[96] As previously discussed with hemophilia, patients with vWD should avoid drugs that interfere with platelet function.

■ Rare Inherited Congenital Clotting Disorders Requiring Transfusion Therapy

Fibrinogen Deficiencies

Congenital afibrinogenemia is a rare disorder with an estimated incidence of 1 to 2 per 1,000,000 that is inherited as an autosomal recessive trait with the gene located on chromosome 4.[100, 101] It is characterized by virtual absence of fibrinogen secondary to deficient liver cell synthesis. Symptoms range from minimal bleeding to life-threatening hemorrhage. Symptoms are commonly seen in the newborn period and include hematomas or intracranial hemorrhage from birth trauma, bleeding from the umbilicus, and excessive bleeding after circumcision. Similar to hemophilia, spontaneous hemorrhage and excessive post-traumatic and post-surgical bleeding are seen and can result in excessive ecchymoses, hemarthroses, gastrointestinal bleeding, and intracranial hemorrhage.[100, 102] In addition, menstrual bleeding can be severe, and first-trimester spontaneous abortion is common.[100, 103] Laboratory screening tests that use clot formation as an endpoint, including the thrombin, prothrombin, and partial thromboplastin times, are markedly prolonged. Definitive diagnosis is made by measurement of plasma fibrinogen, which is undetectable by both functional and immunologic assays.

Dysfibrinogenemia is characterized by structural fibrinogen defects causing alterations in the conversion of fibrinogen to fibrin. Approximately 250 cases have been reported, and the disorder is inherited as an autosomal dominant trait.[104] Dysfibrinogenemias can be associated with either hemorrhage or thromboses, or they can be asymptomatic.[101, 104] The bleeding symptoms most commonly seen are ecchymoses, epistaxis, menorrhagia, and mild to moderate postoperative or post-traumatic bleeding. Symptoms are generally mild, although they can be more severe in patients with homozygous gene mutations. Results of screening tests are variable; the prothrombin time and partial thromboplastin time can be normal or prolonged. The thrombin time is prolonged in dysfibrinogenemias associated with hemorrhage, whereas it can be shortened or prolonged in those conditions associated with thromboses. More definitive diagnosis is made by measurement of fibrinogen; levels are normal or increased by immunologic assay, but they are reduced by functional assays.[102, 104, 105]

For both quantitative and qualitative fibrinogen deficiencies, cryoprecipitate can be used as replacement therapy for significant episodic bleeding. Cryoprecipitate should be administered at a dose to raise the fibrinogen level to between 50 and 100 mg/dL.[100] A typical bag of cryoprecipitate contains 200 to 300 mg of fibrinogen in a volume of 10 to 20 mL.[3] Because the half-life of fibrinogen is 80 hours, dosing is required only every other day.[102] Prophylactic replacement of fibrinogen, practical because of the long half-life of fibrinogen, should be considered for patients with severe symptoms.[106]

Prothrombin Deficiency

Prothrombin deficiency is a very rare autosomal recessive disorder that results from either an absolute protein deficiency or production of an abnormal protein.[107] It is characterized by mild symptoms including mucocutaneous bleeding and hemorrhage after surgery or trauma. The prothrombin time is moderately prolonged, the partial thromboplastin time is normal or mildly prolonged, and the thrombin time is normal. Definitive diagnosis is made by immunologic and functional prothrombin assays.[102, 107]

Therapy is usually not required. Fresh frozen plasma or PCCs can be used to treat clinically significant bleeding. The half-life of prothrombin is 48 to 120 hours.[101] Plasma prothrombin levels greater than 20 to 30 U/dL are generally sufficient to stop bleeding.[107]

Factor V Deficiency

FV deficiency occurs in less than 1 per 1,000,000 persons and is associated with a mild to moderate bleeding tendency.[102] It is inherited as an autosomal recessive disease. Symptoms, generally only seen in homozygotes, consist mainly of mucocutaneous bleeding, including menorrhagia, and ecchymoses. Both the prothrombin and partial thromboplastin times are prolonged with a normal thrombin time. Definitive diagnosis is made by a specific FV assay with deficiency defined as FV levels lower than 20 U/dL.[108]

Fresh frozen plasma should be used to treat severe bleeding episodes and trauma and as prophylaxis for major surgery. For treatment, the FV level should be initially raised to 25% to 30% using a 20 mL/kg dose of plasma followed by infusions of 6 mL/kg every 12 hours.[107] FV is more labile in frozen plasma than other hemostatic factors, and therefore fresh frozen plasma that is less than 1 to 2 months old should be used.[107]

Several families with combined deficiency of FV and FVIII have been reported.[109] Symptoms are usually milder than in hemophilia A because of higher baseline levels of FVIII. Treatment should include fresh frozen plasma in addition to FVIII concentrates.

Factor VII Deficiency

FVII deficiency, resulting from either a protein deficiency or production of a nonfunctional protein, occurs in 1 in 1,000,000 persons and is inherited in an autosomal recessive pattern with high penetrance and variable expressivity.[110] Laboratory evaluation of patients with FVII deficiency

reveals a prolonged prothrombin time with a normal partial thromboplastin time and thrombin time, a pattern that distinguishes FVII deficiency from other inherited clotting disorders. The diagnosis is confirmed by measuring FVII activity using a tissue factor–dependent one-stage technique. The clinical expression of the disease is generally correlated with the degree of factor deficiency, although reports exist of patients with extremely low FVII levels who present without a history of bleeding.[111] Patients with FVII levels greater than 10% to 15% rarely have significant bleeding problems, whereas patients with levels lower than 1% can have severe bleeding symptoms.[110] The most serious complication of FVII deficiency is intracranial hemorrhage, which occurs most frequently during the first year of life, particularly in the first postnatal week.[112] Mucous membrane bleeding, including excessive bruising, epistaxis, gastrointestinal bleeding, and menorrhagia, is the most common manifestation of FVII deficiency. Hemarthroses, in a pattern similar to what is seen in hemophilia, also occur occasionally.[112]

Treatment is required for severe bleeding episodes and before surgical procedures. PCCs have been the mainstays of therapy for FVII deficiency. Replacement doses are calculated to raise the FVII level to more than 15%. FVII concentrations vary among commercially available PCCs and among different lots produced by a single manufacturer, so it is important to monitor the patient's prothrombin time and FVII level carefully.[110] As discussed previously, patients receiving PCCs need to be monitored for an increased risk of developing thromboses. More recently, recombinant FVIIa (Novo Nordisk) has become available and has been shown to be effective as a more specific treatment without an accompanying risk of thrombosis.[113] Studies have shown efficacy of rFVIIa as treatment for intracranial hemorrhage and as prophylaxis for surgical procedures in patients, and these features make rFVIIa the likely treatment of choice for FVII deficiency in the future.[114, 115]

Factor X Deficiency

FX deficiency results from either a protein deficiency or production of a functionally abnormal protein.[107] It is inherited as an autosomal recessive trait, although some heterozygotes can have bleeding with severe trauma or major surgery. Symptoms generally correlate with the severity of the deficiency and consist mainly of mucocutaneous and post-traumatic bleeding. Hemarthrosis and intracranial hemorrhage have been reported in severely affected patients. Laboratory evaluation reveals prolonged prothrombin and partial thromboplastin times. Diagnosis is confirmed with FX immunologic and functional assays.

FX replacement should be given as needed for severe bleeding and trauma as well as before major surgical procedures. The half-life of transfused FX is between 24 and 48 hours, and FX is found in both fresh frozen plasma and PCC.[102] Fresh frozen plasma is given at an initial dose of 10 to 20 mL/kg, followed every 12 hours by a dose of 3 to 6 mL/kg to reach a target plasma FX level of 20 to 30 IU/dL.[107] PCCs contain a variable concentration of FX that can be measured in a specific preparation before elective use.[107] PCCs are more practical to use in situations such as major surgery, when sustained hemostasis is necessary and would require large volumes of plasma infusions. As previously mentioned, when using PCCs, the risk of thrombosis should be considered and monitored.

Factor XI Deficiency

FXI deficiency, sometimes called hemophilia C, is a relatively rare disorder distinguished by a variable bleeding tendency in affected individuals. It is inherited as an autosomal trait and is seen most commonly among persons of Ashkenazi Jewish descent with an 8% frequency of heterozygosity.[116] Three different point mutations in the FXI gene account for nearly all cases of FXI deficiency among the Ashkenazi Jews.[117] FXI deficiency is most often detected in association with a positive family history or secondary to a prolonged partial thromboplastin time found during a routine presurgical evaluation. The diagnosis is confirmed with a plasma FXI assay.

FXI levels correlate with the genotype. Severe deficiency (FXI levels lower than 15 to 20 IU/dL) is seen in homozygotes or compound heterozygotes, and partial deficiency (FXI levels 20 to 60 IU/dL) is seen in heterozygotes. Bleeding tendency, however, does not correlate with genotype.[118] Excessive bleeding is most commonly seen in association with severe deficiency, but it can also be seen in patients with partial deficiency. A compilation of studies shows abnormal bleeding in 30% to 50% of patients with partial deficiency.[119] In general, bleeding symptoms are mild or absent, only occurring in association with trauma or surgery, particularly tonsillectomy. Epistaxis, soft tissue hemorrhage, bleeding after dental extractions, and menorrhagia can also be seen in affected persons.

Fresh frozen plasma is most commonly given as treatment for severe bleeding episodes or as prophylaxis for major surgery. The half-life of FXI in plasma is approximately 45 hours. As an alternative treatment, two specific FXI concentrates are available in Europe.[116] Both have been shown to be hemostatically effective and virally safe, but they have been associated with an increased occurrence of thrombotic events, particularly in older patients with preexisting vascular disease and when these concentrates are given at very high doses.[120, 121] These products may be useful in selected patients without preexisting hypercoagulable states at doses less than 30 IU/kg.[116] Bleeding from minor procedures such as dental extraction can be controlled with local measures or antifibrinolytic agents (ε-aminocaproic acid and tranexamic acid) at the same doses that are used for hemophilia and vWD.[116]

Contact Factor Deficiencies

Deficiencies of the contact factors, FXII, prekallikrein, and high-molecular-weight kininogen, are not associated with bleeding symptoms.[102] Because these factors are necessary for the initiation of the intrinsic pathway, the partial thromboplastin time is markedly prolonged, frequently beyond what is seen in hemophilia, whereas the prothrombin time is normal. Both FXII and prekallikrein deficiencies are inherited as autosomal recessive traits.[102] Patients are usually identified during routine preoperative screening, and definitive diagnosis is made with specific contact factor assays. Treatment is not necessary.

Factor XIII Deficiency

FXIII deficiency is an autosomal recessive disorder. FXIII is also known as fibrin-stabilizing factor and is responsible for cross-linking of the fibrin polymer. Deficiency of FXIII is associated with reduced clot stability, and therefore

ecchymoses or hematomas are usually seen 24 to 36 hours after trauma. FXIII deficiency is associated with severe bleeding, particularly delayed intracranial hemorrhage with minimal trauma. Other symptoms of FXIII deficiency include delayed separation of the umbilical stump in the neonatal period (at more than 3.5 to 4 weeks), poor wound healing, and recurrent spontaneous abortions in women secondary to severe decidual bleeding. Screening tests are normal including bleeding, prothrombin, partial thromboplastin, and thrombin times. Clots from affected persons appear more friable than normal. When the condition is suspected clinically, diagnosis of homozygous patients is made using a urea clot solubility assay or by measuring plasma levels of FXIII subunit proteins.[122]

Fresh frozen plasma is usually used for hemostasis in FXIII deficiency.[107] It is given at a dose of 5 to 10 mL/kg. Because the half-life of FXIII is very long (3 to 6 days), one dose is generally sufficient. Cryoprecipitate also contains FXIII and can also be used to treat acute bleeding episodes.[107] Patients with severe bleeding symptoms can receive either product as prophylaxis every 2 to 4 weeks. In addition, two plasma-derived FXIII concentrates are currently produced (Centeon, King of Prussia, PA, and Bio Products Laboratory, Elstree, UK).[123] These are not yet available for general distribution in the United States.

■ Conclusion

Accurate and early diagnosis, comprehensive clinical care, and the availability of factor concentrates that are manufactured with limited risk of transmitting blood-borne viruses have all contributed to improved outcome for patients with congenital bleeding disorders. Despite these advances, patients with severe hemophilia require tremendous dedication and support for successful management of their disease. The promise of gene transfer, which could allow for amelioration or elimination of the phenotypic abnormalities seen in severe hemophilia, is still in the future.

REFERENCES

1. DiMichele D: Hemophilia 1996. New approach to an old disease. Pediatr Clin North Am 43:709–736, 1996.
2. Soucie JM, Evatt B, Jackson D: Occurrence of hemophilia in the United States: The Hemophilia Surveillance System Project Investigators. Am J Hematol 59:288–294, 1998.
3. Kasper CK: Hereditary plasma clotting factor disorders and their management. Haemophilia 6:13–27, 2000.
4. Goodeve AC: Advances in carrier detection in haemophilia. Haemophilia 4:358–364, 1998.
5. Lillicrap D: Molecular diagnosis of inherited bleeding disorders and thrombophilia. Semin Hematol 36:340–351, 1999.
6. Tedgard U: Carrier testing and prenatal diagnosis of haemophilia: Utilisation and psychological consequences. Haemophilia 4:365–369, 1998.
7. Andrew M, Brooker LA: Blood component therapy in neonatal hemostatic disorders. Transfus Med Rev 9:231–250, 1995.
8. DiMichele D, Neufeld EJ: Hemophilia: A new approach to an old disease. Hematol Oncol Clin North Am 12:1315–1344, 1998.
9. Hoyer LW: Hemophilia A. N Engl J Med 330:38–47, 1994.
10. Hoag MS, Johnson FF, Robinson JA, Aggeler PM: Treatment of hemophilia B with a new clotting-factor concentrate. N Engl J Med 280:581–586, 1969.
11. Mannucci PM: Modern treatment of hemophilia: From the shadows towards the light. Thromb Haemost 70:17–23, 1993.
12. Centers for Disease Control and Prevention: Update on acquired immune deficiency syndrome (AIDS) among patients with hemophilia A. MMWR Morb Mortal Wkly Rep 31:644–646, 652, 1982.

13. Berntorp E: Impact of replacement therapy on the evolution of HIV infection in hemophiliacs. Thromb Haemost 71:678–683, 1994.

14. Brettler DB: Comments on the development of inhibitor antibodies in patients using recombinant factor VIII concentrates. Semin Hematol 28:45–46, 1991.

15. Kasper CK, Lusher JM: Recent evolution of clotting factor concentrates for hemophilia A and B: Transfusion Practices Committee. Transfusion 33:422–434, 1993.

16. Lusher JM: Transfusion therapy in congenital coagulopathies. Hematol Oncol Clin North Am 8:1167–1180, 1994.

17. Mannucci PM: Clinical evaluation of viral safety of coagulation factor VIII and IX concentrates. Vox Sang 64:197–203, 1993.

18. Horowitz MS, Rooks C, Horowitz B, Hilgartner MW: Virus safety of solvent/detergent–treated antihaemophilic factor concentrate. Lancet 2:186–189, 1988.

19. Ludlam CA: Viral safety of plasma-derived factor VIII and IX concentrates. Blood Coagul Fibrinolysis 8(Suppl):S19–S23, 1997.

20. Toole JJ, Knopf JL, Wozney JM, et al: Molecular cloning of a cDNA encoding human antihaemophilic factor. Nature 312:342–347, 1984.

21. Wood WI, Capon DJ, Simonsen CC, et al: Expression of active human factor VIII from recombinant DNA clones. Nature 312:330–337, 1984.

22. Schwartz RS, Abildgaard CF, Aledort LM, et al: Human recombinant DNA-derived antihemophilic factor (factor VIII) in the treatment of hemophilia A: Recombinant Factor VIII Study Group. N Engl J Med 323:1800–1805, 1990.

23. White GC, McMillan CW, Kingdon HS, Shoemaker CB: Use of recombinant antihemophilic factor in the treatment of two patients with classic hemophilia. N Engl J Med 320:166–170, 1989.

24. Lusher JM, Arkin S, Abildgaard CF, Schwartz RS: Recombinant factor VIII for the treatment of previously untreated patients with hemophilia A: Safety, efficacy, and development of inhibitors. Kogenate Previously Untreated Patient Study Group. N Engl J Med 328:453–459, 1993.

25. Bray GL, Gomperts ED, Courter S, et al: A multicenter study of recombinant factor VIII (recombinate): Safety, efficacy, and inhibitor risk in previously untreated patients with hemophilia A. The Recombinate Study Group. Blood 83:2428–2435, 1994.

26. Manno CS: Treatment options for bleeding episodes in patients undergoing immune tolerance therapy. Haemophilia 5:33–41, 1999.

27. Mannucci PM, Tuddenbam EG: The hemophilias: Progress and problems. Semin Hematol 36:104–117, 1999.

28. Hilgartner MW, Manno CS, Nuss R, Di Michele DM: Pediatric issues in hemophilia. In Proceedings of the American Society of Hematology. San Diego, American Society of Hematology, 1997, pp 46–60.

29. Abshire TC, Brackmann HH, Scharrer I, et al: Sucrose formulated recombinant human antihemophilic factor VIII is safe and efficacious for treatment of hemophilia A in home therapy: International Kogenate-FS Study Group. Thromb Haemost 83:811–816, 2000.

30. Berntorp E: Second generation, B-domain deleted recombinant factor VIII. Thromb Haemost 78:256–260, 1997.

31. Sandberg H, Almstedt A, Brandt J, et al: Structural and functional characteristics of the B-domain-deleted recombinant factor VIII protein, r-VIII SQ. Thromb Haemost 85:93–100, 2001.

32. Kohler M, Hellstern P, Lechler E, et al: Thromboembolic complications associated with the use of prothrombin complex and factor IX concentrates. Thromb Haemost 80:399–402, 1998.

33. Goldsmith JC, Kasper CK, Blatt PM, et al: Coagulation factor IX: Successful surgical experience with a purified factor IX concentrate. Am J Hematol 40:210–215, 1992.

34. Shapiro AD, Ragni MV, Lusher JM, et al: Safety and efficacy of monoclonal antibody purified factor IX concentrate in previously untreated patients with hemophilia B. Thromb Haemost 75:30–35, 1996.

35. Bond M, Jankowski M, Patel H, et al: Biochemical characterization of recombinant factor IX. Semin Hematol 35:11–17, 1998.

36. Brinkhous KM, Sigman JL, Read MS, et al: Recombinant human factor IX: Replacement therapy, prophylaxis, and pharmacokinetics in canine hemophilia B. Blood 88:2603–2610, 1996.

37. Choo KH, Gould KG, Rees DJ, et al: Molecular cloning of the gene for human anti-haemophilic factor IX. Nature 299:178–180, 1982.

38. Kurachi K, Davie EW: Isolation and characterization of a cDNA coding for human factor IX. Proc Natl Acad Sci U S A 79:6461–6464, 1982.

39. White G, Shapiro A, Ragni M, et al: Clinical evaluation of recombinant factor IX. Semin Hematol 35:33–38, 1998.

40. White GC 2nd, Beebe A, Nielsen B: Recombinant factor IX. Thromb Haemost 78:261–265, 1997.

41. Furie B, Limentani SA, Rosenfield CG: A practical guide to the evaluation and treatment of hemophilia. Blood 84:3–9, 1994.

42. Mannucci PM: Desmopressin (DDAVP) in the treatment of bleeding disorders: The first 20 years. Blood 90:2515–2521, 1997.

43. Logan LJ: Treatment of von Willebrand's disease. Hematol Oncol Clin North Am 6:1079–1094, 1992.

44. Manno CS, Butler RB, Cohen AR: Low recovery in vivo of highly purified factor VIII in patients with hemophilia. J Pediatr 121:814–818, 1992.

45. Kelly KM, Butler RB, Farace L, et al: Superior in vivo response of recombinant factor VIII concentrate in children with hemophilia A. J Pediatr 130:537–540, 1997.

46. Lusher JM: Prophylaxis in children with hemophilia: Is it the optimal treatment? Thromb Haemost 78:726–729, 1997.

47. Ahlberg A: Haemophilia in Sweden. VII. Incidence, treatment and prophylaxis of arthropathy and other musculo-skeletal manifestations of haemophilia A and B. Acta Orthop Scand Suppl 3:132, 1965.

48. Aronstam A, Kirk PJ, McHardy J, et al: Twice weekly prophylactic therapy in haemophilia A. J Clin Pathol 30:65–67, 1977.

49. Gruppo RA: Prophylaxis for hemophilia: state of the art or state of confusion [editorial]? J Pediatr 132:915–917, 1998.

50. Nilsson IM, Berntorp E, Lofqvist T, Pettersson H: Twenty-five years' experience of prophylactic treatment in severe haemophilia A and B. J Intern Med 232:25–32, 1992.

51. Liesner RJ, Khair K, Hann IM: The impact of prophylactic treatment on children with severe haemophilia. Br J Haematol 92:973–978, 1996.

52. Lofqvist T, Nilsson IM, Berntorp E, Pettersson H: Haemophilia prophylaxis in young patients: A long-term follow-up. J Intern Med 241:395–400, 1997.

53. Aledort LM, Haschmeyer RH, Pettersson H: A longitudinal study of orthopaedic outcomes for severe factor-VIII–deficient haemophiliacs: The Orthopaedic Outcome Study Group. J Intern Med 236:391–399, 1994.

54. Ljung RC: Prophylactic infusion regimens in the management of hemophilia. Thromb Haemost 82:525–530, 1999.

55. Manco-Johnson MJ, Nuss R, Geraghty S, et al: Results of secondary prophylaxis in children with severe hemophilia. Am J Hematol 47:113–117, 1994.

56. Aledort L: Inhibitors in hemophilia patients: Current status and management. Am J Hematol 47:208–217, 1994.

57. Manco-Johnson MJ, Nuss R, Geraghty S, Funk S: A prophylactic program in the United States: Experience and issues. Semin Hematol 31:10–12, 1994.

58. Smith PS, Teutsch SM, Shaffer PA, et al: Episodic versus prophylactic infusions for hemophilia A: A cost-effectiveness analysis. J Pediatr 129:424–431, 1996.

59. Carlsson M, Berntorp E, Bjorkman S, Lindvall K: Pharmacokinetic dosing in prophylactic treatment of hemophilia A. Eur J Haematol 51:247–252, 1993.

60. Blanchette VS, Al-Musa A, Stain AM, et al: Central venous access devices in children with hemophilia: An update. Blood Coagul Fibrinolysis 8(Suppl):S11–S14, 1997.

61. Bollard CM, Teague LR, Berry EW, Ockelford PA: The use of central venous catheters (Portacaths) in children with haemophilia. Haemophilia 6:66–70, 2000.

62. Ragni MJ, Hord JD, Blatt J: Central venous catheter infection in haemophiliacs undergoing prophylaxis or immune tolerance with clotting factor concentrate. Haemophilia 3:90–95, 1997.

63. Conway JH, Hilgartner MW: Initial presentations of pediatric hemophiliacs. Arch Pediatr Adolesc Med 148:589–594, 1994.

64. Baehner RL, Strauss HS: Hemophilia in the first year of life. N Engl J Med 275:524–528, 1966.

65. Buchanan GR: Factor concentrate prophylaxis for neonates with hemophilia. J Pediatr Hematol Oncol 21:254–256, 1999.

66. Kulkarni R, Lusher JM, Henry RC, Kallen DJ: Current practices regarding newborn intracranial haemorrhage and obstetrical care and mode of delivery of pregnant haemophilia carriers: A survey of obstetricians, neonatologists and haematologists in the United States, on behalf of the National Hemophilia Foundation's Medical and Scientific Advisory Council. Haemophilia 5:410–415, 1999.

67. Hoyer LW: Why do so many haemophilia A patients develop an inhibitor? Br J Haematol 90:498–501, 1995.

68. Hoyer LW: Factor VIII inhibitors. Curr Opin Hematol 2:365–371, 1995.

69. Hay CR: Why do inhibitors arise in patients with haemophilia A? Br J Haematol 105:584–590, 1999.

70. Tuddenham EG, McVey JH: The genetic basis of inhibitor development in haemophilia A. Haemophilia 4:543–545, 1998.

71. Kasper CK, Aledort L, Aronson D, et al: Proceedings: A more uniform measurement of factor VIII inhibitors. Thromb Diath Haemorrh 34:612, 1975.

72. Leissinger CA: Use of prothrombin complex concentrates and activated prothrombin complex concentrates as prophylactic therapy in haemophilia patients with inhibitors. Haemophilia 5:25–32, 1999.

73. Green D: Complications associated with the treatment of haemophiliacs with inhibitors. Haemophilia 5:11–17, 1999.

74. Santagostino E, Gringeri A, Mannucci PM: Home treatment with recombinant activated factor VII in patients with factor VIII inhibitors: The advantages of early intervention. Br J Haematol 104:22–26, 1999.

75. Teitel JM: Recombinant factor VIIa versus aPCCs in haemophiliacs with inhibitors: Treatment and cost considerations. Haemophilia 5:43–49, 1999.

76. DiMichele DM: Immune tolerance: A synopsis of the international experience. Haemophilia 4:568–573, 1998.

77. Kay MA, High K: Gene therapy for the hemophilias. Proc Natl Acad Sci U S A 96:9973–9975, 1999.

78. Herzog RW, High KA: Adeno-associated virus-mediated gene transfer of factor IX for treatment of hemophilia B by gene therapy. Thromb Haemost 82:540–546, 1999.

79. Kay MA, Manno CS, Ragni MV, et al: Evidence for gene transfer and expression of factor IX in haemophilia B patients treated with an AAV vector. Nat Genet 24:257–261, 2000.

80. Rodeghiero F, Castaman G, Dini E: Epidemiological investigation of the prevalence of von Willebrand's disease. Blood 69:454–459, 1987.

81. Werner EJ, Broxson EH, Tucker EL, et al: Prevalence of von Willebrand disease in children: A multiethnic study. J Pediatr 123:893–898, 1993.

82. Ginsburg D: Molecular genetics of von Willebrand disease. Thromb Haemost 82:585–591, 1999.

83. Werner EJ: von Willebrand disease in children and adolescents. Pediatr Clin North Am 43:683–707, 1996.

84. Batlle J, Torea J, Rendal E, Fernandez MF: The problem of diagnosing von Willebrand's disease. J Intern Med Suppl 740:121–128, 1997.

85. Mancuso DJ, Tuley EA, Westfield LA, et al: Structure of the gene for human von Willebrand factor. J Biol Chem 264:19514–19527, 1989.

86. Mancuso DJ, Tuley EA, Westfield LA, et al: Human von Willebrand factor gene and pseudogene: Structural analysis and differentiation by polymerase chain reaction. Biochemistry 30:253–269, 1991.

87. Schneppenheim R, Thomas KB, Sutor AH: Von Willebrand disease in childhood. Semin Thromb Hemost 21:261–275, 1995.

88. Phillips MD, Santhouse A: von Willebrand disease: Recent advances in pathophysiology and treatment. Am J Med Sci 316:77–86, 1998.

89. Sadler JE: A revised classification of von Willebrand disease: For the Subcommittee on von Willebrand Factor of the Scientific and Standardization Committee of the International Society on Thrombosis and Haemostasis. Thromb Haemost 71:520–525, 1994.

90. Sadler JE, Matsushita T, Dong Z, et al: Molecular mechanism and classification of von Willebrand disease. Thromb Haemost 74:161–166, 1995.

91. Federici AB: Diagnosis of von Willebrand disease. Haemophilia 4:654–660, 1998.

92. Schwarz HP, Turecek PL, Pichler L, et al: Recombinant von Willebrand factor. Thromb Haemost 78:571–576, 1997.

93. Werner EJ, Abshire TC, Giroux DS, et al: Relative value of diagnostic studies for von Willebrand disease. J Pediatr 121:34–38, 1992.

94. Gill JC, Endres-Brooks J, Bauer PJ, et al: The effect of ABO blood group on the diagnosis of von Willebrand disease. Blood 69:1691–1695, 1987.

95. Mannucci PM: Treatment of von Willebrand's disease. J Intern Med Suppl 740:129–132, 1997.

96. Mannucci PM: Treatment of von Willebrand disease. Int J Clin Lab Res 28:211–214, 1998.

97. Mannucci PM: Desmopressin: A nontransfusional form of treatment for congenital and acquired bleeding disorders. Blood 72:1449–1455, 1988.

98. Menache D, Aronson DL: New treatments of von Willebrand disease: Plasma derived von Willebrand factor concentrates. Thromb Haemost 78:566–570, 1997.

99. Lubetsky A, Schulman S, Varon D, et al: Safety and efficacy of continuous infusion of a combined factor VIII–von Willebrand factor (vWF) concentrate (Haemate-P) in patients with von Willebrand disease. Thromb Haemost 81:229–233, 1999.

100. al-Mondhiry H, Ehmann WC: Congenital afibrinogenemia. Am J Hematol 46:343–347, 1994.

101. Hilgartner M, Corrigan JJ: Coagulation disorders. In Miller DR, Baehner RL (eds): Blood Diseases of Infancy and Childhood, 7th ed. Philadelphia, Mosby, 1995, pp 924–986.

102. Blanchette VS, Dean J, Lillicrap D: Rare congenital hemorrhagic disorders. In Lilleyman JS, Hann IM, Blanchette VS (eds): Pediatric Hematology, 2nd ed. Philadelphia, Churchill Livingstone, 1999, pp 611–628.

103. Kobayashi T, Kanayama N, Tokunaga N, et al: Prenatal and peripartum management of congenital afibrinogenaemia. Br J Haematol 109:364–366, 2000.

104. Haverkate F, Samama M: Familial dysfibrinogenemia and thrombophilia: Report on a study of the SSC Subcommittee on Fibrinogen. Thromb Haemost 73:151–161, 1995.

105. Martinez J: Congenital dysfibrinogenemia. Curr Opin Hematol 4:357–365, 1997.

106. Rodriguez RC, Buchanan GR, Clanton MS: Prophylactic cryoprecipitate in congenital afibrinogenemia. Clin Pediatr 27:543–545, 1988.

107. Bauer KA: Rare hereditary coagulation factor abnormalities. In Nathan DG, Orkin SH (eds): Nathan and Oski's Hematology of Infancy and Childhood, vol 2, 5th ed. Philadelphia, WB Saunders, 1998, pp 1660–1675.

108. Mammen EF: Factor V deficiency. Semin Thromb Hemost 9:17–18, 1983.

109. Seligsohn U, Ramot B: Combined factor-V and factor-VIII deficiency: Report of four cases. Br J Haematol 16:475–486, 1969.

110. Ingerslev J, Kristensen HL: Clinical picture and treatment strategies in factor VII deficiency. Haemophilia 4:689–696, 1998.

111. Triplett DA, Brandt JT, Batard MA, et al: Hereditary factor VII deficiency: Heterogeneity defined by combined functional and immunochemical analysis. Blood 66:1284–1287, 1985.

112. Ragni MV, Lewis JH, Spero JA, Hasiba U: Factor VII deficiency. Am J Hematol 10:79–88, 1981.

113. Bauer KA: Treatment of factor VII deficiency with recombinant factor VIIa. Haemostasis 26:155–158, 1996.

114. Mariani G, Testa MG, Di Paolantonio T, et al: Use of recombinant, activated factor VII in the treatment of congenital factor VII deficiencies. Vox Sang 77:131–136, 1999.

115. Wong WY, Huang WC, Miller R, et al: Clinical efficacy and recovery levels of recombinant FVIIa (NovoSeven) in the treatment of intracranial haemorrhage in severe neonatal FVII deficiency. Haemophilia 6:50–54, 2000.

116. Bolton-Maggs PH: The management of factor XI deficiency. Haemophilia 4:683–688, 1998.

117. Asakai R, Chung DW, Ratnoff OD, Davie EW: Factor XI (plasma thromboplastin antecedent) deficiency in Ashkenazi Jews is a bleeding disorder that can result from three types of point mutations. Proc Natl Acad Sci U S A 86:7667–7671, 1989.

118. Asakai R, Chung DW, Davie EW, Seligsohn U: Factor XI deficiency in Ashkenazi Jews in Israel. N Engl J Med 325:153–158, 1991.

119. Bolton-Maggs PH, Young Wan-Yin B, McCraw AH, et al: Inheritance and bleeding in factor XI deficiency. Br J Haematol 69:521–528, 1988.

120. Bolton-Maggs PH, Colvin BT, Satchi BT, et al: Thrombogenic potential of factor XI concentrate. Lancet 344:748–749, 1994.

121. Mannucci PM, Bauer KA, Santagostino E, et al: Activation of the coagulation cascade after infusion of a factor XI concentrate in congenitally deficient patients. Blood 84:1314–1319, 1994.

122. Anwar R, Miloszewski KJ: Factor XIII deficiency. Br J Haematol 107:468–484, 1999.

123. Gootenberg JE: Factor concentrates for the treatment of factor XIII deficiency. Curr Opin Hematol 5:372–375, 1998.

Chapter 26

Transfusion of the Patient with Acquired Coagulation Defects

Barbara Alving*

Individuals with recognized congenital bleeding disorders usually have immediate access to coagulation factor concentrates for prophylaxis or for treatment of unexpected bleeding episodes. However, patients in whom a bleeding disorder develops because of underlying systemic disease, autoantibody formation, or use of anticoagulants are often more difficult to manage as the cause of their coagulopathy may not be readily apparent and may require a combination of hemostatic agents. This chapter discusses the diagnosis and treatment of the following acquired coagulopathies: those related to underlying systemic disorders such as liver disease and renal failure; disseminated intravascular coagulation (DIC); formation of autoantibodies to coagulation factor VIII, V, II, or XIII; and coagulopathies associated with anticoagulants and the newer antiplatelet agents.

■ Approach to the Patient with a Coagulopathy

The evaluation of the patient with an apparent or possible coagulopathy includes a review of the past and present illness, use of medications, and completion of a physical examination. Any one of these aspects may be limited by the clinical setting, the urgency of the consultation, or the patient's lack of knowledge about prescribed or over-the-counter medications. Patients who have a sufficiently severe systemic disorder to induce a coagulopathy, such as liver failure, usually have other manifestations of the disease. However, patients who have developed autoantibodies to a clotting factor such as factor VIII may have no complaints other than easy bruising or unexpected excessive bleeding with minor trauma. For these patients, laboratory data may be the first indication of the etiology of a bleeding disorder.

Screening tests are an integral part of the initial evaluation (Table 26.1). These include a complete blood count along with evaluation of the peripheral smear for abnormalities in the platelets or white blood cells; toxic granulations and Döhle bodies in the neutrophils may reinforce the possibility of sepsis. The smear may also reveal whether or not an

Table 26.1 Laboratory Testing for Patients with an Acquired Coagulopathy

Perform complete blood count, PT, aPTT, and thrombin time, measurement of fibrinogen concentration, and test for D-dimer as appropriate.

If thrombin time is prolonged, evaluate for heparin (perform reptilase time, add heparinase to sample). If heparin is present, check to be sure that the patient is not excessively anticoagulated or has developed a heparin-like inhibitor.

If aPTT is prolonged, perform "correction" studies. Mix equal volumes of patient and normal plasma and repeat the aPTT immediately and after 1 hour incubation at 37°C. The values for the mixing study should be within 5 seconds of the control value of the normal plasma aPTT.

An aPTT that becomes more prolonged with incubation is suggestive of an inhibitor to a specific factor. An aPTT that is initially prolonged and remains prolonged to the same degree at 1 hour is suggestive of a lupus anticoagulant.

Measure factor levels to be sure that a true deficiency of a coagulation factor is recognized, even if the diagnosis is "lupus anticoagulant."

Consider the presence of an inhibitor to factor XIII if bleeding persists and the screening studies are normal. This requires a special test for the solubility of the clot in urea and monochloroacetic acid.

aPTT, activated partial thromboplastin time; PT, prothrombin time.

*This chapter was written by Dr. Alving in her private capacity. The views expressed in this article do not necessarily represent the views of the National Institutes of Health, Department of Health and Human Services, or the United States. All material in this chapter is in the public domain, with the exception of any borrowed figures or tables.

apparent thrombocytopenia is real or due to platelet clumping in ethylenediaminetetraacetic acid (EDTA). Baseline coagulation studies include the activated partial thromboplastin time (aPTT) and prothrombin time (PT). If they are prolonged, then mixing studies to assess for the presence of an inhibitor and measurement of coagulation factor levels are appropriate. If DIC is suspected, measurement of fibrinogen levels and D-dimer should be done. D-dimer is a late plasmin digest of fibrin that has undergone cross-linking by factor XIIIa. Increased levels indicate that thrombin has been generated in sufficient quantities to activate factor XIII, which induces cross-linking of fibrin, and that plasmin has also been generated to degrade the fibrin. This process is consistent with the generalized activation of the coagulation and fibrinolytic system that occurs in DIC.

In the surgical setting, a realistic goal is to provide sufficient hemostatic support to allow the patient to undergo surgery or other invasive procedures without undue risk. Thus, complete correction of coagulation laboratory abnormalities may not be possible or even desirable. For example, replacement of factor VII, which has a half-life of 2 to 6 hours, by infusion of plasma could lead to excessive volume expansion and pulmonary edema. A critical factor for patients who require invasive procedures such as line placement is the skill of the operator. In one retrospective review of patients who had received arterial, pulmonary artery, or central venous lines, the authors found that hemostatic complications were rare and were related more to the experience of the operator than to the underlying hemostatic defect.[1] They concluded that only patients with severe hemostatic defects require correction of the abnormalities before line placement.

For major surgery in patients with coagulopathies, hemostasis is best managed if there is close communication among the consultants, the surgeons, the personnel of the coagulation laboratory, and the staff of the blood bank (or pharmacy) who are responsible for supplying the products.[2] Table 26.2 provides a list of products that should be readily available in a tertiary hospital to allow rapid treatment of acquired coagulopathies.

Products, such as *fibrin sealant*, that provide localized hemostasis can be used as adjuvants for systemic therapy in patients with coagulopathies. In the United States, one commercial product is now available (Tisseel, produced by Baxter-Immuno in Vienna, Austria and marketed in the United States by Baxter Healthcare and Haemacure Biotech). The indication is for patients who are undergoing reoperative coronary artery bypass surgery or who have bleeding from sites not controlled by sutures, such as in splenic trauma. The product is composed of human fibrinogen (75 to 115 mg/mL) and human thrombin (500 IU/mL), both of which are virally inactivated.[3] The thrombin is solubilized in calcium chloride (40 mM), which stimulates cross-linking of the clot by factor XIII in the product (or patient). The product also contains aprotinin, a bovine-derived protein that directly inhibits plasmin, which is included to increase clot stability.

A much less expensive form of this product can be made by mixing cryoprecipitate in one syringe (fibrinogen concentration, 10 to 15 mg/mL) and bovine thrombin (1000 IU/mL) in the second syringe. This preparation contains a lower concentration of fibrinogen and has not undergone viral inactivation. Furthermore, the bovine thrombin may be contaminated with bovine factor V, which can stimulate production of antibodies in the recipient that cross-react with human factor V, inducing a potentially severe bleeding disorder several days after surgery.[4-6] Currently, the bovine thrombin preparation with the lowest degree of contamination with factor V is that produced for Jones Medical Industries, St. Louis, MO.[7]

Efficacy data for the commercial fibrin sealant were derived in part from a study in which 333 patients from 11 centers in the United States who were undergoing reoperative cardiac surgery or emergency resternotomy were randomly assigned to receive fibrin sealant or conventional hemostatic agents; the endpoint for efficacy was the number of bleeding episodes controlled at 5 minutes.[8] The success rate for fibrin sealant was 92.6% compared with 12.4% for conventional topical agents ($p < .001$). Fibrin sealant also rapidly controlled bleeding episodes that did not initially respond to conventional hemostatic agents in 82% of patients.

In addition to use in cardiac surgery and trauma, fibrin sealants have been used as adhesives to seal dural leaks in neurosurgery, to promote union of middle ear bones in otolaryngology, and as a matrix to repair bone defects.[3] Although randomized, blinded studies have not been done, fibrin sealant has been applied to sites of dental extractions in hemophiliacs; this treatment, combined with the use of an antifibrinolytic agent, has reduced or eliminated the need for systemic factor VIII replacement.[9, 10] This combined therapy would potentially be efficacious in patients with coagulation factor inhibitors as well as those with severe thrombocytopenia who require dental extraction. The sealants can also potentially be used outside the operating room to provide local hemostasis in the critical care setting in patients with coagulopathies who have a localized site of bleeding. In a randomized, prospective evaluation of fibrin sealant in neonates undergoing extracorporeal membrane oxygenation, application of fibrin sealant at the cannulation sites reduced the risk for any bleeding and was associated with a shorter duration of hemorrhage with less blood loss.[11]

Fibrin sealants produced by several manufacturers (in both the United States and Europe) are undergoing or will be undergoing clinical trials in the United States. Differences may include methods of viral inactivation and presence or

Table 26.2   Generic Products for Hemostasis*

Hemophilia A
  Recombinant factor VIII

Hemophilia B
  Recombinant factor IX

Inhibitor to factor VIII (one or more of the following)
  Activated prothrombin complex concentrates
  Recombinant factor VIIa
  Porcine factor VIII

Warfarin overdose
  Prothrombin complex concentrates

Antifibrinolytic agents
  ε-Aminocaproic acid or tranexamic acid

Localized hemostasis
  Fibrin sealant

*These are products that may be needed on an emergent basis in any large tertiary hospital and which should be readily available through the pharmacy and/or blood bank. Some products, because of restricted availability, may require substitutions.

absence of a fibrinolytic inhibitor in the product. In addition, companies are developing other forms of sealants or adhesives composed of collagen and thrombin and devices that allow production of autologous fibrin sealant in the operating room. In the sections that follow, the management of patients with specific acquired bleeding disorders is discussed in greater detail.

■ Coagulopathies in Systemic Disorders

Liver Disease

Patients with liver disease may have a complex coagulopathy consisting of impaired coagulation factor synthesis, increased fibrinolytic activity, and thrombocytopenia.[12] In patients with splenomegaly related to cirrhosis and portal hypertension, 90% of the circulating platelets can be sequestered in the spleen with platelet counts decreasing to as low as 30,000 to 40,000/μL. The thrombocytopenia may be due in part to decreased platelet production because of reduced levels of circulating thrombopoietin, which is synthesized in the liver.[13] In one study of 44 patients with cirrhosis and thrombocytopenia, thrombopoietin levels were undetectable in 89%; however, after undergoing liver transplantation, 94% had detectable levels of thrombopoietin and all had resolution of the thrombocytopenia.[13] In patients undergoing portal decompression or splenectomy, thrombocytopenia often persists, indicating that a defect in thrombopoietin production is present in addition to splenic sequestration. A further reduction in platelet counts is usually due to additional factors such as coexisting immune thrombocytopenia.[12]

The liver is essentially the site of production of all coagulation factors, including the inhibitors protein C, protein S, and antithrombin. Von Willebrand factor and tissue-type plasminogen activator (tPA) are produced by endothelial cells. The factor VIII activity is usually increased in liver disease, which may reflect activation of the molecule or increased synthesis at sites other than the liver.[12] Factor VII, which has the shortest half-life of the coagulation factors (2 to 6 hours), is the first to be decreased in liver disease. In order to be functional, factors II, VII, IX, and X as well as protein S and protein C must undergo γ carboxylation, which is mediated by vitamin K. However, liver disease causes impairment of γ carboxylation that cannot be reversed with vitamin K_1.[14]

Patients with liver disease, including those with hepatomas, may have an acquired dysfibrinogenemia that is due to the synthesis of a fibrinogen molecule that has impaired polymerization because of an increased sialic acid content.[15] The fibrinogen levels are usually normal; however, the PT, aPTT, and thrombin time are prolonged. One case has been reported in which acquired dysfibrinogenemia was part of a paraneoplastic manifestation of renal cell carcinoma and resolved after the tumor was removed.[16] The acquired dysfibrinogenemia is not associated with a bleeding diathesis, and patients with this abnormality do not need any treatment before invasive procedures.

Although inhibitors of the coagulation system are decreased in patients with hepatic disease, a thrombotic state does not usually occur. Liver disease is associated with hyperfibrinolysis as defined by increased activity of tPA and elevation of D-dimer. Using these criteria for hyperfibrinolysis, in one study of cirrhotic patients, those with elevated

tPA and D-dimer had a significantly higher rate of gastrointestinal bleeding than those who did not have these laboratory findings.[17] Patients with ascites and hyperfibrinolysis were also at higher risk for bleeding than those without ascites. The authors postulated that hyperfibrinolysis results in part from activation of the coagulation system, resulting in release of tPA in the presence of fibrin. Decreased clearance of tPA as well as reduced levels of α_2-antiplasmin, which is synthesized in the liver and is the major inhibitor of plasmin, could result in continued plasmin generation and a bleeding diathesis.

The assessment of bleeding risk in a patient with liver disease includes measurement of the platelet count, PT, aPTT, fibrinogen level, and D-dimer. Although measurement of tPA or the euglobulin clot lysis time is desirable, these tests are usually not available in a hospital setting. The PT is also reported as an International Normalized Ratio (INR), which was originally developed to standardize anticoagulation among patients taking warfarin. A study of 29 patients with liver impairment (INR 1.5 to 3.5) was conducted with three different thromboplastin reagents (International Sensitivity Index, 0.86 to 2.53).[18] The mean INR for the three reagents ranged from 1.88 to 2.63, depending on the reagent. In contrast, the three reagents gave the same results for patients taking warfarin. Thus, INRs are not well standardized for patients with liver disease and can vary depending on the reagent. However, this is also true for the measurement of the PT with the different reagents. Patients with liver disease may have only a prolonged PT (normal aPTT and thrombin time), reflecting a decrease in factor VII, which is the first to be reduced in liver disorders because of its short half-life of 2 to 6 hours.

The bleeding time does not predict gastrointestinal bleeding in patients with cirrhosis.[19] Furthermore, mild to moderate coagulopathy is not associated with prolonged bleeding after liver biopsy as assessed by measurement of the bleeding time at the biopsy site; even if the studies are normal, patients may still bleed at the biopsy site.[20] Although controlled studies in 21 patients with cirrhosis (whose platelet counts were 45,000 to 286,000/μL) have shown that desmopressin (DDAVP) at a dose of 0.3 μg/kg significantly shortens the prolonged bleeding time for up to 4 hours, its role in prophylaxis has not been well defined.[21] Nonetheless, it would be a reasonable choice for a hemostatic agent if there were concerns about the platelet function.[21, 22]

Guidelines for prophylaxis in patients with liver disease who are undergoing invasive procedures are summarized in Table 26.3. These suggestions are empirical and are based on many factors as described in the following. In a retrospective study of patients undergoing percutaneous liver biopsy, McVay and Toy[23] found that mild elevations of the PT or aPTT were not associated with bleeding. Risk factors for bleeding were malignancy (hepatoma) and multiple passes. These authors concluded that PT and aPTT that are prolonged to less than 1.5 times the midnormal range do not require treatment and that a platelet count above 50,000/μL is satisfactory.

For patients in whom standard percutaneous biopsy is contraindicated, such as those who have ascites, portal hypertension, and coagulopathy, laparoscopic liver biopsy can be performed successfully using direct pressure and topical Gelfoam and thrombin to achieve hemostasis.[24] In these

Table 26.3   Management of Patients with Liver Disease*

Prophylaxis Before Procedures	
Platelet count < 50,000/μL:	administer platelets to increase to 50,000–75,000/μL
Fibrinogen < 100 mg/dL:	administer cryoprecipitate to maintain fibrinogen > 100 mg/dL
Coagulation factor deficiency	
Prolonged PT and aPTT:	vitamin K, 10 mg daily subcutaneously for 3 days, then FFP if factor VII < 10% or other factors < 50%
Prolonged PT, normal aPTT:	no treatment beyond vitamin K, if factor VII is > 10%.
Prolonged thrombin time (dysfibrinogenemia):	no treatment if fibrinogen > 100 mg/dL

*Prothrombin complex concentrates and ε-aminocaproic acid are not recommended because they may increase the risk for thrombosis. DDAVP (desmopressin) can be used to shorten the bleeding time, but its clinical significance in reducing bleeding in patients with liver disease has not been demonstrated.
aPTT, activated partial thromboplastin time; PT, prothrombin time.

patients there appears to be no correlation between the risk of bleeding and the prophylactic administration of fresh frozen plasma (FFP) or platelets. The advantage of laparoscopic liver biopsy technique is the ability to place direct pressure along with hemostatic agents.

There is usually little or no need to infuse FFP in an individual who has only a prolonged PT and a normal aPTT because factor VII levels of 10% or greater are sufficient for hemostasis. If the PT and aPTT are prolonged and the patient has not responded to empirical treatment with vitamin K at a dose of 10 mg/day subcutaneously for 3 days,[12] measurement of levels of factors IX, X, and V (a non–vitamin K–dependent factor) provides a good assessment of liver function with respect to synthesis of coagulation factors. On occasion, abnormalities are simply due to dysfibrinogen, which can be detected by a prolonged thrombin time and reptilase time. If the latter is the case, no plasma treatment is needed.[16] Preoperative replacement for patients with severe factor VII deficiency consists of infusion of plasma at a dose of 5 to 10 mL/kg beginning preoperatively (in time to achieve a level of 10%) and continued during and after surgery for at least 1 to 2 days.

For patients who have hemostatic defects and are bleeding or are to undergo a major procedure, the goal of therapy is to maintain the platelet count greater than 50,000 to 75,000/μL and the fibrinogen concentration greater than 100 mg/dL. This is achieved by infusion of cryoprecipitate. The quantity of fibrinogen in each bag of cryoprecipitate is approximately 250 mg, and the volume of distribution for the fibrinogen is 30% greater than the intravascular volume. Thus, to increase the fibrinogen level by 50 mg/dL in a 70-kg individual, seven bags of cryoprecipitate would be required.

In patients undergoing rapid blood loss, recombinant factor VIIa (NovoSeven, NovoNordisk, Princeton, NJ), which is approved for use in hemophiliacs with inhibitors, can be combined with FFP. In one preliminary study, factor VIIa was effective in transiently reversing the prolonged PT in a group of nonbleeding cirrhotic patients.[25] However, it is expensive and has not been tried in a larger clinical trial. Prothrombin complex concentrates are not recommended, nor is the antifibrinolytic agent ε-aminocaproic acid, because they may be associated with thrombosis.[12]

Uremia

One of the most common sources of bleeding in uremia is the gastrointestinal tract. Studies have shown, however, that the causes of gastrointestinal bleeding in patients with uremia are not different from the causes in those who are not uremic,[26] and the frequency of rebleeding is similar for both groups. Patients who have occult gastrointestinal blood loss may develop iron deficiency and have a reduced response to erythropoietin. Thus, adequate attention should be given to iron replacement in an anemic patient who appears to be erythropoietin resistant.

Patients who are uremic usually have a normal PT and aPTT and platelet count. However, they may have prolonged bleeding times; the degree of prolongation appears to correlate with clinical bleeding.[27] The platelet dysfunction has multiple causes, including excess formation of nitric oxide, which inhibits platelet function.[28, 29] In addition, platelets may have a storage pool defect, reduced production of prostaglandin, and decreased adhesion because of a decrease in expression of the receptor glycoprotein IIb/IIIa (GPIIb/IIIa), which is a binding site for von Willebrand factor as well as fibrinogen.[30] The vessel wall in patients with uremia may produce an increased amount of prostaglandin I_2, which impairs platelet adhesion.[31] Plasma factors, not well characterized, may also inhibit platelet adhesion and aggregation in vivo.[32]

Multiple strategies can be used to reduce the excessive bleeding associated with uremia (Table 26.4). Platelet function in patients with uremia can be maximized rheologically by maintaining the hematocrit at 30%.[33] The prolonged bleeding time can also be corrected by administration of desmopressin at a dose of 0.3 μg/kg intravenously or subcutaneously. The effect persists for approximately 4 hours and begins 1 hour after onset.[33, 34] Desmopressin should not be used more frequently than once in 24 hours; repeated doses are not efficacious and can result in hyponatremia and seizures.

A double-blind randomized trial of intravenous conjugated estrogens administered at a dose of 0.6 mg/kg/day for 5 days to six patients with uremia and a prolonged bleeding time found that the bleeding time was partially corrected by 6 to 48 hours after the first dose with a peak effect at 5 to 7 days and a duration as long as 14 days.[35] Transdermal estrogen was efficacious in reducing or stopping bleeding in a series of six patients with renal failure, prolonged bleeding times, and excessive bleeding from telangiectasia of the gastrointestinal tract.[36] The estrogen was administered as 17β-estradiol (Estraderm, CIBA-GEIGY, Woodbridge, NJ) in a skin patch that delivered 50 or 100 μg/day. In these patients, the mean bleeding time decreased from 14 to 7 minutes. The effects

Table 26.4 Hemostatic Options for Patients with Uremia

Goal	Treatment	Comments
Maintain hematocrit 27%–32%	Erythropoietin	Monitor for hypertension; maintain adequate iron stores; check iron stores if patient resistant to erythropoietin.
Acutely enhance platelet function	DDAVP, 0.3 µg/kg IV	Administer no more frequently than once in 24 hours. Monitor for hyponatremia to avoid seizures.
Chronic enhancement of platelet function	Conjugated estrogens (0.6 mg/kg/day IV for 4–5 days or transdermal 17β-estradial 50–100 µg/24 hours applied as patch every 3–5 days for 2 months	Adverse effects: fluid retention, hot flashes.

DDAVP, desmopressin.

were noted at 24 hours and persisted at 17 days (total duration of administration was 2 months). No adverse effects were noted.[36] Vigano and colleagues[37] postulate that the prolonged effect of estrogens is due to their ability to enter endothelial cells, which are known to have estrogen receptors, and alter their function so that improved hemostasis occurs. Other studies have shown that administration of estrogen inhibits nitric oxide production.[29]

Disseminated Intravascular Coagulation (DIC)

DIC is associated with clinical conditions, such as sepsis, acute brain injury, or abruptio placentae, that induce expression of tissue factor and overwhelming activation of the coagulation system with a resulting fibrinolytic response. The clinical manifestations of DIC are variable and depend on whether microvascular thrombosis with fibrin formation is the prominent feature or the major component is the fibrinolytic response to fibrin formation.[38, 39] The clinical manifestations determine which hemostatic therapy, if any, is needed. In general, the most critical factor in the resolution of DIC is the ability to control the condition responsible for the initiation of the process.

The laboratory evaluation of DIC includes measurement of the platelet count, PT, aPTT, and D-dimer and examination of the peripheral blood smear for schistocytes. Abnormalities in any one of these tests is not specific for DIC. Rather, the test results are combined with the clinical setting to make a diagnosis. Three conditions frequently associated with DIC are described next.

Sepsis

The coagulopathy of sepsis, which is mediated by a variety of cytokines, is complex. Thrombocytopenia may be a prominent aspect of the coagulopathy and can be due to DIC or to hemophagocytosis.[40, 41] The cytokine macrophage colony-stimulating factor has been shown to be associated with hemophagocytosis,[40, 41] which is characterized by bone marrow findings of greater than 2% histiocytes and more than one hemophagocytic cell per high-power field; other laboratory features include elevated levels of ferritin and lactate dehydrogenase in addition to thrombocytopenia. Hemophagocytosis resolves with treatment of the underlying condition.

DIC in sepsis is due in part to interleukin-6 (IL-6)–induced expression of tissue factor, which generates procoagulant activity. The fibrinolytic response to fibrin formation is reduced because IL-6 also increases the expression of plasminogen activator inhibitor-1, the major inhibitor of tPA.

Thus, the major manifestation in sepsis may be microvascular fibrin deposition. The efficacy of heparin in this setting has not been demonstrated, and anticoagulation is not usually used in these patients. A meta-analysis of four controlled trials (chosen for their well-described methodology) of the effect of antithrombin III concentrates on mortality in patients with DIC and sepsis showed a reduction in mortality of 0.63 (95% confidence interval [CI] 0.39 to 1.00).[39] However, the treatment is costly and it is not known which patients are most likely to benefit from antithrombin III concentrates. Thus, some authors recommend that their use be limited to patients who are likely to die as a result of DIC and to those in whom DIC is expected to cause high morbidity.[39]

Acute Leukemia and DIC

Although DIC can be associated with any type of leukemia, it is most frequently a prominent feature of acute promyelocytic leukemia because the promyelocytes are rich in releasable tissue factor. During activation of the coagulation system, the fibrinolytic response is activated as well and plasmin is initially inhibited by α_2-antiplasmin, its major inactivator.[38, 39] However, with time, the α_2-antiplasmin is depleted, allowing plasmin activity to remain unchecked. This results in ongoing fibrinolysis and excessive bleeding.

The laboratory diagnosis of α_2-antiplasmin deficiency can be confirmed by a specific assay for α_2-antiplasmin that consists of measuring the rate at which plasmin added to patient's plasma undergoes inhibition. However, treatment is usually empirical and consists of administration of an antifibrinolytic agent such as oral ε-aminocaproic acid at a dose of 2 to 3 g every 6 hours or tranexamic acid.[42, 43] Although the antifibrinolytic agents can be used alone, most investigators prefer to use them with heparin as an adjunctive agent at a dose of 300 to 500 units per hour to prevent continued generation of thrombin. A critical aspect of treatment of DIC in patients with acute promyelocytic leukemia is to maintain a platelet count of 50,000/µL. A combination of heparin and antifibrinolytic agents is also useful in patients with DIC related to solid tumors such as prostatic carcinoma. Efficacy of treatment can be monitored clinically and by the increase in fibrinogen levels followed by an increase in platelets in 24 to 48 hours.

Obstetrical Conditions

DIC can occur with abruptio placentae, amniotic fluid embolism, retained placenta, preeclampsia, acute fatty liver, and in utero fetal death.[44] These processes are all associated with the release of tissue factor from the dead fetus or necrotic placenta. DIC is clinically noted by excessive or spontaneous bleeding combined with decreases in fibrinogen and platelet counts and increases in D-dimers. The best treatment is to accomplish delivery as soon as possible. Blood products are given as needed until this can be achieved. The contraction of the myometrium and removal of the source of tissue factor are the two most important factors in controlling the DIC.[44] With proper treatment, the coagulopathy reverses in hours and no further treatment is required. The only obstetrical condition associated with DIC for which heparin has been efficacious is the rare condition in which fetal death has occurred in one of two or more fetuses carried by the mother. Full-dose intravenous heparin has been administered to allow the maturation and delivery of the other viable fetuses.[45, 46]

■ Autoantibodies against Coagulation Factors

Acquired antibodies to specific blood coagulation factors have been reported in association with a variety of conditions including infections, malignancy, pregnancy, and autoimmune disorders.[47, 48] The antibodies, which are usually of the immunoglobulin G (IgG) isotype, may not be detected until the patient undergoes a hemostatic challenge such as surgery, or they may develop in the postoperative period, causing increased morbidity and even mortality. Inhibitors should be suspected in patients who have sustained trauma or who have undergone a surgical procedure and yet continue to bleed excessively for no apparent reason. The first manifestation of an inhibitor may not be apparent for 4 to 5 days after surgery. A review of serial coagulation studies may show an increasingly prolonged aPTT or both PT and aPTT with no apparent explanation (i.e., not corrected by empirical use of vitamin K or FFP or, in the case of hemophiliacs, worsening recovery and shortened half-life of infused factor VIII). Evaluation of coagulation screening studies and measurement of appropriate factor levels can establish the diagnosis so that appropriate blood product replacement can be provided and immunosuppressive therapy initiated.

The antibodies most commonly associated with excessive bleeding are those that develop against factor VIII in a patient with or without hemophilia A. Postoperative patients may also develop an antibody against factor V, which may be due to exposure to bovine thrombin preparations that contain factor V. Patients may also develop lupus anticoagulants (LAs); in the critical care setting, these are usually IgM antibodies that are directed against phospholipid-binding proteins such as prothrombin. They are not associated with excessive bleeding unless the patient also has a true deficiency of prothrombin in association with the LA. The essential goals for the successful treatment of patients with inhibitors are to establish the initial diagnosis and then plan for appropriate factor replacement as well as for immunosuppression to eliminate the inhibitor.

For patients who are not known to have hemophilia but who have a progressive prolongation of the aPTT and continued or excessive bleeding with surgery, a mixing study for the presence of an inhibitor and measurement of coagulation factors XII, XI, IX, and VIII are essential. These measures can be followed by a Bethesda titer, which is not as accurate a measurement of inhibitor titers in patients who do not have hemophilia (i.e., who have an autoantibody to factor VIII) as in those with an alloantibody (severe hemophilia). One

Bethesda unit (BU) is the reciprocal of the dilution of patient's plasma that destroys 50% of the factor VIII in normal plasma after incubation for 2 hours at 37°C. For example, a titer of 40 BU indicates that at a 1:40 dilution the patient's plasma can inhibit 50% of the factor VIII in normal plasma.

Factor VIII Deficiency

In the case of hemophiliacs with inhibitors, exposure to factor VIII during the surgical procedure stimulates antibody titers, resulting in a poor response to factor VIII by the fourth or fifth postoperative day. In these patients, serial aPTT and factor VIII measurements can be performed so that appropriate changes in therapy can be made if necessary. Depending on the clinical setting and the inhibitor titer, treatment choices include human factor VIII, porcine factor VIII, activated prothrombin complex concentrates, or recombinant factor VIIa.

Acquired antibodies to factor VIII generally occur in patients older than 50 years and are first suspected when the patients present with a complaint of new-onset bruising, soft tissue bleeding, or gastrointestinal bleeding.[47] In approximately 50% of the patients, no other medical disorders are identified; rheumatoid arthritis, the postpartum period, allergies, asthma, autoimmune disorders, and malignancy may be associated conditions.[47, 48] In 1981, Green and Lechner[47] reported that major bleeding occurred in as many as 87% of patients with an acquired factor VIII antibody and resulted in death in 22%. With the advent of improved recognition and treatment of inhibitors, in terms of both treatment of bleeding episodes and use of immunosuppression, these data should now be improved.

Although antibodies to factor VIII can disappear spontaneously, the general approach is to begin immunosuppressive therapy to increase the factor VIII level to normal levels. Several therapies have been used with different degrees of success (Table 26.5). Green and coworkers[49] reported a response rate of 30% to oral prednisone alone at a dose of 1 mg per kg of body weight administered daily for 3 to 6 weeks. The responders tended to have lower Bethesda titers than nonresponders (median, 3 BU vs. 50 BU), although responses did occur in three patients with titers of 33, 52, and 240 BU. They also concluded that cyclophosphamide at an oral dose of 2 mg/kg daily is an efficacious therapy for

Table 26.5　Approach to Immunosuppression in Nonhemophiliacs with an Inhibitor

Approaches listed below must be evaluated according to toxicity, especially in older patients. If eradication is impossible, patients can nonetheless do well if they and their families are educated to report all bleeding episodes immediately and even have factor concentrate at home for self-infusion if possible.

Success of immunosuppression with be monitored by Bethesda titer and by measurable factor VIII activity.

Begin oral prednisone daily at a dose of 1mg/kg for 2 weeks. If titer remains unchanged, add oral cyclophosphamide at a dose of 100 to 200 mg daily. Once the inhibitor titer is no longer detectable, slowly taper both agents.

If inhibitor titer remains high, consider combined chemotherapy with factor VIII, cyclophosphamide, vincristine and prednisone (see text for doses).

Cyclophosphamide and cyclosporine have also been used successfully as single agents in some patients with inhibitors (e.g., those who could not tolerate prednisone). Rituximab may also prove to be an effective agent.

patients who cannot tolerate prednisone.[49] In a follow-up publication, Green[50] reported an 80% response rate in 10 patients treated only with prednisone; their initial titers ranged from less than 1 to 27 BU. Patients who did not respond to steroids or had adverse effects all responded to single-agent cyclophosphamide.

In a report of nine consecutive patients (ages 50 to 79) with inhibitor titers ranging from 2.5 to 1040 BU, Shaffer and Phillips[51] described complete remission in 2 to 10 weeks with combined treatment with oral cyclophosphamide (100 to 200 mg/day) and prednisone (50 to 80 mg/day) with slow tapering of these doses when the inhibitor titer was no longer detectable. Cyclosporine has also been used successfully in a limited number of patients at a dose that provides therapeutic serum levels (150 to 350 ng/mL).[52]

Lian and associates[53] reported a good outcome in 11 of 12 patients with acquired hemophilia after one to three courses of the following therapy repeated every 3 to 4 weeks: a single infusion of factor VIII concentrate (50 to 100 U/kg), cyclophosphamide (500 mg intravenously on day 1 and 200 mg orally on days 2 through 5), vincristine (2 mg intravenously on day 1), and prednisone (100 mg/day orally on days 1 to 5). The patients generally tolerated the therapy well, although neutropenia and infection occurred in three.

For treatment of bleeding episodes in patients with an inhibitor, factor VIII concentrates can still be used to neutralize the antibody and achieve a hemostatic level of factor VIII activity if the inhibitor titer is less than 5 BU.[54] For those with a higher titer, other options exist, such as porcine factor VIII (HYATE:C, Speywood Pharmaceuticals) if the patient does not have a high titer of neutralizing antibodies to porcine factor VIII, activated prothrombin complex concentrates (FEIBA, Baxter/Hyland, Immuno Division and Autoplex T, NABI), and recombinant factor VIIa (NovoSeven, NovoNordisk Pharmaceuticals).

In one descriptive study of patients with acquired hemophilia (median titer, 38 BU) who were infused with porcine factor VIII, the response to infusion was good to excellent in 78% of patients who received a mean initial factor VIII dose of 84 IU/kg.[55] Therapy was continued for 8.5 days with 11 infusions. In a retrospective study of use of FEIBA in France in 60 patients with inhibitors (most of whom had congenital hemophilia), efficacy was rated as excellent in 81% of bleeding episodes, which included surgical procedures, and poor in 17%.[56] The treatment was well tolerated in

98% of episodes; the doses infused were 65 to 100 U/kg at 6- to 12-hour intervals (total 65 to 510 U/kg/day).

In patients with high-titer inhibitors, recombinant factor VIIa has been efficacious at a dose of 90 μg/kg administered intravenously every 2 hours during surgery and for 48 hours postoperatively followed by every 2 to 6 hours for the next 3 days.[57] Factor VIIa has also been tested for home use in the treatment of mild to moderately severe bleeding episodes in the joints, muscles, or mucocutaneous tissues in patients with hemophilia A or B with inhibitors.[58] In this study, patients received recombinant factor VIIa (90 μg/kg) intravenously at 3-hour intervals within 8 hours of the onset of the episode. If the dose was considered effective after one to three applications, one additional injection was provided. Recombinant factor VIIa was considered effective in 92% of bleeding episodes after a mean of 2.2 injections. The time from onset of bleeding to the first injection in the successfully treated episodes was 1.1 ± 2 hours (standard deviation). A general approach to the use of coagulation factor components in patients with acquired factor VIII inhibitors is summarized in Table 26.6.

Factor V Deficiency

Antibodies to factor V are rare and are first manifested clinically as unexpected bleeding or bruising in a patient with a prolonged PT and aPTT. Multiple reports have described postoperative patients who have experienced significant bleeding related to factor V antibodies.[48] The coagulopathy develops as a result of exposure of the patient to bovine thrombin during surgery. Bovine thrombin, which is a commonly used hemostatic agent, contains multiple impurities, including bovine factor V. Patients develop antibodies to the bovine factor V, which then cross-react with their endogenous factor V, causing a marked inhibition of factor V activity.[5] Patients may also develop antibodies to the bovine thrombin. However, these antibodies do not cross-react with human thrombin and are of no clinical significance.

Patients who have antibodies to factor V have a prolonged PT and aPTT that are not corrected when the tests are repeated with a 1:1 mix of normal and patient's plasma. The prolongation of the PT and aPTT becomes even greater when the tests are repeated after incubation of patient's and normal plasma for 1 or 2 hours at 37°C. Measurement of coagulation factors shows a decrease in factor V. An antibody to bovine thrombin is detected by a prolongation of the thrombin time if

Table 26.6 Treatment of Bleeding Episodes in Patients with Inhibitors to Factor VIII

If Bethesda titer is <5 U, use recombinant factor VIII concentrates; monitor factor VIII activity. Because Bethesda titers are not highly accurate in nonhemophiliac patients with an inhibitor, recombinant factor VIII may also be effective if the titer is greater than 5 BU. The factor VIII activity is the best guide for treatment. An initial high dose may be required to neutralize the inhibitor in vivo, and then lesser doses may provide satisfactory activity. If possible, factor VIII should be the first choice for treatment.

If factor VIII administration does not result in satisfactory factor VIII activity, then treatment options are porcine factor VIII (can be used in patients who do not have antibodies to porcine factor VIII and can be monitored with factor VIII activity).

Activated prothrombin complex concentrates (FEIBA 75–100 U/kg every 8–12 hours or Autoplex 50–75 U/kg every 8–12 hours) can be used for soft tissue bleeds and other bleeding episodes. Efficacy is judged by patient's response. For soft tissue bleeds, patients can be treated every 8 hours for 48 hours followed by every 12 hours for the next 48 hours.

Recombinant factor VIIa can be used instead of activated prothrombin concentrates at a dose of 90 μg/kg every 2 hours for the duration of bleeding and for several days thereafter. Choice of recombinant factor VIIa over activated prothrombin complex concentrates may be based on experience of the physician, cost, and availability. The two treatments have not been directly compared. Disadvantage of the activated prothrombin complex concentrates is potential for inducing thrombosis.

bovine thrombin is used in the test system. The test remains abnormal when repeated with a 1:1 mix of normal and patient's plasma. The thrombin time is normal, however, if human thrombin is used in the test system.

The majority of patients in whom an antibody to factor V develops do not have clinical symptoms and the PT and aPTT become normal within 3 to 6 weeks after exposure to thrombin. For patients who are actively bleeding, FFP is the first choice for replacement of factor V. Infusion of platelets is a second option because they contain approximately 20% of the body stores of factor V, although they may not provide hemostasis in all situations.[59]

Corticosteroids, cyclophosphamide, and vincristine have been used alone or in combination for suppression of antibodies. Corticosteroids have mostly been used alone as first-line therapy with success. Methylprednisolone at an initial dose of 1 to 1.5 mg/kg is usually given for 2 to 3 weeks and then tapered slowly over the next several weeks.[7] Cyclophosphamide and vincristine have been added to prednisone to suppress the antibody production successfully in cases with acquired factor VIII inhibitors; similar success has been achieved in some cases with factor V inhibitors. Plasmapheresis has also been used to reduce the titer of factor V inhibitors either with or without adjunctive immunosuppression.[5]

Factor II Deficiency

Autoantibodies to prothrombin usually occur in association with lupus anticoagulants (LAs), which are antibodies to phospholipid-binding proteins such as prothrombin or β_2-glycoprotein I.[60] LAs are associated with the antiphospholipid syndrome, systemic lupus erythematosus (SLE), and infections as well as medications, such as procainamide (Pronestyl). In some patients with LA, a true deficiency of prothrombin has also been recognized; this appears to be due to IgG antibodies that selectively bind prothrombin without neutralizing its activity. The antibodies do not interfere with the proteolytic cleavage of prothrombin or with the activity of thrombin. They appear to induce true prothrombin deficiency by binding to prothrombin in vivo and causing increased clearance.[61–63]

The majority of patients with LA and SLE or other autoimmune connective tissue disorders may have IgG autoantibodies to prothrombin, although only 30% of patients with antibodies have a detectable prothrombin deficiency.[60] Antiprothrombin antibodies are more likely to occur in patients with an aPTT that is significantly prolonged (at least 50 seconds with a normal range, 22 to 30 seconds).[62] Bleeding symptoms are correlated with the level of functional prothrombin and occur in patients with a prothrombin activity of 10% or lower.[62] In some cases, the first manifestation of lupus is the development of an LA with true prothrombin deficiency. A significant decrease in the prothrombin activity related to antibody formation can occur at any time in a patient who has an LA and underlying SLE or primary antiphospholipid syndrome. For patients with an LA who are receiving warfarin, the first manifestation of an antibody to prothrombin that induces a significant decrease in the prothrombin activity may be a gradually increasing INR with no other apparent etiology.

LAs and clinically significant hypoprothrombinemia have been associated with viral illnesses in children.[64] In these cases, the antibody disappeared spontaneously. The antibody production can usually be suppressed by administration of corticosteroids with or without adjunctive agents such as azathioprine; with this treatment, the PT can become normal as soon as 7 days after initiation of treatment.[61, 63] For example, a 3-year-old girl with a viral illness and severe hypoprothrombinemia that resulted in epistaxis and gastrointestinal hemorrhage was treated successfully with intravenous methylprednisolone daily for 3 days followed by oral prednisone.[65] For a patient who is actively bleeding and has a severe prothrombin deficiency, treatment options are FFP or prothrombin complex concentrates.

Factor XIII Deficiency

Factor XIII deficiency may be due to the formation of autoantibodies that occur spontaneously or in association with drugs such as penicillin, isoniazid, or diphenylhydantoin or with autoimmune disorders.[66, 67] The inhibitor is not detected on routine screening tests and can be confirmed only by finding rapid lysis of a clot that has been prepared from recalcified plasma and placed in 1% monochloroacetic acid or urea. Treatment consists of immunosuppressive agents and administration of cryoprecipitate if the patient is actively bleeding, with qualitative monitoring performed by assessing solubility of the clot in urea or monochloroacetic acid.[68, 69]

■ Coagulopathies Related to Anticoagulant Administration

Warfarin

The frequency of bleeding in patients who are receiving warfarin ranges from 8 to 16 per hundred patient-years, with major bleeding occurring in 1.3 to 2.7 patients per hundred years.[70] The main strategies for treating warfarin overdose, depending on the degree of overanticoagulation and the clinical site of bleeding, include administration of vitamin K, prothrombin complex concentrates, or FFP. Prothrombin complex concentrates, which contain factors II, VII, and X in addition to factor IX (Table 26.7)[71] and are virally inactivated, were originally developed for treatment of individuals with hemophilia B; although no longer used for this purpose, they are efficacious for use in the emergency correction of coagulation factor deficiencies in individuals who have major bleeding and are anticoagulated with warfarin. Table 26.8 provides guidelines for use of vitamin K and blood products in patients who are excessively anticoagulated with warfarin.

Table 26.7 Coagulation Factor Concentrations of Prothrombin Complex Concentrates (PCCs)

Prothrombin Complex Concentrates*	Coagulation Factor Units/Unit Factor IX		
	II	VII	X
Konyne 80 (Bayer)	1.0	0.2	1.4
Profilnine HT (Alpha)	1.48	0.11	0.64
Proplex T (Baxter)	0.5	4.0	0.5
Bebulin VH (Immuno)	1.2	0.13	1.4

*The activated prothrombin complex concentrates (Autoplex, Nabi and FEIBA, Immuno) contain VIIa, IXa, and Xa, in addition to factors II, VII, IX, and X.
Modified from Roberts HR, Bingham MD: Other coagulation factor deficiencies. In Loscalzo J, Schafer AI (eds): Thrombosis and Hemorrhage, 2nd ed. Philadelphia, Williams and Wilkins, 1998, pp 773–802.

Table 26.8   Guidelines for Reversal of Warfarin Anticoagulation

Major bleeding (INR > 2)	Stop warfarin Infuse PCC* (50 U/kg) of FFP† (15 mL/kg) Give vitamin K 5 mg (SC)‡
INR > 6 (with no or minor bleeding)	Stop warfarin Restart with INR < 5 Give 0.5–2.5 mg vitamin K SC (or oral dose) if reversal within 24–48 hr needed

*PCC, prothrombin complex concentrates.
†FFP, fresh frozen plasma.
‡SC, subcutaneous (original guidelines recommend intravenous, but this is usually not necessary)
Adapted from Baglin T: Management of warfarin (coumarin) overdose. Blood Rev 1998; 12:91–98.

One way to prevent bleeding is to use warfarin only for appropriate indications and to recognize that the risk factors for bleeding are increasing age, fluctuations in the INR, an elevated INR, recent initiation of oral anticoagulation, and the presence of comorbid conditions such as cardiac, renal, or liver failure as well as cerebrovascular disease.[72] Approximately 50% to 90% of intracranial hemorrhages in patients receiving warfarin anticoagulation occur at a time when the INR is within the target range.[72] The mortality associated with intracranial bleeding is 16% to 68% and is influenced by the rapidity with which normalization of the coagulation factor deficiencies occurs.

The preferred replacement therapy in intracranial hemorrhage is PCCs (25 to 50 U/kg). When this dose was compared with infusion of 800 mL of FFP in a small study of patients with intracranial hemorrhage who were also anticoagulated with warfarin, the coagulation factor levels were raised into the normal range with the PCCs but not with FFP. The INR can be corrected four to five times more quickly with the PCCs than with FFP. The elimination half-lives of the coagulation factors are as follows: II (58 hours), VII (5 hours), IX (19 hours), and X (35 hours); thus, repeated infusion may be necessary if the factor deficiency has not been reversed by the administration of vitamin K in 24 hours. Factor VII is in low concentration in some PCCs relative to the other coagulation factors, and it has a short half-life. The importance of replacing the factor VII level to values greater than 10% is unknown. FFP can be used to achieve minimal levels of 10% if this is deemed necessary.

Another issue concerns the duration of time for which warfarin can be safely discontinued after a major bleeding episode in patients with mechanical heart valves. In one study, 15 patients with mechanical heart valves and intracranial bleeding underwent discontinuation of warfarin for a median of 8 days (range, 2 days to 3 months).[73] During this time none developed transient ischemic attacks or ischemic stroke, valve thrombosis, or evidence of systemic embolization. There was no recurrence of intracranial hemorrhage with reinstitution of anticoagulation.

For patients who have ingested rat poison containing a superwarfarin such as brodifacoum, prolonged treatment with daily oral vitamin K is needed because the half-life of the superwarfarin is 16 to 36 days.[74] Oral vitamin K has a bioavailability of 10% to 60% and is therefore given at a dose three to five times greater than the parenteral dose. Initially,

oral vitamin K may have to be taken every 6 to 8 hours and then tapered to a daily dose.

Heparin Preparations (Unfractionated Heparin, Low-Molecular-Weight Heparin, and Heparinoid)

According to one study, risk factors for bleeding are the same for patients receiving *unfractionated heparin* or *low-molecular-weight (LMW) heparin* and include the performance status of the patient as determined by World Health Organization criteria, history of a bleeding tendency, cardiopulmonary resuscitation, recent trauma or surgery, body surface area, and total dose of anticoagulant administered in 24 hours.[75] The bleeding risk may also be increased in older patients (>70 years).[76, 77]

For unfractionated heparin, reversal of anticoagulant activity can be achieved by slow infusion (over 10 minutes) of protamine sulfate, which neutralizes 100 units of heparin for every milligram of protamine administered. Assuming that heparin has a half-life of 60 minutes, the protamine dose can be calculated by adding the heparin dose infused in the last hour to 50% of the dose in the previous hour and 25% of the dose infused 3 hours earlier.[78] The risk for anaphylaxis with protamine sulfate is approximately 1% and may be higher in diabetics who have taken neutral protamine Hagedorn (NPH) insulin. For LMW heparin, protamine does not neutralize the anti–factor Xa activity, and at present there is no satisfactory neutralizing agent for LMW heparin.[79]

One way in which to use LMW heparin safely is to understand its pharmacology, especially with respect to its use in patients in the intensive care setting or in the postoperative state. LMW heparin, when administered subcutaneously, has a plasma half-life of 3 to 6 hours. Since the approval of enoxaparin (Lovenox, Aventis) in 1993 for prophylaxis after total hip or knee replacement at a dose of 30 mg subcutaneously every 12 hours, the Food and Drug Administration (FDA) has received reports of more than 30 patients who experienced spinal or epidural hematomas in conjunction with LMW heparin prophylaxis and spinal or epidural anesthesia. The mean age of the patients was 74 years, and 75% were women. The procedures were predominantly orthopedic (hip or knee replacement), and more than 80% of the patients were receiving LMW heparin twice daily. Published guidelines have emphasized that in patients receiving LMW heparin preoperatively, needle placement for epidural or spinal anesthesia should occur no sooner than 12 hours after the last dose.[80–82] Subsequent dosing should be delayed for at least 2 hours after needle placement. Epidural catheters should be removed 12 to 24 hours after the last LMW heparin dose, with subsequent dosing delayed by at least 2 hours.[80, 81] In addition, enoxaparin should be used whenever possible as a once-daily dose[82] and other antiplatelet or anticoagulant agents should not be administered at the same time.

Danaparoid (Orgaran, Organon, Inc.) is a LMW heparinoid composed of heparan sulfate, dermatan sulfate, and chondroitin sulfate.[83] The FDA-approved indication for danaparoid is prophylaxis of venous thromboembolism, usually at a dose of 750 anti-factor Xa units twice daily subcutaneously.[84] However, it is used primarily in patients suspected of having heparin-induced thrombocytopenia (HIT). Danaparoid has an anti-factor Xa/anti-factor II activity of 28:1 (compared with a 1:1 ratio for heparin). Thus, it cannot be neutralized by protamine. The elimination half-life of the anti-factor Xa activity is 24 hours and that of the minor component of anti-factor II is approximately 4 hours (Table 26.9).[83] The steady state of anti-factor Xa activity is reached after 4 to 5 days of dosing. Because approximately 40% to 50% of the plasma clearance is by the renal route, after an initial dose in patients with renal insufficiency, the subsequent doses should be reduced. Danaparoid can be monitored by its anti-factor Xa activity; however, the assay for the anti-factor Xa activity should contain danaparoid as the standard.

Danaparoid has been used in many different clinical settings with adjustment of the dose. For example, it has been used as a continuous infusion in patients undergoing hemofiltration with an initial bolus of 2500 units followed by a dose of 200 to 600 U/hr.[85] However, even lower doses such as 50 to 100 U/hr may be safer in the critically ill patient. Danaparoid has also been used at a dose of 3750 units for patients undergoing hemodialysis.[85] Ideally, if danaparoid is to be used at doses higher than those used for prophylaxis in the intensive care setting, assays should be readily available for monitoring anticoagulation and the lowest effective dose should be used to reduce the risk of bleeding. Furthermore, a minimum of 24 hours should be allowed between the last dose and a planned invasive procedure.

For prophylaxis against venous thromboembolism in patients with suspected HIT, a dose of 750 anti-factor Xa units twice daily subcutaneously could be used. For treatment of active thrombosis in a patient with normal renal function, the dose could be increased to 1500 units intravenously as a bolus followed by 1500 units subcutaneously twice daily. This recommendation, which is a middle ground, represents a simple doubling of the packaged dose. The support for this dose is based on a randomized study which showed that in patients with normal renal function who had venous thromboembolism, danaparoid at an intravenous bolus dose of 1250 units followed by 1250 units twice daily subcutaneously was similar in efficacy to unfractionated heparin.[86] Even greater efficacy was achieved with a higher dose. Danaparoid administered at an intravenous bolus of 2000 units followed by 2000 units subcutaneously twice daily was associated with a significantly lower risk of recurrence or extension of thrombosis compared with heparin (13% vs. 28%, with a relative risk of 0.45; 95% CI 0.21 to 0.90).[86]

Danaparoid has been used in the bypass setting and in some cases has been associated with excessive bleeding. One way in which to reduce the bleeding is to administer doses that maintain the anti–factor Xa level at 0.7 to 1.5 U/mL and to use newer hemostatic agents such as fibrin sealant at the sternotomy site.[87]

Thrombin Inhibitors (Hirudin and Argatroban)

Lepirudin (Refludan, Hoechst Marion Roussel), which is a recombinant protein, is approved for use in patients with HIT and associated thrombosis to prevent further complications (see Table 26.9). It is similar to the 65-amino-acid natural thrombin inhibitor known as hirudin; however, lepirudin has a leucine instead of isoleucine at the amino terminal of the molecule and lacks a sulfate group on the tyrosine in position 63.

Published data on the use of thrombin-specific inhibitors in patients with HIT are not extensive. One study described the use of lepirudin in 82 patients with laboratory-confirmed HIT.[88] Patients received 0.4 mg/kg as a bolus followed by continuous infusion of 0.15 mg/kg/hr or a lower dose with thrombolysis (0.2 mg/kg bolus followed by 0.1 mg/kg/hr continuous infusion) or for prophylaxis (continuous infusion, 0.1 mg/kg/hr). The treated patients were compared with historical controls; the combined endpoint of mortality, limb amputation, and new thromboembolic events was reduced by 50% ($p = .014$) at day 7 and at day 35 in the group receiving lepirudin. Bleeding events and transfusions were not

Table 26.9   Properties of Anticoagulants Used in Patients with Heparin-Induced Thrombocytopenia

Property	Danaparoid	Argatroban	Lepirudin
Composition	Dermatan sulfate Heparin sulfate Chondroitin sulfate	Synthetic arginine analogue	Recombinant protein
Molecular weight	6000	506	6979
Action	Inhibits factor Xa and thrombin through antithrombin III	Direct thrombin inhibitor	Direct thrombin inhibitor
Half-life	22 hr	40 min	1.5 hr
Monitoring	None or anti–factor Xa assay	aPTT	aPTT
Effect on PT	None	Prolongation	Prolongation
Neutralization	None	None	None
Excretion	Renal	Liver	Renal
Caution	Prolonged half-life in renal disease	Prolonged half-life in liver disease	Prolonged half-life in renal disease

aPTT, activated partial thromboplastin time; PT, prothrombin time.

increased in the treated group compared with the historical controls. Current dosing recommendations are 0.4 mg/kg as a bolus with 0.15 mg/kg/hr (up to weight of 110 kg). The dose can be monitored with the aPTT, and recommendations are to maintain the aPTT at 1.5 to 2.5 times the median value for the normal range.

In normal volunteers, lepirudin, which is excreted and perhaps metabolized by the kidneys, has a half-life of approximately 2 hours. Pharmacokinetic studies in patients with renal failure who were undergoing dialysis showed that after a single dose of lepirudin (0.08 to 0.2 mg/kg) followed by five additional dialyses without further dosing, the half-life was increased to 52 hours.[89] The distribution volume was also lower in hemodialysis patients than in normal volunteers. Lepirudin has been used successfully to maintain anticoagulation during dialysis when given once before dialysis at a dose of 0.08 mg/kg.[90] However, subsequent dosing would require adjustment because of the prolonged half-life. The manufacturer recommends that dosing be reduced by 50% for both bolus and infusion for patients with a creatinine value of 1.5 to 2.0 mg/dL. Reductions would be even greater for those with more severe renal impairment.

The use of lepirudin in five patients who required bypass surgery has also been reported.[91] In these patients the dose was monitored by a coagulation-based assay, and infusions were given to maintain the plasma levels above 2 μg/mL. In patients receiving lepirudin for deep venous thrombosis, the plasma level at steady state was approximately 0.6 μg/mL.[92]

Argatroban (Smith-Kline Beecham), a thrombin-specific inhibitor that has been used in more than 300 patients with HIT, is an arginine-based synthetic molecule.[93] Argatroban has a half-life of 40 minutes in normal individuals. Unlike lepirudin, argatroban does not require dose adjustment in patients with renal disease (see Table 26.9).[94] Argatroban, which is cleared by the liver, requires dose reduction in patients with significant hepatic dysfunction. It is administered in weight-based doses and is monitored with the aPTT with the goal of maintaining the aPTT at 1.5 to 3 times the baseline value. Argatroban has been used successfully in one patient with HIT who required repeated dialysis[95] and in a patient with HIT and thrombosis who required coronary stent implantation.[96]

The thrombin-specific inhibitors, unlike unfractionated heparin, prolong the PT as well as the aPTT. In patients who are undergoing conversion to warfarin while receiving argatroban or hirudin, these agents can be discontinued several hours before a PT is determined to ensure an accurate indication of the INR. Clinical experience with these agents in critically ill patients who are receiving multiple other drugs as well as anesthetic agents is limited and is not well described in the literature. Thus, dosing in critically ill patients should be established with caution.

■ Bleeding Induced by Antiplatelet Agents

Agents That Inhibit the Platelet GPIIb/IIIa Receptor (Abciximab, Tirofiban, and Eptifibatide)

The most potent antiplatelet agents in clinical practice today are those that block the interaction between fibrinogen and platelet GPIIb/IIIa, thus mimicking the bleeding diathesis seen in patients with Glanzmann thrombasthenia. Abciximab (Rheopro, Centocor) is a Fab fragment of chimeric human-murine monoclonal antibody c7E3, which is used in patients undergoing percutaneous transluminal angioplasty (PTCA) and those with unstable angina with PTCA planned in 24 hours.[97] Treatment of patients undergoing angioplasty or stent procedures with abciximab significantly reduced the combined endpoint of death, repeated myocardial infarction, and need for urgent revascularization during 30 days compared with those undergoing stent procedures in the absence of abciximab.[97] Two newer GPIIb/IIIa inhibitors have also been licensed. One is tirofiban (Aggrastat, Merck), a nonpeptide tyrosine derivative that is indicated for patients with unstable angina or non–Q wave myocardial infarction (with or without PTCA).[98, 99] The other drug is eptifibatide (Integrelin, COR Therapeutics, Inc.), a cyclic heptapeptide that is indicated for patients with unstable angina or non–Q wave myocardial infarction (with or without PTCA) and for patients undergoing PTCA.[100]

The risk for bleeding with these agents is in part due to their pharmacokinetics. Abciximab, which has a high affinity for GPIIb/IIIa, has a biologic half-life of 8 hours; in comparison, after completion of the infusion of eptifibatide, the bleeding time becomes normal within 1 hour.[101] The antiplatelet effect of tirofiban is also short-lived after completion of infusion, although in patients with renal failure the biologic effect is more prolonged. Platelet function is inhibited when more than 80% of the GPIIb/IIIa receptors are blocked. For patients who are bleeding, the drugs should be discontinued immediately and 8 to 10 units of platelets administered. The drug redistributes to the receptors of the infused platelets, thus lowering the occupancy of the receptors of the entire platelet pool and resulting in normalization of platelet function.

In patients who have received abciximab within 12 hours of requiring an emergent bypass procedure, platelet infusions should be administered prophylactically to prevent excessive bleeding.[102] This recommendation is based on the observation that patients who underwent bypass surgery within 12 hours of abciximab experienced threefold greater blood loss than those who underwent surgery more than 12 hours after receiving the drug (1300 vs. 400 mL).[103] These patients required platelet infusions, red blood cells, and FFP. The recommendation for preoperative platelet infusions probably does not apply for tirofiban or eptifibatide because of their shorter duration of action.

All of the agents that interact with the GPIIb/IIIa receptor have been associated with induction of thrombocytopenia, with the incidence ranging from 1% to 5.6% in published reports.[104] The mechanism may be that binding of the agents to the receptors induces exposure of an epitope that can be recognized by preexisting anti-GPIIb/IIIa antibodies. Berkowitz and colleagues[104, 105] developed an algorithm and recommendations for evaluation and treatment of thrombocytopenia. They recommend monitoring the platelet count within 2 to 4 hours of starting treatment; if thrombocytopenia is found, a pseudothrombocytopenia needs to be ruled out by examination of the peripheral smear. The drug should be discontinued (although aspirin can be continued) and platelet infusions should be given for platelet counts less than 20,000/μL to decrease the risk of intracranial hemorrhage or other major bleeding episodes.

Agents That Inhibit the Platelet ADP Receptor (Clopidogrel and Ticlopidine)

The thienopyridines ticlopidine and clopidogrel inhibit platelet function by blocking the adenosine diphosphate (ADP) receptor.[106] Although ticlopidine has been widely employed to prevent stent closure after angioplasty and as secondary prevention against stroke in patients with cerebrovascular disease, its relatively poor safety profile has resulted in diminished use. Adverse events in patients receiving ticlopidine have included neutropenia, agranulocytosis, aplastic anemia, and thrombotic thrombocytopenic purpura.[107] In contrast, clopidogrel appears to have an excellent safety profile. In a large, randomized, blinded control trial in patients with atherosclerotic vascular disease, clopidogrel reduced the combined risk of ischemic stroke, myocardial infarction, and vascular death by 8.7% compared with aspirin ($p < .05$).[108] Patients treated with clopidogrel had fewer gastrointestinal ulcers and fewer gastrointestinal bleeding episodes than those treated with aspirin. Clopidogrel is indicated for the reduction of atherosclerotic events (myocardial infarction, stroke, and vascular death) in patients with atherosclerosis documented by recent stroke, myocardial infarction, or peripheral vascular disease.

Both clopidogrel and ticlopidine require metabolism by the hepatic cytochrome P450-1A enzyme system to acquire activity.[106] When clopidogrel was given at a dose of 300 to 400 mg orally, it caused maximal inhibition of platelet function within 2 hours.[109] With a daily dose of 75 mg, the same degree of inhibition was achieved at 3 to 7 days. Recovery of platelet function occurs over 3 to 5 days after discontinuation of either drug. Specific treatment for bleeding related to these agents is not well described. Administration of desmopressin, however, may shorten the bleeding time and provide temporary hemostasis.[110] Otherwise, supportive care and infusion of platelets may be needed in patients who are taking clopidogrel or ticlopidine and have a major bleeding episode.

■ Summary

Acquired coagulation disorders range from subtle to catastrophic. Most can be quickly diagnosed by the history and appropriate laboratory testing, which is usually available in a tertiary hospital. Measurement of specific coagulation factors is much more useful than random infusion of FFP. A major problem is having the appropriate blood components available for the patient. If a hospital does not routinely stock coagulation factor concentrates, the patient should be transferred to hospitals where the specialty care can be provided; in addition, the hospital should know how to arrange for a core of specialty products that may be required on an emergent basis. Communication and collaboration among the services involved in the diagnosis and management of bleeding disorders provide cost-effective, efficient care of patients and maximize the potential for good outcomes.

REFERENCES

1. DeLoughery TG, Liebler JM, Simonds V, Goodnight SH: Invasive line placement in critically ill patients: do hemostatic defects matter. Transfusion 1996;36:827–831.
2. Alving B, Alcorn K: How to improve transfusion medicine: A treating physician's perspective. Arch Pathol Lab Med 1999;123:492–495.
3. Alving BA, Weinstein MJ, Finlayson JS, et al: Fibrin sealant: summary of a conference on characteristics and clinical uses. Transfusion 1995;35:783–790.
4. Rapaport SI, Zivelin A, Minow RA, et al: Clinical significance of antibodies to bovine and human thrombin and factor V after surgical use of bovine thrombin. Am J Clin Pathol 1992;97:84–91.
5. Zehnder JL, Leung LK: Development of antibodies to thrombin and factor V with recurrent bleeding in a patient exposed to topical bovine thrombin. Blood 1990;76:2011–2016.
6. Ortel TL, Charles LA, Keller FG, et al: Topical thrombin and acquired factor coagulation inhibitors: clinical spectrum and laboratory diagnosis. Am J Hematol 1994;45:128–135.
7. Christie RJ, Carrington L, Alving BA: Postoperative bleeding induced by topical bovine thrombin: report of two cases. Surgery 1997;121:708–710.
8. Rousou J, Levitsky S, Gonzalez-Lavin L, et al: Randomized clinical trial of fibrin sealant in patients undergoing resternotomy or reoperation after cardiac operations: A multicenter study. J Thorac Cardiovasc Surg 1989;97:194–203.
9. Martinowitz U, Schulman S: Fibrin sealant in surgery of patients with hemorrhagic diathesis: Thromb Haemost 1995;74:486–492.
10. Rakocz M, Mazar A, Varon D, et al: Dental extractions in patients with bleeding disorders. The use of fibrin glue. Oral Surg Oral Med Oral Pathol 1993;75:280–282.
11. Atkinson JB, Gomperts ED, Kang R, et al: Prospective, randomized evaluation of the efficacy of fibrin sealant as a topical hemostatic agent at the cannulation site in neonates undergoing extracorporeal membrane oxygenation. Am J Surg 1997;173:479–484.
12. Martinez J, Barsigian C: Coagulopathy of liver failure and vitamin K deficiency. In Loscalzo J, Schafer AL (eds): Thrombosis and Hemorrhage, 2nd ed. Philadelphia, Williams & Wilkins, 1998, pp 987–1004.
13. Martin TG III, Somberg KA, Meng YG, et al: Thrombopoietin levels in patients with cirrhosis before and after orthotopic liver transplantation. Ann Intern Med 1997;127:285–288.
14. Blanchard RA, Furie BC, Jorgensen M: Acquired vitamin K–dependent carboxylation deficiency in liver disease, N Engl J Med 1981;305:242–248.
15. Gralnick HR, Givelber H, Abrams E: Dysfibrinogenemia associated with hepatoma: increased carbohydrate content of the fibrinogen molecule. N Engl J Med 1978;299:221–226.
16. Dawson NA, Barr CF, Alving BM: Acquired dysfibrinogenemia. Paraneoplastic syndrome in renal cell carcinoma. Am J Med 1985;78:682–686.
17. Violi F, Basili S, Ferro D, et al: Association between high values of D-dimer and tissue-plasminogen activator activity and first gastrointestinal bleeding in cirrhotic patients. Thromb Haemost 1996;76:177–183.
18. Kovacs MJ, Wong A, MacKinnon K, et al: Assessment of the validity of the INR system for patients with liver impairment. Thromb Haemost 1994;71:727–730.
19. Basili S, Ferro D, Leo R: Bleeding time does not predict gastrointestinal bleeding in patients with cirrhosis. J Hepatol 1996;24:574–580.
20. Dillon JF, Simpson KJ, Hayes PC: Liver biopsy bleeding time: an unpredictable event. J Gastroenterol Hepatol 1994;9:269–271.
21. Mannucci PM, Vicento V, Vianello L, et al: Controlled trial of desmopressin in liver cirrhosis and other conditions associated with a prolonged bleeding time. Blood 1986;67:1148–1153.
22. Burroughs AK, Matthews K, Qadiri M, et al: Desmopressin and bleeding time in patients with cirrhosis. Br Med J 1985;291:1377–1381.
23. McVay PA, Toy PTCY: Lack of increased bleeding after liver biopsy in patients with mild hemostatic abnormalities. Am J Clin Pathol 1990;94:747–753.
24. Inabet WB, Deziel DJ: Laparoscopic liver biopsy in patients with coagulopathy, portal hypertension, and ascites. Am Surg 1995;61:603–606.
25. Bernstein DE, Jeffers L, Erhardtsen E, et al: Recombinant factor VIIa corrects prothrombin time in cirrhotic patients: a preliminary study. Gastroenterology 1997;113:1930–1937.
26. Alvarez L, Puleo J, Balint JA: Investigation of gastrointestinal bleeding in patients with end stage renal disease. Am J Gastroenterol 1993;88:30–33.
27. Steiner RW, Coggins SC, Carvalho ACA: Bleeding time in uremia: a useful test to assess clinical bleeding. Am J Hematol 1979;7:107–117.
28. Noris M, Benigni A, Boccardo P, et al: Enhanced nitric oxide synthesis in uremia: implications for platelet dysfunction and dialysis hypotension. Kidney Int 1993;44:445–450.

29. Noris M, Remuzzi G: Uremic bleeding: closing the circle after thirty years of controversies. Blood 1999;94:2569–2574.
30. Sreedhara R, Itagaki I, Hakim RM: Uremic patients have decreased shear-induced platelet aggregation mediated by decreased availability of glycoprotein IIb-IIIa receptors. Am J Kidney Dis 1996;27:355–364.
31. Zachee P, Vermylen J, Boogaerts MA: Hematologic aspects of end-stage renal failure. Ann Hematol 1994;69:33–40.
32. Rabelink TJ, Zwaginga JJ, Koomans HA, Sixma JJ: Thrombosis and hemostasis in renal disease. Kidney Int 1994;46:287–296.
33. Bolan CD, Alving BM: Pharmacologic agents in the management of bleeding disorders. Transfusion 1990;30:541–551.
34. Mannucci PM: Desmopressin (DDAVP) in the treatment of bleeding disorders: the first 20 years. Blood 1997;90:2515–2521.
35. Livio M. Mannucci PM, Vigano G, et al: Conjugated estrogens for the management of bleeding associated with renal failure. N Engl J Med 1986;315:731–735.
36. Sloand JA, Schiff MS: Beneficial effect of low-dose transdermal estrogen on bleeding time and clinical bleeding in uremia. Am J Kidney Dis 1995;26:22–26.
37. Vigano G, Gaspari F, Locatelli M, et al: Dose-effect and pharmacokinetics of estrogens given to correct bleeding time in uremia. Kidney Int 1988;34:853–858.
38. Levi M, ten Cate H: Disseminated intravascular coagulation. N Engl J Med 1999;341:586–592.
39. Levi M, de Jonge E, van der Poll T, ten Cate H: Disseminated intravascular coagulation. Thromb Haemost 1999;82:695–705.
40. Francois B, Trimoreau F, Vignon P, et al: Thrombocytopenia in the sepsis syndrome: role of hemophagocytosis and macrophage colony-stimulating factor. Am J Med 1997;103:114–120.
41. Baker GR, Levin J: Transient thrombocytopenia produced by administration of macrophage colony-stimulating factor: investigations of the mechanism. Blood 1998;91:89–99.
42. Schwartz BS, Williams EC, Conlan MG, Mosher DF: Epsilon-aminocaproic acid in the treatment of patients with acute promyelocytic leukemia and acquired alpha-2-plasmin inhibitor deficiency. Ann Intern Med 1986;105:873–877.
43. Avvisati G, ten Cate JW, Buller HR, Mandelli F: Tranexamic acid for control of haemorrhage in acute promyelocytic leukemia. Lancet 1989;2:122–124.
44. Bern MM: Acquired and congenital coagulation defects encountered during pregnancy and in the fetus. In Bern MM, Frigoletto FD Jr (eds): Hematologic Disorders in Maternal-Fetal Medicine. New York, Wiley-Liss, 1990, pp 395–447.
45. Romero R, Duffy TP, Berkowitz RL, et al: Prolongation of a preterm pregnancy complicated by death of a single twin in utero and disseminated intravascular coagulation. Effects of treatment with heparin. N Engl J Med 1984;310:772–774.
46. Skelly H, Marivate M, Norman R, et al: Consumptive coagulopathy following fetal death in a triplet pregnancy. Am J Obstet Gynecol 1982;142:595–596.
47. Green D, Lechner K: A survey of 215 non-hemophilic patients with inhibitors to factor VIII. Thromb Haemost 1981;45:200–203.
48. Michiels JJ, Hamulyak K, Nieuwenhuis HK, et al: Acquired haemophilia A in women postpartum: management of bleeding episodes and natural history of the factor VIII inhibitor. Eur J Haematol 1997;59:105–109.
49. Green D, Rademaker AW, Briet E: A prospective, randomized trial of prednisone and cyclophosphamide in the treatment of patients with factor VIII autoantibodies. Thromb Haemost 1993;70:753–757.
50. Green D: Oral immunosuppressive therapy for acquired hemophilia [letter]. Ann Intern Med 1998;128:325.
51. Shaffer LG, Phillips MD: Successful treatment of acquired hemophilia with oral immunosuppressive therapy. Ann Intern Med 1997;127:206–209.
52. Schulman S, Langevitz P, Livneh A, et al: Cyclosporine therapy for acquired factor VIII inhibitor in a patient with systemic lupus erythematosus. Thromb Haemost 1996;76:344–346.
53. Lian EC-Y, Larcada AF, Chiu AY-Z: Combination immunosuppressive therapy after factor VIII infusion for acquired factor VIII inhibitor. Ann Intern Med 1989;110:774–778.
54. Gordon EM, Al-Batniji F, Goldsmith JC: Continuous infusion of monoclonal antibody–purified factor VIII: rational approach to serious hemorrhage in patients with allo-/auto-antibodies to factor VIII. Am J Hematol 1994;45:142–145.
55. Morrison AE, Ludlam CA, Kessler C: Use of porcine factor VIII in the treatment of patients with acquired hemophilia. Blood 1993;81:1513–1520.
56. Negrier C, Goudemand J, Sultan Y, et al: Multicenter retrospective study on the utilization of FEIBA in France in patients with factor VIII and factor IX inhibitors. Thromb Haemost 1997;77:1113–1119.
57. Shapiro AD, Gilchrist GS, Hoots WK, et al: Prospective, randomised trial of two doses of rFVIIa (NovoSeven) in haemophilia patients with inhibitors undergoing surgery. Thromb Haemost 1998;80:773–778.
58. Key NG, Aledort LM, Beardsley D, et al: Home treatment of mild to moderate bleeding episodes using recombinant factor VIIa (Novoseven) in haemophiliacs with inhibitors. Thromb Haemost 1998;80:912–918.
59. Chediak J, Ashenhurst JB, Garlick I, Desser RK: Successful management of bleeding in a patient with factor V inhibitor by platelet transfusions. Blood 1980;56:835–841.
60. Edson JR, Vogt JM, Hasegawa DK: Abnormal prothrombin crossed-immunoelectrophoresis in patients with lupus inhibitors. Blood 1984;64:807–816.
61. Bajaj SP, Rapaport SI, Fierer DS, et al: A mechanism for the hypoprothrombinemia of the acquired hypoprothrombinemia-lupus anticoagulant syndrome. Blood 1983;61:684–692.
62. Fleck RA, Rapaport SI, Rao VM: Anti-prothrombin antibodies and the lupus anticoagulant. Blood 1988;72:512–519.
63. Bajaj SP, Rapaport SI, Barclay S, Herbst KD: Acquired hypoprothrombinemia due to nonneutralizing antibodies to prothrombin: mechanism and management. Blood 1985;65:1538–1543.
64. Lee MT, Nardi MA, Hu G, et al: Transient hemorrhagic diathesis associated with an inhibitor of prothrombin with lupus anticoagulant in an 12-year-old girl: report of a case and review of the literature. Am J Hematol 1996;51:307–314.
65. Bernini JC, Buchanan GR, Ashcroft J: Hypoprothrombinemia and severe hemorrhage associated with a lupus anticoagulant. J Pediatr 1993;123:937–939.
66. Lorand L: Acquired inhibitors of fibrin stabilization: a class of hemorrhagic disorders of diverse origins. In Green D (ed): Anticoagulants: Physiologic, Pathologic, and Pharmacologic. Boca Raton, Fla, CRC Press, 1994, pp 169–191.
67. McDonagh J: Hereditary and acquired deficiencies of activated factor XIII. In Beutler E, Lichtman MA, Coller BS, Kipps TJ (eds): Williams' Hematology, 5th ed. New York, McGraw-Hill, 1995, pp 1455–1458.
68. Abbondanzo SL, Gootenberg JE, Lofts RS, McPherson RA: Intracranial hemorrhage in congenital deficiency of factor XIII. Am J Pediatr Hematol Oncol 1988;10:65–68.
69. Larsen PD, Wallace JW, Frankel LS, Crisp D: Factor XIII deficiency and intracranial hemorrhage in infancy. Pediatr Neurol 1990;6:277–278.
70. Baglin T: Management of warfarin (coumarin) overdose. Blood Rev 1998;12:91–98.
71. Roberts HR, Bingham MD: Other coagulation factor deficiencies. In Loscalzo J, Schafer AI (eds): Thrombosis and Hemorrhage, 2nd ed. Philadelphia, Williams & Wilkins, 1998, pp 773–802.
72. Butler AC, Tait RC: Management of oral anticoagulant–induced intracranial haemorrhage. Blood Rev 1998;12:35–44.
73. Wijdicks EFM, Schievink WI, Brown RD, Mullany CJ: The dilemma of discontinuation of anticoagulation therapy for patients with intracranial hemorrhage and mechanical heart valves. Neurosurgery 1998;42:769–773.
74. Babcock J, Hartman K, Pedersen A, et al: Rodenticide-induced coagulopathy in a young child: A case of Munchausen syndrome by proxy. Am J Pediatr Hematol Oncol 1993;15:126–130.
75. Nieuwenhuis HK, Albada J, Banga JD, Sixma JJ: Identification of risk factors for bleeding during treatment of acute venous thromboembolism with heparin or low molecular weight heparin. Blood 1991;78:2337–2343.
76. Campbell NRC, Hull RD, Brant R, et al: Aging and heparin-related bleeding. Arch Intern Med 1996;156:857–860.
77. Levine MN, Raskob G, Landefeld S, Kearon C: Hemorrhagic complications of anticoagulant treatment. Chest 1998;114:511s–523s.
78. Hirsh J, Warkentin KE, Raschke R, et al: Heparin and low-molecular-weight heparin. Mechanisms of action, pharmacokinetics, dosing considerations, monitoring, efficacy, and safety. Chest 1998;114:489s–510s.
79. Wolzt M, Weltermann A, Nieszpaur-Los M, et al: Studies on the neutralizing effects of protamine on unfractionated and low molecular weight heparin (Fragmin®) at the site of activation of the coagulation system in man. Thromb Haemost 1995;73:439–443.

80. Vandermeulen EP, Van Aken H, Vermylen J: Anticoagulants and spinal-epidural anesthesia. Anesth Analg 1994;79:1165–1177.

81. Horlocker TT, Heit JA: Low molecular weight heparin: biochemistry, pharmacology, perioperative prophylaxis regimens, and guidelines for regional anesthetic management. Anesth Analg 1997;85:874–875.

82. Horlocker TT, Wedel DJ: Spinal and epidural blockade and perioperative low molecular weight heparin: smooth sailing on the *Titanic*. Anesth Analg 1998;86:1153–1156.

83. Danhof M, deBoer A, Magnani HN, Stiekema JCJ: Pharmacokinetic considerations on Orgaran (Org 10172) therapy. Hemostasis 1992;22:73–84.

84. Med Lett 1997;39:94.

85. Chong BH, Magnani HN: Orgaran in heparin-induced thrombocytopenia. Hemostasis 1992;22:85–91.

86. deValk HW, Banga JD, Wester WJ, et al: Comparing subcutaneous danaparoid with intravenous unfractionated heparin for the treatment of venous thromboembolism (a randomized controlled trial). Ann Intern Med 1995;123:1–9.

87. Jackson MR, Danby CA, Alving BA: Heparinoid anticoagulation and topical fibrin sealant in heparin-induced thrombocytopenia. Ann Thorac Surg 1997;64:1815–1817.

88. Greinacher A, Volpel H, Janssens U, et al: Recombinant hirudin (lepirudin) provides safe and effective anticoagulation in patients with heparin-induced thrombocytopenia: A prospective study. Circulation 1999;99:73–80.

89. Vanholder R, Camez A, Veys N, et al: Pharmacokinetics of recombinant hirudin in hemodialyzed end-stage renal failure patients. Thromb Haemost 1997;77:650–655.

90. Vanholder R, Camez A, Veys N, et al: Recombinant hirudin: a specific thrombin inhibiting anticoagulant for hemodialysis. Kidney Int 1994;45:1754–1759.

91. Potzsch B, Riess FC, Volpel H, et al: Recombinant hirudin as anticoagulant during open-heart surgery. Thromb Haemost 1995;73:1456a.

92. Parent F, Bridey F, Dreyfus M, et al: Treatment of severe venous thromboembolism with intravenous hirudin (HBW 023): an open pilot study. Thromb Haemost 1993;70:386–388.

93. Hijikata-Okunomiya A, Okamoto S: A strategy for a rational approach to designing synthetic selective inhibitors. Semin Thromb Hemost 1992;18:135–149.

94. Hursting MJ, Joffrion JL, Brooks RL, Swan SK: Effect of renal function on the pharmacokinetics and pharmacodynamics of argatroban (a direct thrombin inhibitor). Blood 1996;88:167a.

95. Matsuo T, Kario K, Chikahira Y, et al: Treatment of heparin-induced thrombocytopenia by use of argatroban, a synthetic thrombin inhibitor. Br J Haematol 1992;82:627–629.

96. Lewis BE, Iaffaldano R, McKiernan TL, et al: Report of successful use of argatroban as an alternative anticoagulant during coronary stent implantation in a patient with heparin-induced thrombocytopenia and thrombosis syndrome. Cathet Cardiovasc Diagn 1996;38:206–209.

97. The EPISTENT Investigators: Randomised placebo-controlled and balloon-angioplasty-controlled trial to assess safety of coronary stenting with use of platelet glycoprotein-IIb/IIIa blockade. Lancet 1998;352:87–92.

98. PRISM-Plus Study Investigators: Inhibition of the platelet glycoprotein IIb/IIIa receptor with tirofiban in unstable angina and non–Q-wave myocardial infarction. N Engl J Med 1998;338:1488–1497.

99. The RESTORE Investigators: Effects of platelet glycoprotein IIb/IIIa blockade with tirofiban on adverse cardiac events in patients with unstable angina or acute myocardial infarction undergoing coronary angioplasty. Circulation 1997;96:1445–1453.

100. The PURSUIT Trial Investigators: Inhibition of platelet glycoprotein IIb/IIIa with eptifibatide in patients with acute coronary syndromes. N Engl J Med 1998;339:436–443.

101. Kleiman NS: Pharmacokinetics and pharmacodynamics of glycoprotein IIb-IIIa inhibitors. Am Heart J 1999;13:S263–S275.

102. Ferguson JJ, Kereiakes DJ, Adgey AAJ, et al: Safe use of platelet GP IIb/IIIa inhibitors. Am Heart J 1998;135:s77–s89.

103. Gammie JS, Zenati M, Kormos RL, et al: Abciximab and excessive bleeding in patients undergoing emergency cardiac operations. Ann Thorac Surg 1998;65:465–469.

104. Madan M, Berkowitz SD: Understanding thrombocytopenia and antigenicity with glycoprotein IIb-IIIA inhibitors. Am Heart J 1999;138:S317–S326.

105. Berkowitz SD, Harrington RA, Rund MM, Tcheng JE: Acute profound thrombocytopenia after c7E3 Fab (abciximab) therapy. Circulation 1997;95:809–813.

106. Quinn MJ, Fitzgerald DJ: Ticlopidine and clopidogrel. Circulation 1999;100:1667–1672.

107. Bennett CL, Weinberg PD, Rozenberg-Ben-Dror K, et al: Thrombotic thrombocytopenic purpura associated with ticlopidine. A review of 60 cases. Ann Intern Med 1998;128:541–544.

108. Gent M, Beaumont D, Blanchard J, et al: A randomised, blinded, trial of clopidogrel versus aspirin in patients at risk of ischaemic events (CAPRIE). Lancet 1996;348:1329–1339.

109. Savcic M, Hauert J, Bachmann F, et al: Clopidogrel loading dose regimens: kinetic profile of pharmacodynamic response in healthy subjects. Semin Thromb Hemost 1999;25(Suppl 2):15–19.

110. Cattaneo M, Gachet C: ADP receptors and clinical bleeding disorders. Arterioscler Thromb Vasc Biol 1999;19:2281–2285.

Chapter 27

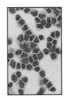

Obstetric and Intrauterine Transfusion

Nancy C. Rose

Transfusion therapy in obstetrics affects the pregnant woman, the developing fetus, and the neonate. Although various hematologic diseases can predispose a pregnant woman to the need for transfusion, healthy pregnant women at term can experience significant blood loss that also requires transfusion. Furthermore, various hematologic disorders may require that transfusions be given to the developing fetus during pregnancy or to the neonate after delivery. Within the context of this chapter, the reader should become familiar with the concepts of obstetric hemorrhage and the physiologic changes in pregnancy that protect the patient from the need for transfusion, as well as the manner in which some hematologic diseases can affect both the patient and her offspring, necessitating transfusion.

■ Gestational Physiology

A rigorous understanding of the normal physiologic changes in pregnancy and their effect on the mother and developing fetus is essential when evaluating and giving care during pregnancy. These changes are designed to protect the parturient from obstetric hemorrhage either before or during labor and delivery. Hemorrhage is the third leading cause of maternal mortality in the United States and causes 30% of maternal mortality worldwide.[1] The expected mean blood loss from a spontaneous vaginal delivery is about 500 mL, whereas the mean blood loss from a routine cesarean section is about 1000 mL. Cesarean hysterectomy, a procedure most often performed due to maternal hemorrhage, has a mean blood loss of 1500 mL or more.[2] At term, 600 mL/min of blood circulates through the placental bed.

At approximately 10 weeks of gestation, the maternal plasma volume begins to increase until it plateaus at 30 to 34 weeks' gestation. The mean increase in plasma volume is about 50%, with a greater increase occurring in multiple gestations. The erythrocyte (RBC) mass also begins to increase at about 10 weeks and continues until term. The increase in RBC mass helps provide for the increase in oxygen transport to the fetus. The total iron requirement is 700 to 1400 mg, with the majority used for RBC mass expansion. The fetus derives its iron solely by active transport across the placenta. It is recommended that women be supplemented with 30 mg of elemental iron daily, which is 100% higher than the recommendation for a nonpregnant woman.[3]

In contrast, platelet volume and function in pregnancy do not change. Because the increase in plasma volume is so much greater than the increase in RBC mass, the hematocrit decreases during gestation, causing the so-called physiologic anemia of pregnancy. This decrease reaches nadir at about 34 weeks' gestation. It is important to note that patients who develop preeclampsia have a smaller amount of plasma volume expansion during gestation but also a greater degree of blood loss at delivery. This is the result of the laboratory changes associated with preeclampsia (e.g., thrombocytopenia), the higher risk for placental abruption secondary to hypertension, and the increased risk for uterine atony secondary to the therapeutic use of magnesium sulfate for this diagnosis.

■ Obstetric Hemorrhage

Antepartum Hemorrhage

Antepartum causes of obstetric bleeding include placenta previa or placental abruption most commonly, although these conditions can also occur at term. The most important information needed for the effective management of obstetric hemorrhage is usually obtained before delivery. An ultrasound is performed to evaluate for placenta previa. Placental abruptions are not generally diagnosed by ultrasound, but by the clinical signs of contractions, pain, and vaginal bleeding. Fetal heart rate monitoring is performed concurrently to evaluate the fetus for tachycardia secondary to blood loss, as well as tocodynometry to evaluate for uterine contractions. A speculum examination is performed to look for signs of vaginal infection or labor causing rapid cervical dilation and resultant bleeding.

Patients identified antenally to be at a higher risk for postpartum hemorrhage should be offered prophylactic autologous blood donation during pregnancy. These include patients with a placenta previa, patients with an anterior placenta that is also covering a prior uterine scar (increasing the risk for placenta accreta and possible hysterectomy), and patients with a history of prior placenta accreta or prior postpartum hemorrhage. These patients should be treated with aggressive iron supplementation, consisting of ferrous sulfate two to three times daily throughout gestation. Blood is donated at least 2 weeks before delivery, and a hematocrit of at least 34% is required.[4] However, it is often difficult for pregnant women to achieve this blood count, owing to the physiologic dilution of RBCs in their increased plasma volume. Autologous blood donation is considered safe during gestation.

Postpartum Hemorrhage

Postpartum hemorrhage is defined as a 10% change in hematocrit or the need for transfusion.[5] Early postpartum hemorrhage is defined as that occurring within the first 24 hours after delivery; late hemorrhage occurs between 24 hours and 6 weeks postpartum.[6] Estimation of blood volume deficit at delivery is sometimes extremely difficult, especially because blood loss may not be obvious from, for example, a high cervical laceration after vaginal delivery. Retroperitoneal bleeding can occur in which there is no evidence of bleeding externally but indirect signs, such as an unstable blood pressure or tachycardia, are present.

Early postpartum hemorrhage is far more common than late postpartum hemorrhage, and it is associated with a greater degree of blood loss and morbidity. The most common cause is uterine atony, which occurs either before or after delivery of the placenta. Atony, or the failure of adequate uterine contraction to decrease blood loss, can be caused by overdistention of the uterus (polyhydramnios, multiple gestation), macrosomia, oxytocin usage, uterine relaxants such as magnesium sulfate, terbutaline, or infectious causes such as chorioamnionitis. Other causes of early postpartum hemorrhage include retained products of conception, genital tract lacerations, uterine rupture or inversion, placenta accreta, and hereditary coagulopathy. Causes of late postpartum hemorrhage include endometritis, retained products of conception, and hereditary coagulopathy.

All patients admitted for labor and delivery should have a blood type and screening determination and a complete blood count performed. Patients with antepartum bleeding should also have a Kleihauer-Betke test performed to assess for the presence and quantity of a fetomaternal hemorrhage (FMH). If the suspicion is great enough that the patient may need a transfusion, as in patient laboring with a history of prior low transverse cesarean section or a patient with placenta previa admitted for cesarean section, blood is typed and cross-matched on admission.

Perhaps the most important issue regarding postpartum bleeding is its recognition. Blood loss is often clinically underestimated by 30% to 50%, and therapeutic interventions can be delayed and complications increased if it is not recognized.[6] After it is observed that the postpartum bleeding is heavier than expected, concurrent steps are performed to evaluate and treat the patient. Intravenous access should be established or maintained. The cause of the blood loss is sought by physical inspection of the lower genital tract for lacerations and by an examination of the placenta to be certain that it was removed intact. Atony is recognized by a flaccid, unresponsive uterus in response to standard postpartum oxytocin infusion.

A speculum examination is performed to evaluate the patient for retained products of conception—which, if present, is treated by manual extraction or curettage with concomitant antibiotic therapy—and for evidence of obstetric trauma such as lacerations of the cervix or uterine rupture, with repairs made as needed. A bimanual examination is then performed to evaluate the patient for uterine atony. If uterine atony is present, the patient is examined for retained products of conception and bimanual massage is begun. Concurrent medical therapy for atony includes continuous intravenous oxytocin, with an initial dose consisting of 20 mU/L in 1000 mL normal saline or lactated Ringer's solution. If the condition does not resolve, 15-methyl prostaglandin $F_{2\alpha}$, 0.25 mg intramuscularly into uterus or muscle, is administered every 15 to 90 minutes, to a maximum of eight doses. Contraindications for prostaglandin therapy include asthma and other active pulmonary, renal, or hepatic disease. Methylergonovine, 0.2 mg intramuscularly, can be given every 2 to 4 hours; this treatment is contraindicated by preeclampsia or chronic hypertension. More aggressive surgical therapies include uterine arterial ligation or hypogastric arterial ligation; both are designed to decrease pulse pressure to the uterine vessels. Uterine packing and selected arterial embolization have been performed in selected cases. Hysterectomy is employed if all other modalities fail to arrest the bleeding.

Blood Component Therapy

Blood component therapy is an integral part of the management of postpartum hemorrhage. The assessment as to when to begin blood product replacement is tailored to the clinical assessment, including the cause of the blood loss, the baseline hemoglobin and hematocrit, the patient's age, the amount of estimated blood loss, and the rapidity with which the blood loss will be controlled. For example, the ratio of infused crystalloid to estimated blood loss should be about 3:1, with urine volume to be maintained at greater than 0.5 mL/kg/hr (or, about 30 mL/hr).

Fresh frozen plasma (FFP) is used only if the patient demonstrates a clotting factor deficiency or if a specific factor concentrate is unavailable. Indications include the reversal of warfarin effects, disseminated intravascular coagulation (DIC), hepatic disease causing a factor deficiency, hemolytic uremic syndrome (HUS), and massive transfusion. A general guideline is that FFP is indicated if the prothrombin time is more than 1.5 times greater than normal. The starting dose is usually 2 bags of FFP. In contrast, cryoprecipitate is indicated only if there is a deficiency of factor VIII, fibrinogen, von Willebrand factor, or factor XIII. The standard dose is 1 bag per 10 kg of body weight. One unit increases fibrinogen by 10 mg/dL. If a coagulopathy is present, FFP should be used empirically, and not cryoprecipitate.

Transfusion with packed RBCs may be appropriate if the baseline hemoglobin is 7 to 9 g/dL, ongoing active bleeding is occurring, or the patient has decreased oxygen-carrying capacity due to chronic lung disease. Packed RBCs are the treatment of choice for acute obstetric hemorrhage, beginning with 1 to 2 units. Each unit increases the hemoglobin concentration by approximately 1 g/dL in a 70-kg woman.[7] FFP is used for massive obstetric hemorrhage (ratio of packed RBCs to FFP, roughly 4:1) and for patients who have a demonstrated factor deficiency or have developed DIC. The usual starting dose is 2 bags of FFP.

Platelets are given to control or prevent bleeding if there is a deficiency in either the volume or function of platelets. If an operative delivery is planned, platelet transfusion may be indicated if the platelet count is less than 50,000/μL. One unit of platelet concentrate increases the count of a 70-kg woman by 5000 to 10,000/μL. Therefore, the usual dose is 1 unit per 10 kg of body weight, beginning with 6 to 8 units. Because small amounts of RBCs (enough to sensitize an Rh-negative woman) can be present in platelet concentrates, platelets must be Rh-specific. If type-specific platelets are unavailable, a standard 300-μg dose of Rh immune globin should be administered to prevent sensitization in an Rh-negative woman.

■ Approach to Fetal Hemolytic Disease

Fetomaternal Hemorrhage

Approximately 75% of women demonstrate evidence of FMH during gestation or at parturition.[8] In 60% of cases, the amount of fetal blood in the maternal circulation is less than 0.1 mL. In fewer than 1% of cases is more than 5 mL transferred, and only 0.25% of women have more than 30 mL of fetal blood in the maternal circulation. The incidence and size of FMH increases as a pregnancy advances. Although FMH can occur spontaneously, complications and procedures that increase a patient's risk include vaginal bleeding due to placenta previa, placental abruption, or other cause; prenatal diagnostic procedures such as chorionic villous sampling, amniocentesis, and umbilical blood sampling; external podalic version; multiple gestations; manual extraction of the placenta; and cesarean section. However, the majority of cases occur in patients without risk factors who have an uncomplicated spontaneous vaginal delivery.

Hemolytic Disease of the Newborn

Hemolytic disease of the newborn (HDN) is defined as neonatal anemia and hyperbilirubinemia, caused by an incompatibility between maternal and fetal RBCs. More than 60% of the cases of HDN are caused by ABO incompatibility, although many other fetoantibodies can initiate this disease. Clinically apparent HDN is mostly confined to the situation in which the mother is type O, generating both anti-A and anti-B antibodies, and the fetus is either type A or type B. Approximately 20% to 25% of all pregnancies are ABO-incompatible. Most ABO-incompatible pregnancies are mild in manifestation, because these antibodies are generally of the immunoglobulin M (IgM) class and therefore do not cross the placenta. Because ABO incompatibility does not cause fetal anemia, it is regarded as a neonatal rather than an obstetric disease. A and B antigens occur on other cell membranes in addition to RBCs, and type A or B sensitization does not

require a prior exposure to RBCs via gestation or transfusion. Therefore, in contrast to Rh sensitization, ABO hemolytic disease can affect a first pregnancy.

The clinical manifestations of HDN occur most often in the first 24 to 48 hours of life and usually include mild to moderate anemia and hyperbilirubinemia. Very high levels of bilirubin can cause kernicterus, with preterm infants being the most susceptible. The natural history of kernicterus was described in relation to Rh hemolytic disease by Bowman and colleagues[9] in 1965. Of those neonates who develop kernicterus, 90% will die, and the survivors will develop severe neurologic complications such as mental retardation, choreoathetosis, and sensory-neural deafness. Phototherapy is the first line of treatment, with exchange transfusions rarely indicated. Because ABO incompatibility can occur in subsequent gestations, it should be documented in the patient's medical record. However, because its severity is limited, checking of maternal antibody titers or analysis of amniotic fluid for hemolysis is not indicated.

Erythroblastosis Fetalis

Erythroblastosis fetalis is the intrauterine manifestation of HDN. It is defined by intrauterine fetal edema and subsequent neonatal hyperbilirubinemia and anemia, caused by maternal antibodies that cross the placenta and hemolyze fetal RBCs. Although many RBC antigens have been described (Table 27.1),[10] only a few are clinically important causes of maternal isoimmunization. The most common of these are the Rh, Kell, Kidd, and Duffy series. Of the minor antigens, the vast majority cause sensitivity via exposure from a prior blood transfusion. The same management plan, including serial Coombs titers and often amniocenteses, is used for the irregular antibodies as described later for Rh sensitization. Like the Rh locus, Kell has been genetically characterized; therefore, the fetus' phenotype for the Kell antigen can be determined antenally by molecular diagnosis.[11] This information cannot yet be obtained for most of the other known RBC antigens.

Rhesus Sensitization

The Rh antigen, the most common cause of erythroblastosis fetalis, has been genetically characterized on the short arm of chromosome 1.[12] The genes coding for the Rh locus lie in tandem, with the first coding for Rh CcEe, followed by Rh D. Patients who are Rh D–negative lack the D locus on both alleles. The Rh gene complex is described by various combinations of these genes. Multiple allelic variations of the Rh gene exist, but perhaps the most clinically common is the Du variant, also known as "weak D positive." The RBCs of most Du-positive individuals have a quantitative decrease in the amount of D antigen sites. Therefore, some of the D antigen is expressed, so these patients are treated as if they were Rh D–positive and are not given RhoGAM (Rh immune globulin) prophylaxis.

The genotypes for the Rh locus are described as pairs of gene complexes, with each chromosome contributing a combination of one of the five CcDEe genes. The most common Rh genotypes are CDe/cde and CDe/CDe, with approximately 55% of all Caucasians having the phenotype of the CcDE or CDe Rh proteins.[13] About 15% of Caucasians are Rh-negative, as are 8% of African Americans and 1% to 2% of Asian Americans. About 60% of those who are Rh-positive are heterozygous for the Rh factor, and 40% are homozygous.

Table 27.1   Non-Rh Blood Group Antigens That Can Cause Isoimmunization

Blood Group System	Antigens Related to Hemolytic Disease of the Newborn	Severity of Hemolytic Disease	Proposed Management
Lewis*			
Kell	K	Mild to severe with hydrops fetalis	Amniotic fluid bilirubin studies
	k	Mild only	Expectant
	K$_0$	Mild only	Expectant
	Kp^a	Mild only	Expectant
	Kp^b	Mild only	Expectant
	Js^a	Mild only	Expectant
	Js^b	Mild only	Expectant
Duffy	Fy^a	Mild to severe with hydrops fetalis	Amniotic fluid bilirubin studies
	Fy^{b+}		
Kidd	Jk^a	Mild to severe	Amniotic fluid bilirubin studies
	Jk^b	Mild to severe	Amniotic fluid bilirubin studies
MNSs	M	Mild to severe	Amniotic fluid bilirubin studies
	N$^+$		
	S	Mild to severe	Amniotic fluid bilirubin studies
	s	Mild to severe	Amniotic fluid bilirubin studies
	U	Mild to severe	Amniotic fluid bilirubin studies
	Mi^a	Moderate	Amniotic fluid bilirubin studies
	Mt^a	Moderate	Amniotic fluid bilirubin studies
	Vw	Mild only	Expectant
Lutheran	Lu^a	Mild only	Expectant
	Lu^b	Mild only	Expectant
Diego	Di^a	Mild to severe	Amniotic fluid bilirubin studies
	Di^b	Mild only	Expectant
Xg	Xg^a	Mild only	Expectant
Public antigens	Yt^a	Moderate to severe	Amniotic fluid bilirubin studies
	Lan	Mild only	Expectant
	Ge	Mild only	Expectant
	Co^a	Severe	Amniotic fluid bilirubin studies
Private antigens	Batty	Mild only	Expectant
	Becker	Mild only	Expectant
	Berrens	Mild only	Expectant
	Biles	Moderate	Amniotic fluid bilirubin studies
	Evans	Mild only	Expectant
	Gonzales	Mild only	Expectant
	Good	Severe	Amniotic fluid bilirubin studies
	Heibel	Moderate	Amniotic fluid bilirubin studies
	Hunt	Mild only	Expectant
	Jobbins	Mild only	Expectant
	Radin	Moderate	Amniotic fluid bilirubin studies
	Rm	Mild only	Expectant
	Ven	Mild only	Expectant
	Wright	Severe	Amniotic fluid bilirubin studies
	Zd	Moderate	Amniotic fluid bilirubin studies

*Not a proven cause of hemolytic disease.
+Not a cause of hemolytic disease.
From Weinstein L: Irregular antibodies causing hemolytic disease of the newborn: A continuing problem. Clin Obstet Gynecol 1982;25:321, with permission.

Theoretically, an Rh-negative Caucasian woman has about a 60% chance of carrying an Rh-positive fetus. However, as many as 30% of Rh-negative women are physiologic non-responders; that is, they do not become sensitized when exposed to Rh-positive blood. Also, ABO incompatibility is protective against Rh sensitization. It has been suggested that ABO-incompatible cells are more rapidly cleared and therefore are not available to develop an antigen-mediated reaction.

Rh Immune Globulin Before the use of Rh immune globulin, about 0.5% to 1% of all women were isoimmunized.[14] According to the Centers for Disease Control and Prevention, the incidence of HDN in 1984 was 10.6 per 10,000 total births, a ratio that has remained relatively constant.[15] Rh immune globulin is a passively administered antibody that prevents active immunization. Although the precise mechanism of this antibody-mediated immune suppression (AMIS) is not understood, it is thought to involve central inhibition. Theoretically, fetal RBCs become covered with anti-D immune globulin and are filtered out of the circulation. This suppresses the primary immune response. The usual dose of Rh immune globulin is 300 μg, which should protect against 30 mL of an FMH. However, for first-trimester pregnancy losses or terminations and for chorionic villous sampling, 50 μg Rh immune globulin can be used. Once the second trimester is reached, only the 300-μg dose should be used. Routine Rh prophylaxis can be given up to 72 hours after exposure. This information is derived from early prison studies,[16] in which patients were evaluated every 3 days after an exposure to Rh-positive blood cells. To be effective, the immune globulin must be given before the primary immune response from the exposure occurs. If, for some reason, Rh immune globulin is not given to the patient when it is indicated, it can be given up to 28 days after delivery to avoid sensitization.[17]

Management of Pregnancy in the Rh-Negative, Unsensitized Woman At the first prenatal visit, every pregnant patient should have her blood type and antibody status determined. These tests should be repeated with each new pregnancy, because antibody status can change. An Rh-negative, Du-negative, antibody-negative patient should receive Rh immune globulin prophylaxis at 28 weeks of gestation and again immediately postpartum. When the patient is admitted for delivery, her antibody status and then the blood type of the neonate are determined. If the patient has no antibodies and the fetus is Rh-positive, 300 μg of RhoGAM is given. After delivery, the mother is screened for excessive FMH by the RBC rosette test. If the result is positive, a Kleihauer-Betke test is used to quantitate the amount of fetal cells in the maternal circulation. Up to 1% of deliveries have greater than 30 mL of whole blood in a FMH, and RhoGAM doses are modified by the degree of hemorrhage.

Fetal Assessment in the Rh-Immunized Gestation If a patient's antibody screen is positive, an indirect determination of the Coombs titer is performed. The so-called critical titer—the titer at which the fetus is at risk for severe fetal hemolysis from isoimmunization—differs slightly by laboratory but is generally considered to be 1:8 or higher. If the titer is less than 1:8, the determinations are repeated monthly. Paternal zygosity testing is simultaneously performed to determine whether the father is Rh-positive or -negative, and, if positive, whether he is homozygous or heterozygous for the D allele. If the father is Rh-negative, no further testing is indicated. If he is heterozygous for the D allele, the couple has a 50% chance of carrying an Rh-negative fetus. If he is a homozygote for the D allele, then all offspring will be Rh-positive.

Once a titer of about 1:8 is reached, the patient is offered amniocentesis to test for fetal hemolysis. If she is undergoing prenatal diagnosis for another indication, Rh typing by DNA analysis can be performed at the same time, by obtaining either chorionic villi or amniocytes. If the patient has no other indication for early prenatal diagnosis, then DNA analysis can be performed at the time of the first amniocentesis for hemolysis. If the fetus is Rh-negative by DNA analysis, no further invasive testing is required, although serial scans are still performed every 2 to 4 weeks to evaluate for hydrops in case of a laboratory error. If the fetus is Rh-positive, serial amniocenteses are performed to evaluate the degree of hemolysis. The obstetric history is essential in the management of these patients: those who have had an affected child usually exhibit earlier hemolysis with subsequent gestations. If there is a history of a prior hydropic fetus, then the chance that the next fetus will be hydropic is greater than 80%.[18]

Amniotic Fluid Analysis Bevis,[19] in 1956, originally noted that spectrophotometric determinants of amniotic fluid bilirubin correlated with the degree of hemolysis. On a semilogarithmic plot, the optical density curve of normal amniotic fluid is linear

between 525 and 375 nm. Bilirubin causes a shift in the spectophotometric density, with a wavelength peak at 450 nm (called the ΔOD450).

Liley[20] retrospectively correlated ΔOD450 measurements with neonatal outcome by dividing the graph into three zones.[21] Unaffected and mildly affected fetuses plot in zone 1; those moderately affected plot in zone 2, and those severely affected in zone 3 (Fig. 27.1). Liley's data began at about 28 weeks' gestation, and other groups have extrapolated the curve to earlier gestations, with varied success. Therefore, the majority of amniocenteses to evaluate for hemolysis begin in the third trimester.

For patients with low titers who are at low risk for fetal hydrops, management includes ultrasound examinations every 2 to 4 weeks until 26 to 28 weeks, followed by an amniocentesis for a baseline ΔOD450 value and for Rh typing if it has not already been done. The timing of repeat procedures depends on the severity of the hemolysis. Intravascular transfusion by umbilical blood sampling is indicated if the value is in zone 3 or if the fetus exhibits hydrops, ensuring a hemoglobin concentration of less than 5 g/dL. However, half of fetuses with a hemoglobin value lower than 5 g/dL are not hydropic, so ultrasound is not necessarily an accurate indicator of fetal well-being. The graphs are determined for Rh-sensitized patients and not from other antigens. Therefore, the data when used to evaluate patients with Kell, Kidd, or Duffy isoimmunization should always be interpreted with caution. As with ΔOD450 values obtained before 26 weeks' gestation, the Liley curves for other types of isoimmunization should be used to evaluate trends from serial procedures and not to interpret individual values.

Fetal Transfusion Fetal intravascular transfusion corrects anemia, increases fetal oxygenation, and downregulates the hematopoietic system, thereby decreasing extramedullary demand, decreasing portal venous pressure, and increasing blood circulation. Both intraperitoneal and intravascular

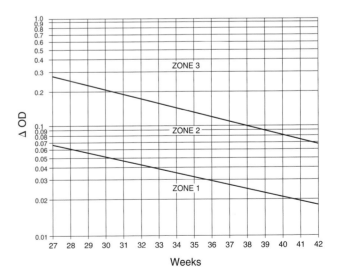

Figure 27.1 Liley graph used to plot degree of isoimmunization. (From American College of Obstetrics and Gynecology. Management of isoimmunization in pregnancy. ACOG Technical Bulletin 227. Washington, DC: ACOG, 1996, with permission.)

transfusion techniques have been described. In the absence of hydrops, 80% to 100% survival rates have been reported with each method.[22] Hydropic fetuses do show increased survival with an intravascular transfusion.[23] Furthermore, because the intravascular approach is used for other procedures, clinicians have better proficiency with it and use it more readily. Further advantages of the intravascular approach include the following: a direct measurement of fetal hematocrit can be obtained, the fetal blood type can be determined if not already assessed, and accurate calculations can be used to determine the amount of blood that needs to be transfused.

In general, O-negative, cytomegalovirus-negative, irradiated donor blood or maternal blood is used for transfusion. The RBCs are washed to remove antibody and are packed to achieve a hematocrit of 0.75 to 0.85, then filtered through a leuko-reduction filter before use. Once the hematocrit of the blood is known, the blood volume to be transfused can be determined from a Nomogram by Nicolaides[24] (Fig. 27.2), with the goal being a post-transfusion hematocrit of 40% to 45%.

After transfusion, the decline in RBCs depends on the lifespan of the RBCs—that is, the ratio of donor to fetal RBCs. MacGregor and colleagues[25] used the following equation to predict the fetal hematocrit:

$$Hct\ predicted = HctF \times \left(\frac{EFW1}{EFW2}\right) \times \left(\frac{120 - days\ elapsed}{120}\right)$$

where HctF is the post-transfusion hematocrit, EFW1 is the fetal weight at the index transfusion, and EFW2 is the weight at the subsequent transfusion.

On average, the drop in fetal hematocrit after the first transfusion is about 1.5% per day. After multiple transfusions, this decrease is 1.0% to 1.2% per day. From such calculations, the interval between transfusions is scheduled to maintain the hematocrit at 25% to 30% or higher.

The procedure carries serious risk for morbidity and mortality.[26] The mortality rate is about 1% to 5% for each transfusion, and morbidity is approximately 10% to 15%, including fetal bradycardia, premature labor, and premature leakage of fluid.

■ Thrombocytopenia

Thrombocytopenia is a disorder that involves either decreased production or accelerated destruction of platelets; it is defined as a platelet count less than normal for the laboratory used (usually about 150,000 platelets/μL). Maternal thrombocytopenia may or may not affect the fetus, and a thorough understanding of the cause of the thrombocytopenia is essential for appropriate antenatal and postnatal management. Neonatal passive immune thrombocytopenia depends on the type of maternal disease generating the antibodies—most commonly, the alloimmune and autoimmune thrombocytopenias.

Benign Thrombocytopenia of Pregnancy

Incidental, or benign, thrombocytopenia of pregnancy (BTP) is the most common cause of thrombocytopenia during gestation, occurring in 60 to 70 women for every 1000 live births.[27] The maternal platelet counts typically return to normal in about 6 weeks after delivery. This entity was originally

described in 1993 by Burrows and Kelton,[27] who identified it in healthy women with no other obvious signs of systemic disease. This disorder has a mild presentation, with most platelet counts between 70,000 to 150,000/μL.[28] The mechanism of BTP is unknown. It has been suggested that this

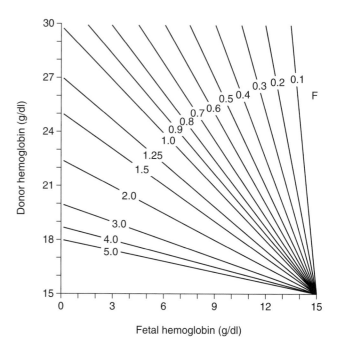

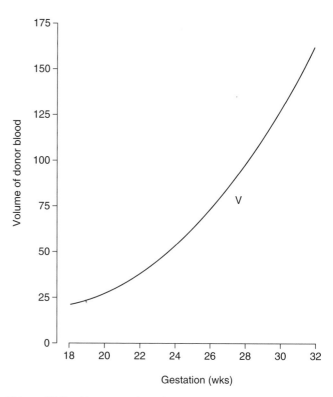

Figure 27.2 Nomogram for calculating volume of donor blood (in milliliters) necessary to correct fetal anemia. The value F (obtained from the top graph) is multiplied by the value V (bottom graph). (From Nicolaides KH, Clewell WH, Mibashan RS, et al: Fetal haemoglobin measurement in the assessment of red cell isoimmunization. Lancet 1988;1:1073, with permission.)

disorder results from a more rapid destruction of platelets during gestation or from the dilutional effect of the normal increase in maternal blood volume (40% to 60%).

Management of BTP includes repeating the platelet count each trimester as a method of identifying another cause for the thrombocytopenia. If the platelet count at initial presentation is lower than about 100,000/μL, a thorough search for systemic diseases that might be causing the thrombocytopenia is performed, including a detailed drug history; evaluation for lupus, other autoimmune disorders (e.g., antiphospholipid syndrome), other medical conditions (e.g., human immunodeficiency virus [HIV] infection), and the leukemias, as well as viral and protozoal infections through a travel history; a family history regarding autosomal dominant inherited disorders such as the May-Hegglin anomaly; and evaluation of current conditions such as preeclampsia or, in an ill patient, HUS. Included in the history are questions regarding easy bruisability and a physical examination for petechiae.

There is often a significant overlap of platelet counts in BTP and in idiopathic thrombocytopenic purpura (ITP), which can occur regardless of pregnancy and can also result in counts in the range of 70,000 to 100,000/μL. These two disorders at times may be indistinguishable. However, because the neonatal outcomes for BTP and for mild ITP are both benign, the ability to differentiate between these disorders during gestation is less meaningful. Patients may undergo regional anesthesia, and they require no special alteration in pregnancy and delivery management. A neonatal platelet count is performed on cord blood at delivery, and no other invasive testing is required.

Idiopathic Thrombocytopenia Purpura and Pregnancy

ITP is the most common immunologically mediated thrombotic condition during gestation.[29] The majority of these patients who present are women of reproductive age: 72% of patients older than 10 years are women, and 70% of those women are younger than 40 years of age.[30] In women, symptoms include refractory menorrhagia, petechiae, gingival bleeding, epistaxis, or a history of easy bruising. The platelets that remain in circulation function normally, but decreased numbers of them are available secondary to autoantibodies directed against platelet surface antigens. In order to establish this diagnosis, a thorough history is obtained to exclude other causes of thrombocytopenia. Immune conditions that may be associated with thrombocytopenia include the antiphospholipid syndrome, lymphoproliferative diseases, systemic lupus erythematosus, HIV, and other viral syndromes. A review of medication usage is essential, because many therapeutic as well as illicit drugs can cause thrombocytopenia. In pregnancy, the overlap with gestational thrombocytopenia has already been mentioned, and the association with hypertension is discussed later. Repeated platelet counts are usually persistently less than 100,000/μL; coagulation studies are normal; and an increased number of megakaryocytes are noted on bone marrow biopsy. The presence of antiplatelet antibodies is not required for the diagnosis of ITP but can contribute to its determination. They are present in approximately 80% of these patients[30] and do not affect the clinical management. Most autoantibodies are directed against epitopes on glycoprotein (GP) IIb-IIIa, which is also the most ubiquitous and immunogenic platelet surface antigen.[31]

Significant bleeding requiring transfusion is unusual unless the platelet count is less than 10,000/μL.[32] Platelet counts persistently greater than 50,000/μL are rarely associated with significant bleeding and are usually managed expectantly. Steroids, given either intravenously or orally, are added if counts are significantly lower than 50,000/μL, and medication use is tailored to the clinical situation as well as the patient's age and health status. About 25% of patients given glucocorticoids respond to therapy, defined as achieving a platelet count greater than 100,000/μL during the therapeutic course.[29] Patients who need prolonged steroid courses or who do not respond to treatment are offered splenectomy.

The disease course is unaffected by pregnancy. However, antenatal management, because of the largely theoretical risk of fetal intracranial hemorrhage (ICH), has been extremely controversial. The autoantibodies generated are of the IgG class, so they readily cross the placenta. Fetuses can develop a decreased platelet count, and the various modalities used to indirectly assess the degree of fetal thrombocytopenia (including the presence of autoantibodies and the degree of maternal disease) are notoriously inaccurate. The neonatal platelet count is decreased in up to 70% of neonates whose mothers had ITP[34] and reaches a nadir at 4 to 6 days after delivery. Although breast-feeding is also associated with thrombocytopenia, owing to the passage of IgG through colostrum,[33] it is not discouraged in these patients. In a population-based study of 15,932 pregnancies, no child born to a woman with ITP had a bleeding complication, and the three infants with ICH all had mothers with alloimmune thrombocytopenia (ATP).[34] In a review of studies of ITP by Silver and colleagues,[35] 14 (3.1%) of 447 neonates had a bleeding complication, and 0.9% (4 patients) had an ICH. In a review of 288 cases in which the mother had ITP and the fetal platelet count was determined at delivery, there were no instances of ICH.[36]

Cook and colleagues,[38] in 1991, reviewed 31 patients with ITP at their institution for the risk of neonatal ICH by mode of delivery. Eighteen of the 31 patients were delivered by cesarean section and the remainder by vaginal delivery. In all, 6 neonates had significant thrombocytopenia, but no episodes of ICH were noted. The authors then reviewed the literature of the previous 20 years and evaluated 474 cases, finding only 4 instances of ICH, with no statistical difference between the two modes of delivery. The extremely low rate of intracranial bleeding makes evaluation of the data very difficult. Furthermore, there is no documented case to date of antenatal ICH resulting from ITP. Antenatal therapy for this disorder is directed at treatment of the patient, and there is no clear evidence that it is of any benefit to the fetus.

It is not certain whether ITP causes significant fetal or neonatal complications such as ICH. The main risk for the parturient is the risk of hemorrhage at delivery if she is severely thrombocytopenic. Steroids are begun if the platelet counts decline to less than 50,000/μL, with the goal of keeping the count higher than 50,000/μL. Nonpregnant patients with refractory ITP undergo splenectomy.

Fetal scalp sampling during labor has been used to try to identify fetal thrombocytopenia. This technique requires that there be some cervical dilation as well as ruptured membranes and a commitment to delivery. With a transvaginal approach, a small incision is made in the fetal scalp and a sample is obtained from a free flow of blood into a heparinized capillary tube.

Scalp sampling can be very inaccurate, which can result in unnecessary cesarean sections.

Fetal umbilical blood sampling has been performed before delivery to assess the fetal platelet count, but this technique requires significant skill and equipment, and sometimes for technical reasons it cannot be performed late in gestation owing to fetal position or decreased amniotic fluid volume. Procedure-related complications were reported in 2.8% of cordocenteses in patients with ITP,[35] including two of three women who required urgent cesarean section for complications of the procedure with a normal platelet count.

Finally, invasive testing such as fetal scalp sampling and umbilical blood sampling were originally offered on the premise that, if a fetal thrombocytopenia could be identified antenatally, then the patient could be offered an elective cesarean section as a preventive measure against an ICH. However, vaginal delivery has never been proven to be an etiologic factor in intracranial bleeding. Among 474 infants of mothers with ITP, there was no association between route of delivery and neonatal bleeding complications.[37] Furthermore, the baseline risks for cesarean delivery in a thrombocytopenic patient are elevated and include increased risks for maternal hemorrhage requiring transfusion of various types of blood products and resultant secondary infections. Although some cases are still managed with invasive antenatal testing, multiple eloquent arguments have been put forth supporting delivery by cesarean section for obstetric indications only, with no determination of a fetal platelet count at any time during gestation. The risk of neonatal hemorrhage is extremely low, and the benefit of invasive testing probably does not outweigh the risk of significant morbidity and mortality from procedures that do not prevent neonatal bleeding complications.

Thrombocytopenia Associated with Hypertension in Pregnancy

Hypertensive disease affects 7% to 10% of all pregnancies, contributing to substantial perinatal morbidity and mortality. The McMaster study, a prospective analysis of pregnant women in Canada, noted that hypertensive disorders were responsible for 21% of thrombocytopenia in their patients, representing an incidence of 13 to 15 per 1000 live births, or approximately 1% to 2% of all pregnancies.[34] Although the clinical manifestations of hypertension may be similar, it can result from a variety of underlying causes, such as renal disease, chronic essential hypertension, pregnancy-induced hypertension, and preeclampsia.

Second in incidence only to BTP, thrombocytopenia during gestation that is related to hypertension is most commonly associated with preeclampsia[34, 38] and is the most common hematologic abnormality associated with that disorder. Preeclampsia is defined by hypertension (a change of varying severity over the baseline screening antenatal blood pressure), proteinuria, and edema during gestation, and it may be superimposed on chronic hypertension. Although most patients have the usual associated symptoms of preeclampsia, including edema, proteinuria, and hypertension, some have normal or minimally elevated blood pressure and absent proteinuria. Approximately 50% of patients who develop severe preeclampsia manifest thrombocytopenia.[39] Typically the thrombocytopenia noted in the preeclamptic woman is mild to moderate, with platelet counts of 50,000 to 100,000/μL.[40]

A subset of preeclamptic patients may also present with other associated findings, known as the HELLP syndrome, an acronym first described by Weinstein in 1982[41]: **h**emolysis, **e**levated **l**iver functions, and **l**ow **p**latelet count. HELLP syndrome is caused by microangiopathy and is associated with endothelial injury. Intimal injury, caused by a vaso-constricted vascular endothelium, stimulates fibrin deposition, which activates platelets, releasing vasoconstrictive substances including serotonin and thromboxane A_2. In a series of 442 patients with HELLP syndrome, Sibai and colleagues[42] detected laboratory evidence of DIC in 21%. Furthermore, 16% of patients experienced a placental abruption. The cause of the thrombocytopenia in such cases is unknown; it may be a response to platelet consumption or destruction. Bone marrow analysis reveals increased megakaryocytes.[43]

Preeclampsia, depending on gestational age and severity, is treated by delivery. However, delivery management depends on the gestational age at presentation. Patients carrying preterm gestations should be stabilized and transferred to a tertiary care center. Magnesium sulfate is administered for seizure prophylaxis. Blood pressure is controlled by intravenous hydralazine or labetalol. Steroids are given if the gestational age is 34 weeks or less, to enhance fetal maturity and decrease the risk of respiratory distress syndrome and ICH. Monitoring of urine output and intravenous fluids is essential. If the platelet count is extremely low (20,000 to 50,000/μL), platelets should be available for transfusion. However, delivery is usually (but not always) curative, because up to 30% of patients develop manifestations of HELLP within 2 days after delivery.[44]

Maternal platelet counts commonly reach their nadir after delivery. In the series of Martin and associates,[45] 13% of 158 patients experienced a nadir in platelet count on admission, 29% at delivery, 30% on postpartum day 1, and 21% by postpartum day 2. The maternal platelet count usually returns to normal within days after delivery, and thrombocytopenia is not identified in neonatal cord blood sampling of these patients.[46] If the neonatal platelet count is low, then a search for other neonatal causes, such as sepsis or complications of prematurity, is indicated.

Thrombotic Thrombocytopenic Purpura and the Hemolytic Uremic Syndrome

Thrombotic thrombocytopenic purpura (TTP) and HUS are characterized by a microangiopathic hemolytic anemia with severe accompanying thrombocytopenia; the risk for development is not increased by pregnancy. Often these disorders are indistinguishable in presentation, and the cause is unknown. However, because thrombocytopenia is so common in pregnant women, these two disorders must be considered in the evaluation of any woman who presents with severe thrombocytopenia. The classic pentad of findings in TTP occur in approximately 40% of affected patients; about 75% present with the triad of a microangiopathic hemolytic anemia, thrombocytopenia, and neurologic findings,[47] whereas the other two characteristics, fever and renal dysfunction, are seen less commonly. Multiple organ systems develop thrombotic occlusions of arterioles and capillaries. Although the pathophysiology of TTP is unclear, diffuse endothelial damage and fibrinolytic changes are seen in these patients. Weiner[48] reviewed a series of 45 pregnant patients, reporting that the mean gestational age at onset of TTP was 23 weeks and the fetal and maternal mortality rates were 80% and 44%, respectively. However, many of the patients included in this series were treated before the modern therapy of exchange transfusion became available. Although there are no current series reviewing therapy in pregnancy, current management includes plasma infusion and exchange therapy at any gestational age.

In contrast, women with HUS, who usually manifest the triad of microangiopathic hemolytic anemia, acute nephropathy, and thrombocytopenia, most often present in the postpartum period. In Weiner's series,[48] only 9 of 62 cases of HUS developed before delivery. HUS is rarer in adults than in children, and often a milder thrombocytopenia is seen. The majority of HUS cases associated with pregnancy occur at least 2 days after delivery.[49] Supportive therapies such as dialysis, platelet transfusion, and fluid resuscitation are used in the treatment of HUS, with mixed results. Plasma exchange transfusions have been less successful in HUS than in TTP.[50] Perhaps the major difference between these disorders is that 15% to 25% of patients with HUS develop chronic renal disease.[49]

Alloimmune Thrombocytopenia

ATP, with an incidence of 1 in every 2000 deliveries, is the analogue of HDN but affects platelets and not RBCs. The overall mortality rate is 6.5% to 14%.[51] Perhaps the most important distinction between ATP and HDN is that the former can occur in a first pregnancy with serious neonatal consequences. Like Rh sensitization, it is caused by maternal alloimmunization to a paternally transmitted fetal human platelet-specific antigens (HPAs) not present on maternal platelets. This stimulates maternal IgG antibodies, which cross the placenta and coat fetal platelets, which are then either destroyed or removed from the circulation. Whether antibodies attack and alter megakaryocytes is uncertain.[52] However, in contrast to Rh alloimmunization, antibody titers are not predictive of the degree of fetal thrombocytopenia.

Expression of the antigens occurs by 19 weeks' gestation.[53] The antigens that cause ATP are generated from platelet glycoproteins, and there are marked racial differences in the expression of HPAs (Table 27.2),[52] perhaps because of a genetic founder effect. Although many different antigens can cause ATP, about 75% of cases are caused by the human platelet-specific alloantigen HPA-1a, which is almost always seen in Caucasians and is located on GPIIIa.[54] In contrast, HPA-1a never occurs in patients of Asian descent, who most often carry HPA-4. It has been suggested that antibodies to human leukocyte antigen (HLA) class I antigens also cause this disorder in some cases, including one managed at our own institution, but this remains unproven, and the cause may be an HPA not yet defined.

The existence of an HPA incompatibility is necessary but not sufficient for antibody development. Although 2% of Caucasian women are at risk for ATP, a far smaller percentage develop the disorder. It is possible that a specific immune response gene is required as well. Antibodies to HPA-1a are significantly associated with specific HLA phenotypes, most strongly the DR52a allele, which is found in almost all HPA-2a mothers who produce HPA-1 antibodies.[55]

The severity of the thrombocytopenia caused by ATP is quite variable and may relate to the density of the target molecules on the fetal platelets. The most densely represented antigens on the platelet surface are HPA-1 and HPA-4: both are found on GPIIIa, with approximately 20,000 sites per platelet on the heterozygous affected fetus.[56] HPA-3 sites are located on GPIIb, and there are 10,000 to 20,000 sites on a heterozygous platelet. In contrast, both HPA-5a and HPA-5b, located on GPIa-IIa, are present at only 1000 to 2000 sites per platelet. This may explain the increase in disease severity in the HPA-1, HPA-3, and HPA-4 systems. However, some of the lower-density HPAs have resulted in severely affected neonates through the HPA-5 system, so density is not the only factor in severity of ATP (Box 27.1).

The diagnosis of a fetal thrombocytopenia is initially made in the neonate during the postpartum period. Approximately 81% have clinical signs at birth, such as petechiae, purpura, or overt bleedings.[57] Laboratory findings include a uniformly low neonatal platelet count and may also include a low hemoglobin level due to fetal or neonatal bleeding, followed by an elevated bilirubin concentration at 72 to 96 hours after delivery, secondary to passive resorption of extravasated blood. This type of thrombocytopenia usually lasts 2 to 3 weeks and resolves spontaneously. The differential diagnosis for thrombocytopenia in the newborn includes infection of bacterial or viral origin, so an evaluation for sepsis is necessary. DIC related to a primary sepsis or another underlying cause is diagnosed by coagulation assays. The maternal platelet count is evaluated to rule out maternal autoimmune thrombocytopenia with passive transfer of IgG antibodies. Rarer causes of neonatal thrombocytopenia include maternal drug exposure (e.g., thiazide diuretics, quinidine), congenital leukemia, thrombocytopenia–absent radius (TAR) syndrome, and Wiskott-Aldrich syndrome.

The most devastating consequence of this diagnosis is the 10% to 15% incidence of ICH, which occurs antenatally in approximately one half of the cases. The type of ICH in this disorder is typically intraparenchymal, unlike the more common hemorrhages caused by prematurity, which are usually intraventricular. This event can lead to structural brain abnormalities such as porencephaly, with subsequent permanent neurologic sequelae such as seizures, mental retardation, and learning disabilities. ICHs have been identified as early as 13 weeks of gestation by ultrasound.[58]

If a neonate has an unexplained thrombocytopenia, platelet incompatibility testing is performed on the neonate and the parents, usually by molecular methods. There are significant limitations to serologic typing of anti-platelet antibodies, especially with testing performed in a subsequent gestation. An antibody to HPA-1a is identified by its ability to bind to HPA-1a-positive and not HPA-1a-negative controls, or by its ability to bind to paternal and not maternal platelets. However, as many as 10% to 20% of patients with HPA-1a are antibody-negative for at least part of the gestation.[59] Further, the finding of an antibody-positive mother or an increase in her antibody titer does not indicate that the fetus is antigen-positive. Therefore, antigen typing is now performed mostly by DNA testing for the five most common HPA antigens. Approximately 1% to 3% of individuals are negative homozygotes for the most common antigen, HPA-1a. Fetal thrombocytopenia is more severe if the fetus is HPA-1a-incompatible. In a review of previously studied patients by Bussel and colleagues,[60] 97 (90.6%) of 107 fetuses with ATP were HPA-1a-incompatible; the median initial platelet

Table 27.2 Laboratory and Clinical Features of Alloimmune Thrombocytopenia

HPA Name	Other Names	Glycoprotein	DNA Allele (amino acid changes)	Gene Frequency (white)	Serologic Frequency		Frequency of Fetal Disease*	Severity*	Antenal ICH
					White	Japanese			
HPA-1a	$ZW^a,P1^{a1}$	GPIIIa	$Leu_{33}Arg_{143}Pro_{407}Arg_{489}Arg_{636}$	0.85	97.9	99.9	1 in 1000–2000	Severe	Yes
HPA-1b	$ZW^b,P1^{A2}$	GPIIIa	$Pro_{33}Arg_{143}Pro_{407}Arg_{489}Arg_{636}$	0.15	26.5	3.7			
HPA-2a	Ko^b	GPIb	Thr_{145}	0.93	99.3	NT			
HPA-2b	Ko^a Sib^a	GPIb	Met_{145}	0.07	14.6	35.4			
HPA-3a	Bak^a,Lek^a	GPIb	Ile_{843}	0.61	87.7	78.9			
HPA-3b	Bak^b	GPIIb	Ser_{843}	0.39	64.1	NT	Rare, <10 published cases	Unknown	
HPA-4a	Pen^a,Yuk^b	GPIIIa	Same as HPA-1a	0.85	99.9	99.9			
HPA-4b	Pen^b,Yuk^a	GPIIIa	$Leu_{33}Gln_{143}Pro_{407}$ $Arg_{489}Arg_{636}$	<0.01	0.2	1.7	Rare in Asians	? severe	Yes
HPA-5a	Br^b,Zav^b	GPIa	Glu_{505}	0.89	99.2	NT			
HPA-5b	Br^a,Zav^a,Hc^a	GPIa	Lys_{505}	0.11	20.6	NT	Uncommon >50 cases	Somewhat milder	Yes
HPA-6a	Ca^b,Tu^b	GPIIIa	Same as HPA-1a	0.85	?	?			
HPA-6b	Ca^a,Tu^a	GPIIIa	$Leu_{33}Arg_{143}Glu_{407}Arg_{489}Arg_{6365}$	<0.01	?	?			
HPA-7a	Mo^b	GPIIIa	Same as HPA-1a	0.85	<1	?			
HPA-7b	Mo^a	GPIIIa	$Leu_{33}Arg_{143}Glu_{407}Arg_{489}Arg_{636}$	<0.01	?	?			
HPA-8a	Sr^b	GPIIIa	Same as HPA-1a	0.85	?	?			
HPA-8b	Sr^a	GPIIIa	$Leu_{33}Arg_{143}Pro_{407}Arg_{489}Cys_{636}$	<0.01	?	?			

NT, not tested; ICH, intracranial hemorrhage.
*Clinical severity and frequency are well defined only for HPA-1a (PIA[1]).
From Skupski DW, Bussel JW: Alloimmune thrombocytopenia. Clin Obstet Gynecol 1999;42:335–348.

Box 27.1   Preferred Approach: Diagnostic Evaluation and Management of Alloimmune Thrombocytopenia (HPA-1a)

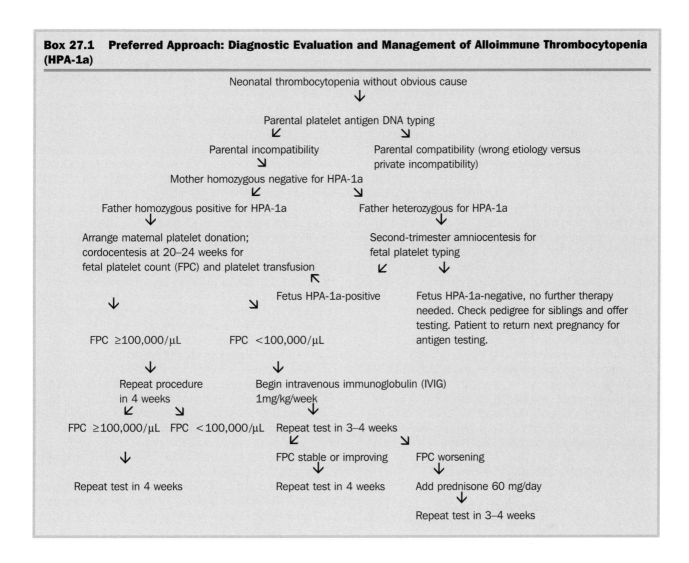

count was 18,000/µL in those fetuses and 60,000/µL in the 10 fetuses with other platelet incompatibilities. A total of eight additional antigens have received HPA numbers, but their incidence and the clinical relevance for several of them are unknown.

HPAs are polymorphisms of surface glycoproteins. Because their DNA sequences are known, any tissue can be used for prenatal diagnosis of the fetal platelet type, including chorionic villi, amniocytes, and fetal blood. The most frequent polymorphism affecting the HPA-1a antigen results from a base pair change from cytosine to thymine at position 196 of the gene for GPIIIa. This change causes the substitution of proline for leucine as amino acid 33 of the resultant protein.[61]

If the family is incompatible for an HPA antigen and the partner is homozygous for the antigen, the recurrence rate in any subsequent gestation is 100%. If the father is heterozygous the recurrence rate is 50%, and in any subsequent pregnancy an amniocentesis can be performed in the second trimester to ascertain fetal status. If the fetus demonstrates the antigen, or if the father is homozygous and paternity is clearly defined, then umbilical blood sampling is usually performed at 20 to 24 weeks' gestation to determine the fetal platelet count.

At the time of umbilical blood sampling, platelets are always kept available for transfusion at the end of the procedure. Because about 98% of the population is HPA-1a-positive, maternal platelets are often harvested to be used for fetal transfusion. Their advantages are multiple: they are readily accessible, they decrease the risk of exposures to blood-borne diseases, and they eliminate the risk of further sensitization. The use of maternal platelets is avoided if the mother tests positive for hepatitis or human immunodeficiency virus (HIV) infection. Platelets are apheresed 24 to 48 hours before use, centrifuged to remove the supernatant plasma (which contains most of the anti-HPA-1a antibody), resuspended, and irradiated. Because at least 10% to 20% of whole blood IgG is found within platelets, there are limits to the reduction in anti-platelet antibodies that can be achieved.[52] Platelet concentrates contain about 55 billion platelets in an average volume of 40 mL, providing about 1 billion platelets per milliliter. The Nicolaides nomogram[62] (see Fig. 27.2) indicates that the average fetal blood volume before 30 weeks' gestation is 150 mL. Because a platelet count of 100,000/µL is equivalent to 100,000,000 platelets per milliliter, 10 mL of platelet concentrate would increase the platelet count by 100,000/µL in a fetus with a blood volume of 100 mL.[51] During cordocentesis, platelets are transfused slowly over 3 to 5 minutes. Platelets that are transfused are functional for only 5 to 7 days. The median drop in fetal platelets per day is approximately 23.6×10^9/L. This value was derived from early procedures in which patients underwent serial intrauterine platelet transfusion for therapy.[63]

Paidas and colleagues,[64] as part of a multicenter treatment program, reported five cases of fetal or neonatal death that was believed to have been caused by exsanguination with ATP, and compared those patients with 44 affected fetuses who survived the procedure. The mean platelet count was significantly lower in the study group than in the survivors at the time of the procedure controls (5800 versus 32,800/μL, respectively; $P = .005$). Furthermore, the incidence of an antenatal hemorrhage in an untreated sibling was higher in the affected group (2 of 5 patients, or 40%) compared with controls (1 of 42 patients, or 2.3%). Because the diagnosis of severe thrombocytopenia can be made only at the time of umbilical blood sampling, most institutions routinely begin platelet transfusion before needle removal, or they give platelets if a rapid platelet count can be performed and the fetal count is less than 50,000/μL. The short platelet half-life (4 to 7 days) requires weekly transfusions to maintain an adequate platelet count in a thrombocytopenic fetus.

Under continuous ultrasonographic guidance, a 20- or 22-gauge spinal needle is directed into the umbilical vessel through the anterior abdominal wall (Fig. 27.3).[65] After 1 to 2 mL has been removed and set aside to preclude the possibility of dilution of the sample by amniotic fluid, multiple 1-mL heparinized syringes are used to withdraw 3 to 5 mL of blood from the umbilical cord. The larger RBC size is used to confirm the fetal origin of the blood from the complete blood count sent for evaluation, as is a Kleihauer-Betke test for fetal cells. Platelet volume for fetal transfusion at the close of the procedure is calculated by the following formula[66]:

$$V = VSF (C3 - C1) / C2$$

where V represents the volume of platelets transfused, VSF is the fetal blood volume at the week of gestation (determined from the nomogram[62] in Fig. 27.2), C1 is the platelet count before transfusion, C2 is the concentration of donor platelets, and C3 is the desired platelet count after transfusion. Because the actual platelet count of the fetus is unknown at the time of the procedure, many physicians empirically transfuse a quantity of platelets derived from this formula before removal of the needle. In such cases, an original count is obtained and platelets are given; then, after about 60 seconds of circulation time, a final platelet count is obtained and the needle is withdrawn. The procedure is performed with continuous ultrasound guidance, and the umbilical cord site is monitored for several minutes to watch for bleeding after the procedure. The fetal heart rate is also observed for bradycardia. If fetal viability has been achieved (24 weeks of gestation or longer), fetal monitoring is done to observe for contractions and bradycardia for approximately 1 hour before discharge.

The only controlled trials for the treatment of ATP involve the use of intravenous immune globulin (IVIG).[67, 68] Lynch and colleagues[67] demonstrated in 1992 the efficacy of the use of IVIG and steroids to increase the fetal platelet count at delivery to greater than $50 \times 10^9/L$ in 11 of 18 affected cases. No cases of ICH occurred in the treated cohort, but 33% of their antecedent affected siblings experienced ICH.

Bussel and colleagues[68] performed a pilot study of 18 patients in which IVIG with or without steroids was found to significantly increase the fetal platelet count, and none of the subjects had any evidence of ICH. Dexamethasone was also given to the first five patients in this series, and four of these five developed oligohydramnios. However, a relatively high dose (3 to 5 mg) was used, and later analysis did note that steroids may have augmented the effect of the IVIG. This report was followed by a multicenter, randomized, controlled trial[69] in which 54 women with ATP and thrombocytopenic fetuses (platelet count <100,000/μL) were randomly assigned to receive IVIG with or without 1.5 mg/day of dexamethasone. Patients who were nonresponders received salvage therapy in the form of 60 mg/day of prednisone. No differences were noted in outcomes between the patients treated with IVIG and those who received IVIG plus dexamethasone. Two patients taking dexamethasone developed oligohydramnios. No fetuses developed an ICH, despite the

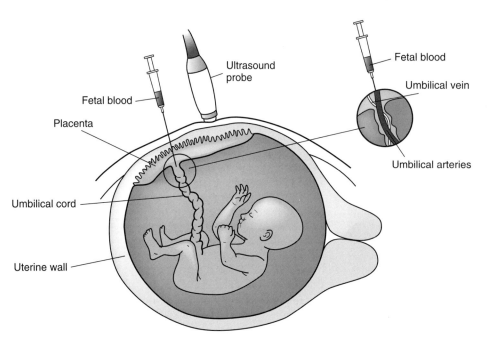

Figure 27.3 Schematic diagram of percutaneous umbilical blood sampling with continuous ultrasound guidance. (From Greenwood Genetic Center: Counseling Aids for Geneticists, 3rd ed. Auburn, NY: Jackobs Press, 1995, p 69, with permission.)

fact that 10 fetuses had siblings who had been affected in a previous pregnancy and had not received medical therapy. Twelve patients did not improve their platelet counts, and three were delivered electively. Of the remaining nine, plus one other subject who was enrolled just for salvage treatment, five improved their fetal platelet count with the use of prednisone. This highlights the importance of obtaining a fetal platelet count before the initiation of therapy, because to empirically use IVIG without a baseline platelet assessment precludes the ability to monitor its success.

Therefore, if the fetal count is less than approximately 100,000/μL, maternal IVIG is given at a dose of 1 g/kg weekly. Repeat cordocentesis and platelet transfusion is performed in 3 to 6 weeks to re-evaluate effectiveness of this therapy. Weekly ultrasound examinations are performed to evaluate for antenatal ICH. If the fetal platelet count is significantly decreased or the fetus is refractory to therapy, prednisone (60 mg/day) is added; this has been effective in increasing the fetal platelet count in about 50% of the patients. Term management of these patients includes a final cordocentesis at about 37 weeks, with fetal lung maturity testing from amniotic fluid obtained before cord puncture. After fetal transfusion with lung maturity has been documented, therapeutic induction of labor can begin. However, delivery timing needs to be individualized according to the clinical circumstances. For example, if the patient has unremitting refractory thrombocytopenia that is severe (i.e., <20,000/μL), delivery could be offered at or after 34 weeks' gestation.

As in HDN, there is some evidence that birth order is related to severity of the disease. In contrast to HDN, in which first pregnancies are not affected and sensitization occurs at delivery, first pregnancies are affected by ATP. The rate of recurrence of ATP is virtually 100% among antigen-positive siblings. Subsequent gestations are at least as severely affected as the index case, if not more severely.[68] Conversely, later siblings often have a better prognosis owing to preventive measures undertaken after diagnosis in the index case. However, the natural history of this disease is progressively worsening thrombocytopenia with each gestation. In fact, a prior history of an antenatal ICH is the only known reliable predictor of severe disease in a subsequent pregnancy.[68]

Unlike HDN, routine screening for ATP has not been instituted into clinical practice, partially because determination of the best test for screening is a complex issue. Screening of mothers for anti-platelet antibodies is costly and has a high rate of false-positive results during gestation. Another approach would be to screen solely for HPA-1a, because lack of this antigen is associated with the most cases of morbidity and mortality. The neonatal platelet count has been calculated to be the least expensive screening modality.[70] However, postpartum neonatal screening precludes the ability to screen affected index cases. In current practice, most cases are detected by the identification of thrombocytopenia in the newborn. However, once a case is identified, a thorough family history should be obtained regarding the reproductive status of siblings of the mother. At our own institution, a patient diagnosed with this disorder was found to have a fraternal twin who had not yet reproduced. The twin underwent HPA typing and was found to be HPA-1a negative, and her partner was found to be homozygous HPA-1a positive. She was treated in her index pregnancy, with an uneventful outcome (unpublished data).

■ Conclusion

The physician managing the parturient needs to have a thorough understanding of the hematologic disorders that may necessitate maternal or fetal transfusion. Obstetric hemorrhage is still an extremely common problem, especially during the postpartum period, and often occurs without warning. Although some of the fetal disorders requiring transfusion are relatively rare, their effect on the current or subsequent pregnancies is dramatic. Rigorous maternal surveillance and a thorough medical history can help prepare both the patient and the medical team for the prevention of maternal or fetal disease.

REFERENCES

1. Abouzahr C, Royston E, (eds): The global picture: The causes of maternal death. In Maternal Mortality: A Global Factbook. Geneva: World Health Organization, 1991, pp 7–11.
2. Pritchard JA, Baldwin RM, Dickey JC, et al: Blood volume changes in pregnancy and the puerperium: II. Red blood cell loss and changes in apparent blood volume during and following vaginal delivery, cesarean section, and cesarean section plus total hysterectomy. Am J Obstet Gynecol 1962;84:1271–1282.
3. American College of Obstetricians and Gynecologists: Nutrition during pregnancy. ACOG Technical Bulletin 179. Washington, DC: ACOG, 1993.
4. American College of Obstetricians and Gynecologists: Blood Component Therapy. ACOG Technical Bulletin 199. Washington, DC: ACOG, 1994, p 4.
5. Combs CA, Murphy EL, Laros RK Jr: Factors associated with postpartum hemorrhage with vaginal birth. Obstet Gynecol 1991;77:69–76.
6. American College of Obstetricians and Gynecologists: Postpartum Hemorrhage. ACOG Technical Bulletin 243. Washington, DC: ACOG, 1990.
7. American College of Obstetricians and Gynecologists: Blood Component Therapy. ACOG Technical Bulletin 199. Washington, DC: ACOG, 1994, p 2.
8. Bowman JM, Pollack JM, Penston LE: Fetomaternal transplacental hemorrhage during pregnancy and after delivery. Vox Sang 1986;51:117.
9. Bowman JM, Pollock JM: Amniotic fluid spectrophotometry and early delivery in the management of erythroblastosis fetalis. Pediatrics 1965;35:815–835.
10. Weinstein L: Irregular antibodies causing hemolytic disease of the newborn: a continuing problem. Clin Obstet Gynecol 1982;25:321.
11. Lee S, Wu X, Reid M, Zelinksi T, Redman C: Molecular basis of the Kell (K1) phenotype. Blood 1995;85:912–916.
12. Le Van Kim C, Mouro I, Cherif-Lazar B, et al: Molecular cloning and the primary structure of the human blood group RhD polypeptide. Proc Natl Acad Sci U S A 1990;89:10.
13. Rote NS: Pathophysiology of Rh isoimmunization. Clin Obstet Gynecol 1982;25:243.
14. Bowman JM: Maternal blood group immunization. In Creasy RK, Resnik R (eds): Maternal-Fetal Medicine: Principles and Practice, 2nd ed. Philadelphia: WB Saunders, 1989, pp 613–649.
15. Chavez GF, Mulinare J, Edmonds LD: Epidemiology of Rh hemolytic disease of the newborn in the United States. JAMA 1991;265:3270–3274.
16. Freda VJ, Gorman JG, Pollack W, et al: Prevention of Rh hemolytic disease: Ten years clinical experience with Rh immune globulin. N Engl J Med 1975;292:1014.
17. Jackson M, Branch DW: Isoimmunization in pregnancy. In Gabbe S (ed): Obstetrics: Normal and Problem Pregnancies. New York: Churchill Livingstone, 1996, p 904.
18. Jackson M, Branch DW: Isoimmunization in pregnancy. In Gabbe S (ed): Obstetrics: Normal and Problem Pregnancies. New York: Churchill Livingstone, 1996, p 908.
19. Bevis DCA: Blood pigments in haemolytic disease of the newborn. J Obstet Gynecol Br Emp 1956;63:65.
20. Liley AW: Liquor amnii analysis in the management of pregnancy complicated by rhesus sensitization. Am J Obstet Gynecol 1961;82:1359.
21. American College of Obstetricians and Gynecologists: Management of Isoimmunization in Pregnancy. ACOG Technical Bulletin 227. Washington, DC: ACOG, 1996.

22. Harman CR, Bowman JM, Manning FA, Menticoglou SM: Intrauterine transfusion—intraperitoneal versus intravascular approach: A case-control comparison. Am J Obstet Gynecol 1990;162:1053.

23. Grannum PA, Copel JA, Plaxe SC, et al: In utero exchange transfusion by direct intravascular injection in severe erythroblastosis fetalis. N Engl J Med 1986;314:1431.

24. Nicolaides KH, Clewell WH, Mibashan RS, et al: Fetal haemoglobin measurement in the assessment of red cell isoimmunization. Lancet 1988;1:1073.

25. MacGregor SN, Socol ML, Pielet BW, et al: Prediction of hematocrit decline after intravascular fetal transfusion. Am J Obstet Gynecol 1989;161:1491.

26. Ghidini A, Sepulveda W, Lockwood CJ, Romera R: Complications of fetal blood sampling. Am J Obstet Gynecol 1993;168:1339–1344.

27. Burrows RF, Kelton JG: Fetal thrombocytopenia and its relationship to maternal thrombocytopenia. N Engl J Med 1993;329:1463–1466.

28. Shehata N, Burrows R, Kelton JG: Gestational thrombocytopenia. Clin Obstet Gynecol 1999;42:327–334.

29. Johnson JR, Samuels P: Review of autoimmune thrombocytopenia: Pathogenesis, diagnosis and management in pregnancy. Clin Obstet Gynecol 1999;42:317–326.

30. George JN, El-Harake MA, Aster RH: Thrombocytopenia due to enhanced platelet destruction by immunologic mechanisms. In Beutler E, Lichtman MA, Coller BS, Kipps TJ (eds): Williams' Hematology, 5th ed. New York: McGraw-Hill, 1994, pp 1315–1355.

31. Berchtold P, Wenger M: Autoantibodies against platelet glycoproteins in autoimmune thrombocytopenia purpura: Their clinical significance and response to treatment. Blood 1993;81:1246–1250.

32. George JN, El-Harake MA, Raskob GE: Chronic idiopathic thrombocytopenic purpura. N Engl J Med 1994;1331:1207–1211.

33. Lacey JV, Penner JA: Management of idiopathic thrombocytopenic purpura in the adult. Semin Thromb Hemost 1977;3:160–174.

34. Klemen E, Szalay F, Petefy M: Autoimmune thrombocytopenic purpura in pregnancy and the newborn. Br J Obstet Gynecol 1978;85:239.

35. Burrows RF, Kelton JG: Fetal thrombocytopenia and its relation to maternal thrombocytopenia. N Engl J Med 1993;329:1463–1466.

36. Silver RM, Branch DW, Scott JR: Maternal thrombocytopenia in pregnancy: time for a reassessment. Am J Obstet Gynecol 1995;173:479–482.

37. Burrows RF, Kelton JG: Pregnancy in patients with idiopathic thrombocytopenic purpura: Assessing the risks for the infant at delivery. Obstet Gynecol Surv 1993;48:471–478.

38. Cook RL, Miller RC, Katz VL, et al: Immune thrombocytopenia purpura in pregnancy: A reappraisal of management. Obstet Gynecol 1991;78:578–582.

39. Burrows RF, Kelton JG: Incidentally detected thrombocytopenia in healthy mothers and their infants. N Engl J Med 1988;319:142–145.

40. Shehata N, Burrows R, Kelton JG: Gestational thrombocytopenia. Clin Obstet Gynecol 1999;42:327–334.

41. Weinstein L: Syndrome of hemolysis, elevated liver enzymes, and low platelets platelet count: A severe consequence of hypertension in pregnancy. Am J Obstet Gynecol 1982;142:159–167.

42. Sibai BM, Ramadan MK, Usta I, et al: Maternal morbidity and mortality in 442 pregnancies with hemolysis, elevated liver enzymes, and low platelets (HELLP syndrome). Am J Obstet Gynecol 1993;169:1000–1006.

43. Thiagarajah S, Bourgeois FJ, Harbert GM, Caudle MR: Thrombocytopenia in preeclampsia: Associated abnormalities and management principles. Am J Obstet Gynecol 1984;150:1.

44. Sibai BM, Taslimi MM, El-Nazar A, et al: Maternal-perinatal outcome associated with the syndrome of hemolysis, elevated liver enzymes, and low platelets in severe preeclampsia-eclampsia. Am J Obstet Gynecol 1986;155:501–509.

45. Martin JN, Blake PG, Perry GK, et al: The natural history of HELLP syndrome: Patterns of disease progression and regression. Am J Obstet Gynecol 1991;164:1500–1513.

46. Burrows RF, Andrew M: Neonatal thrombocytopenia in the hypertensive disorders of pregnancy. Obstet Gynecol 1990;26:234–238.

47. Ridolfi RL, Bell WR: Thrombotic thrombocytopenic purpura: Report of 25 cases and review of the literature. Medicine (Baltimore) 1981;60:413.

48. Weiner CP: Thrombotic microangiopathy in pregnancy and the postpartum period. Semin Hematol 1987;24:119.

49. Miller JM, Pastorek JG: Thrombotic thrombocytopenic purpura and hemolytic uremic syndrome in pregnancy. Clin Obstet Gynecol 1991;34:64.

50. Olah KS, Gee H: Postpartum haemolytic uremic syndrome precipitated by antibiotics. Br J Obstet Gynaecol 1990;97:83.

51. Kaplan C, Daffos F, Forestier F, et al: Current trends in neonatal alloimmune thrombocytopenia: Diagnosis and therapy. In Kaplanj-Gouet C, Schlegel N, Salmon CH, McGregor J (eds): Platelet Immunology: Fundamental and Clinical Aspects. Paris: Colloque INSERM/John Liffey Erotext, 1991, pp 267–278.

52. Skupski DW, Bussel JB: Alloimmune thrombocytopenia. Clin Obstet Gynecol 1999;42:335–348.

53. Kaplan C, Patereau C, Reznikoff-Etievant MF, et al: Antenatal PIA 1 typing and detection of GPIIb-IIIa complex. Br J Haematol 1984;60:568.

54. Muller-Eckhardt C, Kiefel V, Grubert A, et al: 348 Cases of suspected neonatal alloimmune thrombocytopenia. Lancet 1989;1:363–366.

55. Valentin N, Vergracht A, Bignon JD, et al: HLA-DRw52 is involved in alloimmunization against PLA-1 antigen. Hum Immunol 1990;27:73.

56. McFarland JG: Prenatal and perinatal management of alloimmune cytopenias. In Nance ST (ed): Alloimmunity: 1993 and Beyond. Bethesda, MD: American Association of Blood Banks, 1993, p 176.

57. Deaver JE, Leppert PC, Zaroulis CG: Neonatal alloimmune thrombocytopenic purpura. Am J Perinatol 1986;3:127–131.

58. Giovangrandi Y, Daffos F, Kaplan C, et al. Very early intracranial hemorrhage in alloimmune fetal thrombocytopenia. Lancet 1990;335:310.

59. Kaplan C, Daffos F, Forestier F, et al: Current trends in neonatal alloimmune thrombocytopenia: Diagnosis and therapy. In Kaplanj-Gouet C, Schlegel N, Salmon CH, McGregor J (eds): Platelet Immunology: Fundamental and Clinical Aspects. Paris: Colloque INSERM/John Liffey Erotext, 1991, pp 267–278.

60. Bussel JB, Zabusky MR, Berkowitz RL, McFarland JG: Fetal alloimmune thrombocytopenia. N Engl J Med 1997;337:22–26.

61. Newman PJ, Derbes RS, Aster RH: The human platelet alloantigens, PLA1 and PLA2 are associated with a leucine/proline amnio acid polymorphism in membrane glycoprotein IIIA, and are distinguishable by DNA typing. J Clin Invest 1989;83:1778–1781.

62. Nicolaides KH, Clewell WH, Rodeck CH: Measurement of human fetoplacental volume in erythroblastosis fetalis. Am J Obstet Gynecol 1987;157:50–53.

63. Nicolini U, Tannirandorn Y, Gonzalez P, et al: Continuing controversy in alloimmune thrombocytopenia: Fetal hyperimmunoglobulinemia fails to prevent thrombocytopenia. Am J Obstet Gynecol 1990;163:1144–1146.

64. Paidas MJ, Berkowitz RL, Lynch L, et al: Alloimmune thrombocytopenia: Fetal and neonatal losses related to cordocentesis. Am J Obstet Gynecol 1995;172:475–479.

65. Greenwood Genetic Center: Counseling Aids for Geneticists, 3rd ed. Auburn NY: Jackobs Press, 1995, p 69.

66. Moise KJ: Intrauterine transfusion with red cells and platelets. In Fetal Medicine [Special issue]. West J Med 1993;159:318–324.

67. Lynch L, Bussel JB, McFarland JG, et al: Antenatal treatment of alloimmune thrombocytopenia. Obstet Gynecol 1992;80:67–71.

68. Bussel J, Berkowitz R, McFarland J, et al: Antenatal treatment of neonatal alloimmune thrombocytopenia. N Engl J Med 1988;319:1374–1378.

69. Bussel J, Berkowitz RL, Lynch L, et al: Antenatal management of alloimmune thrombocytopenia with intravenous gamma globulin: A randomized trial of the addition of low dose steroids to IVIG in 55 maternal-fetal pairs. Am J Obstet Gynecol 1996;174:1414–1423.

70. Durand-Zaleski I, Schlegel N, Blum-Noisgard C, et al: Screening primiparous women and newborn for fetal/neonatal alloimmune thrombocytopenia: A prospective comparison of effectiveness and costs. Immune Thrombocytopenia Working Group. Am J Perinatol 1996;13:423–431.

Chapter 28

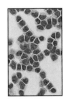

Transfusion of the Neonate and Pediatric Patient

*Ronald G Strauss**

Transfusions of blood components are mandatory for modern management in many premature infants, children with cancer, recipients of hematopoietic progenitor transplants and organ allografts, and children undergoing many surgical procedures. Although transfusions can be lifesaving, they are not without risks. Accordingly, they should be given only when true benefits are likely—for example, to correct a deficiency or functional defect of a blood component that has caused or threatens to cause a clinically significant problem. Because of the extended lifespan of children after transfusions, it is critical to avoid post-transfusion complications that may lead to progressive morbidity and mortality and to considerable expense over the years (e.g., hepatitis).

The principles of transfusion support for older children and adolescents are similar to those for adults, but infants have many special needs. Therefore, each of these two age groups is discussed separately within each section. Because many issues dealing with transfusion therapy in adults, as discussed in other chapters, apply to older children, the bulk of information in this chapter deals with transfusion in infants. Because of space limitations, only red blood cell (RBC), platelet (PLT), and neutrophil (granulocyte) transfusions are discussed. General guidelines and recommendations are given for pediatric blood component transfusions. However, it is important that they be adapted to fit local standards of practice. In particular, terms used to describe clinical conditions, such as "severe" and "symptomatic," must be defined by local physicians.

■ Red Blood Cell Transfusions

Older Children and Adolescents

RBCs, the most frequently transfused blood component, are given to increase the oxygen-carrying capacity of the blood, the goal being to maintain satisfactory tissue oxygenation. Guidelines for RBC transfusions in older children and adolescents are similar to those for adults (Table 28.1). However, transfusions may be given more stringently to children, because normal hemoglobin levels are lower in healthy children than in adults, and most children do not have the underlying cardiorespiratory and vascular diseases that develop with aging in adults. Therefore, children generally have greater abilities to compensate for anemia and may be transfused at lower hemoglobin or hematocrit levels.

In the perioperative period, it is unnecessary for most children to maintain hemoglobin levels of 8.0 g/dL or higher, a level frequently desired for adults. There should be a compelling reason to administer any postoperative RBC transfusion, because most children (without continued bleeding) can quickly restore their RBC volume if given iron therapy. As is true for adults, the most important measures in the treatment of acute hemorrhage occurring with surgery or injury in children are to control the hemorrhage and to restore blood volume and tissue perfusion with crystalloid and/or colloid solutions. Then, if the estimated blood loss is greater than 25% of the circulating blood volume (i.e., >17 mL/kg body weight) and the patient's condition remains unstable, RBC transfusions may be indicated. In acutely ill children with severe cardiac or pulmonary disease—and particularly in those who require assisted ventilation—it is common practice to maintain the hemoglobin level close to the normal range. Although this practice seems logical, its efficacy has not been documented by controlled scientific studies of children. Such studies are needed, because liberal RBC transfusion practices in critically ill adults have been reported to have detrimental effects.[1]

With anemias that develop slowly, the decision to transfuse RBCs should not be based solely on the blood hemoglobin

*This work was supported in part by National Institutes of Health Program Project Grant P01 HL46925.

Table 28.1   Author's Guidelines for Transfusing Children and Adolescents[a]

Red blood cells

Hemoglobin < 13.0 g/dL (HCT < 40%) with *severe* cardiopulmonary disease
Hemoglobin < 8.0 g/dL (HCT < 24%) in the perioperative period
Hemoglobin < 8.0 g/dL (HCT < 24%) with *symptomatic* chronic anemia
Hemoglobin < 8.0 g/dL (HCT < 24%) with marrow failure
Acute loss > 25% estimated blood volume.

Platelets

Blood platelets < 50 × 10⁹/L and *significant* bleeding
Blood platelets < 50 × 10⁹/L and invasive procedure
Blood platelets < 20 × 10⁹/L prophylaxis with bleeding risk factors
Blood platelets < 10 × 10⁹/L prophylaxis without bleeding risk factors
Platelet dysfunction with bleeding or invasive procedure

Neutrophils

Blood neutrophils < 0.5 × 10⁹/L and bacterial infection unresponsive to antibiotics
Blood neutrophils < 0.5 × 10⁹/L and yeast or fungal infection progressing or appearing during treatment with antimicrobials
Neutrophil dysfunction with bacterial, yeast, or fungal infection unresponsive to antimicrobials

[a]Words in italics must be defined according to local practices.
HCT, hematocrit.

concentration, because children with chronic anemias may be asymptomatic despite very low hemoglobin levels. Children with iron deficiency anemia, for example, often are treated successfully with oral iron alone, even at hemoglobin levels lower than 5.0 g/dL. Factors other than hemoglobin concentration that must be considered in the decision to transfuse RBCs include (1) the patient's symptoms, signs, and functional capacities; (2) the presence or absence of cardiorespiratory and central nervous system disease; (3) the cause and anticipated course of the underlying anemia; and (4) alternative therapies such as iron or recombinant human erythropoietin (EPO) therapy, the latter of which has been demonstrated to reduce the need for RBC transfusions and to improve the overall condition of children with chronic renal insufficiency. In anemias that are likely to be permanent (e.g., thalassemia, hemoglobinopathies), the effects of anemia on growth and development (which might be ameliorated by RBC transfusions) must be balanced against the potential toxicities of repeated transfusions.

Infants

Pathophysiology of the Anemia of Prematurity

All infants experience a decline in circulating RBC volume during the first weeks of life. This decline results both from physiologic factors and, in sick preterm infants, from phlebotomy blood losses for laboratory monitoring. In healthy full-term infants, the nadir hemoglobin value rarely is lower than 9.0 g/dL at an age of 10 to 12 weeks. The decline is more rapid (i.e., nadir at 4 to 6 weeks of age) and the blood hemoglobin falls to lower levels in infants born prematurely—to approximately 8.0 g/dL in infants with birth weights of 1.0 to 1.5 kg and to approximately 7.0 g/dL in infants with birth weights lower than 1.0 kg.[2-4] Because this postnatal drop in hemoglobin level in full-term infants is well tolerated, it is commonly referred to as the *physiologic anemia of infancy*. However, the pronounced decline in hemoglobin concentration that occurs in many extremely preterm infants is associated with abnormal clinical signs and need for RBC transfusions. Therefore, the *anemia of prematurity* is not accepted to be a normal, benign event.[5, 6]

Many interacting physiologic factors are responsible for the anemia of prematurity. A key reason that the hemoglobin nadir is lower in preterm than in full-term infants is the former group's diminished plasma EPO level in response to anemia.[4, 7–10] Although anemia provokes EPO production in premature infants, the plasma levels achieved in anemic infants, at any given hematocrit, are lower than those observed in comparably anemic older persons.[9] Erythroid progenitor cells in blood[11] and bone marrow[12] of preterm infants are quite responsive to EPO in vitro—a finding suggesting that inadequate production of EPO is the major cause of physiologic anemia, not marrow unresponsiveness.

The mechanisms responsible for the diminished EPO output by preterm neonates are only partially defined. One factor is that the primary site of EPO production in preterm infants is in the liver, rather than the kidneys.[13, 14] Because the liver is less sensitive to anemia and tissue hypoxia, a relatively sluggish EPO response occurs to the falling hematocrit. The timing of the switch from liver to kidney is set at conception and is not accelerated by preterm birth. Viewed from a teleologic perspective, decreased hepatic production of EPO under in utero conditions of tissue hypoxia may be an advantage for the fetus. If this were not the case, normal levels of fetal hypoxia could trigger high levels of EPO and produce marked erythrocytosis and consequent hyperviscosity in utero. After birth, however, diminished EPO responsiveness to tissue hypoxia is disadvantageous and leads to anemia because of impaired compensation for the falling hematocrit.

Diminished EPO production cannot entirely explain low plasma EPO levels in preterm infants, however. Extraordinarily high plasma levels of EPO were reported in some fetuses of postconceptional age, comparable to those of neonates treated in intensive care settings,[15, 16] and macrophages from human cord blood were found to produce normal quantities of EPO messenger RNA and protein.[17] These studies documented intact synthetic capability, at least under some circumstances. Therefore, additional mechanisms are likely to contribute to diminished EPO plasma levels. For example, plasma levels of EPO undoubtedly are influenced by metabolism (clearance) as well as by production. Data obtained in human infants[18, 19] and in neonatal monkeys[20] demonstrate that low plasma EPO levels may result from increased plasma clearance and volume of distribution and from shorter fractional elimination and mean residence times for EPO in neonates compared with adults. Therefore, accelerated catabolism may contribute to the low plasma levels—with the low plasma EPO in infants possibly representing the combined effects of decreased synthesis and increased metabolism.

Phlebotomy blood losses play a key role in the anemia of prematurity. The modern practice of neonatology requires critically ill neonates to be monitored closely with serial laboratory studies such as blood gases, electrolytes, blood counts, and cultures. Small preterm infants are the most critically ill, require the most frequent blood sampling, and suffer the greatest proportional loss of RBCs because their circulating RBC volumes are smallest. Promising "in-line" devices that withdraw blood, measure multiple analytes, and then reinfuse the sampled blood are being investigated. However, until these devices are proven effective and safe for infants, the replacement of blood losses due to phlebotomy will remain a critical factor responsible for multiple RBC transfusions in critically ill neonates.

Recommendations for RBC Transfusions During Infancy

Guidelines for transfusing RBCs to neonates are controversial, and practices vary.[2, 21–23] The lack of a consistent approach stems from incomplete knowledge of the cellular and molecular biology of erythropoiesis during the perinatal period as well as incomplete understanding of the infant's compensation for anemia and the physiologic response to RBC transfusions. Generally, RBC transfusions are given to maintain the level of hemoglobin or hematocrit believed to be most desirable for each neonate's clinical condition. Broad guidelines for RBC transfusions during early infancy are listed in Table 28.2.[24] These guidelines are very general, and it is important that terms used to describe clinical conditions, such as "severe" and "symptomatic," be defined to fit local practices.

Table 28.2 Author's Guidelines for Transfusing Infants[a]

Red blood cells

Hemoglobin < 13.0 g/dL (HCT < 40%) with *severe* cardiopulmonary disease
Hemoglobin < 10.0 g/dL (HCT < 30%) with *moderate* cardiopulmonary disease
Hemoglobin < 10.0 g/dL (HCT < 30%) with *major* surgery
Hemoglobin < 8.0 g/dL (HCT < 24%) with *symptomatic* anemia
Acute loss > 25% estimated blood volume

Platelets

Blood platelets < 50 to < 100 × 10⁹/L and *significant* bleeding
Blood platelets < 50 × 10⁹/L and invasive procedure
Blood platelets < 20 × 10⁹/L prophylaxis and clinically *stable*
Blood platelets < 50 to < 100 × 10⁹/L prophylaxis and clinically *unstable*

Neutrophils

Blood neutrophils < 3 × 10⁹/L and *fulminant* sepsis during first week of life
Blood neutrophils < 1 × 10⁹/L and *fulminant* sepsis after first week of life

[a]Words in italics must be defined according to local practices.
HCT, hematocrit.

Most RBC transfusions given to infants are small in volume (10 to 15 mL/kg) and are repeated frequently to replace blood drawn for laboratory studies. There is no proven benefit to routine replacement of phlebotomy blood losses "milliliter for milliliter." Instead, RBCs should be transfused to maintain a hematocrit level deemed appropriate for the clinical condition of the infant. In neonates with severe respiratory disease, such as those requiring high volumes of oxygen with ventilator support, it is customary to maintain the hematocrit at greater than 40% (hemoglobin concentration > 13.0 g/dL)—particularly if blood is being drawn frequently for testing. This practice is based on the belief that transfused donor RBCs containing adult hemoglobin will provide optimal oxygen delivery throughout the period of diminished pulmonary function that requires mechanical ventilation. Consistent with this rationale for ensuring optimal oxygen delivery in neonates with pulmonary failure, it seems logical—although unproven by controlled studies—to maintain the hematocrit at greater than 40% in infants with congenital heart disease that is severe enough to cause either cyanosis or congestive heart failure.

Definitive studies are not available to establish the optimal hemoglobin level for infants facing major surgery. However, it seems reasonable to maintain the hemoglobin at greater than 10.0 g/dL (hematocrit >30%) because of the limited ability of the infant heart, lungs, and vasculature to compensate for anemia. Additional factors include the inferior off-loading of oxygen by neonatal RBCs that results from the diminished interaction between fetal hemoglobin and 2,3-diphosphoglycerate and from the developmental impairment of neonatal renal, hepatic, and neurologic function. This transfusion guideline is simply a recommendation for perioperative management, not a firm indication, and it should be applied with flexibility to individual infants who are facing surgical procedures of varying complexity.

The clinical indications for RBC transfusions in preterm infants who are not critically ill but nonetheless develop moderate anemia (hematocrit <24% or blood hemoglobin concentration < 8.0 g/dL) are extremely variable.[2, 23] In general, infants who are clinically stable despite modest anemia do not require RBC transfusions unless they exhibit significant problems that either are ascribed to the presence of anemia or are predicted to be corrected by RBC transfusions. To illustrate, proponents of RBC transfusions to treat disturbances of cardiopulmonary rhythms believe that a low hematocrit contributes to tachypnea, dyspnea, apnea, and tachycardia or bradycardia because of decreased oxygen delivery to the respiratory center of the brain. If this theory is true, transfusions of RBCs should decrease the number of apneic spells by improving oxygen delivery to the central nervous system. However, results of clinical studies have been contradictory.[2, 23]

In practice, the decision whether to transfuse RBCs is based on the desire to maintain the hematocrit at a level judged to be most beneficial for the infant's clinical condition. Investigators who believe that this "clinical" approach is too imprecise have suggested the use of "physiologic" criteria for transfusions, such as RBC mass,[25] available oxygen,[26] mixed venous oxygen saturation, or measures of oxygen delivery and utilization,[27] to develop guidelines for transfusion decisions. In one study of 10 human infants with severe (oxygen-dependent) bronchopulmonary dysplasia, improvement in physiologic endpoints (increased systemic oxygen transport and decreased oxygen use) was shown to be a consequence of small-volume RBC transfusions.[27] However, these promising but technically demanding methods are, at present, difficult to apply in the day-to-day practice of neonatology, and studies conducted directly in human infants are needed. Application of data obtained from studies of animals and adult humans that correlate tissue oxygenation with the clinical effects of anemia and the need for RBC transfusions is confounded by the differences between infants and adults in hemoglobin oxygen affinity, ability to increase cardiac output, and regional patterns of blood flow.

Another physiologic factor to be considered in the transfusion decision is the use of circulating RBC volume rather than blood hematocrit or hemoglobin level.[6, 25, 28] Although circulating RBC volume is a potentially useful index of the blood's oxygen-carrying capacity, it cannot be predicted accurately by measurement of the hematocrit in infants.[29] Low circulating RBC volume identifies, better than hemoglobin or hematocrit, those infants who will respond to transfusion with a decrease in cardiac output.[30] At present, circulating RBC volume measurements are not widely available. However, promising techniques using nonradioactive biotin to tag RBCs may be adapted for infant studies.[30, 31]

Selecting an RBC Product to Transfuse an Infant

The RBC products usually chosen for small-volume transfusions given to infants are RBCs suspended either in citrate-phosphate-dextrose-adenine solution (CPDA) or in extended storage media (AS-1, AS-3, AS-5) at a hematocrit ranging from 55% to 70%. Some centers prefer to centrifuge RBC aliquots before transfusion, to prepare packed RBCs at a hematocrit of 80% to 90%. Most RBC transfusions are infused slowly over 2 to 4 hours at a dose of about 15 mL/kg body weight. Because of the small quantity of RBC preservative fluid infused and the slow rate of transfusion, the type of anticoagulant/preservative medium selected is believed not to pose risks for the majority of premature infants given small-volume transfusions.[32] Accordingly, the traditional use of relatively fresh RBCs (<7 days of storage) has been challenged, and it has been shown by many investigators[33–36] that donor exposure of multiply transfused infants can be diminished safely by the exclusive use of a dedicated unit of stored RBCs (i.e., 21 to 42 days after collection) for each infant.

Neonatologists who object to stored RBCs and continue to insist on transfusing infants with fresh RBCs generally raise three objections: the rise in plasma potassium (K^+) and the drop in RBC 2,3-diphosphoglycerate that occur during extended storage and the possible dangers of additives present in extended-storage media. After 42 days of storage, plasma K^+ levels in RBC units approximate 50 mEq/L (0.05 mEq/mL), a value that, at first glance, seems alarmingly high. By simple calculations, however, the dose of bioavailable K^+ transfused (i.e., ionic K^+ in the extracellular fluid) is shown to be very small. An infant weighing 1 kg who is given a 15 mL/kg transfusion of packed RBCs (hematocrit, 80%) will receive 3 mL of extracellular fluid, containing only 0.15 mEq of K^+, which will be infused slowly. Even if RBCs are not packed but are removed from the blood bag and directly infused at a hematocrit of 60%, the K^+ dose will be only 0.3 mEq. These doses are quite small compared with the usual daily K^+ requirement of 2 to 3 mEq/kg. However, this rationale does not apply to large-volume transfusions (>25 mL/kg), in which larger doses of K^+ may be harmful, especially if the infusion is rapid.

As for the second objection, 2,3-diphosphoglycerate is totally depleted from RBCs by 21 days of storage, and this is reflected by a decrease in the oxygen half-saturation pressure (P_{50}) from about 27 mm Hg in fresh blood to 18 mm Hg at the time of outdate. The last value of older transfused RBCs corresponds to the "physiologic" P_{50} obtained from the RBCs of many normal preterm infants at birth, reflecting the relatively high affinity for oxygen normally exhibited by infant RBCs. Therefore, the P_{50} of older transfused RBCs is no worse than that of RBCs produced endogenously by the infant's own bone marrow. Moreover, these older adult RBCs provide a benefit to the infant because the 2,3-diphosphoglycerate and the P_{50} of transfused RBCs (but not of endogenous infant RBCs) increase rapidly after transfusion.

Regarding the third objection, the quantity of additives present in RBCs stored in extended-storage media is believed not to be dangerous to neonates given small-volume transfusions ($\leq$15 mL/kg).[32] A comparison of CPDA with three types of extended-storage media is presented in Table 28.3. Regardless of the type of suspending solution, the quantity of additives is quite small in the clinical setting in which infants are given small-volume transfusions of RBCs transfused over

Table 28.3   Formulation of Anticoagulant-Preservative Solutions Present in Blood Collection Sets

Constituent	CPDA	AS-1	AS-3	AS-5
Volume(mL)	63[a]	100[b]	100[b]	100[b]
Sodium chloride (mg)	None	900	410	877
Dextrose (mg)	2000	2200	1100	900
Adenine (mg)	17.3	27	30	30
Mannitol (mg)	None	750	None	525
Trisodium citrate (mg)	1660	None	588	None
Citric acid (mg)	206	None	42	None
Sodium phosphate (monobasic) (mg)	140	None	276	None

[a]Approximately 450 mL of donor blood is drawn into 63 mL of CPDA. A unit of red blood cells (hematocrit, approximately 70%) is prepared by centrifugation and removal of most plasma.
[b]When AS-1 or AS-5 is used, 450 mL of donor blood is first drawn into 63 mL of CPD, which is identical to CPDA except that it contains 1610 mg of dextrose per 63 mL and has no adenine. When AS-3 is used, donor blood is drawn into CP2D, which is identical to CPD except that it contains double the amount of dextrose. After centrifugation and removal of almost all plasma, red blood cells are resuspended in 100 mL of the additive solution (AS-1, AS-3, or AS-5) at a hematocrit of approximately 55%–60%.
AS-1, AS-3, and AS-5, extended storage media; CPDA, citrate-phosphate-dextrose-adenine solution.

Table 28.4 Constituents Infused (mg/kg) in 10 mL/kg Red Blood Cells (Hematocrit, 60%)

Additive	CPDA	AS-1	AS-3	Toxic Dose[a]
NaCl	0	28	5	137 mg/kg/day
Dextrose	13	86	15	240 mg/kg/hr
Adenine	0.2	0.4	0.4	15 mg/kg/dose
Citrate	12	6.5	8.4	180 mg/kg/hr
Phosphate	9	1.3	3.7	> 60 mg/kg/day
Mannitol	0	22	0	360 mg/kg/day

[a]Actual toxic dose is difficult to predict accurately because the infusion rate usually is slow, permitting metabolism and distribution from blood into extravascular sites, and dextrose, adenine, and phosphate enter red blood cells and are somewhat sequestered. Potential toxic doses are based on Luban, Strauss, and Hume (1990).[32]
Data from Luban NLC, Strauss RG, Hume HA. Commentary on the safety of red blood cells preserved in extended storage media for neonatal transfusions. Transfusion 1990; 30:229.
AS-1 and AS-3, extended storage media; CPDA, citrate-phosphate-dextrose-adenine solution.

2 to 4 hours, and it is far lower than doses believed to be toxic (Table 28.4). Importantly, the efficacy and safety of these theoretical calculations have been confirmed by clinical experience. Many investigators have reported the successful transfusion of stored, rather than fresh, RBCs for small-volume transfusions in infants.[33–36]

Recombinant Erythropoietin in the Anemia of Prematurity

Recognition of the low plasma EPO levels in preterm infants provides a rational basis for the use of recombinant human EPO (rHuEPO) as therapy for the anemia of prematurity. More than 20 controlled trials have tested several doses and treatment schedules in preterm infants, and results are mixed, making consensus impossible on the optimal role of rHuEPO treatment in the anemia of prematurity.[2, 37, 38]

Unquestionably, proper doses of rHuEPO and iron effectively stimulate erythropoiesis in preterm infants, as evidenced by increased marrow erythroid activity and blood reticulocyte counts. However, the efficacy of rHuEPO in substantially diminishing the number of RBC transfusions—the major goal for which it is prescribed—has not been convincingly demonstrated for all groups of preterm infants.[38] In many trials, the subjects were relatively large preterm infants and those in stable clinical condition; such infants currently receive few RBC transfusions when given only standard supportive care (i.e., not given rHuEPO).[22, 39] Currently, even without use of rHuEPO, fewer than 50% of infants with birth weights greater than 1.0 kg receive RBC transfusions. Almost all infants weighing less than 1.0 kg at birth are given RBCs, and most transfusions are given during the first 3 to 4 weeks of life.[39] To illustrate the difficulty of avoiding RBC transfusions, the multicenter, randomized North American trial, in which infants received either rHuEPO or placebo during a 6-week study period, reported statistically significant but only modest success.[40] Although significantly fewer RBC transfusions were given to rHuEPO-treated infants during the study phase (1.1 transfusions, vs. 1.6 for placebo), all infants required multiple transfusions during the 3-week prestudy phase. Therefore, rHuEPO exerted only a modest effect on total RBC transfusions given throughout the entire study (4.4 for rHuEPO vs. 5.3 for placebo) and did not resolve the problem of severe neonatal anemia.[40]

Physicians wishing to prescribe rHuEPO are faced with a dilemma. The relatively large or stable preterm infants who respond best to rHuEPO plus iron are given relatively few RBC transfusions and, accordingly, have little need for rHuEPO to avoid transfusions. Extremely preterm infants, who are sick and have the greatest need for RBC transfusions shortly after birth, have not consistently responded to rHuEPO plus iron, again questioning the efficacy of rHuEPO therapy.[37] However, extremely preterm infants are being evaluated in therapeutic trials of rHuEPO and iron, both given intravenously shortly after birth.[41, 42] Although preliminary review of these promising studies suggests success in avoiding transfusions early in life, the data are limited and are insufficient to clearly establish efficacy or to detect potential toxicity. Therefore, firm guidelines for the use of rHuEPO in the treatment of the anemia of prematurity cannot be offered at this time.

■ Platelet Transfusions

Older Children and Adolescents

Guidelines for PLT support of children and adolescents with quantitative and qualitative PLT disorders are similar to those for adults (see Table 28.1), in whom the risk of life-threatening bleeding that occurs after injury or spontaneously can be related to the severity of thrombocytopenia (when low blood PLT counts are caused by diminished marrow production). Thrombocytopenia caused by accelerated turnover (e.g., in immune thrombocytopenia) usually is not treated with PLT transfusions. PLT transfusions should be given to patients with PLT counts lower than 50×10^9/L due to marrow failure if they are bleeding or are scheduled for an invasive procedure. Studies of patients with thrombocytopenia caused by poor marrow production indicate that spontaneous bleeding increases markedly when PLT levels fall to less than 20×10^9/L, particularly in patients who are ill with infection, anemia, or dysfunction of the liver, kidneys, or lungs. For this reason, many pediatricians recommend prophylactic PLT transfusions to maintain the PLT count at greater than 20×10^9/L in children with thrombocytopenia due to bone marrow failure. This threshold has been challenged, and some favor a PLT transfusion trigger of 5 to 10×10^9/L for patients with uncomplicated conditions. However, many severely thrombocytopenic oncology and transplantation patients are too ill to be confidently transfused at these very low PLT counts, and in actual practice blood PLT counts are frequently maintained at 20×10^9/L or higher.

Qualitative PLT disorders may be inherited or acquired (e.g., in advanced hepatic or renal insufficiency, after cardiopulmonary bypass procedures). In such patients, PLT transfusions are justified only if significant bleeding actually occurs. Because PLT dysfunction may be present in the long term and repeated transfusions may lead to alloimmunization and refractoriness, prophylactic PLT transfusions are rarely justified unless an invasive procedure is planned. In such cases, a bleeding time greater than twice the upper limit of laboratory normal may be taken as diagnostic evidence that PLT dysfunction exists, but this test is poorly predictive of hemorrhagic risk or the need to transfuse PLTs. In these patients, alternative therapies, particularly desmopressin acetate, should be considered to avoid PLT transfusions.

Infants

Pathophysiology of Neonatal Thrombocytopenia

Blood PLT counts of 150×10^9/L or greater are present in normal fetuses (≥ 17 weeks of gestation) and neonates. Lower PLT counts indicate potential problems, and preterm infants exhibit thrombocytopenia commonly.[43, 44] In one neonatal intensive care unit, 22% of infants had blood PLT counts lower than 150×10^9/L during hospitalization.[43] Although multiple pathogenic mechanisms probably are involved in these sick neonates, a predominant one is accelerated PLT destruction, as shown by shortened PLT survival time, increased PLT-associated immunoglobulin G, increased PLT volume, a normal number of megakaryocytes, and an inadequate increment in blood PLT values after PLT transfusion.[43, 45] Another major mechanism contributing to neonatal thrombocytopenia is diminished PLT production, as evidenced by decreased numbers of clonogenic megakaryocyte progenitors[46, 47] and relatively low levels of thrombopoietin[47, 48] in response to thrombocytopenia, when compared with children and adults. Similar to the situation with EPO and the anemia of prematurity, thrombopoietin is produced by thrombocytopenic preterm infants, but at relatively low levels. Controlled clinical trials are needed to determine the possible role and potential toxicity of recombinant thrombopoietin therapy in infants.

Blood PLT counts lower than 100×10^9/L pose significant clinical risks for premature neonates. In one study, infants with birth weights lower than 1.5 kg and blood PLT counts lower than 100×10^9/L were compared with nonthrombocytopenic control infants of similar size.[44] The bleeding time was prolonged when PLT counts were lower than 100×10^9/L, and in many infants PLT dysfunction was suggested by bleeding times that were disproportionately long for the degree of thrombocytopenia present. Hemorrhage was more frequent in the thrombocytopenic infants, with the incidence of intracranial hemorrhage being 78% in those weighing less than 1.5 kg at birth, compared with 48% for nonthrombocytopenic infants of similar size. Moreover, the extent of hemorrhage and neurologic morbidity was greater in the group of thrombocytopenic infants.[44]

Recommendations for Platelet Transfusions During Infancy

The use of prophylactic PLT transfusions in an attempt to prevent bleeding in preterm neonates has been studied systematically.[49] However, no randomized clinical trials have been reported of therapeutic PLT transfusions in bleeding thrombocytopenic neonates. Therefore, basic questions regarding the relative risks of different degrees of thrombocytopenia in various clinical settings during infancy remain largely unanswered. However, it seems logical to transfuse

PLTs to thrombocytopenic infants, and guidelines acceptable to many neonatologists are listed in Table 28.2. Two firm indications for neonatal PLT transfusions are to treat hemorrhage that has already occurred and to prevent hemorrhage from complicating an invasive procedure. Little disagreement exists regarding the use of a blood PLT count lower than 50×10^9/L as a "transfusion trigger" in these instances. However, PLT transfusions are given to infants by some physicians to treat bleeding that occurs at higher PLT counts (between 50 and 100×10^9/L) or to diminish the threat of intracranial hemorrhage in high-risk preterm infants whenever the PLT count is lower than 100×10^9/L.[44]

Prophylactic PLT transfusions can be given under two circumstances: to prevent bleeding when severe thrombocytopenia is present and poses a risk of spontaneous hemorrhage; and to maintain the presence of a normal PLT count to prevent the infant from slipping into high-risk situations. Regarding the first circumstance, most agree that it is reasonable to give PLTs to any neonate whose blood PLT count is lower than 20×10^9/L. There is broad acceptance that spontaneous hemorrhage is a risk with PLT counts below this level. Also, severe thrombocytopenia occurs most commonly in sick infants who, because of their illnesses, receive medications that may further compromise PLT function. Because all of these factors are pronounced in extremely preterm infants, some neonatologists favor prophylactic PLT transfusion whenever the PLT count falls to less than 50×10^9/L, or even 100×10^9/L, in critically ill infants.[44]

Regarding the second circumstance, the need to maintain a completely normal PLT count ($\geq 150 \times 10^9$/L) or even higher in preterm infants without bleeding is unproven. Intracranial hemorrhage occurs commonly in sick preterm infants, and, although the etiologic role of thrombocytopenia and the therapeutic benefit of PLT transfusions have not been conclusively established in this disorder, it seems logical to presume that thrombocytopenia is a risk factor.[50] However, a randomized trial designed to address this issue—in which transfusion of PLTs whenever the PLT count fell to less than 150×10^9/L so as to maintain the average PLT count at greater than 200×10^9/L was compared with transfusion of PLTs only when the PLT count fell to less than 50×10^9/L—did not detect a difference in the incidence of intracranial hemorrhage (28% versus 26%, respectively).[49] Therefore, there is no documented benefit to transfusing "prophylactic PLTs" to maintain a completely normal PLT count, compared with transfusing "therapeutic PLTs" in response to thrombocytopenia when it actually occurs.

Currently, there are no alternatives to PLT transfusions to treat thrombocytopenia in neonates. Recombinant thrombopoietin (i.e., c-*mpl* ligand or megakaryocyte growth and differentiation factor) and interleukin-11 are promising agents. However, neither is recommended for use during infancy, and both have potential toxicities that might preclude their use in sick preterm infants. Clearly, they must not be prescribed at present, except in experimental settings.

Selecting a Platelet Product to Transfuse an Infant

The ideal goal of most PLT transfusions is to raise the PLT count to greater than 50×10^9/L or, for sick preterm infants, to greater than 100×10^9/L. This goal can be achieved consistently by the infusion of 5 to 10 mL/kg of standard PLT concentrates, collected by centrifugation of fresh units of whole blood or by automated plateletpheresis. PLT concentrates should be transfused as rapidly as the overall condition permits, certainly within 2 hours.

Routinely reducing the volume of PLT concentrates for infants by additional centrifugation steps is both unnecessary and unwise. Transfusion of 10 mL/kg PLT concentrate provides approximately 10×10^9 PLTs. Assuming that the estimated blood volume of an infant is 70 mL/kg body weight, the PLT dose of 10 mL/kg will increase the PLT count by 143×10^9/L. This calculated increment is consistent with the observed increment after this dose reported in clinical studies.[49] In general, 10 mL/kg is not an excessive transfusion volume, provided that the intake of other intravenous fluids, medications, and nutrients is monitored and adjusted. It is desirable that the infant and the PLT donor be of the same ABO blood group, and it is important to minimize repeated transfusions of group O PLTs to group A or B recipients, because large quantities of passive anti-A or -B can lead to hemolysis. Although proven methods exist to reduce the volume of PLT concentrates when truly warranted (i.e., when many transfusions are anticipated in which multiple doses of passive anti-A or -B might lead to hemolysis, or when there is failure to respond to 10 mL/kg of unmodified PLT concentrate), additional processing should be performed with great care because of probable PLT loss, clumping, and dysfunction caused by the additional handling.

■ NEUTROPHIL TRANSFUSIONS

Older Children and Adolescents

Several methodologic advances—in particular, the use of recombinant granulocyte colony-stimulating factor (G-CSF) to stimulate donors—have made it possible to collect extraordinarily large numbers of normal neutrophils (PMNs) for transfusion into neutropenic patients who have life-threatening infections. Because larger doses of PMNs can be transfused, renewed interest has arisen in the use of PMN (granulocyte) transfusions (GTX) to treat adult oncology patients and progenitor cell transplant recipients, in whom neutropenia complicated by severe infections persists as a significant problem despite combination antibiotic therapy, recombinant cytokines, myeloid growth factors, and use of mobilized peripheral blood progenitor cells to minimize neutropenic infections. If children are suffering significant morbidity and mortality from neutropenic infections despite modern supportive care, it is logical to explore the efficacy, potential toxicity, and cost-effectiveness of GTX therapy through properly designed, randomized clinical trials performed in pediatric subjects.[51]

Serious and repeated infections with bacteria, yeast, and fungi are a consequence of severe neutropenia and PMN dysfunction in some settings. In the multicenter Trial to Reduce Alloimmunization to Platelets (TRAP) study, 7% of adult patients with acute nonlymphocytic leukemia died from infection during first-remission induction therapy, despite the use of modern antibiotic therapy.[52] In another study of patients given intensive chemotherapy, some of whom also received transfusions of autologous hematopoietic stem cells, 7.6% of patients experienced systemic fungal infection.[53] Unless severe neutropenia is reversed fairly quickly in adult patients, the mortality of systemic fungal infections approaches 100%. Therefore, modern "high-dose" GTX is

considered by some experts to be very promising for adult oncology and transplantation patients.[54, 55] However, contrary data suggest that, with appropriate anti-infective therapy, serious infections are rare in patients who are transplanted with adequate numbers of peripheral blood progenitor cells.[56]

Because of these controversial views, pediatricians must survey the outcome of life-threatening infections with bacteria, yeast, and fungi in children who are undergoing intense chemotherapy or progenitor cell transplantation in their own institutions to determine whether there is a need for therapeutic GTX. If infections in neutropenic children respond promptly to antibiotics plus standard supportive care and survival approaches 100%, GTX is unnecessary. Moreover, GTX should not be used if there is no apparent need, because the lack of demonstrable benefit would not outweigh the potential risks. However, if significant numbers of infected high-risk patients fail to respond to antibiotics alone, or if the intensity of therapy is compromised because it is limited by fear of neutropenia, the addition of GTX should be considered, along with other modifications of therapy intended to reduce infections, such as selection of different antibiotics, closer monitoring of antibiotic blood levels, and use of intravenous immunoglobulin (IVIG), G-CSF, other recombinant cytokines, and immune-modulating agents.

The role of GTX added to antibiotics for patients with severe neutropenia ($<0.5 \times 10^9$/L) caused by bone marrow failure is similar in adults and children (see Table 28.1). Infected neutropenic patients usually respond to antibiotics alone, provided bone marrow function recovers early in infection. Because children with newly diagnosed leukemia respond rapidly to induction chemotherapy, only rarely are they candidates for GTX. In contrast, infected children with sustained bone marrow failure (e.g., malignant neoplasms resistant to treatment, aplastic anemia, bone marrow transplantation) may benefit from the addition of GTX to antibiotic therapy. The use of GTX for bacterial sepsis that is unresponsive to antibiotics in patients with severe neutropenia ($<0.5 \times 10^9$/L) is supported by most of the controlled studies.[51, 54]

Children with qualitative neutrophil defects (neutrophil dysfunction) usually have adequate numbers of blood neutrophils but are susceptible to serious infections because their cells kill pathogenic microorganisms inefficiently. Neutrophil dysfunction syndromes are rare, and no definitive studies have established the efficacy of GTX. However, several patients with progressive life-threatening infections have improved strikingly with the addition of GTX to antimicrobial therapy. These disorders are chronic, and because of the risk of inducing alloimmunization, GTX is recommended only if the infections are clearly unresponsive to antimicrobial drugs.

Infants

Pathophysiology of Neonatal Neutropenia and Neutrophil Dysfunction

Neonates are unusually susceptible to severe bacterial infections, and several defects of neonatal body defenses have been reported as possible contributing factors. PMNs isolated from the blood of neonates exhibit both quantitative and qualitative abnormalities that may be related to the increased incidence, morbidity, and mortality of bacterial infections. Abnormalities of neonatal PMNs include absolute and relative neutropenia, diminished chemotaxis, abnormal adhesion and aggregation, defective cellular orientation and receptor capping, decreased deformability, inability to alter membrane potential during stimulation, imbalances of oxidative metabolism, and a diminished ability to withstand oxidant stress.[57] A complete discussion of neonatal PMN physiology is beyond the scope of this chapter, and only aspects that are particularly relevant to PMN transfusions and alternative therapies are reviewed here.

Neutropenia can occur during neonatal bacterial infections, particularly with fulminant sepsis. Because a physiologic neutrophilia occurs in normal neonates, it is considered quite abnormal for the absolute blood PMN count to fall below $3.0 \times 10^9/L$ during the first week of life. Although an abnormally low PMN count can occur in neonates with disorders as diverse as sepsis, asphyxia, and maternal hypertension, suspicion of severe bacterial infection must always be high whenever relative neutropenia (PMN count, $<3.0 \times 10^9/L$) occurs. The mechanisms responsible are only partially defined, but abnormalities of neonatal granulopoiesis frequently are involved. As one factor, the postmitotic marrow PMN storage pool (metamyelocytes and mature, segmented PMNs) is small. The PMN storage pool accounts for 26% to 60% of all nucleated cells in the bone marrow of normal neonates. Neonates with sepsis may exhibit a storage pool numbering less than 10% of nucleated marrow cells and are considered to have severely diminished marrow PMN reserves.[58] Second, storage pool PMNs are released at an excessively rapid and, apparently, poorly regulated rate from the marrow during stress. Third, PMN production in response to infection is decreased. The number of committed (clonogenic) PMN precursors in neonatal marrow is lower in neonates than in older patients, and a high percentage of these cells are proliferating even when studied at an apparently basal state.[58, 59] Therefore, neonatal marrow is functioning at capacity and is unable to rapidly expand production to meet the increased demands of infection.[60] For this reason, it is logical to consider PMN transfusions until the marrow recovers.

Recommendations for Neutrophil Transfusions During Infancy

Because both quantitative and qualitative abnormalities of neonatal PMNs have been reported, PMN transfusions have been used to treat neonatal sepsis with or without neutropenia. Neonates exhibiting fulminant sepsis, relative neutropenia (PMN count, $<3.0 \times 10^9/L$ during the first week of life or $<1.0 \times 10^9/L$ thereafter), and a severely diminished PMN marrow storage pool (less than 10% of nucleated marrow cells being postmitotic PMNs) are at increased risk of death if treated only with antibiotics. Results of 11 studies[61–71] on the use of PMN transfusions to treat infected neonates, 6 of which were designed as controlled studies,[61–64, 69, 70] have been reported. The fact that four of the six controlled studies noted significant benefit from PMN transfusions is encouraging.[61–64] However, the controlled studies contained several experimental flaws.[72]

Because of these scientific imperfections, firm recommendations for the role of PMN transfusions in the treatment of neonatal sepsis cannot be made at this time. Guidelines for PMN transfusions are presented in Table 28.2. Although antibiotics are the key to successful treatment of neonatal sepsis, antibiotic therapy is not 100% successful, and attempts to bolster body defenses are warranted. PMN transfusions have not provided a complete answer; although they are efficacious for infants with neutropenia and fulminant sepsis,[72] only PMN

transfusions obtained by automated leukapheresis have demonstrated effectiveness.[71, 72] Moreover, in many instances, standard supportive care with antibiotics seems adequate. Each institution must assess its own experience with neonatal sepsis. If almost all infants survive without apparent long-term morbidity when treated only with antibiotics, PMN transfusions are unnecessary, and attention should be focused on prompt diagnosis and optimal antibiotic therapy. If the outcome of standard therapy is not optimal, alternative therapies such as PMN transfusions must be considered to improve the outlook.

Alternatives to Neonatal Neutrophil Transfusions

Not all neonatologists prescribe PMN transfusions. Their proper role has not been irrefutably established by controlled clinical trials. Moreover, the preparation of PMN concentrates by leukapheresis can be cumbersome and expensive, and the process of collecting and transfusing PMNs can pose risks for both neonates and donors. Accordingly, alternative therapies have been suggested. However, their efficacy has not been clearly established, their risks are only partially defined, and they require extensive study before they can be widely accepted. Two modalities that have been suggested are IVIG and myeloid cytokines or growth factors.

Most studies evaluating IVIG to prevent infections have found little or only modest benefit.[73–84] However, results are inconsistent. Only a few studies have suggested prophylactic benefit.[73, 74, 76] In contrast, several therapeutic studies have demonstrated a benefit from the addition of IVIG to antibiotics in the treatment of neonatal infections.[85–89] In a meta-analysis, prophylactic IVIG studies were found to demonstrate only minimal benefit, whereas therapeutic IVIG exhibited unequivocal benefit.[90] Overall, the data are insufficient to justify the use of IVIG routinely in all preterm neonates to prevent or treat sepsis. However, modest "physiologic" doses (0.3 to 0.4 mg/kg) may lessen the severity of bacterial sepsis in newborns with very low birth weights, who are likely to be hypogammaglobulinemic as a result of extremely premature birth (i.e., before the major placental transport of immunoglobulin G has taken place). However, caution must be used when prescribing IVIG therapy to prevent or treat neonatal sepsis. IVIG therapy, particularly at high dose, can impair body defense mechanisms.[91–93]

To date, properly designed clinical studies of recombinant myeloid growth factors given to human neonates are limited. In a controlled study,[94] 42 neonates with presumed bacterial sepsis, recognized within the first 3 days of life, were randomly assigned to receive three doses of either G-CSF or a placebo. Although the outcome of sepsis was not reported, G-CSF induced a significant increase in the blood PMN count, an increase in the marrow PMN storage pool, and an increase in PMN membrane C3bi expression—the last being an indication of enhanced functional capability.

In a controlled study of granulocyte-macrophage colony-stimulating factor (GM-CSF),[95] 20 premature neonates were randomly assigned within 72 hours after birth to receive either GM-CSF or a placebo for 7 days. GM-CSF increased the blood PMN count, the marrow PMN storage pool, and C3bi receptor expression. In addition, neonates receiving GM-CSF exhibited an increase in blood monocyte and PLT counts. The study was not designed to assess efficacy in the prevention or treatment of infections.

Two additional randomized clinical trials have been conducted to assess the efficacy of G-CSF and GM-CSF. Neither demonstrated clear clinical benefit. In the G-CSF trial, 20 infants with neutropenia and sepsis received either G-CSF (10 mg/kg/day) or placebo for 3 days.[96] Acknowledging that the number of study subjects was too small for definitive conclusions, G-CSF did not significantly improve severity of illness, morbidity, or mortality. In a preliminary report of the GM-CSF trial,[97] preterm infants received either GM-CSF (8 µg/kg/day) or placebo for the first 28 days of life in an attempt to reduce the incidence of infections. Although GM-CSF was well tolerated and significantly increased blood leukocyte counts, it did not significantly decrease infection rates. Therefore, firm guidelines cannot be made at this time regarding the proper role of myeloid growth factors in the management of neonatal neutropenia or sepsis.

Clearly, there is no universally accepted role for PMN transfusions, IVIG, or myeloid growth factors in the treatment of neonatal sepsis. However, it seems reasonable to treat fulminant sepsis in neonates with neutropenia (blood PMN counts $<3 \times 10^9$/L during the first week of life or $<1 \times 10^9$/L thereafter) as follows. For infants born <30 weeks gestation, give one dose of 500 mg/kg of IVIG plus 5 µg/kg of G-CSF on three consecutive days. For infants born ≥ 30 weeks gestation, give 5 µg/kg of G-CSF on three consecutive days. This therapy should be adjunctive to optimal antibiotic and supportive care.

REFERENCES

1. Hebert PC, Wells G, Blajchman MA, et al., and the Transfusion Requirements in Critical Care Investigators for the Canadian Critical Care Trials Group. A multicenter, randomized, controlled clinical trial of transfusion requirements in critical care. N Engl J Med 1999;340:409.
2. Strauss RG: Red blood cell transfusion practices in the neonate. Clin Perinatol 1995;22:641.
3. Strauss RG, Sacher RA, Blazina JF, et al: Commentary on small-volume red cell transfusions for neonatal patients. Transfusion 1990;30:565.
4. Stockman JA: Anemia of prematurity: current concepts in the issue of when to transfuse. Pediatr Clin North Am 1986;33:111.
5. Wardrop CA, Holland BM, Veale KE, et al: Nonphysiological anaemia of prematurity. Arch Dis Child 1978;53:855.
6. Holland BM, Jones JG, Wardrop CA: Lessons from the anemia of prematurity. Hematol Oncol Clin North Am 1987;1:355.
7. Stockman JA III, Garcia JF, Oski FA: The anemia of prematurity: factors governing the erythropoietin response. N Engl J Med 1977;296:647.
8. Brown MS, Phibbs RH, Garcia JF, Dallman PR: Postnatal changes in erythropoietin levels in untransfused premature infants. J Pediatr 1983;103:612.
9. Stockman JA III, Graeber JE, Clark DA, et al: Anemia of prematurity: determinants of the erythropoietin response. J Pediatr 1984;105:786.
10. Brown MS, Garcia JF, Phibbs RH, Dallman PR: Decreased response of plasma immunoreactive erythropoietin to "available oxygen" in anemia of prematurity. J Pediatr 1984;105:793.
11. Shannon KM, Naylor GS, Torkildson JC, et al: Circulating erythroid progenitors in the anemia of prematurity. N Engl J Med 1987;317:728.
12. Rhondeau SM, Christensen RD, Ross MP, et al: Responsiveness to recombinant human erythropoietin of marrow erythroid progenitors from infants with the "anemia of prematurity." J Pediatr 1988;112:935.
13. Zanjani ED, Ascensao JL, McGlave PB, et al: Studies on the liver to kidney switch of erythropoietin production. J Clin Invest 1981;67:1183.
14. Dame C, Fahnenstich H, Freitag P, et al: Erythropoietin mRNA expression in human fetal and neonatal tissue. Blood 1998;92:3218.
15. Widness JA, Susa JB, Garcia JF, et al: Increased erythropoiesis and elevated erythropoietin in infants born to diabetic mothers and in hyperinsulinemic rhesus fetuses. J Clin Invest 1981;67:637.
16. Snijders RJ, Abbas A, Melby O, et al: Fetal plasma erythropoietin concentration in severe growth retardation. Am J Obstet Gynecol 1993;168:615.
17. Ohls RK, Li Y, Trautman MS, Christensen RD: Erythropoietin production by macrophages from preterm infants: implications regarding the cause of the anemia in prematurity. Pediatr Res 1994;35:169.
18. Widness JA, Veng-Pedersen P, Peters C, et al: Erythropoietin pharmacokinetics in premature infants: developmental, nonlinearity, and treatment effects. J Appl Physiol 1996;80:140.
19. Ruth V, Widness JA, Clemons G, Raivio KO: Postnatal changes in serum immunoreactive erythropoietin in relation to hypoxia before and after birth. J Pediatr 1990;116:950.
20. George JW, Bracco CA, Shannon KM, et al: Age related difference in erythropoietic response to recombinant human erythropoietin: comparison of adults and infants rhesus monkeys. Pediatr Res 1990;28:567.
21. Ringer SA, Richardson DK, Sacher RA, et al: Variations in transfusion practice in neonatal intensive care. Pediatrics 1998;101:194.
22. Bednarek FJ, Weisberger S, Richardson DK, et al, for the SNAP II Study Group: Variations in blood transfusions among newborn intensive care units. J Pediatr 1998;133:601.
23. Ramasethu J, Luban NL: Red blood cell transfusions in the newborn. Semin Neonatol 1999;4:5.
24. Blanchette VS, Hume HA, Levy GJ, et al: Guidelines for auditing pediatric blood transfusion practices. Am J Dis Child 1991;145:787.
25. Phillips HM, Holland BM, Abdel-Moiz A, et al: Determination of red-cell mass in assessment and management of anaemia in babies needing blood transfusion. Lancet 1986;1:882.
26. Jones JG, Holland BM, Veale KE, Wardrop CA: "Available oxygen," a realistic expression of the ability of the blood to supply oxygen to tissues. Scand J Haematol 1979;22:77.
27. Alverson DC, Isken VH, Cohen RS: Effect of booster blood transfusions on oxygen utilization in infants with bronchopulmonary dysplasia. J Pediatr 1988;113:722.
28. Hudson IR, Cavill IA, Cooke AD, et al: Biotin labeling of red cells in the measurement of red cell volume in preterm infants. Pediatr Res 1990;28:199.
29. Hudson I, Cooke A, Holland B, et al: Red cell volume and cardiac output in anaemic preterm infants. Arch Dis Child 1990;65:672.
30. Mock DM, Lankford GL, Widness JA, et al: Measurement of circulating red blood cell volume using biotin labeled red cells: validation against ^{51}Cr labeled red cells. Transfusion 1999;39:149.
31. Mock DM, Lankford GL, Widness JA, et al: Measurement of red cell survival using biotin labeled red cells: validation against ^{51}Cr labeled red cells. Transfusion 1999;39:156.
32. Luban NLC, Strauss RG, Hume HA: Commentary on the safety of red blood cells preserved in extended storage media for neonatal transfusions. Transfusion 1990;30:229.
33. Liu EA, Mannio FL, Lane TA: Prospective, randomized trial of the safety and efficacy of a limited donor exposure transfusion program for premature neonates. J Pediatr 1994;125:92.
34. Lee DA, Slagle TA, Jackson TM, Evans CS: Reducing blood donor exposures in low birth weight infants by the use of older, unwashed packed red blood cells. J Pediatr 1995;126:280.
35. Wood A, Wilson N, Skacel P, et al: Reducing donor exposure in preterm infants requiring blood transfusions. Arch Dis Child Fetal Neonatal Ed 1995;72:F29.
36. Strauss RG, Burmeister LF, Johnson K, et al: AS-1 red blood cells for neonatal transfusions: a randomized trial assessing donor exposure and safety. Transfusion 1996;36:873.
37. Strauss RG: Recombinant erythropoietin for the anemia of prematurity: still a promise, not a panacea. J Pediatr 1997;131:653.
38. Widness JA, Strauss RG: Recombinant erythropoietin in treatment of the premature newborn. Semin Neonatol 1998;3:163.
39. Widness JA, Seward VJ, Kromer IJ, et al: Changing patterns of red blood cell transfusion in very low birthweight infants. J Pediatr 1996;129:680.
40. Shannon KM, Keith JF III, Mentzer WC, et al: Recombinant human erythropoietin stimulates erythropoiesis and reduces erythrocyte transfusions in very-low-birth-weight preterm infants. Pediatrics 1995;95:1.
41. Ohla RK, Veerman MW, Christensen RD: Pharmacokinetics and effectiveness of recombinant erythropoietin administered to preterm infants by continuous infusion in total parenteral nutrition solution. J Pediatr 1996;128:518.

42. Ohls RK, Harcum J, Schibler KR, Christensen RD: The effect of erythropoietin on the transfusion requirements of preterm infants weighing 750 grams or less: a randomized, double-blind, placebo-controlled study. J Pediatr 1997;131:661.

43. Castle V, Andrew M, Kelton J, et al: Frequency and mechanism of neonatal thrombocytopenia. J Pediatr 1986;108:749.

44. Andrew M, Castle V, Saigal S, et al: Clinical impact of neonatal thrombocytopenia. J Pediatr 1987;110:457.

45. Castle V, Coates G, Kelton JG, Andrew M: ^{111}In-oxine platelet survivals in thrombocytopenic infants. Blood 1987;70:652.

46. Murray NA, Roberts IA: Circulating megakaryocytes and their progenitors in early thrombocytopenia in preterm neonates. Pediatr Res 1996;40:112.

47. Wolber E-M, Dame C, Fahnenstich H, et al: Expression of the thrombopoietin gene in human fetal and neonatal tissues. Blood 1999;94:97.

48. Murray NA, Watts TL, Roberts IA: Endogenous thrombopoietin levels and effect of recombinant human thrombopoietin on megakaryocyte precursors in term and preterm babies. Pediatr Res 1998;43:148.

49. Andrew M, Vegh P, Caco C, et al: A randomized trial of platelet transfusions in thrombocytopenic premature infants. J Pediatr 1993;123:285.

50. Lupton BA, Hill A, Whitfield MF, et al: Reduced platelet count as a risk factor for intraventricular hemorrhage. Am J Dis Child 1988;142:1222.

51. Strauss RG: The rebirth of granulocyte transfusions: should it involve pediatric oncology and transplant patients? Am J Pediatr Hematol Oncol 1999;21:475.

52. The Trial to Reduce Alloimmunization to Platelets Study Group. Leukocyte reduction and ultraviolet B irradiation of platelets to prevent alloimmunization and refractoriness to platelet transfusions. N Engl J Med 1997;337:1861.

53. Peters BG, Adkins DR, Harrison BR, et al: Antifungal effects of yeast-derived rhu-GM-CSF in patients receiving high-dose chemotherapy given with or without autologous stem cell transplantation: a retrospective analysis. Bone Marrow Transplant 1996;18:93.

54. Vamvakas EC, Pineda AA: Meta-analysis of clinical studies of efficacy of granulocyte transfusions in the treatment of bacterial sepsis. Journal of Clinical Apheresis 1996;11:1.

55. Adkins D, Spitzer G, Johnson M, et al: Transfusions of granulocyte-colony-stimulating factor-mobilized granulocyte components to allogeneic transplant recipients: analysis of kinetics and factors determining posttransfusion neutrophil and platelet counts. Transfusion 1997;37:737.

56. Kolbe K, Domkin D, Derigs HG, et al: Infectious complications during neutropenia subsequent to peripheral blood stem cell transplantation. Bone Marrow Transplant 1997;19:143.

57. Rosenthal J, Cairo MS: Neonatal myelopoiesis and immunomodulation of host defenses. In Petz LD, Swisher SN, Kleinman S, Spence RK, Strauss RG (eds): Clinical Practice of Transfusion Medicine, 3rd ed. New York: Churchill Livingstone, 1995, p 685.

58. Christensen RD, MacFarlane JL, Taylor NL, et al: Blood and marrow neutrophils during experimental group B streptococcal infection: quantification of the stem cell, proliferative, storage and circulating pools. Pediatr Res 1982;16:549.

59. Erdman SH, Christensen RD, Bradley PP, Rothstein G: Supply and release of storage neutrophils: a developmental study. Biol Neonate 1982;41:132.

60. Christensen RD, Harper TE, Rothstein G: Granulocyte-macrophage progenitor cells in term and preterm neonates. J Pediatr 1986;109:1047.

61. Christensen RD, Rothstein G, Anstall HB, Bybee B: Granulocyte transfusions in neonates with bacterial infection, neutropenia and depletion of mature marrow neutrophils. Pediatrics 1982;70:1.

62. Laurenti F, Ferro R, Isacchi G, et al: Polymorphonuclear leukocyte transfusion for the treatment of sepsis in the newborn infants. J Pediatr 1981;98:118.

63. Cairo MS, Rucker R, Bennetts GA, et al: Improved survival of newborns receiving leukocyte transfusions for sepsis. Pediatrics 1984;74:887.

64. Cairo MS, Worcester C, Rucker R, et al: Role of circulating complement and polymorphonuclear leukocyte transfusion in treatment and outcome in critically ill neonates with sepsis. J Pediatr 1987;110:935.

65. DeCurtis M, Romano G, Scarpato N, et al: Transfusions of polymorphonuclear leukocytes (PMN) in an infant with necrotizing enterocolitis (NEC) and a defect of phagocytosis. J Pediatr 1981;99:665.

66. Christensen RD, Anstall H, Rothstein G: Neutrophil transfusion in septic neutropenic neonates. Transfusion 1982;22:151.

67. Laing IA, Boulton FE, Hume R: Polymorphonuclear leukocyte transfusion in neonatal septicemia. Arch Dis Child 1983;58:1003.

68. Laurenti F, LaGreca G, Ferro R, Bucci G: Transfusion of polymorphonuclear neutrophils in a premature infant with *Klebsiella* sepsis. Lancet 1978;2:111.

69. Baley JE, Stork EK, Warkentin PI, Shurin SB: Buffy coat transfusions in neutropenic neonates with presumed sepsis: a prospective, randomized trial. Pediatrics 1987;80:712.

70. Wheeler JC, Chauvenet AR, Johnson CA, et al: Buffy coat transfusions in neonates with sepsis and neutrophil storage pool depletion. Pediatrics 1987;79:422.

71. Newman RS, Waffarn F, Simmons GE, et al: Questionable value of saline prepared granulocytes in the treatment of neonatal septicemia. Transfusion 1988;28:196.

72. Strauss RG: Current status of granulocyte transfusions to treat neonatal sepsis. J Clin Apheresis 1989;5:25.

73. Haque KN, Zaidi MN, Haque SK, et al: Intravenous immunoglobulin for prevention of sepsis in preterm and low birth weight infants. Pediatr Infect Dis 1986;5:622.

74. Chirico G, Rondini G, Plebani A, et al: Intravenous gammaglobulin therapy for prophylaxis of infection in high-risk neonates. J Pediatr 1987;110:437.

75. Clapp DW, Kliegman RM, Baley JE, et al: Use of intravenously administered immune globulin to prevent nosocomial sepsis to low birth weight infants: report of a pilot study. J Pediatr 1989;115:973.

76. Conway SP, Ng PC, Howel D, et al: Prophylactic intravenous immunoglobulin in preterm infants: a controlled trial. Vox Sang 1990;59:6–11.

77. Stabile A, Miceli Sopo S, et al: Intravenous immunoglobulin for prophylaxis of neonatal sepsis in premature infants. Arch Dis Child 1988;63:441.

78. Magny JF, Bremard-Oury C, Brault D, et al: Intravenous immunoglobulin therapy for prevention in high-risk premature infants: report of a multicenter, double-blind study. Pediatrics 1991;88:437.

79. Baker CJ, Melish ME, Hall RT, et al: Intravenous immune globulin for the prevention of nosocomial infection in low-birth-weight neonates. The Multicenter Group for the Study of Immune Globulin in Neonates. N Engl J Med 1992;327:213.

80. Bussel JB: Intravenous gammaglobulin in the prophylaxis of late sepsis in very-low-birth-weight infants: preliminary results of a randomized, double-blind, placebo-controlled trial. Rev Infect Dis 1990;12:S457.

81. Fanaroff AA, Korones SB, Wright LL, et al, for the National Institute of Child Health and Human Development Neonatal Research Network: A controlled trial of intravenous immune globulin to reduce nosocomial infections in very-low-birth-weight infants. N Engl J Med 1994;330:1107.

82. van Overmeire B, Bleyaert S, van Reempts PJ, van Acker KJ: The use of intravenously administered immunoglobulins in the prevention of severe infection in very low birth weight neonates. Biol Neonate 1993;64:110.

83. Weisman LE, Stoll BJ, Kueser TJ, et al: Intravenous immune globulin prophylaxis of late-onset sepsis in premature neonates. J Pediatr 1994;125:922.

84. Christensen RD, Hardman T, Thornton J, Hill HR: A randomized, double-blind, placebo-controlled investigation of the safety of intravenous immune globulin administration to preterm neonates. J Perinatol 1989;9:126.

85. Sidiropoulos D, Boehme U, von Muralt G, et al: Immunoglobulin supplementation in prevention or treatment of neonatal sepsis. Pediatr Infect Dis J 1986;5:S193.

86. Haque KN, Zaidi MH, Bahakim H: IgM-enriched intravenous immuno-globulin therapy in neonatal sepsis. Am J Dis Child 1988;142:1293.

87. Friedman CA, Wender DG, Temple DM, Rawson JE: Intravenous gamma globulin as adjunct therapy for severe group B streptococcal disease in the newborn. Am J Perinatol 1990;7:1.

88. Weisman LE, Stoll BJ, Kueser TJ, et al: Intravenous immune globulin therapy for early-onset sepsis in premature neonates. J Pediatr 1992;121:434.

89. Haque KN, Remo C, Bahakim H: Comparison of two types of intravenous immunoglobulins in the treatment of neonatal sepsis. Clin Exp Immunol 1995;101:328.

90. Jenson HB, Pollock BH: Meta-analyses of the effectiveness of intravenous immune globulin for prevention and treatment of neonatal sepsis. Pediatrics 1997;99:E2.

91. Cross AS, Siegel G, Byrne WR, et al: Intravenous immune globulin impairs anti-bacterial defenses of a cyclophosphamide-treated host. Clin Exp Immunol 1989;76:159.

92. Weisman LE, Lorenzetti PM: High intravenous doses of human immune globulin suppress neonatal group B streptococcal immunity in rats. J Pediatr 1989;115:445.

93. Cross AS, Alving BM, Sadoff JC, et al: Intravenous immune globulin: a cautionary note. Lancet 1984;1:912.

94. Gillan ER, Christensen RD, Suen Y, et al: A randomized, placebo-controlled trial of recombinant human granulocyte colony-stimulating factor administration in newborn infants with presumed sepsis: significant induction of peripheral and bone marrow neutrophilia. Blood 1994;84:1427.

95. Cairo MS, Christensen R, Sender LS, et al: Results of a phase I/II trial of recombinant human granulocyte-macrophage colony-stimulating factor in very low birthweight neonates: significant induction of circulatory neutrophils, monocytes, platelets, and bone marrow neutrophils. Blood 1995;86:2509.

96. Schibler KR, Osborne KA, Leung LY, et al: A randomized, placebo-controlled trial of granulocyte colony-stimulating factor administration to newborn infants with neutropenia and clinical signs of early-onset sepsis. Pediatrics 1998;102:6.

97. Cairo MS, Agosti J, Ellis R, et al: A randomized, double-blind, placebo-controlled trial of prophylactic recombinant human granulocyte-macrophage colony-stimulating factor to reduce nosocomial infections in very low birth weight neonates. J Pediatr 1999;134:64.

Chapter 29

Transfusion in the Hemoglobinopathies

Krista L. Hillyer
James R. Eckman

■ Sickle Cell Disease

Pathogenesis and Clinical Pathology

Eight percent of African Americans are heterozygous carriers of hemoglobin S (HbS), and 1 in every 300 has sickle cell disease (SCD). The homozygous state (HbSS), also known as sickle cell anemia, is the most common type of SCD in the United States; 1 in 600 African Americans has HbSS.[1, 2] Compound heterozygote states, such as sickle cell hemoglobin C (HbSC) disease, together with the combination of HbS and β-thalassemia (sickle cell β-thalassemia), account for most of the remaining African American cases of SCD.[1, 2] Other types of SCD arise from the interaction of HbS with rarer hemoglobin variants; these account for a small number of SCD cases in North America.

Patients with SCD have HbS levels greater than 50% of the total hemoglobin concentration. This abnormal sickle hemoglobin, when deoxygenated, forms polymers within the erythrocyte that distort its shape and decrease its deformability, leading to vaso-occlusive phenomena. A detailed description of the molecular pathogenesis of SCD is beyond the scope of this text; the reader is referred to Bunn[3] and Steinberg[4] for recent extensive reviews of this topic.

The vaso-occlusive events, abnormal blood rheology, complex cellular interactions, and other poorly understood factors resulting from the polymerization of HbS cause hemolytic anemia and increased susceptibility to infection, infarctive organ damage, and recurrent episodes of severe pain (Table 29.1). As a result of these complications, patients with HbSS (in developed countries) have a reduced life span.[5] Many of the complications of SCD can be abrogated, ameliorated, or prevented by transfusion of donor red blood cells (RBCs). Because of the numerous proven clinical benefits from transfusion and the complex rheologic properties of

Table 29.1 Clinical Features of Sickle Cell Disease

Central Nervous System

Cerebrovascular accidents

Skeletal System

Bone pain
Bony abnormalities
Delayed growth
Osteonecrosis
Dactylitis
Osteomyelitis

Cardiopulmonary System

Tachycardia
Pulmonary infarctions
Acute chest syndrome

Genitourinary System

Renal failure
Priapism

Hepatobiliary System

Jaundice
Hepatomegaly
Intrahepatic cholestasis

Spleen

Splenomegaly
Autosplenectomy

Eye

Retinopathy
Visual loss

Skin

Leg ulcers

sickle blood, there are a number of unique goals, indications, and methods for transfusion in SCD.

Goals of Transfusion Therapy

The goals of RBC transfusion in SCD patients are (1) to improve oxygen-carrying capacity by increasing the total hemoglobin concentration; (2) to decrease blood viscosity and improve blood flow by diluting RBCs containing sickle hemoglobin; and (3) to suppress endogenous erythropoiesis by increasing tissue oxygenation.[6, 7] The first goal is common to many clinical indications for RBC transfusion to any patient. The latter two goals lead to indications for RBC transfusion that are required only in individuals with hemoglobinopathies. They also provide unique potential benefits, as well as associated complications, when compared with standard methods of transfusion.

Indications for Transfusion Therapy

RBCs may be administered to patients with SCD by simple RBC infusion or by RBC exchange, either episodically, for the relief of acute symptoms, or chronically, for the prevention of long-term complications. A summary of indications for transfusion of RBCs in SCD patients is shown in Table 29.2. These indications are characterized in the following sections as "generally indicated" or "controversial," based on a recently published consensus of a panel of sickle cell experts.[8]

Indications for Episodic Transfusion

ACUTE SYMPTOMATIC ANEMIA

Because patients with SCD are chronically anemic, they are often asymptomatic despite very low hemoglobin levels. Biochemical and physiologic factors that decrease symptoms during the chronic anemia include increased levels of 2,3-diphosphoglycerate, decreased oxygen–hemoglobin affinity, increased plasma volume, and increased cardiac stroke volume and output.[9] Patients may become acutely symptomatic, making simple transfusion necessary, if they experience a rapid decrease in hemoglobin, hypoxia, or acute

Table 29.2 Clinical Indications for Transfusion in Patients with Sickle Cell Disease

Type of Transfusion	Indication
Episodic	Acute symptomatic anemia
	Aplastic crisis
	Acute chest syndrome
	Acute splenic sequestration
	Acute hepatic sequestration
	Stroke
	Prior to surgery requiring general anesthesia
	Prior to eye surgery
	Acute multiorgan system failure
	Severe infection
Chronic	Prevention of recurrent strokes in children
	Prevention of first stroke in children
	Complicated pregnancy
	Chronic organ failure
	Frequent severe pain episodes
Controversial or not indicated	Recurrent acute chest syndrome
	Priapism
	Acute pain crisis
	Normal pregnancy
	Leg ulcers

cardiac decompensation. Acute anemia can result from bleeding, suppression of erythropoiesis by infection, sequestration, or increased hemolysis. Pulmonary or cardiac disease can cause decompensation, requiring acute transfusion to increase the hemoglobin level above the patient's stable baseline.

APLASTIC CRISIS

Aplastic crisis, typically defined as a decrease in hemoglobin of more than 3.0 g/dL with reticulocytopenia, is a relatively common occurrence in SCD.[10] Aplastic crisis occurs in SCD patients after marked suppression of erythropoiesis for 7 to 10 days, usually as a result of infection of RBC precursors in the bone marrow by human parvovirus B19. In a sample group of 308 children with SCD, human parvovirus B19 accounted for all cases of aplastic crisis that occurred during an 8-year observation period.[11] Because mean RBC survival time in many SCD patients is only 12 to 15 days, the acute and life-threatening anemia caused by human parvovirus B19 infection necessitates immediate RBC transfusion in order to sustain oxygen delivery to the tissues until the bone marrow recovers. Simple RBC transfusion is usually administered slowly (1 mL/kg/hr), because these patients have expanded plasma volumes due to chronic anemia and care must be taken to avoid volume-induced congestive heart failure.[12, 13] Partial exchange transfusion, performed by manually removing whole blood and returning RBCs to the patient without replacing the plasma, is a method that may be preferred if heart failure from acute volume overload is of significant concern.[14]

ACUTE CHEST SYNDROME

According to a report by the Cooperative Study of Sickle Cell Disease, acute chest syndrome (ACS) occurs at least once in approximately 30% of SCD patients, and half of these patients will experience one or more recurrent episodes.[8] ACS is the second most common reason for hospital admission among SCD patients,[15] and it is responsible for 25% of all deaths in this population.[16] Transfusion therapy is vital to the treatment of ACS early in its course,[17] and exchange transfusion has been shown to result in rapid improvement of ACS if instituted within 48 hours after diagnosis.[18] Simple transfusion causes dramatic improvement of symptoms in children with ACS (compared with nontransfused children) if it is begun within 24 hours after diagnosis;[19] therefore, in patients with less serious compromise, simple transfusion is preferred.[20] For those patients with either a progressive decline in arterial oxygen pressure (PaO$_2$ <60 mm Hg in adults, <70 mm Hg in children) or a rapid clinical deterioration, exchange transfusion is recommended.

ACUTE SPLENIC OR HEPATIC SEQUESTRATION

Acute splenic sequestration occurs in SCD patients when sickled RBCs are trapped within splenic sinusoids. As the spleen enlarges, it traps a significant proportion of the circulating RBCs, leading to increased anemia and circulatory failure.[21] The fatality rate from acute splenic sequestration approaches 10%, and approximately 50% of those who survive a first episode will experience another.[21] Immediate simple RBC transfusion has been shown to produce rapid resolution of acute splenic sequestration.[21, 22] Splenic sequestration occurs in HbSS patients early in life. It occurs less frequently, but at all ages, in patients with HbSC or sickle cell β-thalassemia.

Older patients may develop acute hepatic sequestration, which responds well to a similar transfusion strategy.[23]

STROKE

Approximately 3.75% of patients with SCD will experience one or more cerebrovascular accidents, according to a longitudinal clinical trial published by the Cooperative Study of Sickle Cell Disease in 1998.[24] The occurrence of infarctive stroke is greatest in children and older patients, whereas the occurrence of hemorrhagic stroke is greatest in patients age 20 to 29 years. Because the neurologic sequelae of strokes are often devastating, immediate RBC exchange transfusion is indicated upon diagnosis of stroke.[25] Dramatic recovery of neurologic function has been documented after exchange therapy in SCD patients with acute stroke.[24, 26]

Transfusion in the Perioperative Period

BEFORE SURGERY REQUIRING GENERAL ANESTHESIA

Hypoxia, volume depletion, hypotension, hypothermia, and acidosis are all complications of general anesthesia that can lead to intravascular sickling and vascular occlusion, resulting in high rates of morbidity and mortality among SCD patients undergoing general anesthesia.[27] In a prospective study of 717 SCD patients including 1079 surgical procedures, those patients undergoing low-risk surgeries who received perioperative RBC transfusions had a 4.8% rate of SCD-related postoperative complications, compared with a significantly higher complication rate of 12.9% among similar patients who were not transfused.[28] For minor procedures and tonsillectomies, many patients did not receive transfusions and complication rates were very low.[28] Similarly, in a prospective trial of 364 SCD patients undergoing cholecystectomy, the most common surgical procedure among pediatric and adult SCD patients,[28] those who were not transfused perioperatively had a higher incidence of sickle cell events (32%) than transfused patients did.[29]

In a controlled, randomized trial, Vichinsky and colleagues[27] compared "aggressive" versus "conservative" transfusion regimens in the perioperative management of 604 operations in 551 patients with SCD. The aggressive transfusion regimen was designed to maintain a preoperative hemoglobin level of 10 g/dL and an HbS level at or below 30%. The conservative transfusion regimen only maintained a preoperative hemoglobin level of 10 g/dL, regardless of the percentage of HbS. Results showed that the frequency of serious perioperative complications was similar in the aggressive and conservative transfusion groups (31% and 35%, respectively), whereas the transfusion-related complication rates were 14% and 7%, respectively. The authors concluded that a conservative transfusion regimen is as effective in preventing perioperative complications as an aggressive transfusion regimen.

Conversely, Adams and associates[30] published a retrospective review of 92 children with SCD who underwent 130 surgical procedures using an aggressive transfusion regimen, with most RBC units phenotypically matched to recipients for Rh and Kell antigens. Major perioperative complications occurred in only 12% of surgical procedures, compared with 31% to 35% in Vichinsky's study.[27] The transfusion-related complication rate in Adams' pediatric study (8%) was similar to the rate observed in the conservative arm of Vichinsky's adult and pediatric study (7%). Although Adams suggested that the more aggressive approach with phenotypically matched blood is superior, it is difficult to directly compare the results of this small, retrospective study with those of a large, randomized, controlled clinical trial.

For adults and pediatric patients with SCD who are to undergo general anesthesia, simple transfusion to increase the preoperative hemoglobin level to 10 g/dL, together with intraoperative or postoperative RBC replacement for blood loss, appears appropriate based on the studies published to date.

BEFORE EYE SURGERY

The use of transfusions in patients undergoing eye surgery is controversial. Although early studies advocated the use of aggressive exchange transfusion for patients undergoing retinal or vitreous surgery, more recent studies have documented that this approach may not be necessary.[31] Although eye surgery is typically performed under local anesthesia, the microvascular nature of the surgery and the importance of avoiding permanent damage to the eye justify the use of blood transfusion for this indication. Until further data are available, it is reasonable to follow guidelines similar to those used for transfusion of SCD patients undergoing surgical procedures performed under general anesthesia.

ACUTE MULTIORGAN SYSTEM FAILURE

Acute multiorgan failure syndrome may occur after some episodes of severe pain crisis in SCD patients and affects at least two of the following three organs: lung, liver, or kidney. Immediate initiation of RBC transfusion is recommended for the treatment of acute multiorgan failure syndrome.[25, 32] Dramatic clinical improvement and rapid reversal of organ dysfunction have been observed after prompt, aggressive transfusion therapy. Simple transfusion is indicated for patients with severe anemia and rapidly falling hemoglobin levels. Exchange transfusion is indicated for those with higher hemoglobin levels or more severe organ failure.[32]

SEVERE INFECTION

Bacterial and malarial infections are common, and life-threatening complications occurring in SCD patients worldwide. Some experts do consider it acceptable medical practice to transfuse individuals with severe anemia who have concomitantly serious infections.[25] Infection without concomitant anemia is not a widely accepted indication for transfusion in SCD patients.

Indications for Chronic Transfusion

PREVENTION OF RECURRENT STROKES IN CHILDREN

Approximately 3.75% of SCD patients will experience one or more cerebrovascular accidents, or strokes.[24] Without therapeutic intervention, strokes will recur in more than two thirds of this patient group within 2 to 3 years.[33] Chronic RBC transfusions provide a reduction of up to 90% in the risk of recurrent stroke in these SCD patients (10% risk of recurrent stroke while undergoing a chronic RBC transfusion regimen).[34, 35]

The chronic transfusion regimen recommended for prevention of recurrent stroke, in the 3.75% of SCD patients who have experienced a stroke, is simple RBC transfusion every 3 to 4 weeks, with a goal of maintaining HbS at less than 30% and hematocrit at 30% or less.[34, 36] Cohen and colleagues[37] reported no increased risk of recurrent stroke in a small group of patients in whom the desired HbS level was modified to 50% after they had been neurologically stable for 3 years with chronic transfusion maintaining a 30% HbS level. The major benefit of this modified regimen was a 31% decrease in blood requirements for simple transfusions, which reduced cost, decreased inconvenience, and mitigated the development of alloimmunization and iron overload. Although the sample size was too small to conclude that this method is absolutely effective at preventing recurrent stroke, many experts allow the HbS percentage to increase to 50% in patients who have been stable neurologically for 3 years with chronic transfusion.[25]

The optimal duration of chronic transfusion for prevention of recurrent stroke is not known. Wang and coworkers[38] reported that 5 of 10 patients had recurrent strokes within 1 year after discontinuation of chronic transfusions, after a median period without recurrence (since first stroke) of 9.5 years. This rate is significantly greater than the 10% estimated risk of recurrent stroke among patients receiving chronic transfusion therapy. Therefore, most centers recommend continuation of chronic transfusion therapy indefinitely to prevent recurrent stroke.[25, 37]

PREVENTION OF FIRST STROKE IN CHILDREN

High blood-flow velocity in the internal carotid and middle cerebral arteries, detected by transcranial Doppler ultrasonography, has been found to be predictive of subsequent stroke in children with SCD.[39, 40] Adams and associates[30] used transcranial Doppler ultrasonography to identify children at high risk for stroke, randomly assigned them to receive either standard care or chronic transfusion therapy, and then compared the incidence of stroke between the two groups. There were 11 strokes in the standard-care group but only 1 stroke in the transfusion group, a 92% difference in the risk of stroke ($p < .001$). The authors concluded that transfusion greatly reduces the risk of first stroke in children with SCD who have abnormal transcranial Doppler ultrasonography results.[30] Because this diagnostic method is safe and noninvasive and the prevention of stroke in these patients can greatly reduce the morbidity and mortality of this complication, many sickle cell centers have implemented regular transcranial Doppler screening and subsequent chronic transfusion in children with repeated high flow rates, in order to prevent first strokes in children with SCD.[8, 25]

COMPLICATED PREGNANCY

Although normal pregnancy in SCD patients is not an indication for prophylactic transfusion (see later discussion),[41-43] certain complications of either the pregnancy itself or the underlying disease process are indications for simple or exchange transfusion (see Table 29.2). These include preeclampsia/eclampsia, twin pregnancy, previous perinatal mortality, acute renal failure, sepsis, bacteremia, severe anemia with reduction in hemoglobin of more than 20% from baseline or a hemoglobin concentration lower than 5 g/dL, ACS, hypoxemia, anticipated surgery, and preparation for infusion of angiographic dye.[44] For all of these indications, simple transfusion is most often used if the hemoglobin concentration is lower than 5 g/dL and the reticulocyte count is less than 3%. If the hemoglobin is 8 to 10 g/dL or greater, then exchange transfusion is indicated, with the goal of a post-transfusion hemoglobin concentration of 10 g/dL and a post-transfusion HbS of 50% or less.[44]

CHRONIC ORGAN FAILURE

Patients with renal failure develop progressive anemia because of the loss of erythropoietin production by the kidney.[45] Many of these patients need regular transfusions to avoid severe symptomatic anemia. Older patients with pulmonary disease causing either chronic hypoxia or cardiac disease with chronic congestive heart failure also may require chronic transfusion to prevent symptoms.[25]

FREQUENT PAIN EPISODES

Patients with frequent severe pain episodes who have a very poor quality of life or who are unable to engage in activities of normal daily living may benefit from chronic transfusion.[25] The transfusion programs used for stroke prevention will usually prevent recurrent pain episodes.[12]

Controversial Indications for Acute or Chronic Transfusion

RECURRENT ACUTE CHEST SYNDROME

Repeated episodes of ACS in SCD patients have been associated with worsening pulmonary function and restrictive lung disease, which may lead to severe pulmonary fibrosis, pulmonary hypertension, and cor pulmonale by adulthood.[46-48] Some authors have advocated the use of chronic transfusion protocols for the prevention and management of pulmonary and cardiac complications,[48] but currently no definitive evidence exists to support the efficacy of such programs.

PRIAPISM

Case studies have suggested improvement in some patients with acute priapism after exchange[49, 50] or simple transfusion therapy.[51, 52] However, no controlled trial has been performed to establish the effectiveness of transfusion therapy in comparison with hydration, analgesia, stilbestrol,[11] or hydralazine[53, 54] therapies for the treatment of acute priapism. In fact, an *a*ssociation among *S*CD, *p*riapism, *e*xchange transfusion, and subsequent *n*eurologic events has been described in several patients and has been given the eponym *ASPEN syndrome.*[55] As a result, many centers conservatively manage priapism, using hydration and analgesia, and do not transfuse until a single episode has persisted for longer than 24 to 48 hours.[53] The indications for and the preferred method of transfusion in SCD patients with priapism require further study.

ACUTE PAIN CRISES

Episodes of severe pain, also known as pain crises, are the most common reason for hospital admission of SCD patients. Platt and colleagues[56] showed that occurrences of pain crises have a direct correlation with hematocrit levels: the more severe the anemia (i.e., the lower the hemoglobin concentration), the less frequent the occurrence of pain crises. There is no evidence that transfusion reduces the severity or duration of pain during acute pain episodes.[25] Therefore, simple transfusion is not indicated for the treatment of acute pain crises and could actually worsen symptoms.

NORMAL PREGNANCY

A randomized, controlled trial was performed by Koshy and coworkers[41] to assess the benefits, if any, of prophylactic transfusion during pregnancy in women with SCD.

$$\text{Volume of replacement RBCs (mL)} = \frac{[(\text{desired \% Hct} - \text{initial \% Hct}) \times \text{TBV}]}{\text{\% Hct of replacement RBCs}}$$

Figure 29.1   Volume of red blood cells (RBCs) to be transfused to sickle cell patients using the acute simple transfusion method. Hct, hematocrit. (From Wayne AS, Kevy SV, Nathan DG: Transfusion management of sickle cell disease. Blood 1993;81:1109.)

Table 29.3   Methods of Transfusion for the Patient with Sickle Cell Disease

Acute simple transfusion

Chronic simple transfusion

Erythrocytapheresis

Manual red blood cell exchange transfusion

Pregnant patients with SCD who were prophylactically transfused were compared with similar patients who were not transfused. No significant differences in perinatal outcome or in medical or obstetric complications between these two groups were identified. The authors concluded that prophylactic transfusion of the pregnant SCD patient, a practice common at the time their study was conducted, could be omitted without harm to mother or fetus. Therefore, normal pregnancy is not considered an indication for prophylactic RBC transfusion.

LEG ULCERS

Statistical analysis of various methods for the treatment of leg ulcers in SCD patients (including transfusion) did not detect any differences in rate of ulcer healing.[57] Therefore, the routine use of transfusion for the treatment of leg ulcers in SCD patients is not justified, given the long- and short-term complications of transfusion therapy.

Methods of Transfusion Therapy

Unique Considerations in Sickle Cell Disease

Several methods of RBC transfusion therapy are used for SCD patients (Table 29.3) because of the potential limitations of acute simple transfusions, including acute volume overload and reduction in blood flow from increased blood viscosity.[58] Patients with SCD have normal or increased total blood volume because the plasma volume is increased in response to chronic anemia. Acute increases in total blood volume after transfusion of RBCs may increase cardiac work to the point of precipitating congestive heart failure.

Perhaps a more important consideration in SCD is related to changes in blood viscosity from the transfusion of RBCs.[13] Viscosity of deoxygenated or oxygenated sickle blood is increased, when compared with normal blood, at any hematocrit.[58] Because of the opposing effects of hematocrit on oxygen content and blood viscosity, the optimal hematocrit is approximately 40% for normal arterial blood. The optimal

hematocrit for sickle blood is strongly dependent on oxygen tension, varying from 18% at a PO_2 of 18 mm Hg to 31% for fully oxygenated arterial blood.[58]

Transfusion of normal RBCs significantly increases sickle blood viscosity when there are greater than 60% HbS-containing cells.[7] The increase in viscosity is minimal when the proportion of HbS-containing cells is less than 40%.[58] These in vitro observations translate into clinically relevant reductions in tissue oxygenation in SCD patients who are transfused to a hematocrit greater than 30%. This forms the rationale for the use of acute exchange transfusion in many sickle complications.[13] Chronic erythrocytapheresis is primarily used to decrease iron overload.[13]

Acute Simple Transfusion

In simple transfusion, normal donor RBCs are infused into the patient without removal of the patient's own RBCs. In general, acute simple transfusion is indicated when the immediate need for oxygen-carrying capacity is increased but no dramatic decrease in the percentage of HbS in the patient's blood is necessary.[14] The volume of RBCs to be transfused can be calculated by the formula shown in Figure 29.1.

When transfusing patients with SCD, it is desirable to maintain the hematocrit at 30% or less. Once the hematocrit rises above 30%, oxygen delivery to the tissues decreases, owing to increases in viscosity.[59] Because the primary goal of RBC transfusion is to rapidly improve oxygen delivery to tissues to prevent ongoing ischemia, the maximum beneficial hematocrit to be achieved by transfusion is 30%.

For simple transfusion, donor RBCs may be infused through an 18- to 23-gauge needle or catheter, depending on the size of the patient and the accessibility of his or her peripheral veins, using a standard blood infusion set.[60]

Chronic Simple Transfusion

Chronic simple transfusion is indicated for a variety of clinical situations in which it is desirable to increase oxygen-carrying capacity and to chronically depress the percentage of HbS in the patient's blood.[14] When a specific decrease in HbS percentage is desired, the calculation shown in Figure 29.2 estimates the dilutional effects of transfusion on HbS.

As for acute simple transfusion, the typical goal of chronic transfusion therapy is to maintain the HbS percentage at less than 30% of the total hemoglobin concentration.[14, 61] In average-size adults, maintenance of less than 30% HbS

$$\text{\% HbS desired} = \frac{[1 - (\text{transfused RBC volume} \times \text{Hct of replacement RBCs})]}{[(\text{TBV} \times \text{initial Hct}) + (\text{transfused RBC volume} \times \text{Hct of replacement RBCs})] \times (\text{initial \% HbS})}$$

Figure 29.2   Volume of red blood cells (RBCs) to be transfused to sickle cell patients using the chronic simple transfusion method. HbS, sickle hemoglobin; Hct, hematocrit; TBV, total blood volume. (Wayne AS, Kevy SV, Nathan DG: Transfusion management of sickle cell disease. Blood 1993;81:1109.)

usually requires transfusion of 2 to 3 units of RBCs every 3 to 5 weeks. For children, the amount may be calculated from the formula in Figure 29.2. The total volume of RBCs to be transfused at each regular interval in a chronic simple transfusion protocol is determined by the pretransfusion level of hemoglobin A (HbA). If the HbA percentage is too low (in most cases, 70% HbA or higher is the goal), either the volume of RBCs to be transfused is increased or the time interval between transfusions is decreased.

In the case of chronic simple RBC transfusion therapy, peripheral catheters may be surgically implanted and used for multiple transfusion events. This allows for improved venous access and less patient discomfort. Peripheral veins may also be used for chronic transfusion.

Red Blood Cell Exchange Transfusion

Donor RBCs are infused while the patient's own RBCs are removed simultaneously in the method of transfusion known as RBC exchange therapy. The major benefits of RBC exchange are the rapid adjustments in the patient's hematocrit and HbS levels. This is a critically important factor during acute sickling episodes, the major indication for RBC exchange; during certain acute ischemic crises, the replacement of sickled RBCs with normal donor RBCs (improving oxygen delivery to ischemic tissues) must be accomplished quickly to prevent further tissue damage.[14] In addition, unlike simple transfusion, RBC exchange allows for removal of the same volume of RBCs as that replaced, decreasing the risk of iron overload associated with chronic simple transfusion.

The usual measurable endpoints of RBC exchange therapy are HbA level, 70%; HbS level, 30%; and overall hematocrit, 30% or less.[25] The reasons for maintaining the hematocrit at 30% or less that related to viscosity and were explained in the previous section on simple transfusion.

RBC exchange transfusion is typically performed with the use of an automated apheresis instrument (erythrocytapheresis). This instrument removes the patient's blood, separates the RBCs from the platelet-rich plasma by centrifugation, returns the plasma to the patient, and discards the patient's sickled RBCs. At the same time, donor RBCs are infused, maintaining a stable blood volume throughout the procedure. In the past, RBC exchange transfusion could be performed only manually, and a variety of formulas were used to estimate the appropriate exchange volumes. Today, indications still exist for manual RBC exchange (see later discussion), but erythrocytapheresis is currently the most common method of RBC exchange.

The automated apheresis instrument has an internal programmable computer that precisely calculates both the volume of the patient's RBCs to be removed and the volume of the donor's RBCs to be infused. First, the patient's total blood volume and RBC volume are calculated by entering into the computer the patient's gender, height, weight, and current hematocrit. Next, the desired HbS percentage, the desired final hematocrit, and the hematocrit of the donor RBC preparation are entered, and the appropriate volumes for exchange are determined. However, the formula shown in Figure 29.3 provides a general, practical estimate of the number of RBC units to be used in automated RBC exchange transfusion. Having an estimate of the number of units to be exchanged before initiation of the procedure is important, because the blood bank may need extra time to procure the appropriate RBC units.

$$\text{Exchange RBC volume (mL)} = \text{desired \% Hct} \times \text{TBV}$$

Figure 29.3 Practical estimate of the volume of red blood cells (RBCs) to be transfused to sickle cell patients using the automated RBC exchange transfusion method. Hct, hematocrit; TBV, total blood volume. (Wayne AS, Kevy SV, Nathan DG. Transfusion management of sickle cell disease. Blood 1993;81:1109.)

The process of erythrocytapheresis is as follows. In most cases, central venous access is established, typically in the subclavian vein or the internal jugular vein, using a hemodialysis-grade, rigid-wall, large-lumen, double-bore catheter that can withstand high flow rates. In adults and larger children with easily accessible peripheral veins, the antecubital veins may be acceptable for use, with 16- to 18-gauge needles used for blood removal and 18- to 20-gauge catheters for blood return. The apheresis instrument, after being programmed with the appropriate patient data and the desired endpoints for therapy, is used by a trained operator to remove the patient's RBCs and replace them with donor RBCs. Of note, it is desirable to replace the patient's sickled RBCs with HbS-negative (sickle trait–negative) donor RBCs in an exchange procedure, primarily to appropriately calculate and achieve the desired percentages of HbS and HbA.[61]

In infants and small children, the amount of blood in the extracorporeal circuit of the automated apheresis machine represents a significant percentage of the child's total blood volume, which may lead to hypotension or a critically low hematocrit, or both, if the machine is primed with saline. Instead, the automated apheresis instrument should be primed with RBCs if (1) the extracorporeal circuit represents 12% or more of the child's blood volume, (2) the child weighs less than 20 kg, or (3) the child is anemic or unstable.[62]

Occasionally, certain patients require manual RBC exchange transfusions. Potential cases include those infants who have very small total blood volumes and emergency situations involving children or adults for which the additional time required to establish appropriate venous access or to mobilize the apheresis team would be deleterious to the patient's health. A rapid manual partial RBC exchange, for adults or children, may be performed by withdrawing blood from a peripheral (usually antecubital) vein and infusing RBCs via a stopcock into the same vein (or directly into a different peripheral vein), using the methods outlined in Figure 29.4.

In the past, RBC units were reported to have average hematocrits of 80% or more, and it was recommended that RBCs be "reconstituted" to the volume and hematocrit of whole blood (30% to 40%) by adding albumin or saline to the blood bag or syringe before manual exchange transfusion to the SCD patient.[131] However, the current average hematocrit of an RBC unit is approximately 50% to 65%,[60, 130] and the alternating administration to an SCD patient of RBCs and saline in equal volumes (see Fig. 29.4) should theoretically deliver a product essentially identical to "reconstituted" whole blood, as described previously. The requirements that must be honored to ensure a safe and effective manual exchange transfusion are the following: (1) marked increases in blood viscosity should be avoided; (2) blood volume should be maintained throughout the exchange; and (3) the exchange

Children

1. Calculate exchange volume, using 60 mL/kg as a practical estimate.
2. Divide the calculated exchange volume of RBCs into four equal aliquots.
3. Withdraw blood from the patient equal to one exchange aliquot.
4. Infuse saline equal to one exchange aliquot.
5. Withdraw blood from the patient equal to one exchange aliquot.
6. Transfuse a volume of RBCs equal to two exchange aliquots.
7. Repeat steps 3–6.

Adults

1. The exchange volume is 6–8 RBC units, depending on the size of the patient (an average 70-kg man requires approximately 6 RBC units).
2. Withdraw 500 mL of blood from the patient.
3. Infuse 500 mL of saline.
4. Withdraw 500 mL of blood from the patient.
5. Transfuse two units of RBCs.
6. Repeat until 6–8 RBC units have been transfused.

Figure 29.4 Method for rapid manual red blood cell (RBC) exchange transfusion in sickle cell patients, using practical exchange volume estimates, for children and adults. RBC units and saline infused in this alternating manner should theoretically deliver a blood product that is essentially "reconstituted" (within the patient) to the volume and hematocrit of whole blood (30% to 40%), because the current estimated average hematocrit of an RBC unit is 50% to 60%.[60, 130] However, if a known exact percent hematocrit of the blood product to be infused is desired, RBCs may be reconstituted to the volume and hematocrit of whole blood (30% to 40%) within a blood bag or syringe, by the addition of saline or other diluents.[131] (From Reid CD, Charache S, Lubin B (eds): Management and Therapy of Sickle Cell Disease, 3rd ed. Bethesda, MD: National Institutes of Health Publication, 1995, p 62.)

should be completed in the shortest length of time possible.[131] These three important factors must be evaluated and balanced, based on the unique clinical circumstances of the individual patient in need of exchange transfusion.

Chronic Erythrocytapheresis

Iron overload is one of the serious, long-term complications of chronic transfusion in SCD patients.[63] As a result, certain investigators[64–68] have suggested that chronic erythrocytapheresis should be used in place of chronic simple transfusion for the prevention of complications of SCD, in order to decrease long-term iron accumulation in these patients.

The procedure for chronic erythrocytapheresis is the same as that for acute erythrocytapheresis. Similarly, target postpheresis HbS levels for chronic erythrocytapheresis are usually less than 30%, with desirable postpheresis hematocrits of 30% or less. Currently, chronic erythrocytapheresis is not universally used in the United States for SCD patients, although recent reports suggest that the potential benefits of this method may outweigh its risks and costs. A detailed review of the current literature regarding the role of chronic erythrocytapheresis is provided later in this chapter (see "Iron Overload").

Adverse Effects of Transfusion Therapy and Strategies for Their Prevention and Management

Although transfusion is in many ways beneficial and is often necessary for treatment of SCD, adverse effects resulting from transfusion of donor blood can lead to serious long- and short-term complications in SCD patients (Table 29.4). Both immune and nonimmune complications may occur. These adverse effects, as well as recommended strategies for their prevention and management, are discussed in the following sections.

Immune-Related Adverse Effects

FEBRILE NONHEMOLYTIC TRANSFUSION REACTIONS

White blood cells synthesize and release various cytokines during storage of cellular blood products that may cause fever and chills (febrile nonhemolytic transfusion reactions, or FNHTRs) in the transfusion recipient.[69] Current technologies in leukoreduction filtration (LR) of the leukocyte count in cellular blood products to less than 5×10^6 WBC/unit, prevent the development of FNHTRs in recipients of LR blood products.[69] Because SCD patients typically receive large numbers of transfusions and FNHTRs occur in association with 0.5% to 1% of transfusions,[70] most experts recommend use of LR blood products for all SCD patients. In addition, an acute infection or a pain crisis can manifest with the same symptoms (i.e., fever, chills, malaise) as an FNHTR, confounding the clinical picture and possibly delaying appropriate treatment of underlying disorders in SCD patients. In our center, all SCD patients receive LR cellular blood products for the prevention of FNHTRs and for other reasons as well (see later discussion).

ALLOIMMUNIZATION TO RBC ANTIGENS AND DELAYED HEMOLYTIC TRANSFUSION REACTIONS

Alloimmunization to RBC antigens is a common problem in transfused SCD patients, leading both to difficulty in obtaining compatible RBC units and to the development of delayed hemolytic transfusion reactions (DHTRs).[71–75] DHTRs are especially problematic in SCD patients, in that the symptoms of a DHTR can mimic those of a pain crisis and can even lead to a pain crisis,[74] complicating both the clinical diagnosis and the subsequent appropriate treatment of these patients.

Table 29.4 Common Immune and Nonimmune Adverse Effects of Transfusion Therapy in Patients with Sickle Cell Disease and Strategies for Their Prevention and Management

Adverse Effect	Management Strategy
Immune-related	
Febrile nonhemolytic transfusion reactions	*Prevention*: Transfuse leukoreduced blood products *Treatment*: Administer antipyretic medication
Alloimmunization to RBC antigens and delayed hemolytic transfusion reactions	*Prevention*: Transfuse RBC units matched for antigens most commonly associated with alloimmunization *Treatment*: Transfuse RBC units matched for antigens to which antibodies have been made; supportive therapy for delayed reactions
Autoimmunization to RBC antigens	*Prevention*: None known *Treatment*: Administer corticosteroids with or without intravenous immune globulin (IVIG)
Alloimmunization to platelet or HLA-specific antigens	*Prevention*: Transfuse leukoreduced blood products *Treatment*: Transfuse crossmatched or HLA-matched platelet products, if needed
Non–immune-related	
Iron overload	*Prevention*: Chronic erythrocytapheresis *Treatment*: Administer deferoxamine (DFO)
Transfusion-transmitted infection (minimal risk)	*Prevention*: Use the most advanced screening tests for donated blood products; do not transfuse unnecessarily

The most comprehensive study of the frequency of and risk factors associated with alloimmunization in SCD patients was performed by Vichinsky and colleagues.[76] They prospectively determined the transfusion history, RBC antigen phenotype, and alloantibody development of 107 transfused African American patients with SCD. These results were compared with those from similar studies in 51 nontransfused African American SCD patients and in 19 white patients who had undergone multiple transfusions for other forms of chronic anemia. The results showed that the average alloimmunization rate for transfused SCD patients was 30%, compared with only 5% for the multiply transfused patients with other forms of anemia ($p < .001$). None of the nontransfused SCD patients developed alloantibodies, and the alloimmunization rate in individual SCD patients increased exponentially with increasing numbers of transfusions. Of the 32 patients who developed alloantibodies, 17 developed multiple antibodies, and 12 of these 17 patients had more than three different alloantibodies. After conducting an RBC phenotyping study of local blood bank donors and comparing

these phenotypes with those of SCD patients and of white patients with other forms of chronic anemia, the authors suggested that the increased alloimmunization rate in SCD patients most likely resulted from RBC antigenic differences between the SCD patients (African Americans) and the blood donors (the majority of whom were white). Such antigenic differences did not exist between blood donors and the multiply transfused white patients who had other forms of chronic anemia.

Because of this lack of phenotypic compatibility in antigen profile between the majority of donor RBCs and those of SCD patients, many centers have suggested that SCD patients receive RBC units matched for antigens most commonly associated with alloimmunization (see Table 29.4).[72, 74, 76] In Vichinsky's study, comparable to reports by other researchers,[72, 75, 77, 78] 66% of all alloantibodies that formed in transfused SCD patients were directed against C, E, and K RBC antigens.[76] See Table 29.5 for a summary of the most common antigens to which antibodies are made by SCD patients. Tahhan and coworkers[79] reported that none (0%) of 40 patients studied who received matched transfusions for C, E, K, Fy^a, Fy^b, and S antigens developed alloantibodies, whereas 16 (34.8%) of 46 patients who received both matched and nonmatched transfusions became alloimmunized against one or more of these antigens.

In our center, all SCD patients undergo extensive RBC antigen phenotyping before their first transfusion, a policy supported by most experts.[75, 78–80] Those SCD patients who have not yet made RBC alloantibodies routinely receive RBC units phenotypically matched for C, E, and K antigens. Once an SCD patient has made an RBC alloantibody, he or she receives RBC units matched for C, E, K, Fy^a, Jk^b, and S antigens, the six most common and most clinically significant antibodies made by SCD patients.[76] These concepts are supported by most centers, and antigen-matched transfusion results in an alloimmunization rate of approximately 1% to 5%, a significant decrease compared with the rates observed among SCD patients transfused with RBCs not matched for these common RBC antigens.[14, 72, 75, 76, 79, 81]

Limited donor pool programs offer a similar approach to preventing, or at least limiting, alloimmunization in SCD patients. The strategy to combat RBC alloimmunization is to

Table 29.5 Average Frequencies of the Most Common Red Blood Cell Alloantibodies Made by Patients with Sickle Cell Disease

Antibody	Average frequency (%)
E	21
K	18
C	14
Le^a	8
Fy^a	7
Jk^b	7
D	7
Le^b	7
S	6
Fy^b	5
M	4
e	2
c	2

Data from references 75–78.

transfuse RBCs from donors who are ethnically or antigenically closely matched with the SCD patient, most often for the four RBC antigens (C, D, E, and K) to which antibodies are most commonly made. Ambruso and associates[81] reported that such a limited donor antigen-matching program can diminish by tenfold the incidence of alloimmunization in transfused SCD patients. However, administrative problems reported in Ambruso's study included difficulties in recruiting eligible donors from the African American community, inventory management, and distribution and transfusion of the matched blood, as well as increased expense of the program. Tahhan and coworkers[79] reported that the cost of operating an antigen-matching (not a limited donor) program was 1.5 to 1.8 times that of a standard transfusion protocol.

The American Red Cross, Southern Region, in Atlanta, Georgia, has for several years partnered with its area hematologists to supply chronically transfused SCD patients (18 years of age or younger) with RBCs matched for common RBC antigens, using a group of dedicated donors. This program is entitled "Partners for Life" (PFL). PFL donors are chosen based on ethnicity (51% African American, 49% white, Hispanic American, or other) and a history of regular blood donation. Chronically transfused SCD patients enrolled in PFL without prior RBC antibody formation are antigen-matched with their dedicated donors for C, D, E, and K antigens. Patients who enter the program with antibodies already formed and those who develop antibodies during the program are matched with their donors for C, E, K, Fy^a, and Jk^b, as well as any other antigens to which they have formed antibodies. If RBC units from the patient's own pool of dedicated donors are not available when transfusion is necessary, similarly antigen-matched units from random donors are supplied.

Hillyer and colleagues[126] conducted a retrospective review of the records of 85 patients who were enrolled in PFL between January 1993 and August 2000 and reported the following data. The average number of donors per PFL patient was 9.5. The average number of RBC units transfused before PFL was 17.8, and the average number of RBC units transfused during participation in PFL was 39.4. The overall alloimmunization rate for PFL patients was 7% (6/85 developed new RBC antibodies while enrolled in PFL). Of the six patients who developed new antibodies, three had previously identified antibodies on enrollment in PFL, and three had no previously identified antibodies. One patient with previously identified antibodies developed anti-V, another developed anti-Go^a, and the third developed anti-Cw and anti-Kp^a (all antigens not routinely matched in PFL). Two of the three patients without previously formed antibodies developed anti-Fy^a (an antigen not matched in PFL for patients without previously formed alloantibodies). The other patient without previously formed antibodies developed an anti-E after being in PFL for 1.5 years with no antibody formation; however, she was known to have received non–antigen-matched RBCs at a nonparticipating institution immediately before her anti-E formation.

Although the PFL program was successful in mitigating RBC alloimmunization (7% overall rate) for this group of patients, it was not successful in limiting the exposure of SCD patients to a small, dedicated blood donor pool of 9 to 10 donors. Only 6% of PFL patients received all of their RBC units from their dedicated donors. The majority (57%) received a combination of RBC units from their dedicated donors and antigen-matched RBC units from the general volunteer donor pool. The 7% alloimmunization rate for patients enrolled in the antigen-matching, dedicated donor PFL program is significantly lower than the published 30% rate observed in SCD patients who routinely received non–antigen-matched RBCs, but it is similar to rates observed in other antigen-matching programs without the dedicated donor aspect.[75, 79, 81, 127] Based on Hillyer's review and the fact that the program was very expensive and labor-intensive (with respect to recruitment, collection, inventory management, and distribution of dedicated RBC units), the PFL program was changed to an antigen-matching program only, using primarily African American donors from the general volunteer donor pool.

AUTOIMMUNIZATION TO RBC ANTIGENS

Development of autoantibodies to RBC antigens in association with transfusions in SCD patients has been described in multiple case reports and small series of patients.[81–85] In 1999, Castellino and associates[86] reported on the frequency, characteristics, and significance of erythrocyte autoantibodies in a large group of multiply transfused children with SCD.[86] The rate of warm (immunoglobulin G) RBC autoantibody formation in this group was 7.6%; 29% of patients with erythrocyte autoantibodies had clinically significant hemolysis thought to be caused by the autoantibody. All patients with clinically significant hemolysis had both immunoglobulin G and complement detected on the surface of their RBCs. There was a strong association between autoantibody formation and the presence of RBC alloantibodies: 86% of patients with autoantibodies also had one or more alloantibodies.

The phenomenon of RBC autoantibody formation in association with blood transfusion is not well understood, but several theories exist. Alloantibodies may bind to transfused cells and cause conformational changes in the RBC antigenic epitopes, leading to stimulation of autoantibody formation.[86] Alternatively, some SCD patients may simply have a predisposition to develop RBC autoantibodies, perhaps because of an overall dysfunction of their immune systems.[86, 87] For example, the loss of a functional spleen in patients with SCD could lead to immune dysregulation, because some experimental evidence suggests that the spleen is important in the regulation of RBC autoantibody formation.[86, 88]

Whatever the cause, physicians should be aware that a syndrome of clinically significant post-transfusion hemolysis may occur in SCD patients in which both autologous and transfused RBCs are destroyed (bystander hemolysis) and that hemolysis may be exacerbated by further transfusions.[89] Serologic findings may be negative or simply not helpful in identification of the autoantibody.[86] In most cases, corticosteroids with or without intravenous immunoglobulin are beneficial in slowing hemolysis and allowing for successful continuation of necessary transfusions.[89]

ALLOIMMUNIZATION TO HUMAN LEUKOCYTE ANTIGEN- OR PLATELET-SPECIFIC ANTIGENS

As bone marrow/stem cell transplantation (BMT) becomes a viable option for selected patients with SCD,[90–96] alloimmunization to platelets will present more serious problems for this group. Friedman and coworkers[97] reported that 85% of SCD patients receiving 50 or more transfusions, 48% of SCD patients receiving 1 to 49 transfusions, and no nontransfused

SCD patients demonstrated alloimmunization to human leukocyte antigen (HLA)– or platelet-specific antigens. Because platelet refractoriness is a serious complication during BMT, prevention of platelet alloimmunization appears prudent in this group of patients. We support the use of LR of cellular blood products to prevent or reduce platelet allo-immunization and refractoriness in SCD patients, a practice employed for a variety of multiply transfused patient groups.[98–101] In our center, all children (i.e., potential BMT recipients) receive LR cellular blood products.

Non–Immune-Related Adverse Effects

IRON OVERLOAD

Iron overload resulting in hemosiderosis is a serious long-term complication of chronic transfusion in SCD patients. The most informative data regarding transfusion-associated iron overload were described in patients with thalassemia, and a discussion of the pathophysiology of iron overload is included in the thalassemia section of this chapter. Patients who develop iron overload may be treated with long-term chelation therapy in the form of deferoxamine (DFO); however, this therapy is expensive, and because of multiple side effects the compliance rate is poor.[102]

One potential transfusion methodology for the prevention of iron overload currently being investigated in SCD patients is chronic erythrocytapheresis (see previous discussion). Chronic erythrocytapheresis procedures may be performed at 3- to 4-week intervals. In contrast to simple additive transfusions, the patient's own sickled RBCs are removed while an equal volume of normal donor RBCs is infused. The obvious potential benefit of chronic erythrocytapheresis compared with simple transfusion is the prevention of long-term iron accumulation and hemosiderosis.

Although it is not universally implemented, chronic erythrocytapheresis appears to be clinically effective in reducing iron overload in chronically transfused SCD patients. Four investigative teams[64–67] have described their individual experiences with chronic erythrocytapheresis transfusion protocols for SCD patients. All suggested that erythrocytapheresis does limit iron accumulation in SCD patients, but three of the four groups reported that erythrocytapheresis does not obviate the need for chelation therapy in those patients with previously accumulated iron.[65–67] In general, ferritin levels decreased in patients with chronic erythrocytapheresis who received concurrent chelation therapy, and they either mildly decreased or stabilized in patients who were not receiving chelation therapy. However, at-risk patients who were started on erythrocytapheresis without a long history of previous chronic simple transfusions maintained very low serum ferritin levels not requiring chelation therapy.[65–67] Therefore, it appears that chronic erythrocytapheresis may be most beneficial when it is initiated early in the course of chronic transfusion therapy, before significant iron accumulation occurs. Nevertheless, chronic erythrocytapheresis does appear to stabilize or decrease serum ferritin levels in patients who have already developed significant iron overload and continue on chelation therapy.[65–67]

The primary potential problems with the chronic erythrocytapheresis transfusion protocol (compared with chronic simple transfusion protocols) are (1) increased blood product exposure, with concomitant increased risks of alloimmunization to RBCs and platelets and of transfusion-transmitted infection, and (2) the increased cost.

The four published reports[64–67] indicated that SCD patients' blood product exposures do increase in chronic erythrocytapheresis protocols, with reported increases in blood utilization rates ranging from 52% to almost 100% (i.e., one to two times more RBC units transfused than with previous simple transfusions of the same patients). However, of the combined 43 patients studied, only 1 patient developed an alloantibody[65] during the period of erythrocytapheresis treatment. Three of these centers used antigen-matched RBC units for the erythrocytapheresis procedures: Singer and associates[67] matched for C, E, and K; Hilliard and colleagues[66] for C, E, K, Fy^a, and Jk^b; and Adams and associates[65] for C, E, K, and Jk^b. When evaluating the very low alloimmunization rates that have been reported for chronic erythrocytapheresis protocols, it is important to realize that the majority of SCD patients studied received RBC units matched for at least the C, E, and K antigens.

The high cost of erythrocytapheresis is also an important issue. Hilliard and colleagues[66] compared the total cost of 1 year of erythrocytapheresis ($36,085) with the total annual cost for simple transfusion ($26,058) and found an economically significant difference. They suggested that the added cost of chelation therapy ($29,480) with simple transfusion (for a total of $62,143) makes erythrocytapheresis without chelation a much less expensive alternative. However, for patients who have significant iron accumulation at the time erythrocytapheresis therapy is initiated, chelation therapy must be continued to achieve serum ferritin level reduction or stabilization.[64–66] This cost comparison provides further evidence that, if it is technically feasible, early initiation of chronic erythrocytapheresis in SCD patients, before significant iron accumulation occurs, may be preferable to long-term chronic simple transfusion and the resulting complications of iron overload and chelation therapy.

TRANSFUSION-TRANSMITTED INFECTIONS

The risk of transmission via transfusion of infectious agents, particularly viruses, has become substantially reduced since the 1990s,[103] largely owing to improved screening tests for donated blood products. Because the risk of contracting a transfusion-transmitted disease is very low, blood products should not be withheld (if an appropriate clinical indication for transfusion exists) for the sole purpose of preventing a transfusion-transmitted disease. However, the risks of all adverse effects of transfusion (see Table 29–4) should be balanced against the clinical need for transfusion on a case-by-case basis.

■ Thalassemias

Pathogenesis and Clinical Pathology

Thalassemias are among the most prevalent genetic disorders caused by a single gene, occurring in high frequency in Southeast Asia, Southern China, Indonesia, India, the Middle East, Africa, and the Mediterranean basin.[104] α-Thalassemias are caused by mutations that reduce the synthesis of the α globin chain of hemoglobin, and β-thalassemias from mutations that reduce β globin synthesis. The complex molecular genetics of these disorders is beyond the scope of this discussion and have been reviewed elsewhere.[105–107]

By definition, chronic transfusion is required to maintain wellness in homozygous individuals and compound heterozygotes with β-thalassemia major. Individuals with β-thalassemia intermedia have complex genetics and may have severe anemia that requires episodic transfusion. Hemoglobin H disease is caused by structural or functional loss of globin synthesis from three of the normal four α globin genes. Individuals usually are not transfusion dependent, but they may require transfusion support for complications. Compound heterozygotes with β-thalassemia and hemoglobin E disease, which is very common in individuals from East Asia, can have clinical manifestations ranging from mild microcytic anemia to severe transfusion-dependent β-thalassemia major.[108]

Clinical manifestations of severe β-thalassemias include transfusion-dependent anemia, expansion of medullary bone and extramedullary hematopoiesis, severe iron overload, increased infections, retarded growth and development, and osteopenia.[106] Anemia results from severe ineffective erythropoiesis and hemolysis. The excess α globin chain from unbalanced globin chain synthesis leads to arrested development and accelerated intramedullary apoptosis. Erythropoietic activity may be increased tenfold, but more than 95% of the erythropoietin produced may be ineffective. Precipitated α globin in mature erythrocytes alters membrane proteins and causes oxidant damage, shortening RBC survival time. Progressive hypersplenism further reduces RBC survival.

A primary consequence of the ineffective erythropoiesis is increased iron absorption and progressive accumulation of iron in tissues. Anemia, increased erythropoiesis, and hypersplenism also cause marked expansion of the plasma volume and blood volume. Extramedullary hematopoiesis can cause pressure symptoms from perivertebral masses. Expanded marrow activity causes skeletal changes including osteopenia and characteristic changes in the skull and face.[109]

Individuals with β-thalassemia major are transfusion dependent from early life. Chronic transfusion support has markedly improved the prognosis. Transfused children develop iron overload from increased absorption caused by ineffective erythropoiesis and iron administered during transfusion. Cardiac, hepatic, and endocrine failure results in death in the second or third decade without effective therapy to remove excess iron. Although no ideal approach to treatment of transfusion-related iron overload exists, subcutaneous infusion of DFO over 8 to 12 hours, 5 to 7 days a week, appears to control iron accumulation and prevent cardiac and liver damage, thereby improving life expectancy. Bone marrow transplantation has cured more than 1000 individuals with β-thalassemia major worldwide and is considered in all children with a suitable donor.

Goals of Transfusion Therapy

The goals of therapy in β-thalassemia major are to increase oxygen-carrying capacity by correcting the anemia, preventing progressive hypersplenism, suppressing erythropoiesis, and reducing increased gastrointestinal absorption of iron.[106] Transfusion therapy is begun early in life to ameliorate the symptoms and signs of anemia and to support normal growth and development. Adequate transfusion reduces progression of hypersplenism, delaying the need for splenectomy.[110] Suppression of erythropoiesis prevents skeletal changes, prevents complications of extramedullary hematopoiesis, and reduces pathologic fractures and other complications from osteopenia.[111] Suppression of ineffective erythropoiesis decreases transfusion requirements by reducing blood volume[112] and suppresses the increased intestinal absorption of iron.[113]

Indications for Transfusion

Transfusion therapy is initiated in childhood when the symptoms and signs of anemia are present, including growth retardation and failure to thrive. Transfusions are occasionally initiated in β-thalassemia intermedia and hemoglobin H disease to prevent facial and skull deformity from expansion of the medullary bone space. Progressive hypersplenism may require transfusion to postpone splenectomy in β-thalassemia intermedia. Splenectomy is indicated to prevent excessive transfusion requirements.[111]

Methods of Transfusion

Simple transfusion of leukoreduced RBCs to maintain a hemoglobin level greater than 9.5 g/dL is the standard approach to transfusion in thalassemia.[106] The older practice of maintaining higher pretransfusion hemoglobin levels[110–112] has been associated with excessive iron loading and generally is not advocated.[106, 114, 115] Splenectomy is recommended when hypersplenism increases the transfusion requirement beyond 200 to 250 mL/kg/yr.[110, 115]

Another approach to reducing iron loading has been the use of neocytes prepared by cell separators, cell processors, or other density means.[116–123] The use of "neocyte" transfusions was shown to allow a 15% extension in transfusion interval while maintaining the same pretransfusion hemoglobin level.[123] The costs of this approach are increased blood use, increased donor unit exposure, and an estimated fivefold increase in the cost of transfusion.[123] This approach is not presently advocated by most thalassemia experts.

Erythrocytapheresis has also been applied to thalassemia transfusion therapy. The use of automated RBC exchange, returning patient and donor "neocytes" and removing the "gerocytes," resulted in a 30% reduction in RBC transfusion requirement and a 43% increase in transfusion interval.[124, 125] Further clinical trials of this approach are warranted.

REFERENCES

1. Heller P, Best WR, Nelson RB, et al: Clinical implications of sickle cell trait and glucose-6-phosphate dehydrogenase deficiency in hospitalized black male patients. N Engl J Med 1979;300:1001–1005.
2. Beutler E: The sickle cell diseases and related disorders. *In* Beutler E, Lichtman MA, Coller BS, et al (eds): Williams Hematology, 6th ed. New York: McGraw-Hill, 2001, p 585.
3. Bunn HF: Mechanisms of disease: pathogenesis and treatment of sickle cell disease. N Engl J Med 1997;337:762–769.
4. Steinberg MH: Management of sickle cell disease. N Engl J Med 1999;340:1021–1030.
5. Platt OS, Brambilla DJ, Rosse WF, et al: Mortality in sickle cell disease: life expectancy and risk factors for early death. N Engl J Med 1994;330:1639–1644.
6. Reed W, Vichinsky EP: New considerations in the treatment of sickle cell disease. Annu Rev Med 1998;49:461–474.
7. Davies SC, Roberts-Harewood M: Blood transfusion in sickle cell disease. Blood Rev 1997;11:57–71.
8. Vichinsky EP: Current issues in blood transfusion in sickle cell disease. Semin Hematol 2001;38:14–22.
9. Embury SH: The clinical pathophysiology of sickle cell disease. Ann Rev Med 1986;37:361–376.
10. Goldstein AR, Anderson MJ, Serjeant GR: Parvovirus-associated aplastic crisis in homozygous sickle cell disease. Arch Dis Child 1987;62:585–588.

11. Serjeant GR, de Ceulaer K, Maude GH: Stilboestrol and stuttering priapism in homozygous sickle-cell disease. Lancet 1985;2:1274.

12. Vichinsky E: Transfusion. *In* Embury SH, Hebbel RP, Mohandas N, et al: (eds). Sickle Cell Disease: Basic Principles and Clinical Practice. New York: Raven Press, 1994, pp 261–283.

13. Eckman JR: Techniques for blood administration in sickle cell patients. Semin Hematol 2001;38:23–29.

14. Wayne AS, Kevy SV, Nathan DG: Transfusion management of sickle cell disease. Blood 1993;81:1109–1123.

15. Castro W, Brambilla DJ, Thorington B, et al: The acute chest syndrome in sickle cell disease: incidence and risk factors. Blood 1994;84:643–649.

16. Gray J, Anionwu EN, Davies SC, et al: Patterns of mortality in sickle cell disease in the United Kingdom. J Clin Pathol 1991;44:459.

17. Dreyer ZE: Chest infections and syndromes in sickle cell disease of childhood. Semin Respir Infect 1996;11:163–172.

18. Davies SD, Luce PJ, Win AA, et al: Acute chest syndrome in sickle-cell disease. Lancet 1984;1:36–38.

19. Mallouh AA, Asha M: Beneficial effect of blood transfusion on children with sickle cell chest syndrome. Am J Dis Child 1988;142:178–182.

20. Emre U, Miller ST, Gutierez M, et al: Effect of transfusion in acute chest syndrome of sickle cell disease. J Pediatr 1995;127:901–904.

21. Emond AM, Collis R, Darvill D, et al: Acute splenic sequestration in homozygous sickle cell disease: natural history and management. J Pediatr 1985;107:201–206.

22. Seeler RA, Shwiaki MZ: Acute splenic sequestration crises (ASSC) in young children with sickle cell anemia. Clin Pediatr 1972;11:701–704.

23. Sheehy TW, Law DE, Wade BH: Exchange transfusion for sickle cell intrahepatic cholestasis. Arch Intern Med 1980;140:1364–1366.

24. Ohene-Frempong K, Weiner SJ, Sleeper LA, et al: Cerebrovascular accidents in sickle cell disease: rates and risk factors. Blood 1998;91:288–294.

25. Ohene-Frempong K: Indications for red cell transfusion in sickle cell disease. Semin Hematol 2001;38:5–13.

26. Russell MO, Goldberg HI, Reis L, et al: Transfusion therapy for cerebrovascular abnormalities in sickle cell disease. JAMA 1979;242:2317–2318.

27. Vichinsky EP, Haberkern CM, Neumayr L, et al: A comparison of conservative and aggressive transfusion regimens in the perioperative management of sickle cell disease. N Engl J Med 1995;333:206–213.

28. Koshy M, Weiner SJ, Miller ST, et al: Surgery and anesthesia in sickle cell disease. Blood 1995;86:3676–3684.

29. Haberkern CM, Neumayr LD, Orringer EP, et al: Cholecystectomy in sickle cell anemia patients: perioperative outcome of 364 cases from the National Preoperative Transfusion Study. Blood 1997;89:1533–1542.

30. Adams RJ, McKie VC, Hsu L, et al: Prevention of a first stroke by transfusions in children with sickle cell anemia and abnormal results on transcranial Doppler ultrasonography. N Engl J Med 1998;339:5–11.

31. Sergeant GR: Sickle Cell Disease, 2nd ed. Oxford: Oxford Medical Publishers, 1992, p 332.

32. Hassell KL, Eckman JR, Lane PA: Acute multiorgan failure syndrome: a potentially catastrophic complication of severe sickle cell pain episodes. Am J Med 1994;96:155–162.

33. Powars D, Wilson B, Imbus C, et al: The natural history of stroke in sickle cell disease. Am J Med 1978;65:461–471.

34. Russell MO, Goldberg HI, Hodson A, et al: Effect of transfusion therapy on arteriographic abnormalities and on recurrence of stroke in sickle cell disease. Blood 1984;63:162–169.

35. Peglow CH, Adams RJ, McKie V, et al: Risk of recurrent stroke in patients with sickle cell disease treated with erythrocyte transfusion. J Pediatr 1995;126:896–899.

36. Williams J, Goff JR, Anderson HR Jr, et al: Efficacy of transfusion therapy for one to two years in patients with sickle cell disease and cerebrovascular accidents. J Pediatr 1980;96:205–209.

37. Cohen AR, Martin MB, Silber JF, et al: A modified transfusion program for prevention of stroke in sickle cell disease. Blood 1992;79:1657–1661.

38. Wang WC, Kovnar EH, Tonkin IL, et al: High risk of recurrent stroke after discontinuance of five to twelve years of transfusion therapy in patients with sickle cell disease. J Pediatr 1991;118:377–382.

39. Adams R, McKie V, Nichols F, et al: The use of transcranial ultrasonography to predict stroke in sickle cell disease. N Engl J Med 1992;326:605–610.

40. Adams RJ, McKie VC, Carl EM, et al: Long-term stroke risk in children with sickle cell disease screened with transcranial Doppler. Ann Neurol 1997;42:699–704.

41. Koshy M, Burd L, Wallace D, et al: Prophylactic re-cell transfusions in pregnant patients with sickle cell disease. N Engl J Med 1988;319:1447–1452.

42. El-Shafei AM, Dhaliwal JK, Sandhu AK, et al: Indications for blood transfusion in pregnancy with sickle cell disease. Aust N Z J Obstet Gynaecol 1995;35:405–408.

43. Tuck SM, James CE, Brewster EM, et al: Prophylactic blood transfusion in maternal sickle cell syndromes. Br J Obstet Gynecol 1987;94:121–125.

44. Koshy M: Sickle cell disease and pregnancy. Blood Rev 1995;9:157–164.

45. Morgan AG, Gruber CA, Serjeant GR: Erythropoietin and renal function in sickle cell disease. BMJ 1982;285:1686–1688.

46. Weil JV, Castro O, Malik AR, et al: Pathogenesis of lung disease in sickle hemoglobinopathies. Am Rev Respir Dis 1993;148:249–256.

47. Yong RC, Castro O, Baxter RP: The lung in sickle cell disease: a clinical overview of common vascular infections and other problems. J Natl Med Assoc 1981;73:19–26.

48. Collins FS, Orringer E: Pulmonary hypertension and cor pulmonale in sickle hemoglobinopathies. Am J Med 1982;73:814–821.

49. Rifkind S, Waisman J, Thompson R, et al: RBC exchange pheresis for priapism in sickle cell disease. JAMA 1979;242:2317–2318.

50. Walker EM, Mitchum EN, Rous SN, et al: Automated erythrocytapheresis for relief of priapism in sickle cell hemoglobinopathies. J Urol 1983;130:912–916.

51. Seeler RA: Intensive transfusion therapy for priapism in boys with sickle cell anemia. J Urol 1973;110:360–361.

52. Seeler RA: Priapism in children with sickle cell anemia. Clin Pediatr 1971;10:418–419.

53. Miller ST, Rao SP, Dunn KE, et al: Priapism in children with sickle cell disease. J Urol 1995;154:844–847.

54. Baruchel S, Rees J, Bernstein ML, et al: Relief of sickle cell priapism by hydralazine: report of a case. Am J Pediatr Hematol Oncol 1993;15:115.

55. Siegel JF, Rich MA, Brock WA: Association of sickle cell disease, priapism, exchange transfusion and neurological events: ASPEN syndrome. J Urol 1993;150:1480–1482.

56. Platt OS, Thorington BD, Brambilla DJ, et al: Pain in sickle cell disease. N Engl J Med 1991;325:11–16.

57. Koshy M, Entsuah R, Koranda A, et al: Leg ulcers in patients with sickle cell disease. Blood 1989;74:1403–1408.

58. Schmalzer EA, Lee JO, Brown AK, et al: Viscosity of mixtures of sickle and normal red cells at varying hematocrit levels. Transfusion 1987;27:228–233.

59. Sharon BI: Transfusion therapy in congenital hemolytic anemias. Hematol Oncol Clin North Am 1994;8:1053–1086.

60. Vengelen-Tyler V (ed). AABB Technical Manual, 13th ed. Bethesda, Md: American Association of Blood Banks, 1999, p 486.

61. Embury SH, Vichinsky EP: Sickle Cell Disease. *In* Hoffman R, Benz EJ Jr, Shattil SJ, et al: (eds). Hematology: Basic Principles and Practice, 3rd ed. Philadelphia: Churchill Livingstone, 2000, p 539.

62. Kevy SV: Extracorporeal therapy for infants and children. *In* Petz LD, Swisher SN, Kleinman S, et al: (eds). Clinical Practice of Transfusion Medicine, 3rd ed. New York: Churchill Livingstone, 1996, p 734.

63. Cohen A, Kron E, Brittenham G: Toxicity of transfusional iron overload in sickle cell disease. Blood 1984;64(Suppl 1):47a.

64. Kim H, Dugan N, Silber J: Erythrocytapheresis therapy to reduce iron overload in chronically transfused patients with sickle cell disease. Blood 1994;83:1136–1142.

65. Adams D, Schultz W, Ware R, et al: Erythrocytapheresis can reduce iron overload and prevent the need for chelation in chronically transfused pediatric patients. J Pediatr Hematol Oncol 1996;18:46–50.

66. Hilliard LM, Williams BF, Lounsbury AE, et al: Erythrocytapheresis limits iron accumulation in chronically transfused sickle cell patients. Am J Hematol 1998;59:28–35.

67. Singer ST, Quirolo K, Nishi K, et al: Erythrocytapheresis for chronically transfused children with sickle cell disease: an effective method for maintaining a low hemoglobin S level and reducing iron overload. J Clin Apheresis 1999;14:122–125.

68. Lawson SE, Oakley S, Smith NA, et al: Red cell exchange in sickle cell disease. Clin Lab Haematol 1999;21:99–102.

69. Miller JP, AuBuchon JP: Leukocyte-reduced and cytomegalovirus-reduced-risk blood components. *In* Mintz PD (ed). Transfusion

Therapy: Clinical Principles and Practice. Bethesda, Md: AABB Press, 1999, p 313.

70. Stack G, Judge JV, Snyder EL: Febrile and nonimmune transfusion reactions. *In* Rossi EC, Simon TL, Moss GS, et al: (eds). Principles of Transfusion Medicine, 2nd ed. Baltimore: Williams & Wilkins, 1996, p 773–784.

71. Orlina AR, Unger PJ, Koshy M: Post-transfusion alloimmunization in patients with sickle cell disease. Am J Hematol 1978;5:101–106.

72. Davies SC, McWilliam AC, Hewitt PE, et al: Red cell alloimmunization in sickle cell disease. Br J Hematol 1986;63:241–245.

73. Reisner EG, Kostyo DD, Phillips G, et al: Alloantibody responses in multiply transfused sickle cell patients. Tissue Antigens 1987;30:161–166.

74. Cox JV, Steane E, Cunningham G, et al: Risk of alloimmunization and delayed hemolytic transfusion reactions in patients with sickle cell disease. Arch Intern Med 1988;148:2485–2489.

75. Rosse WF, Gallagher D, Kinney T: Transfusion and alloimmunization in sickle cell disease. Blood 1990;76:1431–1437.

76. Vichinsky EP, Earles A, Johnson RA, et al: Alloimmunization in sickle cell anemia and transfusion of racially unmatched blood. N Engl J Med 1990;322:1617–1621.

77. Coles SM, Klein HG, Holland PV: Alloimmunization in two multitransfused patient populations. Transfusion 1981;21:462–466.

78. Luban NL: Variability in rates of alloimmunization in different groups of children with sickle cell disease: effect of ethnic background. Am J Pediatr Hematol Oncol 1989;11:314–319.

79. Tahhan HR, Holbrook CT, Braddy LR, et al: Antigen-matched donor blood in the transfusion management of patients with sickle cell disease. Transfusion 1994;34:562–569.

80. Sarnaik S, Schornack J, Lusher JM: The incidence of development of irregular red cell antibodies in patients with sickle cell anemia. Transfusion 1986;26:249–252.

81. Ambruso DR, Githens JH, Alcorn R, et al: Experience with donors matched for minor blood group antigens in patients with sickle cell anemia who are receiving chronic transfusion therapy. Transfusion 1987;27:94–98.

82. Wenz B, Gurtlinger A, Wheaton D, et al: A mimicking red blood cell autoantibody accompanying transfusion and alloimmunization. Transfusion 1982;22:147–150.

83. Orlina AR, Sosler SD, Koshy M: Problems of chronic transfusion in sickle cell disease. J Clin Apheresis 1991;6:234–240.

84. Sosler SD, Perkins JT, Fong K, et al: The prevalence of immunization to Duffy antigens in a population of known racial distribution. Transfusion 1989;29:505–507.

85. Chaplin H, Mischeaux JR, Inkster MD, et al: Frozen storage of 11 units of sickle red cells for autologous transfusion of a single patient. Transfusion 1986;26:341–345.

86. Castellino SM, Combs MR, Zimmerman SA, et al: Erythrocyte autoantibodies in paediatric patients with sickle cell disease receiving transfusion therapy: frequency, characteristics, and significance. Br J Haematol 1999;104:189–194.

87. Test ST, Woolworth VS: Defective regulation of complement by the sickle erythrocyte: evidence for a defect in control of membrane attack complex formation. Blood 1994;83:842–852.

88. Cox KO, Finlay-Jones JJ: Impaired regulation of erythrocyte autoantibody production after splenectomy. Br J Exp Pathol 1979;60:466–470.

89. Cullis JO, Win N, Dudley TM, et al: Post-transplant hyperhaemolysis in a patient with sickle cell disease: use of steroids and intravenous immunoglobulin to prevent further red cell destruction. Vox Sang 1995;69:355–357.

90. Vermylen C, Cornu G: Bone marrow transplantation in sickle cell anaemia. Blood Rev 1993;7:1–3.

91. Vermylen C, Cornu G, Ferster A, et al: Haematopoietic stem cell transplantation for sickle cell anaemia: the first 50 patients transplanted in Belgium. Bone Marrow Transplant 1998;22:1–6.

92. Walters MC, Patience M, Leisenring W, et al: Bone marrow transplantation for sickle cell disease. N Engl J Med 1996;335:369–376.

93. Platt OS, Guinan EC: Bone marrow transplantation in sickle cell anemia: the dilemma of choice. N Engl J Med 1996;335:426–428.

94. Brichard B, Vermylen C, Ninane J, et al: Persistence of fetal hemoglobin production after successful transplantation of cord blood stem cells in a patient with sickle cell anemia. J Pediatr 1996;128:241–243.

95. Ferster A, Corazza F, Vertongen F, et al: Transplanted sickle-cell disease patients with autologous bone marrow recovery after graft

96. Souillet G: Indications and results of progenitor cell transplant in congenital haemopathies (except Fanconi anaemia). Bone Marrow Transplant 1998;21:S28–S33.

97. Friedman D, Lukas M, Jawad A, et al: Alloimmunization to platelets in heavily transfused patients with sickle cell disease. Blood 1996;88:3216–3222.

98. Slichter SJ: Platelet transfusion therapy. Hematol Oncol Clin North Am 1990;4:291–311.

99. Sniecinski I, O'Donnell MR, Nowicki B, et al: Prevention of refractoriness and HLA-alloimmunization using filtered blood products. Blood 1988;71:1402–1407.

100. Saarinen UM, Kekomaki R, Simes MA, et al: Effective prophylaxis against platelet refractoriness in multitransfused patients by use of leukocyte-free blood components. Blood 1990;75:512–517.

101. Brand A, Claas FHJ, Voogt PJ, et al: Alloimmunization after leukocyte-depleted multiple random donor platelet transfusions. Vox Sang 1988;54:160–166.

102. Cohen AR, Martin MB: Iron chelation therapy in sickle cell disease. Semin Hematol 2001;38(Suppl 1):69–72.

103. Schrieber G, Busch M, Kleinman S, et al: The risk of transfusion-transmitted viral infections. N Engl J Med 1996;334:1685–1690.

104. Weatherall DJ, Clegg JB: Thalassemia: a global public health problem. Nat Med 1996;2:847–849.

105. Higgs DR: Molecular mechanisms in α thalassemia. *In* Steinberg MH, Forget BG, Higgs DR, et al: (eds). Disorders of Hemoglobin: Genetics, Pathophysiology, and Clinical Management. Cambridge: Cambridge University Press, 2001, p 405.

106. Oliveri NF: The β-thalassemias. N Engl J Med 1999;341:99–100.

107. Higgs DR: α-Thalassemia. Baillieres Clin Haematol 1993;6:117–150.

108. Weatherall DJ: Hemoglobin E beta-thalassemia: an increasingly common disease with some diagnostic pitfalls. J Pediatr 1998;132:765–767.

109. Rioja L, Girot R, Garabedian M, et al: Bone disease in children with homozygous beta-thalassemia. Bone Miner 1990;8:69–86.

110. Piomelli S, Graziano J: Reduction in iron overload in thalassemia. Birth Defects 1982;18:339–346.

111. Fosburg MT, Nathan DG: Treatment of Colley's anemia. Blood 1990;76:435–444.

112. Propper R, Button L, Nathan D: New approach to the transfusion management of thalassemia. Blood 1980;55:55–60.

113. Pootrakul P, Kitcharoen K, Yansukon P, et al: The effect of erythroid hyperplasia on iron balance. Blood 1988;71:1124–1129.

114. Cazzola M, Borgna-Pignatti C, Locatelli F, et al: A moderate transfusion regimen may reduce iron loading in β-thalassemia major without producing excessive expansion of erythropoiesis. Transfusion 1997;37:135–140.

115. Olivieri NF, Brittenham GM: Iron-chelation therapy and treatment of thalassemia. Blood 1997;89:739–761.

116. Piomeli S, Seaman C, Reibman J, et al: Separation of younger red cells with improved survival in vivo: an approach to chronic transfusion therapy. Proc Natl Acad Sci U S A 1978;74:3473–3478.

117. Corash L, Klein H, Deisseroth A, et al: Selective isolation of young erythrocytes for transfusion support of thalassemia major patients. Blood 1981;57:599–606.

118. Bracey AW, Klein HG, Chambers S, et al: Ex-vivo selective isolation of young red blood cells using the IBM-2991 cell washer. Blood 1983;61:1068–1071.

119. Cohen AR, Schmidt JM, Martin MB, et al: Clinical trial of young red cell transfusions. J Pediatr 1984;104:865–868.

120. Marcus RE, Wonke B, Bantock HM, et al: A prospective trial of young red cells in 48 patients with transfusion-dependent thalassemia. Br J Haematol 1985;60:153–159.

121. Kevy SV, Jacobson MS, Fosburg M, et al: A new approach to neocyte transfusion: preliminary report. J Clin Apheresis 1988;4:194–197.

122. Simon TL, Sohmer P, Nelson EF: Extended survival of neocytes produced by a new system. Transfusion 1989;29:221–225.

123. Collins AF, Dias GC, Haddad S, et al: Evaluation of a new neocyte transfusion preparation vs. washed cell transfusion in patients with homozygous beta thalassemia. Transfusion 1994;34:517–520.

124. Berdoukas VA, Moorew RC: A study of the value of red cell exchange transfusions in transfusion dependent anemias. Clin Lab Haematol 1986;8:209–220.

125. Cohen AR, Porter JB: Transfusion and iron chelation therapy in thalassemia and sickle cell anemia. *In* Steinberg MH, Forget BG, Higgs DR, et al: (eds). Disorders of Hemoglobin: Genetics, Pathophysiology, and Clinical Management. Cambridge: Cambridge University Press, 2001, p 982.

126. Hillyer KL, Hare VW, Eckman JR, et al: Decreased alloimmunization rates in chronically-transfused sickle cell disease patients in a directed-donor, red blood cell antigen-matching program entitled "Partners for Life" (PFL). Blood 2001;98:2274.

127. Vichinsky EP, Luban NL, Wright E, et al: Prospective red blood cell phenotype matching in a stroke-prevention trial in sickle cell anemia: a multicenter transfusion trial. Transfusion 2001;41:1086–1092.

128. Reid CD, Charache S, Lubin B (eds): Management and Therapy of Sickle Cell Disease, 3rd ed. Bethesda, Md: National Institutes of Health Publication, 1995, p 62.

129. Linderkamp O, Versmold HT, Riegel KP, et al: Estimation and prediction of blood volume in infants and children. Eur J Pediatr 1977;125:227–234.

130. Hillyer KL, Hillyer CD: Packed red blood cells and related products. *In* Hillyer CD, Hillyer KL, Strobl FJ, et al: (eds). Handbook of Transfusion Medicine. Philadelphia: Academic Press, 2001, p 29.

131. Piomelli S, Seaman C, Ackerman K, et al: Planning an exchange transfusion in patients with sickle cell syndromes. Am J Pediatr Hematol Oncol 1990;12:268–276.

Chapter **30**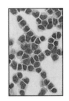

Transfusion to Bone Marrow or Solid Organ Transplant Recipients and HIV-Positive Patients

Keren Osman

Raymond L. Comenzo

David Wuest

With respect to blood component therapy, hematopoietic stem cell (HSC) and solid organ transplant recipients and human immunodeficiency virus (HIV)-positive patients have many features in common. All share defects in T-cell immunity to various degrees, whether as the result of immunosuppressive drugs as in solid organ transplant recipients, or of chemotherapy and radiation as in autologous and allogeneic HSC transplant recipients, or of acquired viral effects as in HIV-positive patients. All these patients are at increased risk of bacterial, fungal, and viral infections. Among the viral infections, cytomegalovirus (CMV) has played a large role in transfusion medicine and has required the use of CMV-seronegative blood and, more recently, leukoreduced blood components to avoid CMV infection in patients who are CMV negative.

Advances in the transplantation of HSCs and solid organs have been made possible by a deeper understanding of immune reconstitution and immunomodulation. Crossover from this field has also contributed to our understanding of HIV disease and has enabled the development of therapeutic approaches for this otherwise fatal illness. Many immunodeficient patients are living longer and are requiring new approaches to continued care. Among these are requirements for blood products and for blood conservation technologies. The complex immunology of these categories of patients has posed challenges to the practice of transfusion medicine that have resulted in the recognition of potential complications of transfusion as well as the development of new transfusion technologies.

Cytopenias play a major role in the transfusion requirements of these categories of patients. Cytopenias may result from bone marrow suppression and decreased production of cells or from syndromes of increased destruction, as may be the case in patients with advanced malignant disease, marrow infiltrative processes such as infection with *Mycobacterium*

avium (in HIV-infected patients), or autoimmune processes. Hemolytic anemia and thrombocytopenia, for instance, may occur in patients after allogeneic or autologous transplantation as well as in HIV-infected patients and, with autoimmune neutropenia, they are major causes of cytopenias in these patients. In this chapter we review the use of blood and adoptive immunotherapy components, the major complications of transfusion, and new developments relevant to these patients with complex immune deficiencies.

■ Transfusion Components

Red Blood Cells

Recipients of HSC and solid organ transplants and HIV-infected patients frequently become anemic. Anemia may occur because of decreased red blood cell production as a result of marrow infiltration, shortened survival of red blood cells, or increased blood loss secondary to coagulation disorders or thrombocytopenia. The indications for red blood cell transfusion are the standard ones, including symptomatic anemia and active bleeding. The estimated risks of transmission of transfusion-related diseases are lower than ever before.[1] This does not mean, however, that the risks are zero. Furthermore, other complications from red blood cell transfusion are more common in this population. Patients may develop human leukocyte antigen (HLA) antibodies and alloantibodies to red blood cell antigens.

To ameliorate some of these problems, certain changes have taken place in the practice of transfusion medicine. Leukocyte reduction (leukoreduction) of red blood cells, for example, is commonly used to avoid allosensitization and HLA antibody formation, as well as to provide CMV-safe components, as noted earlier.[2] Moreover, the use of erythropoietin may accelerate erythroid recovery after bone marrow transplantation and is an important adjuvant therapy to reduce blood transfusions for patients with anemia related to cancer or chronic illness.[3]

Platelets

Prolonged periods of thrombocytopenia after allogeneic bone marrow transplantation, a high incidence of immune thrombocytopenic purpura in patients with cancer and HIV, and the long-term use of drugs that may depress marrow platelet production in solid organ transplant recipients make platelet transfusion an important mainstay of therapy for all these patients. Platelet transfusion in this group of patients raises two issues: the first is the controversy over the threshold for prophylactic platelet transfusion, and the second is the problem of refractoriness to platelet transfusion secondary to alloimmunization.

The indications for prophylactic platelet transfusion have been a source of controversy and active investigation. Increased awareness of transfusion-transmitted viruses and concerns over alloimmunization have led to attempts to decrease the use of prophylactic platelet transfusions. To that end, studies have been conducted to establish a threshold for prophylactic platelet transfusion. These studies indicate that the threshold for prophylactic platelet transfusions can be as low as 10×10^9/L in stable patients. However, in patients with platelet dysfunction or hemorrhagic and coagulation disorders, the threshold should be higher.[3]

Platelet alloimmunization is a major problem in patients who are thrombocytopenic and who have received multiple transfusions. The incidence of this complication is between 30% and 70% and is thought to be mediated through the development of HLA- and platelet-specific alloantibodies. The mechanism, however, is not completely understood. Primary alloimmunization is thought to occur through the presentation of both classes I and II HLA antigens to leukocytes. The antibodies formed in response to this event are transient. Thus, a secondary encounter occurs, provoking a more long-lasting immune response. Nevertheless, it is clear that alloimmunization is independent of the number of transfusions, and, therefore, limiting donor exposures through the use of apheresis platelets is not sufficient. Numerous approaches to improving the outcome of platelet transfusion in refractory patients have been used. One is to improve HLA matching whenever possible, and another is to identify the platelet antibody specificity and to select platelet donors who are negative for the identified antigens. Other approaches have been tried to reverse the established immune process or underlying clinical condition through such measures as splenectomy, plasmapheresis, administration of steroids or γ globulin, and the use of antifibrinolytic agents. These measures have proven ineffective. Finally, current investigational approaches to prevent antigenic exposure and to reduce the frequency of alloimmunization include leukoreduction and ultraviolet B irradiation to inhibit antigen presentation.[3]

Hematopoietic Stem Cells

Both autologous and allogeneic stem and progenitor cells have become more widely used cytotherapeutic components in treating a broad spectrum of diseases. Their use has been established for treatment of primary bone marrow failure syndromes as well as for rescue therapy after high-dose chemotherapy for numerous malignant diseases. The components

used in HSC transplantation include bone marrow, blood mononuclear cells collected after mobilization (peripheral blood stem cells [PBSCs]) and umbilical cord blood stem cells. Until the early 1990s, the most commonly used component was bone marrow. After harvesting marrow from the donor, the marrow was either immediately infused (allogeneic) or cryopreserved for later use (autologous). Since that time, the use of leukapheresis to collect HSCs from the peripheral blood for autologous transplantation has become a more common practice and may eventually replace the use of bone marrow for allogeneic transplantation.

Autologous stem and progenitor cell mobilization and collection are often associated with the recovery phase after myelosuppressive salvage therapy. After chemotherapy, patients receive hematopoietic growth factors such as granulocyte colony-stimulating factor or granulocyte-macrophage colony-stimulating factor to enhance rebound hematopoiesis. Stem cell mobilization can also be performed with growth factors alone. The mechanism for HSC peripheralization or mobilization involves enzymatic digestion of adherent molecules (VCAM-1, CD 106) by neutrophil enzymes.[4] Another source of stem cells is umbilical cord blood. To date, more than 600 transplant procedures have been performed using umbilical cord blood, and the preliminary reports are encouraging. However, technical and ethical aspects of umbilical cord blood collection, storage, and use are not yet comprehensively delineated.

With increasing use of PBSCs, issues that have become salient include the dose of stem cells adequate for hematopoietic reconstitution, the contribution of PBSCs to long-term hematopoietic reconstitution, and tumor contamination of autografts. Because a practical assay for the totipotent HSC does not exist, some variability has existed in the definition of an adequate dose of PBSCs for hematopoietic reconstitution. Parameters that have been shown to correlate with engraftment potential include nucleated and mononuclear cell counts, the quantity of granulocyte-macrophage colony-forming units, and the number of CD34+ cells per kilogram of the recipient weight. The most commonly used guide for dosing is the number of CD34 cells per kilogram because evaluation of this parameter is rapid, amenable to standardization, and a reliable predictor of time to engraftment. It is generally agreed that the minimum dose of CD34+ cells required to provide an adequate rescue dose is 2×10^6/kg. Some studies have compared engraftment time of PBSCs with bone marrow. PBSCs provide faster engraftment in both the allogeneic and autologous settings. Limitations of autologous stem cell transplantation include the potential for relapse secondary to contamination of stem cell components by clonal tumor cells and the lack of an alloreactive graft-versus-disease effect. Although purging or the selection of CD34+ HSC may reduce tumor cells in autologous grafts, a clear-cut benefit for such manipulations has not been defined prospectively in randomized trials.

Adoptive Immunotherapy

Granulocytes

Although the use of stem cells provides effective rescue therapy after high-dose myeloablative chemotherapy for various malignant diseases, many circumstances remain in which patients are at increased risk of succumbing to bacterial or fungal infections because of severe prolonged neutropenia or abnormal granulocyte function. An approach to these patients has been the use of *granulocyte transfusion support.*

Granulocyte transfusion involves collection of polymorphonuclear neutrophil (PMN) concentrates using apheresis technology, often from a donor primed with granulocyte colony-stimulating factor. Some early studies demonstrated the efficacy of granulocyte transfusion with regard to survival and resolution of infection in neutropenic patients with persistent bacteremia who were likely to recover marrow function.[5, 6] The advent of therapy with growth factors to prevent or shorten the duration of neutropenia, the high cost and limited availability of granulocyte transfusion, and the risk of complications such as alloimmunization to HLA antigens, CMV transmission, and the development of the adult respiratory distress syndrome negatively influenced the use of this technology. Some of the studies that did not demonstrate clinical benefit were hampered by the collection of relatively small doses of PMNs, PMNs with defective function secondary to the use of filtration leukapheresis, and lack of provisions to provide HLA-matched products. Although granulocyte transfusions have become less common because of the availability of growth factors, in some patients with severe persistent neutropenia who have active, life-threatening infection, granulocyte transfusion is a reasonable therapy. In these patients, efforts should be made to provide daily infusions of components containing a minimum of 2 to 3×10^{10} PMNs. Whenever possible, granulocytes should be collected from CMV- and HLA-compatible donors. Granulocytes for allogeneic transfusion should always be irradiated and often may require red blood cell or plasma depletion because of ABO incompatibility.[7]

Donor Lymphocytes

The use of lymphocytes for adoptive immunotherapy is of relevance to solid organ and HSC transplant recipients and to HIV-positive patients. The use of donor lymphocytes has been studied most extensively in patients with relapsed leukemia after allogeneic bone marrow transplantation as a method to induce a graft-versus-leukemia effect. Kolb and colleagues[8] studied the effects of donor lymphocyte infusions in 135 patients who had relapses of chronic myelogenous leukemia (CML), acute myelogenous leukemia (AML), or acute lymphoblastic leukemia (ALL) after allogeneic bone marrow transplantation (ABMT). These investigators demonstrated 73% complete remission in patients with chronic myelogenous leukemia but only 29% complete remission in patients with acute myelogenous leukemia and no response in patients with acute lymphoblastic leukemia.

The complications of donor lymphocyte infusion (DLI) include graft-versus-host disease (GVHD) and severe myelosuppression. The number of lymphocytes infused influences both the graft-versus-leukemia (GVL) effect and the rates of GVHD. However, it has not yet been possible to distinguish which subpopulations of lymphocytes are responsible for which effect. The delay between the infusion of lymphocytes and the development of the graft-versus-leukemia effect suggests that only a few of the cells infused recognize the tumor cells as foreign and must therefore undergo clonal expansion to achieve the desired effect.[8] Taking advantage of this mechanism, laboratory studies are under way to develop cytotoxic T lymphocytes (CTLs) for infusion that may decrease the time delay for graft-versus-leukemia effect and

may make this a technology that may then be applicable to less indolent leukemias. Whether ex vivo expanded cells will have shortened survival in vivo, or impaired function, remains an area of concern for the development of such approaches.

Another indication for donor lymphocytes is in treatment of latent Epstein-Barr virus (EBV) infection, which can cause lymphoproliferative disease (LPD) in recipients of solid organ or allogeneic HSC transplants. EBV-LPD occurs in approximately 1% to 10% of solid organ transplant recipients. HSC transplant recipients are at risk of EBV-LPD if their transplant was T-cell depleted or was from a mismatched family donor or a closely matched unrelated donor or if they require extremely high doses of immunosuppressive drugs. Most cases of EBV-LPD are B-cell lymphomas or high-grade immunoblastic or undifferentiated large cell non-Hodgkin lymphomas that do not respond to cytotoxic chemotherapy. Thus, strategies for treating these lymphomas have been developed using donor CTLs.

Two studies were done using CTLs for prophylaxis against EBV-LPD. In one study, 39 patients were treated with infusions of CTLs after T-cell–depleted allogeneic transplants and were compared with historical controls. None of the 39 patients treated with CTLs developed LPD, whereas 11.5% of the historical controls had done so.[9] In another study, EBV-specific CTLs were used, and EBV-DNA was measured after transplantation. For as long as 60 months after the transplant, viral load remained low, and EBV-specific CTLs persisted in the blood of these patients.

When patients develop overt lymphoma, antigen-specific CTLs can be used for treatment. Rooney and colleagues reported that two of three patients who were treated with CTLs for overt lymphoma responded to the infusion, and one died of progressive disease. Alternative approaches such as the use of monoclonal antibodies, namely rituximab, are still being actively investigated.[10, 11]

Investigators have also reported experience in treating EBV-LPD in recipients of solid organ transplants by using allogeneic T cells from HLA-matched siblings. One report described successful treatment in a lung transplant recipient who developed LPD in the central nervous system. A renal transplant recipient was treated with haploidentical EBV-specific CTLs and experienced a transient regression of disease. The transient nature of the response can best be explained by the fact that CTLs are eliminated because of recognition of major histocompatibility complex antigens from the unshared haplotype. Prophylactic therapy was also studied in recipients of solid organ transplants. Three patients received prophylactic infusions of autologous EBV-specific CTLs. All three patients had decreases in EBV load for as long as 3 months after infusion.

Finally, the role of CTLs in the treatment of HIV infection is being actively investigated. Two studies were performed to investigate the ability of CTLs to decrease viremia and to augment CD4 recovery in the early stages of HIV infection. In the first study, autologous HIV envelope-specific CTLs that had been transduced with a Tk-Hyg fusion gene were infused into patients. However, the fusion gene was too immunogenic, and thus the CTLs were destroyed before their action could be adequately evaluated.[12] In a follow-up study, unmodified HIV Gag-specific CD8+ CTLs were infused into HIV-positive patients. These cells localized to areas of viral replication and produced a decrease in the number of HIV-infected cells for a short period.[13] Lieberman and colleagues[14] reviewed the role of CD8+ CTLs in HIV infection and attempted to explain the impaired function of these cells. The molecular basis is multifactorial, including incomplete T-cell signaling, reduced perforin expression, and inadequate tracking to lymphoid areas of infection. These investigators showed that interleukin-2 can partially alter this dysfunction, a finding implicating a role for CD4 helper T cells in early disease.[14]

■ Complications of Transfusion

Transfusion-Transmissible Diseases

Cytomegalovirus Infection

CMV is one of the most common agents transmitted by blood transfusion. Infection may be either primary, related to transfusion of leukocytes in the allogeneic blood, or secondary, resulting from reactivation of latent virus. CMV virions are carried to the host in either mononuclear or polymorphonuclear cells. In most cases, patients with intact immune systems are not at risk of developing severe or significant disease as a result of CMV transmission. Those who are thought to be at risk are patients with either immature or compromised immune systems. This group includes recipients of solid organ transplants in the early months after the transplant procedure, HSC transplant recipients, and patients with acquired immunodeficiency syndrome (AIDS), as well as oncology patients receiving aggressive chemotherapy and neonates with very low birth weights. The risk of transfusion-transmitted CMV infection among these different groups depends on the degree of T-cell dysfunction, on native CMV immune status and possibility for viral inactivation, and on the number of leukocytes contained in the transfusion component.[15] Because of the varied nature of the risk of infection and because CMV-seronegative blood is a limited and expensive resource, attempts have been made to establish guidelines for the use of CMV-seronegative blood.

In the case of both solid organ and allogeneic bone marrow transplantation, the risk of CMV infection from blood products for a CMV-seronegative patient receiving a CMV-seronegative graft is high (30%). The use of CMV-seronegative or CMV-negative–equivalent (filtered or leukocyte-depleted) blood in these patients has been shown to reduce this risk significantly. This finding was confirmed in a retrospective study from the MD Anderson Cancer Center in which data were collected over 2 years from patients undergoing allogeneic transplantation. These data support the findings of prior studies that the use of filtered blood components (CMV-negative–equivalent components) is effective in CMV-seronegative marrow transplant recipients.[16] However, in CMV-seronegative patients receiving CMV-positive grafts, the use of CMV-seronegative blood products does not alter the risk of infection and is therefore not warranted.[17] Among CMV-seropositive recipients, the rate of infection is high (70%) regardless of the status of the donor, likely because of reactivation of endogenous virus. Therefore, CMV-seronegative–equivalent blood components are recommended for CMV-negative patients who are potential allotransplant recipients.[18]

Hepatitis, Including TT Virus Infection

Although transmission of hepatitis B and C was of great concern from the 1960s through the 1980s, advances in serologic testing allowed for successful prevention of post-transfusion infections. Major interventions included hepatitis B virus vaccine, screening and testing of donor blood, and postexposure prophylaxis such as specific hepatitis B virus immunoglobulin. Implementation of a test for a hepatitis C virus antibody had a significant impact on the frequency of transfusion-related hepatitis. Since the recognition of hepatitis C, however, there continue to be a few cases of post-transfusion hepatitis that are not attributable to known viruses. In 1997, a transfusion-transmissible hepatitis virus was described, called *TT virus* after the index patient. It is thought to be a non-enveloped, single-stranded DNA virus of the Parvovirus family.

Preliminary data from England and Japan have shown TT virus to be present in the blood of healthy persons with normal transaminases. In some studies, TT virus sequences were detected in 25% to 45% of patients with hepatitis of unclear origin and in 27% to 68% of patients with hemophilia. One study from Italy demonstrated TT virus (detected by polymerase chain reaction) in 93% of patients with β-thalassemia and in 22% of healthy donors. No correlation was found between levels of viremia and elevations in serum transaminases.[19] TT virus was also studied in bone marrow transplant recipients in Japan because of suggestions that it could be replicated in hematopoietic cells. However, even though TT virus infection was found in numerous patients with hematologic disorders who regularly required blood transfusion, most of the infections did not cause liver injury.[20] Thus, although the finding of TT virus is informative, no correlation has yet been found between viremia and liver disease.[21]

Human Parvovirus B19 Infection

Parvovirus B19 causes erythema infectiosum, normally a benign and self-limited disease commonly found in children. However, it is also a transfusion-transmissible virus that has been shown to cause aplastic crises in patients with chronic hemolytic anemias. Furthermore, evidence indicates that it can do so in patients with AIDS as well, in whom it causes profound reticulocytopenia resulting from infection of pronormoblasts.[22] Human parvovirus B19 does not cause persistent infection in immunocompetent hosts and is likely transmitted during the acute phase of infection. Although it is not susceptible to inactivation using organic solvents because it lacks a lipid coat, parvovirus B19 has been found to be susceptible to inactivation using heat. Although the prevalence of this virus is relatively low (1 per 20,000 donations), it should be recognized as a possible cause of transfusion-related morbidity in patients with AIDS,[23] as well as in solid organ transplant recipients.[24] Currently, evidence is insufficient to recommend universal testing of blood products for parvovirus B19.[25]

Transfusion-Associated Graft-Versus-Host Disease

Transfusion-associated GVHD (TA-GVHD) is a devastating complication of allogeneic blood component transfusion caused by the introduction of immunocompetent lymphocytes into susceptible hosts. The recipient does not reject these allogeneic lymphocytes, and therefore they can engraft, proliferate, and destroy host cells. The result is pancytopenia caused by bone marrow hypoplasia and, because of the lack of effective therapies, the ultimate outcome is usually death within 3 to 4 weeks. Given this profile, the only effective strategy has been to identify which patients are at risk before transfusion. The mechanism of TA-GVHD is thought to depend on three variables: (1) the degree of genetic (HLA) difference between the donor and the recipient, (2) the number of viable lymphocytes that are transfused, and (3) the immunocompetence of the recipient or, in other words, the ability of the recipient to reject these viable lymphocytes. Patients at risk are those with hematologic malignant diseases or some solid tumors, patients with congenital immunodeficiencies, and neonates. Kruskall and colleagues[26] studied HIV-infected recipients to determine whether they were at risk for TA-GVHD. Blood samples from 93 women were studied before and after transfusion from male donors. A Y chromosome–specific polymerase chain reaction assay was done to look for detectable male lymphocytes in the recipients' blood after transfusion. Although some of the patients had evidence of male leukocytes early after transfusion, this effect diminished with time. None of the patients who received leukoreduced blood had evidence of microchimerism after transfusion. Thus, patients with HIV infection do not appear to be at increased risk of TA-GVHD.[26]

TA-GVHD has also been reported in apparently immunocompetent adults in whom there has been a "one-way" HLA match. Such cases of TA-GVHD have been reported to occur when directed donations from immediate family members are used for transfusion in populations with limited heterogeneity. In these instances, the donor is homozygous for an HLA haplotype, whereas the recipient is heterozygous for that haplotype. The donor lymphocytes have no foreign HLA haplotype for the recipient lymphocytes to recognize and reject. The donor lymphocytes recognize the host HLAs that are encoded by the unshared haplotype as being foreign, undergo clonal expansion, and establish TA-GVHD. Such TA-GVHD is not dependent on host immunosuppression because the failure to eliminate donor lymphocytes is not dependent on defects in the host immune system but rather on idiosyncrasies in the HLA system.

Preclinical evidence suggests a role of CD4 and CD8 cells in the control of TA-GVHD. In mouse models, the effect of selective depletion of host CD4 and CD8 cells on TA-GVHD was studied. Depletion of host CD4 cells increased the number of donor lymphocytes needed to cause TA-GVHD, and depletion of CD8 and NK (natural killer) cells decreased the number of donor lymphocytes needed to induce TA-GVHD. This model may explain why patients with HIV (impaired CD4) function are apparently not at increased risk of TA-GVHD.[27]

Numerous treatments for TA-GVHD have been attempted anecdotally, including glucocorticoids, antithymocyte globulin, cyclosporine, cyclophosphamide, and anti–T-cell monoclonal antibodies.[28] A small study conducted by the Japanese Red Cross reported effective use of a serine protease inhibitor, nafamostat mesylate, in four patients. The patients who received this drug demonstrated improvement of skin rash, diminished fever, and normalization of liver function tests.[29] However, prevention remains the most important strategy to combat this condition.

The number of lymphocytes needed for TA-GVHD is unknown, but is thought to be a minimum of 10^6/kg. Irradiation eliminates or reduces the blastic or proliferative potential of lymphocytes; therefore, irradiation of blood components is used routinely to prevent TA-GVHD.

The current recommendation by the American Association of Blood Banks is that each component receive 25 Gy to the central midplane of the irradiation field, with no area receiving less than 15 Gy. Currently, these recommendations apply only to cellular blood components and fresh plasma and not to frozen or thawed plasma or cryoprecipitate, because TA-GVHD associated with transfusion of these latter components has not been reported.

Leukoreduction of blood components is a prevention strategy that is currently being investigated. It is based on the theory that decreasing viable lymphocytes in blood components will decrease the incidence of TA-GVHD.[30] Chang and colleagues[31] also examined the molecular changes that occur during the storage of blood to explain the paucity of TA-GVHD that occurs with the transfusion of older units of blood (more than 4 days old). These investigators found that whereas leukocyte number and viability were the same, the expression of cell surface antigens decreased over time. This decrease in CD antigen expression correlated with decreasing ability to induce the cellular signaling pathway.[31] Thus, another approach to the prevention of TA-GVHD in the future may involve the use of stored blood. It is still unclear whether the currently available technologies to decrease contaminating leukocytes will be sufficient to prevent TA-GVHD.

Transfusion Immunomodulation

The literature on the immunomodulatory effects of allogeneic blood transfusion, particularly as a downregulator of host immune function, is growing. Much of the evidence is relevant to the patient groups discussed in this chapter: bone marrow transplant recipients, organ transplant recipients, and HIV-infected patients. The current understanding of transfusion immunomodulation is that transfusions may cause changes in immune function and may alter clinical outcomes. It is believed that allogeneic leukocytes may be responsible for such effects. In vitro, certain effects on recipient immune function have been found to be related to allogeneic blood transfusion. These include decreased T-helper subset 1 (Th1) and increased Th2 cytokine production, decreased proliferative response to mitogens, decreased NK and CD4 helper cell number and activity, decreased monocyte and macrophage function, decreased cell-mediated cytotoxicity (lymphokine-activated killer cells) against target cells, and enhanced production of anti-idiotypic antibodies suppressive of mixed lymphocyte response. These modulations of immune function and response may be clinically relevant.

Animal models have demonstrated that blood transfusion can enhance organ allograft acceptance in kidney and heart transplants likely mediated through a prostaglandin E–interleukin-2 pathway. Cecka and colleagues[32] reported that transfusions from organ donors were effective in mediating renal allograft acceptance. Moreover, transfusions from third parties were also successful in mediating this effect. In patients with cancer, transfusions may contribute to cancer recurrence through suppression of the immune system.[32] Support for this hypothesis comes from retrospective studies of patients with prostate, colorectal, and cervical cancer. In these studies, even when tumor stage, preoperative anemia, age, and duration of surgery were taken into account, transfusion with whole blood was an independent predictor of earlier tumor recurrence. Certain factors, such as surgical technique, other medications, or the types of transfusion components, were not taken into account. Even though this effect has not been detected in all studies done on this patient population, the effect is suggestive, although not conclusive, of the role of transfusion in accelerating cancer recurrence.

Studies have investigated the role of transfusion immuno-modulation in HIV-infected patients. Busch and colleagues[33] demonstrated in vitro evidence that transfusions containing leukocytes activated HIV-1 replication in infected cell lines. Transfusion of allogeneic peripheral blood mononuclear cells induced a dose-related activation of HIV-1 expression in the in vivo infected cells, followed by dissemination of HIV-1 to previously uninfected cells. No such effect was observed with transfusion of leukocyte-depleted red blood cells, platelets, or plasma.[33] The Transfusion Safety Study Group evaluated data from six clinical centers to ascertain the effect of clotting factor therapy on the progression of HIV infection in patients with hemophilia. These investigators determined that the rate of decline of CD4 cells was related to transfusion of factor concentrates or cryoprecipitates. Their results counter the assertions that clotting factor products accelerate CD4 decrease.[34] Most recently, Collier and colleagues[35] of the Viral Activation Transfusion Study Group found no evidence of HIV, CMV, or cytokine activation after blood transfusion in HIV-infected patients. Although an immunosuppressive effect of transfusion in patients infected with HIV may be present, its clinical relevance is yet to be elucidated.

■ Modifications of Blood Components and Use of Blood-Sparing Approaches

Leukoreduction

Given the transfusion-related complications discussed earlier, it is no surprise that interest in the use of leukoreduced blood products has been increasing. Leukoreduction is beneficial in preventing CMV transmission, allograft rejection, allosensiti-zation causing refractoriness to platelet transfusions, and febrile nonhemolytic transfusion reactions. Based in part on large clinical trials, leukoreduced blood components have been shown to be advantageous to bone marrow transplant recipients, solid organ transplant recipients, and HIV-positive patients. Investigators have expressed concerns regarding the use of leukoreduced components in patients with leukemia because of the loss of a possible graft-versus-leukemia effect through the use of allogeneic blood products. Some groups reported an advantage in remission duration for patients who received standard blood products. However, others failed to demonstrate a difference in either disease-free survival or time to relapse related to the use of leukoreduced blood products. Unfortunately, none of these studies were random-ized, controlled prospective trials, so conclusions are difficult to draw regarding the use of leukoreduced blood in this patient population.[3]

Blood-Sparing Technologies

An important aspect of transfusion medicine is also the use of blood-sparing technologies to reduce the need for blood products. One of the most important developments in this field has been the red blood cell growth factor erythropoietin. *Erythropoietin* is a glycoprotein that is normally produced by the kidneys in a feedback control system. The renal oxygen-sensing mechanism enhances the production of erythropoietin in response to hypoxia. Erythropoietin then interacts with erythroid progenitor cells in the bone marrow through a specific receptor site on erythroid colony-forming units, facilitating the production of new red blood cells. The use of erythropoietin has become a useful supportive measure in patients with cancer who suffer from either cancer-related or treatment-related anemia.[36] It has also been approved for patients with chronic renal failure (and therefore serves as an important supportive therapy in the peritransplant period), for patients undergoing dialysis, and for HIV-infected patients with anemia as a result of zidovudine (AZT) use. New areas of research are also focusing on developing red blood cell substitutes.

New Technologies

Viral Clearance

Whereas the safety of the blood supply has improved dramat-ically since the 1980s because of screening and testing of blood donors, transmission of viruses (especially by blood obtained during the "window period" of viral infection) is still of concern. A field in which research has been expanding rapidly is that of *viral clearance* of blood products. This term refers to both the technology of viral inactivation through the use of chemicals or solvents to disrupt viruses in blood products and the process of viral clearance in which viruses are actually removed from the blood. Viral removal is accom-plished by either filtration or purification methods. Nanofiltration is a technology that uses small-pore filters to remove viruses from plasma products. It has been employed in clearing such products as factor IX and immunoglobulin, but because its effectiveness depends on pore size, it may not be applicable to clearing larger proteins such as factor VIII, fibrinogen, or von Willebrand factor.[37] Chromatography and partitioning methods such as ethanol fractionation and precipitation methods are the other available technologies that are currently used for viral clearance. These technologies, although effective for plasma products, have not been devel-oped for clearing cellular components of blood.

Viral inactivation can be accomplished using numerous approaches, chemical or physical. Chemical methods are based on the characteristic of the virus targeted for inactiva-tion. Ethyl alcohol and isopropyl alcohol are effective against enveloped viruses, as are chlorine-based disinfectants. These methods target viruses through destruction of membrane lipids.[38] Alkylating agents accomplish inactivation through destruction of nucleic acids. Chemical approaches have been effective in plasma products. Physical methods of inactivating viruses include heat, radiation, and photosensitization. These have been applied to both plasma products and cellular com-ponents of blood. The challenge in using these approaches is to achieve viral clearance without destroying activity and function of the transfused blood or introduction of toxic byproducts together with blood components. Thus, research into viral inactivation of cellular blood products continues to reduce the risk to the recipients imparted by use of chemical or physical treatments of blood. This must be balanced against the risk of transmission of viruses in these products.

Gene Therapy

With the understanding of the genetic basis for disease and the growth of recombinant DNA technology, the possibility for treating disease on a genetic level has become a reality.

This investigational approach to disease treatment is becoming an important aspect of transfusion medicine. Obvious targets for gene therapy are inherited diseases, but the use of gene therapy has reached clinical trials in oncology and is being developed in AIDS as well. The principle of *gene therapy* is to replace defective genes or to complement defects in genes by introducing new genetic material into cells in stable fashion. This can be accomplished using physical and chemical methods or biologic methods through the use of viral vectors. Although chemical and physical methods such as liposome-mediated gene transfer or electroporation have been developed, viral vectors remain a more efficient technology.

In HSC transplant recipients, preliminary studies suggest that gene therapy may be an approach to control the severity of GVHD disease. Animal models provided the scientific basis for such approaches. Retroviral producer cells for the herpes simplex thymidine kinase gene were injected in vivo into murine tumors. Expression of thymidine kinase made these cells sensitive to ganciclovir. Thus, treatment with ganciclovir after this gene therapy caused regression of the tumors. For patients with GVHD after allogeneic transplantation, the TK gene was introduced into ex vivo T lymphocytes from the graft. Subsequent treatment of these patients with ganciclovir ameliorated GVHD in two of the three patients treated.[39]

Gene therapy has also been investigated as a therapy for AIDS, although it has not yet reached clinical trials. The preliminary laboratory work has been targeted at disrupting the function of important HIV-encoded gene products in infected cells. For example, in vitro models are being developed in which gene-encoding ribosomes are delivered that specifically cleave HIV RNA and thereby disrupt important post-transcriptional gene regulation in HIV-infected cells.[40] So far, HIV-infected cells have not been targeted in vivo. Results must first be demonstrated in animal models before this therapy is ready for clinical trials in patients.

■ Conclusion

With improvements in therapeutic regimens, advances in transplantation biology, and a better understanding of immunology, transfusion medicine has attempted to face growing challenges in dealing with these categories of immunodeficient patients. This has meant providing novel components for transfusion, improving the safety of the blood supply, recognizing unanticipated transfusion complications and designing new technologies to overcome them, and bringing groundbreaking cytotherapies into clinical trials. Although the biology of solid organ and HSC transplantation and the biology of HIV infection have led to new approaches in transfusion medicine, these changes have been based on a fuller understanding of hematopoiesis, immune function, infectious disease, and tumor biology.

REFERENCES

1. Goodnough LT, Brecher ME, Kanter MH, AuBuchon JP: Transfusion medicine. N Engl J Med 1999;340:438–447.
2. Comenzo RL, Wuest DL: Irradiated components. In Hillyer et al (eds): Handbook of Transfusion Medicine. San Diego, Academic Press, 2001, pp 143–145.
3. Wuest DL: Transfusion and Stem Cell Support in Cancer Treatment. Hematol Oncol Clin North Am 1996;10:397–429.
4. Levesque JP, Takamatsu Y, Nilsson SK, et al: Vascular cell adhesion molecule-1 (CD 106) is cleaved by neutrophil proteases in the bone marrow following hematopoietic progenitor cell mobilization by granulocyte colony-stimulating factor. Blood 2001;98:1289–1297.
5. Bensinger WI, Price TH, Dale FR, et al: The effects of daily recombinant human granulocyte colony-stimulating factor administration on normal granulocyte donors undergoing leukapheresis. Blood 1993;81:1883–1888.
6. Strauss RG: Therapeutic granulocyte transfusions in 1993 [editorial]. Blood 1993;81:1675–1678.
7. Price TH, Bowden RA, Boeckh M, et al: Phase I/II trial of neutrophil transfusions from donors stimulated with G-CSF and dexamethasone for treatment of patients with infections in hematopoietic stem cell transplantation. Blood 2000;95:3302–3309.
8. Kolb HJ, Schattenberg A, Goldman JM: Graft-versus-leukemia effect of donor lymphocyte transfusions in marrow grafted patients. Blood 1995;86:2041.
9. Rooney CM, Smith CA, Ng CYC, et al: Infusion of cytotoxic T cells for the prevention and treatment of Epstein-Barr virus-induced lymphoma in allogeneic transplant recipients, Blood 92:1549–1555, 1998.
10. Milpied N, Vasseur B, Parquet N, et al: Humanized anti-CD20 monoclonal antibody (rituximab) in post transplant B-lymphoproliferative disorder: a retrospective analysis on 32 patients. Ann Oncol 2000;11:113–116.
11. Kuehnle I, Huls MH, Liu Z, et al: CD20 monoclonal antibody (rituximab) for therapy of Epstein-Barr virus lymphoma after hemopoietic stem-cell transplantation. Blood 2000;95:1502–1555.
12. Riddell SR, Greenberg PD, Overell RW, et al: Phase I study of cellular adoptive immunotherapy using genetically modified CD8$^+$ HIV-specific T cells for HIV seropositive patients undergoing allogeneic bone marrow transplant. Hum Gene Ther 1992;3:319–338.
13. Brodie SJ, Lewinsohn DA, Patterson BK: In vivo migration and function of transferred HIV-1-specific cytotoxic T cells. Nat Med 1999;5:34–41.
14. Lieberman J, Shankar P, Manjunath N, Andersson J: Dressed to kill? A review of why antiviral CD8 T lymphocytes fail to prevent progressive immunodeficiency in HIV-1 infection. Blood 2001;98:1667–1677.
15. Boeckh M, Boivin G: Quantitation of cytomegalovirus: Methodologic aspects and clinical applications. Clin Microbiol Rev 2001;11:533–554.
16. Narvios AB, Lichtiger B: Bedside leukoreduction of cellular blood components in preventing cytomegalovirus transmission in allogeneic bone marrow transplant recipients. Haematologica 2001;86:749–752.
17. Laupacis A, Brown J, Costello B, et al: Prevention of postransfusion CMV in the era of universal WBC reduction: A consensus statement. Transfusion 2001;41:560–569.
18. Blajchman M, Goldman M, Freedman J, Sher G: Proceedings of a consensus conference: Prevention of post-transfusion CMV in the era of universal leukoreduction. Transfus Med Rev 2001;15:1–20.
19. Prati D, Lin YH, De Mattei C, et al: A prospective study on TT virus infection in transfusion dependent patients with β-thalassemia. Blood 1999;93:1502–1505.
20. Kanda Y, Hirai H: TT virus in hematological disorders and bone marrow transplant recipients. Leuk Lymphoma 2001;40:483–489.
21. Conroy-Cantilena C, Menitove JE: Hepatitis. In Anderson K, Ness P (eds): Scientific Basis of Transfusion Medicine. Philadelphia, WB Saunders, 2000, pp 472–489.
22. Frickhofen N, Abkowitz JL, Safford M, et al: Persistent B19 parvovirus infection in patients infected with human immunodeficiency virus type 1 (HIV-1): A treatable cause of anemia in AIDS. Ann Intern Med 1990;113:926.
23. Dodd RY: Epidemiology of transfusion transmitted diseases. In Anderson K, Ness P (eds): Scientific Basis of Transfusion Medicine. Philadelphia, WB Saunders, 2000, pp 455–469.
24. Ahsan N, Holman MJ, Gocke JA, Yang HC: Pure red cell aplasia due to parvovirus B19 infection in solid organ transplantation. Clin Transplant 1997;11:265–270.
25. Brown KE, Young NS, Alving BM, Barbosa LH: Parvovirus B19: Implications for transfusion medicine. Summary of a workshop. Transfusion 2001;41:130–135.
26. Kruskall MS, Lee TH, Assmann SF, et al: Survival of transfused donor white blood cells in HIV-infected recipients. Blood 2001;98:272–279.
27. Fast LD, Valeri CR, Crowley JP: Immune responses to major histocompatibility complex homozygous lymphoid cells in murine F1 hybrid recipients: Implications for transfusion associated graft-versus-host disease. Blood 1995;86:3090–3096.
28. Saigo K, Ryo R: Therapeutic strategy for post-transfusion graft-vs-host disease. Int J Hematol 1999;69:147–151.

29. Juji T, Nishimura M, Tadokoro K: Treatment of post transfusion graft-versus-host disease. Vox Sang 2000;78:277–279.
30. Dykewicz C: Guidelines for preventing opportunistic infections among hematopoietic stem cell transplant recipients: Recommendations of the CDC, the Infectious Disease Society of America, and the American Society of Blood and Marrow Transplantation. Biol Blood Marrow Transplant: 195–225, 2001.
31. Chang H, Voralia M, Bali M, et al: Irreversible loss of donor blood leukocyte activation may explain a paucity of transfusion-associated graft-versus-host disease from stored blood. Br J Haematol 2000;111:146–156.
32. Cecka M, Toyotome A: The transfusion effect. In Teraski PI (ed): Clinical Transplants 1989. Los Angeles, UCLA Tissue Typing Laboratory, 1989, pp 335–341.
33. Busch MP, Lee TH, Heitman J: Allogeneic leukocytes but not therapeutic blood elements induce reactivation and dissemination of latent human immunodeficiency virus type 1 infection: Implications for transfusion support of infected patients. Blood 1992;80:2128–2135.
34. Gjerst GF, Pike MC, Mosley JW, et al: Effect of low-and intermediate-purity clotting factor therapy on progression of human immunodeficiency virus infection in congenital clotting disorders: Transfusion Safety Study Group. Blood 1994;84:1666–1671.
35. Collier AC, Kalish LA, Busch MP, et al: Leukocyte-reduced red blood cell transfusions in patients with anemia and human immunodeficiency virus infection. The viral activation transfusion study: A randomized controlled trial. JAMA 2001;285:1592–1600.
36. Klaesson S: Clinical use of rHuEPO in bone marrow transplantation. Med Oncol 1999;16:2–7.
37. Burnouf-Radosevich M, Appourchaux P, Huart JJ, et al: Nanofiltration, a new specific virus elimination method applied to high purity factor IX and factor XI concentrates. Vox Sang 1994;67:132–138.
38. Horowitz B, Prince AM, Horowitz MS, Watklevicz C: Viral safety of solvent-detergent treated blood products. Dev Biol Stand 1993;81:147–161.
39. Bonin C, Ferrari G, Verzeletti S, et al: HSV-TK gene transfer into donor lymphocytes for control of allogeneic graft-versus-leukemia. Science 1997;276:1719–1729.
40. Sullenger BA, Gallardo HF, Ungers GE, Gilboa E: Overexpression of TAR sequences renders cells resistant to human immunodeficiency virus replication. Cell 1990;63:601.

Chapter 31

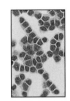

Transfusion of the Platelet-Refractory Patient

Thomas S. Kickler

Three decades ago, platelet transfusion therapy was available principally in tertiary hospitals. The development of potentially curable, myelosuppressive chemotherapeutic regimens necessitated intensive research into the biology of platelets, methods for their procurement and storage, and platelet transfusion practices. This research led to the widespread availability of platelet transfusions. Unlike the surgery patient who receives platelet transfusions during the perioperative period, medical patients frequently receive longer courses of platelet transfusions. Consequently, platelet alloimmunization and refractoriness to platelet transfusions can occur. This is especially true for patients undergoing myelosuppressive therapy or allogeneic marrow transplantation and for those with aplastic anemia. Nonimmune refractoriness and alloimmune-mediated refractoriness are the most important factors limiting the hemostatic effectiveness of platelet transfusions. The purpose of this chapter is to describe the use of platelet transfusions in patients who are receiving supportive care after chemotherapy or marrow transplantation and the methods used to prevent or circumvent platelet refractoriness.[1]

■ Indications for Platelet Transfusions

In patients with thrombocytopenia, the risk of hemorrhage increases progressively once the platelet count drops below 100,000/μL.[2, 3] Many studies have attempted to define the bleeding time or platelet count necessary to achieve hemostasis in surgical patients, with conflicting results.[3–7] Some generalities do exist, however. With normally functioning platelets, most major surgery can be performed safely if the count is maintained in the range of 50,000 to 75,000/μL. A higher range may be necessary for longer and more technically difficult procedures involving extensive incisions or exposure of large surface areas. Performance of surgery on the central nervous system should be done only with platelet counts greater than 100,000/μL.[3]

In amegakaryocytic thrombocytopenia, platelet transfusions are given prophylactically or therapeutically and for the performance of invasive procedures. There is considerable interest in trying to define the lowest safe platelet concentration, so that fewer donor exposures occur and limited blood resources are conserved. Physicians have been generally aware that hemorrhage is more common during the most severe stages of thrombocytopenia. A study of 92 consecutive patients treated for acute leukemia between 1956 and 1959 at the National Cancer Institute led to the current prophylactic guidelines. Platelet counts lower than 100,000/μL were associated with an increased risk of bleeding. Patients with platelet counts of 5,000/μL or less manifested gross hemorrhage on approximately one third of days at risk. A platelet count of 20,000/μL or less was associated with moderate bleeding manifestations such as epistaxis and petechiae. Based on these studies, a prophylactic platelet transfusion strategy, using a platelet count of 20,000/μL as the transfusion trigger, has been commonly employed.[8]

More recently, in a randomized study of prophylactic platelet transfusion, Rebulla and coworkers[5] showed that giving transfusions only when the platelet count dips below 10,000/μL can decrease platelet use with only a small adverse effect on bleeding and no effect on mortality. It therefore appears that, with amegakaryocytic thrombocytopenia, prophylactic transfusions should be given if the count falls below 5,000/μL. At values between 5,000 and 10,000/μL, transfusion may be withheld if the patient is stable and if no other conditions make spontaneous bleeding likely.[5] Such conditions include blast crisis, rapidly falling platelet count, anticoagulation with heparin for disseminated intravascular coagulation (DIC), drugs that affect platelet function, uremia, and recent invasive procedures, including spinal taps or placement of central venous catheters.[9]

■ Platelet Transfusion Refractoriness

Failure to achieve an expected increment with a platelet transfusion is called *platelet transfusion refractoriness*. Refractoriness may be caused by an immune or a nonimmune condition. Clinically, one can assess the response to a platelet transfusion by measuring the increment in platelet count 1 to 18 hours after the transfusion. The post-transfusion platelet response should be calculated on the basis of the patient's body surface area (BSA) in square millimeters and corrected for the number of platelets transfused. The corrected platelet count increment (CCI) is calculated by the following formula:

$$CCI = (Post \text{-} Transfusion\ Count - Pre \text{-} Transfusion\ Count)$$
$$\times BSA \div No.\ Platelets\ Transfused$$

In general, a successful CCI should be greater than 7500 within 10 to 60 minutes after a transfusion and greater than 4500 if measured 18 to 24 hours after transfusion. It has been suggested that the CCI determined 1 hour after platelet transfusion is a useful indirect measure to document allo-immunization.[2] However, human leukocyte antigen (HLA) antibodies are only one of many factors that influence the CCI at 1 hour. Furthermore, even if platelet antibodies are present, excellent 1-hour CCIs may be achieved.[10] This latter phenomenon may be seen after platelets with weak expression of HLA-B–locus antigens are given.[2, 3, 9]

Immunologic Basis of Platelet Transfusion Refractoriness

Soon after the introduction of prophylactic platelet transfusions, it became apparent that serial transfusion results in decreasing effectiveness in many patients.[10] Through the work of Yankee and others[11], it is now recognized that transfusion failures result from the induction of alloantibodies to HLA and other antigens. Yankee and coworkers[11] were able to show that most cases of platelet refractoriness could be reversed by the use of platelet transfusions phenotypically matched at the HLA-A and -B loci. It was also recognized that the development of HLA antibodies, as measured by lymphocytotoxic activity, correlated with the development of the immune refractory state.[12] It is now well recognized that response to HLA-A and -B locus antigens (Table 31.1) is the major cause of post-transfusion alloimmune transfusion failure.

Antibodies to the human platelet-specific antigens (HPAs, Table 31.2) are only rare causes of platelet transfusion refractoriness. In a large series of patients who received platelet transfusions, only 2% had detectable antibodies to HPAs. Most of these antibodies were found in patients who were also alloimmunized to class I HLA antigens. If HLA-identical platelet transfusions fail, antibodies to the HPAs should be considered. Antibody specificity to the HPAs can be identified by enzyme-linked antiglobulin assay and isolated platelet glycoproteins of different phenotypes.[13, 14] In general, few donor centers have a donor population typed for the HPAs, except for those in the HPA-1 system. The recent introduction of DNA-based typing for HPAs permits accurate typing of donors and even thrombocytopenic patients, because lymphocyte-derived DNA is used.[15]

Table 31.1 Listing of Recognized Human Leukocyte Antigen Class I Specificities

A Locus	B Locus
A1	B5
A2	B7
A3	B8
A9	B12
A10	B13
A11	B14
Aw19	B15
A23	B16
A24	B17
A25	B18
A26	B21
A28	Bw22
A30	B27
A31	B35
A32	B37
Aw33	B38
Aw34	B39
Aw36	B40
Aw43	Bw41
Aw66	Bw42
Aw68	B44
Aw69	B45
Aw74	Bw46
A29	Bw47
	Bw48
	Bw49
	Bw50
	Bw51
	Bw52
	Bw53
	Bw54
	Bw55
	Bw56
	Bw57
	Bw58
	Bw59
	Bw60
	Bw61
	Bw62
	Bw63
	Bw64
	Bw65
	Bw67
	Bw71
	Bw73
	Bw75
	Bw76
	Bw77
	Bw4
	Bw6

Detection of Antibodies in Platelet Transfusion Refractoriness

Specific identification of alloimmunization can be done by measurement of HLA antibodies using lymphocytotoxicity testing.[16] Serial lymphocytotoxic antibody measurements are helpful in the management of alloimmunization. Some patients have decreases or a loss of lymphocytotoxic antibody, either permanently or transiently, and can be successfully transfused with platelet concentrates.[17] It should be noted that some patients have antibodies to HLA class I and yet do not have platelet transfusion failures. Kao and coworkers[18] developed a solid-phase enzyme-linked immunoassay that detects the presence of immunoglobulin G (IgG) anti-HLA antibodies with the use of purified HLA antigens prepared from platelet concentrates. This test is now widely used to screen

Table 31.2 Human Platelet Alloantigens

HPA-Antigen	Other Names	Glycoprotein	Protein Polymorphism	DNA Polymorphism
1a1b	Zw(a), Pl(A1)Zw(b), Pl(A2)	IIIa	Leu33Pro33	T196C196
2a2b	Ko(b)Ko(a), Sib	Ibalpha	Thr145Met145	C524T524
3a3b	Bak(a), Lek(a)Bak(b)	IIb	Ile843Ser843	T2622G2622
4a4b	Yuk(b), PenYuk(a)	IIIa	Arg143Gln143	G526A526
5a5b	Br(b)Br(a), Zav, Hc	Ia	Glu505Lys505	G1648A1648
6bW	Tu, Ca	IIIa	Gln489Arg489	A1564G1564
7bW	Mo	IIIa	Ala407Pro407	G1317C1317
8bW	Sr(a)	IIIa	Cys636Arg636	T2004C2004
9bW	Max(a)	IIb	Met837Val837	A2603G2603
10bW	La(a)	IIIa	Gln62Arg62	A281G281
11bW	Gro(a)	IIIa	His633Arg633	A1996G1996
12bW	Iy(a)	Ibbeta	Glu15Gly15	A141G141
13bW	Sit(a)	Ia	Met799Thr799	T2531C2531
	Oe(a)	IIIa		
	Va(a)	IIbIIIa		
	Gov(a), Gov(b)	CD109		

for HLA antibodies in a variety of transfusion and transplantation conditions.

HLA Alloantigens and Antibodies

Understanding the HLA system is important so that compatible platelet transfusions may be selected for alloimmunized patients.[19] Only HLA-A and -B antigens have been shown to be important in causing immune-mediated platelet transfusion refractoriness. There are two broad types of HLA antibodies made in response to platelet transfusions. The first type recognizes epitopes unique to a particular HLA allele, referred to as antibodies to private specificities. Antibodies to HLA-A2 and HLA-B12 fall into this group. The second type of HLA antibody recognizes more than one gene product. These antibodies recognize structural similarities between gene products (cross-reactive epitopes) or identical epitopes present on gene products of different alleles and are referred to as antibodies to public epitopes. Traditionally, HLA serology has placed the greatest emphasis on classification of the private antigens. Recently, more importance has been placed on the clinical importance of public HLA specificities. The best known examples of public specificities are HLA-Bw4 and -Bw6. These antigens are encoded by a diallelic system and are associated with two different groups of HLA-B class I antigens. Other public antigens carried by HLA-B class I antigens have been divided into four cross-reactive groups: HLA-B5, -B7, -B8, and -B12 (Table 31.3). The observation that the specificity of HLA antibodies in multiply transfused individuals is usually against public epitopes suggests that matching for these public antigens is important. With improved serologic approaches to the identification of specificities to class I HLA antigens, selection of platelets for transfusion may be simplified by relying on public specificities.

Clinical Features of Alloimmune Refractoriness

In a series reported by Dutcher and colleagues,[20] 42% of 114 patients developed lymphocytotoxic antibody within the first 8 weeks after transfusion. Approximately one fourth of these patients developed antibody within 1 week, suggesting the presence of an amnestic response. Seventy-five percent of responders appeared to have a de novo response. Of those patients who manifested lymphocytotoxic antibody, 17 ultimately lost antibody despite further transfusions. Of those initial patients who did not respond by developing lymphocytotoxic antibody in the first 8 weeks, 92% remained unresponsive despite continued transfusion therapy. Therefore, the development of an alloimmune response after transfusion seems to be an early event in transfusion therapy. Responsiveness or nonresponsiveness to HLA antigens develops during the first weeks of therapy, and this pattern is apparently maintained throughout subsequent therapy.[20]

ANTIPLATELET GLYCOPROTEIN ANTIBODIES

In addition to the phenotypic differences that arise because of polymorphisms in platelet glycoproteins, patients may form antibodies to the entire platelet glycoprotein molecule. For example, individuals who have the Bernard-Soulier syndrome may become immunized to glycoprotein Ib, and those with Glanzmann thrombasthenia may become immunized to glycoprotein IIb-IIIa. Patients who lack these important

Table 31.3 Class I Cross-Reactive Human Leukocyte Antigen Groups

HLA Group	Associated Private Epitopes
A1C	1, 3, 11, 10, W19, 9, 28
A2C	2, 28, 9, 17, 10, 33
B5C	5, 53, 35, 18, 15, 17, 70, 49
B7C	7, 27, 22, 42, 48, 40, 41, 13, 47
B8C	8, 14, 16, 22, 42, 48, 40, 41, 13, 47
B8C	8, 14, 16, 22, 52
B12C	12, 21, 40, 41, 13

membrane glycoproteins and require platelet transfusions may become immunized to normal platelets. This results in transfusion refractoriness and significantly complicates the transfusion management of qualitative platelet disorders.[21]

ABH BLOOD GROUP ANTIGENS

Platelets have ABH antigens on their surface; some are intrinsically present, and some are adsorbed from the plasma. Although platelets are usually regarded as having only weak expression of A and B antigens, some donors have strong A or B antigen expression that may result in refractoriness to isolated units. The importance of platelet ABH antigens in platelet recovery was clearly demonstrated in 1965 by Aster.[22] After group A platelets were transfused to group O volunteers, the average recovery was 19%, whereas after transfusion with ABO-compatible platelets it was 63%, similar to recovery after autologous platelets. In general, however, less striking differences are seen in practice: increments are only about 20% lower for transfusion with ABO-incompatible compared with ABO-compatible units.[22–25]

Nonimmune Refractoriness

Platelet transfusions may not result in an increment if the stored platelets are defective. This result should be relatively uncommon, given the close scrutiny devoted to quality control of blood products. However, one should not fail to consider freshness of a given platelet transfusion as the cause of a single instance of platelet transfusion failure.[2]

COAGULOPATHY

DIC has classically been associated with platelet refractoriness. This syndrome is associated with bacterial sepsis, which is common in transfused patients, and with acute progranulocytic leukemia. The quantitative role of DIC in the platelet refractory state has not been well characterized.[2, 3]

Splenic Sequestration

Splenomegaly has been shown to be a major cause of platelet transfusion failure. Normally some 30% of a patient's platelet mass is contained within the spleen. With increases in splenic size, up to 90% of circulating platelets can be sequestered in this organ. Characteristically, splenic sequestration is associated with a reduced 1-hour platelet recovery but normal survival.[2, 3]

Fever and Infection

Studies by several groups have implicated both fever and infection as a cause for decreased platelet survival. One study noted that platelet transfusion requirements were increased by 50% in febrile patients. This increase may be greater in patients with major infections, particularly DIC.[26, 27]

Hepatic Dysfunction and Veno-occlusive Disease

Several authors have reported hepatic sequestration of platelets in association with a wide spectrum of liver diseases. A syndrome of veno-occlusive disease (VOD) of the liver has been described and is characterized by deposition of platelets in the hepatic venules and development of an intrahepatic thrombosis with hepatomegaly, right upper quadrant pain, and ascites. This organ dysfunction has been observed after administration of a wide variety of cytotoxic agents, including total body irradiation, alkylating agent therapy, and *Vinca* alkaloids.[2]

Other Factors

Platelet refractoriness has been reported with a number of medications. Amphotericin in particular has been implicated in decreasing platelet recovery and survival. Similarly, vancomycin has been reported to be a major cause of platelet refractoriness, as have antithymocyte globulin, granulocyte-macrophage colony-stimulating factor (GM-CSF), granulocyte-CSF, and other interferons. In view of the large number of drugs cancer patients characteristically receive, it would not be surprising if a number of additional agents were implicated in accelerated platelet destruction.[2, 26, 27]

■ Management in the Alloimmunized Patient

Because alloimmunization to HLA antigens accounts for the majority of cases of alloimmune platelet transfusion refractoriness, platelets can be selected on the basis of HLA matching.[2, 3] Depending on the HLA type of an individual, there may be little difficulty in locating platelets that are identical. In some patients with unusual HLA types, such as in diverse ethnic groups, HLA matching may be more difficult.

Kickler and coworkers[28] studied the effectiveness of HLA matching as the sole method of platelet selection for alloimmunized patients. Of 50 HLA-identical platelet transfusions, 20% were unsuccessful. Of transfusions selected on the basis of cross-reactivities without regard to matching of public specificities, 41% (23 of 56) were failures. One third of those transfusions in which one or two antigen-mismatched platelets were used were failures. These observations indicated that matching of platelets on the basis of HLA private antigens is frequently unreliable as a sole criterion. On the other hand, even if patients are alloimmunized, they may receive mismatched platelets and have successful transfusions.[28]

For these reasons, refining the selection process of platelets for alloimmunized patients has been the subject of much investigation. Table 31.4 outlines a practical approach to selection of platelets for the alloimmunized patient that takes into account of the importance of HLA matching and platelet compatibility testing. Numerous investigators have evaluated the usefulness of cross-matching a recipient's platelets with those of potential donors. This approach can be readily followed because pheresis platelets are stored for 5 days. By analyzing aliquots of platelets taken from integrally attached tubing segments, compatible platelets can be found in the inventory of stored platelets. Compatible donors may be found even if a patient is broadly alloimmunized. A variety

Table 31.4 Non–Antibody-Specific Approach to Selection of Platelets for Alloimmunized Patients

Determine human leukocyte antigen (HLA) phenotype and ABO type of the recipient.

Screen patient's serum for lymphocytotoxic antibody, or antibodies to human platelet antigens if there is a history of failing HLA-identical platelets.

Select from the donor pool those units with the most compatible HLA antigens and, if possible, ABO systems; alternatively, cross-match available platelet units without regard to patient or donor HLA type.

Cross-match the recipient's serum with the sera of selected potential donors and select the most compatible unit.

Table 31.5 Antibody-Specific Approach to Selection of
Platelets for Alloimmunized Patients

Identify human leukocyte antigen (HLA) specificity in patient's serum
using an extended panel of HLA-typed lymphocytes.

Identify platelet donors negative for HLA antigens reactive with the
patient's serum.

Cross-match recipient's serum with platelets to check serologic work
and to detect antibodies to non-HLA antigens.

of techniques exist for platelet cross-matching, most of which
involve a labeled antiglobulin technique. Many referral
centers have developed techniques that have been validated
in their own patient populations. The commercial availability
of platelet compatibility tests has resulted in wider use of
platelet cross-matching.[29, 30]

Because providing cross-matched platelets may be difficult or impractical given frequent transfusions and the need to
cross-match against a large number of potential donors, there
is much interest in developing methods of pretransfusion
testing, similar to those used to select compatible red blood
cells. These procedures are well known to transfusion services
and involve phenotyping of donors and recipients and identification of the specificity of antibodies present in a patient's
serum. Specifically for platelets, HLA phenotyping of donors
and recipients and identification of the HLA antibody
specificities are required. Petz and coworkers[29] extensively
evaluated this approach, and it appears to be highly reliable
and successful in identifying donors who would ordinarily be
excluded if only exact HLA matches were considered. These
investigators coined the phrase *antibody specificity prediction*
(ASP) method to describe these procedures (Table 31.5).

Petz and coworkers[29] reported data on the utility of ASP
for 1621 platelet transfusions in 114 persons with platelet
transfusion refractoriness. They compared the effectiveness of
platelets selected by the ASP method with that of platelets
selected on the basis of HLA matching or cross-matching or,
if selected components were not available, on a random basis.
They concluded that the ASP method was as effective as HLA
matching or cross-matching, and that all three methods were
superior to the random selection of platelets. Further, in a file
of HLA-matched donors, many more potential donors were
identifiable by the ASP method than by HLA matching,
which makes the acquisition of compatible platelets for
alloimmunized refractory patients much more feasible. This
approach appears to be logistically simple on a regional basis
when the testing is offered by blood centers, and it promises
to harmonize the selection of platelets with the selection
process used for red blood cell transfusions.

Management of Platelet Transfusion Refractoriness and Bleeding

A variety of approaches have been attempted when no compatible platelets can be found for a patient who is alloimmunized
and continues to bleed or may be undergoing invasive
procedures.[2, 3] Therapeutic modalities have included splenectomy, corticosteroids, plasmapheresis, administration of
intravenous gammaglobulin (IVIG), and repeated platelet
transfusions. Except for IVIG, there is little evidence that
any of these treatments work.

Kickler and coworkers[31] performed a randomized, placebo-
controlled clinical trial investigating the use of IVIG in

alloimmunized thrombocytopenic patients. In this trial, IVIG
was administered at a dose of 400 mg/kg for 5 days. An
incompatible platelet transfusion from the same donor was
used before and after the administration of IVIG or placebo.
Although platelet recovery in 1 to 6 hours was satisfactory in
five of seven patients after IVIG treatment, 24-hour survival
was not improved in most of them. It could not be excluded that
this poor 24-hour survival result was unrelated to nonimmune
causes of shortened platelet survival. None of the placebo
group (five patients) achieved a satisfactory 1-hour CCI. By
Student's *t* test, the post-treatment mean 1-hour CCI values
were significantly greater in those who received IVIG than in
the control group.[31]

If all conventional methods fail to increase the platelet count
to hemostatic levels, the only remaining alternative that has
been tried is continuous transfusion of platelets (massive
transfusion). It has been argued that, although the platelet count
is not increased, transfused platelets still exert some effect,
permitting platelet plug formation or maintenance of endothelial integrity. These arguments are based on clinical observations. In one well-established animal model of alloimmune
thrombocytopenia, if the platelet count did not increase above
$60,000/mm^3$, capillary leakage of bleeding still persisted.[2, 3]

Other Approaches

In uncontrolled studies and in small controlled studies, the
antifibrinolytic agents, ε-aminocaproic acid and tranexamic
acid, have been used.[32] The results have been mixed in terms
of reduction of microvascular hemorrhage and reduction of
platelet transfusion requirements. The differing results probably are related to the small number of patients studied.
Immunosuppressive agents, splenectomy, and plasma
exchange have not been proven effective.[2, 3]

■ Prevention of Alloimmunization

Reduction of Donor Exposures

Several studies have shown a direct relationship between the
number of platelet transfusions and alloimmunization.[33, 34]
Others have not documented a dose-response relationship.[2]
The reasons for these contradictory conclusions are not clear.
In part, clinical differences in the study populations, such as
the multiparous state of transfusion recipients, may be the
main explanation. Another problem in the literature has been
the definition of alloimmunization, including the laboratory
endpoint and the method used to measure HLA antibodies.
For a primary immune response, 2 to 3 weeks may be
required. If sera are not collected over a sufficient interval, an
antibody response may not be measured. Alternatively, some
patients may lose antibody by the time of testing, contributing
to negative responses. The published data are also consistent
with the hypothesis that the alloimmune response has a
threshold effect. Over a low range of exposure, there may be
a dose-response effect. With larger numbers of exposures,
further alloimmunization may not develop if tolerance has
been established.

Preventive Measures

Results of early animal studies showed that depletion of
contaminating leukocytes from donor blood components was
effective in preventing alloantibody response to the major
histocompatibility complex (MHC).[33] Other approaches, such

as inactivation of donor leukocytes by ultraviolet irradiation, provided further evidence of the important role of donor leukocytes in eliciting immune responses to class I MHC antigens. With the development of highly efficient methods to remove leukocytes from blood products, a number of clinical trials were instituted. In general, if fewer than 1×10^6 contaminating leukocytes remained, alloimmunization was reduced by 30% to 50%. Many of these studies in thrombocytopenic patients also showed some success in the use of leukocyte-poor blood components to prevent HLA alloimmunization or platelet transfusion refractoriness. However, the results obtained from a variety of clinical trials have been inconclusive and not reproducible, perhaps because of variability in blood product preparation and heterogeneity in the patient populations studied.

Because of the confusing data, a large multicenter clinical trial was done in the United States. This Trial for the Reduction of Alloimmunization to Platelets (TRAP) tested the efficacy of transfusion with platelets modified by leukocyte reduction or ultraviolet irradiation or with leukocyte-depleted, single-donor platelets.[34] The results obtained with these modified platelet products were compared with transfusion of platelet concentrates. All patients received leukocyte-depleted red blood cells. A total of 534 patients with acute myeloid leukemia were studied during an 8-week period for the development of platelet alloantibodies. Forty-five percent of patients in the control group developed HLA antibodies compared with 22% of those in the ultraviolet-irradiated group, 18% in the filtered platelet concentrate group, and 17% in the filtered apheresis group. All three types of treated platelets were associated with a significant reduction in the development of HLA antibodies and alloimmune platelet refractoriness compared with the control group. These maneuvers were effective even though 26% of the patients had received previous transfusions of nontreated blood products. Importantly, none of the treatment maneuvers reduced the rate of alloimmunization to HPAs (6% to 10%). Therefore, this large study documented the usefulness of either leukocyte removal or inactivation by ultraviolet irradiation in the chronically transfused platelet recipient. The use of platelet concentrates derived from whole blood did not increase the risk of alloimmunization compared with single-donor platelets. Several other studies have confirmed these findings.[35]

REFERENCES

1. Kickler TS: The platelet transfusion refractory state: Transfusion practices and clinical management. In Kurtz SR, Brubaker DB (eds): Clinical Decisions in Platelet Therapy. Bethesda, MD: American Association of Blood Banks, 1992, pp 87–104.
2. Benson K: Criteria for diagnosing refractoriness to platelet transfusions. In Kickler TS, Herman JH (eds): Current Issues in Platelet Transfusion Therapy and Platelet Alloimmunity. Bethesda, Md: American Association of Blood Banks Press, 1999, pp 33–63.
3. Freidburg RC, Gaupp B: Platelet indications, considerations, and specific clinical settings. In Kickler TS, Herman JH (eds): Current Issues in Platelet Transfusion Therapy and Platelet Alloimmunity. Bethesda, MD: American Association of Blood Banks Press, 1999, p 1.
4. Hersh EM, Mbodey GP, Nies BA, et al: Causes of death in acute leukemia: a ten year study of 414 patients. JAMA 1965;193:99–103.
5. Rebulla P, Finazzi G, Marangoni F, et al: A multicenter randomized study of the threshold for prophylactic platelet transfusions in adults with acute leukemia. N Engl J Med 1997;337:1870–1875.
6. Higby DJ: The prophylactic treatment of thrombocytopenic leukemic patients. Transfusion 1974;14:440–446.
7. Roy AJ, Jaffe N, Djerassi I: Prophylactic platelet transfusions. Transfusion 1973;13:283–290.
8. Gaydos LA, Freirich EJ, Mantel N: The quantitative relation between platelet count and hemorrhage in acute leukemia. N Engl J Med 1962;266:905–909.
9. National Institutes of Health. Consensus conference: Platelet transfusion therapy. JAMA 1987;257:1777–1780.
10. Bishop JF, Matthews JP, Yuen K, et al: The definition of refractoriness to platelet transfusion. Transfus Med 1992;2:35–41.
11. Yankee RA, Grumet D, Rogentine GN: Platelet selection by HLA matching. N Engl J Med 1973;288:760–767.
12. Hogge DE, Dutcher JP, Aisner J, Schiffer CA: Lymphocytotoxic antibody is a predictor of response to random donor platelet transfusion. Am J Hematol 1983;14:363–369.
13. Kickler TS, Kennedy SD, Braine HG: Alloimmunization to platelet specific antigens on glycoprotein IIB-IIIA and IB/IX in multitransfused thrombocytopenic patients. Transfusion 1990;30:622–625.
14. Kiefel V, Santoso S, Weisheit M, Mueller-Eckhardt C: Monoclonal antibody-specific immobilization of platelet antigens (MAIPA): A new tool for the identification of platelet-reactive antibodies. Blood 1987;70:1722–1726.
15. Kim HO, Jing Y, Kickler TS, et al: Immunogenetic studies on the genotypic differences in platelet antigens. Transfusion 1995;35:863–867.
16. Fuller TC, Cosimi AB, Russell PS: Use of an antiglobulin-ATG reagent for detection of low levels of alloantibody: Improvement of allograft survival in presensitized recipients. Transplant Proc 1978;10:463–468.
17. Lee EJ, Schiffer CA: Serial measurement of lymphocytotoxic antibody and response to nonmatched platelet transfusions in alloimmunized patients. Blood 1987;70:1727–1729.
18. Kao KJ, Scornik JC, Small S: Enzyme linked immunoassay for anti-HLA antibodies: An alternative to panel studies by lymphocytotoxicity. Transplantation 1993;55:192–196.
19. Rodey GE: Class I antigens: HLA A, B, C and cross reactive groups. In Moulds J (ed): Scientific and Technical Aspects of the Major Histocompatibility Complex. Arlington, Va: American Association of Blood Banks Press, 1989, p 23.
20. Dutcher JP, Schiffer CA, Aisner J, Wiernik PH: Long-term followup of patients with leukemia receiving platelet transfusions: Identification of a large group of patients who do not become alloimmunized. Blood 1981;58:1007–1011.
21. Shulman NR, Marder VJ, Hiller MC, Collier EM: Platelet and leucocyte isoantigens and their antibodies: Serologic, physiologic, and clinical studies. Prog Hematol 1964;4:222–304.
22. Aster RH: Effect of anticoagulant and ABO incompatibility on recovery of transfused human platelets. Blood 1965;26:732–743.
23. Dunstan RA, Simpson MB, Knowles RW, Rosse WF: The origin of ABH antigens on human platelets. Blood 1985;65:615.
24. Ogasawara K, Ueki J, Takenaka M, Furihata K: Study on the expression of ABH antigens on platelets. Blood 1993;82:993–999.
25. Heal JM, Masel D, Rowe JM, Blumberg N: Circulating immune complexes involving the ABO system after platelet transfusion. Br J Haematol 1993;85:566.
26. Bishop JF, McGrath K, Wolf MM, et al: Clinical factors influencing the efficacy of pooled platelet transfusions. Blood 1988;71:383–387.
27. Klingemann H-G, Self S, Banaji M, et al: Refractoriness to random donor platelet transfusions in patients with aplastic anaemia: A multivariate analysis of data from 264 cases. Br J Haematol 1987;66:115–121.
28. Kickler TS, Braine HG, Ness PM: The predictive value of platelet crossmatching. Transfusion 1985;25:385–389.
29. Petz LD, Garratty G, Calhoun L, et al: Selecting donors of platelets for refractory patients on the basis of HLA antibody specificity. Transfusion 2000;40:1446–1456.
30. Rachel JM, Summers TC, Sinor LT, Plapp FV: Use of a solid phase red blood cell adherence method for pretransfusion platelet compatibility testing. Am J Clin Pathol 1989;90:63–68.
31. Kickler TS, Ness PM, Herman JH, et al: A randomized double-blinded study on the effectiveness of high dose gammaglobulin in ameliorating platelet transfusion refractoriness. Blood 1990;75:313–316.
32. Sarkodee-Adoo CB, Heyman MR: Alternative management strategies in alloimmunized thrombocytopenic patients. In Kickler TS, Herman JH (eds): Current Issues in Platelet Transfusion Therapy and Platelet Alloimmunity. Bethesda, MD: American Association of Blood Banks Press, 1999, pp 135–160.

33. Semple J, Freedman J: The basic immunology of platelet induced alloimmunization. In Kickler TS, Herman JH (eds): Current Issues in Platelet Transfusion Therapy and Platelet Alloimmunity. Bethesda, MD: American Association of Blood Banks Press, 1999, pp 77–101.

34. The Trial to Reduce Alloimmunization to Platelets (TRAP) Study Group: Leukocyte reduction and ultraviolet B irradiation of platelets to prevent alloimmunization and refractoriness to platelet transfusions. N Engl J Med 1997;337:1861–1869.

35. Kao KJ: A critical analysis of clinical trials to prevent platelet alloimmunization. In Kickler TS, Herman JH (eds): Current Issues in Platelet Transfusion Therapy and Platelet Alloimmunity. Bethesda, MD: American Association of Blood Banks Press, 1999, pp 103–134.

Chapter 32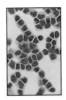

Autoimmune Hemolytic Anemias

Leslie E. Silberstein
Melody J. Cunningham

■ Spectrum of Autoimmune Hemolytic Syndromes

Autoimmune hemolytic anemias refer to a spectrum of disorders in which autoantibodies against antigens on the erythrocyte membrane cause shortened survival of native as well as transfused red blood cells (RBCs). Three categories of antierythrocyte autoantibodies exhibit distinctive serologic properties and result in characteristic clinical disorders (Table 32.1). Immunoglobulin (Ig) G warm autoantibodies attach to erythrocytes at 37°C, IgM cold autoantibodies clump RBCs at cold temperatures, and IgG Donath-Landsteiner antibodies bind to RBC membranes in the cold and cause hemolysis at 37°C; in this chapter, the associated clinical entities are referred to as *warm autoimmune hemolytic anemia* (AIHA), *cold agglutinin disease* (CAD), and *paroxysmal cold hemoglobinuria* (PCH), respectively. All of these antibodies are capable of simply attaching to the RBC membrane without having any pathologic effect or inducing

fulminant hemolysis.[1] The antibodies may be idiopathic or may develop secondary to another disease process or in response to exposure to a drug.

■ Historical Background

The first recognized form of hemolytic anemia was PCH, probably because its clinical manifestation, the passage of black urine after exposure to cold, is so striking. Reports of apparent cold-induced hematuria began to appear in medical literature in the mid-1800s. By 1884, the association of PCH with syphilis was noted. In 1904, Donath and Landsteiner determined that an autolysin fixed to the patient's RBCs in the cold and that a heat-labile serum factor lysed the erythrocytes at 37°C.

The first report of CAD appeared in 1918, but the fact that cold-agglutinating serum antibodies were found in healthy individuals obscured the significance of cold autolysins. In 1937, these cold-reactive antibodies were discovered to occur

Table 32.1 Characteristics of Autoimmune Hemolytic Anemia (AIHA)

Characteristic	Type of AIHA		
	Warm-Reactive	Cold Agglutinin Disease	Paroxysmal Cold Hemoglobinuria
Antibody isotype	IgG Rare IgA, IgM	IgM	IgG
Direct antiglobulin test (DAT) result	IgG Rare C3	C3	C3
Antigen specificity	Multiple, primarily Rh	I/i, Pr	P
Hemolysis	Primarily extravascular	Primarily extravascular	Intravascular
Common disease associations	B-cell neoplasia, lymphoproliferative, collagen-vascular	Viral, neoplastic	Tertiary syphilis, viral

Ig, Immunoglobulin.

Direct Antiglobulin Test (DAT)

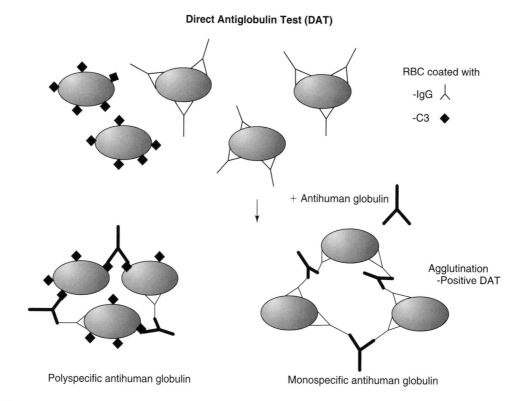

Figure 32.1 Direct antiglobulin test (DAT). C3, complement component 3; IgG, immunoglobulin G; RBC, red blood cell.

in much higher, thus pathologic, levels in affected patients. Dameshek and Schwartz established the first experimental model of immune hemolytic anemia, inducing hemolysis by injection of heterologous antierythrocyte antibodies into guinea pigs. Yet the idea of an "autoimmune" form of hemolytic anemia was resisted for several reasons, punctuated by the difficulty in making the diagnosis.

The antiglobulin test, designed to detect nonagglutinating anti-erythrocyte antibodies, was introduced into clinical medicine by Coombs and associates[2] in 1945. Within one year, this test was used to diagnose autoimmune hemolytic anemia.[3] In 1954, autoimmune hemolytic anemia in dogs was reported,[4] and in 1958, the first easily bred animal model of the disease, the NZB mouse, was described.[5] This last discovery was a turning point in the development of a scientific basis for the study of autoimmunization.

Warm Autoimmune Hemolytic Anemia

Epidemiology in Children and Adults

The incidence of AIHA is estimated to be approximately 1 in 100,000 in adults and less than 0.2 in 100,000 in children. The disorder is less common than immune thrombocytopenia.[6] In teenagers and adults, AIHA is more common in women than in men. In children, boys are somewhat more affected than girls. AIHA occurs at all ages but more commonly in midlife. In pediatric cases, the mortality is less than 10% and primarily occurs in adolescents with a chronic refractory course.[7]

About half of cases of AIHA are idiopathic. In children, AIHA in patients younger than 2 years and older than 12 years is more likely to have a chronic unremitting course.[8] Some

cases are induced by drugs, and others occur concomitantly with another autoimmune disease or malignancy. A substantial proportion of cases develop in patients with systemic lupus erythematosus (SLE), B-cell lymphomas, or chronic lymphocytic leukemia (CLL). A number of other diseases have also been complicated by AIHA, but only as unusual exceptions.[9] Treatment of the underlying process can often resolve the AIHA. In other instances, presumably by affecting T cells more than B cells, drugs induce a disturbance in immunoregulatory T cells and trigger the onset of hemolytic anemia.[10, 11]

Pathophysiology

Attachment of autoantibody to the surface of the RBC may lead to intravascular, extravascular, or no hemolysis. The pathologic effect is determined by the class or subclass as well as the avidity of the antibody attached and the extent to which complement is activated. IgA, IgM, IgG1, and IgG3 can all fix complement, although IgA is a rare cause of AIHA.[12] If complement is activated through the C5 to C9 membrane attack complex, intravascular hemolysis occurs.[13] The RBCs coated with simply antibody or complement component C3b are phagocytized by macrophages and destroyed extravascularly in the spleen or liver, respectively. Cells coated with IgG are destroyed primarily in the spleen, and those with IgM, in the liver.[14]

The interaction of macrophages with RBCs coated with IgG or C3b (or both) occurs through receptors specific for the Fc portion of IgG (especially IgG1 and IgG3) and for C3b.[15, 16] The presence on the erythrocyte membrane of both IgG and C3b accelerates immune clearance,[17–19] suggesting that the Fc and C3b macrophage receptors act synergistically.

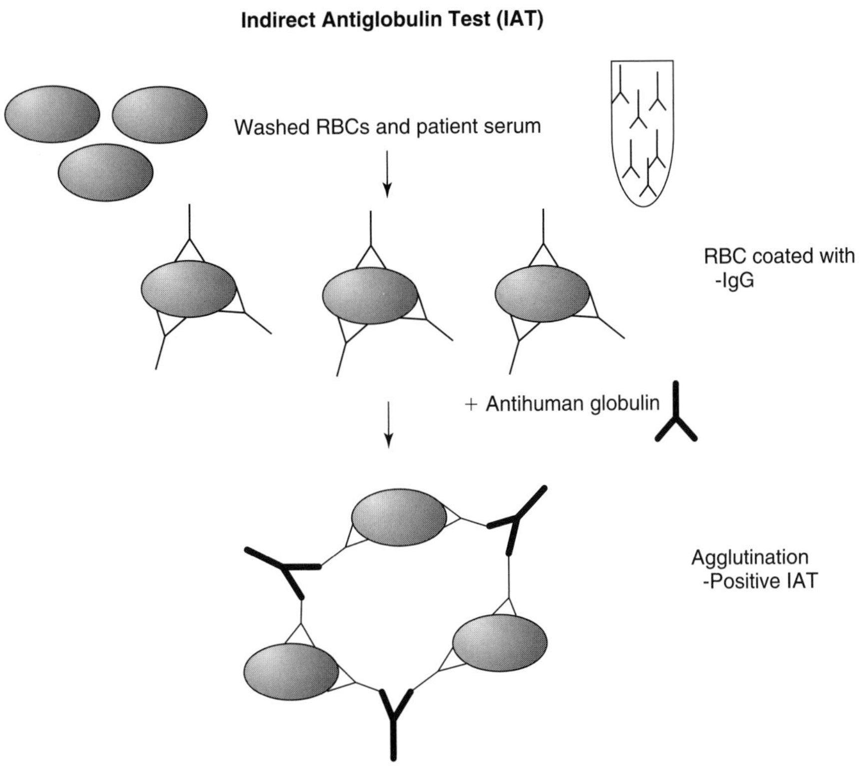

Indirect Antiglobulin Test (IAT)

Washed RBCs and patient serum

RBC coated with -IgG

+ Antihuman globulin

Agglutination -Positive IAT

Figure 32.2   Indirect antiglobulin test (IAT). IgG, immunoglobulin G; RBC, red blood cell.

Red Blood Cell Injury

The opsonized RBC may be phagocytosed and destroyed entirely by macrophages. Alternatively, proteolytic enzymes may digest part of the membrane surface, producing spherocytes. The spherocytes are less deformable and consequently are hemolyzed in the spleen. The predominant mechanism of destruction of erythrocytes coated with IgG with or without C3b occurs extravascularly in AIHA. The amount of immune clearance is also mediated by the entire reticuloendothelial system, and thus, viral or bacterial infections may exacerbate hemolysis.[20] In vitro assays of the ability of blood monocytes from patients with viral infections to phagocytose immunoglobulin-coated RBCs have shown marked deviations from normal.[21, 22]

Clinical Findings

The clinical findings in AIHA are variable. They are determined by the rate of hemolysis and by the abilities of the body to process breakdown products and of the bone marrow to mount a reticulocytosis. Some of the signs are associated with hyperdynamic circulation secondary to anemia and a concomitant decrease in oxygen-carrying capacity. They include hepatomegaly and, in more severe cases, pulmonary edema, lethargy, and obtundation. Splenomegaly can also occur from an increase in white pulp. Other signs and symptoms, such as jaundice, fever, and renal insufficiency, are caused by the breakdown products, and subsequent vasoconstriction. It has now been demonstrated that decreased renal perfusion, not injury due to free hemoglobin, is the mechanism leading to renal insufficiency.

AIHA may have a fulminant presentation, with rapid onset of profound anemia, or may develop gradually, with concomitant physiologic compensation. Occasionally, unsuspected AIHA is diagnosed through a positive direct antiglobulin test (DAT) result in an anemic patient who has been referred for transfusion. The presence of lymphadenopathy, fever, hypertension, renal failure, a rash, petechiae, or ecchymoses necessitates careful investigation for an underlying malignancy or collagen vascular disease.

Laboratory Evaluation

Direct and Indirect Antiglobulin Tests

It can be difficult to distinguish AIHA from other forms of hemolytic anemia on the basis of laboratory data. The positive result of a DAT, also known as the Coombs test, is considered pathognomonic of immune-mediated hemolysis. The test detects the presence of IgG or complement bound to the RBC membrane (Fig. 32.1). Severe disease usually produces a strong DAT response, but this finding does not always correlate with the degree of hemolysis.[1] The indirect antiglobulin test (IAT; indirect Coombs test), which detects the presence of antibodies in the patient's serum, usually has a positive result in AIHA (Fig. 32.2).

A positive DAT result is occasionally noted in a healthy person without anemia or evidence of hemolysis.[23] Conversely, patients with known AIHA may have a negative DAT result; this latter finding can be caused infrequently by laboratory error or by the presence of IgA, IgM, or low-affinity IgG autoantibodies.[24]

More commonly, the test is not sensitive enough to detect small numbers of erythrocyte-bound IgG molecules; this occurs most often in AIHA associated with lymphoma or CLL. If the DAT result is positive, specific reagents are required to identify the erythrocyte-bound protein.

In approximately 80% of patients with AIHA, the autoantibodies are present in serum as well as on RBC membranes.[25] IAT detects the presence of these serum antibodies in the patient's serum. These may be autoantibodies in a patient with AIHA or they may be alloantibodies induced by blood transfusion or maternal-fetal incompatibility. Alloantibodies, present only in the serum, have specificity for RBC antigens not present on the patient's erythrocytes. The DAT result is therefore negative in alloimmunization as long as the patient has not recently been transfused with RBCs that have the target antigen. In the setting of a recent transfusion, the alloantibodies may bind to recently transfused RBCs, yielding a positive DAT result.

Other Supportive Laboratory Investigations

It is very difficult to distinguish intravascular from extravascular hemolysis. The hemoglobin, hematocrit, lactate dehydrogenase (LDH), bilirubin, and haptoglobin values are similarly affected in both types of hemolysis. A significant urine hemosiderin level can indicate intravascular hemolysis yet often appears too late to be a helpful clinical tool. An unchanged hemoglobin or hematocrit value obtained within 4 hours after a transfusion of RBCs is an indicator of intravascular hemolysis. The intravascular destruction occurs so rapidly that no evidence of transfusion is reflected in the laboratory values. Intravascular hemolysis is important to recognize, because the patient may require greater supportive care to treat the anemia and consequent organ injury from intravascular hemolysis.

Like clinical symptoms, laboratory findings reflect the intensity of the hemolytic process as well as the abilities of the body to process the RBC breakdown products and of the bone marrow to respond to the anemia. In fulminant cases, with an RBC life span of less than 5 days, the anemia is severe and erythropoiesis increases eight- to ten-fold. As a result, the reticulocyte count rises, sometimes to levels greater than 40% of RBCs. If the regenerative capacity of the bone marrow lags only slightly behind the rate of RBC destruction, a mild anemia with an elevated reticulocyte count results. Between these extremes are many variations. Inspection of the blood smear in a typical case reveals polychromatophilia, spherocytes, a few fragmented RBCs, nucleated RBCs, and, occasionally, erythrophagocytosis. Examination of the bone marrow, which is rarely indicated, shows erythroid hyperplasia, often with megaloblastoid features. Occasionally, RBC autoantibodies or parvovirus B19[26] cause reticulocytopenia and dyserythropoiesis, thereby contributing to the severity of anemia.[27]

Patients with severe hemolytic anemia and markedly increased erythropoiesis occasionally experience folate deficiency and frank megaloblastosis. The growth of hematopoietic tissue in the bone marrow also leads to moderate increases in the white blood cell (WBC) and platelet counts. The absence of reticulocytosis does not exclude the diagnosis of AIHA but portends a serious prognosis.[28–31] In addition, reticulocytopenia may represent excessive apoptosis of erythroblasts.[28, 29, 31, 32] Presumably as a result of destruction of young erythrocytes by the autoantibody, the reticulocytopenia aggravates the severity of the anemia and increases the need for RBC transfusions.

Therapy

General Principles

The severity of AIHA may range from indolent to life-threatening. The impetus to initiate treatment, as well as the determination whether the treatment required is immediate transfusion or an attempt to modulate the immune system's production of autoantibody, must be based on a thorough appraisal of symptoms and the extent of the clinical compromise.

Rapidly developing anemia with a hematocrit less than 20% requires urgent management. In less aggressive forms of the disease, however, it may be prudent to allow physiologically compensated anemia rather than to institute treatment. The management of AIHA depends in part on whether the disease is primary or is secondary to such disorders as a B-cell malignancy or systemic lupus erythematosus.[33, 34] This, too, demands a careful assessment before any treatment begins. In some cases of AIHA secondary to lymphoma or CLL, the pathogenic autoantibody (usually monoclonal) is secreted by the neoplastic B cells. Combination chemotherapy or irradiation of the underlying malignancy often brings the hemolytic anemia under control.[35–37]

In other cases, however, the autoantibodies (usually polyclonal) do not originate from the B-cell neoplasm but probably result from abnormal immune regulation instigated by the neoplastic B cells. Treatment of the latter type of secondary AIHA with immunosuppressive agents may improve the anemia but may also trigger an exacerbation.[38] Multiple chemotherapeutic agents and immunosuppressive medications interfere with T-cell function and can thus trigger autoimmune processes in general and autoimmune hemolytic anemia specifically. Fludarabine and cladribine given as therapy for CLL have been demonstrated to precipitate autoimmune processes by interfering with the balance of T- and B-cell functions.[11]

The ultimate goal of therapy is control of the B-cell populations that secrete pathogenic autoantibodies. However, so little is known about such cells[39, 40] that the currently available therapy is, by default, nonspecific and often aimed at reducing RBC clearance by macrophages. The desired therapeutic effect is eradication of the abnormal hemolytic process, not reversal of the serologic abnormalities. Indeed, DAT results often remain positive in the presence of a hematologic response.

Transfusion

Some cases of AIHA may be life-threatening and may necessitate transfusion with RBCs (Box 32.1). It is important to recognize that, in the majority of cases, the patient receives crossmatch-incompatible blood.[41–44] The presence of autoantibodies complicates and prolongs the evaluation performed by the blood bank. In situations of fulminant hemolysis, transfusion of incompatible blood or transfusion performed on an emergency basis before completion of the evaluation may be imperative and lifesaving. Severe anemia may cause high-output cardiac failure and subsequent pulmonary edema, somnolence, and even obtundation, which require immediate intervention with RBC transfusion. The hemoglobin level at which these symptoms occur varies according to the rate of fall of the hemoglobin level, the capacity for cardiac compensation, and other underlying clinical features. Occasionally (1% to 2% of cases), relative specificity of the

Box 32.1   Transfusion Therapy and Autoimmune Hemolysis

There are times when a patient requires transfusion of incompatible RBCs or transfusion prior to completion of the blood bank evaluation. Autoimmune hemolytic anemia always complicates and prolongs the blood bank evaluation, which may take up to 24 to 48 hours to complete. It is imperative, however, that the patient receive RBCs expeditiously, *even though they are crossmatch incompatible,* if the hematocrit is not stabilized or cardiac or cerebral function is compromised. In these situations, the patient should be very closely monitored and should receive the smallest volume of blood necessary to alleviate the life-threatening symptoms.

autoantibodies can be demonstrated. This specificity usually occurs within the Rh system, and RBCs lacking the corresponding Rh antigen survive better in vivo than those that express the antigen.[45–48]

Specificities of IgG autoantibodies for multiple other blood groups have been described.[49] In addition, the blood bank must look for alloantibodies that may be masked by the autoantibodies. Alloantibodies, usually with specificity for the Rh or Kell blood group systems, occur in approximately 30% of patients with AIHA who have a history of blood group immunization by maternal-fetal incompatibility or previous transfusions.[50–52] The nonspecific serum autoantibodies that react with nearly all normal RBCs must be removed to ensure that no concomitant alloantibodies are present. An adsorption test is performed, using either the patient's cells or cells of known phenotype to absorb the autoantibodies from the serum—a process known as autologous adsorption or heterologous adsorption, respectively.

These tests are not performed by all laboratories and should not be required before transfusion of a patient in need. However, standard antibody detection and identification tests with both the patient's serum and an eluate prepared from the patient's cells should be performed whenever possible. Titration of the eluate and the serum against RBCs of various Rh phenotypes can indicate an autoantibody specificity (or preference) within the Rh system. Any such specificity should be respected in the selection of donor units.[53, 54]

RBC substitutes have been transfused in a few situations of severe hemolytic anemia and have demonstrated benefit to the patients.[55, 56] These substitutes require further investigation to determine their efficacy and safety. They could potentially be of benefit in the short-term emergent situation when the presence of underlying alloantibodies cannot be ruled out or when the hemolysis is so brisk that transfusion of least incompatible cells does not result in any increase in hemoglobin and, thus, in oxygen-carrying capacity.[57]

Corticosteroids

Corticosteroids are the first line of treatment for most patients with symptomatic, unstable AIHA, either idiopathic or secondary. The clinical response to prednisone results primarily from its ability to disable macrophages from clearing IgG- or C3b-coated erythrocytes. Corticosteroids interfere with both the expression and function of macrophage Fc receptors. This interference is probably the earliest, and perhaps even the primary, mechanism in the ability of steroids to diminish the immune clearance of blood cells.[58–61] Prednisone can also reduce autoantibody production, but only after several weeks of therapy.

The side effects of corticosteroids often preclude the long-term use of high-dose therapy. The cushingoid features that develop can lead to noncompliance, especially in adolescents. The associated osteoporosis and immunosuppression as well as the risk of gastric bleeding may warrant discontinuation of therapy.

Intravenous Immune Globulin

Intravenous immune globulin (IVIG) has been found effective in management of selected cases of AIHA. The soluble IgG in the material may lengthen the life span of IgG-coated RBCs by saturating Fc receptors on macrophages. In a study of patients who had AIHA associated with lymphoproliferative disorders, a long-term benefit was observed with a maintenance dose schedule of intravenous IgG every 21 days. A decrease in antiglobulin titer was found in these patients, suggesting a mechanism other than blockade of Fc receptors by intravenous IgG.[62]

The mechanism of action of IVIG has been further elucidated by Samuelsson and colleagues.[63] They investigated the mechanism of protection in a murine model of immune thrombocytopenia that may have relevance to mechanism of action in other autoimmune diseases. Their model demonstrated that the inhibitory Fc receptor FcγRIIB was necessary for IVIG to confer protection against platelet destruction.[63] This finding suggests that modulation of inhibitory signals in macrophages could possibly be involved in autoimmunity and could be investigated as therapeutic targets in other autoimmune diseases, such as AIHA.

Splenectomy

Splenectomy has been used as therapy for AIHA for many years.[64] Indications for splenectomy include failure to respond to prednisone, need for prednisone dosages higher than 10 to 20 mg/day, and intractable corticosteroid side effects. The procedure can be highly effective, presumably through removal of the major reticuloendothelial site of RBC destruction; an animal model demonstrated that IgG-coated RBCs are removed almost exclusively by the spleen.[58] In addition, the procedure eliminates many phagocytosing macrophages and autoantibody-producing B cells.

In most young adults with chronic AIHA, the question of splenectomy arises almost inevitably. However, in an elderly patient with a stable but incomplete remission, maintenance therapy with prednisone at a dose of 10 mg/day for an indefinite period may be the better alternative. There is a slight risk that overwhelming sepsis by encapsulated organisms may develop immediately and up to 25 years after splenectomy.[65] The risk is higher in children, especially those younger than 6 years, so a conservative approach to splenectomy is prudent in this age group. The risk of overwhelming sepsis is lessened by immunization with pneumococcal and meningococcal vaccines, which are optimally administered at least 2 weeks preoperatively, and by the prompt use of antibiotics for febrile illness.[66] The *Haemophilus influenzae* series of vaccines should also be completed in children prior to splenectomy.

The response to splenectomy does not correlate with the age of the patient, the presence or absence of an underlying B-cell disorder, the strength of the antiglobulin test result, a prior response to prednisone, or the pattern of sequestration of chromium 51 (^{51}Cr)–labeled RBCs. Between 50% and 60% of patients with classic AIHA have a good to excellent initial response to splenectomy. They will need less than 15 mg/day of prednisone to maintain an adequate level of hemoglobin.[67] Information regarding the clinical implications of an accessory spleen in AIHA is meager. Faced with such a rare finding in a patient with relapse, many hematologists would recommend its removal. The role of splenectomy in patients with mixed IgG, IgM, or mixed cold- and warm-reactive IgG antibodies is unclear.

Immunosuppressive Therapy

Most experience with immunosuppressive drugs in the treatment of autoimmune hemolytic anemia has been with alkylating agents (cyclophosphamide and chlorambucil) and thiopurines (azathioprine and 6-mercaptopurine).[68] The basis for the clinical use of these drugs is their inhibitory effect on the immune system, possibly affecting both B cells and T cells.[69, 70]

Cyclophosphamide and azathioprine, like prednisone, can induce numerous side effects. The early side effects include bone marrow suppression and impairment of the immune response (particularly T-cell–mediated immunity) that occur concomitantly with therapy. After sustained administration, cyclophosphamide may damage ovarian function, inhibit spermatogenesis,[71–74] and cause bladder fibrosis.[75] Acute myeloid leukemia can develop years after administration of this drug.[69] By contrast, the prolonged use of azathioprine has not been associated with a statistically significant increase in malignant diseases. All of these considerations mandate careful monitoring of any patient treated with either cyclophosphamide or azathioprine.

Cyclosporine, a powerful T-cell modulator, has been used alone and in combination to elicit successful and sometimes durable remission in patients with AIHA and Evans syndrome.[76] Cyclosporine and other immunosuppressive agents are discussed here and have been reported in the literature. However, their long-term use is not recommended, because the benefits do not usually offset the side effects inherent in the prolonged use of these agents.

Rituximab Therapy

Rituximab, a chimeric anti–CD20 monoclonal antibody with a well-established, favorable safety profile, has exciting possibilities for widespread clinical application in autoimmune disease in general and AIHA specifically.[77, 78] Rituximab induces cell death through complement-dependent lysis, antibody-dependent cellular toxicity, and cellular apoptosis.[77] Although plasma cells, fully differentiated B cells, are CD20 negative, the response rates of patients with AIHA and thrombocytopenia suggest that earlier CD20-positive B cells are producing antibody or that other as yet not clearly delineated effects of rituximab are effecting the disease remission. Reports that rituximab induces remission in patients with ITP within 1 week of first infusion suggest that the mechanism of action may involve more than elimination of B cells.[78]

The efficacy and safety of rituximab have been demonstrated in multiple large trials in adult patients with non-Hodgkin lymphomas.[78] Infusion-related side effects, including fever, respiratory distress, and hypotension, are reported to occur in a small population of lymphoma patients.[79, 80] No side effects have precluded completion of planned therapy in patients with autoimmune disease.[81] The occurrence and severity of side effects seem to be related to B-cell level and, thus, tumor burden.[80] It is anticipated and has been demonstrated that the side-effect profile will be even more favorable in patients with autoimmune disease who have a lower level of B cells.[82]

No large trials have studied the efficacy and safety of rituximab in patients with autoimmune disease. The results, however, of multiple case reports, case series, pilot studies, and small therapeutic trials indicate that rituximab warrants further study in patients with autoimmune disease. The literature reveals successful use of anti-CD20 treatment in multiple autoimmune diseases.[6, 7, 83–89]

Response to rituximab has been reported in a patient with Evans syndrome secondary to interleukin-2 (IL-2) therapy and in another with Evans syndrome secondary to CLL.[83, 90] Treatment with rituximab was initiated after failure of multiple modalities, including splenectomy, high-dose corticosteroids, splenectomy, and chemotherapy (with alkylating agents). In both cases, the patients demonstrated complete remission. Six patients with AIHA, one of whom had undergone bone marrow transplantation, were treated with anti-CD20 monoclonal antibody and remained in complete remission 15 to 22 months after the start of the rituximab infusions.[84, 91] They have either stopped corticosteroid therapy or are taking markedly reduced doses.

Plasma Exchange

Because a single-volume plasma exchange replaces only about 60% of the patient's plasma volume, its therapeutic advantage lies in the removal of plasma antibodies to IgG, IgM, or both, which mediate the hemolysis. Unfortunately, continuous antibody production and the large extravascular distribution of IgG limit the long-term efficacy of plasma exchange in IgG-mediated autoimmune hemolytic anemia. On cessation of therapy, the rate of return to pretreatment levels of autoantibody depends on the rate of autoantibody production.[92] However, there are some reports that this modality is efficacious in IgG-mediated disease.[93] Occasional dramatic responses have been reported in patients being prepared for surgery or when plasma exchange was used as a temporizing measure after initiation of immunosuppressive therapy.[93, 94] This therapy is reserved for patients in critical condition whose AIHA is unresponsive to transfusion because of rapid destruction and clearance of the RBCs.

■ Cold Agglutinin Disease

Cold agglutinin disease refers to a group of disorders caused by anti-erythrocyte autoantibodies (e.g., cold agglutinins) that preferentially bind RBCs at cold temperatures (4° to 18°C) and may or may not induce hemolysis. Virtually all sera from healthy individuals contain low-titer cold agglutinins, which are regarded as benign or harmless RBC autoantibodies and are considered polyclonal. Similarly, cold agglutinins that arise after certain infections are also polyclonal and usually benign; in rare cases, a transient form of cold agglutinin disease ensues. By contrast, monoclonal cold agglutinins are generally pathogenic and are derived from clonal B-cell expansions (as in idiopathic or chronic cold agglutinin disease), which may be a prelude to frank lymphoma.

Chronic Cold Agglutinin Disease

The most common type of cold agglutinin disease, a chronic form characterized principally by a stable anemia of moderate severity and attacks of acrocyanosis precipitated by exposure to cold, constitutes about one third of all cases of immuno-hemolytic anemia. Cold agglutinins cause the cardinal abnormalities of the disease. The acrocyanosis stems from intra-arteriolar agglutination of erythrocytes in the relatively cool tips of the fingers, feet, ear lobes, and nose. The occurrence of this hemolytic anemia depends on the capacity of the cold agglutinins to initiate activation of the complement cascade on the surface of the RBC. Most patients with chronic cold agglutinin disease are in the fifth to eighth decade of life and have a B-cell neoplasm or lymphoma, Waldenström macroglobulinemia, or CLL. The cold agglutinin in cases secondary to such diseases is monoclonal, almost always IgMκ, and may show up as a monoclonal band in the γ region of the serum protein electrophoretic pattern. In the absence of a B-cell neoplasm, the spleen and lymph nodes are rarely enlarged; therefore, the finding of splenic and lymph node enlargement warrants a search for the neoplasm.

Transient Cold Agglutinin Disease

A second type of cold agglutinin disease, usually acute and always self-limited, occurs as a rare complication of several infectious diseases, most notably *Mycoplasma pneumoniae* infection and infectious mononucleosis. Patients with this form of cold agglutinin disease are therefore much younger than those with chronic cold agglutinin disease. The onset is abrupt, occurring as the infection wanes, and the anemia can be severe. Cold agglutinin titers are moderately elevated, and the cold agglutinins are polyclonal. Often these polyclonal cold agglutinins coincide with high-titer warm-reactive IgG RBC autoantibodies.

Antigenic Targets of Cold Agglutinin Disease

The antigenic specificity of cold agglutinins is usually identified from their degree of reactivity with RBCs from adults (blood group I) and from cord blood (blood group i). The cold-reactive autoantibody produced after some cases of *M. pneumoniae* infection has anti-I specificity,[102] whereas the antibody in infectious mononucleosis frequently, but not always, has anti-i specificity.[103, 104] Additional specificities have been identified by tests with rare adult RBCs that lack the I antigen or with enzyme-treated erythrocytes. Rarely, cold agglutinins are specific for the A blood group antigen.[44]

Laboratory Evaluation

The usual laboratory findings in hemolytic anemia (i.e., anemia, reticulocytosis, polychromatophilia, spherocytosis, erythroid hyperplasia in the bone marrow, and elevations in serum bilirubin and lactate dehydrogenase levels) are generally not striking in chronic cold agglutinin disease. Hemagglutination may be visible to the unaided eye in blood drawn from a patient with cold agglutinin disease and can interfere with automated blood counts. The anemia is often mild and stable, because the C3b inactivator in serum limits the extent of cold agglutinin–induced complement activation

on the erythrocyte membrane. Exposure to cold may greatly augment the binding of cold agglutinins, however, exceeding the restraints of the inactivator system. This occurrence can lead to a sudden drop in hematocrit value, with complement-mediated intravascular hemolysis and renal failure.

In a distinctive subset of patients with aggressive cold agglutinin disease, the cold agglutinin titer is relatively low but the autoantibody has a high thermal amplitude. Recognition that a patient has this variant of cold agglutinin disease is important because it may respond to prednisone,[61] whereas high-titer cold agglutinin disease usually does not.

In typical cases of chronic cold agglutinin disease, the cold agglutinin titer is very high ($>1{:}10^5$, and occasionally $>1{:}10^6$). The antibodies are most reactive in the cold, and hemagglutination disappears as the temperature rises toward 37°C. In some cases, however, the antibody is reactive at relatively high temperatures, and occasionally even at 37°C. The reactivity of the cold agglutinin at high temperatures (i.e., its thermal amplitudes), not the titer of the antibody, most accurately predicts the severity of the disease. The DAT result is positive because of erythrocyte-bound C3d (see later discussion of pathophysiology), but results of tests with anti-IgG reagents are negative. The result of the IAT, which is conducted at 37°C, is negative. In addition to monoclonal IgM cold agglutinins, IgG-IgM mixed cold agglutinins have been reported.[95–97] Besides the usual high titers of IgM cold agglutinins, some patients with cold agglutinin disease have low titers of IgG and IgA cold agglutinins.

Cold agglutinins are not cryoglobulins. The latter are most often monoclonal IgM immunoglobulins that, in the cold, either self-associate and precipitate from solution (type I cryoglobulinemia) or precipitate as complexes with poly-clonal IgG molecules (type II cryoglobulinemia, often due to a monoclonal IgM rheumatoid factor). Type III cryoglob-ulins consist of a mixture of polyclonal IgM and polyclonal IgG immunoglobulins. The clinical manifestations of the cryoglobulinemic syndromes are highly variable: Type I and type II cryoglobulinemias occur in B-cell neoplasms (Waldenström macroglobulinemia, multiple myeloma, lymphoma, and CLL); type II and type III cryoglobulinemias can produce a picture of immune complex-mediated vasculitis, with vascular purpura, arthritis, and nephritis as the dominant complications. In occasional patients, the cryoglobulin can also be a cold agglutinin.[98–101]

Pathophysiology

The pathogenic IgM autoantibody in cold agglutinin disease is highly efficient in activating the classic complement pathway on the erythrocyte membrane.[34, 105] However, the thermal dependency of the antibody constrains its pathogenic effects. The autoantibody rapidly elutes off RBCs at 37°C, the temperature of the visceral circulation, but in the cool peripheral circulation of the hands and feet, the cold agglutinin remains on the erythrocyte membrane for at least a few seconds. That amount of time is sufficient to activate the complement cascade to the stage of C3b, which adheres to the RBC after it reenters the central circulation. In the hepatic circulation, C3b-positive RBCs encounter macrophages with receptors specific for C3b;[17, 106, 107] however, C3b sensitization is only a weak signal for the activation of phagocytosis—the hepatic clearance of C3b-coated RBCs requires 500 to 800 C3b molecules per RBC. As a result, many C3b$^+$ RBCs escape unharmed into the systemic circulation, where they come under the influence of the regulatory proteins of the complement system. The C3b inactivator system degrades C3b into C3dg, C3d, or both. The result is a cohort of erythrocytes coated with C3d but not with the IgM autoantibody.[108] Because macrophages bind to C3d with even lower avidity than to C3b, the C3d$^+$ erythrocytes tend to have near-normal survival in vivo despite a heavy coating with that degradation product of C3.[109, 110] It is important to recognize that if transfusion is necessary, the transfused cells will not have the protection conferred by C3d and therefore may be rapidly lysed.[110]

These limits on the pathogenicity of cold agglutinins account for the subdued hematologic picture in most patients with cold agglutinin disease. If, however, the regulatory C3b inactivator proteins are impaired, limiting cleavage of RBC-bound C3b, or if the production of IgM autoantibodies with a high thermal amplitude is impaired, permitting completion of the complement cascade in the visceral circulation, severe extravascular hemolysis can occur. Several patients with high titers of IgA cold agglutinins have been reported. Such cases are not associated with cold agglutinin disease, which may relate to the lack of complement activation by IgA antibodies.[111–119]

Therapy

Chronic Cold Agglutinin Disease

Therapy for the cold agglutinin syndromes depends on the gravity of the symptoms, the serologic characteristics of the autoantibody, and any underlying disease. In the idiopathic, or primary, form of chronic cold agglutinin disease, prolonged survival and spontaneous remissions and exacerbations are not unusual. The anemia is generally mild, and the simple measure of avoiding exposure to cold temperatures can avoid exacerbations, especially if the cold agglutinin responsible has a low thermal amplitude. Prednisone has been beneficial in rare cases in which there are relatively low titers of cold agglutinins of a high thermal amplitude or an IgG cold-reactive antibody is produced. However, prednisone is not useful therapy in most patients with primary IgM-induced cold agglutinin disease, and its administration should not be undertaken lightly, given the chronicity of the disease.[120, 121] Plasma exchange may help as a temporary measure in acute situations.[94] Splenectomy is usually ineffective because the liver is the dominant site of sequestration of RBCs heavily sensitized with C3b. However, rare cases in patients with enlarged spleens have responded to splenectomy; in some of these patients, a localized splenic lymphoma was found, whereas in others, only lymphoid hyperplasia was evident.

It is essential to seek evidence of a B-cell neoplasm before therapy for chronic cold agglutinin disease is initiated. Oral alkylating agents (chlorambucil or cyclophosphamide) help many patients with the secondary form of cold agglutinin disease because of their effect on the B-cell neoplasm, but only occasionally do they benefit patients with the primary form of the disease.[122, 123] When cold agglutinin disease is part of an established B-cell malignancy, the severity of hemolysis often waxes and wanes parallel with the activity of the neoplasm.

Patients with IgM-mediated hemolysis can be dramatically helped with plasma exchange. Because of its large size, the antibody is located primarily in the intravascular space and is efficiently removed by plasma exchange. Some patients with Waldenström macroglobulinemia are maintained over the long term with this therapy.

Transient Cold Agglutinin Disease

Transient cold agglutinin disease is a rare form that is always self-limited. Supportive measures, including transfusions and avoidance of cold, may suffice to tide the patient over the episode of hemolysis. Corticosteroids are usually not helpful, and splenectomy is almost never indicated.

■ Paroxysmal Cold Hemoglobinuria

Clinical Features

Paroxysmal cold hemoglobinuria (PCH) was historically associated with tertiary syphilis, which is rarely seen today. PCH is now more commonly seen primarily in children after a viral or, much less commonly, bacterial illness.[124] Most commonly, the viral etiology is not known but is associated with an upper respiratory tract infection. However, case reports in both adults and children have reported an association of PCH with varicella.

Although the Donath-Landsteiner antibody often occurs in tertiary or congenital syphilis, it generally does not cause hemolytic disease in this situation. On exposure to cold, an occasional patient experiences paroxysms of hemoglobinuria and constitutional symptoms (fever, back pain, leg pain, abdominal cramps, and rigors) followed by hemoglobinuria. In contrast, the postviral form of PCH[125–127] is characterized by constitutional symptoms with fulminant intravascular hemolysis and its associated signs of hemoglobinemia, hemoglobinuria, jaundice, severe anemia, and, sometimes, renal failure. The disease is self-limited, usually lasting 2 to 3 weeks, although it can be life-threatening because of the severity of the hemolysis and consequent anemia.

Laboratory Evaluation

The IgG antibody responsible for paroxysmal cold hemoglobinuria is found in the patient's serum through incubation of normal erythrocytes, fresh normal serum as a source of complement, and the patient's serum, first at 4°C and then at 37°C, with appropriate controls. The Donath-Landsteiner antibody fixes the first two components of complement in the cold and completes the cascade upon warming to 37°C.[128] The DAT result is almost always negative, but occasionally, weak reactions for erythrocyte-bound complement are manifested. The IAT result is negative. Most Donath-Landsteiner antibodies have specificity for the P blood group system,[129, 130] but other specificities have been described.[131–133] The diagnosis depends on recognition of the clinical picture, because tests for the Donath-Landsteiner antibody are not routinely performed.

Therapy

No specific treatment for PCH has been found. Unlike the effectiveness of steroids in most IgG-mediated autoimmune diseases, prednisone is not useful for PCH. The best approach consists of supportive care, transfusions to alleviate symptoms, and avoidance of cold temperatures. The patient should be kept in a warm room, and transfusions should be given through a blood warmer.

■ Drug-Associated Immune Hemolytic Anemia

Drug-associated immune hemolytic anemia can be either induced by or dependent on a drug. Four distinct mechanisms are associated with the disorder. The first involves any drug that can bind to the RBC membrane. The patient then makes antibodies against the drug (e.g., penicillin), which combine with the erythrocyte-bound drug, opsonizing and preparing the RBC for destruction. Discontinuation of the drug brings the hemolytic anemia to a rapid halt, because the antibodies have no specificity for antigens on the RBC membrane. Clues to the diagnosis are the appropriate clinical setting, a positive DAT result, a negative IAT result, and failure of antibodies eluted from the patient's RBCs to bind to normal erythrocytes. The diagnosis is established when both the eluate and the patient's serum, contain antibodies directed against the drug-coated cells. In the case of penicillin,[134] hemolytic anemia occurs only when large amounts are administered; in patients treated with lower doses, a positive DAT result without hemolytic anemia is not unusual, because the production of low-avidity IgG antipenicillin antibodies is a common event.

The second mechanism involves immune complexes. The offending drug, or drug metabolite, binds to a plasma protein, forming an immunogenic conjugate. If the patient develops an antibody to the conjugate, it is usually IgM. This antibody then binds to the immunogenic conjugate, forming an immune complex that adheres to RBCs. The resulting clinical picture consists of intravascular hemolysis and concomitant hemoglobinemia, hemoglobinuria, and even renal failure through efficient activation of complement on the erythrocyte membrane. This chain of events accounts for most reported examples of drug-induced immune hemolytic anemia. Reports concerning the nonsteroidal drug diclofenac have shown that autoimmune hemolytic anemia is induced by sensitization to the glucuronide conjugate of the drug.[135]

Serologic findings in erythrocyte-bound immune complexes are similar to those of the first mechanism, except that the DAT reveals only complement bound to the RBC; the IgM antibody is presumed to be no longer present after complement activation. The patient's serum reacts with RBCs (lacking antidrug antibody) in the presence of the offending drug, and the eluate from the patient's RBCs generally does not react with normal erythrocytes.

The third mechanism involves in vivo sensitization to drugs through the formation of immunogenic drug-RBC complexes. In these cases, the specificity of the drug-induced antibodies is contributed to not only by the drug (or its metabolites) but also by defined RBC antigens, particularly those of the Rhesus and I/i systems.[136]

The first mechanism of drug-associated immune hemolytic anemia involves the induction of authentic autoantibodies against RBCs by a drug; methyldopa is the classic example.[137] In as many as 20% of patients treated with methyldopa, the DAT result turns positive, but few demonstrate hemolytic anemia. The antiglobulin test result may take several months to a year or more after the start of drug therapy to become positive. In patients with hemolytic anemia, discontinuation of the drug results in only gradual cessation of the hemolytic anemia and disappearance of the autoantibody, because the drug itself is not required for the hemolytic process, only for the initiation of antibody production. Curiously, the autoantibody is usually specific for antigens of the Rh system. The serologic findings are indistinguishable from those in primary autoimmune hemolytic anemia; they consist of a positive DAT result, usually a positive IAT result, and an eluate that reacts with normal erythrocytes. Patients taking methyldopa often have other antibodies in addition to the RBC autoantibodies. The mechanism by which methyldopa induces autoantibodies is unknown but may involve effects on immunoregulatory T cells.

Drug-induced immune hemolytic anemia was commonly seen when penicillin was administered in large doses (i.e., >20 million U/day) and when methyldopa was widely used in the treatment of hypertension.[138, 139] However, the disease is unusual in present-day clinical practice.[140] Numerous drugs can induce hemolytic anemia.

■ Animal Models of Autoimmune Hemolytic Anemia

Insights into Pathogenesis and Therapeutic Targets

NZB Mice

The inbred NZB mouse is genetically programmed to develop autoimmune hemolytic anemia at around the age of 6 to 8 months (the life span of a normal mouse is about 2 years). Anti-erythrocyte autoantibodies begin to appear at around the age of 3 months, and by 9 months, the DAT result is positive in 60% to 80% of animals. Typical signs of hemolytic anemia develop—reticulocytosis, spherocytosis, a shortened RBC survival time, and splenomegaly.[141]

Okamoto and colleagues[142] developed a transgenic murine model of autoimmune hemolytic anemia. The symptoms in this model range from unaffected to severe anemia. The B-1 subpopulation has been demonstrated to mediate the autoimmune hemolytic anemia.[143] They are activated in both T cell–dependent and T cell–independent ways.[144] These cells are unique from B-2, the more prevalent B cells, in several ways. B-1 cells preferentially locate in the peritoneal and pleural cavities, produce 50% of the natural serum IgM, and escape clonal deletion in these immunoprivileged sites. IL-10 influences T cell–dependent proliferation of B-1 cells, and continuous administration of anti–IL-10 monoclonal antibody depletes B-1 but not B-2 cells in murine models. The influence of this T_h2 cytokine on the behavior of the B-1 cells in vivo[145] suggests possible avenues for treatments.

Origins of Anti-erythrocyte Autoantibodies

The vast improvement in our understanding of what prevents autoimmunization has not yet informed us of the mechanism that causes autoimmunization. Virtually nothing is known of the origins of warm-reactive IgG anti-erythrocyte autoantibodies, despite the availability of a thoroughly investigated, spontaneous animal model of the disease (the NZB mouse) and stocks of pathogenic autoantibodies, which are readily obtained from patients with the disease. A major impediment to advances in our understanding of how autoimmune hemolytic anemia originates is that the autoantigens are for the most part unknown. Even in those cases in which blood group specificity of the autoantibodies has been identified, the relevant structures have not been elucidated. Leddy and associates[146] have succeeded in identifying four proteins on the RBC membrane that bind to anti-erythrocyte autoantibodies; they are the band 3 anion transporter, glycophorin A, and two polypeptides, probably related to the Rh family of antigens. Various combinations of those four autoantibody specificities were found in a group of 20 patients with autoimmune hemolytic anemia.

The association of autoimmune hemolytic anemia with systemic lupus erythematosus and with immune thrombocytopenia (Evans syndrome), the induction of the disease by drugs that seem to perturb immune regulation, and the graft-versus-host model of autoimmune hemolytic anemia all suggest that, at least in some cases, there is antigen-independent activation of clones of B cells with the capacity to produce IgG anti-RBC autoantibodies. Such polyclonal B-cell activation may account for the production of anti-erythrocyte autoantibodies in patients with acquired immunodeficiency syndrome (AIDS).[102, 147, 102] Hypergamma-globulinemia and other signs of nonspecific activation of B cells are prominent in human immunodeficiency virus infection.[148]

The immunologic basis of autoimmune hemolytic anemia in patients with CLL or a B-cell lymphoma is equally obscure.[149] In CLL, the autoantibodies are IgG and often polyclonal,[150] whereas the malignant CD5[+] B cells of that disease generally produce only IgM antibodies that are monoclonal. It is therefore likely that B cells other than those constituting the leukemia produce the autoantibodies. The large mass of CD5[+] B cells in CLL might induce non-neoplastic CD5-negative B cells to produce IgG autoantibodies, perhaps through a disturbance of immunoregulatory idiotypic networks. The demonstration of the simultaneous presence of autoantibodies and anti-idiotypic antibodies on RBCs in autoimmune hemolytic anemia[151] suggests that such networks may indeed have a role in the disease.

In contrast to the antigens that incite warm-reactive autoantibodies, the structures of the autoantigens of cold agglutinin disease, the I/i system, are known;[152] this knowledge has clarified our thinking about the immunology of this group of disorders. There is little reason to doubt that the very high levels of monoclonal cold agglutinins found in some patients with B-cell neoplasms are produced by the malignant cells. The demonstration that an idiotypic marker on monoclonal cold agglutinins could be detected not only on the patients' neoplastic B cells but also on 3% to 10% of normal B cells[153] supports the view that these autoantibodies are part of the normal immune repertoire; malignant transformation of a cold agglutinin–producing B cell results in a lymphoma complicated by chronic cold agglutinin disease.

The basis of the association of paroxysmal cold hemoglobinuria with syphilis may be antigenic mimicry, in which structural similarities between a microbial antigen and a self-antigen trigger an autoantibody response. In the case of paroxysmal cold hemoglobinuria, the infecting organism, *Treponema pallidum*, should possess two antigenic determinants (epitopes), one recognized by T cells (the foreign epitope) and the other by self-reactive B cells (the mimicking epitope). Donath-Landsteiner antibodies would be produced only by syphilitic patients whose class II major histocompatibility complex (MHC) glycoproteins could present the foreign epitope in an immunogenic form to T cells. A similar mechanism could apply to postinfectious acute cold agglutinin disease, in which a cross-reaction involving antigenic determinants of *M. pneumoniae* and the I blood group substance has been incriminated.[154]

Structural analyses of monoclonal anti-I and anti-i autoantibodies from patients with B-cell neoplasms are beginning to yield important clues about the origins of chronic cold agglutinin disease. A striking observation is the repetitive use of the same immunoglobulin V_H gene, V_{H4-34}, in monoclonal IgM cold agglutinins, regardless of the anti-I or anti-i specificity of the autoantibody.[155, 156] In each case, the V_{H4-34} heavy chain gene had a different CDR3 (complementarity-determining region 3); the light chains of cold agglutinins with anti-I or anti-i specificity differed as well. The V_{H4-34} genes of these cold agglutinins contained few or no somatic mutations of the type that would lead to amino acid substitutions (replacement mutations). This finding, together with the variations in their CDR3s and in the light chains, implies that the V_{H4-34} germline gene segment itself encodes a binding site for the I and i antigens. In contrast to the heavy chain gene, the light chain genes of the cold agglutinins do contain replacement mutations, especially in their hypervariable regions.[156]

It appears from these results that (1) the germline V_{H4-34} heavy chain encodes the dominant specificity of monoclonal cold agglutinins, (2) the somatic mutations of the light chain genes of the cold agglutinins are the result of an immune response, and (3) the V_H CDR3 and the light chain confer fine specificity (e.g., for I or i) on the cold agglutinin and influence its affinity. These data make a convincing case that monoclonal cold agglutinins arise as the result of an immune response, perhaps an autoimmune response to an autoantigen on erythrocytes. The results of these molecular studies of cold agglutinins complement other evidence favoring a role for antigen-mediated clonal selection in some types of B-cell neoplasms.

In contrast to monoclonal cold agglutinins associated with chronic cold agglutinin disease, the naturally occurring IgM cold agglutinins that are present in low titers in normal serum are not restricted to the V_{H4-34} gene segment. They are associated with different genes of the V_{H3} family as well as the V_{H4-34} gene.[156] It therefore appears that B-cell neoplasia is an important, but not exclusive, element in the association between V_{H4-34} and cold agglutinins. The correlation with lymphomas has additional interest, because V_{H4-34} has been independently linked to B-cell lymphomas that do not secrete cold agglutinins.[157]

◾ Perspective

In previous years, there have been many debates concerning the factors that contribute to the severity of autoimmune hemolytic anemia. Previous studies have focused to a large extent on the humoral aspect of the autoimmune response. The antibodies were easily available from peripheral blood allowing for many serologic investigations. However, none of the serologic parameters by itself—the quantity of serum RBC autoantibodies, titer, thermal amplitude, or allotype—has proved useful in predicting severity of the disease in patients. This fact is perhaps not surprising, because RBC clearance in both cold and warm autoimmune hemolytic anemias occurs predominantly extravascularly through the actions of macrophages rather than intravascularly through antibody-mediated complement lysis. Also, membrane receptors on macrophages, such as FcγIIRB and SIRPα (signal regulation protein-α), have been identified that have the ability to modulate RBC clearance and, thus, severity of hemolysis. Therefore, it is possible that the activity of these receptors may vary among patients as well, contributing to the severity of disease expression. Moreover, these macrophage receptors may prove to be viable targets for the development of more specific immunotherapy than the methods currently used (i.e., corticosteroid therapy and IVIG). Another potentially exciting therapeutic approach is targeting of the humoral immune response, either through direct targeting of the B cells, such as with anti-CD20 antibody, or through interference with the interactions between B and T lymphocytes, such as with co-stimulatory molecule blockade (e.g., anti-CD40 antibody).

REFERENCES

1. Sloan SR, Silberstein L: Transfusion in the face of autoantibodies. In Reid ME, Nance SJ (eds): Red Cell Transfusion: A Practical Guide. Totowa, NJ, Humana Press, 1998.
2. Coombs RRA, Mourant AE, Race RR: A new test for the detection of weak and incomplete Rh agglutinins. Br J Exp Pathol 1945;26:255.
3. Boorman KE, Dodd BE, Loutit JF: Hemolytic icterus (acholuric jaundice): Congenital and acquired. Lancet 1946;1:812.
4. Lewis RM, Henry WB, Thornton GW, et al: A syndrome of autoimmune hemolytic anemia and thrombocytopenia in dogs. Proc J Am Vet Med Assoc 1963;1:140.
5. Bielschowsky M, Helyer BJ, Howie JB: Spontaneous hemolytic anemia in mice of the NZB/Bl strain. Proc Univ Otago Med Sch 1959;37:9.
6. Petschner F, Walker UA, Schmitt-Graff A, et al: ["Catastrophic systemic lupus erythematosus" with Rosai-Dorfman sinus histiocytosis: Successful treatment with anti-CD20/Rituximab]. Dtsch Med Wochenschr 2001;126:998.
7. Stasi R, Pagano A, Stipa E, Amadori S: Rituximab chimeric anti-CD20 monoclonal antibody treatment for adults with chronic idiopathic thrombocytopenic purpura. Blood 2001;98:952.
8. Sackey K: Hemolytic anemia: Part 1. Pediatr Rev 1999;20:152.
9. Pirofsky B: Autoimmunization and the Autoimmune Hemolytic Anemias. Baltimore, Williams & Wilkins, 1969.
10. Myint H, Copplestone JA, Orchard J, et al: Fludarabine-related autoimmune haemolytic anaemia in patients with chronic lymphocytic leukaemia. Br J Haematol 1995;91:341.
11. Robak T, Blasinska-Morawiec M, Krykowski E, et al: Autoimmune haemolytic anaemia in patients with chronic lymphocytic leukaemia treated with 2-chlorodeoxyadenosine (cladribine). Eur J Haematol 1997;58:109.
12. Beckers EA, van Guldener C, Overbeeke MA, van Rhenen DJ: Intravascular hemolysis by IgA red cell autoantibodies. Neth J Med 2001;58:204.
13. Janeway CA, Travers P, Walport M, Capra JD: Immunobiology: The Immune System in Health and Disease, 4th ed. New York, Garland Publishing, 1999.
14. Domen RE: An overview of immune hemolytic anemias. Cleve Clin J Med 1998;65:89.
15. Huber J, Polley MJ, Linscott WD, Müller-Eberhard HJ: Human monocytes: Distant receptor sites for the third component of complement and for immunoglobulin G. Science 1962;162:1281.
16. LoBuglio AF, Cotran RS, Jandl JH: Red cells coated with immunoglobulin G: Binding and sphering by mononuclear cells in man. Science 1967;158:1582.
17. Fleer A, van der Meulen FW, Linthout E, et al: Destruction of IgG-sensitized erythrocytes by human blood monocytes: Modulation of inhibition by IgG. Br J Haematol 1978;39:425.
18. Schreiber AD, Frank MM: Role of antibody and complement in the immune clearance and destruction of erythrocytes. I: In vivo effects of IgG and IgM complement-fixing sites. J Clin Invest 1972;51:575.
19. Schreiber AD, Frank MM: Role of antibody and complement in the immune clearance and destruction of erythrocytes. II: Molecular nature of IgG and IgM complement-fixing sites and effects of their interaction with serum. J Clin Invest 1972;51:583.
20. Meite M, Leonard S, Idrissi ME, et al: Exacerbation of autoantibody-mediated hemolytic anemia by viral infection. J Virol 2000;74:6045.
21. Brown DL, Lachmann PJ, Dacie JV: The in vivo behaviour of complement-coated red cells: Studies in C6-deficient, C3-depleted and normal rabbits. Clin Exp Immunol 1970;7:401.
22. Munn LR, Chaplin H Jr: Rosette formation by sensitized human red cells: Effects of source of peripheral leukocyte monolayers. Vox Sang 1977;33:129.
23. Gorst DW, Rawlinson VI, Merry AH, Stratton F: Positive direct antiglobulin test in normal individuals. Vox Sang 1980;38:99.
24. Unger LJ: A method for detecting Rh₀ antibodies in extremely low titer. J Lab Clin Med 1951;37:825.
25. Issitt PD, Pavone BG, Goldfinger D, et al: Anti-Wrb and other autoantibodies responsible for positive direct antiglobulin tests in 150 individuals. Br J Haematol 1976;34:5.
26. Smith MA, Shah NS, Lobel JS: Parvovirus B19 infection associated with reticulocytopenia and chronic autoimmune hemolytic anemia. Am J Pediatr Hematol Oncol 1989;11:167.
27. Roush GR, Rosenthal NS, Gerson SL, et al: An unusual case of autoimmune hemolytic anemia with reticulocytopenia, erythroid dysplasia, and an IgG2 autoanti-U. Transfusion 1996;36:575.
28. Conley CL, Lippman SM, Ness PM, et al: Autoimmune hemolytic anemia with reticulocytopenia and erythroid marrow. N Engl J Med 1982;306:281.
29. Conley CL, Lippman SM, Ness P: Autoimmune hemolytic anemia with reticulocytopenia: A medical emergency. JAMA 1980;244:1688.
30. Crosby WH, Rappaport H: Reticulocytopenia in autoimmune hemolytic anemia. Blood 1956;11:929.
31. Mangan KF, Besa EC, Shadduck RK, et al: Demonstration of two distinct antibodies in autoimmune hemolytic anemia with reticulocytopenia and red cell aplasia. Exp Hematol 1984;12:788.
32. Van De Loosdrecht AA, Hendriks DW, Blom NR, et al: Excessive apoptosis of bone marrow erythroblasts in a patient with autoimmune haemolytic anaemia with reticulocytopenia. Br J Haematol 2000;108:313.
33. Frank MM, Schreiber AD, Atkinson JP, Jaffe CJ: Pathophysiology of immune hemolytic anemia. Ann Intern Med 1977;87:210.
34. Pruzanski W, Shumak KH: Biologic activity of cold-reacting autoantibodies (first of two parts). N Engl J Med 1977;297:538.
35. Crisp D, Pruzanski W: B-cell neoplasms with homogeneous cold-reacting antibodies (cold agglutinins). Am J Med 1982;72:915.
36. Silberstein LE, Robertson GA, Harris AC, et al: Etiologic aspects of cold agglutinin disease: Evidence for cytogenetically defined clones of lymphoid cells and the demonstration that an anti-PR cold autoantibody is derived from a chromosomally aberrant B cell clone. Blood 1986;67:1705.
37. Silberstein LE, Goldman J, Kant JA, Spitalnik SL: Comparative biochemical and genetic characterization of clonally related human B-cell lines secreting pathogenic anti-Pr2 cold agglutinins. Arch Biochem Biophys 1988;264:244.
38. Rosenthal MC, Pisciotta AV, Komninos ZD, et al: The auto-immune hemolytic anemia of malignant lymphocytic disease. Blood 1955;10:197.
39. Hamblin TJ, Oscier DG, Young BJ: Autoimmunity in chronic lymphocytic leukaemia. J Clin Pathol 1986;39:713.
40. Sikora K, Krikorian J, Levy R: Monoclonal immunoglobulin rescue from a patient with chronic lymphocytic leukemia and autoimmune hemolytic anemia. Blood 1979;54:513.
41. Petz LD: Transfusing the patient with autoimmune hemolytic anemia. Clin Lab Med 1982;2:193.
42. Plapp FV, Beck ML: Transfusion support in the management of immune haemolytic disorders. Clin Haematol 1984;13:167.
43. Rosenfield RE, Jagathambal: Transfusion therapy for autoimmune hemolytic anemia. Semin Hematol 1976;13:311.
44. Sokol RJ, Hewitt S, Booker DJ, Morris BM: Patients with red cell autoantibodies: Selection of blood for transfusion. Clin Lab Haematol 1988;10:257.
45. Dacie JV, Cubush M: Specificity of auto-antibodies in acquired haemolytic anemia. J Clin Pathol 1954;7:18.
46. Hogman C, Killander J, Sjolin S: A case of idiopathic auto-immune haemolytic anemia due to anti-e. Acta Paediatr 1960;49:270.
47. Sachs V: Anti-C as a sole autoantibody in autoimmune hemolytic anemia. Transfusion 1985;25:587.
48. Weiner W, Battey DA, Cleghorn TE, et al: Serological findings in a case of haemolytic anaemia with some general observations on the pathogenesis of this syndrome. Br Med J 1953;2:125.
49. Issitt PD, Anstee DJ: Applied Blood Group Serology, 4th ed. Montgomery, Durham, NC, Scientific Publications, 1998.

50. James P, Rowe GP, Tozzo GG: Elucidation of alloantibodies in autoimmune haemolytic anaemia. Vox Sang 1988;54:167.

51. Laine ML, Beattie KM: Frequency of alloantibodies accompanying autoantibodies. Transfusion 1985;25:545.

52. Wallhermfechtel MA, Pohl BA, Chaplin H: Alloimmunization in patients with warm autoantibodies: A retrospective study employing three donor alloabsorptions to aid in antibody detection. Transfusion 1984;24:482.

53. Mollison PL: Measurement of survival and destruction of red cells in haemolytic syndromes. Br Med Bull 1959;15:59.

54. Petz LD, Garratty G: Acquired Immune Hemolytic Anemias. New York, Churchill Livingstone, 1980.

55. Gould SA, Rosen AL, Sehgal LR, et al: Fluosol-DA as a red-cell substitute in acute anemia. N Engl J Med 1986;314:1653.

56. Mullon J, Giacoppe G, Clagett C, et al: Transfusions of polymerized bovine hemoglobin in a patient with severe autoimmune hemolytic anemia. N Engl J Med 2000;342:1638.

57. Klein HG: The prospects for red-cell substitutes. N Engl J Med 2000;342:1666.

58. Atkinson JP, Schreiber AD, Frank MM: Effects of corticosteroids and splenectomy on the immune clearance and destruction of erythrocytes. J Clin Invest 1973;52:1509.

59. Fries LF, Brickman CM, Frank MM: Monocyte receptors for the Fc portion of IgG increase in number in autoimmune hemolytic anemia and other hemolytic states and are decreased by glucocorticoid therapy. J Immunol 1983;131:1240.

60. Schreiber AD, Parsons J, McDermott P, Cooper RA: Effect of corticosteroids on the human monocyte IgG and complement receptors. J Clin Invest 1975;56:1189.

61. Schreiber AD: Clinical immunology of the corticosteroids. Prog Clin Immunol 1977;3:103.

62. Besa EC: Rapid transient reversal of anemia and long-term effects of maintenance intravenous immunoglobulin for autoimmune hemolytic anemia in patients with lymphoproliferative disorders. Am J Med 1988;84:691.

63. Samuelsson A, Towers TL, Ravetch JV: Anti-inflammatory activity of IVIG mediated through the inhibitory Fc receptor. Science 2001;291:484.

64. Collins PW, Newland AC: Treatment modalities of autoimmune blood disorders. Semin Hematol 1992;29:64.

65. Schwartz SI, Bernard RP, Adams JT, Bauman AW: Splenectomy for hematologic disorders. Arch Surg 1970;101:338.

66. Committee on Infectious Disease, American Academy of Pediatrics: Red Book: Report of the Committee on Infectious Diseases, 24th ed. Elk Grove Village, Il, American Academy of Pediatrics, 1997.

67. Parker AC, MacPherson AI, Richmond J: Value of radiochromium investigation in autoimmune haemolytic anaemia. Br Med J 1977;6055:208.

68. Murphy S, LoBuglio AF: Drug therapy of autoimmune hemolytic anemia. Semin Hematol 1976;13:323.

69. Fauci AS, Dale DC, Wolff SM: Cyclophosphamide and lymphocyte subpopulations in Wegener's granulomatosis. Arthritis Rheum 1974;17:355.

70. Steinberg AD, Plotz PH, Wolff SM, et al: Cytotoxic drugs in treatment of nonmalignant diseases. Ann Intern Med 1972;76:619.

71. Fahey JL: Cancer in the immunosuppressed patient. Ann Intern Med 1971;75:310.

72. Floersheim GL: A comparative study of the effects of anti-tumour and immunosuppressive drugs on antibody-forming and erythropoietic cells. Clin Exp Immunol 1970;6:861.

73. Miller JJ III, Williams GF, Leissring JC: Multiple late complications of therapy with cyclophosphamide, including ovarian destruction. Am J Med 1971;50:530.

74. Qureshi MS, Pennington JH, Goldsmith HJ, Cox PE: Cyclophosphamide therapy and sterility. Lancet 1972;7790:1290.

75. Johnson WW, Meadows DC: Urinary-bladder fibrosis and telangiectasia associated with long-term cyclophosphamide therapy. N Engl J Med 1971;284:290.

76. Emilia G, Messora C, Longo G, Bertesi M: Long-term salvage treatment by cyclosporin in refractory autoimmune haematological disorders. Br J Haematol 1996;93:341.

77. Gopal AK, Press OW: Clinical applications of anti-CD20 antibodies. J Lab Clin Med 1999;134:445.

78. Grillo-Lopez AJ, White CA, Varns C, et al: Overview of the clinical development of rituximab: First monoclonal antibody approved for the treatment of lymphoma. Semin Oncol 1999;26(Suppl 14):66.

79. Dillman RO: Monoclonal antibodies in the treatment of malignancy: Basic concepts and recent developments. Cancer Invest 2001;19:833.

80. Dillman RO: Infusion reactions associated with the therapeutic use of monoclonal antibodies in the treatment of malignancy. Cancer Metastasis Rev 1999;18:465.

81. Waldmann TA, Levy R, Coller BS: Emerging therapies: Spectrum of applications of monoclonal antibody therapy. Hematology (Am Soc Hematol Educ Program) 2000;394.

82. Hagberg H, Holmbom E: Risk factors for side effects during first infusion of rituximab: Definition of a low risk group. Med Oncol 2000;17:218.

83. Abdel-Raheem MM, Potti A, Kobrinsky N: Severe Evans's syndrome secondary to interleukin-2 therapy: Treatment with chimeric monoclonal anti-CD20 antibody. Ann Hematol 2001;80:543.

84. Ahrens N, Kingreen D, Seltsam A, Salama A: Treatment of refractory autoimmune haemolytic anaemia with anti-CD20 (rituximab). Br J Haematol 2001;114:244.

85. Berentsen S, Tjonnfjord GE, Brudevold R, et al: Favourable response to therapy with the anti-CD20 monoclonal antibody Rituximab in primary chronic cold agglutinin disease. Br J Haematol 2001;115:79.

86. Borradori L, Lombardi T, Samson J, et al: Anti-CD20 monoclonal antibody (Rituximab) for refractory erosive stomatitis secondary to CD20(+) follicular lymphoma-associated paraneoplastic pemphigus. Arch Dermatol 2001;137:269.

87. Heizmann M, Itin P, Wernli M, et al: Successful treatment of paraneoplastic pemphigus in follicular NHL with Rituximab: Report of a case and review of treatment for paraneoplastic pemphigus in NHL and CLL. Am J Hematol 2001;66:142.

88. Quartier P, Brethon B, Philippet P, et al: Treatment of childhood autoimmune haemolytic anaemia with Rituximab. Lancet 2001;358:1511.

89. Zecca M, De Stefano P, Nobili B, Locatelli F: Anti-CD20 monoclonal antibody for the treatment of severe, immune-mediated, pure red cell aplasia and hemolytic anemia. Blood 2001;97:3995.

90. Seipelt G, Bohme A, Koschmieder S, Hoelzer D: Effective treatment with Rituximab in a patient with refractory prolymphocytoid transformed B-chronic lymphocytic leukemia and Evans syndrome. Ann Hematol 2001;80:170.

91. Seeliger S, Baumann M, Mohr M, et al: Autologous peripheral blood stem cell transplantation and anti-B-cell directed immunotherapy for refractory auto-immune haemolytic anaemia. Eur J Pediatr 2001;160:492.

92. Orlin JB, Berkman EM: Partial plasma exchange using albumin replacement: Removal and recovery of normal plasma constituents. Blood 1980;56:1055.

93. Silberstein LE, Berkman EM: Plasma exchange in autoimmune hemolytic anemia (AIHA). J Clin Apheresis 1983;1:238.

94. Kutti J, Wadenvik H, Safai-Kutti S, et al: Successful treatment of refractory autoimmune haemolytic anaemia by plasmapheresis. Scand J Haematol 1984;32:149.

95. Szymanski IO, Teno R, Rybak ME: Hemolytic anemia due to a mixture of low-titer IgG lambda and IgM lambda agglutinins reacting optimally at 22 degrees C. Vox Sang 1986;51:112.

96. Silberstein LE, Shoenfeld Y, Schwartz RS, Berkman EM: A combination of IgG and IgM autoantibodies in chronic cold agglutinin disease: Immunologic studies and response to splenectomy. Vox Sang 1985;48:105.

97. Tschirhart DL, Kunkel L, Shulman IA: Immune hemolytic anemia associated with biclonal cold autoagglutinins. Vox Sang 1990;59:222.

98. Deutsch HF: Properties and modifications of a cryomacroglobulin possessing cold agglutinin activity. Biopolymers 1969;7:21.

99. Kuenn JW, Weber R, Teague PO, Keitt AS: Cryopathic gangrene with an IgM lambda cryoprecipitating cold agglutinin. Cancer 1978;42:1826.

100. Tsai CM, Zopf DA, Yu RK, et al: A Waldenström macroglobulin that is both a cold agglutinin and a cryoglobulin because it binds N-acetylneuraminosyl residues. Proc Natl Acad Sci U S A 1977;74:4591.

101. Umlas J, Kaufman M, MacQueston C, et al: A cryoglobulin with cold agglutinin and erythroid stem cell suppressant properties. Transfusion 1991;31:361.

102. Rapoport AP, Rowe JM, McMican A: Life-threatening autoimmune hemolytic anemia in a patient with the acquired immune deficiency syndrome. Transfusion 1988;28:190.

103. Capra JD, Dowling P, Cook S, Kunkel HG: An incomplete cold-reactive gamma G antibody with i specificity in infectious mononucleosis. Vox Sang 1969;16:10.

104. Rosenfield RE, Schmidt PJ, Calvo RC, McGinniss MH: Anti-i, a frequent cold agglutinin in infectious mononucleosis. Vox Sang 1965;10:631.

105. Ruddy S, Gigli I, Austen KF: The complement system of man I. N Engl J Med 1972;287:489.

106. Borsos T, Rapp HJ: Complement fixation on cell surfaces by 19S and 7S antibodies. Science 1965;150:505.

107. Konig AL, Kather H, Roelcke D: Autoimmune hemolytic anemia by coexisting anti-I and anti-Fl cold agglutinins. Blut 1984;49:363.

108. Sokol RJ, Booker DJ, Stamps R: The pathology of autoimmune haemolytic anaemia. J Clin Pathol 1992;45:1047.

109. Abramson N, Gelfand EW, Jandl JH, Rosen FS: The interaction between human monocytes and red cells: Specificity for IgG subclasses and IgG fragments. J Exp Med 1970;132:1207.

110. Atkinson JP, Frank MM: Studies on the in vivo effects of antibody: Interaction of IgM antibody and complement in the immune clearance and destruction of erythrocytes in man. J Clin Invest 1974;54:339.

111. Shulman IA, Branch DR, Nelson JM, et al: Autoimmune hemolytic anemia with both cold and warm autoantibodies. JAMA 1985;253:1746.

112. Silberstein LE, Berkman EM, Schreiber AD: Cold hemagglutinin disease associated with IgG cold-reactive antibody. Ann Intern Med 1987;106:238.

113. Tonthat H, Rochant H, Henry A, et al: A new case of monoclonal IgA kappa cold agglutinin with anti-Pr1d specificity in a patient with persistent HB antigen cirrhosis. Vox Sang 1976;30:464.

114. Garratty G, Petz LD, Brodsky I, Fudenberg HH: An IgA high-titer cold agglutinin with an unusual blood group specificity within the Pr complex. Vox Sang 1973;25:32.

115. Pruzanski W, Cowan DH, Parr DM: Clinical and immunochemical studies of IgM cold agglutinins with lambda type light chains. Clin Immunol Immunopathol 1974;2:234.

116. Angevine CD, Andersen BR, Barnett EV: A cold agglutinin of the IgA class. J Immunol 1966;96:578.

117. Dellagi K, Brouet JC, Schenmetzler C, Praloran V: Chronic hemolytic anemia due to a monoclonal IgG cold agglutinin with anti-Pr specificity. Blood 1981;57:189.

118. Moore JA, Chaplin H Jr: Autoimmune hemolytic anemia associated with an IgG cold incomplete antibody. Vox Sang 1973;24:236.

119. Ambrus M, Bajtain G: A case of an IgG-type cold agglutinin disease. Haematologia 1969;3:225.

120. Andrzejewski C Jr, Gault E, Briggs M, Silberstein L: Benefit of a 37 degree C extracorporeal circuit in plasma exchange therapy for selected cases with cold agglutinin disease. J Clin Apheresis 1988;4:13.

121. Park JV, Weiss CI: Cardiopulmonary bypass and myocardial protection: Management problems in cardiac surgical patients with cold autoimmune disease. Anesth Analg 1988;67:75.

122. Hippe E, Jensen KB, Olesen H, et al: Chlorambucil treatment of patients with cold agglutinin syndrome. Blood 1970;35:68.

123. Schubothe H: The cold hemagglutinin disease. Semin Hematol 1966;3:27.

124. Godder K, Pati AR, Abhyankar SH, et al: De novo chronic graft-versus-host disease presenting as hemolytic anemia following partially mismatched related donor bone marrow transplant. Bone Marrow Transplant 1997;19:813.

125. Gottsche B, Salama A, Mueller-Eckhardt C: Donath-Landsteiner autoimmune hemolytic anemia in children: A study of 22 cases. Vox Sang 1990;58:281.

126. Heddle NM: Acute paroxysmal cold hemoglobinuria. Transfus Med Rev 1989;3:219.

127. Nordhagen R, Stensvold K, Winsnes A, et al: Paroxysmal cold haemoglobinuria: The most frequent acute autoimmune haemolytic anaemia in children? Acta Paediatr Scand 1984;73:258.

128. Hinz DF, Picken MD, Lepow IH: Studies on immune human hemolysis II: The Donath-Landsteiner reaction as a model system for studying the mechanism of action of complement and the role of C1 and C1 esterase. J Exp Med 1961;113:193.

129. Levine P, Celano MJ, Falkowski F: The specificity of the antibody in paroxysmal cold hemoglobinuria (PCH). Transfusion 1963;3:278.

130. Worlledge SM, Rousso C: Studies on the serology of paroxysmal cold haemoglobinuria (PCH) with special reference to its relationship with the P blood group system. Vox Sang 1965;10:293.

131. Engelfriet CP, Borne AV, Moes M, van Loghem JJ: Serological studies in autoimmune haemolytic anaemia. Bibl Haematol 1968;29:473.

132. Judd WJ, Wilkinson SL, Issitt PD, et al: Donath-Landsteiner hemolytic anemia due to an anti-Pr-like biphasic hemolysin. Transfusion 1986;26:423.

133. Weiner W, Gordon EG, Rowe D: A Donath-Landsteiner antibody (non-syphilitic type). Vox Sang 1964;9:684.

134. Petz LD, Fudenberg HH: Coombs-positive hemolytic anemia caused by penicillin administration. N Engl J Med 1966;274:171.

135. Bougie D, Johnson ST, Weitekamp LA, Aster RH: Sensitivity to a metabolite of diclofenac as a cause of acute immune hemolytic anemia. Blood 1997;90:407.

136. Salama A, Mueller-Eckhardt C: On the mechanisms of sensitization and attachment of antibodies to RBC in drug-induced immune hemolytic anemia. Blood 1987;69:1006.

137. Carstairs KC, Breckenridge A, Dollery CT, Worlledge SM: Incidence of a positive direct Coombs test in patients on alpha-methyldopa. Lancet 1966;7455:133.

138. Petz LD: Drug-induced immune haemolytic anaemia. Clin Haematol 1980;9:455.

139. Worlledge SM: Immune drug-induced hemolytic anemias. Semin Hematol 1973;10:327.

140. Danielson DA, Douglas SW III, Herzog P, et al: Drug-induced blood disorders. JAMA 1984;252:3257.

141. Theofilopoulos AN, Dixon FJ: Murine models of systemic lupus erythematosus. Adv Immunol 1985;37:269.

142. Okamoto M, Murakami M, Shimizu A, et al: A transgenic model of autoimmune hemolytic anemia. J Exp Med 1992;175:71.

143. Sakiyama T, Ikuta K, Nisitani S, et al: Requirement of IL-5 for induction of autoimmune hemolytic anemia in anti-red blood cell autoantibody transgenic mice. Int Immunol 1999;11:995.

144. Nisitani S, Honjo T: Breakage of B cell tolerance and autoantibody production in anti-erythrocyte transgenic mice. Int Rev Immunol 1999;18:259.

145. Nisitani S, Sakiyama T, Honjo T: Involvement of IL-10 in induction of autoimmune hemolytic anemia in anti-erythrocyte Ig transgenic mice. Int Immunol 1998;10:1039.

146. Leddy JP, Falany JL, Kissel GE, et al: Erythrocyte membrane proteins reactive with human (warm-reacting) anti-red cell autoantibodies. J Clin Invest 1993;91:1672.

147. Bloy C, Blanchard D, Lambin P, et al: Human monoclonal antibody against Rh(D) antigen: Partial characterization of the Rh(D) polypeptide from human erythrocytes. Blood 1987;69:1491.

148. Lane HC, Masur H, Edgar LC, et al: Abnormalities of B-cell activation and immunoregulation in patients with the acquired immunodeficiency syndrome. N Engl J Med 1983;309:453.

149. Kipps TJ, Carson DA: Autoantibodies in chronic lymphocytic leukemia and related systemic autoimmune diseases. Blood 1993;81:2475.

150. Leddy JP, Bakemeier RF: Structural aspects of human erythrocyte autoantibodies. J Exp Med 1965;121:1.

151. Masouredis SP, Branks MJ, Victoria EJ: Antiidiotypic IgG crossreactive with Rh alloantibodies in red cell autoimmunity. Blood 1987;70:710.

152. Hakomori S: Blood group ABH and Ii antigens of human erythrocytes: Chemistry, polymorphism, and their developmental change. Semin Hematol 1981;18:39.

153. Stevenson FK, Smith GJ, North J, et al: Identification of normal B-cell counterparts of neoplastic cells which secrete cold agglutinins of anti-I and anti-i specificity. Br J Haematol 1989;72:9.

154. Costea N, Yakulis VJ, Heller P: Inhibition of cold agglutinins (Anti-I) by M. pneumoniae antigens. Proc Soc Exp Biol Med 1972;139:476.

155. Pascual V, Victor K, Lelsz D, et al: Nucleotide sequence analysis of the V regions of two IgM cold agglutinins: Evidence that the VH4-21 gene segment is responsible for the major cross-reactive idiotype. J Immunol 1991;146:4385.

156. Silberstein LE, Jefferies LC, Goldman J, et al: Variable region gene analysis of pathologic human autoantibodies to the related i and I red blood cell antigens. Blood 1991;78:2372.

157. Stevenson FK, Spellerberg MB, Treasure J, et al: Differential usage of an Ig heavy chain variable region gene by human B-cell tumors. Blood 1993;82:224.

i. Transfusion Reactions

Chapter **33**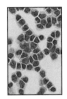

Hemolytic Transfusion Reactions

◼ ACUTE

Daniel R. Ambruso

Although rare, acute hemolytic transfusion reactions (AHTRs) are among the most dramatic and challenging adverse events of blood transfusions to manage. The most common circumstances leading to AHTR are situations in which red blood cells (RBCs) are infused that are incompatible with an antibody preexisting in the recipient's circulation, resulting in intravascular destruction of the cells. Subsequent complications of the hemolysis may lead to hypotension and shock, consumptive coagulopathy, and acute renal failure. Prompt diagnosis and treatment are required to reverse these complications and avoid the high mortality rate.

◼ Definition

Acute hemolytic transfusion reaction is rapid destruction of blood cells immediately after or within 24 hours of a transfusion.[1] Most commonly, such reactions occur with transfusion of whole blood or RBCs. However, transfusion of platelets, fresh frozen plasma, or other plasma-derived products may contain antibodies incompatible with the recipient's RBCs and may cause AHTR.[2-6] Because of the variability in clinical presentation, recognition, and reporting, the precise incidence of AHTR is unknown. A general risk may be estimated as the number of reactions per units transfused. Various studies have estimated this rate as 1 in 12,000 to 1 in 35,000.[7-9] Although the rate of this adverse event is low, mortality is high and depends on the amount of incompatible blood infused—ranging from 25% for infusion of 500 to 1000 mL of blood to 44% for infusion of more than 1000 mL.[10, 11] The incidence of fatal AHTR is estimated to be 1 per 100,000 to 1 per 600,000 units transfused.[11-14] Some investigators have suggested that these reported rates may be too low because of failure to recognize or report some cases.

◼ Pathophysiology

The most common sequence of events leading to AHTR is transfusion of whole blood or RBCs that are immunologically incompatible with antibodies preexisting in the recipient (Table 33.1). The antibodies most commonly involved are

Table 33.1 Causes of Hemolysis Associated with Acute Hemolytic Transfusion Reactions

Conditions that destroy donor cells	Naturally occurring or stimulated alloantibodies (anti-A, -Kell, -Jk^a, -Fy^a)
	Autoantibodies
	Drug-associated antibodies
	Bacterial contamination
	Mechanical trauma associated with infusion
	Thermal trauma: (heat or cold)
	Reconstitution of red blood cells with hypotonic solutions
	Equipment that damages blood cells extracorporeally
Conditions that destroy recipient cells	Incompatible (ABO) platelets, plasma, cryoprecipitate, or plasma-derived products
	Infusion of large amounts of hypotonic solutions
	Mechanical trauma (mechanical heart valves, high-pressure jet lesions, microangiopathic syndromes)

those to A, Kell, Jk^a, and Fy^a.[15] ABO incompatibility accounts for 74% of all fatal reactions. Although severe acute hemolysis is less common, it can occur if antibodies, primarily ABO, from a transfused component other than whole blood or RBCs results in destruction of recipient cells.[2–6] Reported components associated with these episodes of AHTR include infusion of platelets and plasma, usually from patients with high anti-A titers. Non–immune-mediated acute hemolysis of donor cells may occur before or during the transfusion of blood components and can produce reactions that mimic immune-mediated hemolysis (see Table 33.1). Causes of non–immune-mediated hemolysis include bacterial contamination, mechanical trauma during the infusion, thermal hemolysis from overheating or freezing of the unit, and osmotic lysis of RBCs associated with reconstitution of blood components with hypotonic solutions.[16]

The sequence of events subsequent to the infusion of incompatible RBCs centers on binding of antibody to the surface of the transfused cells followed by activation of complement and intravascular lysis of the cells with release of hemoglobin, RBC stroma (cytoskeleton and plasma membrane), and enzymes. Although hemolysis is primarily intravascular, there may be an extravascular component of hemolysis when cells that were not lysed by complement activation are coated with antibodies and complement components and are then ingested by mononuclear phagocytes of the reticuloendothelial system.

Immune hemolysis with complement activation leads to the following three major complications: (1) hypotension, (2) vasoconstriction and renal ischemia, and (3) activation of platelets and the coagulation cascade, which results in disseminated intravascular coagulation (DIC).[1, 16] Activation of complement results in complete assembly of the membrane attack complex and intravascular destruction of RBCs, releasing plasma membrane and stroma, hemoglobin, and enzymes into the vascular space.[16–18] Potent anaphylotoxins, including the complement fragments C_{3a} and C_{5a}, are also released;[1, 17, 18] these products contribute directly to the hypotension and, through their interaction with mast cells, cause degranulation and release of histamine and serotonin, both of which are potent vasoactive amines.[19] The amines cause constriction of small arteries and arterioles and increased vascular permeability, contributing to renal ischemia.[19, 20] The kallikrein system is activated through the effects of Hageman factor, producing bradykinin, a potent vasodilator that also induces greater capillary permeability.[20] Finally, hypotension can be effected through the activity of cytokines such as tumor necrosis factor-α (TNF-α) and interleukins IL-1 and IL-8, which are known to be produced in response to immune hemolysis, particularly ABO hemolysis.[21–24] Hypotension relates directly to some of the signs and symptoms of AHTR and also contributes to renal ischemia and renal failure.

Immune hemolysis has dramatic effects on coagulation. The process of antigen-antibody interaction may trigger the platelet release reaction as well as the release of serotonin and histamine, further enhancing vasoconstriction in the kidneys and the release of platelet factor 3, a phospholipid that supports the activity of the procoagulant cascade.[25] The primary antibody-antigen interaction also activates Hageman factor, which initiates activity of the intrinsic clotting cascade, leading to consumption of procoagulant clotting factors with resultant prothrombin activation and cleavage of fibrinogen to fibrin and activation of fibrinolysis.[26, 27] Activation of platelets

and procoagulant activity in the kidney results in platelet and fibrin microthrombi, further exacerbating renal damage. Diffuse consumption of hemostatic constituents may be severe enough to produce DIC and pathologic bleeding.

Production of TNF-α and IL-1 in response to immune destruction of RBCs has dramatic effects on endothelial cells, causing increased expression of adhesive procoagulant and proinflammatory molecules. This expression may further tip the hemostatic balance by producing microthrombi in the kidney and supporting the diffuse consumptive coagulopathy. Additional cytokines, such as IL-8, which has powerful priming, activating, and chemoattractant effects on neutrophils, and MCP-1, which exerts similar effects on monocytes, are produced during immune hemolysis. They have dramatic proinflammatory effects with the potential to enhance kidney damage.[23, 24]

■ Signs and Symptoms

The clinical presentation of AHTR varies depending on the antigen involved, the quantity of RBCs infused, and the titer of the antibody as well as the thermal range of its activity. Common symptoms and signs include fever or fever and chills, chest pain, hypotension, flushing, dyspnea, pallor, jaundice, diffuse bleeding, hemoglobinuria, and oliguria or anuria (Table 33.2).[1, 7, 28] Patients may also have pain in the abdomen, flanks, back, and head or at the infusion site. An overwhelming feeling of dread or anxiety may accompany other complaints. Patients with a severe reaction may present in shock with severe hypotension, disorientation, or an altered state of consciousness. Atypical presentations may occur in patients with a variety of clinical states.[1, 16] In patients who sustain AHTR under anesthesia, early symptoms are not recognized, and changes in blood pressure, diffuse bleeding, and hemoglobinuria may be the only signs. Chills and rigors are not seen with paralysis. Concurrent medications may mask the signs and symptoms of hypotension.

■ Differential Diagnosis

Acute hemolysis from any cause can be confused with AHTR.[1, 16] Microbial contamination as well as physical,

Table 33.2 Common Signs and Symptoms of Acute Hemolytic Transfusion Reaction

Fever
Chills/rigors
Anxiety, feeling of dread
Facial flushing
Chest pain
Abdominal pain
Back and flank pain
Nausea
Vomiting
Diarrhea
Dyspnea
Hypotension
Hemoglobinuria
Hemoglobinemia
Pallor
Icterus
Oliguria/anuria
Pain at the transfusion site
Diffuse bleeding
Jaundice

chemical, and drug-related damage to stored RBCs must be considered. In patients who have autoimmune hemolytic anemia (AIHA) with either warm or cold autoantibodies, some of the presenting signs and symptoms and clinical laboratory findings may be the same as those found in AHTR. To further confound the clinical picture, patients with AIHA who have received transfusions of RBCs may develop alloantibodies to minor blood group antigens, making complete antibody detection difficult and raising the risk for AHTR with subsequent transfusions. Congenital hemolytic anemias, such as hereditary spherocytosis, glucose-6-phosphate dehydrogenase deficiency, and sickle cell anemia, can also manifest as acute hemolysis and exacerbations of chronic hemolysis that, if temporally related to a transfusion, may mimic AHTR. Conditions associated with microangiopathic hemolytic anemia, including hemolytic uremic syndrome, thrombotic thrombocytopenic purpura, DIC and mechanical fragmentation (as seen with mechanical heart valves) may also be confused with AHTR. Episodes of acute hemolysis are also seen with paroxysmal nocturnal hemoglobinuria and a variety of infections.

Laboratory Diagnosis

In conjunction with a number of actions to document and treat the AHTR, specific laboratory tests are required to confirm the suspicion of a hemolytic transfusion reaction (Table 33.3). The first group of tests confirms the existence of hemolysis and includes a drop in oxygen-carrying capacity (hematocrit, hemoglobin concentration). Hemoglobinuria or hemoglobinemia is invariably associated with AHTR, because hemolysis is mostly intravascular and acute. Unconjugated hyperbilirubinemia may be reflected in elevated total and fractionated bilirubin levels. Decreased levels of serum haptoglobin and elevations of serum methemalbumin, lactate dehydrogenase, and aspartate transaminase may be associated with the hemolysis but are not usually required to define the process.

A direct Coombs test should be performed. It usually yields a mixed-field reaction, representing the combination of patient and donor RBCs, only one of which is sensitized with antibodies. Antibody detection should be performed, and the specificity of the offending antibody or antibodies should be determined. Renal function studies as well as coagulation studies to define the status of the procoagulant cascade and platelet numbers aid in management of the effects of hemolysis.

Table 33.3 Laboratory Investigations for Acute Hemolytic Transfusion Reaction

Product Samples	Reconfirmation of ABO, Rh type, and antibody screen results
Patient Samples	Reconfirmation of ABO type, antibody screen, and direct Coombs test, and antibody identification results Complete blood count, platelet count Urinalysis to document hemoglobinuria Serum bilirubin (fractionated/total) Blood urea nitrogen, creatinine, quantitation of urine output Coagulation screen: prothrombin time, partial thromboplastin time, thrombin time, fibrin split products, fibrinogen; evaluation of fibrinolytic system as necessary (euglobulin lysis time, plasminogen)

Prevention and Management

The best way to prevent AHTR is to avoid transfusion. Defining clear-cut and defendable indications for transfusion is the first step in avoiding adverse events of transfusion. Careful determination of the hemoglobin concentration or hematocrit level that will be the "trigger" for ordering a blood transfusion is critical to this process. Blood substitutes offer a potentially safer alternative to transfusions in urgent situations, in which clerical errors and patient-donor identification problems have the greatest impact. Currently, however, blood substitutes can be used only in research protocols and are not approved for general use.

Of course, autologous blood is always safer than homologous components, but there is still a significant risk that an incorrect unit will be transfused. If homologous blood must be used, ensuring the most sensitive antibody screening for donors and recipients is the hallmark of safety. Active programs to effect accurate clerical function relating to patient identification, sample collection, sample and unit labeling, unit identification, patient testing, component handling, and infusion at the bedside minimize the risk of adverse events of transfusion. A strong quality assurance program provides control over the processes involved in testing, processing, selecting, and transfusing blood components and minimize errors leading to AHTRs.

Physical, mechanical, chemical, and thermal damage to component cells can be avoided through strict adherence to a process designed to ensure that (1) blood is stored only in carefully monitored and certified refrigerators, (2) blood is not exposed to temperatures greater than 37°C or allowed to freeze, (3) no medications are added to the blood, and (4) reconstitution of blood components is performed under strict protocols and is completed within the carefully controlled environment of the blood bank or center. Following procedures for specimen collection, labeling, testing, and issuing blood enhances safe transfusions and minimizes the risk of AHTR.

If a transfusion reaction is suspected because of an acute change in the clinical status of a patient, the transfusion must be stopped immediately, intravenous access must be maintained, and patient assessment must be initiated (Table 33.4). Such an assessment includes a rapid evaluation of symptoms and a physical examination to determine physiologic status. Any of the transfused blood units, empty containers, and tubing should be collected for transfer back to the transfusion service. Identification of the unit or units and of the patient should be reconfirmed. Patient blood samples collected for laboratory tests as described previously should be submitted to the diagnostic laboratory.

Treatment of AHTR is best determined by the clinical status of the patient. If symptoms and signs are mild, minimal support is necessary. If the hemolysis is severe, more aggressive measures must be initiated. Acute cardiopulmonary support must be provided according to standard protocols (the ABCs of resuscitation). If hypotension is present, infusion fluids, the use of vasopressors, or both must be initiated early. The amount of fluid given depends on the patient's renal status. Dopamine at a low dose may be indicated, but higher doses may unfavorably restrict renal blood flow and enhance pathologic processes affecting the kidney, results that outweigh the agent's beneficial effect on blood pressure.[1]

Table 33.4 Management of Acute Hemolytic Transfusion Reaction

1. Stop the transfusion and maintain intravenous access.
2. Make initial rapid assessment of patient and requirements for basic and advanced support.
3. Notify transfusion service, collect transfused units (full or partially), tubing, etc., and return them to blood bank.
4. Reconfirm identity of blood units and patient.
5. Collect appropriate patient blood specimens (see also Table 33.3).
6. Pending results of initial evaluation, consider the following supportive approaches:
   a. IV fluid resuscitation to treat hypotension.
   b. Maintenance intravenous fluids at 3000 mL/M^2/day with administration of sodium bicarbonate to keep pH > 7.0.
   c. Diuretics: mannitol (20%), 100 mL/M^2 given over 30–60 min, then 30 mL/M^2/hr for text 12 hours; furosemide (adults 20–80 mg; infants and children 1–2 mg/kg up to an adult dose).
   d. Low-dose dopamine, 1–5 mcg/kg/min.
   e. Replacement of procoagulant factors and fibrinogen with fresh frozen plasma and cryoprecipitate and of platelets with platelet concentrate.
   f. Heparin: 50–100 U/kg, (unfractionated heparin) and infusion 15–25 U/kg/hr to keep heparin level 0.4–0.7 U/mL.

Renal failure may be averted by the infusion of fluids and the use of vasopressors to reverse hypotension. Renal function and urine output are maintained with intravenous fluids and diuretics, either furosemide or mannitol.[29-31] Consultation with a nephrologist in severe cases can be important.

Treatment of DIC may be one of the most important strategies in the management of AHTR with renal involvement. However, the approach to this complication remains controversial. Once cells are transfused into the patient, the rate of hemolysis cannot be controlled; thus, the first strategy in treating this complication, reversal of the trigger, may be thwarted. All of the other supportive care already mentioned aid in reversing the effects of processes occurring "downstream" of the hemolytic event and may help control DIC related to these events.

For severe DIC, manifesting as consumption of platelets and procoagulant factors along with severe bleeding, accepted therapy consists of replacement of lost components with platelet concentrates, fresh frozen plasma, and cryoprecipitate. Although some experts state that such a replacement maneuver merely adds "fuel to the fire," worsening of DIC associated with AHTR after replacement of platelets and clotting factors has not been documented.[32]

Finally, in severe cases, heparin has also been advocated as treatment for DIC. By enhancing the effect of antithrombin III–neutralizing serine proteases, heparin may decrease the inappropriate diffuse activation of procoagulant activity.[32,33] In addition, heparin may also have a direct anti-complement activity, thereby decreasing hemolysis.[34] Concern has been raised about the bleeding risk of heparin therapy. Because most patients with AHTR may be bleeding from consumption coagulopathy, use of heparin may not pose an additional risk and may control the diffuse consumption of procoagulant activity.

The basic pathophysiology of AHTR is related to incompatible RBCs. Exchange transfusion with antigen-negative blood washes out sensitized or potentially sensitized cells. This approach should be evaluated carefully, however, because the chance to reduce morbidity must be balanced by the added risk of the procedure. Simple direct transfusions

to correct ensuing anemia may be considered but should be delayed until the etiology of the AHTR has been established and the antibody causing immune-mediated hemolysis has been determined.[1,16] No patient should be allowed to suffer significant morbidity and higher risk of mortality because of anemia, but great care should be taken in selection of appropriate units for RBC transfusion. Platelets and fresh frozen plasma should be selected so as not to aggravate hemolysis.

REFERENCES

1. Davenport RD: Hemolytic transfusion reactions. In Popovsky MA (ed): Transfusion Reactions. Bethesda, MD, American Association of Blood Banks, 1996, p 1.
2. Inwood MJ, Zuliani B: Anti-A hemolytic transfusion with packed O cells. Ann Intern Med 1978;89:515.
3. Chipping PM, Lloyd E, Goldman JM: Haemolysis after granulocyte transfusions. Br Med J 1980;281:1529.
4. Reis MD, Coovadia AS: Transfusion of ABO-incompatible platelets causing severe haemolytic reaction. Clin Lab Haematol 1989;113:237.
5. Murphy MF, Hook S, Waters AH, et al: Acute haemolysis after ABO-incompatible platelet transfusions. Lancet 1990;335:974.
6. Pierce RN, Reich LM, Mayer K: Hemolysis following platelet transfusions from ABO-incompatible donors. Transfusion 1985;25:60.
7. Pineda AA, Brzica SM Jr, Taswell HF: Hemolytic transfusion reaction: Recent experience in a large blood bank. Mayo Clin Proc 1978;53:378.
8. Lichtiger B, Perry-Thornton E: Hemolytic transfusion reactions in oncology patients: Experience in a large cancer center. J Clin Oncol 1984;25:438.
9. Moore SB, Taswell HF, Pineda AA, et al: Delayed hemolytic transfusion reactions: Evidence of the need for an improved protransfusion compatibility test. Am J Clin Pathol 1980;74:94.
10. Bluemle LW Jr: Hemolytic transfusion reactions causing acute renal failure: Serologic and clinical considerations. Postgrad Med 1965;38:484.
11. Sazama K: Reports of 355 transfusion-associated deaths: 1976 through 1985. Transfusion 1990;30:583.
12. National Institutes of Health Consensus Conference: Perioperative red blood cell transfusion. JAMA 1988;260:2700.
13. Honig CL, Bove JR: Transfusion-associated fatalities: Review of Bureau of Biologics reports 1976–1978. Transfusion 1980;20:653.
14. Linden JV, Paul B, Dressler KP: A report of 104 transfusion errors in New York State. Transfusion 1992;32:601.
15. Taswell HF: Hemolytic transfusion reactions: Frequency and clinical and laboratory aspects. In Bell CA (ed): A Seminar on Immune Mediated Cell Destruction. Washington, DC, American Association of Blood Banks, 1981, p 71.
16. Brecher ME, Taswell HF: Hemolytic transfusion reactions. In Rossi EC, Simon TL, Moss GS (eds): Principles of Transfusion Medicine. Baltimore, Williams & Wilkins, 1991.
17. Goldfinger D: Acute hemolytic transfusion reactions—a fresh look at pathogenesis and considerations regarding therapy. Transfusion 1974;27:171.
18. Rother K, Till GO (eds): The Complement System. Berlin, Springer Verlag, 1988.
19. McKay DG: Vessel wall and thrombogenesis-endotoxin. Thromb Diath Haemorrh 1973;29:11.
20. Morat HZ, DiLorenzo NL: Activation of plasma kinin system by antigen-antibody aggregates. I: Generation of permeability factor in guinea pig serum. Lab Invest 1968;19:187.
21. Butler J, Parker D, Pillai R, et al: Systemic release of neutrophil elastase and tumour necrosis factor alpha following ABO incompatible blood transfusion. Br J Haematol 1991;79:525.
22. Davenport RD, Strieter RM, Kunkel SL: Red cell ABO incompatibility and production of tumour necrosis factor-alpha. Br J Haematol 1991;78:540.
23. Davenport RD, Strieter RM, Standiford TJ, et al: Interleukin-8 production in red blood cell incompatibility. Blood 1990;76:2439.
24. Davenport RD, Burdick MD, Strieter RM, et al: Monocyte chemoattractant protein production in red cell incompatibility. Transfusion 1994;34:16.
25. Pfueller SL, Luscher EF: Studies of the mechanisms of human platelet release reaction induced by immunologic stimuli. I:

Complement-dependent and complement-independent reactions. J Immunol 1974;112:1201.

26. Davenport RD, Burdick M, Kunkel SL: Endothelial cell activation in hemolytic transfusion reactions. Transfusion 1992;32:53S.

27. Davenport RD, Polak TJ, Schmouder RE, et al: Endothelial cell procoagulant activity induced by red cell incompatibility. Transfusion 1994;34:943.

28. Gralnick HR, Marchesi S, Grivelber H: Intravascular coagulation in acute leukemia: Clinical and subclinical abnormalities. Blood 1972;40:709.

29. Barry KG, Malloy JP: Oliguric renal failure: Evaluation and therapy by the intravenous infusion of mannitol. JAMA 1962;179:510.

30. Wolf CFW, Canale VC: Total pulmonary hypersensitivity reaction to HLA incompatible blood transfusion: Report of a case and review of the literature. Transfusion 1976;16:135.

31. Hammerschmidt DE, Jacob HS: Adverse pulmonary reactions to transfusion. Adv Intern Med 1983;27:511.

32. Hathaway WE, Goodnight S Jr: Disorders of Hemostasis and Thrombosis: A Clinical Guide. New York, McGraw-Hill, 1993, p 227.

33. Rock RC, Bove JR, Nemerson Y: Heparin treatment of intravascular coagulation accompanying hemolytic transfusion reactions. Transfusion 1969;9:57.

34. Gray JM, Oberman HA, Beck ML: Delay in onset of hemolysis in vivo apparently due to heparinization. Transfusion 1973;13:422.

◼ DELAYED

R. Sue Shirey

Karen E. King

Paul M. Ness

As the term implies, a *delayed* hemolytic transfusion reaction (DHTR) is generally not recognized until 3 to 10 days after transfusion of blood that appeared to be serologically compatible. Classically, DHTRs occur in patients who have been previously immunized by transfusion or pregnancy but in whom the antibody was not detected in pretransfusion testing. Stimulated by the transfusion of RBCs that possess the corresponding antigen, the antibody titer rises and sensitizes the transfused donor RBCs, which may then lead to intravascular hemolysis, extravascular hemolysis, or both.[1-3] The clinical symptoms associated with DHTRs, which are generally milder than those observed in acute hemolytic transfusion reactions, include fever, unexplained anemia, and jaundice. Hemoglobinuria may occur and has been associated with a variety of antibody specificities, including Kidd system antibodies.[4,5] Although uncommon, severe complications in DHTRs, such as acute renal failure and disseminated intravascular coagulation (DIC), have been reported.[6-9] Antibodies directed against Rh (CEce) and Kidd system antigens (Jk^a, Jk^b) are the antibodies most commonly implicated in DHTR; however, many other specificities (e.g., anti-K, anti-Fy^a, anti-S, etc.) have been described.[2,3,8]

◼ Traditional Concepts

Mollison[2] credits the first account of DHTR in humans to that by Boorman and colleagues[10] in 1946. Approximately 4 to 7 days after group A_2 transfusion with multiple units of group A blood, the patient became severely jaundiced. Serologic testing revealed that the patient had developed an atypical anti-A_1 antibody that was reactive at 37°C to a titer of 32. None of the group A_1 transfused donor RBCs (most of the transfused units were retrospectively typed as group A_1) could be detected in the patient's post-transfusion sample, whereas transfused group O donor RBCs persisted in the patient's circulation. Boorman and colleagues[10] called this finding "a delayed blood transfusion incompatibility reaction."

Many more reports of DHTR have been described since the 1940s.[11-14] With rare exceptions,[15-19] cases of DHTR have the following common features:

1. The DHTRs have occurred in patients who have been alloimmunized by previous transfusions or pregnancies.

2. Because of the low titer of reactivity, the implicated antibody was not detected in pretransfusion antibody screening or compatibility testing.

3. The DHTR was usually suspected 3 to 10 days after transfusion, when clinical symptoms associated with hemolysis were observed.

4. An antibody not detected in pretransfusion testing was readily identified in the post-transfusion sample.

Two early sequential studies of DHTRs, spanning the years 1964 to 1977, were reported by the Mayo Clinic (Table 33.5).[8-13] In the first series, 22 of 23 patients (96%) had clinical manifestations of hemolysis, and three deaths were attributed to DHTR. In the second series, only 24 of 37 patients (65%) had clinical evidence of hemolysis; the remaining 13 (35%) demonstrated serologic findings consistent with a DHTR, but no clinical or laboratory evidence of

Table 33.5 Early Findings in Delayed Hemolytic Transfusion Reactions (DHTR): Mayo Clinic Series

	DHTRs at the Clinic	
	1964–1973	1974–1977
Incidence*	1:11,650	1:4000
Total number	23	37
Morbidity	22 (96%)	24 (65%)
Mortality	3 (13%)	0

*Incidence of DHTRs expressed as DHTR per red cell units transfused.

hemolysis was associated with transfusion. This trend of higher frequency but less clinical significance may have been related to the manner in which DHTR was defined. If the measured frequency of DHTRs relies on clinical reporting alone, the incidence is lower than the true rate, because the signs and symptoms of hemolysis are nonspecific and may be difficult to distinguish from those in the complicated medical course of patients who undergo multiple transfusions.[6] If DHTR is defined by post-transfusion serologic testing, the frequency may be higher and the rate of clinical findings may diminish, because correlation between serologic results and clinical hemolysis is often poor.[9]

■ Serologic Studies

The serologic findings in classic cases of DHTR include (1) the development of a positive direct antiglobulin test (DAT) result with a mixed field appearance owing to the presence of donor RBCs that have been sensitized by immunoglobulin (Ig) G antibody interspersed with DAT-negative autologous RBCs and (2) a newly identified alloantibody in the RBC eluate, plasma sample, or both 3 to 7 days after the index transfusion.[2, 3] It has generally been accepted that in DHTR, the sensitized donor RBCs are removed from the circulation within approximately 14 days of the putatively responsible transfusion. Thereafter, results of DAT and eluate studies should become negative, coinciding with the in vivo destruction of donor RBCs that provoked the immune response (Table 33.6).

Almost 40 years after the first case of DHTR was presented, Salama and Mueller-Eckhardt[19] published a report that called into question many of the traditionally held concepts of DHTR. The authors studied 26 patients with apparent DHTR due to antibodies of the Rh, Kell, and Duffy systems. Surprisingly, DAT results in all 26 cases showed complement sensitization of the RBCs regardless of the implicated antibody specificities, and none of the DAT samples had a mixed field appearance. The most extraordinary finding in this study was that DAT results were persistently positive for weeks or even months after transfusion, long after the transfused cells should have been removed from the circulation. In some cases, the implicated antibody was recovered in eluates prepared from samples drawn more than 100 days after the index transfusion.

To explain these findings, Salama and Mueller-Eckhardt[19] speculated that complement activation may occur in vivo in all cases of DHTR, regardless of the antibody specificity. Because antibodies implicated in DHTRs were recovered in eluates prepared from samples drawn long after sensitized donor RBCs would have been removed from the circulation, these researchers theorized that alloantibodies not only may sensitize allogeneic donor RBCs but also may nonspecifically sensitize autologous RBCs during these reactions, activating complement via the classical pathway. Therefore, at least hypothetically, both autologous and allogeneic RBCs could be involved in a DHTR, with antibody sensitization and complement activation leading to accelerated destruction of donor RBCs and transient destruction of autologous cells.[20-22]

The long-term serologic findings reported by Ness and colleagues[9] were not in complete agreement with either the classic serologic findings associated with DHTR or with the findings reported by Salama and Mueller-Eckhardt[19] (see Table 33.6). These researchers found that only 2 of the 15 patients with apparent DHTRs who were monitored for 25 to 194 days after the putatively responsible transfusion had serologic findings consistent with what is expected in DHTR. That is, the DAT results in these 2 cases (7%) became negative within 25 days of the transfusion, indicating removal of antibody-sensitized donor RBCs from the circulation. In the remaining 13 cases, the DAT results were persistently positive because of sensitization with IgG, complement, or both. Eluates prepared from samples drawn more than 3 weeks after transfusion demonstrated (1) an implicated alloantibody similar to the findings reported by Salama and Mueller-Eckhardt in 5 cases (38%),[19] (2) panagglutination consistent with the presence of warm-reacting autoantibodies with broad specificity in 4 cases (31%), and (3) no reactivity in 4 cases (31%). From these results, Ness and colleagues[9] concluded that several immunologic mechanisms may be involved in the persistence of a positive DAT result after a DHTR, including the development of post-transfusion autoantibodies.

Table 33.6   Serologic Findings in Delayed Hemolytic Transfusion Reactions

		Reported Findings	
	Traditionally-Expected Findings[3]	Salama and Mueller-Eckhardt[19]	Ness et al.[9]
Initial Findings			
DAT result:	+	+	+
Anti-IgG	+	+/0	+
Anti-C3	+/0	+	+/0
Mixed-field	Usually	Never	Rarely
Eluate	Alloantibody	Alloantibody	Alloantibody
Long-Term Findings			
DAT result:	0	+	+/0
Anti-IgG	0	+/0	+/0
Anti-C3	0	+	+/0
Eluate	0	Alloantibody	Alloantibody, autoantibody, nonreactive

DAT, direct antiglobulin test; Ig, immunoglobulin; +, positive; 0, negative; +/0, test may be positive or negative.

■ Delayed Serologic Transfusion Reactions

The term *delayed serologic transfusion reaction* (DSTR) was introduced by Ness and colleagues[9] to describe cases with serologic evidence of a DHTR (i.e., the development of a positive post-transfusion DAT result and a newly identified alloantibody in eluate studies and/or plasma studies) but no clinical evidence of hemolysis. In their series conducted at the Johns Hopkins Hospital, of 34 consecutive patients with post-transfusion serologic findings consistent with a DHTR, only 6 patients (18%) had clinical evidence of hemolysis attributable to a transfusion reaction. In all 6 patients, there were unexplained drops in hemoglobin and hematocrit values. Anti-Jk[a] was implicated in 5 of the 6 cases. Twenty-eight (82%) of the 34 patients were designated as having DSTR because they had no clinical evidence of hemolysis, as determined by retrospective chart review. Thus, the ratio of DHTR to DSTR could be expressed as 18:82. The combined frequency of DSTR and DHTR was calculated as 1 case per 1605 units transfused (0.06%), or 1 case per 151 patients for whom post-transfusion samples were submitted for evaluation. The frequency of true DHTR (i.e., presence of clinical evidence of hemolysis) was only 1 case per 9094 units transfused, or 0.01%.

In a series spanning the years 1980 through 1992, the Mayo Clinic reported a combined frequency of DHTR and DSTR as 1 case per 1899 allogeneic RBC units transfused, with a DHTR-to-DSTR ratio of 36:64 when patients were evaluated for clinical hemolysis concurrent with the detection of positive post-transfusion serologic results.[23] Comparable to findings reported by Ness and colleagues,[9] anti-Jk[a] was frequently implicated in DHTR in the Mayo Clinic series. The latest study from the Mayo Clinic indicates a decline in DHTR and a concomitant increase in DSTR, which Pineda and associates,[24] the authors of the study, attributed to the implementation of a more sensitive antibody screening method and a decrease in the average length of stay for inpatients.[24] Interestingly, the current rates of observed reactions and DHTR-to-DSTR ratio in their study are similar to those reported by Ness and colleagues[9] in 1990 (Table 33.7).

■ Severe Delayed Hemolytic Transfusion Reactions in Sickle Cell Disease

It is well recognized that patients with sickle cell disease (SCD) have a high rate of alloimmunization compared with other patient groups receiving multiple transfusions.[25]

Table 33.7 Incidence of Delayed Hemolytic Transfusion Reaction (DHTR) and Delayed Serologic Transfusion Reaction (DSTR)

Study	DHTR:DSTR	Incidence*
Ness et al.,[9] Johns Hopkins Hospital (January 1986–August 1987)	18:82	1:1605
Vamvakas et al.,[23] Mayo Clinic (1980–1992)	36:64	1:1899
Pineda et al.,[24] Mayo Clinic (1993–1998)	19:81	1:1300

*Incidence expressed as DHTRs and/or DSTRs per number of red blood cell units transfused.

Alloimmunization rates ranging from 17.6% to 36% have been reported in SCD.[25-31] According to the Cooperative Study of Sickle Cell Disease, the overall rate of alloimmunization was 18.6% for both pediatric and adult patients.[27] Thus, it is not surprising that the rate of DHTR encountered in SCD is higher than the frequency of DHTR in the general hospital population receiving transfusions. The frequency of DHTR in patients with SCD ranges from 4% to 22%,[26, 29, 32, 33] whereas the frequency of true, clinical DHTR in all transfused patients is only 0.04% (1 case per 2537 transfused patients)[34] to 0.1% (1 case per 854 transfused patients).[9] A continually growing number of case reports in the literature indicates that DHTR in SCD may manifest as a painful sickle cell crisis and may often be characterized by severe, life-threatening anemia.[35-39] The causes of severe DHTR in SCD are unclear and controversial.

In some anecdotal cases, patients with SCD have developed not only the alloantibodies implicated in DHTR but also warm-reacting autoantibodies.[40-43] The development of autoantibodies after alloimmunization and DHTR is not uncommon, and the clinical importance of these post-transfusion autoantibodies varies.[9, 40-50] Because autoantibodies may mimic alloantibody specificities, the actual incidence of autoimmunization after alloimmunization and DHTR may be higher than reported.[49, 50] In the patients with SCD, the severe anemia associated with DHTR appears to be due to the development of post-transfusion, pathologic autoantibodies resulting in autoimmune hemolytic anemia.[40-42] Interestingly, there are at least two cases of SCD in which preexisting autoantibodies that were clinically benign appeared to become pathologic autoantibodies after transfusion of RBCs.[51, 52] In a series of pediatric patients with SCD who received long-term RBC transfusion, 14 of 184 (7.6%) developed warm autoantibodies, 4 of whom (28.6%) had clinical hemolysis.[43]

King and associates[52] described five patients who experienced severe DHTR after preoperative exchange transfusions. Alloantibodies against E, S, Fy[a], or Jk[a] were implicated in three of the reactions, although the alloantibodies responsible for apparent DHTR in two of the cases were serologically undetectable. By monitoring the levels of hemoglobin A (transfused allogeneic donor RBCs) and hemoglobin S (autologous sickle cells), these researchers identified one patient who had a substantial loss of autologous as well as transfused donor RBCs during an apparent DHTR. King and associates[52] suggested that the phenomenon of bystander hemolysis might have played a role in the accelerated destruction of autologous RBCs in this severe hemolytic transfusion reaction.

Bystander hemolysis has been defined as the immune destruction of autologous RBCs that may occur during DHTR[52]; the mechanism is unclear. One theory has proposed that activation of complement could occur when alloantibodies react with transfused antigen-positive donor RBCs,[53, 54] leading to destruction of allogeneic and "innocent bystander" autologous red cells. Bystander hemolysis is difficult to document but may be suspected when hemoglobin and hematocrit levels measured after the transfusion reaction are lower than the pretransfusion values; these decreases suggest that there may be simultaneous destruction of transfused donor RBCs and autologous RBCs. Perhaps the most remarkable and best-documented case of bystander hemolysis was described by Polesky and Bove in 1964.[53] The patient had aplastic anemia associated with acute leukemia. Normal autologous RBC survival had been documented by in vivo survival studies using chromium 51–labeled RBCs just 1 week before transfusion. After transfusion of 300 mL of donor RBCs, the patient experienced a hemolytic transfusion reaction with clinical hemolysis due to anti-Jk[a]. RBC survival studies demonstrated that there was acute hemolysis of autologous RBCs during the reaction at a rate of 28% per day. The patient died 3 days after transfusion.

The occurrence of bystander hemolysis in DHTR has been reported in patients without SCD.[53, 55, 56] However, bystander hemolysis may actually be more prevalent in patients with SCD, because sickle cells have a regulatory defect in the formation of the complement membrane attack complex, which makes them more susceptible to complement-mediated hemolysis.[54] In fact, Garratty[34] has suggested that complement activation in these cases may be triggered not only by antibody reacting with transfused RBC antigens but also by antibody reacting with other foreign antigens (e.g., HLA, plasma proteins). Thus, the mechanism of bystander hemolysis during DHTR in patients with SCD may be similar to that of paroxysmal nocturnal hemoglobinuria (PNH), in which immune complex formation may result in hemolysis of "innocent" autologous RBCs.[53] This theory may explain the case reported by King and associates[52] in which no antibody responsible for the severe DHTR and bystander hemolysis could be detected serologically.

Some authorities have used the term *hyperhemolysis* to specifically describe DHTR in SCD in which the ongoing hemolysis of sickle cells appears to be accelerated during the course of a hemolytic transfusion reaction. For example, Win and associates[57] described two cases of hyperhemolytic transfusion reactions in SCD and speculated that the accelerated destruction of autologous sickle cells in these cases was due to hyperactive macrophages that readily sequestered both mature sickle cells and sickle reticulocytes, resulting in profound anemia.

Petz and colleagues[58] found that in five cases of hemolytic transfusion reaction in SCD, the severe anemia appeared to be due to the destruction of transfused donor RBCs coincident with suppression of erythropoiesis. They defined these findings as "the sickle cell hemolytic transfusion reaction syndrome," in which reticulocytopenia coupled with the hemolysis of transfused donor RBCs caused life-threatening anemia. In their series, none of the patients appeared to have accelerated autologous RBC destruction (i.e., bystander hemolysis) or hyperhemolysis.

Regardless of the mechanisms that may be involved, it is important to recognize that severe DHTR in a patient with SCD is not an infrequent finding and may mimic a painful sickle cell crisis. Effective treatment requires prompt diagnosis and transfusion support with appropriate antigen-negative RBCs. Steroid therapy and intravenous immune globulin infusions have been successfully used for the treatment of the most severe cases.[57, 59]

■ Prevention

The implementation of more sensitive pretransfusion antibody screening methods may have reduced the frequency of DHTR.[24, 60] Because antibody titers may diminish over time so as to fall below even sensitive antibody screening thresholds,

it is essential that records of identified antibodies be maintained for patients with clinically significant antibodies, who should also be given personal identification cards containing this information.[61, 62] One must understand that patients diagnosed with DSTR are at risk for severe hemolytic transfusion reaction (i.e., DHTR) with future transfusions and must receive donor blood that is negative for the antigens corresponding to the implicated alloantibodies.[3, 9]

The high rate of alloimmunization and the high risk of DHTR in SCD appears to be due, at least in part, to the disparity in antigen frequencies between the African American recipient and white donor populations (Table 33.8).[26] For example, approximately 70% of white donors have the C antigen, which may cause alloimmunization when transfused to African American recipients, who are most likely to be C negative (approximately 73% of African Americans are C negative). Consequently, increasing the number of African American blood donations, particularly if the donations could be linked to patients with SCD requiring transfusion support, might be of benefit.

Most workers would agree that patients with SCD should undergo extensive phenotyping (e.g., Rh antigens [CEce], K1, MNSs, Fy[a], Fy[b], Jk[a], Jk[b]) so that antibodies that the patients may potentially produce can be easily discerned.[63, 64] Having extensive or complete phenotypes on file for patients with SCD who require multiple transfusions is particularly advantageous in resolving complex antibody problems.

Prophylactic antigen matching of donor RBCs with the recipient's complete phenotype has been advocated for patients with SCD in an effort to reduce the rate of alloimmunization and severe DHTR.[27, 31, 63, 65] Various transfusion protocols, which differ in the number of antigens considered for prophylactic matching, have been proposed. Perhaps the most widely known protocol is one in which donor blood is routinely matched with the recipient's phenotype for C, E, and K RBC antigens.[27, 31, 65] That is, patients who are C-, E-, and K-negative are given donor blood lacking those antigens. Of course, this protocol may prevent alloimmunization to these specific antigens but does not prevent alloimmunization to other blood group specificities that are perhaps more likely to be implicated in DHTR, such as anti-Jk[a] or anti-Jk[b].

Table 33.8 Comparison of Antigen Frequencies in White and African American Populations

Antigen	Frequency in Whites (%)[*]	Frequency in African Americans (%)
C	70	27
E	30	22
c	80	96
e	97	98
K	10	3
Fy[a]	67	11
Fy[b]	80	23
S	55	31
s	89	97
Jk[a]	75	91
Jk[b]	75	43

[*](%) = Percent frequency of antigen.

Ness[65] has proposed that prophylactic antigen matching should be considered only for a patient who has developed one or more RBC alloantibodies, thereby indicating that the patient is a "responder" and may be at greater risk for further alloimmunization and DHTR with subsequent RBC transfusions. This protocol is particularly appealing, because it avoids unnecessary prophylactic antigen matching of donor blood for the approximate 70% of patients with SCD who do not become alloimmunized even after multiple transfusions.

Prophylactic antigen matching may prevent some cases of DHTR. Nevertheless, even protocols calling for extensive prophylactic antigen matching cannot prevent the severe hemolytic reactions due to unusual alloantibody specificities or the development of pathologic warm autoantibodies.[52, 64–68]

In the future, DHTR may be prevented, at least in some instances, by the use of artificial blood substitutes or more sensitive antibody screening methods.[69] The potential use of blood substitutes in SCD rather than preoperative RBC transfusions is particularly intriguing. Research on the pathophysiology of DHTR and the mechanisms and inhibition of in vivo hemolysis using suitable animal models may also provide some answers for the prevention and treatment of DHTR in humans.[70]

REFERENCES

1. Mollison PL: Antibody-mediated destruction of red cells. Clin Immunol Newsl 1985;6:100–103.
2. Mollison PL: Blood Transfusion in Clinical Medicine, 9th ed. Oxford, Black Scientific, 1993, pp 434–542.
3. Shirey RS, Ness PM: New concepts of delayed hemolytic transfusion reactions. In Nance J (ed): Clinical and Basic Science Aspects of Immunohematology . Arlington, VA, American Association of Blood Banks, 1991, pp 179–197.
4. Rauner RA, Tanaka KR: Hemolytic transfusion reactions associated with the Kidd system antibody (JKᵃ). N Engl J Med 1967;276:1486.
5. Kurtides ES, Salkin MS, Widen AL: Hemolytic reaction due to anti-Jkb. JAMA 1966;197:816.
6. Solanki D, McCurdy PR: Delayed hemolytic transfusion reactions: An often missed entity. JAMA 1978;239:729–731.
7. Holland PV, Wallerstein RO: Delayed hemolytic transfusion reaction with acute renal failure. JAMA 1968;204:1007–1008.
8. Pineda AA, Taswell HF, Brzica SM Jr: Delayed hemolytic transfusion reaction: An immunologic hazard of blood transfusion. Transfusion 1978;18:1–7.
9. Ness PM, Shirey RS, Thoman SK, Buck SA: The differentiation of delayed serologic and delayed hemolytic transfusion reactions: Incidence, long-term serologic findings and logical significance. Transfusion 1990;30:688–693.
10. Boorman KE, Dodd BE, Loutit JF, Mollison PL: Some results of transfusion of blood to recipients with 'cold' agglutinins. BMJ 1946;i:751.
11. Fudenberg H, Allen FJ Jr: Transfusion reactions in the absence of demonstrable incompatibility. N Engl J Med 1957;256:1180–1184.
12. Walker PC, Jennings ER, Monroe C: Hemolytic transfusion reactions after the administration of apparently compatible blood. Am J Clin Pathol 1965;44:193–197.
13. Moore SB, Taswell HF, Pineda AA, Sonnenberg CL: Delayed hemolytic transfusion reactions: Evidence of the need for an improved pretransfusion compatibility test. Am J Clin Pathol 1980;74:94–97.
14. Taswell HF, Pineda AA, Moore SB: Hemolytic transfusion reactions: Frequency and clinical and laboratory aspects. In Bell CA (ed): A Seminar on Immune-Mediated Red Cell Destruction. Washington, DC, American Association of Blood Banks, 1981, pp 71–92.
15. Taddie SJ, Barrasso C, Ness PM: A delayed transfusion reaction caused by anti-K6. Transfusion 1982;22:68–69.
16. Patten E, Reddi CR, Riglin H, Edwards J: Delayed hemolytic transfusion reaction caused by a primary immune response. Transfusion 1982;22:248–250.
17. Davey RJ, Gustafson M, Holland PV: Accelerated immune red cell destruction in the absence of serologically detectable alloantibodies. Transfusion 1980;20:348–353.
18. Baldwin ML, Barasso C, Ness PM, Garratty G: A clinically significant erythrocyte antibody detectable only by survival studies. Transfusion 1983;23:40–44.
19. Salama A, Mueller-Eckhardt C: Delayed hemolytic transfusion reactions: Evidence for complement activation involving allogeneic and autologous red cells. Transfusion 1984;24:188–193.
20. Chaplin H Jr: The implication of red cell-bound complement and delayed hemolytic transfusion reactions [editorial]. Transfusion 1984;24:185–187.
21. Salama H, Mueller-Eckhardt C: Binding of fluid phase C3b to non-sensitized bystander human red cells: A model for in vivo effects of complement activation on the blood cells. Transfusion 1985;25:528–534.
22. Devine DV: Complement. In Anderson KC, Ness PM (eds): Scientific Basis of Transfusion Medicine: Implications for Clinical Practice, 2nd ed. Philadelphia, WB Saunders, 2000, pp 107–119.
23. Vamvakas EC, Pineda AA, Reisner R, et al: The differentiation of delayed hemolytic and delayed serologic transfusion reactions: Incidence and predictors of hemolysis. Transfusion 1995;35:26–32.
24. Pineda AA, Vamvakas EC, Gorden LD, et al: Trends in the incidence of delayed hemolytic and delayed serologic transfusion reactions. Transfusion 1999;10:1097–1103.
25. Shirey RS, King KE: Alloimmunization to the blood group antigens. In Anderson KC, Ness PM (eds): Scientific Basis of Transfusion Medicine: Implications for Clinical Practice, 2nd ed. Philadelphia, WB Saunders, 2000, pp 393–400.
26. Vichinsky EP, Earles PNP, Johnson RA, et al: Alloimmunization in sickle cell anemia and transfusion of racially unmatched blood. N Engl J Med 1990;322:1617–1621.
27. Rosse WF, Gallagher D, Kinney TR, et al: Cooperative study of sickle cell disease: Transfusion and alloimmunization in sickle cell disease. Blood 1990;76:1431–1437.
28. Orlina AR, Unger PJ, Koshy M: Post-transfusion alloimmunization in the patients with sickle cell disease. Am J Hematol 1978;5(2):101–106.
29. Cox JV, Steane E, Cunningham G, et al: Risk of alloimmunization and delayed hemolytic transfusion reactions in the patients with sickle cell disease. Arch Intern Med 1998;148:2485–2489.
30. Ambruso DR, Githens JH, Alcorn R, et al: Experience with donors matched for minor blood group antigens in the patients with sickle cell anemia who are receiving chronic transfusion therapy. Transfusion 1987;27:94–98.
31. Rosse WF, Telen M, Ware RE: Transfusion Support for the Patients with Sickle Cell Disease. Bethesda, MD, American Association of Blood Banks Press, 1998, pp 73–92.
32. Koshy M, Burd L, Wallace D, et al: Prophylactic red cell transfusions in pregnant patients with sickle cell disease: A randomized cooperative study. N Engl J Med 1988;319:1447–1452.
33. Diamond WJ, Brown FI Jr, Bitterman P, et al: Delayed hemolytic transfusion reaction presenting as sickle-cell crisis. Ann Intern Med 1980;93:231–234.
34. Garratty G: Severe reactions associated with transfusion of patients with sickle cell disease [editorial]. Transfusion 1977;37:357–361.
35. Heddle NM, Sortar RL, O'Hoski P, et al: A prospective study to determine the frequency and clinical significance of alloimmunization post-transfusion. Br J Haematol 1995;91:1000–1005.
36. Rao KR, Patel AR: Delayed hemolytic transfusion reactions in the sickle cell anemia. South Med J 1989;9:1034–1036.
37. Kalyanaraman M, Heidemann SM, Sarnaik AP, et al: Anti-s antibody-associated delayed hemolytic transfusion reaction in the patients with sickle cell anemia. J Pediatr Hematol Oncol 1999;21:70–73.
38. Fabron JA, Moreira JG, Bordin JO: Delayed hemolytic transfusion reaction presenting as a painful crisis in a patient with sickle anemia. Rev Paul Med 1999;117:385–389.
39. Milner PF, Squires JE, Larison PJ, et al: Posttransfusion crises in the sickle cell anemia: Role of delayed hemolytic reactions to transfusion. South Med J 1985;78:1462–1469.
40. Sosler SD, Perkins JT, Saporito C, et al: Severe autoimmune hemolytic anemia induced by the transfusion in two alloimmunized patients with sickle cell disease [abstract]. Transfusion 1989;29(Suppl):495.
41. Chaplin H Jr, Zarkowsky HS: Combined sickle cell disease and autoimmune hemolytic anemia [abstract]. Arch Intern Med 1981;141:1091.

42. Reed W, Walker P, Haddix T, Perkins HA: Acute anemia events in sickle cell disease. Transfusion 2000;40:267–273.

43. Castellino SM, Combs MR, Zimmerman MA, et al: Erythrocyte autoantibodies in the pediatric patient with sickle cell disease receiving transfusion therapy: Frequency, characteristics and significance. Br J Haematol 1999;104:189–194.

44. Chan D, Poole GD, Binney M, et al: Severe intravascular hemolysis due to autoantibodies stimulated by the blood transfusion. Immunohematology 1996;12:80–83.

45. Worlledge SM: The interpretation of a positive direct antiglobulin test. Br J Haematol 1978;39:157–162.

46. Lalezari P, Talleyrand NP, Wenz B, et al: Development of direct antiglobulin reaction accompanying alloimmunization in a patient with Rh^d (D, category III) phenotype. Vox Sang 1975;28:19–24.

47. Cook IA: Primary rhesus immunization of male volunteers. Br J Haematol 1971;20:369–375.

48. Beard MEJ, Pemberton J, Blagdon J, et al: Rh immunization following incompatible blood transfusion and a possible long-term complication of anti-D immunoglobulin therapy. J Med Genet 1971;8:317–320.

49. Issitt PD, Zellner DC, Rolih SD, et al: Autoantibodies mimicking alloantibodies. Transfusion 1977;17:531–538.

50. Issitt PD, Pavone BG: Critical re-examination of the specificity of auto-anti-Rh antibodies in the patients with a positive direct antiglobulin test. Br J Haematol 1978;38:63–74.

51. Petz LD, Garrantty G: Acquired Immune Hemolytic Anemia. New York, Churchill Livingstone, 1980, pp 318–320.

52. King KE, Shirey RS, Lankiewicz MW, et al: Delayed hemolytic transfusion reactions in sickle cell disease. Transfusion 1997;37:376–381.

53. Polesky HF, Bove JR: A fatal hemolytic transfusion reaction with acute autohemolysis. Transfusion 1964;4;285–292.

54. Wiener AS: Hemolytic reactions following transfusions of blood of the homologous group. II: Further observations on the role of the property Rh, particularly in cases without demonstrable iso-antibodies. Arch Pathol 1941;32:227–250.

55. Petz LD: The expanding boundaries of transfusion medicine. In Nance LST (ed): Clinical and Basic Science Aspects of Immunohematology. Arlington, VA, American Association of Blood Banks, 1991, pp 73–113.

56. Test ST, Woolworth VS: Defective regulation of complement by the sickle erythrocyte: Evidence for defect in the control of membrane attack complex formation. Blood 1994;83:842–852.

57. Win N, Doughty H, Telfer P, et al: Hyperhemolytic transfusion reaction in sickle cell disease. Transfusion 2001;41:323–328.

58. Petz LD, Calhoun L, Shulman IA, et al: The sickle cell hemolytic transfusion reaction syndrome. Transfusion 1977;37:382–392.

59. Cullis JO, Win N, Dudley JM, Kaye T: Post-transfusion hyperhaemolysis in a patient with sickle cell disease: Use of steroids and intravenous immunoglobulin to prevent further red cell destruction. Vox Sang 1995;69:355–357.

60. Bunker ML, Thomas CI, Geyer SJ: Optimizing pretransfusion antibody detection and identification: A parallel, blinded comparison of tube PEG, solid phase, and automated methods. Transfusion 2001;41:621–626.

61. Taswell HF, Pineda AA, Moore SB: Hemolytic transfusion reactions: Frequency and clinical and laboratory aspects. In Bell CA (ed): A Seminar on Immune-Mediated Red Cell Destruction. Washington, DC, American Association of Blood Banks, 1981, pp 71–92.

62. Schonewille H, Haak HL, van Zijl AM: RBC antibody persistence. Transfusion 2000;40:1127–1131.

63. Tahhan HR, Holbrook CT, Braddy LR, et al: Antigen matched donor blood in the transfusion management of patients with sickle cell disease. Transfusion 1994;34:562–569.

64. Vichinsky EP, Luban NLC, Wright E, et al: Prospective RBC phenotype matching in a stroke prevention trial in sickle cell anemia: A multicenter transfusion trial. Transfusion 2001;41:1086–1092.

65. Ness PM: To match or not to match: The question for chronically transferred patients with sickle cell anemia [editorial]. Transfusion 1994;34:558–560.

66. Strupp A, Cash K, Uehlinger J: Difficulties in identifying antibodies in the Dombrock blood group system in multiply alloimmunized patients. Transfusion 1998;38:1022–1025.

67. Campbell SA, Shirey RS, King KE, Ness PM: An acute hemolytic transfusion reaction due to anti-IH in a patient with sickle cell disease. Transfusion 2000;40:828–831.

68. Callahan DL, Kennedy MS, Ranalli MA, et al: Delayed hemolytic transfusion reaction caused by antibody detected by only solid phase technique [abstract]. Transfusion 2000;40(Suppl):113S.

69. Winslow RM: Red cell substitutes. In Anderson KC, Ness PM (eds): Scientific Basis of Transfusion Medicine: Implications for Clinical Practice, 2nd ed. Philadelphia, WB Saunders, 2000, pp 588–598.

70. Ness PM, Shirey RS, Weinstein MH, King KE: An animal model for delayed hemolytic transfusion reactions. Transfusion Med Rev 2001;16:305–317.

Chapter 34

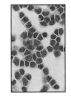

Febrile, Allergic, and Other Noninfectious Transfusion Reactions

Karen S. Roush

Transfusion reactions have been found to occur during or within 24 hours of transfusion for approximately 2% of units.[1] With an incidence of 1 in 50 units of blood products, transfusion reactions are important not only because they can lead to adverse outcomes for patients but also because of the blood product loss incurred when transfusion is discontinued upon recognition of reactions. Although it is appropriate to discontinue transfusions upon recognition of most transfusion reactions, measures may be taken to prevent reactions initially and thereby decrease product loss. In this chapter, noninfectious, nonhemolytic transfusion reactions are discussed in terms of their definition, manifestation, prevalence, pathophysiology (when known), diagnosis, treatment, and prevention. These types of reactions include febrile nonhemolytic transfusion reaction, allergic transfusion reaction, post-transfusion purpura, transfusion-related acute lung injury, circulatory overload, iron overload, and other miscellaneous types of reactions (Table 34.1).

All reactions must be documented in the patient's chart,[2] and reports of all acute transfusion reactions, with the exception of mild allergic reactions and circulatory overload, must include a formal transfusion reaction evaluation.[3] At a minimum, transfusion reaction assessments should include collection of a post-transfusion serum sample, return to the transfusion service of any remaining blood product and associated tubing, and clerical check of the patient's armband with the patient's identification associated with the issued unit.[3] A post-transfusion urine specimen examined for the presence of free hemoglobin and communication to the transfusion service of any intravenous solution that may have been transfused with the blood product may also yield information necessary for the accurate assignment of reaction type.

■ Febrile Transfusion Reactions

Definition/Manifestations/Prevalence

Febrile nonhemolytic transfusion reaction (FNHTR) is defined as a temperature rise of at least 1°C occurring with or without chills in association with transfusion or shortly thereafter (up to 4 hours)[4] that is not attributable to other causes including hemolysis or underlying disease. One study found that chills occurred in approximately 58% of patients.[5]

The incidence of FNHTR during or after receipt of an allogeneic nonleukoreduced red blood cell unit is approximately 0.5% to 1.4%,[6, 7] and FNHTR has been found to constitute approximately 43% to 75% of all transfusion reactions.[1, 6] A 15% recurrence rate in patients who have experienced an initial FNHTR has also been documented.[7]

Pathophysiology

See Figure 34.1. FNHTRs are thought to be caused by white blood cells, white blood cell antibodies, or cytokines elaborated by white blood cells, infused with blood products.[4, 5, 8–14] Granulocyte[5, 9, 10, 15–17] and human leukocyte antigen 5 (HLA5)[15, 17] antibodies have been implicated in these reactions. In one study of 40 patients with FNHTR, 100% were found to have alloantibodies to granulocytes,[5] lymphocytes, or platelets, with HLA antibodies being the most common and granulocyte antibodies the least common.[5, 15] Cytokines including interleukin-1 (IL-1), IL-6, IL-8, and tumor necrosis factor α (TNF-α) have been found to accumulate during storage in platelets, but when these products are leukoreduced before storage, the levels are quite low and do not increase during storage.[18, 19] Some febrile reactions may represent immune responses to infused substances, such as IL-6, which has been found to be elevated in patients who experience an FNHTR.[20, 21]

Table 34.1 Febrile, Allergic, and Other Noninfectious Transfusion Reactions

Reaction	Incidence	Pathophysiology	Symptoms	Treatment	Prevention
Febrile nonhemolytic transfusion reaction (FNHTR)	0.5%–1.4% of nonleuko-reduced red blood cell transfusions with a 15% recurrence rate 43%–75% of all transfusion reactions	Infused white cells, white cell antibodies, or cytokines elaborated by either donor or recipient white cells	Fever and/or chills in absence of other causes of fever	Discontinue transfusion Antipyretics Supportive care	Antipyretics Prestorage leukoreduced blood products, although this does not ameliorate all FNHTR reactions
Uncomplicated allergic transfusion reactions	1%–3% of transfusions 45% of all transfusion reactions	Preformed immunoglobulin E (IgE) antibody directed against soluble donor antigens	Local or diffuse urticaria	Discontinue transfusion Administer antihistamines If urticaria abates, transfusion may be restarted	Pretransfusion antihistamine administration
Anaphylactoid reactions	1%–3% of all transfusion reactions	Subclass, allotypic, or specific anti-IgA in patients who have demonstrable and often normal levels of IgA Rarely, preformed antibodies to other proteins deficient in the recipient	Typically less severe version of anaphylactic reaction (see below)	Discontinue transfusion Antihistamine administration Subcutaneous, intramuscular, or intravenous epinephrine if needed Supportive care	Depends on severity of reactions and etiology May require avoidance of all plasma-containing products as in anaphylactic reactions (see below) Reaction may be prevented by pretransfusion anti-histamine administration
Anaphylaxis	0.002%–0.005%/transfused product	Preformed anti-IgA antibodies in IgA-deficient individuals Rarely, preformed antibodies to other proteins deficient in the recipient	Severe hypotension May also present with chills, fever, nausea, vomiting, diarrhea, and/or urticaria	Discontinue transfusion Subcutaneous, intramuscular, or intravenous epinephrine Antihistamine administration Supportive care	Avoidance of all plasma-containing products unless collected from a known IgG-deficient donor Stringently washed red blood cell and platelet products
Post-transfusion purpura	Rare In excess of 200 cases reported	Transfusion of donor platelets with a platelet antigen lacking in the recipient. This antigen is commonly human platelet-specific alloantigen 1a (HPA-1a). A poorly described innocent bystander phenomenon is thought to lead to recipient platelet destruction.	Severe thrombocytopenia and associated purpura occurring 1–2 weeks after transfusion	Intravenous immunoglobulin Plasma exchange Corticosteriods Avoidance of additional platelet transfusion if possible Supportive care as required	Future transfusion should consist of platelets negative for the antigen against which the antibody is directed (i.e., HPA-1a antigen–negative units)

Reaction	Frequency	Cause	Clinical Manifestations	Treatment	Comments
Transfusion-related acute lung injury (TRALI)	Rare	Infusion of donor antibodies reactive against recipient white cells—most common. Infusion of donor granulocytes to which recipient antibodies are reactive—uncommon. Both of the preceding mechanisms lead to pulmonary leukoagglutinates and resultant typical symptoms.	Respiratory distress manifested radiographically by the presence of bilateral pulmonary infiltrates. Symptoms may also include chills, fever, increased respiratory rate, cough, and tachycardia.	Supportive care only. No specific therapy indicated	Typically, TRALI is a donor-specific phenomenon in which a specific recipient has essentially no risk of recurrence. These donors should be identified and deferred from donating plasma products. If the reaction is thought or proved to be mediated by recipient antibody, provision of leukocyte-containing products should be avoided.
Circulatory overload	May complicate up to 1 in 100 transfusions	Volume infusion that cannot be effectively processed by the recipient because of either high rates and volumes of infusion or underlying heart and pulmonary pathology	Dyspnea, orthopnea, cough, tachycardia, hypertension	Cessation of transfusion or slowed rate of infusion. Diuretics. Oxygen if necessary. Other supportive care as required.	Vigilant assessment of patient's input and output. Slow rates of infusion. Pretransfusion and/or intratransfusion diuretic administration
Iron overload	Unknown	Iron accumulation in liver, heart, and pancreas	Hepatic, cardiac (including arrhythmias), and pancreatic disease	No effective therapy once symptomatic	Iron chelation therapy in chronically transfused patients

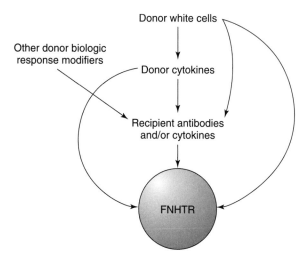

Figure 34.1 Proposed mechanisms leading to febrile nonhemolytic transfusion reactions (FNHTRs).

Cytokines, increased storage time, and white blood cell concentration have all been shown to correlate positively with FNHTR,[13, 14, 22, 23] and it has been known for some time that bedside leukoreduction filtration does not affect the incidence of FNHTR in platelet transfusions.[24, 25] For all of these reasons, leukoreduction of blood products, particularly before storage, has long shown beneficial results as a preventive intervention.[9] Since the Food and Drug Administration (FDA) Blood Products Advisory Committee recommended universal leukoreduction (ULR) in 1998, several collection facilities and hospitals have converted to ULR. Because some FNHTRs are attributed to donor white blood cells or cytokines, a drop in the rate of FNHTR was expected.

At least one large teaching hospital has demonstrated no statistically significant difference in the rate of transfusion reactions when nonleukoreduced versus leukoreduced units were provided.[26] This study compared the rate of FNHTR at Barnes-Jewish Hospital, St Louis, after red blood cell transfusion for 1 year before implementation of prestorage ULR with the rate in a 6-month period after implementation of hospitalwide leukoreduction. Of 31,543 units transfused in 1999 before ULR, 39 or 0.12% of red blood cell transfusions were associated with FNHTR. In the first 6 months of 2000, of 16,093 units, 13 or 0.08% were associated with FNHTR, yielding a statistically insignificant p value of .33.[26] Another study found differences in prestorage and poststorage leukoreduction FHNTR rates of 1.1% and 2.2%, respectively.[27]

In addition to recipient white blood cell antibody–mediated FNHTR are reactions ascribed to passive transfer of white blood cell antibodies. In one case, anti-HLA antibodies were found to be incompatible with a prior donor's bystander white blood cells in the same patient, so-called interdonor incompatibility.[28]

Diagnosis

The diagnosis of FNHTR is initially made by the recognition of newly developed fever or chills, or both, in a recipient during or shortly after transfusion. Upon recognition of fever in a recipient, the transfusion should be discontinued and a transfusion reaction evaluation should be initiated, with the immediate goal of assessing a possible hemolytic transfusion

reaction. It is important to note that patients who are in the midst of a multiunit transfusion sequence could be reacting to a prior transfusion, if the prior transfusion occurred within 4 hours of the reaction. For this reason, all prior transfused units (within approximately 4 hours) should be included in the transfusion reaction evaluation. To avoid confusion, it is recommended that patients receive transfusions during an afebrile period. This may not always be possible, and differentiating fever secondary to underlying disease from FNHTR or other transfusion reaction associated with fever may not always be possible. In any case, a transfusion reaction evaluation should be initiated for temperature increases greater than 1°C. As an apparent oxymoron, patients who receive pretransfusion antipyretics may have chills only and thereby manifest a FNHTR without fever.

The differential diagnosis of acute febrile transfusion reaction includes hemolytic transfusion reactions, reactions to bacterially contaminated blood products, and fever only temporally related to transfusion in addition to FNHTR.

Treatment

When patients manifest fever or chills, or both, during transfusion, the transfusion should be discontinued immediately, an intravenous line should be maintained, and a formal transfusion reaction assessment should be initiated. Fever secondary to FNHTR usually responds to antipyretics such as acetaminophen. Severe shaking chills may rarely necessitate meperidine administration. These symptoms resolve with or without treatment and do not typically lead to additional or long-term adverse sequelae.

Prevention/Recurrence

Pretransfusion antipyretic administration may be beneficial in the prevention of recurrent FNHTR. One concern about this strategy is that fever associated with other types of reactions, that is, hemolytic transfusion reactions and reactions to bacterially contaminated products, may be masked.

Prior to the availability of leukocyte-reduced products, washing red blood cells was a method commonly employed for the prevention of recurrent FNHTR.[12, 29] And at one point, microaggregate filtration was postulated as a method to reduce granulocytes, and thereby FNHTR, in red blood cell units.[30, 31] That was a short-lived method that did not become common practice.

The rate of FNHTR with platelet transfusions may be positively correlated with storage time because of accrual of cytokines including TNF-α, IL-1, and IL-6.[13] Provision of blood products leukoreduced in the early storage period may lead to fewer reactions of this type.

■ Allergic Reactions

Allergic reactions constitute a large proportion of all transfusion reactions. One large study showed that these types of reactions accounted for approximately 45% of all transfusion reactions.[1] Broadly, allergic transfusion reactions may be categorized into a number of reaction types on an overlapping spectrum: (1) uncomplicated allergic reactions consisting of localized or diffuse urticaria, (2) anaphylactoid allergic reactions, and (3) anaphylactic allergic reactions. Anaphylactic reactions have a high potential for adverse outcomes including death; they require immediate recognition and intervention and avoidance of virtually all plasma-containing products. At the other end of the spectrum, an uncomplicated allergic reaction consists only of urticaria (by definition). In addition, there are reactions falling between these two ends of the spectrum that are termed anaphylactoid reactions.

Anaphylaxis/Anaphylactoid Reactions

Definition/Manifestations/Prevalence

Anaphylactic transfusion reactions are characterized by hypotension, typically severe, and are often commonly associated with chills, fever, bronchospasm or dyspnea, nausea, vomiting, diarrhea, and urticaria.[32–38] These severe reactions may occur after infusion of a very small volume (<10 mL) of blood product,[38] and many people found to have anti–immunoglobulin A (anti-IgA) give no history of prior blood exposure.[34] Of note is that anaphylactic reactions have been reported to occur in recipients at a rate of 1 in 20,000 to 1 in 47,000 (0.002% to 0.005%) per transfused product,[39] considerably less than the sector of the population thought to be at risk (0.08%).[40] Canadian figures are even smaller, with an anaphylactic transfusion reaction incidence of 0.00013% per unit transfused.[41] Between 1976 and 1985, three deaths were attributed to transfusion-associated anaphylaxis in the United States.[42]

Anaphylactoid reactions are generally less severe than anaphylaxis. This is not an absolute, however, because severe and even fatal reactions have been reported in patients with detectable levels of IgA and concurrent specific anti-IgA.[32, 39, 43, 44]

Pathophysiology

Anaphylactic reactions are most commonly due to preformed, class-specific, recipient anti-IgA to infused donor IgA proteins in patients with IgA deficiency.[39] See Figure 34.2. However, other case reports have linked anaphylactic reaction to HLA-associated antibodies in platelet transfusion,[45] anti-C4 in a C4-deficient patient,[46] and antihaptoglobin in an ahaptoglobinemic patient.[47] One study involving 32,376 random blood donors found an IgA deficiency incidence of 0.26% (1 in 372).[40] IgA deficiency with associated

anti-IgA in the same study was found to occur at a rate of 0.08% (1 in 1200).[40] From this one may infer that the incidence of anti-IgA in IgA-deficient donors is approximately 31% (0.26/0.08).

Anaphylactoid reactions are typically associated with subclass, allotypic, or specific anti-IgA in patients who have demonstrable and often normal levels of IgA.[32, 39, 40, 43, 44] It is difficult to identify patients who may have a specific anti-IgA because that would involve a seemingly infinite number of specific IgA proteins. These types of reactions may also be due to other transfused products found in donor units, such as peanut allergen transfused to patients who may have peanut allergy.

Diagnosis

Anaphylaxis/anaphylactoid reactions should be recognized immediately when a patient presents with the symptoms just described. When anaphylaxis related to blood transfusion is suspected, administration of any additional plasma-containing blood product should be avoided if possible until an appropriate diagnostic evaluation can be performed. Differential diagnosis of transfusion-related anaphylaxis includes angiotensin-converting enzyme (ACE) inhibitor transfusion-related reactions (discussed later in this chapter), transfusion-related acute lung injury (TRALI, also discussed later), and other events unrelated to transfusion, including myocardial infarction or pulmonary embolus (Fig. 34.3). When anaphylaxis occurs in association with blood transfusion, IgA deficiency with concomitant anti-IgA must be investigated. For a firm diagnosis, this requires demonstration of recipient anti-IgA.[32, 34–36, 39, 41, 44, 48, 49]

The initial investigation may include nephelometry for the detection of IgA. Demonstration of IgA by this method effectively negates a diagnosis of anaphylaxis related to anti-IgA. If no IgA is detected, additional studies should be performed because some patients have IgA levels that are below the limit of detection by nephelometry. To detect anti-IgA in these cases, passive hemagglutination assays (PHA) utilizing IgA-coated red blood cells are performed. Most often, the IgA used to coat these red blood cells is from patients with multiple myeloma whose monoclonal protein is IgA.[32, 34–36, 39–41, 43, 44, 48–50]

Treatment

In addition to immediate discontinuation of product infusion, treatment of anaphylactic reactions related to transfusion is the same as that of anaphylaxis from other causes. Such treatment includes antihistamine; subcutaneous, intramuscular, or intravenous epinephrine; and other supportive care as required.

Prevention

Prevention of anaphylactic reactions in patients who are determined to be IgA deficient with anti-IgA antibodies requires avoidance of transfusion with plasma-containing products or transfusion of such products acquired from IgA-deficient donors.[40] Most often these donors are identified by screening immunodiffusion methods[51] followed by a confirming passive hemagglutination inhibition assay (PHIA).[40, 44, 50, 52] This assay differs from PHA by the addition of a known amount of reagent anti-IgA and the observation of inhibition of agglutination, which is due to the presence of donor IgA; that is, no agglutination inhibition would be observed in donors who lacked IgA.[32, 40, 50, 53] It is important to use a sensitive method

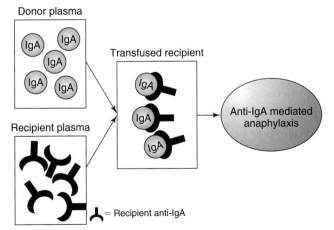

Figure 34.2   Proposed mechanism of anti–immunoglobulin A (anti-IgA)–mediated anaphylaxis. Note that preformed anti-IgA antibody, in addition to lack of IgA, is required for this response.

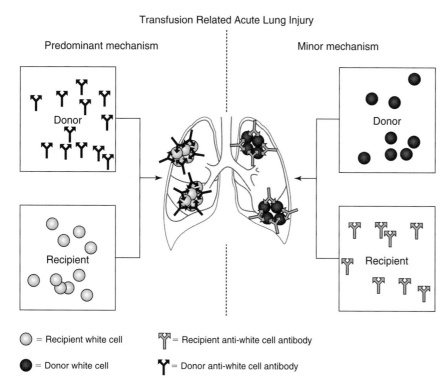

Transfusion Related Acute Lung Injury

Predominant mechanism

Minor mechanism

Donor

Recipient

Donor

Recipient

○ = Recipient white cell   Y = Recipient anti-white cell antibody

● = Donor white cell   Y = Donor anti-white cell antibody

Figure 34.3 Major and minor pathways leading to transfusion-associated acute lung injury (TRALI).

such as PHIA to confirm IgA deficiency in donors. Case reports show that some patients found to be at risk for IgA-deficient anaphylactic reaction were transfused with presumptive IgA-deficient plasma containing products that led to anaphylactic reactions. Retesting of these products by more sensitive methods showed that they contained low levels of IgA.[40]

When red blood cell transfusion is indicated for IgA-deficient patients at risk for anaphylaxis, units may be autologous, washed allogeneic, frozen deglycerolized allogeneic, or IgA-deficient donor units. Because washed red blood cells have been shown to contain low or undetectable amounts of IgA,[19, 36, 37] they are commonly used for these patients simply because they are the easiest to acquire.

Skin-Restricted Allergic Reactions

Definition/Manifestations/Prevalence

These types of reactions, which occur in up to 3% of all transfusions,[54] are recognized by a localized or confluent red, raised rash or itching, or both, collectively termed urticaria. For a reaction to be classified as uncomplicated urticaria, there may be no additional symptoms such as asthma-like attacks, coughing, difficulty in breathing, or other symptoms, apart from urticaria, associated with anaphylactoid or anaphylactic reactions.

Pathophysiology

These reactions presumably occur as a result of cutaneous hypersensitivity in which the recipient has been previously sensitized to soluble allergens found in the donor unit.[54] It is important to note that all allergic reactions occur within a spectrum and that reactions that begin as urticaria may develop into anaphylactoid or anaphylactic reactions, although this is rare.

Diagnosis

Diagnosis of skin-restricted allergy is straightforward and requires recognition of a rash with associated itching but without additional symptoms. The rash resolves with discontinuance of transfusion or antihistamine therapy, or both.

Treatment

Treatment for uncomplicated urticaria requires discontinuation of the blood product infusion and provision of antihistamines. If the symptoms resolve, the transfusion may be restarted, and a formal transfusion reaction assessment is not required. If the symptoms do not regress or if they progress during treatment or upon continuance of the transfusion, the transfusion should be stopped and not restarted.

Prevention

Prevention of urticarial reactions includes pretransfusion and intratransfusion treatment with antihistamines. If this treatment is not effective or if repeated reactions of increasing severity occur, washed cellular products may be beneficial.

In general, the rate of allergic reactions is not thought to be affected by leukoreduction. In fact, allergic reactions were not found to be statistically significantly different at a large hospital when ULR was implemented. Of 31,543 nonleukoreduced red blood cell transfusions, 0.04% were associated with allergic reactions. In the 6 months after adoption of ULR, of 16,093 units leukoreduced before storage, 0.06% were associated with allergic reactions.[26]

■ Post-transfusion Purpura

Definition/Manifestations/Prevalence

Initially described by Shulman and colleagues in 1961,[55] post-transfusion purpura (PTP) consists of profound thrombocytopenia occurring 1 to 2 weeks after transfusion,[56] which makes identification of this entity difficult. Cases have also been described in which both PTP and delayed hemolytic transfusion reaction occurred simultaneously.[57, 58] Cases of PTP are quite rare, although known cases are currently in excess of 200.[38]

Pathophysiology

PTP is most commonly attributed to the effect of antibody directed against donor platelet antigens that the recipient lacks. The most common platelet alloantibody identified in patients with PTP is that against human platelet-specific alloantigen 1a (HPA-1a),[56] although others have also been identified.[57] A poorly characterized phenomenon of platelet destruction ensues that includes autologous platelets as well as donor platelets, leading to a profound thrombocytopenia. This phenomenon is commonly referred to as the "innocent bystander" effect. Possible mechanisms include nonspecific antibody adherence, soluble proteins that are taken up by recipient platelets against which an antibody has been formed, formation of autoreactive or cross-reactive antibody, and immune complex deposition onto platelet surfaces with resultant recipient platelet destruction.[38] A similar clinical picture has been associated with the passive transfer of platelet antibodies with resultant recipient thrombocytopenia.[59, 60]

Treatment

The usual treatment for this reaction is intravenous immunoglobulin (IVIG), followed by plasmapheresis in patients with a poor response to reduce the antibody and possibly soluble antigen titers.[61, 62] The mechanism of action of IVIG is not well understood but may involve reticuloendothelial blockade or nonspecific antibody adherence to the target antigen that blocks access by specific antibody. Corticosteroids, to depress immune system responsiveness, have also been used in the treatment of this disease, but they are no longer generally employed because IVIG with or without plasmapheresis is effective therapy. If PTP does not lead to death resulting from hemorrhage, it is a self-limited disease with recovery typically occurring within 4 to 5 days of therapy. Recovery may be hastened by the use of antigen-negative platelets if the specificity of the antibody has been determined and antigen-negative platelets are available.[63, 64] In general, routine allogeneic platelet transfusion is not recommended because it may exacerbate the reaction process and does not increase the platelet count.

Prevention/Recurrence

Little has been published about the recurrence or prevention of this process, although it seems prudent to avoid antigen-positive platelet transfusion in patients in whom PTP has previously occurred.

■ Transfusion-Related Acute Lung Injury

Definition/Manifestation/Prevalence

TRALI typically occurs during or within 4 hours of transfusion[65] and consists of symptoms of respiratory distress manifested radiographically by the presence of bilateral pulmonary infiltrates.[66–71] Symptoms and signs may also include chills, fever, increased respiratory rate, cough, and tachycardia.[66–71] Urticaria has been reported as an uncommon finding in these patients.[70] Thirty-one deaths related to "acute pulmonary edema" after transfusion were reported between 1976 and 1985,[42] and death is thought to complicate 5% to 7% of reactions.[16, 72] Signs include rales and generalized hypoxia that may require supportive respiratory care such as intubation.[66–71] A few reports in the early literature described pulmonary edema associated with transfusion, although in many of these cases radiographic findings were not reported or were not available.[66–70]

Pathophysiology

TRALI is thought to be the result of antibodies, typically donor, directed against white blood cell antigens. Most donors associated with this type of reaction are multiparous females or other donors who have had multiple exposures to varying HLA types.[65] These antibodies have long been thought to be directed toward granulocytic antigens, including NA2,[73] NB2,[74] and anti-5b,[75] and Popovsky and coworkers[76] found that 89% of patients with TRALI displayed granulocytic or lymphocytotoxic antibodies. The interaction of antigen and antibody leads to agglutinins trapped in the pulmonary circulation with resultant release of toxic substances and pulmonary edema.[10, 73, 75, 77, 78] In at least one reported autopsy case, these pulmonary granulocytic infiltrates and underlying alveolar damage were confirmed by light and electron microscopy.[79] Some have suggested that for this reaction to occur, patients must also have underlying pathology or circumstances, such as those seen in thrombotic thrombocytopenic purpura[74] or patients undergoing general anesthesia,[65] that predispose them to hypoxia. Bioactive lipids found in some blood products have also been implicated in the fulminant granulocytic accumulation in the lungs of patients with TRALI.[80] Yet another theory postulates that complement activation occurs with the release of anaphylatoxins that induce white blood cell entrapment in the pulmonary vasculature with resultant pulmonary edema.[81–83]

Recipient white blood cell antibodies have also been associated with TRALI when sufficient numbers of donor white blood cells have been infused,[10, 16, 84] including those in which HLA antibodies were identified.[85, 86]

Treatment

Treatment is supportive, and intubation may be required.[71] Resolution, if the reaction is not fatal, occurs in approximately 81%[65] and is usually complete within a few days (3 to 5) of onset.[66–71] The findings can usually be distinguished from those of fluid overload by the circumstances of the reactions and by the nature of the radiographic findings. Circulatory overload is typically manifested by a perihilar infiltrate, whereas that ascribed to TRALI involves a diffuse, patchy infiltrate.[71]

One case of TRALI in an adult who was not responsive to other supportive therapeutic efforts was treated successfully with extracorporeal membrane oxygenation.[87]

Prevention/Recurrence

TRALI does not typically recur in the same patient when the reaction is due to recipient antibodies. However, suspected cases of TRALI should be reported with the corresponding unit information and reaction symptoms to the collection facility. Although TRALI is a rare event, investigators have found that 18% of pregnant females have HLA antibodies, with more than half having these antibodies demonstrable up to 3 years later.[88] Antibodies identified in pregnant women include lymphocytotoxic, neutrophil-nonspecific, and neutrophil-specific antibodies.[89] Other investigators exploring the incidence of HLA antibodies in multiparous donors found that they were present in 7%.[76] At least one group has suggested that plasma-containing products (whole blood, plasma, and apheresis platelets) from multiparous donors not be used.[90] In the rarer instances in which recipient antibodies are determined to be the cause of TRALI, infusion of leukocyte-containing products should be avoided.

■ Circulatory Overload

Definition/Manifestation/Prevalence

Circulatory overload complicates up to 1 in 100 transfusions and is often unrecognized.[91] Symptoms and signs of volume overload include dyspnea, hypertension, tachycardia, and cough.

Pathophysiology

The intravascular volume may be overtaxed by either an inappropriate rate of transfusion or an inappropriate volume of transfusion in addition to other infused substances. Patients who have congestive heart failure or other heart or pulmonary disease are predisposed to these types of reactions.

Treatment

Treatment includes cessation or reduction of the rate of blood product infusion, diuretics, and other supportive therapy.

Prevention/Recurrence

Prevention depends on vigilant assessment of input and output, especially in susceptible patients. Slowed infusion rates are effective in many patients. Blood product units may be divided if the transfusion time will exceed the time allotted for infusion (>4 hours after the product has been entered). Pretransfusion and intratransfusion therapy with diuretics is also beneficial. Formal transfusion reaction assessment is not required for these types of reactions.[3]

■ Iron Overload

Iron overload is an uncommon complication that occurs after long periods of time in patients who receive red blood cell transfusions for chronic disease, most commonly sickle cell disease and thalassemia. On average, one unit of packed red blood cells contains 200 mg of iron. Chronic iron overload leads to liver, cardiac, and pancreatic disease and is prevented by iron chelation therapy (deferoxamine). Additional information regarding iron deficiency may be found in Chapter 24.

■ Other

Metabolic Derangements

Metabolic derangements, including those related to hypothermia, are most commonly observed in neonatal or rapid, large-volume transfusions. These derangements include effects of citrate toxicity with effective hypocalcemia, hyperkalemia, and hypothermia. These metabolic effects may interact synergistically to cause a variety of manifestations,[92, 93] the most severe of which include cardiac arrhythmias. Use of an FDA-approved blood warmer may help to prevent hypothermia related to infusion of a large volume of products stored below normal body temperature.

Most cases of hyperkalemia related to large-volume blood product infusion are transient, and most reactions associated with massive transfusion resolve with effective treatment of the underlying process. For neonatal transfusions, slowed infusion rates with the use of a blood warmer may prevent most reactions. For additional information regarding neonatal and pediatric transfusions, see Chapter 28.

Bedside Leukoreduction and Transfusion Reaction

Severe hypotensive reactions, which may include facial flushing, abdominal pain and nausea, loss of consciousness, respiratory distress, and shock,[94] have been noted in patients undergoing ACE inhibitor therapy who were concurrently transfused with blood products that were infused through bedside leukoreduction filters.[95–97] These reactions typically occurred approximately 10 minutes into the transfusion[98] and were usually distinguishable from other types of transfusion reactions that may occur with hypotension. The filters were subsequently noted to be primarily negatively charged,[96, 98–100] although positively charged filters have also been implicated in these types of reactions.

Several mechanisms have been proposed for this reaction phenomenon.[96, 101] The most prevalent theory involves factor XII, prekallikrein, and high-molecular-weight kininogen activation by negatively charged membranes with resultant accumulation of bradykinin and its subsequent retarded metabolism secondary to ACE inhibitor action.[94, 96, 102–104] One study found a significant difference in the half-life of des-Arg^9-bradykinin, which is an active metabolite of bradykinin also partially metabolized by ACE, between sera from patients with documented hypotensive reactions and sera from normal control subjects upon exposure in vitro to ACE inhibitor.[101] There is some evidence that this difference may be due to reduced activity of a metallopeptidase, aminopeptidase P, which is the predominant metabolic pathway for the breakdown of des-Arg^9-bradykinin.[101, 105]

Some of these reactions occur in patients who are not receiving concurrent ACE inhibitor therapy.[106] Of note, all of these reactions, whether or not they are associated with ACE inhibitor therapy, have been documented only with the use of bedside reduction filters, not with prestorage leukoreduction of blood products[104]; the theory is that bradykinin has a temporal opportunity for breakdown before infusion in an otherwise susceptible patient.

Treatment for these reactions consists of cessation of blood product transfusion and supportive care. Resolution of symptoms typically occurs shortly thereafter.[97]

Prevention of this type of reaction includes transfusion of products that are leukoreduced before storage, when available and indicated, and avoidance of transfusion of products leukoreduced at the bedside to patients who are receiving ACE inhibitor therapy.[97]

Other transfusion reactions that have been attributed to leukoreduction filters include ocular reactions, the so-called red-eye syndrome.[107] All of these reactions exhibited bilateral conjunctival injection or hemorrhage, which occurred within 1 day of transfusion and had an average duration of approximately 5 days. Other features of the reaction were eye pain, headache, periorbital edema, arthralgias, nausea, dyspnea, and rash.[107] These reactions were predominantly linked to a specific leukoreduction filter, which has since been taken off the market.

Transfusion-associated graft-versus-host disease, transfusion-induced refractoriness to platelet transfusion, and other transfusion-related immunomodulations also occur and are discussed in detail in other chapters.

Conclusion

The noninfectious, nonhemolytic transfusion reactions discussed in this chapter may lead to significant adverse sequelae and blood product loss. They are also likely to be underreported in many institutions. All of the reactions discussed, with the exception of circulatory overload and uncomplicated allergic reaction, should be evaluated with a formal transfusion reaction investigation that includes at least a clerical check and pretransfusion and post-transfusion serum sample evaluation including a direct antiglobulin test.[3] The transfusion reaction evaluation is performed primarily to assess for evidence of hemolysis; other classifications of reactions may be assigned after the absence of hemolysis has been demonstrated. In most instances the pattern of reaction strongly suggests the reaction type, although there are several overlapping symptoms.

In all cases in which transfusion is thought to be the cause of death, the FDA must be notified by phone within 24 hours after discovery and this must followed up with a written report within 7 days (21 CFR 606.170).

REFERENCES

1. Baker RJ, Moinichen SL, Nyhus LM: Transfusion reaction: a reappraisal of surgical incidence and significance. Proc Inst Med Chic 1969;27:214–215.
2. Menitove JE, Chambers LA, Gjertson DW, et al: Standard 5.18.5. In Standards for Blood Banks and Transfusion Services, 21st ed. Bethesda, Md, AABB Press, 2002.
3. Menitove JE, Chambers LA, Gjertson DW, et al: Standard 7.4.3. In Standards for Blood Banks and Transfusion Services, 21st ed. Bethesda, Md, AABB Press, 2002.
4. Brittingham TE, Chaplin H Jr: Febrile transfusion reactions caused by sensitivity to donor leukocytes and platelets. JAMA 1957;165:819–825.
5. de Rie MA, van der Plas-van Dalen CM, Engelfriet CP, von dem Borne AE: The serology of febrile transfusion reactions. Vox Sang 1985;49:126–134.
6. Ahrons S, Kissmeyer-Nielsen F: Serological investigations of 1,358 transfusion reactions in 74,000 transfusions. Dan Med Bull 1968;15:259–262.
7. Menitove JE, McElligott MC, Aster RH: Febrile transfusion reaction: what blood component should be given next? Vox Sang 1982;42:318–321.
8. Perkins HA, Payne R, Ferguson J, Wood M: Nonhemolytic febrile transfusion reactions. Quantitative effects of blood components with emphasis on isoantigenic incompatibility of leukocytes. Vox Sang 1966;11:578–600.
9. Greenwalt TJ, Gajewski M, McKenna JL: A new method for preparing buffy-coat poor blood. Transfusion 1962;2:221–229.
10. Ward HN: Pulmonary infiltrates associated with leukoagglutination transfusion reactions. Ann Intern Med 1970;73:689–694.
11. Barton JC: Nonhemolytic, noninfectious transfusion reactions. Semin Hematol 1981;18:95–121.
12. Goldfinger D, Lowe C: Prevention of adverse reactions to blood transfusion by the administration of saline-washed red blood cells. Transfusion 1981;21:277–280.
13. Muylle L, Joos M, Wouters E, et al: Increased tumor necrosis factor alpha (TNF-alpha), interleukin 1, and interleukin 6 (IL-6) levels in the plasma of stored platelet concentrates; relationship between TNF-alpha

and IL-5 levels and febrile transfusion reactions. Transfusion 1993;33:195–199.
14. Heddle NM, Klama LN, Griffith L, et al: A prospective study to identify the risk factors associated with acute reactions to platelet and red cell transfusions. Transfusion 1993;33:794–797.
15. Heinrich D, Mueller-Eckhardt C, Stier W: The specificity of leukocyte and platelet alloantibodies in sera of patients with nonhemolytic transfusion reactions. Absorption and elution studies. Vox Sang 1973;25:442–456.
16. Wolf CFW, Canale VC: Fatal pulmonary hypersensitivity reaction to HLA incompatible blood transfusion: report of a case and review of the literature. Transfusion 1976;16:135–140.
17. DeCary F, Ferner P, Giavedoni L, et al: An investigation of nonhemolytic transfusion reactions. Vox Sang 1984;46:277–285.
18. Aye MT, Palmer DS, Giulivi A, Hashemi S: Effect of filtration of platelet concentrates on the accumulation of cytokines and platelet release factors during storage. Transfusion 1995;35:117–124.
19. Yap PL, Pryde EAD, McClelland DBL: IgA content of frozen-thawed-washed red blood cells and blood products measured by radioimmunoassay. Transfusion 1982;22:36–38.
20. Boyle L, McLeskey S, Wolfson A, et al: High circulating interleukin-6 levels associated with acute transfusions reaction-cause or effect [abstract]. Blood 1991;78(Suppl 1):355.
21. Sacher RA, Boyle L, Freter CE: High circulating interleukin 6 levels associated with acute transfusion reaction: cause or effect? [letter]. Transfusion 1993;33:962.
22. Heddle NM, Klama L, Singer J, et al: The role of the plasma from platelet concentrates in transfusion reactions. N Engl J Med 1994;331:625–628.
23. Riccardi D, Raspollini E, Rebulla P, et al: Relationship of time of storage and transfusion reactions to platelet concentrates from buffy coats. Transfusion 1997;37:528–530.
24. Chambers LA, Kruskall MS, Pacini DG, Donovan LM: Febrile reactions after platelet transfusion: the effect of single versus multiple donors. Transfusion 1990;30:219–221.
25. Leukocyte reduction and ultraviolet B irradiation of platelets to prevent alloimmunization and refractoriness to platelet transfusion. The Trial to Reduce Alloimmunization to Platelets Study Group. N Engl J Med 1997;337:1861–1869.
26. Uhlmann EJ, Isgriggs E, Wallhermfechtel M, Goodnough LT: Prestorage universal WBC reduction of RBC units does not affect the incidence of transfusion reactions. Transfusion 2001;41:997–1000.
27. Federowicz I, Barrett BB, Andersen JW, et al: Characterization of reactions after transfusion of cellular blood components that are white cell reduced before storage. Transfusion 1996;36:21–28.
28. Eastlund DR, McGrath PC, Burkart P: Platelet transfusion reaction associated with interdonor HLA incompatibility. Vox Sang 1988;55:157–160.
29. Kurtz SR, Valeri DA, Melaragno AF, et al: Leukocyte-poor red blood cells prepared by the addition and removal of glycerol from red blood cell concentrates stored at 4 degrees C. Transfusion 1981;21:435–442.
30. Wenz B, Gurlinger KF, O'Toole AM, Dugan EP: Preparation of granulocyte-poor red blood cells by microaggregate filtration. Vox Sang 1980;39:282–287.
31. Wenz B: Microaggregate blood filtration and the febrile transfusion reaction. Transfusion 1983;23:95–98.
32. Vyas GN, Perkins HA, Fudenberg HH: Anaphylactoid transfusion reactions associated with anti-IgA. Lancet 1968;2:312–315.
33. Vyas GN, Fudenberg HH: Isoimmune anti-IgA causing anaphylactoid transfusion reactions. N Engl J Med 1969;280:1073–1074.
34. Schmidt AP, Taswell HF, Gleich GJ: Anaphylactic transfusion reactions associated with anti-IgA antibody. N Engl J Med 1969;280:188–193.
35. Miller WV, Holland PV, Sugarbaker E, et al: Anaphylactic reactions to IgA: a difficult transfusion problem. Am J Clin Pathol 1970;54:618–621.
36. Leikola J, Koistinen J, Lehtinen M, Virolainen M: IgA-induced anaphylactic transfusion reactions: a report of four cases. Blood 1973;42:111–119.
37. Koistinen J: Selective IgA deficiency in blood donors. Vox Sang 1975;29:192–202.
38. Vengelen-Tyler V, Brecher ME, Butch SH, et al: Noninfectious complications of blood transfusion. In AABB Technical Manual, 13th ed. Bethesda, Md, AABB Press, 1999, pp 577–600.
39. Pineda AA, Taswell HF: Transfusion reactions associated with anti-IgA antibodies: report of four cases and review of the literature. Transfusion 1975;15:10–15.

40. Sandler SG, Eckrich R, Malamut D, Mallory D: Hemagglutination assays for the diagnosis and prevention of IgA anaphylactic transfusion reactions. Blood 1994;84:2031–2035.

41. Laschinger C, Shepherd FA, Naylor DH: Anti-IgA–mediated transfusion reactions in Canada. Can Med Assoc J 1984;130:141–144.

42. Sazama K: Reports of 355 transfusion-associated deaths: 1976 through 1985. Transfusion 1990;30:583–590.

43. Strauss RA, Gloster ES, Schanfield MS, et al: Anaphylactic transfusion reaction associated with a possible anti-A2m(1). Clin Lab Haemotol 1983;5:371–377.

44. Vyas GN, Holmdahl L, Perkins HA, Fudenberg HH: Serologic specificity of human anti-IgA and its significance in transfusion. Blood 1969;34:573–581.

45. Take H, Tamura J, Sawamura M, et al: Severe anaphylactic transfusion reaction associated with HLA-incompatible platelets. Br J Haematol 1993;83:672–673.

46. Lambin P, LePennec PY, Hauptmann G, et al: Adverse transfusion reactions associated with a precipitating anti-C3 antibody of anti-Rodgers specificity. Vox Sang 1984;47:242–249.

47. Morishita K, Shimada E, Watanabe Y, Kimura H: Anaphylactic transfusion reactions associated with anti-haptoglobin in a patient with ahaptoglobinemia. Transfusion 2000;40:120–121.

48. Wells JV, Buckley RH, Schanfield MS, Fudenberg HH: Anaphylactic reactions to plasma infusion in patients with hypogammaglobulinemia and anti-IgA antibodies. Clin Immunol Immunopathol 1977;8:265–271.

49. Koistinen J, Heikkila M, Leikola J: Gammaglobulin treatment and anti-IgA antibodies in IgA-deficient patients. Br Med J 1978;2:923–924.

50. Eckrich RJ, Mallory DM, Sandler SG: Laboratory tests to exclude IgA deficiency in the investigation of suspected anti-IgA transfusion reactions. Transfusion 1993;33:488–492.

51. Ochterlony O: Diffusion in gel methods for immunological analysis. Prog Allergy 1958;5:1.

52. Holt P, Tandy N, Anstee D: Screening of blood donors for IgA deficiency: a study of the donor population of South West England. J Clin Pathol 1977;30:1007–1010.

53. Fudenberg HH, Koistinen J: Human allotype detection by passive hemagglutination with special reference to immunoglobulin A allotypes. In Rose NR, Friedman H (eds): Manual of Clinical Immunology, 2nd ed. Washington, DC, American Society for Microbiology, 1980, p 767.

54. Vamvakas EC, Pineda AA: Allergic and anaphylactic reactions. In Popovsky MA (ed): Transfusion Reactions. Bethesda, Md, AABB Press, 1996, pp 81–123.

55. Shulman NR, Aster RH, Leitner A, Hiller MC: Immunoreactions involving platelets. V. Post-transfusion purpura due to a complement-fixing antibody against a genetically controlled platelet antigen. J Clin Invest 1961;40:1497.

56. Vogelsang G, Kickler TS, Bell WR: Post-transfusion purpura: a report of five patients and a review of pathogenesis and management. Am J Hematol 1986;21:259–267.

57. Chapman JF, Murphy MF, Berney SI, et al: Post-transfusion purpura associated with anti-Baka and anti-PlA2 platelet antibodies and delayed haemolytic transfusion reactions. Vox Sang 1987;52:313–317.

58. Swanson JL, Pulkrabek S, Scofield T, et al: Simultaneous occurrence of posttransfusion purpura due to anti-HPA-1a and a delayed transfusion reaction due to anti-Jkb [letter]. Transfusion 1997;37:449–450.

59. Ballem PJ, Buskard NA, Cecary F, Coubroff P: Post-transfusion purpura secondary to passive transfer of anti-PlA1 by blood transfusion. Br J Haematol 1987;66:113–114.

60. Scott EP, Moilan-Bergeland J, Dalmasso AP: Posttransfusion thrombocytopenia associated with passive transfusion of a platelet-specific antibody. Transfusion 1988;28:73–76.

61. McLeod BC, Strauss RG, Ciavarella D, et al: Management of hematological disorders and cancers. J Clin Apheresis 1993;8:211–230.

62. Mueller-Eckhardt C, Kiefel V: High-dose IgG for post-transfusion purpura—revisited. Blut 1988;57:163–167.

63. Brecher ME, Moore SB, Letendre L: Posttransfusion purpura: the therapeutic value of PL^A1-negative platelets. Transfusion 1990;30:433–435.

64. Win N, Matthey F, Slater NGP: Blood components—transfusion support in post-transfusion purpura due to HPA-1a immunization. Vox Sang 1996;71:191–193.

65. Popovsky MA, Moore SB: Diagnostic and pathogenetic considerations in transfusion-related acute lung injury. Transfusion 1985;25:573–577.

66. Barnard RD: Indiscriminate transfusion: a critique of case reports illustrating hypersensitivity reactions. NY J Med 1951;51:2399–2402.

67. Gould DM, Torrance DJ: Pulmonary edema following packed cell transfusion. Am J Roentgenol 1955;73:366–374.

68. Hirsch EO, Caracta AR: Pulmonary edema following packed cell transfusion. J Med Soc NJ 1966;83:45–46.

69. Philipps E, Fleischner FG: Pulmonary edema in the course of blood transfusion without overloading the circulation. Dis Chest 1966;50:619–623.

70. Ward HN, Lipscomb TS, Cawley LP: Pulmonary hypersensitivity reaction after blood transfusion. Arch Intern Med 1968;122:362–366.

71. Byrne JP Jr, Dixon JA: Pulmonary edema following blood transfusion reaction. Arch Surg 1970;102:91–94.

72. Eastlund T, McGrath PC, Britten A, Propp R: Fatal pulmonary transfusion reaction to plasma containing donor HLA antibody. Vox Sang 1989;57:63–66.

73. Yomtovian R, Kline W, Press C, et al: Severe pulmonary hypersensitivity associated with passive transfusion of a neutrophil-specific antibody. Lancet 1984;1:244–246.

74. Van Buren NL, Stroncek DF, Clay ME, et al: Transfusion-related acute lung injury caused by an NB2 granulocyte-specific antibody in a patient with thrombotic thrombocytopenic purpura. Transfusion 1990;30:42–45.

75. Nordhagen R, Conradi M, Dromtorp SM: Pulmonary reaction associated with transfusion of plasma containing anti-5b. Vox Sang 1986;51:102–107.

76. Popovsky MA, Abel MD, Moore SB: Transfusion-related acute lung injury associated with passive transfer of antileukocyte antibodies. Am Rev Respir Dis 1983;128:185–189.

77. Thompson JS, Severson CD, Parmely MJ, et al: Pulmonary "hypersensitivity" reactions induced by transfusion of non-HLA leukoagglutinins. N Engl J Med 1971;234:1120–1175.

78. Kernoff PBA, Durrant IJ, Rizza CR, Wright FN: Severe allergic pulmonary edema after plasma transfusion. Br J Haematol 1972;23:777–781.

79. Dry SM, Bechard KM, Milford EL, et al: The pathology of transfusion-related acute lung injury. Am J Clin Pathol 1999;112:216–221.

80. Silliman CC, Paterson AJ, Dickey WO, et al: The association of biologically active lipids with the development of transfusion-related acute lung injury; a retrospective study. Transfusion 1997;37:719–726.

81. Craddock PR, Fehr J, Dalmasso AP, et al: Hemodialysis leukopenia. Pulmonary vascular leukostasis resulting from complement activation by dialyzer cellophane membranes. J Clin Invest 1977;59:879–888.

82. Jacob HS, Craddock PR, Hammerschmidt DE, Moldow CF: Complement-induced granulocyte aggregation. N Engl J Med 1980;302:789–794.

83. Hammerschmidt DE, Weaver J, Hudson LD, et al: Association of complement activation and elevated plasma-C5a with adult respiratory distress syndrome. Pathophysiological relevance and possible prognostic value. Lancet 1980;1:947–949.

84. Higby DJ, Burnett D: Granulocyte transfusions: current status. Blood 1980;55:2–8.

85. Andrews AT, Zmijewski CM. Bowman HS, Reihart JK: Transfusion reaction with pulmonary infiltration associated with HLA-specific leukocyte antibodies. Am J Clin Pathol 1977;66:483–487.

86. Campbell DA, Swartz RD, Waskerwitz JA, et al: Leukoagglutination with interstitial pulmonary edema. A complication of donor-specific transfusion. Transplantation 1982;34:300–301.

87. Worsley MH, Sinclair CJ, Campanella C, et al: Non-cardiogenic pulmonary oedema after transfusion with granulocyte antibody containing blood: treatment with extracorporeal membrane oxygenation. Br J Anaesth 1991;67:116–119.

88. Payne R: The development and persistence of leukoagglutinins in parous women. Blood 1962;19:411–424.

89. Clay M, Kline W, McCullough J: The frequency of granulocyte-specific antibodies in postpartum sera and a family study of the 6B antigen. Transfusion 1984;24:252–255.

90. Popovsky MA, Chaplin HC Jr, Moore SB: Transfusion-related acute lung injury: a neglected, serious complication of hemotherapy. Transfusion 1992;32:289–292.

91. Audet AM, Popovsky MA, Andrzejewski C: Transfusion-associated circulatory overload in orthopedic surgery patients: a multi-institutional study. Immunohematology 1996;12(2):87–89.

92. Iserson KV, Huestis DW: Blood warming: current applications and techniques. Transfusion 1991;31:551–571.

93. Sessler DI: Current concepts: mild perioperative hypothermia. N Engl J Med 1997;336:1730–1737.

94. Sano H, Koga Y, Hamasaki K, et al: Anaphylaxis associated with white-cell reduction filter [letter]. Lancet 1996;347:1053.

95. Hume HA, Popovsky MA, Benson K, et al: Hypotensive reactions: a previously uncharacterized complication of platelet transfusion? Transfusion 1996;36:904–909.

96. Shiba M, Tadokoro K, Sawanobori M, et al: Activation of the contact system by filtration of platelet concentrates with a negatively charged white cell removal filter and measurement of venous blood bradykinin level in patients who received filtered platelets. Transfusion 1997;37:457–462.

97. Hypotension and bedside leukocyte reduction filters. Center for Device and Radiologic Health, 1999. Available at http://www.fda.gov/cdrh/safety/hypoblrf.html.

98. Mair B, Leparc GF: Hypotensive reactions associated with platelet transfusions and angiotensin-converting enzyme inhibitors. Vox Sang 1998;74:27–30.

99. Fried MR, Eastlund T, Christie B, et al: Hypotensive reactions to white cell–reduced plasma in a patient undergoing angiotensin-converting enzyme inhibitor therapy. Transfusion 1996;36:900–903.

100. Owen HG, Brecher ME: Atypical reactions associated with use of angiotensin-converting enzyme inhibitors and apheresis. Transfusion 1994;34:891–894.

101. Cyr M, Hume HA, Champagne M, et al: Anomaly of the des-Arg9-bradykinin metabolism associated with severe hypotensive reactions during blood transfusion: a preliminary study. Transfusion 1999;39:1084–1088.

102. Abe H, Ikebuchi K, Shimbo M, Sekiguchi S: Hypotensive reactions with a white-cell reduction filter: activation of kallikrein-kinin cascade in a patient [letter]. Transfusion 1998;38:411–412.

103. Hild M, Soderstrom T, Egberg N, Lundahl J: Kinetics of bradykinin levels during and after leukocyte filtration of platelet concentrates. Vox Sang 1998;75:18–25.

104. Sweeney JD, Dupois M, Mega AJ: Hypotensive reactions to red cells filtered at the bedside, but not to those filtered before storage, in patients taking ACE inhibitors [letter]. Transfusion 1998;38:410–411.

105. Blais C Jr, Marc-Aurele J, Simmons WH, et al: Des-Arg9-bradykinin metabolism in patients who presented hypersensitivity reactions during hemodialysis: role of serum ACE and aminopeptidase P. Peptides 1999;20:421–430.

106. Belloni M, Alghisi A, Bettini C, et al: Hypotensive reactions associated with white cell–reduced apheresis platelet concentrates in patients not receiving ACE inhibitors [letter]. Transfusion 1998;38:412–413.

107. Adverse ocular reactions following transfusions—United States, 1997–1998. MMWR Morb Mortal Wkly Rep 1998;47:49–50.

Chapter 35

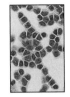

Immunomodulation

Ian S. Gourley
Leslie E. Silberstein

The concept that transfusion of blood or blood products can have an immunomodulatory effect first emerged more than 30 years ago. In this chapter, we discuss three important clinical scenarios in which the transfusion effect has been observed—transplantation, malignancy, and postoperative infection. In addition, we highlight the current theories about the interactions between donor and host that may result in the transfusion effect.

■ The Transfusion Effect in Transplantation

It was noted in 1964 that experimental renal transplants in a canine model survived longer if the recipient had received a blood transfusion from the donor animal.[1] Several years later, a similar effect was observed in human transplantation. The overall 1-year graft survival rate for renal transplantation had risen to around 60% by the early 1970s. This increase was due mainly to improvement in surgical technique, greater experience in the use of steroids as immunosuppressive agents, and the advent of antilymphocyte serum.

In 1973, analysis of U.S. transplant data revealed that the 1-year graft survival rate was significantly higher in patients who had received pretransplantation blood transfusions than in those who had not.[2] Subsequent studies confirmed this finding, and the practice of giving recipients of cadaver renal transplants one or more blood transfusions before transplantation was widely adopted as a means to increase graft survival.[3, 4] Protocols for donor-specific transfusions enabled 1-year survival rates of up to 94%, a figure comparable to that for recipients of HLA-identical related-donor grafts who did not receive transfusions (see later).[5]

This situation continued until the advent of cyclosporine in the early 1980s.[6] With the use of this new immunosuppressive

drug, 1-year graft survival rates of 80% or higher were routinely achieved, and the beneficial effect of pretransplantation blood transfusion was no longer uniformly apparent.[7–9] The use of such a transfusion gradually declined during the late 1980s and 1990s. In 1981, the ratio of transfused to nontransfused recipients was 10:1; in 1990, it was 1:1. Interest in the potential benefits and underlying mechanisms continued, however, and even as late as 1997, studies showing better outcome in transfused patients, independent of cyclosporine use or HLA-DR matching, continued to appear in the literature.[10, 11]

Figure 35.1 illustrates the improvement in 1-year graft survival rate over the last three decades for both transfused and nontransfused patients. The figure also shows that graft survival was better in nontransfused patients in the 1990s than

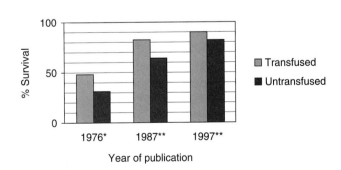

Figure 35.1 Comparison of 1-year first cadaver renal graft survival between transfused and nontransfused recipients in three studies published in 1976, 1987, and 1997. All patients received cyclosporine. *Patients transfused with 1–5 units of blood; **all transfused patients.

it was in transfused patients in the 1970s, demonstrating the effectiveness of other modalities of treatment, especially newer immunosuppressive drugs such as cyclosporine.

Blood Transfusion and Malignancy

Although beneficial in transplantation, blood transfusion may be detrimental in other settings. A 1980 study provided evidence that transfusion of allogeneic washed blood to potential renal allograft recipients caused a suppression of cellular immunity.[12] This effect was more pronounced and longer-lasting after a second transfusion. Autologous blood given to volunteers had no such effect. In 1981, Gantt[13] raised the possibility that this nonspecific immunosuppressive effect might lead to enhanced tumor survival in individuals who had received a blood transfusion. A study published later the same year showed that allogeneic blood transfusions given to rats produced a measurable reduction in immune function compared with autologous transfusion or saline infusion.[14] In transfused rats that were inoculated with a sarcoma homogenate, these effects were associated with a significant increase in the weight and volume of the tumors.

In 1982, two retrospective studies showed that decreased recurrence-free survival and higher recurrence rates were associated with perioperative transfusion in patients undergoing curative resection for colonic carcinoma.[15, 16] Later studies showed a similar effect for patients with cancer of the prostate and cervix.[17] Multivariate analysis in these studies demonstrated that transfusion status was independently associated with outcome. Subsequent reports included patients with cancer of the lung, breast, and kidney as well as colorectal carcinoma. Some studies confirmed the association of poor outcome with transfusion, but others did not.

Blumberg and Heal[18] performed a meta-analysis of the data for colorectal carcinoma, which revealed a marked difference in outcome between transfused and nontransfused patients. As they pointed out, the difference was unlikely to be due to the selection of only positive studies (studies in which transfusion was associated with poor outcome), because an almost equal number of negative studies were included. In a

second meta-analysis of data from 11 retrospective studies, Vamvakas and Moore[19] found that there was an estimated 37% higher risk of cancer recurrence or cancer-related death after transfusion. They estimated a "true" transfusion effect, after further hidden confounding variables are included, of around 10% to 20%. A third group subjected 20 studies, including 2 prospective studies, to meta-analysis, calculating the odds ratios of a negative outcome in transfused patients as 1.69, of recurrence as 1.8, of death from cancer as 1.76, and of death as 1.63.[20] This group was unable to differentiate between a true effect of transfusion and the effects of unknown confounding variables.

Three prospective, randomized trials investigating the role of transfusion in colorectal cancer recurrence have been published.[21-23] Only one of the studies showed a significant association between allogeneic blood transfusion and tumor recurrence, although this association was reduced to borderline status after tumor stage was taken into consideration. The results of these three studies are summarized in Table 35.1.

In summary, most of the evidence for a detrimental effect of transfusion in the setting of malignancy comes from retrospective studies, which are subject to the effects of hidden confounders. Prospective studies have failed to prove conclusively that such an effect exists.

Blood Transfusion and Infection

Many studies have investigated the possible effect of blood transfusion on the susceptibility to infection. Two retrospective studies and one prospective study identified blood transfusion as an independent predictor of infection in patients undergoing treatment for trauma.[24-26] In the largest of these studies, the risk increased with the number of units of blood transfused.[25] Multivariate analysis in two nonrandomized, prospective studies found perioperative transfusion to be a significant predictor of postoperative infection in patients with colonic carcinoma or with Crohn's disease.[27, 28] Six prospective, randomized studies have been published, five looking at infectious complications after colorectal surgery, and the sixth after cardiac surgery.[21, 29-33] The results of

Table 35.1 Summary of Three Prospective, Randomized Studies Looking at Effect of Perioperative Blood Transfusion on Recurrence of Colorectal Carcinoma

	Busch et al (1993)[21]	Houbiers et al (1994)[22]	Heiss et al (1994)[23]
Treatment arms	Allogeneic (PC) vs autologous	Allogeneic (LD) vs allogeneic (BC)	Allogeneic (BC) vs autologous
Outcome parameters	Relapse-free survival at 4 years	Recurrence at 3 years	Recurrence (median follow-up 22 months)
Number of patients in study	475	697	120
Result	34% vs 37% ($P = .93$)	29% vs 27% ($P = .79$)	28.9% vs 16.7% ($P = .11$)
Secondary outcome parameters	Relative rate of recurrence at 4 years in transfused vs nontransfused	Recurrence rates at 3 years, transfused vs nontransfused	Relative risk of recurrence after ≤2 units, allogeneic vs autologous
Result	Allogeneic transfused vs nontransfused, = 2.1 ($P = .01$) Autologous vs non transfused, = 1.8 ($P = .04$).	30% vs 26%, ($P = .22$)	5.16 ($P = .034$) (RR 3.54, $P = .107$, after adjustment for tumor and node stage)

BC, buffy coat–depleted packed red blood cells; LD, leukocyte-depleted (filtered) packed red blood cells; PC, packed red blood cells; RR, relative risk.

Table 35.2 Summary of Six Randomized, Prospective Trials Looking at Effect of Perioperative Transfusion on Postoperative Bacterial Infection Rates after Surgery for Colorectal Carcinoma, and Cardiac Surgery

Trial	Infection as primary or secondary endpoint	Types of transfusions and result	Significance
Jensen et al (1992)[29]	Primary	Whole > LR Whole > nontransfused	$P < .01$ $P < .01$
Busch et al (1993)[21]	Secondary	Allogeneic (PC) vs autologous	$P =$ ns
Heiss et al (1993)[30]	Primary	Allogeneic (BC) vs autologous	$P < .05$
Jensen et al (1996)[31]	Primary	BC > LD BC > nontransfused	$P \le .01^*$ $P < .01^*$
Houbiers et al (1997)[32]	Secondary	BC or LD > nontransfused BC vs LD	$P < .01$ $P =$ ns
van de Watering et al (1997)[†]	Primary	BC vs LD (fresh) vs LD (Stored)	$P =$ ns

*Infection related to surgery (wound infections and intra-abdominal abscess) and nonsurgical infections (pneumonia).
†Cardiac surgery.
BC, buffy coat–depleted red blood cells; LD, leukocyte-depleted red blood cells; PC, packed red blood cells.
Modified from Blajchman MA: Allogeneic blood transfusions, immodulation and postoperative bacterial infecion: Do we have the answers yet? [editorial; comment]. Transfusion 1997;37:121–125.

these studies are summarized in Table 35.2. Although there were differences in design, all of the studies compared infection rates among groups that differed in the allogeneic leukocyte content of transfusions received. Four of the studies found a significantly higher infection rate in patients randomized to receive blood containing more allogeneic leukocytes. In the other two studies, no such association was found.

One of the studies, performed by Houbiers and colleagues,[32] concluded that susceptibility to infection was related to the amount of red blood cells transfused. These researchers also reported a meta-analysis of 11 studies (1 randomized, 4 prospective, and 6 retrospective) of a total of 2779 patients who had undergone abdominal surgery. The group found that the average infection rate for nontransfused patients was 11.9%, versus 27.5% for transfused patients ($P < .01$). A separate meta-analysis of 7 studies comparing infection rates in patients receiving allogeneic transfusion and autologous transfusion found a greater risk of infection after allogeneic transfusion, with an odds ratio of 2.37 (total of 1060 patients).[34]

This evidence does not conclusively support the existence of a transfusion effect either in the setting of cancer recurrence or in postoperative infection. Two issues make interpretation of the preceding studies more difficult. First, studies now suggest that autologous transfusion is not immunologically neutral, at least in patients undergoing surgery for colorectal carcinoma.[35, 36] Rather, it seems to promote cellular immunity, in contrast to some of the effects of allogeneic transfusion, which leads to diminution in cellular immunity (see later). Second, red blood cells differ in their leukocyte content, depending on the method of preparation.[37] Packed red blood cells contain 2×10^9 to 5×10^9 leukocytes (white blood cells [WBCs]) per unit. Buffy coat depletion, which is used in Europe but not elsewhere, results in a product with approximately 1×10^9 WBCs per unit. In contrast, modern leukocyte reduction filters can leave a residual leukocyte content of less than 1×10^6 WBCs per unit. These difficulties have led some researchers to call for further studies or meta-analyses of the available randomized studies before the effect of transfusion on infection in colorectal cancer patients is accepted.[37–39] Others argue that the strength of evidence is enough not only for acceptance of the effect but also to warrant a change in transfusion policy for surgical patients.[40]

Mechanisms of Immunosuppressive Effect

It had been suggested that the immunosuppressive effect of blood transfusion is related to excess iron or of overloading of the reticuloendothelial system by red cell debris, thus leading to decreased macrophage function.[41] It has now become generally accepted that the effect is due to the WBC content of the blood transfusion. As discussed previously, several prospective randomized studies have shown that the immunosuppressive effect of transfusion is reduced when the WBC content of the transfused blood is lower.[29, 31, 33]

Donor-Specific Transfusion

In order to explore some of the current theories about the nature of the immunosuppressive effect of blood transfusion, one must first look at the practice of donor-specific transfusion. By the 1980s, random transfusion of potential renal allograft recipients had become widespread because of the reported association with better graft survival. Donor-specific transfusion had already been shown to improve graft survival in a canine renal transplant model.[1] In 1980, Salvatierra and associates[5] demonstrated a similar benefit in human renal transplantation. Forty-five patients were given three transfusions from their prospective donors, all of whom were relatives with a one-haplotype match. Thirteen patients could not receive renal transplants from their blood donors because of the development of positive serologic crossmatches; 30 of the remainder did receive kidneys from their blood donors. The researchers found that graft survival was significantly better and episodes of rejection were significantly decreased in these patients than in nontransfused recipients of grafts from living related donors.

A later study found that graft survival was significantly enhanced if there was a class II HLA incompatibility between donor and recipient on the unshared haplotype.[42] These findings are in contrast, however, to data presented from the University of California–Los Angeles (UCLA) International Transplant Registry.[43] In this analysis of several hundred transplant procedures after 1980, 1-year graft survival was higher after donor-specific transfusion from an HLA-identical sibling than from (1) a sibling with a one-haplotype match or (2) parents or offspring (who were therefore matched for one haplotype). These clinical studies

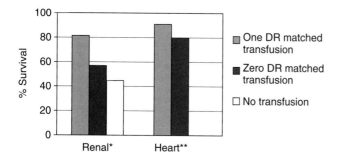

Figure 35.2 Five-year graft survival for renal and heart transplant recipients after random donor transfusions matched for either one or zero HLA-DR antigens, or no transfusion. *Patients given a single pretransplantation transfusion (buffy coat depleted); 32 patients received one HLA-DR antigen–matched blood, 30 blood with no HLA-DR match, and 41 no transfusion. **Patients given a single pretransplant transfusion (buffy coat depleted); 45 received one HLA-DR antigen–matched blood, and 55 blood with no HLA-DR match.

demonstrate that donor-specific transfusion has a beneficial effect on graft outcome, but they are inconclusive as to the degree of HLA matching that is most beneficial.

This issue has also been addressed in the setting of cadaver transplantation, in which the recipients received pretransplantation transfusions from third-party, unrelated blood donors. Beneficial effects of transfusion of blood sharing one HLA-DR antigen have been observed in both renal and heart transplantation.[44, 45] These studies are summarized in Figure 35.2.

On the basis of this evidence, some centers adopted a policy of deliberately transfusing a potential kidney recipient with HLA-typed blood from a third-party donor who shared one HLA-DR antigen with the recipient.[46] Although the evidence is inconclusive, it is possible that sharing of one HLA-DR antigen between patient and blood donor is responsible for a specific immunosuppressive or tolerant effect directed against the donor antigens. This effect then manifests as improved graft survival in the setting of donor-specific transfusion. The same degree of HLA sharing seems to lead to an effect that manifests as better survival of unrelated cadaver grafts, perhaps through a more global immunosuppressive effect.[44, 45]

Several mechanisms have been proposed for the donor-specific transfusion effect. A nonspecific step in which suppressor cells prevent formation of antibodies, including anti–HLA class I, has been proposed.[47] In a subsequent antigen-specific stage, anti-idiotype antibodies develop that prevent activation of recipient T cells by class I antigens on donor blood, or even of the donor kidney.

Others have proposed that pretransplantation donor-specific blood transfusion actually immunized the patient to donor antigens and that subsequent transplantation of the kidney stimulated a strong secondary response.[48] The high level of immunosuppression used would then kill or inactivate the actively proliferating clone of cells specific for the foreign antigens.

It has been hypothesized that this clonal deletion might be modified by the formation of anti-idiotypic antibodies that would suppress recipient anti-donor T cells, or that anti-idiotypic T cells might even be the suppressing force.[49] In this situation, the expansion of donor-specific T cells after transplantation would be matched by expansion of the anti-idiotypic B or T cell, thus blocking the anti-donor response.

Further investigation of this mechanism has revealed evidence of alterations in donor-specific cytotoxic T-lymphocyte precursor (CTLp) activity after transfusion. Complete T-cell nonresponsiveness has been demonstrated after transfusion with blood matched for at least one HLA-B and HLA-DR antigen, but responses did not decline after transfusions of blood that was HLA mismatched.[50] Decreased usage of certain T-cell receptor (TCR) Vβ genes has also been demonstrated after similarly matched random transfusion.[51] In another case, enhanced donor-specific CTL responses were found after transfusion of whole blood to recipients sharing no HLA-DR antigens with the donor.[52] With transfusion of blood between donor and recipient who shared one HLA-DR antigen, there was only a slight but insignificant increase in response.

These findings were not uniformly reported by later studies, however. Only 2 of 14 recipients of buffy coat–depleted blood showed a decrease in donor-specific CTL responses if they shared an HLA haplotype or at least one HLA-DR and B antigen with the donor.[53] No difference was found in blood donor–specific CTL hyporesponsiveness between patients who received transfusions of whole blood with one haplotype or one HLA-B and HLA-DR match and patients given HLA-mismatched blood.[54] In this study, helper T-cell activity (both donor-specific and nonspecific) declined after transfusion, but most of the effect was seen after HLA-mismatched transfusion.

Similarly, no evidence was found for donor-specific CTL or helper T-cell hyporesponsiveness or for restriction in TCR Vβ usage after one transfusion of HLA-DR– or one HLA-B-DR–matched, buffy coat–depleted blood.[55] No decrease in donor-specific CTL responses could be demonstrated after one transfusion of HLA-DR–matched, plasma-reduced blood.[56] Indeed, in this last study, donor-specific CTL responses rose in a majority of patients in both groups given the one HLA-DR–matched blood as well as in a control group given no HLA-DR–matched transfusions.

In summary, several studies have found evidence of donor-specific T cell tolerance after one transfusion of HLA-DR–matched blood, but later studies did not confirm these findings.

Various non–antigen-specific immunologic abnormalities have also been reported after transfusion (Table 35.3).[57] Two groups have found cell-mediated immunity (CMI) to be decreased after allogeneic transfusion to potential renal transplant recipients.[12, 58] CMI was measured as response to mitogen and antigen in one case and through skin rechallenge with dinitrochlorobenzene in the other. In the first study, a dose-related response was observed after a second

Table 35.3 Transfusion-Induced Immunomodulatory Effects on the Immune System of the Recipient

Decreased response in mixed lymphocyte culture assay

Decreased CD4:CD8 ratio

Increased CD8 numbers

Decreased natural killer cell function and number

Decreased cell-mediated immunity (proliferation assays and delayed-type skin hypersensitivity responses)

transfusion. Delayed-type hypersensitivity to recall antigens was found to be decreased after allogeneic transfusion in patients with colorectal cancer.[30] Abnormalities in natural killer (NK) cell function have also been observed after transfusion, in one report to patients with colorectal cancer and in another to patients with sickle cell anemia or hemophilia.[29, 59] Finally, NK cell numbers were significantly lower after allogeneic transfusion in a group of patients undergoing spinal surgery.[60]

Shift in Th1/Th2 System After Transfusion

A shift towards a Th2 (type 2 helper T cell) type of immune response has been proposed to account for the nonspecific immunosuppressive effect of transfusion. The Th1/Th2 system was first described in the mouse when it was noticed that the immune system could respond to antigenic stimulus in one of two ways. Sometimes, helper T cells produced a pattern of cytokines that promoted cell-mediated immunity and activation of macrophages and NK cells, such as interleukin-2 (IL-2), interferon-γ (IFN-γ), and tumor necrosis factor (TNF) (the Th1 response). At other times, however, the helper T cells produced cytokines that promoted humoral immunity, including IL-4 and IL-10 (the Th2 response).

Furthermore, there was a reciprocal downregulation, such that a Th1 response would tend to suppress Th2 cytokine formation, and vice versa. This system has been shown to exist in humans also.[61] Several papers have suggested that transfusion of blood shifts the immune response towards a Th2 phenotype.[62–67] The levels of the cytokines TNF and IL-2 derived from peripheral blood mononuclear cells had fallen by 30% and 26%, respectively, and that of IFN-γ by 70%, by the second week after allogeneic transfusion to patients undergoing hemodialysis.[62] Production of prostaglandin E_2 (PGE_2) by monocytes increased significantly by day 7 but fell to baseline levels by day 14.[63] It is known that production of PGE_2 by monocytes leads to a predominantly Th2 pattern of cytokine secretion, possibly by directly downregulating production of IL-2 from T cells.[64, 65] A later study of patients undergoing dialysis found that production of IL-4, IL-10, and the anti-inflammatory cytokine transforming growth factor-β were all significantly elevated after transfusion with allogeneic packed red cells.[66] In contrast, production of IL-4 and IL-10 was unchanged after transfusion with washed, filtered red cells (97% to 98% leukocyte free). IL-10 secretion was measured in stimulated whole blood cultures after either allogeneic or autologous transfusion to patients undergoing joint surgery.[67] Significantly higher levels were observed after allogeneic transfusion. IL-4 production was also higher, but not significantly so.

Some researchers argue that a leukocyte-mediated shift towards a Th2 response leads to the subsequent downregulation of cell-mediated immunity in favor of humoral immunity. This change favors enhanced allograft survival and also predisposes the patient to infections and recurrence of tumors. The preceding argument would also explain why transfusion of allogeneic blood or lymphocytes is beneficial in the setting of Crohn's disease and repetitive abortion; a Th1 immune response is thought to play a role in the pathogenesis of these two conditions.[68, 69] It has also been argued that successful pregnancy, in which the fetus shares one haplotype with the mother, is characterized by a shift to a Th2 type of immune response, thereby protecting the fetomaternal unit by downregulating cellular immunity.[70, 71]

In summary, one factor involved in the transfusion effect may be a shift toward a Th2 immune response, leading to downregulation of cellular immunity.

Microchimerism

Another factor that may be important to the development of immunosuppression after transfusion is the length of time donor lymphocytes stay in the recipient's circulation (microchimerism). Several methods have been used to detect microchimerism in various settings, such as during pregnancy and after transfusion.[72–79] For example, Y chromosome probes have identified male nucleated erythrocytes in the maternal circulation during pregnancy.[72] Polymerase chain reaction (PCR) amplification of Y chromosome sequence has been used to identify male CD34-positive, CD38-positive progenitor cells in females who either were currently carrying a male fetus or had done so in the past, in one case 27 years previously.[73] A similar technique was used to demonstrate that donor WBCs circulated for a mean of 2 days (range 1 to 6) in women given blood transfusions from male donors.[74] In a similar setting, a quantitative method showed that after an initial clearance, the numbers of donor leukocytes rose again by day 5.[75] These data were reproduced in a canine model, in which it was shown that gamma-irradiation of the blood prevented the secondary expansion phase.

One study has demonstrated a relationship between the degree of HLA matching and the extent of microchimerism after transfusion.[76] Nested PCR amplification of donor-specific HLA sequences was used to detect microchimerism after transfusion of buffy coat–depleted blood in 21 patients waiting for renal transplantation. In recipients of partially HLA-matched blood (at least one HLA-B and HLA-DR) (n = 12), donor signal was found in all patients in the first week, in 88% at 2 to 4 weeks, and in 3 patients up to 8 weeks after transfusion. In contrast, after mismatched transfusion (n = 9), donor signal was detected in 5 of 7 patients in the first week, 3 of 8 at weeks 2 to 4, and only 1 of 5 patients at weeks 5 to 8.

Several studies have found evidence of greater microchimerism in patients with scleroderma than in normal controls.[77–79] In these studies, HLA typing has also revealed more compatibility for class II alleles between either patient and mother or patient and offspring pairs than in normal controls. HLA compatibility was defined as the patient not having a class II allele that was different from those of the mother or offspring. These findings provide some evidence for the theory that scleroderma is a form of graft-versus-host disease due to microchimerism from fetomaternal or maternofetal blood exchange.

Long-term microchimerism, which would be necessary to cause disease years after pregnancy, may be facilitated by complete class II identity between the host and the "foreign" leukocytes, such that immune activation and clearance of these cells do not occur. In contrast, the studies discussed earlier suggest that blood transfusion may lead to short-term microchimerism—that is, microchimerism that lasts a few weeks—with at least preliminary evidence that matching for one haplotype or at least one HLA-DR antigen may be necessary to ensure that microchimerism is established and that it lasts for more than a few days. It is this degree of HLA sharing that seems to be the optimum for the transfusion effect. Therefore, short-term microchimerism may be important, in that it allows interactions between recipient and donor cells that lead to the immunologic changes manifesting as the clinical outcomes previously discussed for transplantation, malignancy, and infection.

Recipient-Donor Interactions

Lagaaij and associates[52] have proposed a possible mechanism whereby one HLA-DR–matched blood transfusion could lead to downregulation of donor-specific helper T-cell responses. They suggest that in transfusions in which there is mismatching for both HLA-DR antigens, donor antigen is presented to host T cells by host antigen-presenting cells (APCs), resulting in activation of donor-directed immunity. In contrast, when there is sharing of one HLA-DR antigen, donor antigens can be presented on this shared antigen on the donor APC. In the setting of an intravenous lymphocyte infusion, the cells most likely to present antigen would be donor B cells or, possibly, activated T cells, which lack the second signal capacity of "professional" APCs such as dendritic cells. Researchers suggest that this scenario leads to either anergy of the T cells specific for these antigens or, perhaps, to a shift toward a Th2 response, owing to lack of IL-12 production by the APCs.[31, 61] This situation may be analogous to the observation that, during a pregnancy in which the mother and fetus share one HLA-DR antigen and are mismatched for the other, the fetus may demonstrate specific unresponsiveness to the noninherited maternal HLA antigens.[80] Studies have demonstrated that an alloimmune response to foreign cells can be characterized by the recognition of, and binding to, foreign major histocompatibility complex (MHC) antigens by up to 10% of recipient T cells.[81] This response is thought to occur in one of the following two ways: (1) the recipient TCRs form a good fit with the peptide/nonself MHC complex or (2) the TCRs simply recognize the MHC molecule itself.

Lack of co-stimulation and consequent anergy or Th2 shift of this much larger population of T cells may be relevant to our understanding of the more global immunosuppressive effect associated with random transfusion.[81] Effectively, in the right circumstances, transfusions associated with a nonspecific immunosuppressive effect may also induce donor-specific tolerance, and vice versa.

The preceding evidence suggests that the immunosuppressive effect of "random" transfusion (1) may be influenced by the extent of MHC compatibility or incompatibility between recipient and donor, (2) perhaps also depends on the length of time donor leukocytes remain in the recipient circulation, and (3) may ultimately be mediated through T-cell anergy or a shift in the recipient's immune response to a Th2 pattern of cytokine production.

The Role of Soluble Factors in Transfusion-Induced Immunosuppression

Although transfused leukocytes are favored as the agents responsible for the transfusion effect, some evidence also suggests that one or more soluble immunosuppressive factors may be present in blood transfusions. For example, placental protein 14 (PP14) is found in amniotic fluid, at highest concentrations in the first trimester of pregnancy. It has been shown to inhibit T-cell proliferative responses by a mechanism believed to involve inhibition of early events in TCR signaling.[82] This molecule is also known to be produced by platelets, suggesting that the presence of PP14 in

transfused blood products could influence the recipient's immune response either specifically to donor antigens or in a nonspecific manner.[83]

Soluble forms of HLA antigens have also been implicated as contributors to the transfusion effect. Synthetic peptides corresponding to certain linear sequences of human HLA molecules have been demonstrated to have immunosuppressive or tolerogenic effects through downregulation of T-cell responses.[84] This finding has led to the evaluation of such peptides for therapeutic use.[85] Soluble HLA antigens of donor origin have been measured in the blood of transplant recipients, but it is possible to detect soluble class I antigens also in the sera of normal individuals.[86, 87] Thus, the presence of soluble HLA antigens in transfused blood products may also influence the recipient's immune response, either in a donor-specific manner or in a more global, nonspecific manner.

■ Conclusion

The existence of an immunomodulatory effect of transfusion in the transplant setting has now been accepted, as both the global immunosuppressive effect of random transfusion and the donor-specific effect seen after transfusion from a prospective organ donor. There is also strong evidence to support a transfusion effect in the surgical patient that leads to higher risk of postoperative infection. Although some studies have suggested that transfusion also leads to earlier tumor recurrence, this area is still controversial, especially because hidden confounding variables may be responsible for much of the effect. We have attempted to discuss not only the evidence for and against the transfusion effect but also the immunologic abnormalities described and the possible mechanisms that have been proposed to explain the effect (Fig. 35.3). Most authorities now believe that transfused WBCs are the responsible agent, although soluble factors such as placental protein 14 and soluble HLA molecules or peptides may play a role. There is also evidence to suggest that the degree of HLA compatibility between recipient and blood donor is key to induction of the effect, with sharing of one haplotype or at

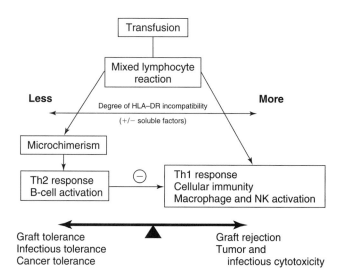

Figure 35.3 Provisional model of mechanisms involved in transfusion-induced immunomodulation. NK, natural killer cells.

least one HLA-DR antigen being optimal. This observation applies to both random and donor-specific transfusions. Strong evidence exists to show that transfusion can shift the recipient's immune response toward a Th2 pattern, a change which is known to upregulate humoral immunity at the expense of cellular responses, thus favoring allograft survival but also leading to a greater susceptibility to infection and, possibly, to tumor recurrence. Specific anergy of selected T-cell populations may also occur. The link between HLA class II antigen sharing and the Th2 shift may well be microchimerism, especially if it can be shown definitively that the level or duration of the microchimerism after transfusion depends on HLA sharing between recipient and donor.

REFERENCES

1. Halasz NA OM, Hirose F: Increased survival of renal homografts in dogs after injection of donor blood. Transplantation 1964;2:453–458.
2. Opelz G, Sengar DP, Mickey MR, Terasaki PI: Effect of blood transfusions on subsequent kidney transplants. Transplant Proc 1973;5:253–259.
3. Opelz G, Terasaki PI: Prolongation effect of blood transfusions on kidney graft survival. Transplantation 1976;22:380–383.
4. Opelz G, Terasaki PI: Dominant effect of transfusions on kidney graft survival. Transplantation 1980;29:153–158.
5. Salvatierra O Jr, Vincenti F, Amend W, et al: Deliberate donor-specific blood transfusions prior to living related renal transplantation: A new approach. Ann Surg 1980;192:543–552.
6. Blood transfusion and allograft survival [editorial]. Lancet 1984;1(8381):830–831.
7. Lundgren G, Groth CG, Albrechtsen D, et al: HLA-matching and pretransplant blood transfusions in cadaveric renal transplantation—a changing picture with cyclosporin. Lancet 1986;2(8498):66–69.
8. Melzer JS, Husing RM, Feduska NJ, et al: The beneficial effect of pretransplant blood transfusions in cyclosporine-treated cadaver renal allograft recipients. Transplantation 1987;43:61–64.
9. Opelz G: Improved kidney graft survival in nontransfused recipients. Transplant Proc 1987;19:149–152.
10. Opelz G, Vanrenterghem Y, Kirste G, et al: Prospective evaluation of pretransplant blood transfusions in cadaver kidney recipients. Transplantation 1997;63:964–967.
11. Sharma RK, Rai PK, Kumar A, et al: Role of preoperative donor-specific transfusion and cyclosporine in haplo-identical living related renal transplant recipients. Nephron 1997;75:20–24.
12. Fischer E, Lenhard V, Seifert P, et al: Blood transfusion-induced suppression of cellular immunity in man. Hum Immunol 1980;1:187–194.
13. Gantt CL: Red blood cells for cancer patients [letter]. Lancet 1981;2(8242):363.
14. Francis DM, Shenton BK: Blood transfusion and tumour growth: Evidence from laboratory animals [letter]. Lancet 1981;2(8251):871.
15. Burrows L, Tartter P: Effect of blood transfusions on colonic malignancy recurrent rate [letter]. Lancet 1982;2(8299):662.
16. Blumberg N, Agarwal MM, Chuang C: Relation between recurrence of cancer of the colon and blood transfusion. BMJ 1985;290(6474):1037–1039.
17. Blumberg N, Heal J, Chuang C, et al: Further evidence supporting a cause and effect relationship between blood transfusion and earlier cancer recurrence. Ann Surg 1988;207:410–415.
18. Blumberg N, Heal JM: Transfusion and host defenses against cancer recurrence and infection. Transfusion 1989;29:236–245.
19. Vamvakas E, Moore SB: Perioperative blood transfusion and colorectal cancer recurrence: A qualitative statistical overview and meta-analysis [see comments]. Transfusion 1993;33:754–765.
20. Chung M, Steinmetz OK, Gordon PH: Perioperative blood transfusion and outcome after resection for colorectal carcinoma [see comments]. Br J Surg 1993;80:427–432.
21. Busch OR, Hop WC, Hoynck van Papendrecht MA, et al: Blood transfusions and prognosis in colorectal cancer [see comments]. N Engl J Med 1993;328:1372–1376.
22. Houbiers JG, Brand A, van de Watering LM, et al: Randomised controlled trial comparing transfusion of leucocyte-depleted or buffy-coat-depleted blood in surgery for colorectal cancer [see comments]. Lancet 1994;344(8922):573–578.
23. Heiss MM, Mempel W, Delanoff C, et al: Blood transfusion-modulated tumor recurrence: First results of a randomized study of autologous versus allogeneic blood transfusion in colorectal cancer surgery [see comments]. J Clin Oncol 1994;12:1859–1867.
24. Dawes LG, Aprahamian C, Condon RE, Malangoni MA: The risk of infection after colon injury. Surgery 1986;100:796–803.
25. Agarwal N, Murphy JG, Cayten CG, Stahl WM: Blood transfusion increases the risk of infection after trauma. Arch Surg 1993;128:171–176.
26. Nichols RL, Smith JW, Klein DB, et al: Risk of infection after penetrating abdominal trauma. N Engl J Med 1984;311(17):1065–1070.
27. Tartter PI, Quintero S, Barron DM: Perioperative blood transfusion associated with infectious complications after colorectal cancer operations. Am J Surg 1986;152:479–482.
28. Tartter PI, Driefuss RM, Malon AM, et al: Relationship of postoperative septic complications and blood transfusions in patients with Crohn's disease. Am J Surg 1988;155:43–48.
29. Jensen LS, Andersen AJ, Christiansen PM, et al: Postoperative infection and natural killer cell function following blood transfusion in patients undergoing elective colorectal surgery. Br J Surg 1992;79:513–516.
30. Heiss MM, Mempel W, Jauch KW, et al: Beneficial effect of autologous blood transfusion on infectious complications after colorectal cancer surgery [published erratum appears in Lancet 1994;343(8888):64] [see comments]. Lancet 1993;342(8883):1328–1333.
31. Jensen LS, Kissmeyer-Nielsen P, Wolff B, Qvist N: Randomised comparison of leucocyte-depleted versus buffy-coat-poor blood transfusion and complications after colorectal surgery [see comments]. Lancet 1996;348(9031):841–845.
32. Houbiers JG, van de Velde CJ, van de Watering LM, et al: Transfusion of red cells is associated with increased incidence of bacterial infection after colorectal surgery: A prospective study [see comments]. Transfusion 1997;37:126–134.
33. van de Watering LM, Hermans J, Houbiers JG, et al: Beneficial effects of leukocyte depletion of transfused blood on postoperative complications in patients undergoing cardiac surgery: A randomized clinical trial. Circulation 1998;97:562–568.
34. Duffy G, Neal KR: Differences in post-operative infection rates between patients receiving autologous and allogeneic blood transfusion: A meta-analysis of published randomized and nonrandomized studies [see comments]. Transfus Med 1996;6:325–328.
35. Heiss MM, Fasol-Merten K, Allgayer H, et al: Influence of autologous blood transfusion on natural killer and lymphokine-activated killer cell activities in cancer surgery. Vox Sang 1997;73:237–245.
36. Heiss MM, Fraunberger P, Delanoff C, et al: Modulation of immune response by blood transfusion: Evidence for a differential effect of allogeneic and autologous blood in colorectal cancer surgery. Shock 1997;8:402–408.
37. Blajchman MA: Allogeneic blood transfusions, immunomodulation, and postoperative bacterial infection: Do we have the answers yet? [editorial; comment]. Transfusion 1997;37:121–125.
38. Lapierre V, Auperin A, Tiberghien P: Transfusion-induced immunomodulation following cancer surgery: Fact or fiction? J Natl Cancer Inst 1998;90:573–580.
39. Jensen LS: Benefits of leukocyte-reduced blood transfusions in surgical patients. Curr Opin Hematol 1998;5:376–380.
40. Blumberg N, Heal JM: Blood transfusion immunomodulation: The silent epidemic [editorial; comment]. Arch Pathol Lab Med 1998;122:117–119.
41. de Sousa M: Blood transfusions and allograft survival: Iron-related immunosuppression? [letter]. Lancet 1983;2(8351):681–682.
42. Lazda VA, Pollak R, Mozes MF, et al: Evidence that HLA class II disparity is required for the induction of renal allograft enhancement by donor-specific blood transfusions in man. Transplantation 1990;49:1084–1087.
43. Iwaki Y, Terasaki PI: Donor-specific transfusion. Clin Transpl 1986:267–275.
44. Lagaaij EL, Hennemann IP, Ruigrok M, et al: Effect of one-HLA-DR-antigen-matched and completely HLA-DR-mismatched blood transfusions on survival of heart and kidney allografts. N Engl J Med 1989;321:701–705.
45. van der Mast BJ, Balk AH: Effect of HLA-DR-shared blood transfusion on the clinical outcome of heart transplantation. Transplantation 1997;63:1514–1519.
46. Middleton D, Martin J, Douglas J, McClelland M: Transfusion of one HLA-DR antigen-matched blood to potential recipients of a renal allograft. Transplantation 1994;58:845–848.
47. van Rood J: Pretransplant blood transfusion. Sure: but how and why? Transplant Proc 1983;15:915–916.

48. Terasaki PI: The beneficial transfusion effect on kidney graft survival attributed to clonal deletion. Transplantation 1984;37:119–125.

49. Burlingham WJ, Sollinger HW: Action of donor-specific transfusions—analysis of three possible mechanisms. Transplant Proc 1986;18:685–689.

50. van Twuyver E, Mooijaart RJ, ten Berge IJ, et al: Pretransplantation blood transfusion revisited [see comments]. N Engl J Med 1991;325:1210–1213.

51. Munson JL, van Twuyver E, Mooijaart RJ, et al: Missing T-cell receptor Vβ families following blood transfusion: The role of HLA in development of immunization and tolerance. Hum Immunol 1995;42:43–53.

52. Lagaaij EL, Ruigrok MB, van Rood JJ, et al: Blood transfusion induced changes in cell-mediated lympholysis: To immunize or not to immunize? J Immunol 1991;147:3348–3352.

53. van Prooijen HC, Aarts-Riemens MI, van Oostendorp WR, et al: Prevention of donor-specific T-cell unresponsiveness after buffy-coat-depleted blood transfusion. Br J Haematol 1995;91:219–223.

54. Young NT, Roelen DL, Iggo N, et al: Effect of one-HLA-haplotype-matched and HLA-mismatched blood transfusions on recipient T lymphocyte allorepertoires. Transplantation 1997;63:1160–1165.

55. van der Mast BJ, Vietor HE, van der Meer-Prins EM, et al: Modulation of the T cell compartment by blood transfusion: Effect on cytotoxic and helper T lymphocyte precursor frequencies and T cell receptor Vβ usage. Transplantation 1997;63:1145–1154.

56. Baudouin V, de Vitry N, Hiesse C, et al: Cytotoxic T lymphocyte changes after HLA-DR match and HLA-DR mismatch blood transfusions. Transplantation 1997;63:1155–1160.

57. Blumberg N, Heal JM: Transfusion and recipient immune function. Arch Pathol Lab Med 1989;113:246–253.

58. Schot JD, Schuurman RK: Blood transfusion suppresses cutaneous cell-mediated immunity. Clin Exp Immunol 1986;65:336–344.

59. Kaplan J, Sarnaik S, Gitlin J, Lusher J: Diminished helper/suppressor lymphocyte ratios and natural killer activity in recipients of repeated blood transfusions. Blood 1984;64:308–310.

60. Triulzi DJ, Vanek K, Ryan DH, Blumberg N: A clinical and immunologic study of blood transfusion and postoperative bacterial infection in spinal surgery. Transfusion 1992;32:517–524.

61. Romagnani S: Biology of human TH1 and TH2 cells. J Clin Immunol 1995;15:121–129.

62. Kalechman Y, Gafter U, Sobelman D, Sredni B: The effect of a single whole-blood transfusion on cytokine secretion. J Clin Immunol 1990;10:99–105.

63. Gafter U, Kalechman Y, Sredni B: Induction of a subpopulation of suppressor cells by a single blood transfusion. Kidney Int 1992;41:143–148.

64. Snijdewint FG, Kalinski P, Wierenga EA, et al: Prostaglandin E2 differentially modulates cytokine secretion profiles of human T helper lymphocytes. J Immunol 1993;150:5321–5329.

65. Walker C, Kristensen F, Bettens F, deWeck AL: Lymphokine regulation of activated (G1) lymphocytes. I: Prostaglandin E2-induced inhibition of interleukin 2 production. J Immunol 1983;130:1770–1773.

66. Gafter U, Kalechman Y, Sredni B: Blood transfusion enhances production of T-helper-2 cytokines and transforming growth factor beta in humans. Clin Sci (Colch) 1996;91:519–523.

67. Kirkley SA, Cowles J, Pellegrini VD Jr, et al: Cytokine secretion after allogeneic or autologous blood transfusion [letter; comment]. Lancet 1995;345(8948):527.

68. Worldwide collaborative observational study and meta-analysis on allogenic leukocyte immunotherapy for recurrent spontaneous abortion. Recurrent Miscarriage Immunotherapy Trialists Group [see comments] [published erratum appears in Am J Reprod Immunol 1994;32:255]. Am J Reprod Immunol 1994;32:55–72.

69. Williams JG, Hughes LE: Effect of perioperative blood transfusion on recurrence of Crohn's disease [see comments]. Lancet 1989;2(8655):131–133.

70. Wegmann TG, Lin H, Guilbert L, Mosmann TR: Bidirectional cytokine interactions in the maternal-fetal relationship: Is successful pregnancy a Th2 phenomenon? [see comments]. Immunol Today 1993;14:353–356.

71. Blumberg N, Heal JM: The transfusion immunomodulation theory: The Th1/Th2 paradigm and an analogy with pregnancy as a unifying mechanism. Semin Hematol 1996;33:329–340.

72. Bianchi DW, Flint AF, Pizzimenti MF, et al: Isolation of fetal DNA from nucleated erythrocytes in maternal blood. Proc Natl Acad Sci U S A 1990;87:3279–3283.

73. Bianchi DW, Zickwolf GK, Weil GJ, et al: Male fetal progenitor cells persist in maternal blood for as long as 27 years postpartum. Proc Natl Acad Sci U S A 1996;93:705–708.

74. Adams PT, Davenport RD, Reardon DA, Roth MS: Detection of circulating donor white blood cells in patients receiving multiple transfusions. Blood 1992;80:551–555.

75. Lee TH, Donegan E, Slichter S, Busch MP: Transient increase in circulating donor leukocytes after allogeneic transfusions in immuno-competent recipients compatible with donor cell proliferation. Blood 1995;85:1207–1214.

76. Vervoordeldonk SF, Doumaid K, Remmerswaal EB, et al: Long-term detection of microchimaerism in peripheral blood after pretransplantation blood transfusion. Br J Haematol 1998;102:1004–1009.

77. Artlett CM, Welsh KI, Black CM, Jimenez SA: Fetal-maternal HLA compatibility confers susceptibility to systemic sclerosis. Immunogenetics 1997;47:17–22.

78. Artlett CM, Smith JB, Jimenez SA: Identification of fetal DNA and cells in skin lesions from women with systemic sclerosis [see comments]. N Engl J Med 1998;338:1186–1191.

79. Nelson JL, Furst DE, Maloney S, et al: Microchimerism and HLA-compatible relationships of pregnancy in scleroderma [see comments]. Lancet 1998;351(9102):559–562.

80. Claas FH, Gijbels Y, van der Velden-de Munck J, van Rood JJ: Induction of B cell unresponsiveness to noninherited maternal HLA antigens during fetal life. Science 1988;241(4874):1815–1817.

81. Janeway CA Jr, Travers P, Hunt S, Walport M: Immunobiology: The Immune System in Health and Disease, 3rd ed. New York, Garland, 1997.

82. Rachmilewitz J, Riely GJ, Tykocinski ML: Placental protein 14 functions as a direct T-cell inhibitor. Cell Immunol 1999;191:26–33.

83. Morrow DM, Xiong N, Getty RR, et al: Hematopoietic placental protein 14: An immunosuppressive factor in cells of the megakaryocytic lineage [see comments]. Am J Pathol 1994;145:1485–1495.

84. Krensky AM, Clayberger C: HLA-derived peptides as novel immunotherapeutics. Clin Immunol Immunopathol 1995;75:112–116.

85. Murphy B, Kim KS, Buelow R, et al: Synthetic MHC class I peptide prolongs cardiac survival and attenuates transplant arteriosclerosis in the Lewis–>Fischer 344 model of chronic allograft rejection. Transplantation 1997;64:14–19.

86. Zavazava N: Soluble HLA class I molecules: Biological significance and clinical implications. Mol Med Today 1998;4:116–121.

87. Zavazava N, Leimenstoll G, Muller-Ruchholtz W: Measurement of soluble MHC class I molecules in renal graft patients: A noninvasive allograft monitor. J Clin Lab Anal 1990;4:426–429.

Chapter 36

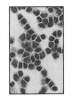

Microchimerism and Graft-Versus-Host Disease

William Reed

Eberhard W. Fiebig

Tzong-Hae Lee

Michael P. Busch

Microchimerism (MC), defined as the stable presence of a minority of nonself cells in a host, and graft-versus-host disease (GVHD), a disorder marked by attack and destruction of recipient cells by engrafted immune cells, may be viewed as related conditions. However, they differ vastly in clinical significance. MC is an expected outcome after transplantation, may be observed under certain conditions after transfusion,[1-6] and is also regularly present during pregnancy as a result of bidirectional trafficking of viable cells between fetus and mother.[7, 8] In and of itself, MC is not a threat to the recipient. Rather, the condition has been viewed by some as a welcome sign of stable graft acceptance in transplant recipients,[9, 10] has attracted attention as a model for investigating immune evasion and development of tolerance,[11, 12] and offers an exciting new venue for fetal diagnosis.[13-16] GVHD, on the other hand, remains a serious and common complication in transplant patients[17-19] and still poses a rare but serious threat to transfusion recipients.[20, 21]

In this chapter we review the discovery and current status of MC and provide a concise overview of transfusion-associated GVHD. The disease process and clinical presentation of transplant-associated GVHD differ in several important aspects from those of transfusion-associated GVHD and are covered briefly to compare and contrast the conditions. A number of current reviews specifically address basic science and clinical issues of GVHD in the transplant setting.[19, 22, 23]

■ Microchimerism

A chimera is a creature that harbors cells or tissues derived from another individual. In Greek mythology the chimera was a beast with a lion's head and foreparts, a goat's body, and a serpent's tail. Medical research on chimerism can be traced to Ray Owen, who was born on a Wisconsin dairy farm in 1915. After studying agriculture and animal husbandry at the University of Wisconsin, he joined the faculty in the department of genetics and turned his attention to the study of bovine blood groups. Owen was fascinated by Lillie's observations,[24] published in 1916, that "demonstrated union of the circulatory systems between twin bovine embryos of the opposite sex." Lillie had shown that hormones from a male fetus could enter the circulation of its female twin, producing developmental abnormalities of the reproductive system in the female twin. This "modified" female twin is called a freemartin and is an early example illustrating the effect of hormones on sexual development.

Owen examined 80 pairs of bovine twins for patterns of twinning, placental vascular anastomosis, and blood group antigens.[25] Finding that the majority of twin pairs displayed identical blood group patterns, Owen reasoned that neither chance nor monozygotic twinning could explain the blood group concordance. He reasoned that only the exchange of erythroid progenitor cells through the same vascular anastomoses that carried Lillie's hormones was likely to be responsible. This remarkable insight, attributable more to Owen's powers of observation than to available technology, changed biology[26] and introduced the notion of blood cell chimerism that was recognized by Dunsford and colleagues[27] in their early description of a human blood group chimera.

At the tissue level, chimerism can occur with solid organ transplantation or, in the research setting, when a portion of an animal embryo is grafted to another species during the early stages of development. This method has been employed extensively to investigate the developmental biology of the nervous system.[28] In humans, organ transplant recipients are tissue chimeras and, because lymphoid tissue often accompanies a solid organ graft, passenger leukocytes may be "cotransplanted" and go on to establish their lineage within the recipient.[29] If the tissue of interest is blood, chimerism of its cellular elements, hematopoietic chimerism, occurs readily when stem cells are transplanted. Hematopoietic chimerism is said to be complete when essentially all of the recipient's hematopoietic cells are replaced with cells derived from donor hematopoiesis; chimerism is said to be partial (or mixed) when a substantial proportion of donor cells is present along with those of the recipient. MC is said to exist when only a small proportion (<2.5%) of hematopoietic donor cells exists within a recipient, although these terms are often used imprecisely in the literature.

MC has been demonstrated during pregnancy and is expected after stem cell transplantation. More recently, stable MC has also been demonstrated years after both blood transfusion and normal pregnancy. In each of these settings, MC has become established in the absence of any overt manipulation of host immunity. Because of these observations, which we explore in detail, a new conceptual relationship is beginning to emerge to describe the relationship between transfusion and transplantation, where transfusion is construed broadly to mean exposure to the viable mononuclear cells of another individual. This relationship acknowledges a potential overlap between transfusion and transplantation.

Neither the conditions that permit stable MC in the setting of transfusion nor the biological consequences of MC are yet understood. In some cases, MC appears to be an incidental finding in otherwise healthy individuals. In other cases, MC has been found in association with significant disease processes including GVHD and adult-onset systemic sclerosis. In still other circumstances, chimerism may be a deliberate therapeutic strategy in transplantation or adoptive immunotherapy. Taken together, these data suggest a complex relationship among allogeneic exposures, the development of MC, and the potential consequences of MC, either pathologic or therapeutic. We review methods for detection of blood cell MC before going on to discuss clinical studies that describe the presence of MC in various circumstances of health and disease, including blood transfusion.

Microchimerism Detection Methods

Karyotype, Microscopy, and Transfer Factor

Early studies of MC utilized karyotype analysis to identify allogeneic material.[30] This technique is convincing when it yields a positive result but is relatively insensitive and depends on laborious analysis of numerous individual cells and on male-female differences. The morphologic state of lymphocytes and the rate at which they take up thymidine have also been used to study transfusion-associated MC.[6] These studies, although relatively insensitive and nonspecific, first showed that transfused leukocytes caused lymphocyte activation in the recipient, and subsequent studies provided evidence that donor cells actually participate in the proliferative response.[2] In 1969 Mohr and colleagues[31] reported on six patients who were shown to lack tuberculin sensitivity but received transfusions from donors with known sensitivity. When these investigators showed that each recipient transiently acquired the donor's tuberculin sensitivity after transfusion, great interest developed in "transfer factor." Transfer factor proved elusive to isolate or characterize but was suspected of being passenger leukocytes. Despite attempts to pursue these intriguing observations, detailed investigation would have to await the development of sensitive molecular methods, most often the polymerase chain reaction (PCR).

Polymerase Chain Reaction

Although PCR has extraordinary sensitivity derived from its ability to amplify a specific genetic sequence exponentially, the detection of a minor population of nucleic acid species against a highly similar genetic background is a technical problem unique to the detection of MC and requires unique PCR strategies to solve it. Several aspects of PCR methodology influence the detection of minor leukocyte populations. These features, summarized and annotated in Table 36.1, include the total amount of nucleic acid entering the assay, the degree and character of sequence difference distinguishing the minor population's nucleic acid, whether the PCR strategy calls for recognition of this sequence difference at the primer level or through probe specificity, whether the preparation procedures isolate leukocytes or total DNA for analysis, whether quantitation is attempted, what methods are employed for detection of amplified products, and finally whether the reaction products are observed at each cycle (real-time or kinetic PCR) or only after the reaction is complete.

We and others[32, 33] have recognized the possibility that primers that do not recognize the minor population as unique may be consumed early in the reaction through amplification of closely related sequences in the major population that vastly outnumber the minor population sought; this would be expected to produce a false-negative MC assay. Thus, in our experience, allele-specific primer pairs that recognize at least a two- to three-base-pair difference in the minor population can usually be optimized for MC detection. Amplification

Table 36.1 Polymerase Chain Reaction Strategies and Assay Characteristics Influencing the Detection of Minor Leukocyte Populations (Microchimerism)

Characteristic	Options for Assay Development		
Degree of genetic, difference between major and minor populations	Single nucleotide polymorphism	Two- to four-base-pair difference	Wholly unique allogeneic sequence (e.g., X vs Y chromosome)
Primer specificity	Allele-specific	Group-specific	Locus-specific
Observation of reaction	End reaction	End reaction labeled probe	Continuous by kinetic PCR (with or without specific hybridization probe)
Detection of amplified product	Sizing gel	Hybridization of amplified product using specific probe	DNA melting probe
Quantitation	None	Autoradiography standard dilutions	Cycle number by kinetic methodology

Table 36.2 Proportion of Chimeric Cell Populations Detected in ex vivo Cell Mixtures as a Function of Amplification Strategy

Amplification Strategy	Percent Allogeneic (Chimeric) Cell Composition			
	10%	1%	0.1%	0.01%
Locus-specific	17/18	0/16	0/18	1/17
Group-specific	21/21	21/21	21/21	16/21
Allele-specific	12/12	21/21	21/21	21/21

strategies with less primer specificity for the minor population are likely to be much less sensitive to the presence of MC. This principle is illustrated with the analysis of ex vivo cell mixtures illustrated in Table 36.2.

Real-time PCR is an important strategy in which the accumulation of amplified product is observed at each amplification cycle rather than at the reaction's termination. This is accomplished by spectrophotometric or fluorometric observation of amplified product at the completion of each cycle. The detection chemistry may include direct intercalation by ethidium bromide or SyBr green. Alternative, TaqMan[34] chemistry or molecular beacons can be used in detection.[35] The result is an information-rich analysis that provides a plot of signal intensity related to reaction product formation versus amplification cycle number. The reaction is said to become positive when the signal exceeds a predefined background level. The advantages of this technique include elimination of the probe hybridization step (ethidium bromide, SyBr green) and ready quantitation; the target copy number in the analyte is directly related to the cycle number at which the reaction becomes positive. Disadvantages include the need for some specialized equipment (sometimes requiring proprietary reagents) and the fact that, without probe hybridization, the reaction product's precise identity may be less certain. Some kinetic PCR equipment can be used to measure melting curve characteristics directly on the reaction products without further handling; this can provide confidence in the reaction's specificity. Alternatively, reaction products may be hybridized using one or more specific probes at additional steps.

Nested PCR methods have also been applied in analyses of MC.[36] Although the possibility for amplicon contamination with this method has led some groups to avoid it, nested PCR may provide some absolute advantage in sensitivity and has been used successfully in MC analysis.[37] Methods such as fluorescence in situ hybridization (FISH) have also been widely applied to the detection of MC. The limited range of sensitivity that derives from the need to analyze laboriously individual cells makes this method more suitable for detection of higher level MC such as in the post-transplantation setting. FISH has also been valuable as an independent method to confirm MC demonstrated by PCR or vice versa. Microsatellite markers and analysis of variable numbers of tandem repeats have also been widely used in chimerism analyses but are generally suited to analysis of the higher level (mixed) chimerism encountered in the stem cell transplantation setting.[38]

Rare Event Analysis and Stochastic Detection Methods

When the minor leukocyte population sought is present only at extremely low levels, detection of MC may become stochastic; that is, allogeneic material may or may not be present in the modest and limited sample volume analyzable with a single PCR reaction. Attempts to amplify much more than 10 µg of DNA in a single reaction predictably lead to PCR inhibition. To approach this problem of stochastic detection, larger volumes of blood must be analyzed in multiple parallel aliquots under identical reaction conditions. Such enhanced input assay methods are probably necessary to give meaning to a negative result in the study of rare events,[39] such as very low level MC.

Clinical Studies of Microchimerism

Bidirectional Microchimerism at the Maternal-Fetal Interface

During pregnancy, exchange of blood across the placenta occurs in both directions. The presence of maternal lymphocytes in units of placental blood collected for transplantation raised early concern about their potential to cause GVHD in the graft recipient;[40, 41] conversely, the presence of fetal lymphocytes and DNA in maternal blood or plasma holds promise for noninvasive prenatal diagnosis. We review and summarize several clinically based studies of MC at the maternal-fetal interface.

Exchange of small amounts of whole blood and lymphocytes across the placenta is a common event during normal human pregnancy. A PCR-based analysis of 66 mother-child pairs studied at the time of parturition by Lo and associates[42] was the first report to emphasize the bidirectional nature of this phenomenon. The investigators used several common polymorphisms as genotypic chimerism markers including Y chromosome, β-globin variants, and glutathione S-transferase genotype; they found fetal cells in the maternal peripheral blood in 26 of 51 informative cases. Maternal cells were detectable in the corresponding placental blood in 16 of 38 informative cases. The authors found no obvious pattern to the directionality of cell trafficking, although relatively few of the cases were informative in both directions and the genetic markers employed were non–human leukocyte antigen (HLA), so maternal-fetal histocompatibility, a factor thought by some to be potentially important in determining cell persistence, could not be examined.

Bianchi and colleagues[43] studied 32 pregnant women and 8 nonpregnant control women who had given birth to a male fetus 6 months to 27 years earlier. Flow sorting was applied to these samples to isolate several immunophenotypic subpopulations, including a stem-progenitor fraction; these were then analyzed for Y chromosome specific sequences using nested or nonnested PCR techniques. Thirteen of 19 currently pregnant women were positive for male DNA in the sorted CD34+ fraction, and 4 of 13 nonpregnant women were also positive. Because the latter women had either a history of male pregnancy or termination of pregnancy of unknown gender, the positive results were interpreted to indicate that male cells can persist as long as 27 years postpartum in some pregnant females. This study, although quite convincing overall, suffered from the absence of control samples from prepubertal females who could not have been pregnant.

Lo and coworkers[44-46] in Hong Kong have studied the presence of fetal DNA in maternal plasma and serum extensively. Studying 43 pregnant women, they found fetal DNA in 24 of 30 (80%) maternal plasma samples and in 21 of 30 (70%) serum samples, whereas no positives occurred among nonpregnant control women or among women carrying female fetuses. These and other findings led Lo's group to approach the clinical problem of determining the Rh D genotype of a fetus being carried by an Rh-negative mother through analysis of circulating DNA in the maternal plasma.[47] Among 42 women in the second or third trimester, they obtained perfect concordance for Rh type compared with serological postnatal Rh typing done by the blood bank. Among the 15 first-trimester women, Rh typing was concordant in 13, with 2 Rh-positive fetuses yielding a false-negative PCR result.

Quantitative study of the time course of fetal DNA in the maternal circulation during pregnancy by our group has shown that much more fetal DNA exists in the plasma than in the leukocyte compartment and that copy number increases to its highest levels during the third trimester before falling precipitously at parturition. Whether this plasma DNA is derived from trophoblast or turnover of fetal leukocytes or parenchymal tissues is not known.

Because plasma DNA from a pregnant woman contains a mixture of maternal and fetal DNA, many groups have pursued the isolation of fetal cells from the maternal circulation as a more definitive source for fetal DNA. Trophoblastic cells are uniquely fetal in origin but have proved difficult to isolate reliably because of the paucity of specific cell surface markers for sorting and because 1% of pregnancies display chorionic mosaicism in which the placenta, but not the fetus, manifests cytogenetic abnormalities. Leukocyte fractions of fetal origin may be isolated from the maternal circulation, but the occasional persistence of cells in the CD34+ progenitor population from a prior pregnancy causes concern about the possibility of an erroneous result. The fetal nucleated erythrocyte has drawn attention as perhaps the cell best suited for prenatal diagnosis. These cells enter the maternal circulation in high numbers (~1000:1 over leukocytes) early in pregnancy carrying a full complement of fetal genomic DNA, and, being terminally differentiated, bystander cells of this type should not persist from prior pregnancies. These cells are just beginning to be isolated and studied systematically for their potential value in prenatal diagnosis.[48, 49]

Fetal Microchimerism and Autoimmune Diseases

A report from France in 1998 examined archival skin biopsy material from 10 women with a skin rash, polymorphous eruption of pregnancy (PEP), who later gave birth to male infants.[48] Male DNA could be demonstrated in the skin of 6 of the 10 women but none of an extensive and appropriate set of control subjects. Investigators used microdissection techniques to separate dermis from epidermis and were able to show that both were positive, strongly arguing that the PCR signal did not originate from trapped circulating blood cells; having no blood vessels, the epidermis' only cellular source is the dermis. Although a PEP rash typically regresses after parturition, this elegant small study provided a precedent for the idea that fetal cells, at least under some circumstances, may infiltrate maternal skin and cause a pathological reaction.

The clear similarities between clinical features of chronic GVHD and adult-onset systemic scleroderma have long led to speculation that the conditions may be somehow related. Although the etiology of scleroderma remains unknown, application of molecular analyses is providing a convincing case that fetal cells are indeed often present in the circulation

and skin lesions of adult females with scleroderma. Although these allogeneic cells exist at very low levels, they have been found more often and in greater number among scleroderma cases than among control subjects.

Nelson and colleagues[50] described their findings in a study of 40 women, all of whom had given birth to at least one male infant. They studied 17 scleroderma patients, 16 healthy controls, and 7 sisters of the scleroderma patients. Histocompatibility between mother and fetus was assessed for an additional 21 patients, 32 controls, and their combined total of 105 offspring. Processing large volumes of whole blood for stochastic detection, these workers found a mean of 0.38 male genomic equivalents per 16 mL of whole blood among controls compared with 11.1 among women with scleroderma ($p = .0007$). In analyzing the histocompatibility data, they found that DR compatibility between mother and fetus was significantly more prevalent among scleroderma mother-child pairs than among control pairs, suggesting that DR compatibility facilitated MC while not providing an absolute requirement. They concluded that MC may be involved in the pathogenesis of scleroderma.

Artlett and colleagues[51] utilized a nonquantitative Y chromosome PCR to study peripheral blood and paraffin-embedded skin biopsy material from 69 women with systemic scleroderma. Thirty-two (46%) of the peripheral blood samples had demonstrable Y chromosome sequences compared with only 1 of 25 (4%) in normal women. FISH was employed as an independent technique to confirm the PCR findings. Nucleated cells displaying a Y chromosome signal on FISH were demonstrable in all skin biopsy material found by PCR to contain Y chromosome sequences. The authors concluded that fetal antimaternal GVHD reactions may be involved in the pathogenesis of scleroderma for some female patients.

To follow up their earlier findings, Nelson's group used Y chromosome PCR to study subpopulations of peripheral blood lymphocytes highly enriched for CD3, CD19, CD14, and CD56/16 by flow cytometric sorting.[52] Allogeneic cells were present in 12 of 20 women with scleroderma and 16 of 48 healthy control women. No significant differences between immunophenotypic subsets were observed. The authors concluded that the finding of persistent, presumably fetal cells in these women suggested the existence of specific immunoregulatory pathways that allowed persistence while preventing effector function.

Blood transfusion has been identified as a significant risk factor for the development of rheumatoid arthritis,[53] and several groups have speculated that MC from pregnancy or transfusion may play a role in other "autoimmune" diseases, including rheumatoid arthritis and multiple sclerosis. Much work remains to be done in the area of MC and autoimmune disease before a definitive causal relationship is established, however. If MC cells are reproducibly present and etiologically involved, it is important to elucidate the mechanism by which so few allogeneic cells contribute to the pathogenesis of complex autoimmune disorders. Such work could lead to novel therapeutic strategies to suppress MC-mediated pathological conditions.

Microchimerism Associated with Solid Organ Transplantation

In solid organ transplantation, MC has been attributed to engraftment of donor hematopoietic stem cells that reside in the transplanted organ.[9] After surgery, the donor cells migrate from the transplanted organ to recipient tissues throughout the body and also enter the circulation, where they may be detected as a minor cell population. In the transplant setting, establishment of MC has been viewed by some as a welcome sign of successful transplantation and a predictor of stable engraftment of the transplanted organ,[9] although others have questioned the validity of this assumption.[54] Fetal cell MC in maternal blood and tissues may similarly play a role in the establishment of immunological tolerance that is required for successful pregnancy.[42, 43, 48] These observations have led to large-scale clinical evaluations of protocols in which allogeneic peripheral blood or bone marrow–derived cells are infused into patients undergoing solid organ transplantation[55, 56] and into women with recurrent spontaneous abortions[57, 58] in an effort to induce tolerance or reverse alloimmunization. There is also interest in development of strategies for establishing MC and immunological tolerance to facilitate novel therapies employing genetically modified allogeneic cells.[59]

Transfusion-Associated Microchimerism

Studies by Schechter and coworkers[2, 6] first demonstrated that transfusion of fresh blood is associated with transient detection of donor leukocytes in recipients (detected by karyotype analyses) with associated recipient immune activation. In their seminal paper, Schechter and colleagues[6] reported the transient appearance (days 3 to 7 after transfusion) of activated, proliferating lymphocytes in the circulation of recipients of fresh whole blood (but not frozen-deglycerolized blood). In a follow-up study, Schechter and coworkers[2] used karyotype analysis to show that whereas the majority of proliferating lymphocytes were recipient cells, occasional donor lymphocytes were also detectable at the time of peak activation. On the basis of these data, they hypothesized that transfusion of blood containing viable donor lymphocytes results in a two-way proliferation reaction, representing an attempted GVH reaction by donor cells and graft rejection by recipient cells.

Adams and colleagues[4] were among the first to deploy molecular methods for detection of donor leukocytes after transfusion. They prospectively studied 20 female patients undergoing major surgical procedures for the presence of male donor leukocytes using Y chromosome specific PCR. The assays were nonquantitative analyses of total extracted DNA and demonstrated male sex-determining region Y (SRY) sequences up to 6 days after transfusion. A Dutch group reported a retrospective study of 21 renal transplant recipients using samples archived from donor-specific transfusions given before renal transplantation. They analyzed the presence of donor DNA using nested PCR based on HLA DRB1 polymorphisms. They found that in some patients, especially those receiving blood from a partially HLA-matched donor, donor leukocytes could be detected up to 8 weeks after transfusion.[5]

Following the work of Schechter and coworkers cited earlier,[2, 6] our group utilized quantitative allele-specific PCR methods developed specifically for the detection of transfusion-associated MC to characterize more precisely the kinetics of donor leukocyte persistence after transfusion. In an initial study of transfused adult women undergoing elective orthopedic surgery, we demonstrated a thousandfold expansion of allogeneic donor leukocytes in the recipient's

circulation 3 to 5 days after transfusion.[60] Each patient had received fresh unmodified packed red blood cells from a male donor; both Y chromosome and class II allele-specific PCR assays were used to detect and quantify donor leukocytes. The allogeneic cells were cleared from the circulation within 2 weeks. The finding was also corroborated in a canine transfusion model in which irradiation of the transfused blood abrogated the donor leukocyte expansion phase.

Building on these findings, our group has now documented high-level and long-lasting leukocyte MC among selected victims of traumatic injury who received a large number of fresh units of blood during their resuscitation.[1] Whereas very low levels of chimeric cells were observed in scleroderma patients or after transfusions in patients having elective surgery, in these trauma patients' peripheral blood, 3% to 4% of leukocytes were of donor origin and the donor cells persisted at high levels for as long as 2 years after transfusion. Analysis of lymphocyte subsets from these recipients using immunomagnetic bead enrichment showed that both lymphoid and myeloid lineage were represented. In some cases, HLA typing of the donor combined with MC assays based on class II polymorphisms showed a single donor to be the sole source of the chimeric leukocytes. When that implicated donor could be recalled, a mixed lymphocyte culture also showed the recipient to have acquired tolerance to that donor while remaining normally reactive to third-party lymphocytes.

These observations suggest that conditions exist, although they remain undefined, under which histocompatibility, immune responsiveness, and blood product characteristics can combine to permit establishment of stable MC even without the conditioning regimens used to create "marrow space" in transplantation. These observations, especially when combined with interest in the deliberate induction of MC as a strategy for transplantation,[61] compel more detailed study of the kinetics and mechanisms that underlie donor leukocyte clearance after infusion of allogeneic material, whether in the setting of transfusion or transplantation. Larger clinical studies of well-characterized populations in various states of health and disease are needed to better understand the prevalence and distribution of MC in the population and the allogeneic exposures that may determine its development. When such populations can be identified, detailed studies of the clonality and function of the chimeric cells will become possible. Finally, the development of animal transfusion models should allow much more systematic investigation of factors influencing donor leukocyte survival and development of transfusion-associated MC.[1, 60-63]

■ Graft-Versus-Host Disease

The current concept of GVH reactions was first formulated in the 1950s when it was recognized that spleen cell transplants in irradiated mice initially resulted in recovery of the animals from radiation injury and marrow aplasia but led to fatal "secondary disease" and "runting syndrome," characterized by wasting, diarrhea, skin lesions, and liver abnormalities.[64] In the 1960s, the term graft-versus-host disease was coined, and Simonsen[65] and later Billingham[66] defined minimum criteria for the condition: (1) presence of immunocompetent cells in the graft, capable of reacting against the recipient; (2) major histocompatibility differences between donor and recipient; and (3) inability of the recipient to reject donor cells. With the exception of the second criterion, which has been revised to include inappropriate recognition of self-antigens (i.e., autoimmunity),[67, 68] Billingham's criteria remain the basis for our understanding of the disease process in GVH reactions. Extensive research efforts have since clarified the mechanisms and conditions that lead to GVHD, although details and causal relationships of the multifactorial process are still incompletely understood.[68–70]

Clinical GVHD was first described by Shimoda[71] in 1955 as "postoperative erythroderma" in a case report of what was later identified as transfusion-associated GVHD. The first accounts of recognized transfusion-associated GVHD were published in the mid-1960s by Hathaway and associates.[72, 73] Subsequently, transfusion-associated GVHD was described in immunosuppressed patients[74] and later also in immunocompetent transfusion recipients who were recognized as being at risk because of a relatedness in HLA antigens to the blood donor.[75, 76] Transfusion-associated GVHD remains a rare but distinct threat to at-risk recipients because of its severe course and resistance to therapy. Recognition of susceptible recipients who can be protected by selecting gamma-irradiated blood for transfusion is essential.

GVHD after transplantation was first recognized in 1959 in a report of "secondary-like disease" afflicting leukemia patients who had received bone marrow transplants.[64] We now recognize acute GVHD and chronic GVHD as clinically distinct entities in transplant patients, although some overlap may occur between the two conditions.[22, 23] GVHD is most common in bone marrow transplant recipients but also occurs in recipients of solid organ transplants, particularly liver transplants.[77, 78] Disease severity is extremely variable, but both acute and chronic GVHD are reasonably responsive to a variety of immunosuppressive and immunomodulatory therapy protocols that have been developed.[19]

Pathophysiology

The simplified model of pathogenesis that has emerged since the pioneering studies of GVHD in the 1950s suggests that immunocompetent donor lymphocytes that are not cleared because of a compromised host immune system go on to proliferate in the recipient. This is followed by attack and destruction of host tissues in target organs, including liver, intestines, skin, and, perhaps, lung.[68] Supporting the validity of this model in transfusion-associated GVHD is a positive correlation between the number of transfused viable donor lymphocytes and the degree of immunosuppression in the host on the one side and the likelihood of occurrence and severity of transfusion-associated GVHD on the other.[64] The threshold dose of lymphocytes to incite transfusion-associated GVHD in humans is not known, but case reports suggest that leukoreduction by current filtration (usually to $< 1\text{-}5 \times 10^6$ white blood cells per 300 mL of blood component) is not sufficient to prevent the disease.[79–81]

Occurrence of transfusion-associated GVHD in immunocompetent recipients has been explained by a so-called one-way HLA match in which the donor cells are homozygous for an HLA type for which the recipient is heterozygous.[76] As a consequence, the recipient immune cells do not recognize the donor cells as foreign and fail to mount an immune response that would normally clear the donor cells. The latter, however, respond to the mismatched haplotype and

incite the GVH reaction, which proceeds as aggressively as in immunocompromised patients.

Refinements in the basic model suggest a complex interaction of recipient and host immune cells and emphasize the notion that the latter is not a mere passive bystander but participates in and maintains the GVH reaction through dysregulated cell activation and cytokine release. Recipient T-helper subset 1 (Th1) cytokines interleukin-2 (IL-2) and interferon-γ and proinflammatory cytokines IL-1 and tumor necrosis factor α (TNF-α) appear to promote the deleterious effects of GVH, whereas Th2 cytokines IL-4 and IL-10 are thought to have a downregulating effect.[69]

New insights into the roles of lymphocyte subpopulations in the pathophysiology of GVHD have also been gained. A mouse model provided evidence that T-cell subsets play opposite roles in the disease process, with recipient CD8 cells providing protection whereas CD4 cells promote a GVH response.[82, 83] According to the authors, patients with impaired CD8 and natural killer cell function are at increased risk for transfusion-associated GVHD, especially if they receive HLA haploidentical blood. Interestingly, this hypothesis provides one explanation for the clinical observation that human immunodeficiency virus (HIV)–infected persons whose CD4 counts drop early but whose CD8 counts remain high until late in the disease do not have GVHD despite markedly impaired cellular immunity. Infection of infused CD4 cells by HIV followed by attack of the infected cells by cytolytic CD8 cells provides an additional explanation for the apparent absence of GVHD in patients with acquired immunodeficiency syndrome (AIDS).[84] The precise role of T-cell subsets in GVH reactions remains controversial, however, and others maintain that reactive CD8 cells are required for the development of GVHD.[85]

With regard to the effector cells that cause tissue damage in GVHD, evidence from studies of patients with transfusion-associated GVHD suggests that T cells participating in the disease process are clonally restricted in expression of T-cell receptor repertoires[86] and are composed of a variety of CD4- and CD8-positive clones that may cause tissue damage through different mechanisms, including direct and indirect cytotoxicity.[87] The latter finding may explain the often characteristically sparse lymphocytic infiltrate of target tissues in GVHD. Indirect cell lysis may occur through an apoptosis-inducing mechanism or through cytokine release (TNF-β, IL-1) followed by attraction of platelets and neutrophils causing cell damage by release of free radicals and elastases.

Clinical Presentation

Patients with transfusion-associated GVHD typically present within 7 to 10 days of the transfusion with fever; a characteristic reddish, raised rash spreading from trunk or face to the extremities; evidence of hepatitis; watery diarrhea; and nonspecific signs including anorexia, nausea, and vomiting.[20, 88] The diarrhea may be profuse, and the skin lesions may progress to bullous lesions and generalized erythroderma. The development of pancytopenia caused by immune destruction of host marrow cells distinguishes transfusion-associated GVHD from GVHD following hematopoietic stem cell transplantation and is the usual cause of death from hemorrhage and overwhelming infection. Most patients die within 1 to 3 weeks after the onset of clinical symptoms.[75]

In neonates, symptoms appear later, approximately a month after transfusion, and the disease tends to run a more prolonged course with survival for up to 3 months.[88] The naive T-cell population in infants and a different cytokine milieu favoring interferon-γ over IL-2 may be responsible for the delayed response.

Few patients survive transfusion-associated GVHD, although spontaneous recovery or development of a chronic form of GVHD has been reported.[88–90]

Epidemiology

Transfusion-associated GVHD is rare in unselected U.S. transfusion recipients and has been almost exclusively observed in immunocompromised patients.[91] In contrast, over 200 cases of transfusion-associated GVHD have been described in Japan alone,[75] with incidence rates reaching 1 in 660 patients undergoing cardiovascular surgery.[92] Greater genetic homogeneity of the Japanese population and frequent use of fresh whole blood from related donors are thought to be the primary reasons for the surprisingly frequent occurrence of transfusion-associated GVHD in Japan before the institution of prophylactic irradiation of blood from related donors.[93, 94] Reports of relatively high rates of transfusion-associated GVHD have also come from other geographic areas with genetically homogeneous populations.[95] Estimates of the risk of transfusion-associated GVHD based on genetic similarities in HLA haplotype frequencies between random blood donor–recipient pairs yielded a risk of 1 in 17,700 to 1 in 39,000 among whites in the United States; the risk in Japan was projected to be 1 in 1600 to 1 in 7900. Directed donations between parents and children increase the risk of histocompatibility 10- to 20-fold.[96, 97]

Diagnosis

Given the rarity of the disease, the diagnosis of transfusion-associated GVHD may be missed and is often not made until late in the course or posthumously unless there is a high degree of suspicion.[97] Other diagnoses such as drug reaction or infections are usually considered first, and routine laboratory studies are not helpful for an etiological diagnosis. Histological findings on skin, liver, or intestinal biopsies may suggest the diagnosis of transfusion-associated GVHD but are not pathognomonic. The only definitive method of diagnosis is the identification of donor-derived lymphocytes in the circulation or tissues of the affected host.

In seeking donor-derived genotypes to support the diagnosis of transfusion-associated GVHD, it is critical to consider the PCR amplification strategy; a strategy with limited primer specificity could result in a false-negative chimerism assay (see Table 36.2).[33] This may be accomplished by detailed HLA typing, cytogenetic analysis, or studies of genomic markers capable of reliably identifying donor and recipient cells.[94, 98, 99] For example, detection of Y chromosome regions by PCR has been used to confirm transfusion-associated GVHD by documenting circulating male cells in female recipients.[98, 100] However, caution must be exercised when seeking donor-derived genotypes by PCR to support the diagnosis of transfusion-associated GVHD because it is critical to select an appropriate amplification strategy; use of primers with limited specificity or other methods of limited sensitivity for detection of a minor population can result in a false-negative chimerism assay.[33]

Therapy

Immunosuppressive therapy with corticosteroids, antithymocyte globulin, cyclophosphamide, methotrexate, and cyclosporine, often used in combination, is usually able to influence transplant-associated GVHD[22, 23] but is mostly ineffective in transfusion-associated GVHD.[21, 69, 100] Hematopoietic stem cell transplantation has been attempted successfully in rare cases.[101] Because of the small number of case reports in which treatment resulted in recovery[89, 102] and uncertainty about whether a milder form of the disease contributed to the success, consensus treatment guidelines have not been formulated.

Prevention

Gamma irradiation of blood components containing viable lymphocytes is virtually 100% effective in preventing transfusion-associated GVHD, although rare failures have been reported with irradiation doses considered suboptimal today.[103–105] Irradiation prophylaxis is recommended for all whole blood, red blood cell, platelet, and granulocyte units transfused to patients at risk.[106] Irradiation prevents proliferation of lymphocytes through cross-linkage of DNA.[107] The required dose is 25 Gy to the midplane of the blood container with a minimum of 15 Gy to any point of the irradiated field.[106] The Food and Drug Administration further mandated that the maximum dose not exceed 50 Gy.[100] In this dosage range, irradiation is considered safe with unlikely harm to the recipient of the treated component.

Adverse effects of irradiation on therapeutic blood components include a moderate decrease in survival of red blood cells[108] and leakage of potassium from intracellular stores.[109, 110] The allowable storage period for irradiated red blood cell units has therefore been reduced to 28 days,[106] and caution is advised in administering stored irradiated red blood cell units to recipients at risk for ill effects of hyperkalemia.[111] These include primarily neonates and premature infants with renal failure or those who receive large-volume transfusions, especially if administered through central venous catheters, or treatment with extracorporeal membrane oxygenation through central venous catheters. Platelets do not appear to be affected by the recommended radiation dose during routine 5-day blood bank storage,[112, 113] and no reduction in storage time is necessary. Frozen thawed red blood cell units, fresh frozen plasma (FFP), and cryoprecipitate are widely viewed as "noncellular" blood components, and no documented cases of transfusion-associated GVHD after administration of these components have been reported;[100] irradiation is therefore not currently recommended. Transfusion-associated GVHD has occurred after transfusion of fresh liquid plasma that had never been frozen,[114] and some concern has been expressed that FFP may contain sufficient viable lymphocytes to cause transfusion-associated GVHD.[115, 116] This issue is currently under investigation.

Experimental methods of lymphocyte inactivation for transfusion-associated GVHD prophylaxis include ultraviolet B (UVB) irradiation[117] and photochemical treatment with UVA-activated psoralens.[118] The latter approach, which has been developed for pathogen inactivation in plasma units and is being evaluated in clinical trials, may be at least equally effective in preventing lymphocyte response to immunological stimulation and proliferation.[118, 119]

Table 36.3 Patient Groups at Risk for Developing Transfusion-Associated Graft-versus-Host Disease

Clear Risk

Patients with selected immunodeficiencies:
Congenital immunodeficiencies
Hodgkin's disease
Chronic lymphocytic leukemia treated with fludarabine

Newborns with erythroblastosis fetalis

Recipients of intrauterine transfusions

Recipients of hematopoietic stem cell transplants

Recipients of blood products donated by relatives

Recipients of human leukocyte antigen (HLA)–selected (matched) platelets or platelets known to be homozygous

Probable Risk

Patients with
Other hematological malignancies
Solid tumors treated with cytotoxic agents

Recipient-donor pairs from genetically homogeneous populations

Premature and possibly full-term neonates

No Defined Risk

Patients with acquired immunodeficiency syndrome (AIDS)

Patients taking immunosuppressive medications.

From Webb IJ, Anderson KC: Transfusion-associated graft-versus-host disease. In Anderson KC, Ness PM (eds): Scientific Basis of Transfusion Medicine, 2nd ed. Philadelphia, WB Saunders, 2000, p 421.

Patients at Risk Who Should Receive Transfusion-Associated GVHD Prophylaxis

Because transfusion-associated GVHD may occur in immunocompetent individuals, any transfusion recipient may be considered at risk and identification of defined risk groups may provide a false sense of security to those not included in the at-risk groups. However, unless it is decided to irradiate all blood components, the categorization of patients who are at particular risk on the basis of experience is useful and practically important. Table 36.3 lists groups of patients at risk for developing transfusion-associated GVHD; for these groups, irradiation of cellular blood components for prevention of GVHD is indicated.

■ Conclusion

In summary, chimerism appears to arise from a variety of different allogeneic exposures such as pregnancy, transplantation, and the transfusion of cellular blood products. Chimerism and GVHD define a continuum for quantity and immunologic behavior of chimeric blood cells within an individual recipient. MC seems to exist in some individuals without apparent clinical effect, but even at extremely low levels it has also been associated with diverse pathologic conditions. In contrast, the chimerism that arises during the evolution of GVHD behaves in a far more aggressive manner, usually leading to tissue destruction and death.

There is a great need for standardization of assays used in the detection of chimerism and for normative data describing the prevalence, magnitude, and immunophenotypic characteristics of chimerism in normal individuals and in various pathologic conditions. Much remains to be learned through clinical investigation and study of animal models regarding the host factors and characteristics of allogeneic exposure favoring establishment of stable chimerism, the factors influencing the behavior of chimeric cells (coexistence versus pathologic effect), and the immunologic mechanisms that underlie all of these.

REFERENCES

1. Lee T-H, Paglieroni T, Ohto H, et al: Survival of donor leukocyte subpopulations in immunocompetent transfusion recipients: Frequent long-term microchimerism in severe trauma patients. Blood 1999;93:3127–3139.
2. Schechter GP, Whang-Peng J, McFarland W: Circulation of donor lymphocytes after blood transfusion in man. Blood 1977;49:651–656.
3. Hutchinson DL, Turner JH, Schlesinger ER: Persistence of donor cells in neonates after fetal and exchange transfusion. Am J Obstet Gynecol 1971;109:281–284.
4. Adams P, Davenport R, Reardon DA, Roth MS: Detection of circulating donor white blood cells in patients receiving multiple transfusions. Blood 1992;80:551–555.
5. Vervoordeldonk SF, Doumaid K, Remmerswaal EBM, et al: Long-term detection of microchimerism in peripheral blood after pretransplantation blood transfusion. Br J Haematol 1998;102:1004–1009.
6. Schechter GP, Soehnlen F, McFarland W: Lymphocyte response to blood transfusion in man. N Engl J Med 1972;287:1169–1173.
7. Bianchi DW, Zickwolf GK, Weil GJ, et al: Male fetal progenitor cells persist in maternal blood for as long as 27 years postpartum. Proc Natl Acad Sci U S A 1996;93:705–708.
8. Lo YM, Lo ES, Watson N, et al: Two-way cell traffic between mother and fetus: Biologic and clinical implications. Blood 1996;88:4390–4395.
9. Starzl TE, Demetris AJ, Murase N, et al: Cell migration, chimerism, and graft acceptance. Lancet 1992;339:1579–1582.
10. Starzl TE: Clinical and basic scientific implications of cell migration and microchimerism after organ transplantation. Artif Organs 1997;21:1154–1155.
11. Ko S, Deiwick A, Dinkel A, et al: Functional relevance of donor-derived hematopoietic microchimerism only for induction but not for maintenance of allograft acceptance. Transplant Proc 1999;31:920–921.
12. Ko S, Deiwick A, Jager MD, et al: The functional relevance of passenger leukocytes and microchimerism for heart allograft acceptance in the rat. Nat Med 1999;5:1292–1297.
13. Lo YM: Fetal RhD genotyping from maternal plasma. Ann Med 1999;31:308–312.
14. Tang NL, Leung TN, Zhang J, et al: Detection of fetal-derived paternally inherited X-chromosome polymorphisms in maternal plasma. Clin Chem 1999;45:2033–2035.
15. Lo YM: Application of PCR for fetal cell detection. Early Hum Dev 1996;47(Suppl):s73–s77.
16. Lo YM: Non-invasive prenatal diagnosis using fetal cells in maternal blood. J Clin Pathol 1994;47:1060–1065.
17. Dey B, Sykes M, Spitzer TR: Outcomes of recipients of both bone marrow and solid organ transplants. A review. Medicine (Baltimore) 1998;77:355–369.
18. Wagner ND, Quinones VW: Allogeneic peripheral blood stem cell transplantation: Clinical overview and nursing implications. Oncol Nurs Forum 1998;25:1049–1055; quiz 1056–1057.
19. Klingebiel T, Schlegel PG: GVHD: Overview on pathophysiology, incidence, clinical and biological features. Bone Marrow Transplant 1998;21(Suppl 2):s45–s49.
20. Rososhansky S, Badonnel MC, Hiestand LL, et al: Transfusion-associated graft-versus-host disease in an immunocompetent patient following cardiac surgery. Vox Sang 1999;76:59–63.
21. Webb IJ, Anderson KC: Transfusion-associated graft-versus-host disease. In Anderson KC, Ness PM (eds): Scientific Basis of Transfusion Medicine. Implications for Clinical Practice, 2nd ed. Philadelphia, WB Saunders, 2000, pp 420–426.
22. Parkman R: Chronic graft-versus-host disease. Curr Opin Hematol 1998;5:22–25.
23. Flowers ME, Kansu E, Sullivan KM: Pathophysiology and treatment of graft-versus-host disease. Hematol Oncol Clin North Am 1999;13:1091–1112, viii–ix.

24. Lillie FR: The theory of the free-martin. Science 1916;43:611–613.
25. Owen R: Immunogenetic consequences of vascular anastomoses between bovine twins. Science 1945;102:400–401.
26. Burlingham WJ, Muller D: Chimerism and tolerance. Hum Immunol 1997;52:73–74.
27. Dunsford I, Bowley C, Hutchinson A, et al: A human blood group chimera. Br Med J 1953;2:81.
28. Teillet MA, Ziller C, Le Douarin NM: Quail-chick chimeras. Methods Mol Biol 1999;97:305–318.
29. Starzl TE, Demetris AJ, Murase N, et al: Cell migration, chimerism, and graft acceptance. Lancet 1992;339:1579–1582.
30. Hutchinson D, Turner J, Schlesinger E: Persistence of donor cells in neonates after fetal and exchange transfusion. Am J Obstet Gynecol 1971;109:281–284.
31. Mohr J, Killebrew L, Muchmore H, et al: Transfer of delayed hypersensitivity: The role of blood transfusions in humans. JAMA 1969;207:517–519.
32. Dzik S: The power of primers [editorial]. Transfusion 1998;38:118–121.
33. Reed W, Lee T-H, Trachtenberg E, et al: Detection of microchimerism by PCR is a function of amplification strategy. Transfusion 2001;41:39–44.
34. Moody A, Sellers S, Bumstead N: Measuring infectious bursal disease virus RNA in blood by multiplex real-time quantitative RT-PCR. J Virol Methods 2000;85:55–64.
35. Marras SA, Kramer FR, Tyagi S: Multiplex detection of single-nucleotide variations using molecular beacons. Genet Anal 1999;14:151–156.
36. Carter AS, Bunce M, Cerundolo L, et al: Detection of microchimerism after allogeneic blood transfusion using nested polymerase chain reaction amplification with sequence-specific primers (PCR-SSR): A cautionary tale. Blood 1998;92:683–689.
37. Carter AS, Cerundolo L, Bunce M, et al: Nested polymerase chain reaction with sequence-specific primers typing for HLA-A, -B, and -C alleles: Detection of microchimerism in DR-matched individuals. Blood 1999;94:1471–1477.
38. Van Deerlin VM, Leonard DG: Bone marrow engraftment analysis after allogeneic bone marrow transplantation. Clin Lab Med 2000;20:197–225.
39. Dzik S: Principles of counting low numbers of leukocytes in leukoreduced blood components. Transfus Med Rev 1997;11:44–55.
40. Scaradavou A, Carrier C, Mollen N, et al: Detection of maternal DNA in placental/umbilical cord blood by locus-specific amplification of the noninherited maternal HLA gene. Blood 1996;88:1494–1500.
41. Petit T, Gluckman E, Carosella E, et al: A highly sensitive polymerase chain reaction method reveals the ubiquitous presence of maternal cells in human umbilical cord blood. Exp Hematol 1995;23:1601–1605.
42. Lo YM, Lo ES, Watson N, et al: Two-way cell traffic between mother and fetus: Biologic and clinical implications. Blood 1996;88:4390–4395.
43. Bianchi DW, Zickwolf GK, Weil GJ, et al: Male fetal progenitor cells persist in maternal blood for as long as 27 years postpartum. Proc Natl Acad Sci U S A 1996;93:705–708.
44. Lo YM, Corbetta N, Chamberlain PF, et al: Presence of fetal DNA in maternal plasma and serum. Lancet 1997;350:485–487.
45. Lo YM: Detection of minority nucleic acid populations by PCR. J Pathol 1994;174:1–6.
46. Lo YM, Tein MS, Lau TK, et al: Quantitative analysis of fetal DNA in maternal plasma and serum: Implications for noninvasive prenatal diagnosis. Am J Hum Genet 1998;62:768–775.
47. Lo YM, Hjelm NM, Fidler C, et al: Prenatal diagnosis of fetal RhD status by molecular analysis of maternal plasma. N Engl J Med 1998;339:1734–1738.
48. Bianchi D: Current knowledge about fetal blood cells in the maternal circulation. J Perinat Med 1998;26:175–185.
49. Aractingi S, Berkane N, Bertheau P, et al: Fetal DNA in skin of polymorphic eruptions of pregnancy. Lancet 1998;352:1898–1901.
50. Nelson JL, Furst DE, Maloney S, et al: Microchimerism and HLA-compatible relationships of pregnancy in scleroderma. Lancet 1998;351:559–562.
51. Artlett C, Smith J, Jimenez S: Identification of fetal DNA and cells in skin lesions from women with systemic sclerosis. N Engl J Med 1998;338:1186–1191.
52. Evans P, Lambert C, Maloney S, et al: Long-term fetal microchimerism in peripheral blood mononuclear cell subsets in healthy women and women with scleroderma. Blood 1999;93:2033–2037.

53. Symmons DPM, Bankhead CR, Harrison BJ, et al: Blood transfusion, smoking, and obesity as risk factors for the development of rheumatoid arthritis. Arthritis Rheum 1997;40:1955–1961.
54. Elwood ET, Larsen CP, Maurer DH, et al: Microchimerism and rejection in clinical transplantation. Lancet 1997;349:1358–1360.
55. Opelz G, Terasaki PI: Improvement of kidney graft survival with increased numbers of blood transfusions. N Engl J Med 1978;299:799–803.
56. Opelz G, Vanrenterghem Y, Kirste G, et al: Prospective evaluation of pretransplant blood transfusions in cadaver kidney recipients. Transplantation 1997;63:964–967.
57. Ober C, Karrison T, Odem RR, et al: Mononuclear-cell immunisation in prevention of recurrent miscarriages: A randomised trial. Lancet 1999;354:365–369.
58. Recurrent Miscarriage Immunotherapy Trialist Group: Worldwide collaborative observational study and meta-analysis on allogenic leukocyte immunotherapy for recurrent spontaneous abortion. Am J Reprod Immunol 1994;32:55–72.
59. Hillyer CD, Klein HG: Immunotherapy and gene transfer in the treatment of the oncology patient: Role of transfusion medicine. Transfus Med Rev 1996;10:1–14.
60. Lee T-H, Donegan E, Slichter S, Busch M: Transient increase in circulating donor leukocytes after allogeneic transfusion in immunocompetent recipients compatible with donor cell proliferation. Blood 1995;85:1207–1214.
61. McSweeney PA, Storb R: Mixed chimerism: Preclinical studies and clinical applications. Biol Blood Marrow Transplant 1999;5:192–203.
62. Lee T-H, Reed W, Mangawang-Montalvo L, et al: Donor WBCs can persist and transiently mediate immunologic function in a murine transfusion model: Effects of irradiation, storage, and histocompatibility. Transfusion 2001;41:637–642.
63. Kao KJ: Mechanisms and new approaches for allogeneic blood transfusion–induced immunomodulatory effects. Transfus Med Rev 2000;14:12–22.
64. Brubaker DB: Transfusion-associated graft-versus-host disease. In Anderson KC, Ness PM (eds): Scientific Basis of Transfusion Medicine. Implications for Clinical Practice. Philadelphia, WB Saunders, 1994, pp 544–579.
65. Simonsen M: Graft versus host reactions: Their natural history and applicability as tools of research. Prog Allergy 1962;6:349–467.
66. Billingham R: The biology of graft-versus-host reactions. Harvey Lect 1966–67;62:21–78.
67. de Arriba F, Corral J, Ayala F, et al: Autoaggression syndrome resembling acute graft-versus-host disease grade IV after autologous peripheral blood stem cell transplantation for breast cancer. Bone Marrow Transplant 1999;23:621–624.
68. Vogelsang GB, Hess AD: Graft-versus-host disease: New directions for a persistent problem. Blood 1994;84:2061–2067.
69. Ferrara JL, Levy R, Chao NJ: Pathophysiologic mechanisms of acute graft-vs.-host disease. Biol Blood Marrow Transplant 1999;5:347–356.
70. Orlin JB, Ellis MH: Transfusion-associated graft-versus-host disease. Curr Opin Hematol 1997;4:442–448.
71. Shimoda T: The case report of post-operative erythroderma. Geka 1955;17:487.
72. Hathaway WE, Brangle RW, Nelson TL, Roeckel IE: Aplastic anemia and alymphocytosis in an infant with hypogammaglobulinemia: Graft-versus-host reaction? J Pediatr 1966;68:713–722.
73. Hathaway WE, Fulginiti VA, Pierce CW, et al: Graft-vs-host reaction following a single blood transfusion. JAMA 1967;201:1015–1020.
74. Brubaker DB: Human posttransfusion graft-versus-host disease. Vox Sang 1983;45:401–420.
75. Ohto H, Anderson KC: Survey of transfusion-associated graft-versus-host disease in immunocompetent recipients. Transfus Med Rev 1996;10:31–43.
76. Thaler M, Shamiss A, Orgad S, et al: The role of blood from HLA-homozygous donors in fatal transfusion-associated graft-versus-host disease after open-heart surgery. N Engl J Med 1989;321:25–28.
77. Schmuth M, Vogel W, Weinlich G, et al: Cutaneous lesions as the presenting sign of acute graft-versus-host disease following liver transplantation. Br J Dermatol 1999;141:901–904.
78. Jamieson NV, Joysey V, Friend PJ, et al: Graft-versus-host disease in solid organ transplantation. Transplant Int 1991;4(2):67–71.
79. Akahoshi M, Takanashi M, Masuda M, et al: A case of transfusion-associated graft-versus-host disease not prevented by white cell–reduction filters. Transfusion 1992;32:169–172.

80. Hayashi H, Nishiuchi T, Tamura H, Takeda K: Transfusion-associated graft-versus-host disease caused by leukocyte-filtered stored blood. Anesthesiology 1993;79:1419–1421.

81. Heim MU, Munker R, Sauer H, et al: [Graft versus host disease with fatal outcome after administration of filtered erythrocyte concentrates]. Beitr Infusionsther 1992;30:178–181.

82. Fast LD, Valeri CR, Crowley JP: Immune responses to major histocompatibility complex homozygous lymphoid cells in murine F1 hybrid recipients: Implications for transfusion-associated graft-versus-host disease. Blood 1995;86:3090–3096.

83. Fast LD: Recipient CD8+ cells are responsible for the rapid elimination of allogeneic donor lymphoid cells. J Immunol 1996;157:4805–4810.

84. Ammann AJ: Hypothesis: Absence of graft-versus-host disease in AIDS is a consequence of HIV-1 infection of CD4+ T cells. J Acquir Immune Defic Syndr 1993;6:1224–1227.

85. Habeshaw JA, Dalgleish AG, Hounsell EF: Absence of GVH diseases in AIDS. J Acquir Immune Defic Syndr 1994;7:1287–1289.

86. Wang L, Tadokoro K, Tokunaga K, et al: Restricted use of T-cell receptor V beta genes in posttransfusion graft-versus-host disease. Transfusion 1997;37:1184–1191.

87. Nishimura M, Uchida S, Mitsunaga S, et al: Characterization of T-cell clones derived from peripheral blood lymphocytes of a patient with transfusion-associated graft-versus-host disease: Fas-mediated killing by CD4+ and CD8+ cytotoxic T-cell clones and tumor necrosis factor beta production by CD4+ T-cell clones. Blood 1997;89:1440–1445.

88. Ohto H, Anderson KC: Posttransfusion graft-versus-host disease in Japanese newborns. Transfusion 1996;36:117–123.

89. Cohen D, Weinstein H, Mihm M, Yankee R: Nonfatal graft-versus-host disease occurring after transfusion with leukocytes and platelets obtained from normal donors. Blood 1979;53:1053–1057.

90. Mori S, Matsushita H, Ozaki K, et al: Spontaneous resolution of transfusion-associated graft-versus-host disease. Transfusion 1995;35:431–435.

91. Vogelsang GB: Transfusion-associated graft-versus-host disease in nonimmunocompromised hosts. Transfusion 1990;30:101–103.

92. Juji T, Takahashi K, Shibata Y, et al: Post-transfusion graft-versus-host disease in immunocompetent patients after cardiac surgery in Japan [letter]. N Engl J Med 1989;321:56.

93. Takahashi K, Juji T, Miyamoto M, et al: Analysis of risk factors for post-transfusion graft-versus-host disease in Japan. Japanese Red Cross PT-GVHD Study Group. Lancet 1994;343:700–702.

94. Wang L, Juji T, Tokunaga K, et al: Brief report: Polymorphic microsatellite markers for the diagnosis of graft-versus-host disease. N Engl J Med 1994;330:398–401.

95. Kfoury-Baz E, Alami SY, Nassif RE, et al: Transfusion-associated graft-versus-host disease: A report of three cases in immunocompetent patients in Lebanon [letter]. Transfusion 1996;36:286–287.

96. Wagner FF, Flegel WA: Transfusion-associated graft-versus-host disease: Risk due to homozygous HLA haplotypes. Transfusion 1995;35:284–291.

97. Shivdasani RA, Anderson KC: Transfusion-associated graft-versus-host disease: Scratching the surface [editorial; comment]. Transfusion 1993;33:696–697.

98. Hayakawa S, Chishima F, Sakata H, et al: A rapid molecular diagnosis of posttransfusion graft-versus-host disease by polymerase chain reaction. Transfusion 1993;33:413–417.

99. Kunstmann E, Bocker T, Roewer L, et al: Diagnosis of transfusion-associated graft-versus-host disease by genetic fingerprinting and polymerase chain reaction. Transfusion 1992;32:766–770.

100. Gorlin J, Mintz P: Transfusion-associated graft-versus-host disease. In Mintz P (ed): Transfusion Therapy: Clinical Principles and Practice. Bethesda, Md, AABB Press, 1999, pp 341–357.

101. Yasukawa M, Shinozaki F, Hato T, et al: Successful treatment of transfusion-associated graft-versus-host disease. Br J Haematol 1994;86:831–836.

102. Prince M, Szer J, van der Weyden MB, et al: Transfusion associated graft-versus-host disease after cardiac surgery: Response to antithymocyte-globulin and corticosteroid therapy. Aust NZ J Med 1991;21:43–46.

103. Sproul AM, Chalmers EA, Mills KI, et al: Third party mediated graft rejection despite irradiation of blood products. Br J Haematol 1992;80:251–252.

104. Lowenthal RM, Challis DR, Griffiths AE, et al: Transfusion-associated graft-versus-host disease: Report of an occurrence following the administration of irradiated blood. Transfusion 1993;33:524–529.

105. Drobyski W, Thibodeau S, Truitt RL, et al: Third-party–mediated graft rejection and graft-versus-host disease after T-cell–depleted bone marrow transplantation, as demonstrated by hypervariable DNA probes and HLA-DR polymorphism. Blood 1989;74:2285–2294.

106. Menitove J (ed): Standards for Blood Banks and Transfusion Services, 19th ed. Bethesda, Md, AABB Press, 1999.

107. Baskaeva IO: [The formation of DNA-protein cross-links in response to gamma radiation, UV irradiation and chemical agents]. Radiobiologiia 1992;32:673–684.

108. Davey RJ, McCoy NC, Yu M, et al: The effect of prestorage irradiation on posttransfusion red cell survival. Transfusion 1992;32:525–528.

109. Arseniev L, Schumann G, Andres J: Kinetics of extracellular potassium concentration in irradiated red blood cells. Infusionsther Transfusionsmed 1994;21:322–324.

110. Moroff G, Holme S, AuBuchon JP, et al: Viability and in vitro properties of AS-1 red cells after gamma irradiation. Transfusion 1999;39:128–134.

111. Strauss RG: Routinely washing irradiated red cells before transfusion seems unwarranted. Transfusion 1990;30:675–677.

112. Duguid JK, Carr R, Jenkins JA, et al: Clinical evaluation of the effects of storage time and irradiation on transfused platelets. Vox Sang 1991;60:151–154.

113. Rock G, Adams GA, Labow RS: The effects of irradiation on platelet function. Transfusion 1988;28:451–455.

114. Park BH, Biggar WD, Good RA: Minnesota experience in bone-marrow transplantation in man, 1968 to June 1973. Transplant Proc 1974;6:379–383.

115. Willis JI, Lown JA, Simpson MC, Erber WN: White cells in fresh-frozen plasma: Evaluation of a new white cell-reduction filter. Transfusion 1998;38:645–649.

116. Gresens CJ, Paglieroni TG, Ward TM, et al: T cells in fresh frozen plasma are viable and can respond to mitogen, superantigen and allogeneic monocytes [abstract S452-030Q]. Transfusion 1999;39 (10 Suppl):99s.

117. van Prooijen HC, Aarts-Riemens MI, Grijzenhout MA, van Weelden H: Ultraviolet irradiation modulates MHC-alloreactive cytotoxic T-cell precursors involved in the onset of graft-versus-host disease. Br J Haematol 1992;81:73–76.

118. Grass JA, Wafa T, Reames A, et al: Prevention of transfusion-associated graft-versus-host disease by photochemical treatment. Blood 1999;93:3140–3147.

119. Fiebig E, Hirschkorn DF, Maino VC, et al: Assessment of donor T cell function in cellular blood components by the CD69 induction assay: Effects of storage, irradiation and photochemical treatment. Transfusion 2000;40:761–770.

Chapter 37

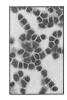

Hepatitis A, Hepatitis B, and Non-A, Non-B, Non-C Viruses

Roger Y. Dodd

Hepatitis was recognized as an adverse consequence almost from the outset of transfusion therapy. In fact, viral hepatitis was originally classified either as "infectious or "serum" hepatitis according to its predominant transmission mode. We now realize that infectious hepatitis was almost entirely accounted for by hepatitis A virus (HAV), whereas serum hepatitis was most likely due to infection with hepatitis B and C viruses. Other hepatitis viruses have been recognized, including hepatitis D virus (previously delta virus) and hepatitis E virus. Other viruses have also been identified in the context of hepatitis, although they do not appear to be primary causative agents of the disease; included in this group are the hepatitis G virus and the TTV/SEN-V complex.

■ Hepatitis A

Hepatitis A is usually a relatively mild disease, and there are no reports of chronic infection or disease. The mortality rate is 0.2% or less. Although symptoms may be severe, most cases are inapparent, as the seroprevalence rates may range from 5% to 74% of subsets of the U.S. population, depending on age. The incubation period averages 25 to 30 days, with a range of about 15 to 45 days. When symptoms are present, there may be a short prodromal phase lasting 2 to 10 days, involving fever, chills, malaise, and arthralgias. During this phase, the alanine aminotransaminase (ALT) levels rise; they peak during the appearance of the more definitive symptoms of hepatitis, namely anorexia, nausea and vomiting, and epigastric tenderness. Laboratory diagnosis is normally based on evaluation of serum ALT levels plus the use of an immunoassay for anti-HAV immunoglobulin (Ig) M.

The virus is typically transmitted by the fecal-oral route. High levels of virus are shed in the feces during the prodromal stage. Uncooked shellfish from contaminated waters is a common source of infection. Food-borne outbreaks are relatively common and the source is usually an infected food-handler. Infection is often transmitted among diapered infants in daycare and in hospital nursery settings.

The hepatitis A virus is a picornavirus, classified in the genus Hepatovirus. As such, it is a nonenveloped virus, about 27 nm in diameter. It was first recognized in the 1970s on immunoelectron microscopy of fecal samples. Unlike other hepatitis viruses, HAV can be readily grown in tissue culture.[1]

Transfusion-transmitted hepatitis A is very uncommon, with about 25 cases reported in the literature, and a risk estimated as considerably less than one case per million transfused component units. Interestingly, some of the reported cases did involve young children, and there were secondary cases as a result of transmission in the nursery.[2–6] The low frequency of transfusion-transmitted HAV is usually attributed to the rather short period of viremia prior to the appearance of symptoms. Bower and colleagues[7] have reported, however, that HAV RNA could be detected in the blood an average of 17 days before and 79 days after the peak of serum ALT. Such findings do not necessarily correlate with infectivity.

In the United States, individuals with a history of viral hepatitis are not permitted to give blood unless they had the disease before the age of 11 years. This practice recognizes the fact that almost all hepatitis occurring prior to this age is due to HAV, which would not offer any risk of transmission. There are no other specific measures in place to prevent transfusion-transmitted HAV infection. However, it is usual to withdraw blood products if it is learned that the donors were recently exposed to HAV (for example, through a known food-borne outbreak).

There has also been concern about transmission of HAV via some specific lots of antihemophilic factor products.[8–11]

Whether the contamination derived from the plasma donors or was introduced elsewhere in the processing is unclear. However, it was clear that the solvent-detergent process failed to inactivate the contaminating virus. This finding is not unexpected for a nonenveloped virus. As a result of these events, additional inactivation steps are used, and manufacturing pools are monitored for HAV RNA. Additionally, it is recommended that certain recipients of plasma products (including solvent-detergent–treated plasma) should receive the hepatitis A vaccine.

■ Hepatitis B

Hepatitis B is the prototypic transfusion-transmitted disease. Until the early 1970s, it was considered the only form of parenterally transmitted hepatitis. Exposure to hepatitis B virus (HBV) may result in a prolonged but asymptomatic infection with the potential for high titers of circulating virus, even in the presence of a vigorous immune response. Indeed, a number of lines of evidence, including early studies of human transmission, animal inoculation, and nucleic acid testing, show that such titers may reach 10^9 to 10^{10} virions per mL.[12]

The essentially serendipitous discovery, by Blumberg and associates,[13, 14] of "Australia Antigen" (hepatitis B surface antigen [HBsAg]) and its subsequent linkage to one form of viral hepatitis can be considered the first seminal event in the development of modern blood donor screening procedures and policies. Not only was HBsAg clearly associated with what was then known as hepatitis B, but some studies had established that blood that was positive for the antigen clearly transmitted hepatitis B to recipients.[15]

Test methods became available around 1969 but were not uniformly adopted until about 1970 or 1971. The very first test to be implemented was Ouchterlony agar gel diffusion (AGD), which used human or animal antibodies to detect the antigen in donor serum. It is important to recognize, however, that the actual level of HBsAg in a highly infectious sample was extraordinarily high—tens to hundreds of micrograms per mL. The AGD test was soon replaced by directed immunoprecipitation systems, such as counterimmunoelectrophoresis, or rheophoresis, in which an electrical potential or evaporative buffer flow forced the antibodies and antigen together, thus increasing the speed and sensitivity of the test. The tests were, however, highly subjective. Some alternative methods, such as reversed passive hemagglutination, were also developed and achieved a limited degree of implementation. A historical footnote is that AGD was (retrospectively) defined as a "first-generation" test, and the agglutination and directed immunoprecipitation tests were defined as "second-generation."

Ling and Overby,[16] working at Abbott Laboratories, soon developed a tube-based, solid-phase radioimmunoassay (RIA) for the detection of HBsAg. This method clearly had greatly improved analytical sensitivity (i.e., around 1 ng/mL) relative to second-generation tests and was formally defined as a "third-generation" test. It was not long before the Bureau of Biologics (the 1970s equivalent of the U.S. Food and Drug Administration [FDA]) published a notice in the *Federal Register*, indicating that licensure of this third-generation test was imminent and "advising" blood establishments to "become familiar" with it.

At the time of implementation of the RIA, a solution to the problem of post-transfusion hepatitis was widely anticipated. It had already been recognized that second-generation tests did not eliminate all post-transfusion hepatitis—indeed, there was only about a 20% decline in reporting rates. However, by what turned out to be a coincidence, RIA generated about fivefold more reactive results that did the second-generation tests. It soon became apparent that most of the additional "detections" represented false-positive results. This finding was a disappointment, but it led directly to the introduction of additional confirmatory tests and an enhanced perception of the rights of the donor to be properly informed about the significance of screening test results. After a relatively short time, RIA was replaced by the enzyme immunoassay (EIA).

Clinical Aspects

The clinical outcomes of hepatitis B vary in terms of severity, from asymptomatic to fatal, and in terms of chronicity, from acute to lifelong. There do not seem to be any very clear predictors of the severity of disease, other than the presence of detectable levels of the viral e antigen (HBeAg) in the circulation of an infected individual. However, it is clear that the likelihood of chronic infection is very much a function of the age of the patient at the time of infection. Chronic infection is very common among persons who were infected in infancy, but the frequency is reduced to 5% or fewer of persons who were infected in adolescence or adulthood.[12]

Hepatitis B differs little from other viral hepatitides in its clinical manifestations, although such manifestations may often be somewhat more severe than those of hepatitis A or C. The incubation period is about 8 to 12 weeks although it may extend to 6 months or longer, particularly if hepatitis B immune globulin has been used for postexposure prophylaxis. The majority of infections appear to be asymptomatic, although up to 30% of infected adults experience some level of jaundice. Hepatitis B may be fulminant and leads to death in about 0.5% to 1% of cases. As previously pointed out, a variable proportion of infections, irrespective of the occurrence of acute disease, resolve without further clinical symptoms with the development of essentially lifelong immunity, as indicated by the development and maintenance of detectable levels of antibodies to HBsAg (anti-HBs). However, it should be noted that such individuals may continue to harbor virus in the liver, as demonstrated by the occurrence of hepatitis B in transplanted livers from anti-HBs–positive donors.[17]

Chronic hepatitis B may be asymptomatic, but there is a wide range of symptomatic outcomes, up to and including fatal disease. As with other chronic hepatitis viruses, a proportion of patients may eventually demonstrate cirrhosis. In addition, chronic hepatitis B infection may result in the development of primary hepatocellular carcinoma, probably as a direct result of viral integration into the host cell genome. Unlike with hepatitis C, liver cancer induced by the hepatitis B virus may occur in the absence of cirrhosis.

There are a number of extrahepatic manifestations of HBV infection, including rashes, arthritis, vasculitis, and glomerulonephritis.[12] Most are related to the formation of immune complexes involving HBsAg.

Treatment

There is no established treatment for acute hepatitis B, but therapies are approved for chronic disease. Currently, a 4- to

6-month course of interferon alfa-2b (5 to 10 million units, three times per week) is recommended. Improvement, as evidenced by HBe seroconversion, normalization of ALT, and sustained loss of HBV DNA in the circulation, may be seen in 20% to 30% of treated patients, although only about 10% lose their HBsAg. Similar results are seen after a 12-month course of lamivudine, and response rates improve with more prolonged therapy.[18]

Epidemiology

Hepatitis B virus is transmitted parenterally, through exposure to blood and other body fluids. Transmission occurs readily, as a consequence of the high titers of infectious virus found during acute and chronic infection. Infection routes include frank skin piercing and more subtle exposure via minor skin abrasion. Transmission by the sexual route is very common for both male-to-male and heterosexual exposure. In addition, infection may be transmitted from a viremic woman to her infant during birth.

In countries such as the United States, which have relatively low prevalence and incidence rates for HBV, most infection occurs horizontally between adults. Because adult infection generally has an acute outcome, opportunities for secondary transmission tend to be limited. Some behavior patterns, however, such as sharing of needles during injection drug use or frequent sexual contact with many partners, do result in a very high incidence of HBV infection. In areas with a high prevalence of chronic infection, both horizontal and perinatal patterns of infection occur, and the latter frequently leads to chronic infection and a prolonged carrier state. Thus, high prevalence rates are maintained; such a situation is seen in parts of the Far East, for example.

The overall prevalence of serologic evidence of HBV infection in the United States is about 5.6%, as indicated by measurements of HBsAg and antibodies to hepatitis B core antigen (anti-HBc).[19] However, infection rates are much higher among groups engaging in risky behaviors, such as male-to-male sex and injection drug use. The national prevalence of active infection, as defined by the presence of HBsAg is much lower, however—0.1% or less. In contrast, some parts of the world have seroprevalence rates of 50% or greater, with correspondingly high rates of active infection. Within the United States, the prevalence and incidence of HBV markers among blood donors are much lower than those seen in the overall population, reflecting the efficacy of measures used for donor selection.[20] Indeed, many of the donor screening questions in current use derived from efforts to minimize the transmission of hepatitis B. Additionally, questions used to reduce the risk of transmission of human immunodeficiency virus (HIV) are also likely to have had a significant impact on the number of infected donors. Key risk factors for HBV are as follows: injection drug use; sexual exposure (both male-to-male and heterosexual); other parenteral exposures to blood and body fluids, including nonsterile tattooing and body piercing; and familial exposure. In addition, there is geographic risk related to residence in areas of high prevalence.

Virology

The human hepatitis B virus is the prototype of a small group of unusual DNA viruses known at the Hepadnaviridae. They have a lipid envelope and a small, partially double-stranded DNA genome, the full-length section of which has about 3200 bases, encoding four overlapping reading frames. DNA replicates in the hepatocyte nucleus by means of a unique mechanism involving a viral DNA polymerase and an RNA intermediate that is reverse-transcribed. The virus itself is about 42 nm in diameter. The outer envelope is lipoprotein, is antigenic, and is known as HBsAg. The virus-specific antigen is termed "a," and there are a variety of antigenic subtypes, broadly and simplistically defined as two pairs of mutually exclusive alleles, d, y and w, r. The w determinant has itself been further characterized into four subspecificities. The major significance of these antigenic subtypes has been their use in epidemiologic studies.

Assessment of genome sequence variation of the virus has led to the recognition of six genotypes, A through F, on the basis of sequence variations of 8% or more. There is no systematic relationship between genotypes and antigenic subtypes. Genotyping may supplant antigenic subtyping for definition of the molecular epidemiology of HBV infection. Additionally, genotypes are more likely to reflect variations in the biology of different viral isolates.

Perhaps the most intriguing characteristic of HBV is that active HBV infection leads to copious overproduction of HBsAg, which is released into the circulation as self-assembled spheres and tubules, 22 nm in diameter. As already mentioned, HBsAg was first recognized (as Australia antigen) by Blumberg and associates.[13, 14] The subsequent finding that HBsAg is associated with hepatitis B led directly to blood donor testing for the antigen in the early 1970s and indirectly to the recognition of other hepatitis viruses.

The inner capsid of the virus has a different immunologic specificity and is known as the hepatitis B core antigen. This antigen was first recognized on immunoelectron microscopy of detergent-treated samples of virus-containing blood.[21] The core antigen is not normally detectable in serum or plasma, because it is located within the virus. It may, however, be detected in the nuclei of liver cells with active viral replication. Also coded by the gene for the core antigen is a smaller polypeptide sequence, masked in the full-length transcript, that includes a separate antigenic specificity termed HBeAg. This smaller peptide can be found free in the circulation during active infection.[22]

Laboratory investigations have clearly demonstrated the sequence of appearance of plasma markers of HBV infection.[23] Some 25 days after exposure to the virus, HBV DNA may be detected at low levels (a few hundreds or thousands of copies per mL). About 25 days later, these levels rise significantly, and at the same time, HBsAg becomes detectable by relatively insensitive techniques such as enzyme immunoassay. Generally, this period coincides with the appearance of symptoms of hepatitis and elevated liver function markers. About 4 to 8 weeks after the initial appearance of HBsAg, anti-HBc may be detected in the circulation.

A specific test for IgM anti-HBc is available and is extremely useful for diagnosis of HBV infection. With use of the available tests, IgM antibody may be detectable for 3 to 6 months. The IgG antibody persists over many years, whether or not the infection is frankly chronic. In the event of self-limited infection, HBsAg may be detected for about 6 to 12 weeks, but its level declines as anti-HBs becomes detectable. The presence of anti-HBs is usually taken to signal resolution of infection and the absence of infectious virus in the circulation. However, as pointed out previously, virus may persist in the liver.

Diagnostic Testing and Donor Screening

The primary diagnosis of hepatitis relies on symptoms and the results of liver function tests. However, such tests do not permit differentiation of the etiology, and serologic testing is required. During the course of infection, a variety of patterns of expression of different markers is seen. To some extent, it is possible to define the stage of infection on the basis of these patterns.[12, 22] The simplest situation is in acute infection (or the early stages of an infection that becomes chronic), in which the most reliable diagnostic marker is IgM anti-HBc. Figures 37.1 and 37.2 illustrate the patterns of marker expression in acute self-limited infection and chronic infection, respectively. Table 37.1 summarizes the interpretation of differing patterns of expression of key diagnostic markers.

In the United States, all whole blood donations are tested for HBsAg and for anti-HBc in order to reduce the risk of transmission of HBV. Interestingly, testing for anti-HBc was initially introduced in 1986 as a surrogate test for infectivity for non-A, non-B hepatitis. In the face of sensitive tests for hepatitis C virus (HCV), there is now no such surrogate value for anti-HBc testing. The actual benefit of anti-HBc testing in prevention of HBV infection is unclear, although it is generally accepted that, among voluntary donations that are anti-HBc positive but HBsAg negative, about 1% may have detectable HBV DNA. Many years ago, the benefit of

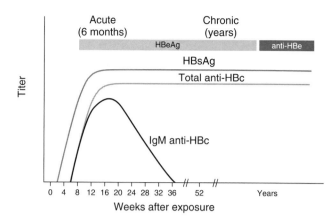

Figure 37.2 Typical serologic course of progression to chronic hepatitis B virus infection. In patients with chronic hepatitis B virus (HBV) infection, both hepatitis B surface antigen (HBsAg) and immunoglobulin (Ig) G antibody to hepatitis B core antigen (anti-HBc) remain persistently detectable, generally for life. Hepatitis B e antigen (HBeAg) is variably present in these patients. The presence of HBsAg for 6 months or longer generally indicates chronic infection. In addition, a negative test result for IgM anti-HBc together with a positive test for HBsAg in a single serum specimen usually indicates that an individual has chronic HBV infection. (Courtesy of Centers for Disease Control and Prevention; From a publicly available slide set.)

anti-HBc testing was thought to lie in its ability to detect infectious samples during a window when HBsAg was no longer detectable and effective levels of anti-HBs had not developed. This window is no longer apparent with HBsAg tests at their current levels of sensitivity.

Estimates of the residual risk of HBV transmission are surprisingly high; in 1996, Schreiber and colleagues[24] suggested a figure of 1:63,000 donations. Some researchers express concern that this figure may be inappropriately high, on the basis of questions about the underlying assumptions and the absence of observed post-transfusion hepatitis B. In 2000, even with the same assumptions made by Schreiber and colleagues,[24] the risk of HBV transmission was estimated to have at least halved as a result of the decreased incidence of HBV among U.S. donors.[20]

At of the middle of 2002, nucleic acid testing (NAT) for HCV and HIV is firmly in place, and one of the two available procedures has been licensed by the FDA. There is speculation that such NAT would be extended to HBV. However, it is clear that the current minipool approach would not have any significant benefits, as NAT has essentially the same sensitivity as the newest of the serologic tests for HBsAg. Such NAT for HBV DNA has, however been implemented in some European locations (where anti-HBc testing is not performed) and by some manufacturers of pooled plasma products.[25] The potential added value of single-unit (i.e., nonpooled) NAT for HBV DNA has not been well-defined.

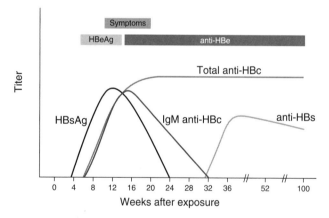

Figure 37.1 Typical serologic course of acute hepatitis B virus infection with recovery. Serologic markers of hepatitis B virus (HBV) infection vary, depending on whether the infection is acute or chronic. The first serologic marker to appear after acute infection is hepatitis B surface antigen (HBsAg), which can be detected as early as 1 or 2 weeks and as late as 11 or 12 weeks (mode, 30–60 days) after exposure to HBV. In persons who recover, HBsAg is no longer detectable in serum after an average of about 3 months. Hepatitis B e antigen (HBeAg) is generally detectable in patients with acute infection; the presence of HBeAg in serum correlates with higher titers of HBV and greater infectivity. A diagnosis of acute HBV infection can be made on the basis of the detection of immunoglobulin (Ig) M class antibody to hepatitis B core antigen (IgM anti-HBc) in serum; IgM anti-HBc is generally detectable at the time of clinical onset and declines to subdetectable levels with 6 months. IgG anti-HBc persists indefinitely as a marker of past infection. Anti-HBs becomes detectable during convalescence after the disappearance of HBsAg in patients who do not experience chronic infection. The presence of anti-HBs after acute infection generally indicates recovery and immunity from re-infection. (Courtesy of Centers for Disease Control and Prevention; From a publicly available slide set.)

Mutants and Vaccines

A number of mutants of HBV have been recognized, and there is evidence that the representation of such mutants is increasing. Perhaps of greatest concern for transfusion medicine are those mutants that do not express HBsAg.[26–28] This group includes those defined as "escape mutants"— a term signifying an ability to evade the protective effects of HBV vaccines

Table 37.1 Interpretation of Results of Hepatitis B Test Panel

Tests	Results	Interpretation
HBsAg Anti-HBc Anti-HBs	Negative Negative Negative	Susceptible
HBsAg Anti-HBc Anti-HBs	Negative Positive Positive	Immune because of natural infection
HBsAg Anti-HBc Anti-HBs	Negative Negative Positive	Immune because of hepatitis B vaccination
HBsAg Anti-HBc IgM anti-HBc Anti-HBs	Positive Positive Positive Negative	Acutely infected
HBsAg Anti-HBc IgM anti-HBc Anti-HBs	Positive Positive Negative Negative	Chronically infected
HBsAg Anti-HBc Anti-HBs	Negative Positive Negative	Four interpretations possible*

*The patient (1) may be recovering from acute HBV infection; (2) may be distantly immune (the test is not sensitive enough to detect very low levels of anti-HBs in serum); (3) may be susceptible with a false-positive anti-Hbc test result; or (4) may have an undetectable level of HBsAg in serum, so is actually a carrier.
Anti-HBc, antibody to hepatitis B core antigen; anti-HBs, antibody to hepatitis B surface antigen; HBsAg, hepatitis B surface antigen; Ig, immunoglobulin.
Courtesy of Centers for Disease Control and Prevention.

(which are currently based on HBsAg). However, infection with these mutants still provokes the formation of detectable levels of anti-HBc, so that most such infections would be detected, at least in the United States and other countries where anti-HBc testing of donations is routine.

Currently available hepatitis B vaccines prepared from recombinant antigens are safe and effective and are recommended for universal use in infants. It is to be hoped that consistent use of these vaccines will eventually lead to significant reduction in HBV infection rates and, thus, to a decline in the prevalence of chronic infection. Current vaccines provoke only anti-HBs and so do not interfere with routine blood donation testing. However, it should be noted that HBsAg itself may be detectable in the circulation for a few days after inoculation. Although there is no need to defer a recent vaccinee for safety reasons, it is wise to avoid collection of blood from such a person for about 7 days after vaccination. Otherwise, there is a risk that the donor will be confirmed positive for HBsAg and will thus be deferred. Finally, although the risk of transmission of HBV by blood components has almost been eliminated and although there should be no cases from manufactured plasma products as a result of careful donor management and viral inactivation of the final product, chronic users of blood and blood products should certainly receive the HBV vaccine.

Hepatitis D

Hepatitis D is caused by a small satellite virus, originally termed the delta virus, that can replicate only in the presence of HBV infection. The virus is an RNA virus, and almost unique among animal viruses, its genome is circular. It codes a single peptide, originally observed in infected hepatocytes

and termed delta antigen. The infectious form of HDV is coated with HBsAg. Co-infection with HBV and HDV results in a more serious disease than does HBV alone. In truth, HDV has little current relevance to transfusion safety, because measures designed to detect infectivity for HBV also detect all individuals co-infected with HDV.[29, 30]

Hepatitis E

Hepatitis E virus (HEV) causes an epidemic form of hepatitis that is self-limited.[31, 32] The disease is somewhat similar to hepatitis A, although it is much more severe in pregnancy. Transmission is by the fecal-oral route and is most often water-borne. The virus is related to the calicivirus group and, as such, is a nonenveloped virus that has an RNA genome. Although there is some evidence (based largely on seroprevalence studies) that HEV is present in the United States, it is found predominantly in tropical countries. Indeed, most cases identified in the United States appear to have resulted from infections that occurred in countries where HEV is endemic. Because of the self-limited and acute nature of HEV infection, there is little risk of transmission by transfusion, and no cases of transfusion-associated HEV infection of disease have been reported.[33]

Hepatitis G Virus/GBV-C

The vast majority of cases of post-transfusion hepatitis have been shown to be caused by HBV or HCV. Nevertheless, there continue to be some cases of hepatitis associated with transfusion. For example, in Harvey Alters's continuing studies at the National Institutes of Health, about 12% of cases of non-A, non-B hepatitis could not be attributed to either of these viruses. These residual cases appear to be mild and self-limited, and some may not even have an infectious etiology. Such cases have, however, led to a continuing search for additional hepatitis viruses. The first of such putative hepatitis viruses was identified by two separate groups in the late 1990s. In one case, scientists at Abbott Laboratories looked for genomic sequences related to those of an existing isolate known as the GB virus (GBV), which had previously been associated with hepatitis in a physician. Three viruses were identified, one of which (termed GBV-C) was found among a number of human sources.[34] Working in parallel, but using a different approach, scientists at Gene-Labs isolated viral RNA sequences and characterized a virus they termed hepatitis G virus (HGV).[35] It is generally accepted that these two isolates were, in fact, representatives of essentially the same virus group, which is now known as HGV.

HGV, like HCV, appears to be closely related to the Flavivirus group. It is found among a relatively high proportion of the normal population, as exemplified by blood donors. Its presence has been demonstrated both by seroprevalence studies, in which the frequency of antibodies is 3% to 15%, and, more interestingly, by detection of viral RNA in the plasma of 1% to 3% of normal subjects.[36] Perhaps not surprisingly, the virus is readily transmissible by transfusion and is found at high prevalence among individuals who have undergone multiple transfusions. However, it has not proved possible to demonstrate that infection with HGV is associated with hepatitis or even with signs of mild liver disease, such as elevated ALT levels. Indeed, HGV appears to be a virus that is currently in search of a disease. The term "hepatitis" in its name may be a misnomer, attributable only to the fact that the virus was found in association with hepatitis in the first place. It is also important to recognize that the worldwide distribution of HGV clearly shows that it is not a new virus but, rather, one that has coexisted with humans for many centuries.

■ TTV and SEN-V

Curiously, another pair of viruses were separately identified among individuals with hepatitis and were also shown to be poorly, if at all, associated with hepatitis. These viruses were also found to cause prolonged viremia and, in some cases, turned out to be present in up to 90% of the population. Like HGV, they were readily transmitted by transfusion. Both viruses were thought to be representatives of the circovirus group: small, nonenveloped viruses with a circular DNA genome. This group of viruses had not previously been described among humans.

Workers in Japan used representational difference analysis to isolate DNA sequences from three patients with unexplained post-transfusion hepatitis. The sequence was established as viral, and the virus was named TTV, reflecting the initials of the patient from whom it was isolated.[37] A considerable amount of research has revealed some of the key features of this virus.[38]

It is a small virus with a covalently closed, circular DNA genome of around 3800 bases. The virus is thought to be nonenveloped. It is most closely related to the circoviruses, which are responsible for a number of diseases in plants and a handful of mammalian or avian disease states. The classification of TTV is currently incomplete, and proposals

have been made to place it in at least two genera. What has become apparent is that TTV is a member of an extremely diverse group of viruses, as demonstrated by considerable variation in genomic sequence.

Epidemiologic studies have confirmed that TTV is a widely distributed virus and have clearly established that it is transmissible by transfusion. Interestingly, it also appears to be transmitted by the vertical, fecal-oral, and, perhaps, other routes.

A key issue is the clinical significance of this group of viruses. Although the original source of the virus and its apparent association with ALT elevations implied that TTV was indeed a hepatitis virus, this identification no longer seems tenable. Indeed, there are far more infections without ALT elevations than with such evidence of liver disease.

Even in clear, transfusion-associated transmission of TTV, the recipients did not manifest ALT elevations in any pattern that could be associated with the infection. At this stage, there is little evidence that this virus expresses any pathogenic potential. However, it is certainly too early to conclude that this entire group of viruses is without any clinical significance.

After the recognition of TTV, the search for hepatitis viruses continued, and Primi and colleagues[39, 40] used degenerate primers derived from TTV to probe samples from selected patients. An isolate was identified and named SEN-V (after the initials of the source patient, an HIV-infected injection drug user). Eventually, at least eight different strains were isolated, termed A through H. The SEN group has been shown to be one branch of the TTV group, seeming to share its epidemiologic characteristics. Although two of the strains (D and H) have been associated with evidence of transfusion-associated hepatitis, a causal relationship has not been established.[39, 40]

Thus, attempts to define the etiology of non-A through E hepatitis do not appear to have been successful to date. The availability of powerful genomic techniques has certainly led to the recognition of previously undescribed viruses, but it has not been possible to associate any particular disease with these remarkably widespread viruses. No doubt other such orphan viruses will be identified; it will be important to avoid an automatic assumption of causality when such viruses are isolated from patients with any given disease state. It may also be important to question whether all residual transfusion-associated hepatitides do indeed have an infectious etiology.

REFERENCES

1. Cuthbert JA: Hepatitis A: Old and new. Clin Microbiol Rev 2001;14:38–58.
2. Hollinger FB, Khan NC, Oefinger PE, et al: Posttransfusion hepatitis type A. JAMA 1983;250:2313–2317.
3. Azimi PH, Roberto RR, Guralnick J, et al: Transfusion-acquired hepatitis A in a premature infant with secondary nosocomial spread in an intensive care nursery. Am J Dis Child 1986;140:23–27.
4. Giacoia GP, Kasprisin DO: Transfusion-acquired hepatitis A. South Med J 1989;82:1357–1360.
5. Lee KK, Vargo LR, Le CT, Fernando L: Transfusion-acquired hepatitis A outbreak from fresh frozen plasma in a neonatal intensive care unit. Pediatr Infect Dis 3 1992;11:122–123.
6. Mosley JW, Nowicki MI, Kasper CK, et al: Hepatitis A virus transmission by blood products in the United States. Vox Sang 1994;67(Suppl)1:24–28.
7. Bower WA, Nainan OV, Han XH, Margolis HS: Duration of viremia in hepatitis A virus infection. J Infect Dis 2000;182:12–17.

8. Soucie JM, Robertson BH, Bell BP, et al: Hepatitis A virus infections associated with clotting factor concentrate in the United States. Transfusion 1998;38:573–579.
9. Mannucci PM, Gdovin S, Gringeri A, et al: Transmission of hepatitis A to patients with hemophilia by factor VIII concentrates treated with organic solvent and detergent to inactivate viruses. Ann Intern Med 1994;120:1–7.
10. Johnson Z, Thornton L, Tobin A, et al: An outbreak of hepatitis A among Irish haemophiliacs. Int J Epidemiol 1995;24:821–828.
11. Lawlor E, Graham S, Davidson F, et al: Hepatitis A transmission by factor IX concentrates. Vox Sang 1996;71:126–128.
12. Lee WM: Hepatitis B virus infection. N Engl J Med 1997;337:1733–1745.
13. Blumberg BS, Alter HJ, Visnich S: A "new" antigen in leukemia sera. JAMA 1965;191:541–546.
14. Blumberg BS, Gerstley BJS, Hungerford DA, et al: A serum antigen (Australia antigen) in Down's syndrome, leukemia and hepatitis. Ann Intern Med 1967;66:924.
15. Gocke DJ, Greenberg HB, Kavey NB: Correlation of Australia antigen with posttransfusion hepatitis. JAMA 1970;212:877–879.
16. Ling CM, Overby LR: Prevalence of hepatitis B virus antigen as revealed by direct radioimmune assay with 125-1-antibody. J Immunol 1972;109:834–841.
17. Dodson SF, Issa S, Araya V, et al: Infectivity of hepatic allografts with antibodies to hepatitis B virus. Trans 1997;64:1582–1584.
18. Lin OS, Keeffe EB: Current treatment strategies for chronic hepatitis B and C. Annu Rev Med 2001;52:29–49.
19. McQuillan GM, Coleman PJ, Kruszon-Moran D, et al: Prevalence of hepatitis B virus infection in the United States: The National Health and Nutrition Examination Surveys, 1976 through 1994. Am J Public Health 1999;89:14–18.
20. Dodd RY: Germs, gels, and genomes: A personal recollection of 30 years in blood safety testing. In Stramer SL (ed): Blood Safety in the New Millenium. Bethesda, MD: American Association of Blood Banks, 2001, pp 97–122.
21. Almeida JD, Rubenstein D, Stott EJ: New antigen-antibody system in Australia-antigen positive hepatitis. Lancet 1971;2:1225–1227.
22. Mahoney FJ: Update on diagnosis, management, and prevention of hepatitis B virus infection. Clin Microbiol Rev 1999;12:351–366.
23. Busch MP: HIV, HBV and HCV: New developments related to transfusion safety. Vox Sang 2000;78:253–256.
24. Schreiber GB, Busch MP, Kleinman SH, Korelitz JJ: The risk of transfusion-transmitted viral infections. N Engl J Med 1996;334:1685–1690.
25. Roth WK, Weber M, Seifried E: Feasibility and efficacy of routine PCR screening of blood donations for hepatitis C virus, hepatitis B virus, and HIV-1 in a bloodbank setting. Lancet 1999;353(9150):359–363.
26. Blum HE: Hepatitis B virus: Significance of naturally occurring mutants. Intervirology 1993;35:40–50.
27. Hsu HY, Chang MH, Liaw SH, et al: Changes of hepatitis B surface antigen variants in carrier children before and after universal vaccination in Taiwan. Hepatology 1999;30:1312–1317.
28. Jongerius IM, Wester M, Cuypers HTM, et al: New hepatitis B virus mutant form in a blood donor that is undetectable in several hepatitis B surface antigen screening assays. Transfusion 1998;38:56–59.
29. Lai MMC: The molecular biology of hepatitis delta virus. Annu Rev Biochem 1995;64:259–286.
30. Liaw YF, Tsai SL, Sheen IS, et al: Clinical and virological course of chronic hepatitis B virus infection with hepatitis C and D virus markers. Am J Gastroenterol 1998;93:354–359.
31. Purcell RH: The discovery of the hepatitis viruses. Gastroenterology 1993;104:955–963.
32. Thomas DL, Yarbough PO, Vlahov D, et al: Seroreactivity to hepatitis E virus in areas where the disease is not endemic. J Clin Microbiol 1997;35:1244–1247.
33. Mateos ML, Camarero C, Lasa E, et al: Hepatitis E virus: Relevance in blood donors and other risk groups. Vox Sang 1998;75:267–269.
34. Leary TP, Muerhoff AS, Simons JN, et al: Sequence and genomic organization of GBV-C: A novel member of the Flaviviridae associated with human non-A-E hepatitis. J Med Virol 1996;48:60–67.
35. Linnen J, Wages J Jr, Zhang-Keck ZY, et al: Molecular cloning and disease association of hepatitis G virus: A transfusion transmissible agent. Science 1996;271:505–508.
36. Allain JP: Emerging viral infections relevant to transfusion medicine. Blood Rev 2000;14:173–181.
37. Nishizawa T, Okamoto H, Konishi K, et al: A novel DNA virus (TTV) associated with elevated transaminase levels in posttransfusion hepatitis of unknown etiology. Biochem Biophys Res Commun 1997;241:92–97.
38. Bendinelli M, Pistello M, Maggi F, et al: Molecular properties, biology, and clinical implications of Tf virus, a recently identified widespread infectious agent of humans. Clin Microbiol Rev 2001;14:98–113.
39. Umemura T, Yeo AE, Sottini A, et al: SEN virus infection and its relationship to transfusion-associated hepatitis. Hepatology 2001;33:1303–1311.
40. Tanaka Y, Primi D, Wang RY, et al: Genomic and molecular evolutionary analysis of a newly identified infectious agent (SEN virus) and its relationship to the TT virus family. J Infect Dis 2001;183:359–367.

Chapter 38

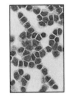

Hepatitis C

Roger Y. Dodd

For many years, hepatitis C was the most common infectious outcome of blood transfusion in the United States. Indeed, a number of studies in the 1970s showed that more than 10% of blood recipients had biochemical evidence of hepatitis, then termed non-A, non-B hepatitis (NANBH).[1, 2] Subsequently, almost all of these cases were shown to be due to infection with the hepatitis C virus (HCV). Implementation of increasingly sensitive tests for HCV infection has reduced the incidence of post-transfusion hepatitis C infection to levels that are essentially undetectable by direct study; by early 2001, the risk was estimated at about one infection per 500,000 component units.[3]

■ The Disease

The symptoms of acute hepatitis C do not differ significantly from those of other viral hepatitides, although they may be somewhat less severe than those of hepatitis B. The incubation period is 7 to 8 weeks, but a wide range has been noted. It has been estimated that about 25% of acute cases may be accompanied by symptoms that, in some cases, may be quite mild. When present, symptoms include fatigue, anorexia, abdominal pain, and weight loss. A proportion (perhaps 20% to 30%) of patients with acute hepatitis C may become jaundiced. Symptoms may last for up to 10 weeks. Alanine aminotransaminase (ALT) levels are elevated during the acute phase; such elevations tend to be moderate (i.e., around 300–400 IU/L) but may be quite high (up to 2000 IU/L). Acute disease is rarely fatal, with mortality rates of 1% or less.

Approximately 20% of acute infections resolve. The remaining 80% (whether symptomatic or not) become chronic. Such chronic infections may last for the lifetime of the patient, although there is growing evidence that 26% to 45% of these cases may eventually resolve, as shown by the disappearance of detectable HCV RNA in the circulation and,

perhaps, by the eventual loss of detectable antibody. The natural history of chronic HCV infection is not completely understood. Many infected individuals may remain completely asymptomatic for many years (perhaps even their whole lives), but a good number have histologic evidence of liver disease, including hepatitis, fibrosis, and cirrhosis. In some cases, hepatocellular carcinoma occurs.

Alter and Seeff[4] have published a framework representing the outcome of HCV infection that is based on a large number of published studies. They conclude that 20% of infected individuals resolve the acute infection. Of the remaining 80% who become chronically infected, 30% demonstrate a stable chronic hepatitis with a favorable outcome. Another 30% have severe, progressive hepatitis, and the remaining 40% may have some variable progression. If these two last groups are treated, 35% would be expected to have a sustained response, and in the remainder, treatment would fail. Thus, overall, perhaps 36% of those infected would have a more or less severe outcome.

Prospective studies have shown, however, that chronic symptomatic hepatitis may take an average of 10 to 14 years (and frequently, much longer) to develop, whereas cirrhosis may take an average of 21 years, and hepatocellular carcinoma almost 30 years. Although life-threatening outcomes may be uncommon, or considerably delayed, it is still true that the consequences of HCV infection are the leading indicator for liver transplantation.

From the perspective of transfusion medicine, this pattern of disease has two important consequences. First, although the immediate consequences of post-transfusion hepatitis C may seem to be largely trivial, the long-term outcomes cannot be ignored. Second, the preponderance of asymptomatic, chronic infection leads to a relatively large population of individuals who are at risk of transmitting the infection via transfusion.

Treatment

In 1997, a National Institutes of Health Consensus Development Conference provided recommendations for treatment of chronic hepatitis C, applicable to individuals with significant histologic findings on biopsy, HCV antibody, elevated ALT, and detectable levels of HCV RNA.[5] In brief, such patients should initially be treated with 3 million units of interferon alfa three times a week for 12 months. In the absence of any response (i.e., normalization of ALT and loss of detectable HCV RNA), this therapy should be discontinued after 3 months, and the patient should be considered for combination therapy with interferon and ribavirin. Overall, it has been recognized that about 50% of patients show temporary improvement with this regimen, but ultimately, only about 25% of all patients show definitive resolution of disease. A subsequent Consensus Development Conference in 2002 updated these recommendations, emphasizing the value of combination therapy.

These treatment recommendations have been updated by Liang and colleagues[6] on the basis of experience with combination therapies. In fact, a review of two studies revealed that a sustained response to interferon alone was observed in 29% of patients after treatment for either 24 or 48 weeks.[6] However, among those receiving combination therapy (interferon plus ribavirin), 33% showed a sustained response at 24 weeks, and 41% showed such a response after 48 weeks of therapy. It was also noted that treatment of patients with HCV subtypes 2 and 3 for more than 24 weeks was unnecessary, because of the greater efficacy of treatment for these subtypes.

Epidemiology

HCV is globally distributed, and with a few notable exceptions, the seroprevalence rate is remarkably constant from one region to another, usually on the order of 1% to 2%.[7] Some countries or localities have startlingly high rates, but these may be attributable to cultural factors, including the use of traditional medicine practices; in Egypt, numerous infections were attributed to a program involving injections for control of schistosomiasis.[8] In the United States, the overall seroprevalence rate has been estimated at 1.8%, and 65% of persons infected with HCV are 30 to 49 years old.[9]

Transmission of HCV seems to be essentially confined to parenteral routes. In the United States, it is clear that many of the currently identified infections are a result of prior exposure via illegal injection of drugs. In addition, many infections are believed to have resulted from blood transfusions given prior to the availability of sensitive tests.[10] Other epidemiologic associations are (1) the use of clotting factor concentrates before the implementation of effective viral inactivation in 1987, (2) exposure in a health care setting, (3) household exposure, (4) multiple sexual partners, and (5) low socioeconomic level.[11]

There has been considerable speculation about the natural transmission routes of HCV, which have presumably been responsible for maintaining the baseline level of transmission over centuries or even millennia. Some evidence exists for sexual transmission, and some for perinatal transmission, but in both cases, it seems likely that transmission may occur only during early acute infection. HCV infection does not show the strong association with male-to-male sex that has been seen for hepatitis B and human immunodeficiency viruses (HIVs).

The incidence of new HCV infections has declined by 80% or more since 1989. Clearly, there has been a major reduction in incidence due to transmission by transfusion, and the majority of new infections (about 60%) are attributable to injection drug use. Even though incidence is declining, it is anticipated that the burden of HCV disease will continue to rise over the foreseeable future because of the large number of chronically infected individuals.[12]

Studies on the epidemiology of HCV infection among blood donors are of considerable importance in the context of strategies for donor selection and questioning. Conry-Cantilena and associates[13] studied a population of 481 blood donors who were found to be reactive in screening tests for anti-HCV. Among the 241 with positive strip immunoassay results, 27% had a history of transfusion, 68% had used cocaine intranasally, 42% had a history of intravenous drug use, 53% reported a history of sexual promiscuity, and ear-piercing among men was also significantly associated with a positive test result. Many of these risk factors were confounded, but these observations resulted in the institution of measures to ask donors about intranasal cocaine use; a formal requirement for this question was subsequently eliminated, however. It is of interest to note that, in a small study performed in blood donors who tested positive for HCV RNA but negative for HCV antibody, 7 of 14 reported a history of recent intravenous drug use.[14] Prevalence of HCV infection in current injection drug users is estimated to be 79%. It is unclear how better to ensure accurate histories from donors, particularly for illicit drug exposures that may have occurred many years ago. Fortunately, individuals with such histories do not contribute to window period risk.

Virology

The hepatitis C virus was first recognized in 1989 as the principal etiologic agent of non-A, non-B hepatitis. A small RNA genome segment was isolated from a presumptive viral pellet prepared from the plasma of an experimentally infected chimpanzee. The encoded peptide was expressed in bacteria, through the use of a lambda phage vector, and the clone was recognized from its reactivity with antibodies present in convalescent serum from a patient with non-A, non-B hepatitis.[15] This genome fragment, termed 5-1-1, was used as a basis for the eventual sequencing of the entire genome of the virus. The 5-1-1 sequence was used as a basis for developing the capture reagent (the c100-3 peptide) used to develop an initial version of an enzyme immunoassay (EIA) for the detection of antibodies to HCV. These peptides represented a portion of the NS3 region of the HCV genome.[16] Subsequently, additional peptides have been expressed and incorporated in improved versions of the HCV antibody test.

The virus itself is an enveloped, single-strand RNA virus now classified as a separate genus (Hepacivirus) within the Flaviviridae. It has positive-strand genome of barely less than 10,000 bases. The functional organization of the genome has been well-defined.

HCV is characterized by considerable genetic variability, expressed at three levels: genotype, subtype, and isolate. There are six major genotypes of HCV, designated by the Arabic numerals 1 to 6. The RNA sequence between genotypes varies by some 25% to 35%, and this level of differentiation has probably emerged over periods of 500 to 2000 years. Subtypes within a genotype, designated by lower-case letters (a, b, etc.), represent RNA sequence variation of 15% to 25% that evolved over about 300 years. Individual isolates within a subtype may vary by 5% to 10% in RNA sequence.[17–21] Overall, these studies indicate that the frequency of major subtypes in the United States is as follows: 1a, 42.6%; 1b, 29.2%; 2a, 2.7%; 2b, 8.1%; 3a, 4.7%.

Additionally, there are hypervariable regions in the genome, and many quasispecies of HCV are likely to develop in an individual patient over time. In general, any variation below the level of subtype is unlikely to be reliable enough to differentiate sources of infection. The distribution of HCV subtypes may change with geography. It has been suggested that the clinical outcome of HCV infection and the response to treatment may vary with subtype. Genotypes 2 and 3 appear to be more responsive to treatment than the more common subtypes 1a and 1b.[5, 22, 23]

The sequence of events after infection with HCV has been well-characterized at the level of detection of markers in the circulation. Antibodies may be detected by version 3.0 tests an average of 70 days after exposure, although this period may be quite variable.[24, 25] However, some 40 to 50 days prior to the appearance of such antibodies, HCV RNA may be detected in the plasma. The HCV levels rise rapidly (over a few days) to 10^5 to 10^7 copies/mL. This level is generally maintained at least until antibody levels are significant. It is now apparent that a soluble viral core antigen is also present and can be detected once the RNA levels exceed about 50,000 copies/mL.[26, 27] Elevated levels of ALT are frequently observed a few days before antibodies are detectable, but always after the steep rise in RNA levels.

Interestingly, there is growing evidence that there may be occasional low levels of RNA in the circulation during the early eclipse phase, after infection and prior to the steep rise to peak levels of RNA.[5, 23] The implementation of widespread nucleic acid testing (NAT) for HCV RNA has been shown to detect a meaningful number of RNA-positive, anti-HCV–negative donations (currently at a frequency of about 1 per 250,000 to 1 per 350,000 among U.S. whole blood donations).[28] It is likely that such testing identifies almost all donations that are from donors whose infection is in the steep rise phase, from the steep rise in RNA through anti-HCV detection. Additionally, almost all such donors display seroconversion on follow-up. In a limited number of cases, however, seroconversion is delayed; in the Red Cross system for example, 1 of 25 donors detected by NAT had not showed seroconversion even after more than a year of observation.[29] Anecdotal reports show that blood components from such "immunosilent" donors are infectious. Given the sensitivities of today's serologic tests, however, such occurrences seem to be rare.

Once antibodies are detectable, RNA levels may decrease or may become variable. In the evaluation of samples from blood donors, HCV RNA is detected in about 80% of samples that are found reactive on a version 3.0 EIA and confirmed reactive on the version 3.0 strip immunoassay (SIA).[30] The frequency of RNA detection declines with the strength of the antibody response (as defined by the number and strength of bands on the SIA).[31] It seems likely that the antibody-positive, RNA-negative samples actually represent resolved infections. In some cases, antibodies may eventually decline to undetectable levels.

There is a vigorous humoral and cytotoxic immune response to HCV, but in most cases, it is clearly unable to eliminate the virus. The mechanisms underlying the ability of the virus to escape the immune response are not well understood. The infecting virus often generates a wide variety of quasispecies, and further, the representation of these variant forms changes rapidly over time.[32] Yet it appears that these changes may contribute only in part to viral persistence.

■ Serologic Tests for HCV Infection

Two licensed EIA tests for HCV antibodies are currently available in the United States. Both use recombinant viral antigens as the solid-phase capture reagent. The two tests differ in their physical format and in the number and nature of viral antigens used (Table 38.1). The test manufactured by Ortho Clinical Diagnostics uses a microplate solid phase and has been designated as a 3.0 version by the manufacturer. The peptides that are coated onto the microplate well are known as c22-3 from the C (core) region, c200 from the NS3-NS4 regions, and an NS-5 peptide. The test manufactured by Abbott Laboratories uses a polystyrene bead solid phase and is designated as a version 2.0 test. The capture reagents for this test are c22-3, and c33, and c100-3 (both from the NS3/NS4 region). Both test procedures use an antiglobulin conjugate to detect the analyte antibodies. The performance characteristics of the tests, representing the manufacturers' claims (see Table 38.1), have been validated by extensive clinical trials, and the tests have been licensed as Biologics by the U.S. Food and Drug Administration (FDA). Most diagnostic reagents are defined as Devices, but those that are used in the preparation of blood and blood products are required to meet the more stringent Biologics requirements, because blood itself is defined as a Biologic.

In the context of clinical trials, the sensitivity of these tests was defined in populations of patients diagnosed with non-A, non-B hepatitis. Because this diagnosis is not specific, the significance of the sensitivity figures is unclear. Of more importance now, at least in the context of blood donor screening, is the ability of the test method to detect infection

Table 38.1 Enzyme Immunoassay Tests for Anti-HCV: Components and Performance Characteristics

Version of Test (manufacturer)	Peptides	Sensitivity*	Specificity*
1.0 (Ortho Clinical Diagnostics)	C100	81%	>99.4%
2.0 (Abbott Laboratories)	HC34 (c22), HC31 (c33), c100	85.7%[†]	99.83%
3.0 (Ortho Clinical Diagnostics)	c22, c200[‡], NS-5	88.1%[†]	99.95%

*Based on manufacturers' claims in product inserts.
[†]Based on a diagnosis of chronic non-A, non-B hepatitis—ALT elevated > 6 months, HBsAg negative.
[‡]Includes c33 and c100 sequences.

at the earliest possible time during the seroconversion period. Studies of seroconversion panels suggest that currently available tests detect antibodies, on average, 70 to 80 days after exposure to the source of infection and 40 to 50 days after the initial detection of HCV RNA in the plasma. In addition, it should be noted that earlier versions of the EIA tests clearly failed to detect some infected individuals.[33] This is not surprising, because only a very limited number of viral epitopes were included in the capture reagent. Current tests for anti-HCV are whole-antibody tests. Currently, no tests are commercially available for immunoglobulin (Ig) M anti-HCV.

Although these EIA tests have high sensitivity and specificity, there is a possibility that some reactive test results are nonspecific. As discussed later, when the EIA is used to screen blood donors, its actual positive predictive value is 70% to 80%.[31] Consequently, it is recommended that all asymptomatic individuals who test as reactive on EIA repeatedly should be further tested with an additional, more specific procedure. Currently, only one such immunologic method is licensed and available in the United States. This is a strip immunoblot assay (SIA; RIBA 3.0™, Chiron) that is constructed by application of recombinant or synthetic viral peptides representing c22, c33, c100, 5-1-1, and NS5 regions to nitrocellulose strips in a fixed pattern. The c-100 and 5-1-1 peptides are present in the same band on the strip. The expression protein for the recombinant viral antigens is also applied (superoxide dismutase, SOD), as are strong and weak positive controls. Patient or donor samples are applied to the strips and, after washing, adherent antibodies are detected by an appropriate enzyme-conjugated antiglobulin and visualization reaction. The number and intensity of bands are scored, and the result is interpreted as follows:

- *Positive:* Two or more bands with an intensity equal to, or greater than, that of the weak positive control band, plus nonreactive SOD band.
- *Negative:* No band with a greater intensity than the weak positive control.
- *Indeterminate:* Only one band reactive or any pattern in association with a reactive SOD band.

Table 38.2 summarizes the results of testing a large number of volunteer blood donations with HCV EIA and SIAs.

Unlike the situation with HIV, there does not seem to be a common pattern of the sequence of appearance of reactive bands in the blot during the process of seroconversion with HCV. However, a number of studies define the relationship between particular bands, or band patterns, and the likelihood that a sample will also contain detectable HCV RNA. For example, Dow and colleagues[30] reviewed data from 177 blood donor specimens that were reactive on EIA and tested positive on the version 3.0 SIA. Among 82 samples with four positive bands, 69 (84.1%) were RNA-positive. Among the 54 samples with three positive bands, 40 (74.1%) were RNA-positive, whereas only 14 (34.1%) of the 41 samples with two positive bands were RNA-positive. Among the samples with indeterminate SIA results, the frequencies of RNA-positive results were 3 of 154 for c22, 1 of 220 for c33, 1 of 191 for c100, and 0 of 380 for NS5.[30] Thus, a few indeterminate patterns may be associated with the presence of RNA and, therefore, of active HCV infection. Similar data were published by Dodd and Stramer.[31]

■ Tests for HCV RNA

Tests for HCV RNA serve an important role in diagnosis and patient management.[34] A variety of procedures is available; as might be expected, all depend on nucleic acid amplification. The reverse transcriptase polymerase chain reaction (RT-PCR) is perhaps the most familiar. Viral RNA is reverse-transcribed to DNA, and two primers are used to define a sequence for repetitive amplification using a temperature-resistant DNA polymerase and a temperature-cycling protocol. A variety of methods may be used to detect the resulting amplified sequence. Such methods vary from visualization in gels to hybridization with labeled probes. Some procedures even allow for the detection of amplicons in real time. Both qualitative and quantitative procedures are available.[5, 35, 36] In most cases, a conserved region of the 5′ untranslated region of the genome is selected for amplification. PCR-based assays are available commercially (e.g., Roche Molecular Systems) as well as from independent reference laboratories; alternatively, they may be developed in-house with the use of standard technologies.

Another technique, known as nucleic acid sequence–based amplification (NASBA; a proprietary technology from Organon-Technika),[37] and the very similar transcription-mediated amplification (TMA; a proprietary technology from

Table 38.2　Results of Testing 19.2 Million Blood Donations with HCV 3.0 EIA and Version 3.0 SIA and Percentage of RNA-Positive Samples among Subgroups of SIA-Positive Subjects

	Number of Subjects with SIA Finding (% RNA +)		
	Positive (% RNA +)	Indeterminate	Negative
HCV EIA RR N = 30,680	19,541	4898	6241
SIA			
> 2 bands	17,139 (82%)*	NA	NA
2 bands only	2402 (42%)†	NA	NA

*Sample of 200 tested.
†2347 tested.
EIA, enzyme immunoassay; NA, not applicable; RR, repeatedly reactive; SIA, Strip immunoblot assay.
Data courtesy Susan L. Stramer, Ph.D (personal communication).

Gen-Probe Inc.) can be performed without temperature cycling. Two enzymes are used to develop an RNA amplicon, which can be detected by a variety of methods, including the hybridization protection assay. It should be noted that Chiron owns patent rights to the HCV genomic sequence.

Sample collection and stability and preparation for amplification are all important and must be properly controlled. HCV RNA is quite labile, and it is preferable, if not essential, to collect specimens in EDTA. Samples should be maintained at refrigerated temperatures and should be tested with minimal delay. A number of different methods may be used to prepare the RNA for testing, including conventional extraction from ultracentrifugal pellets, extraction on silica, and probe-capture techniques.

Finally, in a method known as the branched-chain DNA (B-DNA, Chiron) assay, a probe is labeled with a large branched DNA molecule that carries many copies of the detection label. This method does not amplify the target nucleic acid; rather, it provides a system in which very many label molecules may be associated with a single target sequence. As might be expected, this technique is not as sensitive as amplification. The lack of sensitivity has been exploited in order to differentiate those patients with high levels of circulating RNA.[38, 39]

Within the United States, almost all blood donations have been tested for HCV RNA since 1999. Two methods are in use, PCR (Roche) and TMA (Chiron/Gen-Probe). To date, all such testing has been performed on small pools of samples. Currently, pool sizes are 24 for the Roche procedure and 16 for the Chiron/Gen-Probe method.

A number of methods are available for the determination of genotype and subtype. Not all methods are able to discriminate every genotype or subtype, however. Available methods may be broadly separated into those that depend on immunologic differentiation and those that directly detect variation in nucleic acid sequences. In the former case, specific peptides derived from the NS4 region are used to probe for antibodies in the specimen. Nucleic acid–based techniques include sequencing amplicons from selected genomic areas, PCR using genome-specific primers, DNA-enzyme immunoassay (DEIA), restriction fragment length polymorphism (RFLP) analysis of amplicons, and differential hybridization of amplicons with specific probes. The last two of these approaches are commercially available (GEN-ETI-K DEIA kit, Sorin, Saluggia, Italy, and INNO-LiPA HCV-I and -II, Innogenetics, Zwijnaarde, Belgium); the reader is referred elsewhere for further details.[17, 40]

◼ Diagnostic Algorithm

The Centers for Disease Control and Prevention (CDC) has published an algorithm for diagnostic testing for HCV among asymptomatic individuals (Fig. 38.1).[11] This algorithm is somewhat different from that recommended for blood donor screening, in that it explicitly permits the use of NAT to confirm a repeatedly reactive EIA result. However, NAT-negative samples must be further evaluated by an SIA. This algorithm also provides useful guidance in the context of treatment. Given that blood donors are now routinely evaluated by NAT for HCV RNA, it is hoped that these results may be incorporated into the notification and management of seropositive donors.[32, 40]

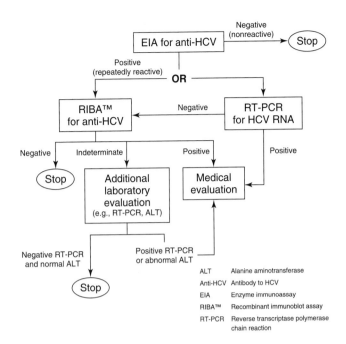

Figure 38.1 Algorithm for hepatitis C virus (HCV) testing among asymptomatic individuals. (From Centers for Disease Control and Prevention: Recommendations for prevention and control of hepatitis C virus (HCV) infection and HCV-related chronic disease. MMWR Morb Mortal Wkly Rep 1998;487[RR-19]:1–39.)

◼ Impact of Blood Donor Screening and Testing for HCV

Results of Testing: Confirmation

In 2001, the frequency of positive results among blood donations was 0.08%, as defined by RIBA. The rate is 0.366% among first-time donations and 0.0074% among repeat donations. These figures translate to a prevalence rate of 386 per 100,000, which is about one fifth of the national prevalence rate of 1800 per 100,000. The incidence of new infections in the donor population is 2.8 new infections per 100,000 person-years; the corresponding national incidence figure is 13.4 per 100,000 person-years. Thus, the donor rate is about one fifth of the national rate. These differences are attributable, at least in part, to the procedures used to recruit safer populations for donation and to the measures used to question presenting donors about their medical and behavioral histories. However, it should be noted that only a very few donors are actually deferred on the basis of their response to risk questions, in part because donors do not always provide complete answers[41] but also perhaps because potential donors make a conscious decision to avoid giving blood so as not to have to answer the questions.

Risk of Post-transfusion HCV Infection

It is clear from a number of published studies that donor screening and testing measures have had a profound impact on the incidence of post-transfusion hepatitis C. Indeed, prospective studies have not demonstrated any infections since the implementation of the so-called multiantigen tests. But there is substantial evidence for the efficacy of a variety of screening approaches used even before this time.

The essentially complete elimination of commercial donation of whole blood had a major effect on the frequency of post-transfusion hepatitis. It is also believed that a further reduction was seen as a result of more stringent donor questioning to reduce the risk of transmission of HIV and acquired immunodeficiency syndrome (AIDS), although subsequent information implies that the major effect would have come from a reduction in the number of injection drug users.

The first study to clearly demonstrate the impact of testing measures on hepatitis C infection was published by Nelson and colleagues.[43] They evaluated samples from a large population of patients undergoing cardiac surgery, using the first-generation test for anti-HCV. These researchers found that the risk of infection was 0.45% per unit prior to the implementation of any testing. After implementation of testing for ALT levels and for anti-HBc, the rate of infection dropped to 0.19%. Finally, once the version 1.0 EIA test was implemented, the rate dropped to 0.03%, or 1 per 3300 units.[42] A subsequent reevaluation using the more sensitive version 2.0 test on the blood recipients suggested that the actual risk was closer to 1:1700.[43] Once the version 2.0 test was introduced for blood donor screening, however, the frequency of residual infection declined profoundly. As pointed out previously, cases of hepatitis C were no longer observed in prospective studies, and risk estimates were developed on the basis of the length of the window period (as determined from post-transfusion infections) and the incidence of new infections within the donor population. In a landmark publication in 1996, Schreiber and colleagues estimated the residual risk of HCV infection at 1 per 103,000 donations, based on a window period of 82 days and an incidence rate of 4.84 per 100,000 person-years.[48] Subsequent evaluations account for a 12- to 13-day reduction in the window period attendant upon the implementation of the version 3.0 EIA and an overall decline in the incidence of HCV infection to 2.8 per 100,000 person-years. Thus, the estimate of residual risk for HCV is approximately 1:233,000.[3] It is projected that NAT for HCV RNA has decreased this risk by at least 50%, to less than 1:500,000 and may be as low as 1 in 1.5 million.

It should be noted that the estimates of the window period are based on the assumption that the incidence of HCV infection is the same for both repeating and first-time donors. Janssen and colleagues, using a sensitive/less sensitive test strategy, showed that this assumption was not true for HIV and that first-time donors had a 2.4-fold greater incidence of new infection than repeating donors.[49] By inspecting the frequency of HCV RNA–positive, antibody-negative donations among first-time donors, Dodd and colleagues[44] similarly estimated that first-time donors had a 3.3-fold greater HCV incidence than repeating donors.

It is interesting to speculate about the higher incidence of infections among first-time donors, but there are no definitive data. One possibility is that there are more test-seekers among people presenting to donate for the first time. It is also possible that the process of giving blood has an educational impact, and that individuals who learn about risk factors for blood-borne infections defer themselves from future donation.

■ Lookback

A positive test result for HCV antibodies does not provide any information about the duration of infection, even if accompanied by a positive finding for HCV RNA. Consequently, if a blood donor is found to be HCV antibody positive, it is possible that prior donations from that individual were infectious for HCV. There are two broad mechanisms by which this could occur. First, a previous donation could have been in the infectious but seronegative window period. Second, the prior donations could have been collected at a time when a less sensitive test was in use, or even before testing was initiated. Accordingly, a focused lookback program has been initiated in order to locate, notify, test, and, if appropriate, treat recipients of such potentially infectious prior donations. Studies in Canada and elsewhere suggest that up to 70% of such recipients may indeed have been infected.[45, 46] However, in the United States, the effort appears to have been less productive.

A team from the CDC reported that an estimated 98,484 blood components were identified as potentially infectious. Of these, 85% had been transfused. This interim study found that lookback had been completed for 80% of the transfused products; 69% of the recipients had died. Of those living, 78% were successfully notified that they had received a potentially infectious blood component. It was estimated that, of recipients notified, 49.5% were tested for anti-HCV; of those, 18.9% were seropositive, but 32% of these individuals were already aware that they were seropositive. Thus, at the time of publication of the study, it was estimated just over 1000 individuals were newly notified of unexpected HCV infection; this estimate translated to a national figure of 1520, on the assumption that the lookback process was to be completed. The figure represents fewer than 1% of all individuals who may have been infected as a result of transfusion.[47] It should be noted that this component of the lookback program was restricted only to donations that were identified as a result of testing with multiantigen tests (i.e., versions 2.0 or 3.0). It is likely that, as lookback is extended to cover donors initially identified by the version 1.0 test, the proportional yield will be greater, but the efficiency of the process will certainly be affected by availability of required records.

■ Comment and Summary

In its way, the history of hepatitis C has been as remarkable as that of HIV and AIDS. In retrospect, hepatitis C was the blood-borne agent most commonly transmitted by transfusion in the United States, right up until the early 1990s. The legacy of this problem will be seen for many years, as the long-term health consequences of HCV infection become manifest. The almost complete solution of the problem of transfusion-transmitted HCV is the result of many years of dedicated study of an intractable problem. There were no simple solutions; the virus was refractory to laboratory study, and there was a truly frustrating inability to identify any serologic markers of infection. Indeed, only at the very end of the 21st century was a naturally occurring, circulating viral antigen recognized, and then only in the few weeks preceding seroconversion.

As with HIV, the solution to transfusion-transmitted HCV infection was the development of serologic tests. In the case of HCV, however, this development was achieved through the combination of years of study of the disease, development of animal models, and the painstaking application of new recombinant technology. It is fitting that Harvey Alter and

Michael Houghton received the 2000 Lasker award for this work, but hundreds of others contributed over many years.

Serologic and nucleic acid testing have essentially eliminated the risk of transfusion-transmitted HCV. Plasma derivatives are prepared from highly tested starting material and are further treated with advanced inactivation procedures. It is of interest to note, however, that the early tests failed to identify all infectious units, while removing a substantial fraction of antibody-positive units, probably leading to the unexpected occurrence of HCV in recipients of some immunoglobulin products.

Despite the success of testing for HCV, there continue to be barriers to other aspects of management of this virus. As with many viral diseases, treatment options for HCV are limited and incomplete. More baffling, however, are the difficulties inherent in understanding and manipulating the interactions between the immune system and HCV. Development of an effective vaccine seems to be a particularly elusive goal.

REFERENCES

1. Aach RD, Szmuness W, Mosley JW, et al: Serum alanine aminotransferase of donors in relation to the risk of non-A, non-B hepatitis in recipients. The Transfusion-Transmitted Viruses Study. N Engl J Med 1981;304:989–994.
2. Alter HJ, Purcell RH, Holland PV, et al: Donor transaminase and recipient hepatitis: Impact on blood transfusion services. JAMA 1981;246:630–634.
3. Dodd RY: Germs, gels, and genomes: A personal recollection of 30 years in blood safety testing. In Stramer SL (ed): Blood Safety in the New Millenium. Bethesda, MD, American Association of Blood Banks, 2001, pp 97–122.
4. Alter HJ, Seeff LB: Recovery, persistence, and sequelae in HCV infection: A perspective on long-term outcome. Semin Liver Dis 2001;20:17–35.
5. Management of Hepatitis C. NIH Consens Statement 1997;15:1–41.
6. Liang TJ, Rehermann B, Seeff LB, Hoofnagle JH: Pathogenesis, natural history, treatment, and prevention of hepatitis C. Ann Intern Med 2000;132:296–305.
7. Purcell RH: Hepatitis viruses: Changing patterns of human disease. Proc Natl Acad Sci U S A 1994;91:2401–2406.
8. Frank C, Mohamed MK, Strickland GT, et al: The role of parenteral antischistosomal therapy in the spread of hepatitis C virus in Egypt. Lancet 2000;355(9207):887–891.
9. Alter MJ, Kruszon-Moran D, Nainan OV, et al: The prevalence of hepatitis C virus infection in the United States, 1988 through 1994. N Engl J Med 1999;341:556–562.
10. Alter MJ: Hepatitis C virus infection in the United States. J Hepatol 1999;31:88–91.
11. CDC: Recommendations for prevention and control of hepatitis C virus (HCV) infection and HCV-related chronic disease. MMWR 1998;47(RR-19):1–39.
12. Alter MJ: Epidemiology of hepatitis C and lookback. Hematology 1999;1999:418–421.
13. Conry-Cantilena C, VanRaden M, Gibble J, et al: Routes of infection, viremia, and liver disease in blood donors found to have hepatitis C virus infection. N Engl J Med 1996;334:1691–1696.
14. Orton SL, Peoples BG, Stramer SL, et al: Identification of recent risk factors among blood donors confirmed to be HCV NAT reactive, anti-HCV nonreactive. Transfusion 2000;40(Suppl 10):3S.
15. Choo Q-L, Kuo G, Weiner AJ, et al: Isolation of a cDNA clone derived from a blood-borne non- A, non-B viral hepatitis genome. Science 1989;244:359–362.
16. Kuo G, Choo Q-L, Alter HJ, et al: An assay for circulating antibodies to a major etiologic virus of human non-A, non-B hepatitis. Science 1989;244:362–364.
17. Lau JYN, Mizokami M, Kolberg JA, et al: Application of six hepatitis C virus genotyping systems to sera from chronic hepatitis C patients in the United States. J Infect Dis 1995;171:281–289.
18. Simmonds P, Holmes EC, Cha T-A, et al: Classification of hepatitis C virus into six major genotypes and a series of subtypes by phylogenetic analysis of the NS-5 region. J Gen Virol 1993;74:2391–2399.
19. McOmish F, Yap PL, Dow BC, et al: Geographical distribution of hepatitis C virus genotypes in blood donors: An international collaborative survey. J Clin Microbiol 1994;32:884–892.
20. Simmonds P, Alberti A, Alter HJ, et al: A proposed system for the nomenclature of hepatitis C viral genotypes. Hepatology 1994;19:1321–1324.
21. Zein NN, Persing DH: Hepatitis C genotypes: Current trends and future implications. Mayo Clin Proc 1996;71:458–462.
22. Martin P: Hepatitis C genotypes: The key to pathogenicity. Ann Intern Med 1995;122:227–228.
23. Cooreman MP, Schoondermark-Van de Ven EME: Hepatitis C virus: Biological and clinical consequences of genetic heterogeneity. Scand J Gastroenterol 1996;31(Suppl 218):106–115.
24. Busch MP, Korelitz JJ, Kleinman SH, et al: Declining value of alanine aminotransferase in screening of blood donors to prevent posttransfusion hepatitis B and C virus infection. Transfusion 1995;35:903–910.
25. Busch MP: HIV, HBV and HCV: New developments related to transfusion safety. Vox Sang 2000;78:253–256.
26. Couroucé AM, Le Marrec N, Bouchardeau F, et al: Efficacy of HCV core antigen detection during the preseroconversion period. Transfusion 2000;40:1198–1202.
27. Tanaka E, Ohue C, Aoyagi K, et al: Evaluation of a new enzyme immunoassay for hepatitis C virus (HCV) core antigen with clinical sensitivity approximating that of genomic amplification of HCV RNA. Hepatology 2000;32:388–393.
28. Stramer SL, Caglioti S, Strong DM: NAT of the United States and Canadian blood supply. Transfusion 2000;40:1165–1168.
29. Peoples BG, Preston SB, Tzeng JL, et al: Prolonged antibody-negative HCV viremia in a US blood donor with apparent HCV transmission to a recipient. Transfusion 2000;40:1280–1281.
30. Dow BC, Buchanan I, Munro H, et al: Relevance of RIBA-3 supplementary test to HCV PCR positivity and genotypes for HCV confirmation of blood donors. J Med Virol 1996;49:132–136.
31. Dodd RY, Stramer SL: Indeterminate results in blood donor testing: What you don't know can hurt you. Transfus Med Rev 2000;14:151–160.
32. Farci P, Shimoda A, Coiana A, et al: The outcome of acute hepatitis C predicted by the evolution of the viral quasispecies. Science 2000;288(5464):339–344.
33. Alter MJ, Margolis HS, Krawczynski K, et al: The natural history of community-acquired hepatitis C in the United States. N Engl J Med 1992;327:1899–1905.
34. Gretch DR, Dela Rosa C, Carithers RL Jr, et al: Assessment of hepatitis C viremia using molecular amplification technologies: Correlations and clinical implications. Ann Intern Med 1995;123:321–329.
35. Lunel F, Mariotti M, Cresta P, et al: Comparative study of conventional and novel strategies for the detection of hepatitis C virus RNA in serum: Amplicor, branched-DNA, NASBA and in-house PCR. J Virol Methods 1995;54:159–171.
36. Hawkins A, Davidson F, Simmonds P: Comparison of plasma virus loads among individuals infected with hepatitis C virus (HCV) genotypes 1, 2, and 3 by Quantiplex HCV RNA assay versions 1 and 2, Roche monitor assay, and an in-house limiting dilution method. J Clin Microbiol 1997;35:187–192.
37. Damen M, Sillekens P, Sjerps M, et al: Stability of hepatitis C virus RNA during specimen handling and storage prior to NASBA amplification. J Virol Methods 1998;72:175–184.
38. Sangiovanni A, Morales R, Spinzi GC, et al: Interferon alfa treatment of HCV RNA carriers with persistently normal transaminase levels: A pilot randomized controlled study. Hepatology 1998;27:853–856.
39. Halfon P, Khiri H, Gerolami V, et al: Impact of various handling and storage conditions on quantitative detection of hepatitis C virus RNA. J Hepatol 1996;25:307–311.
40. Lau JYN, Davis GL, Prescott LE, et al: Distribution of hepatits C virus genotypes determined by line probe assay in patients with chronic hepatitis C seen at tertiary referral centers in the United States. Ann Intern Med 1996;124:868–876.
41. Williams AE, Thomson RA, Schreiber GB, et al: Estimates of infectious disease risk factors in US blood donors. JAMA 1997;277:967–972.

42. Donahue JG, Murioz A, Ness PM, et al: The declining risk of post-transfusion hepatitis C virus infection. N Engl J Med 1992;327:369–373.

43. Nelson KE, Ahmed F, Ness P, Donahue JG: The incidence of post-transfusion hepatitis: Reply. N Engl J Med 1993;328:1280–1281.

44. Dodd RY, Aberle-Grasse JM, Stramer SL, for the ARCNET Program: The yield of nucleic acid testing (NAT) for HIV and HCV RNA in a population of U.S. voluntary donors: Relationship to contemporary measures of incidence. Transfusion 2000;40(Suppl 10):1S.

45. Long A, Spurll G, Demers H, Goldman M: Targeted hepatitis C lookback: Quebec, Canada. Transfusion 1999;39:194–200.

46. Christensen PB, Groenboek K, Krarup HB, Danish HVL: Transfusion-acquired hepatitis C: The Danish lookback experience. Transfusion 1999;39:188–193.

47. Culver DH, Alter MJ, Mullan RJ, Margolis HS: Evaluation of the effectiveness of targeted lookback for HCV infection in the United States—interim results. Transfusion 2000;40:1176–1181.

48. Schreiber GB, Busch MP, Kleinman SH, et al: The risk of transfusion–transmitted viral infections. N Engl J Med 1996; 336:1685–1690.

49. Janssen RS, Satten GA, Stramer SL, et al: New testing strategy to detect early HIV-1 infection for use in incidence estimates and for clinical and prevention purposes. JAMA 1998;280:42–48.

Chapter 39

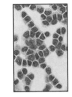

Human Immunodeficiency Virus, Human T-cell Lymphotrophic Viruses, and Other Retroviruses

Eberhard W. Fiebig

Edward L. Murphy

Michael P. Busch

Prior to the outbreak of the acquired immunodeficiency syndrome (AIDS) epidemic in the early 1980s, retroviruses had been identified as a cause of rare malignancies in humans and animals but were not considered a threat to transfusion recipients. The discovery that human immunodeficiency virus (HIV), a transfusion-transmissible retrovirus in the lentivirus group, is the etiologic agent of AIDS changed this perception dramatically. Since then, efforts to keep HIV out of the blood supply has affected virtually every aspect of blood banking and transfusion medicine with dramatic success in improving blood safety.[1,2]

In this chapter, we provide a general overview of retroviruses with emphasis on those aspects of human retrovirus epidemiology and pathophysiology of greatest relevance to specialists in transfusion medicine. The four major known pathogenic human retroviruses—human immunodeficiency virus types 1 and 2 (HIV-1 and HIV-2) and human T-cell lymphotrophic virus types I and II (HTLV-I and HTLV-II) are considered in greater detail. Our discussion closes with a critical outlook on new and emerging strategies to further reduce the risk of transfusion-acquired retroviral infections in industrialized and developing nations.

■ Definition, Life Cycle, and Distribution of Retroviruses

Retroviruses were among the first viruses described in scientific literature. They constitute a major class of membrane-coated, diploid, single-stranded RNA viruses with wide distribution in nature; examples exist in genera ranging from insects to reptiles to virtually all mammals.[3] The human retroviruses HIV and HTLV belong to the lentivirus and oncornavirus groups of the retrovirus family, respectively.[4] Characteristic features of retroviruses are (1) a distinct genomic organization, (2) the presence of viral particle (virion)–associated reverse transcriptase, and (3) a unique replication cycle (Fig. 39.1).

The first step of infection is attachment of virus particles to the cell membrane. In the case of HIV, which has tropism for T cells and macrophages, virus glycoprotein 120 (gp120) attaches to CD4 molecules expressed on the surface of these cells, but efficient infection also requires engagement of viral proteins with chemokine co-receptors identified as CCR5 on macrophages and CXCR4 on T cells.[5] After entry into a host cell, typically by fusion of the virion and host cell membranes, the reverse transcriptase enzyme copies viral DNA into complementary double-stranded DNA (cDNA). Virion-associated integrase then mediates integration of this cDNA into random sites in the host cell's chromosome, forming integrated viral cDNAs termed *proviruses*. Subsequent transcription, processing, and translation of viral genes are mediated principally by host cell enzymes, although both viral and host cell regulatory gene products influence the level and pattern of viral gene expression and replication. The classic retrovirus life cycle is completed when nascent particles associate and bud from the plasma membrane to form progeny virions, which can then infect other cells and other organisms.

Retroviruses can also spread horizontally, by fusion of infected and uninfected cells, or vertically, by replication of integrated viral DNA along with cellular DNA during mitosis or meiosis. Indeed, integrated proviruses have evolved that are passed congenitally through the germline; these so-called endogenous retroviral elements (as contrasted with vertically transmitted exogenous retroviruses) are present in many species, including humans, and in some species account for up to 10% of total genomic DNA.[4]

Disease manifestations of retroviruses are highly variable. Many animal species harbor exogenous or endogenous

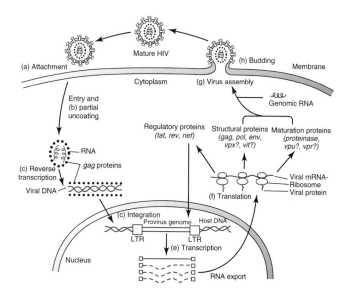

Figure 39.1   Replication cycle of human immunodeficiency virus type 1. (a) After attachment of virus particles to the CD4 receptor molecule, virus enters the cell by a pH-dependent mechanism and/or endocytosis. Not shown is the required interaction of viral proteins and chemokine co-receptors. (b) The outer lipid envelope of the virus is removed when the particle undergoes fusion with cytoplasmic vacuoles. (c) The core particle that remains is the site for reverse transcription of the virion RNA into DNA. (d) After translocation into the nucleus, integration into the DNA of the cell occurs. (e) The integrated provirus genome is transcribed by cellular RNA polymerase II. (f) Translation of viral messenger (m)RNA produces regulatory proteins, which stimulate synthesis of maturation proteins and the structural proteins of the virion. (g) Accumulation of structural proteins in the cell membrane permits the assembly of virus particles. (h) Muturation and release from the cell by budding. (From Mayer and Busch, with permission.)

retroviruses that appear to be benign and may in fact be beneficial in restricting infection by related pathogenic retroviruses. On the other hand, retroviruses became the focus of intense research in the 1960s and 1970s because of their capacity to induce malignancies in a wide range of species. The demonstration that certain retroviruses (termed *acute RNA tumor viruses*) rapidly transform target cells in vitro and induce tumors within days to weeks of inoculation into animals greatly facilitated experimental investigation of viral carcinogenesis.[6] Studies of the molecular differences between these acute retroviruses and genetically related *slow viruses* (which failed to transform cells in vitro and only occasionally caused tumors many months after inoculation) led to the discovery of viral oncogenes, which were responsible for tumorigenesis.

This achievement was followed by the revolutionary discovery that these viral oncogenes had in fact arisen by recombination events between slow viruses and key cellular genes termed *proto-oncogenes*.[6] Thus, investigation of retrovirus-induced cancers in animals led to unparalleled insights into normal cell biology and disease pathogenesis in humans. Retroviruses have also attracted interest from researchers who explore nonpathogenic strains as vehicles for therapeutic gene transfer.

The first report of successful isolation and characterization of a bona fide human retrovirus (later termed HTLV-I) occurred in 1980 and involved a patient with a rare type

of leukemia (now called adult T-cell leukemia/lymphoma [ATL]).[7] Subsequently, HTLV-I was also identified as cause of a rare neurologic condition known as HTLV-associated myelopathy/tropical spastic paraparesis (HAM/TSP).[8] A second, closely related human retrovirus (HTLV-II) was isolated in 1982 from a patient with a somewhat more common type of leukemia (hairy cell leukemia)[9]; however, further surveys failed to show a relationship between HTLV-II and hairy cell leukemia, but established the virus as a causative agent of HAM/TSP.[8, 10]

Both HTLV-I and HTLV-II are thought to be derived from simian T-lymphotropic retroviruses transmitted to humans over the past hundreds to thousands of years. The full pathogenic potential of human retroviruses was not realized until HIV was established as the cause of AIDS in 1984. It is now thought that the virus originated in a chimpanzee species, from where it was introduced to native people of the central African rain forest.[11] There may have been multiple introductions of the virus into humans dating back several centuries; so far, however, the earliest documented evidence of HIV infection in humans comes from a blood sample collected in 1959.[12] Sub-Saharan Africa remains the area worst affected by the epidemic today, with an estimated 70% of the global caseload.[13] According to World Health Organization (WHO) figures, 5.6 million people were newly infected in 1999, raising the projected number of infected people to a staggering 33.6 million worldwide.[13]

■ Human Immunodeficiency Virus

Genomic Organization and Virion Structure

The organization of the HIV RNA genome is shown in Figure 39.2. The products of the *gag*, *pol*, and *env* genes that are shared among all retroviruses give rise to the structural elements of the virion, which is shown in Figure 39.3. Similar to other lentiviruses, HIV contains at least six additional genes, which encode for regulatory proteins and virulence factors that appear to play an important role in pathogenicity. Detection of specific antibodies against viral proteins or identification of viral nucleic acid sequences in infected hosts provides the basis of screening and supplemental assays used in blood donor eligibility testing.

Risk of Transmission by Transfusion Before Blood Donor Screening

Not surprisingly, the majority of HIV transmissions in the United States occurred before discovery of the virus and institution of blood donor screening. A principal lesson learned from the HIV-1 epidemic is how an infectious agent with a prolonged clinical incubation period (i.e., the interval between initial infection and clinically apparent disease; median ≈10 years) can spread silently within a population (and its blood donor base) for years before recognition.[14] In the United States, this early phase was localized primarily to homosexual and bisexual men, groups who were eligible blood donors at the time.

Although we now know that the virus began to spread at an exponential rate in these men in the late 1970s, it was not until 1981 that clusters of Kaposi sarcoma and *Pneumocystis* pneumonia were first recognized among homosexual men in New York and Los Angeles. In late 1982, descriptions of AIDS-like illnesses in hemophiliacs and recipients of blood

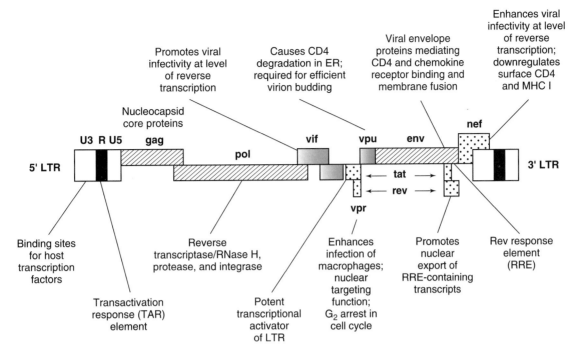

Figure 39.2   Genomic structure of HIV-1. The nine known genes of HIV-1 are shown, and their recognized primary functions are summarized. The 5′ and 3′ long terminal repeats (LTRs) containing regulatory sequences recognized by various host transcription factors are also depicted, and the positions of the Tat and Rev RNA response elements—transactivation response (TAR) element and Rev response element (RRE)—are indicated. ER, endoplasmic reticulum; MHC I, major histocompatibility complex class I. (Reproduced with permission from Geleziunas R, Greene WC: Molecular insights into HIV-1 infection and pathogenesis. In Sande MA, Volberding PA (eds): The Medical Management of AIDS, 6th ed. Philadelphia, WB Saunders, 1999, p 24.)

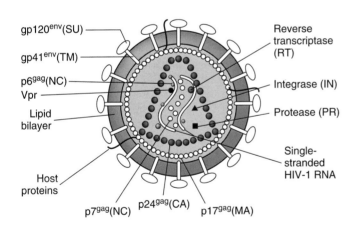

Figure 39.3   Schematic of the HIV-1 virion. Each of the virion proteins making up the envelope (gp120^{env} and gp41^{env}) and inner core (p24^{gag}, p17^{gag}, p7^{gag}, and p6^{gag}) is identified. In addition, the diploid RNA genome is shown associated with reverse transcriptase (RT), an RNA- and DNA-dependent DNA polymerase. Integrase (IN) and protease (PR) are also found in the mature HIV-1 virion. The auxiliary protein Vpr is incorporated into the HIV-1 virion through an interaction with the p6^{gag} protein, which comprises the carboxyl terminus of the p55^{gag} precursor protein. CA, capsid protein; MA, matrix protein; NC, nucleocapsid protein; SU, surface protein; TM, trans-membrane protein. (Reproduced with permission from Geleziunas R, Greene WC: Molecular insights into HIV-1 infection and pathogenesis. In Sande MA, Volberding PA (eds): The Medical Management of AIDS, 6th ed. Philadelphia, WB Saunders, 1999, p 25.)

components first appeared.[15, 16] With these reports, a blood-borne infectious etiology for AIDS became probable, and efforts were initiated to exclude from blood donation persons with symptoms of or risk factors associated with AIDS.[17] Approximately a year later, HIV-1 was discovered, an event soon followed by development of the anti–HIV-1 tests, which were licensed for donor screening in March 1985.

Combining HIV-1 seroincidence data among homosexual men in San Francisco with data from the Transfusion Safety Study (TSS) Donor Repository collected in the city in late 1984[18] enabled researchers to piece together an accurate picture of the risk of HIV-1 transmission by transfusion in the San Francisco Bay area between 1978 and 1985 (Fig. 39.4). The analysis showed that the risk of transfusion-associated (TA) HIV-1 infection rose rapidly from its first occurrence in 1978 to a peak risk of approximately 1.1% per transfused unit in late 1982. Beginning in early 1983 and continuing through implementation of anti–HIV-1 screening, there was a marked, progressive decline in risk as a result of diminishing numbers of blood donations from at-risk or infected individuals. This decline was directly attributable to growing awareness of the infectious nature of AIDS in the homosexual community and to implementation and refinement of donor education and deferral measures by blood banks.[18, 19] In fact, in San Francisco, it was estimated that approximately 90% of high-risk men who were donors between 1980 and 1982 deferred themselves from blood donation prior to implementation of the anti–HIV-1 test in early 1985.[18] These data illustrate dramatically the effectiveness of donor education and self-deferral measures.

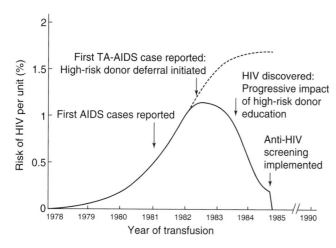

Figure 39.4 Risk of human immunodeficiency virus (HIV-1) infections from transfusions in San Francisco before anti-HIV screening. Solid line represents estimated risk of recipient infection per unit transfused. Dashed line indicates what the risk would have been if high-risk donor deferral measures had not been implemented. The risk in the United States as a whole probably trailed that in San Francisco by approximately 1 year, and the peak risk was of lower magnitude. (Modified from Busch et al., with permission.)

Hemophiliacs, who are exquisitely vulnerable to transfusion-transmitted diseases because of exposure to factor concentrates derived from plasma pooled from thousands of blood donors, were hit especially hard by the early epidemic of transfusion-transmitted AIDS.[20] Incidence and prevalence data from 1978 through 1990 for 16 hemophiliac cohorts in the United States and Europe show that infections began in 1978, peaked in October 1982 at 22 infections per 100 person-years at risk, and declined to 4 per 100 person-years by July 1984. Few new infections occurred among hemophiliacs after 1986, but by that time, 50% of subjects in the combined cohort were infected. Median seroconversion dates for infected hemophiliacs in U.S. cohorts ranged from July 1980, for those treated with high doses of factor VIII, to December 1983, for those treated with low doses of factor IX; corresponding dates for European cohorts were approximately 1 year later, reflecting the delay in importation and use of products manufactured from American plasma. The decline in incidence from the infection peak in late 1982 coincided with health interventions introduced to reduce transmission, including recommendations for reduction in use of factor concentrates in 1982, voluntary donor deferral in 1983, and the availability of heat-treated factor VIII in 1984 and of HIV-1 screening in 1985.

This temporal profile for the risk of HIV from blood components and derivatives was further corroborated in a report from the Centers for Disease Control and Prevention (CDC),[21] in which 4619 cases of TA AIDS reported from 1982 through 1991 were reviewed. (These cases represented 2% of the total of 222,413 U.S. AIDS cases reported during that period.) Analysis by year of AIDS diagnosis (with adjustment for delay between diagnosis and report) showed a steep rise of reported AIDS cases from 14 in 1982 to approximately 800 cases per year from 1987 to 1991. In contrast, when these same cases were plotted by year of implicated transfusion that led to HIV infection, the number of cases rose from 56 in 1978 to 714 in 1984, dropped sharply to 288 by 1985 when screening for

antibody began, and fell to a mean of 20 per year from 1986 through 1991. This difference reflects the incubation period between infection (transfusion) and diagnosis of clinical AIDS. For example, more than 95% of AIDS cases diagnosed in 1991 were attributable to transfusions received before implementation of anti-HIV screening in early 1985. Upon further investigation, the patients in many of the cases diagnosed from post-1985 transfusions were found to be infected from sources other than HIV-seronegative blood transfusions.[21]

Efficiency of Transmission by Transfusion

HIV is not inactivated by blood refrigeration and survives freezing of plasma; the virus is therefore readily passed on by transfusion. Clinical, virologic, and immunologic studies of exposed transfusion recipients and hemophiliacs have yielded important insights into the significance of factors that might influence the transmission of HIV-1 infection and the course of disease. The TSS, which is unique in being the only U.S. study that traced and enrolled recipients of known seropositive units,[22, 23] offers some of the clearest data addressing these issues. In the TSS, 111 (89.5%) of 124 enrolled recipients transfused with anti–HIV-1–positive blood components demonstrated seroconversion (to anti–HIV-1 positivity).[23] Neither characteristics of the donor's infection nor inherent recipient susceptibility factors significantly influenced transmission of HIV-1 by transfusions.[24] Variables that have been identified to correlate with likelihood of HIV-1 transmission are the type of blood component transfused and its duration of storage.[25] Washed red blood cell (RBC) units and RBC units stored more than 26 days had lower transmission rates than other components. This observation as well as experimental evidence[26] suggests that component manipulations that reduce the number of viable leukocytes, free virus, or both in plasma may reduce but not eliminate infectiousness.

With regard to recipients of clotting factor concentrates, an average of approximately 50% of hemophiliacs treated with factor VIII in the early 1980s experienced seroconversion.[20, 27] However, the rate of seroconversion to anti–HIV-1 positivity in hemophiliacs who were treated with very high doses of factor VIII (>500,000 units) approached 100%.[27] This finding indicates that, perhaps with the rare exception of persons lacking HIV-1 co-receptors required for infection (see later), no one is resistant to HIV-1 infection, given a large enough inoculum and repeated exposures. There was early hope that seroconversion in a proportion of seropositive hemophiliacs might have occurred as a result of exposure to denatured HIV-1 proteins rather than infectious virus. Several large studies, however, have confirmed persistent HIV-1 infection in 100% of seropositive hemophiliacs by means of sensitive viral culture and polymerase chain reaction (PCR) techniques.[28, 29] On the other hand, although several early studies using PCR reported detection of HIV-1 DNA in a subset of seronegative exposed hemophiliacs,[30] subsequent studies have refuted these reports[31, 32] as well as the general concept of seronegative (so-called immunosilent) HIV-1 infections.[33]

Clinical Course of Transfusion-Acquired AIDS and the Role of Allogeneic Transfusion in the Progression of HIV Infection

Investigating the course of HIV-1 infection in transfusion recipients not only provides data for counseling and management of affected and at-risk patients but also is of particular medical scientific interest because (1) the date of infection or transfusion is precisely known and (2) recipients lack many cofactors (e.g., other sexually transmitted diseases or intravenous drug use) that might influence disease course in other infected cohorts. In addition, the transfusion setting is unique, in that the disease course in the recipient can be compared with that in a linked donor, thus allowing the study whether a relationship exists between disease progression in a blood donor and his or her recipients.[24, 34, 35] However, blood recipients may have co-morbid diseases related to their transfusion, and they have shortened life expectancy.

Of the 112 infected recipients enrolled in the TSS, 37 had progressed to AIDS (CDC's 1987 revised definition) by 7 years of post-transfusion follow-up.[36] On the basis of Kaplan-Meyer analysis, the actuarial risk of AIDS at 7 years was 51%. This rate is faster than the rate of progression observed for the infected donors and hemophiliacs followed in parallel in that study.[36, 37] As observed by others,[38] an effect of age on rate of disease progression was noted in all three TSS groups, with older patients manifesting symptoms of AIDS earlier than younger individuals. Once age and underlying disease were controlled for, rates of progression to clinical AIDS were virtually identical for TSS recipients and hemophiliacs, whereas the rate of AIDS diagnosis was slightly higher for enrolled donors (most of whom were homosexual men).[36] This finding suggests that the route of infection, inoculum size, and proposed cofactors, such as other viral infections (e.g., cytomegalovirus or hepatitis B virus), are not highly significant in determining the course of HIV disease.

Further analyses of TSS data illustrate the importance of the level of viremia for HIV transmission in cases of transfusion-acquired infection[39] and in heterosexual transmissions from persons infected through transfusion to their sexual partners.[40] With regard to factors influencing disease progression, data from the study point to host factors, rather than to differences in viral strains within B-type HIV-1 (clade B [See below]), as determinants for disease progression.[41] Archived samples from the TSS also served for investigation of the role of the beta-chemokine CCR5, a newly discovered co-receptor for non–syncytium-inducing (NSI) strains of HIV-1, in parenteral transmission of virus. Recipients of HIV-seropositive blood units and coagulation factor concentrates who had a 32–base pair deletion in the CCR5 gene were less susceptible to infection, although disease in those who were infected progressed at the same rate as disease in recipients with a normal CCR5 gene.[42] Finally, the significance of a virulence gene, *nef*, was demonstrated in an Australian cohort of a blood donor and eight transfusion recipients who were infected with an HIV-1 viral strain lacking a functioning *nef* gene. The cohort members had a milder than usual disease course and prolonged disease-free survival without therapy.[43]

Interestingly, transfusion not only provides a mode of transmission for HIV but, according to some evidence, may also affect the course of disease in patients with AIDS. Observations from retrospective studies and small prospective studies suggest that allogeneic transfusions may result in accelerated disease progression and shortened survival in HIV-infected patients.[44] In vitro experiments provided evidence that transfusion of allogeneic leukocytes, presumably through immunologic activation of lymphocytes and macrophages, cause greater replication of HIV, whereas

transfusion of autologous leukocytes and allogeneic red cells, platelets, and plasma did not show this effect.[45] The Viral Activation [by] Transfusion Study (VATS), a multicenter U.S. clinical trial, addressed this issue and investigated the benefits of providing leukocyte-reduced blood to patients in late-stage HIV infection. The study found no evidence of significant activation of HIV replication or accelerated disease progression in recipients of either leukoreduced or non-leukoreduced transfusions.

HIV Diversity: HIV-2 and HIV-1 Subtypes

Extensive genetic diversity is a hallmark of HIV and other lentiviruses. A contributing factor is the high error rate during reverse transcription, which is attributable to the negligible proofreading exonuclease activity of the reverse transcriptase.[46] Nucleotide misincorporations may occur at an astonishingly high rate of 5 to 10 per HIV genome per replication cycle, a phenomenon known as *hypermutation*. Insertions, deletions, and intergeneic recombination add to the trend toward genetic diversification.[47] Within an HIV-1–infected individual, a swarm of quasispecies of HIV variants develops over time,[48] and dual and multiple infections and recombination between the infecting HIV-1 strains have been reported.[49, 50]

On the basis of relatedness of genomic sequences, the HIV-1 family is divided into main (M) and outlier (O) groups, with at least nine distinct subtypes or clades (A through I) recognized within group M.[51] Of note is the currently almost exclusive prevalence of clade B strains in the United States and, to a lesser degree, Europe; other clades are more predominant in South America and Asia. The greatest genetic diversity of HIV-1 strains is found in Central Africa, in keeping with this area's role as the presumed point of origin of the pandemic. The worldwide distribution of HIV-subgroups and clades is depicted in Figure 39.5. A recent survey of 572 U.S. blood donors identified several infected with non-B subtypes. Although these subtypes were detectable by antibody assays used in blood donor screening, the seroconversion window period from beginning of infectiousness to detectability of anti-HIV is prolonged, suggesting that the current assays, which are optimized for subtype B detection, are less sensitive for non-B strains.[52]

Group O viral strains are most common in Cameroon and surrounding West African countries, where an estimated 1% to 2% of HIV infections are caused by these viral strains.[53, 54] Outside this geographic area, group O isolates have rarely been seen. Concern arose in the mid-1990s when studies demonstrated that some group O isolates were not reliably detected by a number of HIV-1 and HIV-1/HIV-2 combination assays,[55] including some that are used for blood donor screening.[56] Antibody assays employing synthetic peptides or recombinant antigens on the solid phase, and those using the so-called third-generation "antigen-sandwich" format, were especially prone to false-negative results. Since then, test manufacturers have moved quickly to enhance their assays' sensitivity to unusual variants like subtype O. As an added precaution, the U.S. Food and Drug Administration (FDA) has recommended permanent deferral of blood and plasma donors who were born, resided, or traveled in West Africa since 1977 or had sexual contact with someone identified by these criteria.[57] The current risk of group O infection in the United States is very low. As of 1997, only two such infections had been reported; both involved immigrants from West

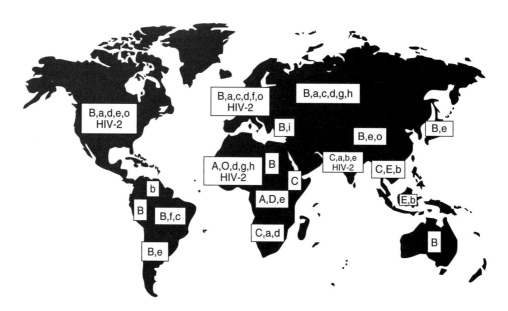

Figure 39.5   Distribution of human immunodeficiency virus (HIV) throughout the world according to the prevalence of its types and subtypes (clades). The distribution of HIV-1 clades is indicated by letters A to I (more prevalent in capital letters). Clades of HIV-2 are not shown separated. (Reproduced with permission from Diaz RS, Busch MP: Human immunodeficiency viruses. In Anderson KC, Ness PM (eds): Scientific Basis of transfusion Medicine: Implications for Clinical Practice, 2nd ed. Philadelphia, WB Saunders, 2000, p 508.)

Africa who had never donated blood or plasma. Furthermore, surveillance testing for HIV-1 divergent strains did not detect any group O viral isolates among 1072 serum samples from high- and low-risk population groups in the United States and Puerto Rico.[58]

HIV-2, discovered in 1985 in several countries in West Africa,[59] was initially called HTLV-IV and lymphadenopathy-associated virus type 2. HIV-2 has now spread throughout Western Europe, where a substantial number of infected blood donors have been detected, and cases of transfusion transmission have been documented.[60] HIV-2 is transmitted in the same manner as HIV-1 (i.e., by sexual contact, intravenous drug use, and, at a lower rate than for HIV-l, from mother to child) and causes progressive immunodeficiency, with susceptibility to an array of opportunistic infections similar to those seen with HIV-1. Rates of disease progression and secondary viral transmission appear to be lower, however, in persons infected with HIV-2 than in those infected with HIV-1, possibly owing to lower viral burden in HIV-2 infection.[61, 62]

HIV-l and HIV-2 are highly (>50%) homologous at the nucleic acid sequence level, and they cross-react immunologically to a great extent (particularly the core and polymerase antigens). For this reason, up to 90% of sera from HIV-2–infected persons have been found to test positive with FDA–licensed anti–HIV-1 assays, with variable reactivity on HIV-1 Western blots.[63, 64] This cross-reactivity undoubtedly prevented transfusion transmission of HIV-2 by blood screened for anti–HIV-1 in areas where the type 2 virus was present prior to implementation of combination HIV-1/HIV-2 screening tests. This high-level cross-reactivity has also facilitated surveillance for HIV-2 in regions where it is currently rare or absent.[65, 66]

In a comprehensive review of the extent of HIV-2 in the United States through the end of 1991, the CDC identified 17 case reports with confirmed HIV-2 infection.[60] Of the 17

persons, 13 had immigrated to the United States from West Africa, a fact that formed the basis for the exclusion of sub-Saharan Africans from blood donation prior to implementation of improved, HIV-2–sensitive screening assays in early 1992. One of the case reports involved an American woman identified as reactive on anti–HIV-1 enzyme immunoassay (EIA) screening (indeterminate Western blot) after a volunteer blood donation in New York City in 1986; she had recently traveled to Africa but denied specific risk factors for infection.[67] From diagnosis in 1987 of the first case of HIV-2 infection in the United States to 1998, a total of 79 persons with HIV-2 infections were documented, of which approximately two thirds had been born in West Africa.[68]

Combination HIV-l/HIV-2 assays were developed in the late 1980s,[69–71] and mandatory implementation of either a combination test or a separate anti–HIV-2 test in the donor screening setting was required by the FDA effective June 1, 1992.[72] From the implementation of HIV-2 screening in 1992 through 1996, three prospective U.S. blood donors were found to be HIV-2 positive at the time of attempted donation.[73] One was a U.S.-born woman without identifiable risks for HIV infection; the other two were men, born in France and Liberia, West Africa, who had resided for years in West Africa. The detection of three cases of HIV-2 infection in more than 50 million whole blood donations, since the beginning of HIV-2 screening in 1992 through the end of 1996, suggests that the U.S. prevalence of HIV-2 is less than 1 in 15 million screened donations. As of 2001, no cases of HIV-2–infected transfusion recipients had been reported in the United States.

Blood Donor Testing for HIV-1 and HIV-2 Antibody

Screening of pooled blood donor samples for HIV based on nucleotide amplification techniques known as nucleic acid testing (NAT) has been in use in Europe since 1998 and in the

United States since 1999 (see later). Routine blood donor screening, however, continues to rely on serologic methods for detection of antibodies to HIV-1 and HIV-2 and antigens for HIV-1, which are performed on individual samples from all units. Initial testing is performed on serum or plasma from "pilot" tubes collected at the time of donation. If the initial test result is reactive, another test is performed on both the originally tested pilot tube serum or plasma and either a second pilot tube or an aliquot of plasma obtained from segmented tubing attached to the blood components. This element of the screening algorithm is designed as an additional safeguard to identify and resolve possible specimen labeling errors. If results of one or both second tests are reactive, the unit is designated "repeat reactive" and discarded. A process is also initiated to identify and quarantine all in-date components from any prior donations from that donor and to notify recipients who received blood components from prior donations.[74]

Developments in test methodology have occurred at a rapid rate, and blood banks have implemented improved assays as soon as possible after FDA licensure. The evolution of antibody assays has been achieved through improvements in the antigens on the solid phase and in assay formats. From crude viral lysates, production moved to viral lysate assays spiked with purified HIV-1 antigens, and then on to the use of cloned (recombinant DNA [rDNA]–derived) and synthetic peptide antigens. Although concerns have been raised about the sensitivity of rDNA-derived and peptide antigen–based EIAs to immunologically variant strains,[55, 56] these assays have been "engineered" to include highly selected antigenic regions of HIV-1 and HIV-2 that maximize sensitivity to infected subjects from around the world. Consequently, rDNA-derived and synthetic peptide antigen–based assays are now in wide use in U.S. blood banks.

Test manufacturers have also developed new assay formats with greater capacity to detect low-titer immunoglobulin (Ig) M antibody produced during early seroconversion. For example, the recombinant "antigen sandwich" EIA format employed in Abbott Laboratories' anti–HIV-1/HIV-2 EIA allows use of lower dilutions of donor sera and detects IgM with better sensitivity.[70, 75] The progressive introduction of assays with increased sensitivity to early infection has led to significant narrowing of the seroconversion window period and concomitant reductions in the risk of receiving screened blood (see later).[75, 76] The realization that HIV-1 subgroup and variant strains may not be reliably detected by current HIV-1/HIV-2 assays has led to demands by the FDA and efforts by kit manufacturers to reengineer standard assay formats to improve detection of unusual viral strains without compromising their sensitivity to main group HIV-1/HIV-2 strains.[77]

Testing for HIV Antigen

Beginning in March 1996, testing for HIV-1 antigens (HIV-1 Ag, in practice p24 Ag) became mandatory in the United States. This decision was based on studies showing that HIV-1 Ag appears in blood early in the course of infection, approximately 1 week before antibody is detectable. Transmission of HIV has been reported from transfusion of seronegative blood that was later shown to contain p24 antigen; the donors subsequently showed seroconversion.[78] Mathematical models, constructed with findings from geographic areas with very high incidence of new HIV infections, suggested that routine antigen testing

would detect one antigen-positive/antibody-negative donation in every 1.6 million tested.[79] In reality, this projection was not achieved. Only seven donations from infected window-phase (p24 Ag positive/anti-HIV negative) volunteer donors were intercepted on the basis of p24 Ag testing alone in the first 5 years of screening,[80] for an observed yield of 1 in 10 million donations. A possible explanation for the under-performance of HIV-1 antigen testing in detecting HIV-1 antibody–negative window period infections is that prospective blood donors in the early phase of HIV-1 infection, who have HIV-1 antigen only, may be experiencing symptoms from acute retroviral infection that deter them from blood donation or result in their rejection during the predonation history and physical examination.

Nucleic Acid Testing

In the U.S., NAT for HIV (and HCV) in blood donor screening began in spring of 1999 in the form of large scale clinical trials conducted under investigational new drug (IND) applications for FDA. Despite the research aspect, NAT quickly became the standard of practice, and by July 2001 essentially the entire U.S. blood supply was screened for HIV and HCV with the new technology.[81] NAT is currently performed on pools of 16 to 24 blood donor samples, known as "minipool NAT." The pooling strategy lowers the sensitivity of the test but allows faster turnaround times which is critically important for on-time blood product release. In over 2 years of practical experience in the U.S., HIV NAT detected 6 HIV-1 RNA-positive, HIV-1 EIA-negative, p24 Ag-negative donors out of 26 million donations tested (approximately 1 in 4 million) and missed no p24-positive, HIV-1 EIA-negative donations.[81] These results are consistent with a modest reduction in the infectious window period of HIV, averaging approximately 10 to 12 days against a sensitive HIV-1 antibody test and 3 days against p24 Ag testing (see discussion of the incidence-window period model below). Rare, unfortunate cases of HIV transmission from NAT screened units have occurred, demonstrating the potential infectiousness of such units.[82, 83] The first NAT test system for blood donor screening was licensed by the FDA in early 2002; facilities that use the licensed test will probably be able to discontinue HIV-1 antigen testing, but HIV antibody testing will continue.

Supplemental Testing

Because of the exquisite sensitivity of HIV EIAs used in blood donor screening and the low pretest probability of HIV infection among blood donors, the majority of positive screening results are false-positive, despite excellent specificity of the tests. Supplemental assays are therefore essential to confirm positive screening results and for donor counseling. Supplemental testing must use FDA-licensed reagents and must rule out both HIV-1 and HIV-2 infection.[72] Although combination HIV-1/HIV-2 supplemental assays using rDNA-derived or synthetic peptide antigens that appear to accurately detect and discriminate anti–HIV-1 and anti–HIV-2 have been developed,[74] they are not yet approved by the FDA. Therefore, current confirmatory algorithms in U.S. blood banks employ HIV-1 viral lysate–based Western blots or immunofluorescence assays, in combination with a licensed anti–HIV-2 EIA and an unlicensed HIV-2 supplemental assay.[72]

Interpretive criteria for Western blots have evolved over time as tests have improved and our understanding of the meaning of various banding patterns has grown (refer to chapter 38). For currently licensed assays, a *positive* interpretation requires antibody reactivity to two of the following three HIV antigens: p24 (the major *gag* protein), gp41 (transmembrane *env* protein), and gp120/160 (external *env* protein/*env* precursor protein). Although these criteria are generally very accurate, it is clear that some donors who show antibody reactivity only to the envelope glycoproteins are not infected with HIV-1.[84] It is important, therefore, that all initial positive Western blot results are confirmed by testing of a separate follow-up sample, both to rule out specimen mix-up or testing errors and to discriminate nonspecific patterns from early seroconversion. A *negative* test result of Western blot is, by definition, the absence of any bands. Any other pattern of reactivity is classified as *indeterminate*. Only a very small proportion of donors who test indeterminate on Western blot are infected with HIV-1.[85, 86] Schochetman and George[87] provide a detailed discussion of interpretive criteria and review of developments in HIV supplemental test technology.

All donors who test "repeat reactive" and those with persistently indeterminate Western blot patterns are deferred from further blood donations and are notified of their screening and supplemental test results. Recipients of prior donations from donors with confirmed positive results are traced, in a process called *lookback*.[73, 88] Donors whose supplemental test results are completely negative are eligible for possible reentry into the donor pool according to an FDA-specified protocol,[72] although in practice, logistical and legal considerations have generally prevented reinstatement of such donors.

Supplemental testing for HIV-1 Ag results relies on neutralization assays. When the EIA screening test result for HIV-1 Ag is repeat reactive, a confirmatory neutralization test should be performed to aid in counseling the donor and to determine the need for product quarantine, lookback, and deferral.[78] Although donors whose serum shows neutralization are classified as confirmed positive for HIV-1 Ag and must be permanently deferred, studies involving reverse transcriptase PCR (RT-PCR) testing and follow-up in such donors have established that only a small proportion are actually infected with HIV—that is, in most cases, the neutralization test results are false-positive.[80]

Donors whose serum does not show neutralization on assay are currently considered "not confirmed" for HIV-1 Ag, but they must be reported as having an HIV-1 Ag indeterminate status; they should be temporarily deferred from donation for a minimum of 8 weeks. Such donors can be reentered into the donor pool if they have been retested after this period and are found to be nonreactive on both the HIV-1-Ag screening test and the HIV antibody test. Unfortunately, at follow-up testing, approximately 70% of donors who had indeterminate results are found to be indeterminate again and must be indefinitely deferred from donation. Like antibody-reactive units, units from donors with repeat reactive HIV-1 Ag results cannot be used for transfusion or for further manufacturing into injectable products; instead, they must be quarantined and destroyed.

Risk of Infection from Screened Donations

Implementation of anti–HIV-1 screening in 1985 resulted in a marked decline of virus transmission by transfusion over the first several years of screening (see Fig. 39.4).[37, 89] However, initial hopes that the newly developed antibody test would lead to eradication of HIV transmission by blood donor screening were not fulfilled.

In the late 1980s, well-documented cases of HIV-1 transmission from screened blood transfusions were reported,[90] and 14 of 106 (13%) of the cases initially reported as due to infections from screened blood transfusions could be confirmed. It was therefore clear that a small number of transmissions continued, despite screening with antibody tests. After adjusting for uninvestigated cases, and assuming an equal distribution of infections from 1986 through 1991, CDC investigators estimated that during that period, approximately five TA AIDS cases due to infections from anti-HIV–screened blood transfusions had occurred per year.[21]

In the United States, two prospective studies estimated the risk of HIV transmission from antibody-screened donations at approximately 1 in 60,000 units between 1985 and 1991.[91, 92] These studies were discontinued in 1992 because of their high cost and the realization that monitoring TA AIDS case reports represents an insensitive and inadequate approach for assessing the small residual risk of HIV transmission from screened transfusions. Since then, an alternative approach has been developed for estimating the risk of HIV infection from transfusions, now known as the incidence–window period model.[79] It is based on the premise that the risk of viral transmission by blood transfusion in a given geographic area is primarily a function of the incidence rate—that is, the number of newly infected blood donors per person-years of observation—and the length of the window period—defined as the time from infectiousness to seroconversion, when screening tests become positive. The risk of HIV-1 transmission from repeat donors and, with some adjustments, from first-time donors can then be calculated. Window period estimates for HIV-1 infection in the United States dropped from a median of 45 days (95% confidence interval, 34–55 days) for the overall period from 1985 to 1990 to approximately 22 to 25 days with routine introduction in 1992 of new format anti–HIV-1/HIV-2 "combi-tests," which detect HIV-specific IgM antibody 10 to 15 days earlier than previously available assays (Fig. 39.6).[74–76] By combining the 25-day window period estimate with data on the frequency of HIV seroconversions in large U.S. donor populations, two independent studies derived at point estimates for the risk for HIV transmission during the period 1992 through 1995 as 1:450,000[93] and 1:495,000.[94]

Introduction of HIV-1 antigen screening in 1995 is likely to have further reduced the risk, but because fewer than expected HIV-1 antigen–positive HIV-1/2 antibody–negative units were intercepted once the test was introduced, the test's contribution to risk reduction seems to have been rather modest. Nevertheless, incorporation of minipool NAT into routine blood donor screening, is estimated to have lowered the risk to approximately 0.5 to 1 per million units. Multiplying the per-unit risk estimates by apppproximately 25 million components transfused to 5 million recipients per year in the United States leads to the expectation that fewer than 10 recipients per year are transfused with HIV-1–infected blood. Furthermore, only a fraction of these infected recipients would be expected to experience AIDS-related diseases prior to dying from other causes; this estimate is thus consistent with findings of the previously cited CDC report by Selik and colleagues.[21] The risk of HIV-2

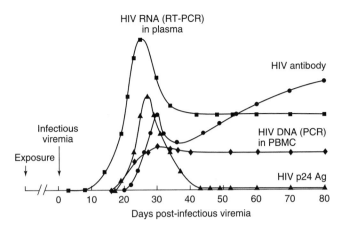

Figure 39.6 Approximate sequence and time course of virological and serological events during primary human immunodeficiency virus (HIV) infection. Following exposure, there is a variable period (usually 1 to 2 weeks, but occasionally up to 6 months) of viral replication in mucosal and lymphoid tissue draining the inoculation site, followed by hematogenous dissemination consistent with an infectious blood donation (day 0 in figure). The subsequent rapid increase in plasma viremia is first detectable by reverse transcriptase polymerase chain reaction (RT-PCR) for HIV RNA in plasma (■) on approximately day 10 and by p24 antigen (Ag) assays (▲) on day 15, with RNA and p24 Ag levels peaking between days 20 and 30. Infected (DNA PCR-positive) peripheral blood mononuclear cells (PBMCs) (♦) are detected later than free virus at approximately day 15 and remain present at stable, low levels through complete seroconversion. HIV antibody (●) appears between days 20 and 30 post viremia, with an early immunoglobulin M spike followed by progressive development of immunoglobulin G over several months. Seroconversion is associated with clearance of viremia to set-points that correlate with long-term outcome of disease, as well as with probability of secondary transmission of virus. (From Busch MP, Satten GA: Time course of viremia and antibody seroconversion following human immunodeficiency virus exposure. Am J Med 1997; 102 [Suppl5B]:117. Reproduced with permission from Diaz RS, Busch MP: Human immunodeficiency viruses. In: Anderson KC, Ness PM (eds): Scientific Basis of transfusion Medicine: Implications for Clinical Practice, 2nd ed, Philadelphia, WB Saunders, 2000, p 504.

transmission has been estimated at less than 1 in 15 million,[73] with other rare subtypes (e.g., HIV-1 subtype O)[55] being of even lesser concern. These combined risks are more than 10,000-fold lower than the risk existing at the peak of the TA AIDS epidemic between 1982 and 1984.[18]

Investigators have frequently used calculations based on the incidence–window period model to project the risk of transmission of HIV and other viruses by transfusion in different geographic areas and at various periods of the epidemic.[95–97] Experience over time has confirmed the validity of the approach, and the risk projections derived from the model are generally accepted as meaningful and reliable estimates of the true risk. Decreasing projections of the magnitude of risk in the same population over time reflect removal of high-risk donors and improvements in blood donor screening.

■ Human T-Cell Lymphotropic Virus

Although eclipsed by concerns about HIV, HTLV is relevant to the safety of blood transfusion. Both HTLV-I and HTLV-II

are transmitted by blood transfusion, cause chronic retroviral infection of humans, and are associated with serious disease outcomes. Serologic testing for HTLV-I in U.S. blood donors has been in place since 1988. This policy has led to the unexpected discovery that at least half of blood donors testing positive for HTLV-I are in fact infected with HTLV-II, for which disease outcomes are less well described.[98–100]

Virology

Both HTLV-I and HTLV-II are human retroviruses of the oncornavirus class. As previously mentioned, the first report of HTLV-I discovery was published in 1980, and that of HTLV-II in 1982.[7, 9] With RNA genomes of approximately 8000 nucleotides in length, the genetic organization of HTLV-I and HTLV-II are similar to those of other retroviruses (Fig. 39.7).[101, 102] The HTLV genome contains *gag* regions coding for viral core proteins, *pol* regions coding for viral reversed transcriptase, protease and integrase *env* regions coding for the viral envelope proteins, and finally the *tax* or *px* region (analogous to the HIV *tat* gene), which is responsible for transcriptional regulation of HTLV-I and HTLV-II. HTLV-I and HTLV-II have approximately 60% nucleotide sequence homology. Many of their viral proteins cross-react serologically, although peptides eliciting specific immune responses and allowing differential serologic diagnosis of HTLV-I versus HTLV-II have been discovered.

HTLV-I predominantly infects CD4+ T lymphocytes, whereas HTLV-II has a broader tropism with preference for CD8+ lymphocytes, and to a lesser degree, CD4+ lymphocytes, B lymphocytes, and macrophages.[103, 104] Neither virus has high levels of cell-free viremia, perhaps accounting for a lower transmissibility than either hepatitis B virus or HIV. Also in contrast to HIV, there is relatively little active replication of HTLV-I and HTLV-II in infected humans. Instead, most expansion of the pool of infected lymphocytes appears to occur by lymphocytic division and the proliferation of clones of infected lymphocytes.[105] Corollaries of these observations are that descriptions of HTLV viral load refer to measurements of proviral DNA in the cellular compartment. There has been only one report of measurable HTLV RNA in cell-free plasma[106]; however, further research will be necessary to exclude the possibility of a significant viremia in cell-free plasma.

Epidemiology and Modes of Transmission

HTLV-I is endemic in sub-Saharan Africa; the Caribbean region and parts of South America including Colombia, Peru, and Brazil as a result of the slave trade; Southwestern Japan; and parts of Melanesia and Australia.[107] HTLV-I has also been reported from Iran, India, and Taiwan as well as in countries containing significant immigrant populations from the main endemic areas. Given the high HTLV-I prevalence in Southwestern Japan, the absence of HTLV-I infection in mainland China and in Korea as well as other parts of Southeastern Asia poses an epidemiologic puzzle. Molecular epidemiologic studies have indicated the presence of at least two viral subtypes in Africa, a cosmopolitan subtype found in Africa, Japan, the Caribbean, and other more recent foci of HTLV-I infection, and a distantly related Melanesian subtype.[108]

HTLV-II has also been found to be endemic in a number of Amerindian tribes throughout South, Central, and North

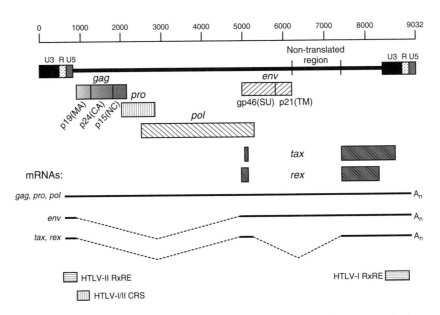

Figure 39.7 Structure and organization of the HTLV genome. The HTLV provirus genome is shown at the top of the figure. Positions of known genes are indicated. Sizes and positions of the proteins encoded by the provirus are shown beneath the provirus. The structure of the three messenger RNA species produced are shown at the bottom of the figure. (Reproduced with permission from Fields BN, Knipe DM, Howley PM (eds): Fields Virology, 3rd ed. Philadelphia, New York, Lippincott-Raven, 1996, p 1850.)

America.[109–111] Not all tribes are infected, and tribes with the least intermingling with Western settlers, such as the Kayapo of Brazil, appear to have the highest prevalence rate.[110] The other endemic focus of HTLV-II infection appears to be among Pygmies in sub-Saharan Africa, again in tribes having relatively little contact with European settlers.[112] HTLV-II infection is also prevalent among injection drug users and their sexual partners in the United States, Brazil, and Europe.[113] Given the relative recency of injection drug use behavior, there appears to have been an epidemic spread of HTLV-II over the past 40 or 50 years as a result of the introduction of endemic HTLV-II into the injection drug use population and subsequent spread through sharing of contaminated needles.[114]

In endemic populations, both HTLV-I and HTLV-II show age-specific seroprevalence rates that rise steadily with age from 1% or less among infected children to 5% to 10% of older individuals.[115, 116] Female seroprevalence is generally greater than male seroprevalence, presumably owing to more efficient sexual transmission from males to females than vice versa.

Among blood donors in the United States, HTLV-I seroprevalence is currently approximately 10 per 100,000 overall, rises steadily with age, and is twice as prevalent in females as in males (Fig. 39.8).[114] In contrast, HTLV-II is found among U.S. blood donors at a rate of 20 per 100,000 overall.[114] Although there is at least a two-fold female excess of infection, the age prevalence curve peaks in persons 30 to 49 years old and falls in older individuals. This apparent birth cohort effect is consistent with the hypothesis of an epidemic of HTLV-II transmitted by injection drug use and secondary sexual transmission beginning in the late 1960s and 1970s.[114]

HTLV-I and HTLV-II have similar modes of transmission. Mother-to-child transmission is important for both viruses, and between 20% and 30% of infants born to infected

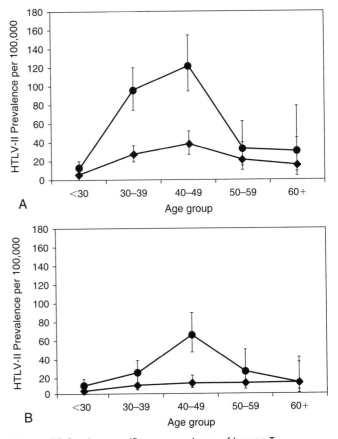

Figure 39.8 Age-specific seroprevalence of human T lymphotropic virus type II among female (A) and male (B) blood donors in 5 U.S. cities participating in multicenter Retrovirus Epidemiology Donor Study, stratified by 2 western (●) and 3 eastern or central (◆) blood centers. Seroprevalence is expressed per 100,000 donors.

mothers become infected themselves.[117] In contrast to HIV, however, the great majority of such transmission appears to occur by means of breast-feeding. Public health intervention studies in Japan have documented a decrease in the transmission rate from 30% to 3% when infected mothers substituted bottle-feeding for breast-feeding.[117]

Sexual transmission also occurs for both HTLV-I and HTLV-II, presumably by means of infected lymphocytes or other cells contained in seminal fluid.[118, 119] Transmission from males to females appears to be more efficient than vice versa. The most important factors determining whether transmission will occur between HTLV-serodiscordant couples (i.e., one seropositive and one seronegative for HTLV) are the total duration of the sexual relationship and the HTLV proviral load in the male.[119] The frequency or type of sexual activities performed appears to have little effect on the risk of transmission, although the predominant behavior in this study was heterosexual vaginal intercourse. The CDC recommends prevention of sexual transmission through the use of condoms by HTLV-serodiscordant couples as well as by HTLV-seropositive single individuals with multiple sexual partners.[120]

HTLV-I and HTLV-II are also transmitted efficiently by the sharing of contaminated needles or other parenteral exposures, leading to high seroprevalence among injection drug users.[113, 121] Data on transmission by blood transfusion are provided in more detail later. There is no data supporting the casual transmission of HTLV-I or HTLV-II within households or between individuals who do not have any of the preceding risk factors for transmission.

Disease Outcomes

Soon after its discovery, HTLV-I was associated with a CD4+ T-lymphocytic lymphoma known as adult T-cell leukemia/lymphoma (ATL).[122, 123] This lymphoma, which has a leukemic phase in one fourth to one third of infected individuals, is also associated with hypercalcemia, skin lesions, and hepatosplenomegaly.[124] Atypical malignant lymphocytes with convoluted nuclei, referred to as "flower cells," are seen in a high number of patients with leukemic-phase ATL and may also be seen in low numbers in asymptomatic persons who are seropositive for HTLV-I.[125, 126] The prognostic implications of having flower cells are not well defined, although individuals with either very high HTLV proviral loads or with relatively high numbers of circulating flower cells appear to be predisposed to a higher risk of ATL.[127] An individual infected with HTLV-I at birth has an estimated 4% lifetime risk of ATL, and the risk is presumably lower for those infected sexually as adults.[128] There are two case reports of ATL occurring after apparent transfusion-related HTLV-I infection.[129] Chemotherapy is often less effective for ATL than for other lymphomas and leukemia, and a high mortality is associated with this hematologic malignancy.[130, 131]

Although both HTLV-I and HTLV-II are known to cause spontaneous lymphocytic proliferation in vitro,[1, 2] HTLV-II does not appear to cause hematologic malignancy. Even though HTLV-II was initially isolated from two cases of atypical T-lymphocytic hairy cell leukemia, subsequent epidemiologic studies of hairy cell leukemia have not revealed an association with HTLV-II infection.[132–135] Similarly, initial case reports of mycosis fungoides and large granular cell

leukemia among HTLV-II–infected persons have not led to confirmed associations after further investigation.[136–138]

The other major disease association of both HTLV-I and HTLV-II is HAM/TSP. Initially described by Gessain and colleagues[139] in Martinique, the association with HAM/TSP was soon confirmed by Japanese and other investigators.[140–143] HAM/TSP is a slowly progressive myelopathy characterized by spastic paraparesis of the lower extremity, hyper-reflexia, bowel and bladder symptomatology, and relative sparing of both upper extremity strength and cognitive function.[144] The disease course is slow but progressive, with 10 years often elapsing between the first signs and severe paraplegia necessitating the use of a wheelchair. Despite the significant disability associated with this disease, it does not appear to be associated with greater mortality. There is no definitive treatment for HAM/TSP, although the use of systemic steroids, immunosuppression with azathioprine, and the use of the androgenic agent danazol have had transient success.[144]

A cohort study has estimated the risk of HAM/TSP to be about 2% in HTLV-I–positive persons.[145] Sexual acquisition of HTLV-I may be a risk factor for HAM/TSP[146]; however, the incubation period may be shortest after transfusion-acquired infection.[147–149] HTLV-II–positive individuals have been less well studied, but the risk appears to be slightly less than or equal to that with HTLV-I.[145] In contrast to some initial reports, there is no association of either HTLV-I or HTLV-II and classic multiple sclerosis.[150–152] Likewise, the implication of HTLV-I and HTLV-II in other neurologic syndromes is controversial, because individuals infected with HTLV-II may have genetic or environmental factors that also cause neurologic disease.[153]

Other immunologic diseases and phenomena have been reported in relation to HTLV-I and HTLV-II. HTLV-I has been associated with lymphocytic pneumonitis and uveitis.[154, 155] HTLV-I–positive cases of polymyositis have also been reported, and both HTLV-I and HTLV-II may be associated with a higher incidence of arthritis.[156, 157] Of particular interest, a cohort study has shown that HTLV-I, and particularly HTLV-II, may be associated with a higher incidence of other infections, including pneumonia, acute bronchitis, and urinary tract infection.[158] This finding is consistent with the association of HTLV-I and infective dermatitis in children.[159] Although the mechanism of immunologic dysfunction has not yet been described, these results do indicate a mild level of immunosuppression. It is not clear whether either HTLV-I or HTLV-II contributes to an increased incidence of other types of malignancy; a study in Japan has reported an increased risk of "viral-associated" malignancy such as hepatoma.[160] However, a study in the United States shows no increase of any nonhematologic malignancy with HTLV-I or HTLV-II.[158]

Transfusion-Related Transmission

Soon after its discovery, HTLV-I was shown to be transmitted by blood transfusion with transmission efficiency in Japan of at least 50%.[161, 162] A cohort study in Jamaica in the late 1980s demonstrated a 25% to 30% risk of HTLV-I infection after transfusion of one unit of HTLV-I–infected blood, with a 50-day mean latency period between the implicated transfusion and the development of de novo anti-HTLV antibodies.[163] Results of the TSS in the United States, with data from the mid-1980s, showed a much lower rate of transmission, only 10% to 20% for HTLV-I and HTLV-II.[164] Differences between these transmission rates may be due to the requirement that HTLV-infected, viable lymphocytes must be present in the transfused unit for it to be classified as infected. A significant inverse correlation between the duration of refrigerated storage (presumably related to lymphocyte viability) and the risk of HTLV transmission was demonstrated in the Transfusion Safety Study (TSS). Although such data were not reported, it is conceivable that blood unit storage times were shorter in the Japanese and Jamaican studies than in the U.S. study, and therefore viable infected lymphocytes were frequently transfused.

A later study of recipients of large-volume transfusions in the United States showed estimated risks of HTLV transmission to be 12 per 100,000 units before and 1.4 per 100,000 units after the 1988 institution of universal screening for HTLV antibodies.[91] The screening was introduced in that year after consideration of early data on HTLV-I prevalence in blood donors, its transfusion transmissibility, and diseases associated with the infection.[165] Studies estimating the current risk of HTLV-I by blood transfusion, similar to those of other low-frequency agents, are hindered by the large sample sizes required to measure low-frequency events. Nonetheless, the Retrovirus Epidemiology Study (REDS) has measured the incidence of HTLV-I and HTLV-II infection among serial blood donors and has used these data, along with estimates of the window period between infection and the development of antibodies, to model the residual risk of HTLV-I infection.[94] This study has estimated a residual risk of 1.6 per million units for HTLV-I, which is comparable to the risk of HIV infection and ten-fold lower than that for hepatitis B or C infection in the early 1990s.

The risk of transmission of HTLV-I by cell-free plasma is controversial. The Jamaican study showed no episodes of transfusion transmission in individuals receiving only plasma transfusions,[166] and laboratory studies have shown that cell-free transmission of HTLV-I is difficult. A report on the detection by RT-PCR of HTLV-I viral RNA in cell-free plasma is of concern, if its findings are replicated.[106] Nonetheless, transfusion of blood products containing residual leukocytes appears to carry a higher risk of HTLV transmission than transfusion of products free of leukocytes.[91]

Also of note in regard to transfusion safety is the definite association between HTLV-II infection and previous injection drug use or sexual relations with an injection drug user. Because injection drug users are more effectively screened out of the blood donor population, the typical HTLV-II–infected individual is a middle-aged woman who reports remote sexual exposure to an injection drug user. These data highlight the need to continue refining behavioral screening criteria, including consideration of banning donors who admit any prior sexual contact with injection drug users.[167]

Laboratory Diagnosis

Screening for HTLV-I and HTLV-II, analogous to HIV screening, is generally performed with EIAs. The earliest assays included only HTLV-I native viral proteins. It soon became apparent, however, that these assays were deficient in the native HTLV envelope proteins because of the viral purification process used to produce the proteins. This problem led to the subsequent addition of recombinant envelope proteins to the EIA antigen mix to improve the test's sensitivity. Because HTLV-I and HTLV-II have 60% nucleotide sequence

homology, there is significant cross-reaction of HTLV-II with HTLV-I EIAs.[102] However, because 10% to 15% of HTLV-II infections were missed by earlier HTLV-I EIAs,[168] subsequent EIAs utilized a recombinant transmembrane envelope glycoprotein, rgp21, that had greater sensitivity for both HTLV-II and HTLV-I, and later generations of EIA assays use recombinant proteins from both HTLV-II and HTLV-I. Thus, the FDA has permitted the labeling of single assays for the combined detection of HTLV-I and HTLV-II.

Supplemental testing for HTLV-I and HTLV-II has continued to be more problematic. The earliest and most common supplemental test used for supplemental testing is the Western blot. Because of a deficiency in viral envelope protein, however, Western blots using only HTLV-I native viral proteins are relatively nonspecific and may also be insensitive to HTLV-II. Western blots supplemented with rgp21, which have greater sensitivity to HTLV-II because of its cross-reactivity with rgp21, soon became available. However, it soon became apparent that false-positive reactivity to rgp21 in combination with nonspecific reactivity with the *gag* p19 or p24 bands could occasionally lead to false-positive Western blot interpretations.[169] Radioimmunoprecipitation (RIPA) has been used in research laboratories over the years to more specifically confirm the presence of antibodies to envelope proteins of HTLV-I and HTLV-II. However, this assay is very labor-intensive and so is not suitable for use as a routine supplemental test in blood banks.

Second-generation Western blots have been developed that contain native HTLV-I proteins supplemented with a refined version of rgp21, to decrease nonspecific reactions, in addition to recombinant peptides specific to both HTLV-I (rgp46-I) and HTLV-II (rgp46-II).[170, 171] In the research setting, these assays have proved to be both sensitive and specific for the diagnosis of HTLV-I and HTLV-II. In addition, because of the presence of the type-specific epitopes, they allow the differentiation of HTLV-I from HTLV-II infection in the great majority of cases.[170, 171] HTLV type-specific peptides are also available in the EIA format; however, these tests should be used for typing specimens that have already been confirmed by other supplemental assays.[172–174] This issue is important, because counseling of the infected donor should be specific to the disease outcomes to be expected with either HTLV-I or HTLV-II, and risk factor profiles have been shown to be specific to either HTLV-I or HTLV-II.[121]

Few of the HTLV supplemental tests described have been licensed by the FDA, however, so they have been used only under provisions for research. Thus, the counseling of infected donors based on the results of such tests has carried potential regulatory risks. In addition, because of the complexity of some of these supplemental assays, proficiency of the laboratories performing them depended on the local expertise and the volume of supplemental testing performed. This situation has led the FDA to ban the use of nonlicensed supplemental assays in the diagnosis of blood donors who test positive on the HTLV EIA. Although the regulatory reasons for this decision are understandable, it has significantly reduced the specificity of the diagnosis of HTLV-infected blood donors, because only 10% to 25% of EIA-positive blood donors are in fact seropositive for HTLV-I or HTLV-II, and donors with indeterminate EIA results are unlikely to be infected with HTLV in the absence of definite risk factors.[175] The lack of accurate licensed supplemental tests means that a large number of HTLV EIA–positive donors are falsely being informed that they are potentially seropositive for HTLV. Thus, there is an urgent need for the development of licensed supplemental assays that would differentiate HTLV-I and HTLV-II infections.

■ Approaches for Further Reducing the Risk of Retroviral Transmission by Transfusions

A 1997 U.S. government report concluded that the safety of the nation's blood supply is greater now than at any earlier time in history,[1] and similar positive assessments of blood safety have been reported from other industrialized countries.[95–97] Yet, despite the exceedingly small likelihood of becoming infected with HIV or HTLV from a screened blood transfusion, there continues to be strong political and regulatory pressure to further reduce the risk in any way possible, seemingly at all costs. Principal avenues that are actively being pursued in the effort to eliminate transfusion-transmitted retroviral infections are (1) the selection of the safest possible donor populations, (2) continuing improvements in blood donor testing, and (3) introduction of safe, effective, and affordable viral inactivation methods into transfusion practice.

Because of the disproportionate impact of the HIV epidemic on poor urban racial minorities and the known higher prevalence of HIV among minority donors, some have argued for what has been termed "demographic recruitment." However, this concept fails to recognize the critical need for a genetically diverse donor base to support the transfusion needs of a similarly diverse recipient population. Others have proposed expanding or modifying the risk factor interview process, for example, by adding questions on recent heterosexual activity (see later), using cartoon depictions of risk behaviors to improve understanding by less educated donors, and implementing computer-based interview strategies to enhance confidentiality.[176] Convincing data to support these proposals have not been generated, however.[177] Risk factor profiles of seropositive donors have changed over time. For example, Petersen and associates[178] compared HIV risk factors among 508 seropositive donors identified at 20 blood centers between May 1988 and August 1989 with those of 472 seropositive donors identified from January 1990 through May 1991. The overall rate of seropositive donations declined slightly over time (from 0.021% to 0.018%), primarily as a result of a decrease in infected donations by homosexual and bisexual men. In contrast, the rate of infected donations by persons probably exposed through heterosexual contact remained stable. Toward the end of the observation period, 56% of infected female donors and 12% of infected male donors had seropositive heterosexual partners; another 41% of infected female donors and 29% of infected heterosexual male donors were probably infected by heterosexual contact (on the basis of serologic studies for sexually transmitted disease markers), even though specific infected sex partners could not be identified. These researchers rejected the option of deferring donors on the basis of recent or lifetime number of heterosexual partners, because numeric cutoffs that would identify only half of the seropositive heterosexual donors would also result in a loss of 7% to 13% of all donations. This study illustrates the significant tradeoffs required to maintain an adequate as well as safe blood supply.

Incentives for blood donors pose a similar dilemma. Paid blood donors have long been identified as having a higher risk for transmissible viral diseases, and a volunteer-only blood donor system is considered a cornerstone in ensuring blood safety.[179] Nonmonetary incentives are widely used to attract volunteer donors, however, and surveys have shown that some of these incentives may also entice high-risk donors to give blood.[180]

Strategies to improve blood donor testing focus on introduction of new tests as well as on enhancing the performance of existing assays. NAT, which has been introduced for HIV and hepatitis C virus, is the most significant advancement in blood donor screening. This technology has already demonstrated in practice that it is capable of intercepting virus-containing blood units that are being missed by serologic assays.[181, 182] The current approach, the testing of pooled blood donor samples, although practical, is not optimal, both because sample dilution reduces assay sensitivity and because of the complexities involved in pooling algorithms and identification of the source of a positive test result in a pool. It is therefore expected that upgrading to single-donation testing with NAT will be phased in as soon as technically and financially feasible.

The rush to fully incorporate NAT into blood donor screening is fueled by the hope of completely preventing transfusion-transmitted HIV infection. Studies have revealed that entry of HIV into a receptive host is followed by an approximately week-long tissue-only phase of viral distribution, the so-called eclipse phase, during which blood and body fluids are not infective. Furthermore, transmission experiments involving chimpanzees showed that blood samples from very recently infected animals that tested negative for HIV RNA on existing NAT assays did not transmit the virus to other animals.[183] NAT may therefore be able to eliminate HIV contamination of the blood supply. The financial costs of its implementation are not trivial, however, and some delays in blood component availability are inevitable. This is a particular concern for platelets, which have a shelf life of only 5 days. In addition, false-positive results, which can be expected with any new screening test, raise concerns about unnecessary deferral of healthy blood donors at a time when blood shortages are becoming more frequent and more severe.

Upgrades of existing HIV assays are continuously being made to ensure optimal sensitivity for the variant viral strains that gain prominence as the epidemic continues globally. Ongoing surveys of HIV viral subtypes in the United States are still detecting subtype B strains almost exclusively; these strains have predominated since the beginning of the epidemic 20 years ago.[52] Worldwide, however, other HIV subtypes are being detected with growing frequency, and overall viral diversity is increasing, necessitating continuous performance monitoring and re-engineering of assay formats as necessary to guarantee reliable detection of variant HIV strains.[51]

An added layer of safety is provided by viral inactivation technology, which has been used for more than a decade in the manufacturing of plasma derivatives and almost as long for treatment of pooled plasma in many European countries.[184] Various methods are being used, with solvent-detergent treatment being the most common principle employed.[184] Effectiveness of the solvent-detergent method is very high for lipid-enveloped viruses, including HIV and HTLV, but the procedure does not reliably inactivate nonenveloped viruses.[185] This problem has raised concern that fresh frozen plasma treated with the solvent-detergent method, which is prepared in the United States from plasma (FFP) donated by a 2500-member pool of donors, could spread such viruses more widely than untreated single-donation FFP.[184]

Newer chemical, photodynamic and photochemical methods, capable to inactivate a wide range of pathogens, including known transfusion-transmissible viruses, bacteria, and parasites, work with single-donation platelets and FFP, thereby avoiding the risks associated with pooling of blood components.[186] One photochemical inactivation system was licensed in Europe in early 2002, and licensing in the U.S. is expected in the near future. Systems of pathogen inactivation of red cell products are at an earlier stage of development and clinical study and are therefore further away from possible implementation.[186] An impediment to the introduction of any new viral inactivation method for blood components is the concern for new threats to transfusion recipients, which may offset the benefits of such a method in comparison with existing strategies.

It is safe to predict that the combined impact of safeguards already implemented and those currently under development will reduce the risk of retrovirus transmission in the highly developed industrialized nations to near zero levels. Unfortunately, this optimistic view does not apply to many developing nations, particularly those in sub-Saharan Africa and parts of Asia. In some of the worst affected areas, up to 50% of the population is infected with HIV, and a significant proportion of HIV infections are due to blood transfusion. Even if blood donor screening is performed in such areas, the risk of HIV transmission due to window period donations and test errors may be as high as 2%, or more than 10,000-fold higher than in the U.S.[187] The countries in these areas often lack the resources and supporting infrastructure to implement or maintain donor selection strategies that were developed in industrialized nations.[187, 188] From a global perspective, prevention of retroviral infection by transfusion will remain a difficult challenge in the foreseeable future, requiring continued vigilance and the support of broad blood safety programs in order to be successful .

REFERENCES

1. U.S. General Accounting Office: Blood Supply: Transfusion-Associated Risks. Washington, DC, United States General Accounting Office. GAO/PEMD-97-2. 1997.
2. AuBuchon JP, Birkmeyer JD, Busch MP: Safety of the blood supply in the United States: Opportunities and controversies. Ann Intern Med 1997;127:904.
3. Zanotto PM, Gibbs MJ, Gould EA, Holmes EC: A reevaluation of the higher taxonomy of viruses based on RNA polymerases. J Virol 1996;70:6083.
4. Levy JA (ed): The Retroviridae. New York, Plenum, 1994.
5. Kahn JO, Walker BD: Acute human immunodeficiency virus type 1 infection. N Engl J Med 1998;339:33.
6. Bishop JM: The molecular genetics of cancer. Science 1987;235:305.
7. Poiesz BJ, Ruscetti FW, Cazdar AF, et al: Detection and isolation of type C retrovirus particles from fresh and cultured lymphocytes of a patient with cutaneous T-cell lymphoma. Proc Natl Acad Sci U S A 1980;77:7415.
8. Blattner WA (ed): Human Retrovirology: HTLV. New York, Raven Press, 1990.
9. Kalyanaraman VS, Sarogatiharan MG, Robert-Groff M, et al: A new subtype of human T-cell leukemia virus (HTLV-II) associated with a T-cell variant of hairy cell leukemia. Science 1982;218:571.
10. Rosenblatt JD, Chen IS, Golde DW: HTLV-II and human lymphoproliferative disorders. Clin Lab Med 1988;8:85.
11. Gao F, Bailes E, Robertson DL, et al: Origin of HIV-1 in the chimpanzee *Pan troglodytes troglodytes*. Nature 1999;397:436.
12. Zhu T, Korber BT, Nahmias AJ, et al: An African HIV-1 sequence from 1959 and implications for the origin of the epidemic. Nature 1998;391:594.
13. Joint United Nations Program on HIV/AIDS: AIDS epidemic update: December 1999. Geneva, World Health Organization, 1999.
14. Kilbourne ED: New viral diseases: A real and potential problem without boundaries. JAMA 1990;264:68.
15. Centers for Disease Control: Update on acquired immune deficiency syndrome (AIDS) among patients with hemophilia A. MMWR Morb Mortal Wkly Rep 1982;31:844.
16. Centers for Disease Control: Possible transfusion-associated acquired immune deficiency syndrome (AIDS)—California. MMWR Morb Mortal Wkly Rep 1982;31:652.
17. American Association of Blood Banks (AABB), Council of Community Blood Centers (CCBC), American Red Cross (ARC): Joint statement on acquired immune deficiency syndrome (AIDS) related to transfusion. Transfusion 1983;23:87.
18. Busch MP, Young MJ, Samson SM, et al, and the Transfusion Safety Study Group: Risk of human immunodeficiency virus transmission by blood transfusions prior to the implementation of HIV antibody screening in the San Francisco Bay Area. Transfusion 1991;31:4.
19. Perkins HA, Samson S, Busch MP: How well has self-exclusion worked? Transfusion 1988;28:601.
20. Kroner BL, Rosenberg PS, Aledort LM, et al, for the Multicenter Hemophilia Cohort Study: HIV-1 infection incidence among persons with hemophilia in die United States and western Europe, 1978–1990. J Acquir Immune Defic Syndr Hum Retrovirol 1994;7:279.
21. Selik RM, Ward JW, Buehler JW: Trends in transfusion-associated acquired immune deficiency syndrome in the United States, 1982 through 1991. Transfusion 1993;33:890.
22. Kleinman SH, Niland JC, Azen SP, et al, and the Transfusion Safety Study Group: Prevalence of antibodies to human immunodeficiency virus type 1 among blood donors prior to screening: The Transfusion Safety Study/NHLBI donor repository. Transfusion 1989;29:572.
23. Donegan E, Stuart M, Niland JC, et al, and the Transfusion Safety Study Group: Infection with human immunodeficiency virus type I (HIV-1) among recipients of antibody-positive blood donations. Ann Intern Med 1990;113:733.
24. Busch M, Donegan E, Stuart M, Mosley JW: Donor HIV-1 p24 antigenaemia and course of infection in recipients. Transfusion Safety Study Group. Lancet 1990;8701:1342.
25. Donegan E, Lenes BA, Tomasulo RA, Mosley JW, and the Transfusion Safety Study Group: Transmission of HIV-l by components type and duration of shelf storage before transfusion. Transfusion 1990;30:851.
26. Rawal BD, Busch MP, Endow R, et al: Reduction of human immunodeficiency virus-infected cells from donor blood by leukocyte filtration. Transfusion 1989;26:460.
27. Kim HC, Nahum K, Raska K Jr, et al: Natural history of acquired immunodeficiency syndrome in hemophilic patients. Am J Hematol 1987;24:168.
28. Jackson JB, Sannerud KJ, Hopsicker JS, et al: Hemophiliacs with HIV antibody are actively infected. JAMA 1988;260:2236.
29. Jackson JB, Kwok SY, Sninsky JJ, et al: Human immunodeficiency virus type I detected in all seropositive symptomatic and asymptomatic individuals. J Clin Microbiol 1990;28:16.
30. Hewlett IK, Laurian Y, Epstein J, et al: Assessment by gene amplification and serological markers of transmission of HIV-1 from hemophiliacs to their sexual partners and secondarily to their children. J Acquir Immun Defic Syndr 3:714,1990.
31. Jason J, Ou C-Y, Moore JL, et al and the Hemophilia-AIDS Collaborative Study Group: Prevalence of human immunodeficiency virus type 1 DNA in hemophilic men and their sex partners. J Infect Dis 1989;160:789.
32. Gibbons J, Cory JM, Hewlett IK, et al: Silent infections with human immunodeficiency virus type 1 are highly unlikely in multitransfused seronegative hemophiliacs. Blood 76:1924, 1990.
33. Sheppard HW, Busch MP, Louie PH, et al: HIV-1 PCR and isolation in seroconverting and seronegative homosexual men: Absence of long-term immunosilent infection. J Acquir Immun Defic Syndr 6:1339, 1995.
34. Ward JW, Bush TJ, Perkins HA, et al: The natural history of transfusion-associated infection with human immunodeficiency virus. N Engl J Med 321:947, 1989.

35. Ashton LJ, Learmont J, Luo K, et al: HIV infection in recipients of blood products from donors with known duration of infection. Lancet 1994;344:718.

36. Operskalski EA, Stram DO, Lee H, et al: Human immunodeficiency virus type 1 infection: Relationship of risk group and age to rate of progression to AIDS. Transfusion Safety Study Group. J Infect Dis 1995;172:648.

37. Busch MP, Operskalski EA, Mosley JW, et al, and the Transfusion Safety Study Group: Epidemiologic background and long-term course of disease in human immunodeficiency virus type 1-infected blood donors identified before routine laboratory screening. Transfusion 1994;34:858.

38. Bluxhelt A, Granath F, Lidman K, Giesecke J: The influence of age on the latency period to AIDS in people infected by HIV through blood transfusion. AIDS 1990;4:125.

39. Busch MP, Operskalski EA, Mosley JW, et al: Factors influencing human immunodeficiency virus type 1 transmission by blood transfusion. Transfusion Safety Study Group. J Infect Dis 1996;174:26.

40. Operskalski EA, Stram DO, Busch MP, et al: Role of viral load in heterosexual transmission of human immunodeficiency virus type 1 by blood transfusion recipients. Transfusion Safety Study Group. Am J Epidemiol 1997;146:655.

41. Operskalski EA, Busch MP, Mosley JW, Stram DO: Comparative rates of disease progression among persons infected with the same or different HIV-1 strains. The Transfusion Safety Study Group. J Acquir Immune Defic Syndr Hum Retrovirol 1997;15:145.

42. Wilkinson DA, Operskalski EA, Busch MP, et al: A 32-bp deletion within the CCR5 locus protects against transmission of parenterally acquired human immunodeficiency virus but does not affect progression to AIDS-defining illness. J Infect Dis 1998;178:1163.

43. Learmont JC, Geczy AF, Mills J, et al: Immunologic and virologic status after 14 to 18 years of infection with an attenuated strain of HIV-1: A report from the Sydney Blood Bank Cohort. N Engl J Med 1999;340:1715.

44. Collier AC, Kalish LA, Busch MP et al., for the Viral Activation Transfusion Study Group: Leukocyte-reduced red blood cell transfusions in patients with anemia and human immunodeficiency virus infection. The Viral Activation Transfusion Study: A randomized controlled trial. JAMA, 2001;285:1592.

45. Busch MP, Lee TH, Heitman J: Allogeneic leukocytes but not therapeutic blood elements induce reactivation and dissemination of latent human immunodeficiency virus type 1 infection: Implications for transfusion support of infected patients. Blood 1992;80:2128.

46. Roberts JD, Bebenek K, Kunkel, TA: The accuracy of reverse transcriptase from HIV-1. Science 1998;242:1171.

47. Vartanian J-P, Meyerhans A, Asjo B, et al: Selection, recombination, and G-A hypermutation of HIV-1 genomes. J Virol 1991;65:1779.

48. Zhu T, Mo H, Wang N, et al: Genotypic and phenotypic characterization of HIV-1 in patients with primary infection. Science 1993;261:1179.

49. Zhu T, Wang N, Carr A, et al: Evidence for coinfection by multiple strains of human immunodeficiency virus type 1 subtype B in an acute seroconverter. J Virol 1995;69:1324.

50. Diaz R, Sabino EC, Mayer A, et al: Dual human immunodeficiency virus type 1 infection and recombination in a dually-exposed transfusion recipient. J Virol 1995;69:3273.

51. Hu DJ, Dondero TJ, Rayfield MA, et al: The emerging genetic diversity of HIV: The importance of global surveillance for diagnostics, research, and prevention. JAMA 1996;275:210.

52. de Oliveira CF, Diaz RS, Machado DM, et al: Surveillance of HIV-1 genetic subtypes and diversity in the US blood supply. Transfusion 2000;40:1399.

53. Nkengasong JN, Janssens W, Heyndrickx L, et al: Genotypic subtypes of HIV-1 in Cameroon. AIDS 1994;8:1405.

54. Peeters M, Gueye A, Mboup S, et al: Geographical distribution of HIV-1 group O viruses in Africa. AIDS 1997;11:493.

55. Loussert-Ajaka I, Ly TD, Chaix ML, et al: HIV-1/HIV-2 seronegativity in HIV-1 subtype 0 infected patients. Lancet 1994;343:1393.

56. Schable C, Zekeng L, Pau CP, et al: Sensitivity of United States HIV antibody tests for detection of HIV-1 group O infections. Lancet 1994;344:1333.

57. U.S. Food and Drug Administration: Interim Recommendations For Deferral of Donors at Increased Risk for HIV-1 Group O Infection. Rockville, MD, 1996.

58. Pau CP, Hu HDJ, Spruill C, et al: Surveillance for human immunodeficiency virus type 1 group O infections in the United States. Transfusion 1996;36:398.

59. Clavel F, Guetard D, Brun-Vezinet F, et al: Isolation of a new human retrovirus from West African patients with AIDS. Science 1986;233:343.

60. O'Brien TR, George JR, Holmberg SD: Human immunodeficiency virus type 2 infection in the United States: Epidemiology, diagnosis, and public health implications. JAMA 1992;267:2775.

61. Marlink R, Kanki P, Thior I, et al: Reduced rate of disease development after HIV-2 infections as compared to HIV-1. Science 1994;265:1587.

62. Poulsen AG, Aaby P, Larsen O, et al: 9-year HIV-2-associated mortality in an urban community in Bissau, West Africa. Lancet 1997;349:911.

63. George JR, Rayfield MA, Phillips S, et al: Efficacies of U.S. Food and Drug Administration licensed HIV-1-screening enzyme immunoassays for detecting antibodies to HIV-2. AIDS 1990;4:321.

64. de Cock KM, Porter A, Kouadio J, et al: Cross-reactivity on Western blots in HIV-1 and HIV-2 infection. AIDS 1991;5:859.

65. Busch MP, Petersen L, Schable C, Perkins HA: Monitoring blood donors for HIV-2 infection by testing anti-HIV-1 reactive sera. Transfusion 1990;30:184.

66. Centers for Disease Control: Surveillance for HIV-2 infection in blood donors—United States, 1987–1989. MMWR Morb Mortal Wkly Rep 1990;39:829.

67. O'Brien T, Polon C, Schable C: HIV-2 infection in an American. AIDS 1991;5:85.

68. CDC Update: Facts About Human Immunodeficiency Virus Type 2. Atlanta, Centers for Disease Control and Prevention, 1998.

69. Parry JV, McAlpine L, Avillez MF: Sensitivity of six commercial enzyme immunoassay kits that detect both anti-HIV-l and anti-HIV-2. AIDS 1990;4:355.

70. Gallarda JL, Henrard DR, Liu D, et al: Early detection of antibody to HIV-1 using an antigen conjugate immunoassay correlates with the presence of IgM antibody. J Clin Microbiol 1992;30:2379.

71. Zaaijer HL, v Exel-Oehlers P, Kraaijeveld T, et al: Early detection of antibodies to HIV-1 by third-generation assays. Lancet 1992;340:770.

72. U.S. Food and Drug Administration, Center for Biologics Evaluation and Research: Revised Recommendations for the Prevention of Human Immunodeficiency Virus (HIV) Transmission by Blood and Blood Products. Rockville, MD, 1992.

73. Sullivan MT, Guido EA, Metler RP, et al: Identification and characterization of an HIV-2 antibody-positive blood donor in the United States. Transfusion 1998;38:189.

74. U.S. Food and Drug Administration: Current Good Manufacturing Practices for Blood and Blood Components: Notification of Consignees Receiving Blood and Blood Components at Increased Risk for Transmitting HIV Infection. Fed Regist 1996;61:47413.

75. Busch MP, Lee LLL, Satten GA, et al: Time course of detection of viral and serological markers preceding HTV- I seroconversion: Implications for blood and tissue donor screening. Transfusion 1995;35:91.

76. Busch MP: Retroviruses and blood transfusions: The lessons learned and the challenge yet ahead. In Nance S (ed): Blood Safety: Current Challenges [transcription of the Emily Cooley Award/AABB 1992 Annual Seminar]. Bethesda, MD, American Association of Blood Banks, 1992, p 1.

77. Dorn J, Masciotra S, Yang C, et al: Analysis of genetic variability within the immunodominant epitopes of envelope gp41 from human immunodeficiency virus type 1 (HIV-1) group M and its impact on HIV-1 antibody detection. J Clin Microbiol 2000;38:773.

78. U.S. Food and Drug Administration: Memorandum: Recommendation for Donor Screening With A Licensed Test for HIV-1 Antigen. Rockville, MD, Congressional and Consumer Affairs, 1995.

79. Kleinman S, Busch MP, Korelitz JJ, Schreiber GB: The incidence/window period model and its use to assess the risk of transfusion-transmitted human immunodeficiency virus and hepatitis C virus infection. Transfus Med Rev 1997;11:155.

80. Busch MP, Stramer SL: The efficiency of HIV p24 antigen screening of US blood donors: Projections versus reality. Presented at Satellite symposium "Sensitivity and Validity of HIV Screening Methods," Joint Congress of the International Society of Blood Transfusion, and the German Society for Transfusion Medicine and Immunohematology, Frankfurt, Oct 1997. Infusionther Transfusionmed 1998;25:5.

81. Implementation of donor screening for infectious agents transmitted by blood by nucleic acid technology. Vox Sang 2002;82:87.

82. Ling AE, Robbins KE, Brown TM, et al: Failure of routine HIV-1 tests in a case involving transmission with preseroconversion blood components during the infectious window period. JAMA 2000;284:210.

83. Delwart E, Kalmin N, Jones T, et al: First case of HIV transmission by an RNA screened blood donation. Submitted to AIDS 2002.

84. Kleinman S, Busch MP, Hall L, et al, for the Retrovirus Epidemiology Donor Study: False-positive HIV-1 test results in a low-risk screening setting of voluntary blood donation. JAMA 1998;280:1080.

85. Busch MP, Kleinman SH, Williams AE, et al., and the Retrovirus Epidemiology Donor Study (REDS): Frequency of human immunodeficiency virus (HIV) infection among contemporary anti-HIV-1 and anti-HIV-1/anti-HIV-2 supplemental test-indeterminate blood donors. Transfusion 1996;36:37.

86. Jackson JB: Human immunodeficiency virus (HIV)-indeterminate Western blots and latent HIV infection. Transfusion 1992;32:497.

87. Schochetman G, George JR (eds): AIDS Testing: Methodology and Management Issues, 2nd ed. New York, Springer Verlag, 1994.

88. Busch MP: Let's look at human immunodeficiency virus lookback before leaping into hepatitis C virus lookback! Transfusion 1991;31:655.

89. Leitman SF, Klein HG, Melpolder JJ, et al: Clinical implications of positive tests for antibodies to human immunodeficiency virus type I in asymptomatic blood donors. N Engl J Med 1989;321:917.

90. Ward JW, Holmberg SD, Allen JR, et al: Transmission of human immunodeficiency virus (HIV) by blood transfusions screened as negative for HIV antibody. N Engl J Med 1988;318:473.

91. Nelson KE, Donahue JG, Munoz A, et al: Transmission of retroviruses from seronegative donors by transfusion during cardiac surgery: A multicenter study of HIV-1 and HTLV-I/II infections. Ann Intern Med 1992;117:554.

92. Busch MP, Eble BE, Khayam-Bashi H, et al: Evaluation of screened blood donations for human immunodeficiency virus type I infection by culture and DNA amplification of pooled cells. N Engl J Med 1991;325:1.

93. Lackritz EM, Satten GA, Aberle-Grasse J, et al: Estimated risk of transmission of the human immunodeficiency virus by screened blood in the United States. N Engl J Med 1995;333:1721.

94. Schreiber GB, Busch MP, Kleinman SH, Korelitz JJ: The risk of transfusion-transmitted viral infections. The Retrovirus Epidemiology Donor Study. N Engl J Med 1996;334:1685.

95. Schwartz DW, Simson G, Baumgarten K, et al: Risk of human immunodeficiency virus (HIV) transmission by anti-HIV-negative blood components in Germany and Austria. Ann Hematol 1995;70:209.

96. Whyte GS, Savoia HF: The risk of transmitting HCV, HBV or HIV by blood transfusion in Victoria. Med J Australia 1997;166:584.

97. Remis RS, Delage G, Palmer RW: Risk of HIV infection from blood transfusion in Montreal. Can Med Assn J 1997;157:375.

98. Lee HH, Swanson P, Rosenblatt JD, et al: Relative prevalence and risk factors of HTLV-I and HTLV-II infection in US blood donors. Lancet 1991;337:1435.

99. Taylor PE, Stevens CE, Pindyck J, et al: Human T-cell lymphotropic virus in volunteer blood donors. Transfusion 1990;30:783.

100. Eble BE, Busch MP, Guiltinan A, et al: Determination of human T-lymphotropic virus type by PCR and correlation with risk factors in northern California blood donors. J Infect Dis 1993;167:954.

101. Cann AJ, Chen ISY: Human T-cell leukemia virus types I and II. In Fields BN, Knipe DM (eds): Virology. New York, Raven Press, 1990.

102. Hall WW, Ishak R, Zhu SW, et al: Human T lymphotropic virus type II (HTLVII): Epidemiology, molecular properties, and clinical features of infection. J Acquir Immun Defic Syndr Hum Retrovirol 1996;13(Suppl 1):s20414.

103. Lal RB, Owen SM, Rudolph DL, et al: In vivo cellular tropism of human T lymphotropic virus type II is not restricted to CD8+ cells. Virology 1995;210:4417.

104. Casoli C, Cimarelli A, Bertazzoni U: Cellular tropism of human T cell leukemia virus type II is enlarged to B lymphocytes in patients with high proviral load. Virology 1995;206:11268.

105. Wattel E, Vartanian JP, Pannetier C, Wain-Hobson S: Clonal expansion of human T cell leukemia virus type I infected cells in asymptomatic and symptomatic carriers without malignancy. J Virol 1995;69:28638.

106. Rios M, Pombo de Oliveira MS, Correa RB, et al: HTLV-I viremia in infected individuals with and without disease [abstract ME 19]. Presented at the Eighth International Conference on Human Retrovirology: HTLV, Rio de Janeiro, June 9–13, 1997.

107. Manns A, Hisada M, La Grenade L: Human T lymphotropic virus type I infection. Lancet 1999;353(9168):19518.

108. Gessain A, Mahieux R, de The G: Genetic variability and molecular epidemiology of human and simian T cell leukemia/lymphoma virus

type I. J Acquir Immun Defic Syndr Hum Retrovirol 1996;13 (Suppl 1):S13245.

109. Black FL, Biggar RJ, Neel JV, et al: Endemic transmission of HTLV type II among Kayapo Indians of Brazil. AIDS Resand Hum Retroviruses 1994;10:116571.

110. Reeves WC, Cutler JR, Gracia F, et al: Human T cell lymphotropic virus infection in Guayami Indians from Panama. Am J Trop Med Hyg 1990;43:410.

111. Hjelle B, Mills R, Swenson S, et al: Incidence of hairy cell leukemia, mycosis fungoides, and chronic lymphocytic leukemia in first known HTLV-II-endemic population. J Infect Dis 1991;163:435.

112. Gessain A, Mauclere P, Froment A, et al: Isolation and molecular characterization of a human T-cell lymphotropic virus type II (HTLV-II), subtype B, from a healthy Pygmy living in a remote area of Cameroon: An ancient origin for HTLV-II in Africa. Proc Nat Acad Sci U S A 1995;92:4041.

113. Khabbaz RF, Onorato IM, Cannon RO, et al: Seroprevalence of HTLV-I and HTLV-II among intravenous drug users and persons in clinics for sexually transmitted diseases. N Engl J Med 1992;326:375.

114. Murphy EL, Watanabe K, Nass CC, et al: Evidence among blood donors for a 30-year old epidemic of HTLV-II infection in the United States. J Infect Dis 1999;180:1777.

115. Murphy EL, Figueroa JP, Gibbs WN, et al: Human T-lymphotropic virus type I (HTLV-I) seroprevalence in Jamaica. I: Demographic determinants. Am J Epidemiol 1991;133:1114.

116. Vitek CR, Gracia FI, Giusti R, et al: Evidence for sexual and mother to child transmission of human T lymphotropic virus type II among Guayami Indians, Panama. J Infect Dis 1995;171:10226.

117. Hino S, Katamine S, Miyata H, et al: Primary prevention of HTLV1 in Japan. Leukemia 1997;11(Suppl 3):579.

118. Murphy EL, Figueroa JP, Gibbs WN, et al: Sexual transmission of human T-lymphotropic virus type I. Ann Intern Med 1989;111:555.

119. Kaplan J, Khabbaz RF, Murphy EL, et al, and the Retrovirus Epidemiology Donor Study Group: Male to female transmission of human T lymphotropic virus types I and II: Association with viral load. J Acquir Immun Defic Syndr Hum Retrovirol 1996;12:193–201.

120. Centers for Disease Control and Prevention (CDC) and the U.S. PHS Working Group: Guidelines for counseling persons infected with human T-lymphotropic virus type I (HTLV-l) and type II (HTLV-II). Ann Intern Med 1993;118:448.

121. Feigal E, Murphy EL, Vranizan K, et al: HTLV-I/II in intravenous drug users in San Francisco: Risk factors associated with seropositivity. J Infect Dis 1991;164:36.

122. Hinuma YK, Nagata K, Hanoaka M, et al: Adult T-cell leukemia: Antigen in an ATL cell line and detection of antibodies to the antigen in human sera. Proc Natl Acad Sci U S A 1981;78:6476.

123. Hinuma YK, Komoda H, Chosa T, et al: Antibodies to adult T-cell leukemia-virus-associated antigens (ATIA) in sera from patients with ATL and controls in Japan: A nationwide seroepidemiologic study. Int J Cancer 1982;29:631.

124. Bunn PA, Schechter GP, Jaffe E, et al: Clinical course of retrovirus-associated adult T-cell lymphoma in the United States. N Engl J Med 1983;309:258.

125. Seiki M, Eddy R, Shows TB, Yoshida M: Non-specific integration of the HTLV provirus into adult T-cell leukemia cells. Nature 1984;309:640.

126. Kinoshita K, Amagasaki T, Ikeda S, et al: Preleukemic state of adult T cell leukemia: Abnormal T lymphocytosis induced by human adult T cell leukemia-lymphoma virus. Blood 1985;66:120.

127. Tachibana N, Okayama A, Ishihara S, et al: High HTLV-I proviral DNA level associated with abnormal lymphocytes in peripheral blood from asymptomatic carriers. Int J Cancer 1992;51:5935.

128. Murphy EL, Hanchard B, Figueroa JP, et al: Modeling the risk of adult T-cell leukemia/lymphoma in persons infected with human T-lymphotropic virus type I. Int J Cancer 1989;43:250.

129. Chen Y-C, Wang C-H, Su I-J, et al: Infection of human T-cell leukemia virus type I and development of human T-cell leukemia/lymphoma in patients with hematologic neoplasms: A possible linkage to blood transfusion. Blood 1989;74:383.

130. Prince H, Kleinman S, Doyle M, et al: Spontaneous lymphocyte proliferation in vitro characterizes both HTLV-I and HTLV-II infection. J Acquir Immun Defic Syndr Hum Retrovirol 3:1199, 1990.

131. Wiktor SZ, Jacobson S, Weiss SH, et al: Spontaneous lymphocyte proliferation in HTLV-II infection. Lancet 1991;337:327.

132. Rosenblatt JD, Giorgi JV, Golde DW, et al: Integrated human T-cell leukemia virus II genome in CD8+ T cells from a patient with

"atypical" hairy cell leukemia: Evidence for distinct T and B cell lymphoproliferative disorders. Blood 1988;71:363.

133. Rosenblatt JD, Gasson JC, Glaspy J, et al: Relationship between human T-cell leukemia virus-II and atypical hairy cell leukemia: A serologic study of hairy cell leukemia patients. Leukemia 1987;1:397.

134. Lion T, Razvi N, Golomb HM, Brownstein RH: B-lymphotropic hairy cells contain no HTLV-II DNA sequences. Blood 1988;72:1428.

135. Katayama I, Maruyama K, Fukushima T, et al: Cross-reacting antibodies to human T cell leukemia virus-I and -II in Japanese patients with hairy cell leukemia. Leukemia 1987;1:401.

136. Zucker-Franklin D, Coutaves EE, Rush MG, Zouzias DC: Detection of human T-lymphotropic virus-like particles in cultures of peripheral blood lymphocytes from patients with mycosis fungoides. Proc Natl Acad Sci U S A 1991;88:7630.

137. Busch MP, Murphy EL, Nemo G: More on HTLV tax and mycosis fungoides. N Engl J Med 1993;329:2035.

138. Loughran TP Jr, Coyle T, Sherman MP, et al: Detection of human T cell leukemia/lymphoma virus, type II, in a patient with large granular lymphocyte leukemia. Blood 1992;80:11169.

139. Gessain A, Vernant JC, Sonan T, et al: Antibodies to human T-lymphotropic virus type-I in patients with tropical spastic paraparesis. Lancet 1985;8452:407.

140. Osame M, Usuku K, Izumo S, et al: HTLV-I associated myelopathy, a new clinical entity. Lancet 1986;8488:1031.

141. Maloney EM, Cleghorn FR, Morgan OS, et al: Incidence of HTLV-I associated myelopathy/tropical spastic paraparesis (HAM/TSP) in Jamaica and Trinidad. J Acquir Immun Defic Syndr Hum Retrovirol 1998;17:16770.

142. Jacobson S, Raine CS, Mingioli ES, McFarlin DE: Isolation of an HTLV-l-like retrovirus from patients with tropical spastic paraparesis. Nature 1988;331:540.

143. Bhagavati S, Ehrlich G, Kula R, et al: Detection of human T-cell lymphoma/leukemia virus type 1 DNA and antigen in spinal fluid and blood of patients of chronic progressive myelopathy. N Engl J Med 1988;318:1141.

144. Gessain A, Gout O: Chronic myelopathy associated with human T-lymphotropic virus type I (HTLV-I). Ann Intern Med 1992;117:933.

145. Murphy EL, Fridey J, Smith JW, et al: HTLV associated myelopathy in a cohort of HTLV-I and HTLV-II infected blood donors. The REDS Investigators. Neurology 1997;48:315.

146. Kramer A, Maloney EM, Morgan OSC, et al: Risk factors and cofactors for HAM/TSP in Jamaica. Am J Epidemiol 1995;142:1212.

147. Gout O, Baulac M, Gessain A, et al: Rapid development of myelopathy after HTLV-I infection acquired by transfusion during cardiac transplantation N Engl J Med 1990;322:383.

148. Kurosawa M, Machii T, Kitani T, et al: HTLV-I associated myelopathy (HAM) after blood transfusion in a patient with CD2+ hairy cell leukemia. Am J Clin Pathol 1991;95:72.

149. Osame M, Janssen R, Kubota H, et al: Nationwide survey of HTLV-I-associated myelopathy in Japan: Association with blood transfusion. Ann Neurol 1990;28:50.

150. Reddy EP, Sandberg-Wollheim M, Mettus R, et al: Amplification and molecular cloning of HTLV-I sequences from DNA of multiple sclerosis patients. Science 1989;243:529.

151. Madden DL, Mundan FK, Tzan NR, et al: Serologic studies of MD patients, controls, and patients with other neurologic diseases: Antibodies to HTLV-I, II, III. Neurology 1988;38:81.

152. Richardson JH, Wucherpfennig KW, Endo N, et al: PCR analysis of DNA from multiple sclerosis patients for the presence of HTLV-I. Science 1989;246:821.

153. Hjelle B, Appenzeller O, Mills R, et al: Chronic neurodegenerative disease associated with HTLV-II infection. Lancet 1992;339:645.

154. Sugimoto M, Nakashima H, Watanabe S, et al: T-lymphocyte alveolitis in HTLV-I-associated myelopathy. Lancet 1987;ii:1220.

155. Mochizuki M, Watanabe T, Yamaguchi K, et al: HTLV-I uveitis: A distinct clinical entity caused by HTLVI. Jpn J Cancer Res 1992;83:2369.

156. Morgan OS, Rodgers-Johnson P, Mora C, Char G: HTLV-I and polymyositis in Jamaica. Lancet 1989;2(8673):11847.

157. Kitajima I, Maruyama I, Maruyama Y, et al: Polyarthritis in human T lymphotropic virus type I-associated myelopathy. Arthritis Rheum 1989;32:1342.

158. Murphy EL, Glynn SA, Fridey J, et al: Increased incidence of infectious diseases and neurologic abnormalities during prospective follow-up of HTLV-II and -I infected blood donors. Arch Intern Med 1999;159:1485.

159. LaGrenade L, Hanchard B, Fletcher V, et al: Infective dermatitis of Jamaican children: A marker for HTLV-I infection. Lancet 1990;336:1345.

160. Stuver SO, Okayama A, Tachibana N, et al: HCV infection and liver cancer mortality in a Japanese population with HTLV-I. Int J Cancer 1996;67:357.

161. Okochi K, Satao H, Hinuma Y: A retrospective study on transmission of adult T cell leukemia virus by blood transfusion: Seroconversion in recipients. Vox Sang 1984;46:245.

162. Kamihira S, Nakasima S, Oyakawa Y, et al: Transmission of human T-cell lymphotropic virus type I by blood transfusion before and after mass screening of sera from seropositive donors. Vox Sang 1987;52:43.

163. Manns A, Wilks RJ, Murphy EL, et al: A prospective study of transmission by transfusion of HTLV-I and risk factors associated with seroconversion. Int J Cancer 1992;51:886.

164. Donegan F, Lee H, Operskalski EA, et al: Transfusion transmission of retroviruses: Human T-lymphotropic viruses types I and II compared with human immunodeficiency virus type 1. Transfusion 1994;34:478.

165. Williams AE, Fang CT, Slamon DJ, et al: Seroprevalence and epidemiologic correlates of HTLV-I infection in U.S. blood donors. Science 1988;240:643.

166. Manns A, Wilks RJ, Murphy EL, et al: A prospective study of transmission by transfusion of HTLV-I and risk factors associated with seroconversion. Int J Cancer 1992;51:886.

167. Kleinman S: Donor selection and screening procedures. In Nance SJ (ed): Blood Safety: Current Challenges. Bethesda, MD, American Association of Blood Banks, 1992, p 169.

168. Hjelle B, Wilson C, Cyrus S, et al: Human T-cell leukemia virus type II infection frequently goes undetected in contemporary U.S. blood donors. Blood 1993;81:1641.

169. Kleinman S, Kaplan J, Khabbaz R, et al: Evaluation of a p21e-spiked western blot (Immunoblot) in confirming human t-cell lymphotropic virus type I and II infection in volunteer blood donors. J Clin Microbiol 1994;32:603.

170. Lal RB, Brodine S, Kuzura J, et al: Sensitivity and specificity of a recombinant transmembrane glycoprotein (rgp21)-spiked Western immunoblot for serologic confirmation of human T-cell lymphotropic virus type I and type II infection. J Clin Microbiol 1992;30:296.

171. Brodine SK, Kaime EM, Roberts C, et al: Simultaneous confirmation and differentiation of human T-lymphotropic virus types I and II infection by modified Western blot containing recombinant envelope glycoproteins. Transfusion 1993;33:925.

172. Lal RB, Heneine W, Rudolph DL, et al: Synthetic peptide-based immunoassays for distinguishing between human T-cell lymphotropic virus type I and type II infections in seropositive individuals. J Clin Microbiol 1991;29:2253.

173. Lal RB, Rudolph DL, Lairmore MD, et al: Serologic discrimination of human T cell lymphotropic virus infection by using a synthetic peptide-based enzyme immunoassay. J Infect Dis 1991;163:41.

174. Viscidi RP, Hill PM, Li S, et al: Diagnosis and differentiation of HTLV-I and HTLV-II infection by enzyme immunoassays using synthetic peptides. J Acquir Immun Defic Syndr Hum Retrovirol 41991:1190.

175. Busch MP, Laycock M, Kleinman SH, et al: Accuracy of supplementary serological testing for human T-lymphotropic virus (HTLV) types I and II in US blood donors. The Retrovirus Epidemiology Donor Study. Blood 1994;83:1143.

176. Mayo DJ, Rose AM, Matchett SE, et al: Screening potential blood donors at risk for human immunodeficiency virus. Transfusion 1991;31:466.

177. Johnson ES, Doll LS, Satten GA, et al: Direct oral questions to blood donors: The impact on screening for human immunodeficiency virus. Transfusion 1994;34:769.

178. Petersen LR, Doll LS, White CR, et al: Heterosexually acquired human immunodeficiency virus infection and the United States blood supply: Considerations for screening of potential blood donors. HIV Blood Donor Study Group Transfusion 1993;33:552.

179. Eastlund T: Monetary blood donation incentives and the risk of transfusion-transmitted infection. Transfusion 1998;38:874.

180. Munsterman KA, Grindon AJ, Sullivan J, et al: Assessment of motivations for return donation among deferred blood donors. Transfusion 1998;38:45.

181. Roth WK, Weber M, Seifried E, et al: Feasibility and efficacy of routine PCR screening of blood donations for hepatitis C virus,

hepatitis B virus, and HIV-1 in a blood-bank setting. Lancet 1999;353:359.

182. Busch MP, Dodd RY: Nucleic acid amplification testing and blood safety: What is the paradigm? Transfusion 2000;40:1157

183. Murthy KK, Henrard DR, Eichberg JW, et al: Redefining the HIV-infectious window period in the chimpanzee model: Evidence to suggest that viral nucleic acid testing can prevent blood-borne transmission. Transfusion 1999;39:688.

184. Klein HG, Dodd RY, Dzik WH, et al: Current status of solvent/detergent-treated frozen plasma. Transfusion 1998;38:102.

185. Pehta JC: Clinical studies with solvent detergent-treated products. Transfus Med Rev 1996;10:303.

186. Council of Europe Expert Committee in Blood Transfusion Study Group on pathogen inactivation of labile blood components: Pathogen inactivation of labile blood products. Transfusion Medicine 2001;11:149.

187. Lackritz EM: Prevention of HIV transmission by blood transfusion in the developing world: Achievements and continuing challenges. AIDS 1998;12(Suppl A):S81.

188. Wake DJ, Cutting WA: Blood transfusion in developing countries: Problems, priorities and practicalities. Trop Doct 1998; 28:4.

Chapter 40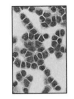

Human Herpesvirus Infections

John D. Roback

The Herpesviridae are a family of approximately 100 viruses with common structural features. Each virus has a linear, 120- to 230-kb, double-stranded DNA genome maintained in a toroidal conformation and surrounded by an icosadeltahedral nucleocapsid. The 100-nm diameter capsid, composed of 162 capsomeres, is encompassed by a dense tegument or matrix and an outer trilaminar lipid envelope that contains proteins of both viral and host cell origin.[1] Herpesviruses share a number of biologic characteristics, including expression of viral enzymes that participate in DNA synthesis and nucleic acid metabolism, confinement of viral DNA synthesis and packaging to the host cell nucleus, destruction of the infected cell during active viral replication, and the capacity to remain in a latent state indefinitely.[1]

Of the herpesviruses, eight are known to infect humans (Table 40.1). Members of the human herpesvirus (HHV) family are categorized into three subfamilies based on biologic properties including cell tropism, genome structure, and sequences of conserved open reading frames (ORFs).

Table 40.1 Human Herpesviruses

Subfamily	HHV Designation	Common Name
Alpha-herpesvirinae	HHV-1	Herpes simplex-1 (HSV-1)
	HHV-2	Herpes simplex-2 (HSV-2)
	HHV-3	Varicella-zoster virus (VZV)
Beta-herpesvirinae	HHV-5	Cytomegalovirus (CMV)
	HHV-6A, -6B	—
	HHV-7	—
Gamma-herpesvirinae	HHV-4	Epstein-Barr virus (EBV)
	HHV-8	Kaposi sarcoma herpesvirus (KSHV)

Although most have a commonly employed name, such as cytomegalovirus (CMV), each is also known by an accompanying HHV designation according to guidelines of the International Committee on Taxonomy of Viruses[2] (e.g., CMV is HHV-5). This chapter focuses primarily on CMV, the herpesvirus with greatest clinical relevance to transfusion medicine, along with some discussion of other leukocytotropic herpesviruses that may contaminate blood components, including the Epstein-Barr virus (EBV or HHV-4) and HHV-6 through -8.

■ Cytomegalovirus (HHV-5)

Molecular and Cellular Virology of CMV

Viral Structure

CMV was the first identified beta-herpesvirus, and it remains the prototype of this group. The CMV virion contains a linear, double-stranded DNA genome approximately 230 kb in length, the largest of the herpesviruses.[3, 4] The genome is divided into unique long (UL) and unique short (US) segments, each flanked by a pair of inverted repeat regions.[4] The UL and US segments can each independently invert with respect to one another, yielding four different genomic isomers. After infection, the termini of the linear genome are joined to produce a circular, or concatemeric, replicative form.[5] Circularized CMV genomes have also been identified in latently infected peripheral blood CD14-positive leukocytes.[6] At least 200 ORFs have been identified within the CMV genome, many of which encode viral proteins of still unknown function.[4] After translation, viral proteins may undergo modifications including phosphorylation, glycosylation, and cleavage. Mature virions range from 150 to 200 nm in diameter[7] and contain approximately 30 viral proteins distributed in the capsid, tegument, and envelope. Recently, viral RNA transcripts have also been identified in infectious virions, although their function is currently unclear.[8]

Biology of Infection

VIRAL–CELLULAR INTERACTIONS

CMV can infect a range of cell types, including those of endothelial, epithelial, mesenchymal, hematopoietic, and neuronal lineages, frequently producing cell enlargement (cytomegalia).[4, 9] Infection appears to involve three sequential steps: viral attachment to the target cell, fusion of the viral and cellular membranes, and penetration of the viral capsid into the cell. Each step may require interactions between multiple viral coat proteins and cellular membrane proteins, the latter serving the role of viral "receptors." The observation that the CMV genome contains at least 54 ORFs that encode putative viral membrane glycoproteins[10] hints at the potential complexity of these processes.

Viral attachment, the formation of a dissociable viral-cellular interaction, involves glycoprotein B, or gB (sometimes called gC-1, UL55, or gp130/55), a disulfide-linked complex composed of 120- to 130-kD and 55- to 60-kD viral glycoproteins. The most abundant protein in the viral envelope, gB is also a prominent target of neutralizing antibodies produced during natural infection.[11] gB binds to two classes of cellular receptors. One receptor has been identified as the protein annexin II, and the other is a yet uncharacterized heparan sulfate proteoglycan (HSPG).[12–15] However, the roles of these putative receptor proteins in viral attachment and infection are still unclear, because annexin II is not required for CMV infection, and HSPGs by themselves are not sufficient for infection.[16]

Although attachment complexes are initially dissociable, they can be stabilized by membrane fusion. After attachment, interactions between gB and its receptors may initiate fusion. In addition, the viral protein complex gp86 (also called gC-III, UL75:UL115, or gH:gL) appears to be involved in these processes.[17] Evidence indicates that gp86 is composed of the viral gH and gL proteins, as well as a third component not yet identified.[18] The cell membrane receptor for gp86 has been identified as a 92.5-kD, constitutively phosphorylated glycoprotein.[19, 20] Binding of gB and gp86 to the target cell initiates signaling processes that may be important to CMV infection. Interactions between gB and its cellular receptor or receptors activate signal transduction through the interferon-response pathway, leading to induction of the interferon-responsive genes *OAS* and *ISG54*,[21] whereas binding of gp86 to the cellular 92.5-kD protein can alter the intracellular calcium concentration.[22]

After fusion, the viral capsid penetrates into the host cell and releases viral DNA. The molecules mediating these processes have not been identified. Additional proteins have also been hypothesized to mediate viral infection. For example, cellular human leukocyte antigen (HLA) class I proteins may promote viral attachment through interactions with β_2-microglobulin attached to the virion membrane.[23]

VIRAL LIFE CYCLE

Active and Latent Infection. After the steps of viral attachment, fusion, and penetration have been completed, active infection occurs if the target cell is permissive for the complete sequence of viral gene expression, viral genome replication, and production of progeny virions. During active infection, viral genes are expressed in coordinated waves. Three distinct kinetic classes of viral genes have been identified: the immediate-early (α), the delayed-early (β), and the late (γ) groups.[4] α-Class gene transcription is controlled by a combination of constitutively expressed host cell proteins and viral proteins present in the infecting virion. Therefore, α genes can be transcribed in the presence of pharmacologic inhibitors of protein synthesis. Viral α proteins, in turn, are required for the expression of viral genes of the β and γ classes.[24–26] The β protein products perform viral DNA replication and metabolic functions, while the γ genes encode structural proteins required for the assembly of progeny virions. Finally, mature virions are transported through the Golgi apparatus and are released from infected cells by exocytosis,[27] eventually resulting in host cell destruction.

CMV may also assume a latent state when it infects target cells that are not permissive for viral replication. Latency, the presence of viral DNA in an infected cell in the absence of active viral replication, can persist indefinitely because the host cell is not destroyed by the virus. The latent CMV genome retains the capacity to reactivate viral gene expression, produce infectious virions, and enter lytic growth at a later time. Studies with human and murine CMV have demonstrated that latency can be established in hematopoietic cells, primarily those of the granulocyte-monocyte lineage, as well as in endothelial cells.[28–34] The possibility of CMV latency in other cell types has not been excluded. The molecular mechanisms regulating CMV latency and reactivation from latency have not been completely elucidated. In the herpesvirus EBV, a clearly defined set of viral proteins controls latency and reactivation.[35] Similarly, CMV latency-associated transcripts (LATs) have been detected in 0.01% to 0.001% of sorted CD33+ lineage-committed hematopoietic progenitors from the peripheral blood of naturally infected individuals.[32, 36] CMV LATs are transcribed from the viral immediate-early gene locus and encode immunogenic viral proteins that are targets of naturally arising antibodies in CMV-seropositive individuals.[28, 36, 37] The function of LATs is currently unknown. Circularization of the CMV genome is associated with latency in CD14+ peripheral blood mononuclear cells (PBMNCs) in CMV-seropositive individuals,[6] a phenomenon also seen during latent infection by other herpesviruses.[38–40] The possibility of persistent viral infection, an intermediate state between active and latent infection in which low levels of virus are produced, remains a topic of considerable debate.[41, 42]

Viral Genes Important to Pathogenesis. In addition to viral proteins that control expression of viral genes and virion assembly and provide structural support for the viral particle, CMV also encodes proteins that favor viral replication at the expense of host cell metabolism and disrupt the host's ability to combat viral infection. For example, CMV infection alters the expression, accumulation, and activity of the cellular tumor suppressor proteins, cyclins, and cyclin-associated kinases. These alterations in the cell cycle machinery act to simultaneously promote progression toward the G_1/S transition but prevent cellular DNA synthesis and cell division, resulting in cell cycle arrest and cellular aneuploidy. It has been hypothesized that in the arrested state cellular DNA synthesis is blocked but the cellular milieu contains abundant nucleotides and other metabolic precursors that can support viral replication.[43–46] One viral protein involved in this process is the immediate-early protein IE1-72, which complexes with the cellular retinoblastoma-related protein p107 and blocks its ability to repress E2F-responsive promoters.[47] The IEl-72–mediated derepression at the level of E2F in turn allows expression of cellular genes that promote cell-cycle progression.[47] CMV infection also activates cyclin-dependent kinase 2 (CDK2), a cellular protein that controls progression through the G_1 and S phases of the cell cycle. The importance of CDK2 to viral replication was illustrated by an experiment in which CDK2 activity was blocked with either a dominant negative mutant or the pharmacologic inhibitor roscovitine. In both cases, inhibition of CDK2 activity prevented CMV replication and production of progeny virus.[46]

CMV has also developed mechanisms to interfere with antiviral immune function (reviewed by Hengel and colleagues[48]). The UL37 ORF of CMV encodes viral mitochondria-localized inhibitor of apoptosis (vMIA), an antiapoptotic protein that localizes to the mitochondria and protects infected cells from immune-mediated apoptosis by blocking the effects of Fas, tumor necrosis factor receptor 1, and granzyme B.[49] Monocytes are a prominent cite of CMV latency, and monocyte-derived macrophages can support active CMV replication. During differentiation to macrophages, CMV in monocytes displays delayed replication kinetics and viral particles are retained in the Golgi apparatus, which may facilitate immune evasion until sufficient progeny virions have been produced.[50] In contrast, in patients with compromised antiviral immunity, CMV can replicate with rapid kinetics, displaying viral doubling times approaching 24 hours.[51]

Despite sophisticated viral mechanisms of immune evasion, clinical and experimental evidence demonstrates that the competent immune system can ultimately suppress viral replication. For example, the murine CMV glycoproteins gp40 and gp48 (ORFs *m152* and *m06*, respectively) can decrease expression of cellular class I major histocompatibility complex (MHC) proteins during infection of fibroblasts, and thus decrease CMV antigen presentation to CD8+ T cells. However, the significance of these mechanisms during natural infection are unclear, because CMV infection does not disrupt class I MHC expression and antigen presentation in macrophages, the professional antigen-presenting cells most important in initiating the anti-CMV immune response.[52] Furthermore, although human CMV has also evolved mechanisms to interfere with antigen presentation by infected cells,[53, 54] the immune system circumvents these obstacles by utilizing structural proteins in the infecting viral particle as immunodominant epitopes for an immune response.[55, 56] Thus, the immune response can be initiated before expression of antiviral proteins that halt antigen presentation by the infected cell. CMV has also developed strategies to interfere with interferon-γ (IFN-γ) signals that normally upregulate MHC expression during viral infection.[57] Interestingly, downregulation of MHC class I cell surface expression by CMV should lead to destruction of the infected cells by host natural killer (NK) cells.[58] However, expression of the viral MHC class I homolog m144 by murine CMV decreases the susceptibility of the infected cell to NK-mediated lysis.[59]

CMV Infection, Immune Response, and Diagnosis

Transmission, Prevalence, and Epidemiology

During CMV infection, active viral replication results in shedding of infectious virions into plasma and bodily fluids, including saliva, tears, breast milk, urine, stool, and semen. Community-acquired CMV infection is usually the result of close contact with a person shedding CMV. The incidence of community-acquired CMV infection varies with the study population. For example, the yearly CMV seroconversion rate among health care workers has been estimated at 0.6% to 3.3%,[60] similar to the rates of 2.0% to 6.3% reported in middle-class women during and between pregnancies.[61] In contrast, rates as high as 13% per year have been observed in adolescents.[62] Among blood donors, the CMV seroconversion rate is estimated to be approximately 1% per year.[63] Most studies have shown that 50% to 80% of the population is CMV seropositive,[4] although the incidence can be higher in some urban populations and lower in some groups of blood donors.[64]

Most individuals contracting community-acquired CMV infection are immunocompetent, and the infection is often asymptomatic. However, a mild, self-limited infectious mononucleosis syndrome can occur, with symptoms including fever, malaise, hepatosplenomegaly, and a rash.[65] CMV can be isolated from bodily secretions during the symptomatic phase. The infected individual mounts both a humoral and a cell-mediated immune response, and viral symptoms rapidly resolve, leading to a complete recovery. However, despite effective control of CMV infection by the competent host immune system, the virus is not completely eliminated but instead becomes latent.

Transplacental transmission of CMV to a developing fetus is an important viral cause of birth defects.[66, 67] Fetal infection occurs in 40% to 50% of cases in which a seronegative mother contracts a primary CMV infection during pregnancy.[68, 69] CMV disease occurs in 5% to 15% of the infected infants, most often resulting in intrauterine growth retardation, deafness, mental retardation, blindness, and thrombocytopenic bleeding.[67, 68] However, if the mother is seropositive before pregnancy, maternal antiviral immunity can limit congenital CMV infection and disease. For example, in one study of seropositive mothers the rate of vertical transmission was approximately 1%.[68] Furthermore, no cases of symptomatic CMV infection were seen among 27 congenitally infected infants born to seropositive mothers.[68]

CMV can also be transmitted by blood transfusion and by transplantation of hematopoietic stem cells or solid organs from infected donors. If the recipient is immunocompromised, CMV transmission through these mechanisms can produce serious clinical consequences. Prevention of CMV infection is an important concern in transfusion medicine; it is discussed in more detail later in this chapter.

CMV Infection of Peripheral Blood and Marrow Cells

CELL TROPISM

From the perspective of transfusion medicine, the most important target cells of CMV infection are white blood cells (WBCs) and their progenitors. Under appropriate conditions, these cell types can either harbor latent CMV or allow active viral replication; therefore, they are well suited to mediate transfusion-transmitted CMV infection (TT-CMV). CMV infection of bone marrow hematopoietic progenitor cells probably occurs during primary infection[70] (Fig. 40.1). Most evidence suggests that these cells restrict viral replication but support viral latency,[28, 29] although some studies have shown low levels of CMV replication in bone marrow–derived cells

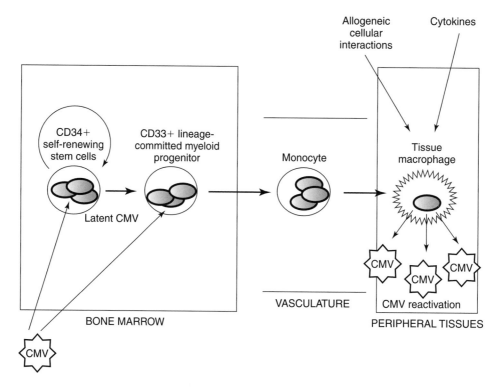

Figure 40.1 Hypothetical model integrating long-term latency of cytomegalovirus (CMV) in the hematopoietic compartment with transmission of CMV by blood transfusion and hematopoietic stem cell transplantation. CMV infects CD34+ multipotent progenitors during primary infection, and latently infected cells retain the viral genome during self-renewal. Committed progenitors in the marrow may also be directly infected with CMV. Either cell type can transmit CMV to a seronegative transplant recipient. CMV remains latent as CD33+ progenitors differentiate into circulating peripheral blood monocytes. Latently infected monocytes subsequently differentiate into tissue macrophages, either in the original host or after transfusion into a recipient. The allogeneic or cytokine-mediated signals monocytes encounter during differentiation render them permissive to CMV reactivation and viral replication. See text for detailed discussion.

in culture.[70, 71] CMV DNA has been identified by polymerase chain reaction (PCR) in sorted multipotent CD34+ progenitor cells from the bone marrow of seropositive donors, and in some cases from seronegative donors.[29, 32, 72, 73] Because of their capacity for self-renewal, latently infected hematopoietic progenitors represent a potential long-term reservoir of latent virus. In fact, when CMV-infected CD34+ cells were grown in long-term suspension cultures, transfer of CMV DNA to progeny cells during mitosis was demonstrated.[30] CMV DNA was also identified in myeloid-lineage–committed CD33+ progenitor cells in the marrow, or mobilized into the peripheral blood by granulocyte-macrophage colony-stimulating factor (GM-CSF). Lineage-committed progenitors appear to be latently infected, as indicated by the presence of CMV LATs in 0.01% to 0.001% of sorted CD33+CD14+ or CD33+CD15+ bone marrow cells from seropositive donors.[32] These findings support a model for latency in which early hematopoietic progenitors are latently infected during primary CMV infection and thereafter serve as viral reservoirs. Furthermore, latently infected marrow progenitor cells are a likely vector for transmission of CMV infection via hematopoietic stem cell transplantation.

As CD33+ progenitors continue to differentiate, they enter the peripheral blood. Monocytes appear to retain latent virus, but as they differentiate into macrophages CMV replication

with production of progeny virus occurs[31, 74] (see Fig. 40.1). Although cells of the monocytic lineage have been hypothesized to mediate TT-CMV, the prevalence of latently infected monocytes in the peripheral blood appears to be low. It has been estimated that 0.004% to 0.01% of granulocyte colony-stimulating factor (G-CSF)–mobilized PBMNCs[34] and 0.01% to 0.12% of PBMNCs from healthy seropositive blood donors[31] contain CMV DNA, with a range of 2 to 13 viral genomes per infected cell.[34] Because about 5% of PBMNCs are monocytes, latently infected monocytes may comprise only 1 to 25 of every 1 million peripheral blood WBCs. The low numbers of latently infected leukocytes in transfused blood components may contribute to the variable incidence of TT-CMV observed clinically.

CMV is also found associated with other cell types in the peripheral blood and marrow. In immunocompromised patients with CMV infection, polymorphonuclear leukocytes phagocytose and contain large amounts of virus.[75] Although these cells do not appear to support the complete viral replication cycle, they can retain CMV in a viable and infectious form under experimental circumstances.[76] CMV can also productively infect megakaryocytic precursors and mature megakaryocytes.[77] Plasma free virus appears to be less stable than intracellular virus, and the presence of free virus in plasma is usually transient.[78, 79] For example, in one study of recently infected adolescents, only a minority (25% to 40%) had plasma viremia, which was rarely identified more than 4 months after seroconversion.[62] These other peripheral blood sources of CMV are unlikely to be as important as latently infected monocytes to the pathogenesis of TT-CMV.

VIRAL LOADS

Quantitation of the peripheral blood CMV load is clinically useful in immunocompromised patients, in whom viral loads can reach 10^8 copies per milliliter of plasma or greater[80] and correlate with the severity of viral disease.[81-86] For example, in liver transplant recipients a 50% probability of CMV disease was associated with a viral load of $10^{5.1}$ genomes per milliliter of blood, and a 90% probability with $10^{5.5}$ genomes per milliliter.[83] Infectious virus can also be cultured readily from the blood of immunocompromised patients with active infection.[87]

In contrast, the peripheral blood viral load in CMV-infected but otherwise healthy individuals is much lower and is rarely quantitated. For example, in a series of published studies CMV could be cultured from only 2 of more than 1500 buffy coat samples from healthy blood donors.[65, 88, 89] Nonetheless, a consideration of CMV loads in healthy individuals who are potential blood donors is useful for understanding the biology of TT-CMV (Fig. 40.2). WBC-associated viremia is often detectable for 6 months after

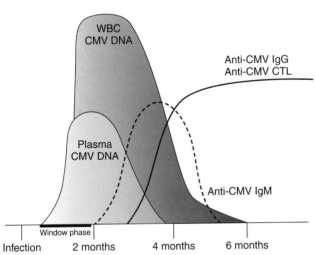

Figure 40.2 Temporal relation between detection of plasma- or white blood cell (WBC)–associated cytomegalovirus (CMV) DNA and the development of an immune response after primary infection. CMV DNA can be detected by polymerase chain reaction in both the plasma and WBC peripheral blood compartments during the first month after infection, with a subsequent decline to undetectable levels over 4 to 6 months. The curves are not meant to be quantitative but rather to illustrate that WBC-associated virus is more frequently detectable than plasma CMV during primary infection, and it also persists for a longer time. A humoral response is usually detectable by 8 weeks after infection and persists indefinitely, along with a cytotoxic T-lymphocyte (CTL) response. The window phase represents the period between the initial presence of CMV in the peripheral blood and the first serologic evidence of CMV infection. Seronegative blood components obtained from donors in the window phase may explain some episodes of breakthrough transfusion-transmitted CMV in patients transfused exclusively with seronegative blood. See text for detailed discussion.

infection,[62, 90] in contrast to plasma free virus, which often disappears by 4 months. In recently seroconverted adolescents, 75% to 80% of WBC samples were positive for CMV DNA by PCR within the first 4 months after infection, compared with 25% to 40% of plasma samples within the same period.[62] A study of 98 seroconverting blood donors similarly identified a low frequency (20%) of transient plasma viremia.[79] In recently infected pregnant women, WBC-associated CMV DNA was detected in 100% of samples during the first month after infection using PCR, and in 90% of samples during the second month after infection. None of the samples was positive 6 months after infection.[90] The WBC-associated viral load decreased substantially during early infection. During the first month, 60% of positive samples had viral loads greater than 10 CMV GEs per 10^5 WBCs (range, 10 to 398 GE), whereas only 3.3% of positive samples during the second month of infection had that many GEs.[90] Therefore, viral load peaks shortly after infection in an immunocompetent host, and the subsequent decline in viral load follows the development of an immune response.

Host Immune Response

HUMORAL IMMUNITY

CMV infection initiates both a humoral and a cellular immune response in the host, although anti-CMV antibodies exert limited control over CMV infection and disease. Antibody expression is typical of other humoral responses: Transient anti-CMV immunoglobulin M (IgM) synthesis is followed by persistent expression of antiviral IgG (see Fig. 40.2). In a study of recently infected adolescents, anti-CMV antibodies were usually detectable by 6 to 8 weeks after infection, a time of high peripheral blood viral loads.[62] However, despite the fact that anti-CMV, anti-gB, and viral neutralizing antibodies could be detected during the humoral response, they were insufficient to produce a precipitous decline in CMV DNA either in the plasma (free virus) or in WBCs. Plasma- and WBC-associated viral DNA was present, respectively, in 25% to 40% and 75% to 80% of individuals during the first 16 weeks after infection and could still be detected in some individuals at 48 weeks. Development of an antibody response likewise failed to immediately suppress viral shedding, because CMV could be isolated from 59% of urine specimens during the first 80 weeks after infection.[62] Consistent with these observations, infectious virus was also identified in saliva and cervical secretions of remotely infected seropositive individuals.[91, 92] These findings indicate that anti-CMV antibodies, including those with neutralizing activities in vitro, may not completely prevent viral infectivity in vivo.

Nonetheless, anti-CMV antibodies can protect against sequelae of CMV infections in some circumstances. In a study of neonatal CMV infection, 5 (50%) of 10 infants who were born to seronegative mothers and subsequently contracted TT-CMV developed serious or fatal CMV disease. In contrast, 32 infants born to seropositive mothers contracted CMV infection, but none developed CMV disease, suggesting that passively acquired maternal CMV antibodies abrogated disease severity.[93] Therapeutic administration of antiviral antibodies, such as those present in intravenous immunoglobulin (IVIG) preparations, can also be efficacious in altering CMV disease course in some circumstances.[94]

Although anti-CMV antibodies generated during natural infection display a spectrum of specificities, among the more important targets is the viral gB glycoprotein. Radioimmunoprecipitation assays using recombinant gB demonstrated the presence of anti-gB antibodies in the serum of all 48 seropositive donors tested.[11] Furthermore, the anti-gB antibodies were a significant component of the CMV neutralizing activity in the serum samples. When anti-gB antibodies were absorbed with recombinant gB protein, the viral neutralizing titer in the serum was reduced by an average of 48%.[11] Similarly, other studies demonstrated that 40% to 88% of serum CMV-neutralizing activity in naturally infected donors was directed against gB.[95, 96] These results lend support for the use of recombinant gB as a subunit CMV vaccine.

CELLULAR IMMUNE RESPONSE

Cellular immune response plays an important role in the control of CMV infection. In bone marrow transplant (BMT) recipients, a patient population at high risk for CMV infection, development of an MHC class I–restricted CD8+ cytotoxic T-lymphocyte (CTL) response to CMV was significantly associated with the effective control of CMV infections.[97–101] In a study of 58 allogeneic BMT recipients with low or absent anti-CMV CTL activity at enrollment, 43 developed CMV infections, which were lethal in 12 of the patients.[97] Detectable anti-CMV CTL activity developed in all survivors of CMV infection, but in only 2 of the 12 patients who died from CMV disease. NK cell activity was also depressed in the patients with fatal CMV infection, but not in those who controlled their infections.[97, 98] In another study, 10 of 20 recipients of allogeneic BMT developed CMV-specific CTL activity by 3 months after transplantation. Six of the 10 patients who failed to develop anti-CMV CTL activity died from CMV pneumonitis, but all of the 10 patients with a detectable CMV CTL response were protected.[99] Similar conclusions regarding the protective effects of CMV CTLs were reached in regard to CMV-seropositive patients who underwent autologous transplantation of peripheral blood stem cells or BMT. In these patients, whose pre-existing CMV-specific CTLs were suppressed by the preparative regimen, the reappearance of anti-CMV CTL activity was positively correlated with control of CMV infections ($P = .002$).[100] The investigators also noted that a CD4+ T-helper cell response to CMV always preceded the reappearance of anti-CMV CTLs and appeared to be obligatory for the CTL response.[100, 101]

Using a murine model, investigators specifically depleted CD4+ and CD8+ T cells from the animals before experimental CMV infection to determine the contribution of each subset to antiviral immunity. These studies showed that CMV-primed CD8+ CTLs were capable of controlling CMV infections in the absence of CD4+ cells, except in salivary glands.[102, 103] Furthermore, the mice deficient in CD4+ cells did not make high levels of anti-CMV antibodies, indicating that when the antiviral CTL response is intact a humoral response is unnecessary for effective control of CMV infection.[102] In the murine model, NK cells are also important for control of acute CMV infection.[59, 104] IFN-γ production appears to be one of the principal mechanisms through which CD8+ and NK cells exert this effect.[104–109] The observation that cellular immunity plays a critical role in controlling CMV infection has led to successful early stage clinical trials in which CMV-immune CTLs were adoptively transferred into immunocompromised BMT recipients.[110]

Laboratory Diagnosis of CMV Infection

Accurate detection of CMV infection enables the identification of transfusion recipients who are at risk for CMV infection, as well as blood donors whose components are potentially infectious. Furthermore, quantitation of the degree of viral replication is important for guiding appropriate use of antiviral therapies such as ganciclovir, cidofovir, or foscarnet in immunocompromised patients. The standard approach for identifying a previously infected individual is through detection of anti-CMV antibodies (Table 40.2). Serologic assays have been developed in multiple configurations, including indirect hemagglutination, complement fixation, solid-phase fluorescence immunoassay, enzyme immunoassay (EIA), latex or particle agglutination, and solid phase red blood cell (RBC) adherence, although the first three of these techniques are no longer frequently used.[111–115] These assays detect anti-CMV antibodies of the IgG, and in some cases IgM and IgA, classes. Direct comparisons of the sensitivities and specificities of the four presently used methodologies have not been published. Some EIA assays have stated sensitivities and specificities of approximately 99%, and because of their objective readouts they may have advantages over techniques such as latex agglutination. However, anti-CMV antibodies may not be detected by serology until 6 to 8 weeks after primary infection,[62] and serology cannot accurately identify or quantitate the extent of active CMV infection. Although viral culture can be used for these purposes, conventional tube cultures can require 2 weeks or longer to yield results, and the more recently implemented shell vial methodology may still require 24 to 48 hours to detect the presence of infectious CMV.[116, 117] Furthermore, these assays are quantitative only in a limiting-dilution format, which is labor-intensive and not suited to routine clinical use.

Table 40.2 Routine Diagnostic Laboratory Methods for Cytomegalovirus

Method	Rapid	Quantitative	Detects Active Infection	Detects Latent Infection	Differentiates Active from Latent Infection
Serology	++	No	Yes	Yes	No
Culture	No	No	Yes	No	Yes
Antigenemia	+	Yes	Yes	No	Yes
Polymerase chain reaction	++	Yes*	Yes	Yes	Yes*

++, <hr turnaround time; +, <24hr turnaround time; *, depending on assay—see text for details.

Introduction of the CMV antigenemia assay, which uses immunostaining to identify and quantitate peripheral blood leukocytes that contain CMV proteins, has solved some of these problems[118–120] as has PCR.[121, 122] The antigenemia assay can be used for both viral diagnosis and surveillance.[123–125] Significantly, this methodology is sensitive enough for early quantitative detection of CMV infections, allowing the institution of preemptive (presymptomatic) antiviral therapies.[126, 127] Qualitative PCR allows even earlier detection of CMV infection than does antigenemia.[82, 124, 128] However, because of its sensitivity, in some earlier studies PCR displayed poor positive predictive value for identifying at-risk patients, because some patients with low but detectable viral loads did not develop CMV disease.[82, 127, 128] Quantitative, PCR assays for CMV may provide a more rapid, sensitive, and specific predictor of patients who are at risk for CMV disease.[129] For example, the results obtained with a moderately sensitive quantitative CMV PCR assay (400 copies of CMV DNA per milliliter) strongly correlated with results from the antigenemia method and with the development of CMV disease.[130] Advantages of the PCR method included reduced turnaround time, smaller sample requirements (200 μL plasma versus 3 to 5 mL blood), simplified specimen processing, improved stability of specimens before processing, and ability to test samples from patients with leukopenia. Turnaround time for PCR testing may be reduced even further by adopting assays to the real-time format.[80]

Alternative nucleic acid testing methodologies, such as nucleic acid sequence-based amplification (NASBA) of CMV immediate-early messenger RNA, may also be useful in CMV diagnosis.[131, 132]

Transfusion-Transmitted CMV Infection

Background

By the mid-1960s, a number of investigators had described an illness with clinical similarities to infectious mononucleosis occurring in patients who were exposed to blood products during cardiopulmonary bypass for open heart surgery.[133, 134] Patients typically presented with fever, splenomegaly, and atypical lymphocytosis within 3 to 8 weeks after surgery but had a negative heterophile antibody test and did not experience exudative pharyngitis or lymphadenopathy. Klemola and Kaariainen[135, 136] subsequently demonstrated an increase in the titer of complement-fixing anti-CMV antibodies concurrent with the illness, suggesting that the cause was CMV infection acquired from transfused blood products. Further support for this hypothesis was provided by culture of CMV shed into the urine or blood of patients experiencing what was then called "cytomegalovirus mononucleosis."[137] In the ensuing years, the disease has come to be known as transfusion-transmitted CMV infection, or TT-CMV. It has been described in a wide variety of clinical circumstances, although it is of most significance in immunocompromised transfusion recipients.[138–142] In most cases the diagnosis of TT-CMV is correlative: evidence of primary CMV infection in a previously seronegative patient who received a cellular blood component (RBCs, platelets, or granulocytes) that was neither CMV-seronegative nor filtered. However, in at least one instance unequivocal molecular evidence for TT-CMV infection was provided by the demonstration of identical restriction endonuclease digestion patterns of CMV isolates from a seropositive blood donor and from the neonates who were transfused with that donor's blood component and subsequently developed CMV infection.[143]

Transfusion can lead to active CMV infection in the recipient by three mechanisms. The term TT-CMV is used to describe a primary CMV infection occurring in a seronegative recipient transfused with an infectious blood component. In contrast, reactivated CMV infection can occur when a seropositive transfusion recipient experiences reactivation of latent CMV infection after blood transfusion from a seronegative donor. The mechanism underlying reactivated CMV infection most likely involves immunomodulatory interactions between MHC mismatched leukocytes of the donor and recipient. Consistent with this mechanism, studies indicate that the incidence of CMV reactivation is independent of donor serostatus and component storage time but increases with the volume of blood transfused.[144, 145] Finally, CMV superinfection (second-strain infection) occurs when a seropositive recipient contracts a new strain of CMV from an infectious blood component.

The diagnosis of both reactivation and superinfection is based on a fourfold or greater rise in the titer of anti-CMV antibodies and/or renewed viral shedding in secretions of seropositive transfusion recipients.[65] Although reactivation and superinfection can be distinguished from one another by restriction endonuclease genotyping of CMV strains,[146] this analysis has no significant clinical implications. The three mechanisms of transfusion-associated CMV infection appear to occur with similar frequencies. A review of five early studies of transfused CMV-seropositive patients calculated a 26% cumulative incidence of CMV reactivation or superinfection (66 of 252 patients), compared with the overall incidence of 31% (99 of 323 patients) for TT-CMV in seronegative recipients that was reported in seven contemporary studies (reviewed by Adler[65]). Nonetheless, the clinical significance of TT-CMV overshadows that of CMV reactivation and superinfection, because TT-CMV results in a primary infection against which the recipient has no immunologic memory. In contrast, CMV reactivation and superinfection are unlikely to cause morbidity in the transfusion recipient.[147] Finally, it should be noted that although most cases of suspected TT-CMV result from the transfused component,[148, 149] a minority of cases may result from community-acquired CMV infection that occurs in temporal proximity to the transfusion.

Patients at Risk and Incidence

Although TT-CMV produces a primary CMV infection, in the immunocompetent transfusion recipient it is of no more clinical significance than community-acquired CMV infection. Furthermore, the risk of TT-CMV is very low in these patients. Early studies showed that 1.2% or fewer of immunocompetent patients experienced TT-CMV.[150, 151] In a more recent study of 76 seronegative children with malignancies, there were no cases of TT-CMV among patients who received either seronegative or unscreened units, resulting in a calculated TT-CMV risk of less than 1 in 698 donor exposures in this population.[152] It should be noted that, for reasons unrelated to study design, some of the units transfused in this study were washed or filtered. Follow-up of these children revealed that 2 of 76 subsequently developed community-acquired CMV infections (1.7% per patient-year), demonstrating the relatively greater incidence of community-acquired CMV infection compared with TT-CMV in this immunocompetent population. Furthermore, even in one early study in which 32% of nonimmunosuppressed patients undergoing tumor resection developed TT-CMV, there was no evidence of CMV disease.[144] Therefore, at present there are no compelling reasons to provide nonimmunosuppressed seronegative transfusion recipients with special components for the purpose of preventing TT-CMV.

In contrast, TT-CMV can be an important cause of morbidity and mortality in immunocompromised patients (Table 40.3). Most studies suggest that 13% to 37% of these patients will contract TT-CMV from transfusion of unscreened and unfiltered cellular blood components.[93, 153–156] The most well-established patient groups at risk for TT-CMV include premature low birth weight infants (<1250 to 1500 g) born to seronegative mothers, seronegative recipients of seronegative allogeneic or autologous BMT, seronegative recipients of seronegative solid organ transplants, and seronegative patients with acquired immunodeficiency syndrome (AIDS).[141, 157] In these patients, the first manifestations of TT-CMV are often a viral syndrome, characterized by a flu-like illness including fever, chills, malaise, leukopenia, thrombocytopenia, and mild abnormalities in liver function tests. The illness can progress to disseminated tissue-invasive CMV disease, including CMV hepatitis, retinitis, interstitial pneumonitis, encephalitis, and gastroenteritis including esophagitis.[158] Progression to disease is more likely in patients with high viral loads. CMV infections are also associated with, and may predispose to, other complications in immunocompromised patients, including graft-versus-host disease (GVHD) in allogeneic BMT recipients,[159–161] accelerated solid organ graft rejection,[162, 163] and other opportunistic infections including invasive fungal disease.[158, 164]

Seronegative infants transfused with unscreened blood products had a 13.5% incidence of TT-CMV.[93] When more than 50 mL of packed RBCs was transfused, the incidence of TT-CMV increased to 24%. Of the infants who acquired TT-CMV, five (50%) developed serious symptoms or fatal disease; all of those infants weighed less than 1200 g.[93] In other studies, seronegative neonates weighing less than 1250 to 1500 g also experienced a high incidence of TT-CMV (reviewed by Preiksaitis[165]), probably owing to their immature immune systems. It should be noted, however, that low-birth-weight infants born to seropositive mothers can also be at risk for lethal CMV infection, despite the transfer of humoral immunity.[166]

BMT recipients are at significant risk for morbidity and mortality from CMV infection. Up to one third of these patients who contract CMV infection develop CMV pneumonitis, a frequently fatal complication.[167] In seropositive BMT recipients, CMV infection is usually caused by viral reactivation, making CMV seropositivity the most important risk factor for CMV infection and disease.[167–170] CMV infection also occurs frequently in seronegative recipients of seropositive marrow.[153–155] However, in seronegative recipients of seronegative marrow or autologous transplants, TT-CMV is the primary mechanism for CMV infection.[153–155] Solid organ transplant recipients are also susceptible to CMV infection and disease. In contrast to BMT, the most important source of CMV infection is the donor organ, with TT-CMV being less significant.[140, 171–174] Among seronegative recipients of seronegative organs, transfusion of unscreened blood products has been associated with an incidence of TT-CMV ranging from 0% to 33%, with a cumulative incidence of approximately 9% (reviewed by Preiksaitis[165] and by Hillyer and colleagues[175]). Among organ transplant recipients, those receiving heart, heart-lung, liver, or pancreas transplants usually require numerous transfusions and therefore have an increased risk of TT-CMV. Early studies showed that even in heavily transfused organ transplant recipients, the

---

Table 40.3 Patients at Risk for Transfusion-Transmitted Cytomegalovirus (TT-CMV)

Category A: Clear morbidity and mortality from TT-CMV; CMV-safe components proven efficacious in decreasing incidence of TT-CMV and should be used for all transfusions
- Low-birth-weight infants (<1500 g) of seronegative mothers
- Seronegative recipients of autologous or seronegative allogeneic bone marrow transplants (BMT)
- Seronegative recipients of seronegative solid organ transplants, excluding renal and cardiac

Category B: Identified risk of morbidity and mortality from TT-CMV; benefit of CMV-safe products is possible or likely but not proven, consider using CMV-safe components when availability allows
- Seronegative pregnant women requiring antepartum blood transfusion or intrauterine transfusion
- Seropositive women requiring intrauterine transfusion
- Low-birth-weight infants or seronegative immunosuppressed patients requiring granulocyte transfusions
- Seronegative patients, infected with human immunodeficiency virus (HIV)
- Children born to HIV-infected mothers
- Low-birth-weight infants of seropositive mothers
- Seronegative patients who may be candidates for BMT

Category C: Morbidity and mortality of TT-CMV low or poorly documented, but probably greater than for category D; consider CMV-safe products on a case-by-case basis
- Infants with birth weight >1500 g born to seronegative mothers
- Neonates receiving extracorporeal membrane oxygenation (ECMO) or extensive transfusion support (e.g., exchange transfusions)
- Seronegative recipients of seronegative renal or cardiac transplants
- Seronegative patients receiving chemotherapy
- Seronegative patients experiencing major trauma or splenectomy

Category D: Low morbidity and mortality of TT-CMV; CMV-safe components not indicated
- Infants with birth weight >1500 g born to seropositive mothers
- All other transfusion recipients not listed

Modified from Preiksaitis JK: The cytomegalovirus-"safe" blood product: Is leukoreduction equivalent to antibody screening? Transfus Med Rev 2000; 14: 112–136, with permission.

use of seronegative blood products could effectively prevent TT-CMV.[175–177]

In addition to these patient populations with well-defined susceptibility to TT-CMV, there are other groups that may be susceptible to TT-CMV and may also benefit from transfusion of CMV-safe blood components (see Table 40.3). For example, it is well documented that primary CMV infection during pregnancy carries a high risk of congenital fetal infection. Although there is no evidence that primary maternal infection resulting from TT-CMV can in turn lead to fetal infection,[63, 151] it is prudent to provide CMV-safe blood components to pregnant women who are seronegative. Because of the high incidence of CMV reactivation and infection in seropositive BMT recipients, 69% in one study,[167] TT-CMV is not a significant concern in these patients. However, special components may be considered for seronegative patients who are candidates for BMT, including immunosuppressed oncology patients, to prevent infection before transplantation.

Blood Components Implicated in TT-CMV

Most evidence suggests that the primary vector for TT-CMV is the CMV-infected leukocyte (Table 40.4). TT-CMV has not been observed in patients who received blood components that were free of WBCs, arguing that plasma free virus is not significantly involved in the pathogenesis of TT-CMV.[178] For example, there was no evidence of TT-CMV in a group of 21 immunosuppressed seronegative recipients of seronegative BMT undergoing total plasma exchange, although they were exposed to an average of 47.6 ± 19.5 units of unscreened fresh frozen plasma (FFP).[179] The absence of TT-CMV after transfusion of FFP may be a result of the scarcity of plasma free virus in healthy seropositive donors, as well as neutralization of virus by anti-CMV antibodies.

In contrast, there is an abundance of evidence that TT-CMV can be mediated by WBCs in blood components and that the incidence of TT-CMV correlates with the WBC load. For example, multiple studies have demonstrated TT-CMV after transfusion of granulocytes, most often seropositive granulocyte preparations transfused to seronegative recipients.[149, 167, 180] RBC and platelet transfusions are also known to transmit TT-CMV[93] (see Table 40.4).

Comparison of data over the last 4 decades reveals a correlation between the decreased use of fresh blood since the 1960s and a decline in the incidence of TT-CMV produced by unscreened units over the same period.[181] Most early evidence suggested that fresh blood (used within 24 hours after donation) from seropositive donors was more infectious than stored blood.[141, 150] For example, in the initial descriptions, TT-CMV typically occurred after open heart surgery in which the patient was exposed to fresh whole blood.[134–136]

In nonimmunosuppressed seronegative transfusion recipients, 6 of 7 patients who seroconverted had received fresh whole blood, compared with 53 of 585 who did not seroconvert ($P < .001$).[150] Similar results were found in a pediatric study in which TT-CMV occurred in 13 (87%) of 15 children who received fresh blood, compared with 1 (17%) of 6 children who received blood that was more than 24 hours old ($P = .01$).[156] In the same study, none of the children who received only CMV-seronegative blood but 36% those who received unscreened blood developed TT-CMV.[156] Overall, the infection rate after transfusion of fresh blood has been documented at between 10% and 59% (reviewed by Lee and associates[156]). A decline in infectivity with storage has also been shown experimentally. When naturally infected blood obtained from AIDS patients with CMV viremia was refrigerated under standard conditions, CMV infectivity was rapidly lost during the first 5 days of storage.[182] However, not all studies have demonstrated an effect of product storage interval on the incidence of TT-CMV.[65, 144, 148, 183]

It is also useful to consider the percentage of donated blood components that can transmit CMV infection. In a review of 10 studies published between 1968 and 1988, including data from 2806 patients, Ho[181] calculated the changing risk of contracting TT-CMV over this period. The risk per unit of unscreened and unfiltered blood was calculated at 11% to 12% in 1968–1970 and remained at greater than 1% per unit until the early 1980s. However, the risk subsequently fell, to 0.4% or less by 1988. Possible reasons for changes in the epidemiology of TT-CMV include decreasing use of fresh blood, improved tools for CMV serologic screening of blood donors and recipients, implementation of improved protocols to screen for other viral infections, and exclusion of blood from homosexual men starting in the mid-1980s.[181] The risk of TT-CMV also varies with the type of transfusion recipient. In studies in which the recipients were immunosuppressed, 2.5% to 12% of unscreened blood components were estimated to be infectious.[65, 93, 140] Adler and colleagues[184] estimated that, although 5% of all units were capable of producing TT-CMV, 15% of seropositive units were potentially infectious. Among nonimmunosuppressed patients, in contrast, the risk may be as low as 0.14% of randomly selected units or 0.38% of seropositive units.

Pathobiology of TT-CMV Infections

Clinical evidence for the involvement of leukocytes in TT-CMV includes the observations that CMV is transmitted with high frequency by granulocyte transfusions from seropositive donors,[149] whereas the incidence of TT-CMV can be attenuated by removing leukocytes from blood components.[142, 185] Furthermore, these WBCs are in almost all cases latently infected.

Table 40.4 Component-Associated Risk of Transfusion-Transmitted Cytomegalovirus (TT-CMV)

Blood Component	TT-CMV Risk	Processing to Abrogate TT-CMV
Red cells	Yes	Screening, filtration, frozen deglycerolized
Platelets	Yes	Screening, filtration
Granulocytes	Yes	Screening
Fresh frozen plasma	No	n/a
Cryoprecipitate	No*	n/a
Clotting factors	No	n/a

*Not specifically tested, but other plasma-derived components have not been shown to be infectious for CMV; n/a, not applicable

When more than 1500 buffy coat samples from healthy blood donors were subjected to viral culture in multiple studies, only 2 samples (both seropositive) grew infectious CMV.[65, 88, 89] These results demonstrated that, when WBC-associated CMV is present, it is almost always in the latent state. Experimental studies have indicated that WBCs of the monocyte lineage are the most likely to carry latent CMV in seropositive donors[32] and therefore are likely to be of most importance for TT-CMV (see Fig. 40.1). Circulating, latently infected monocytes must be able to support viral reactivation from latency in order to mediate TT-CMV. Cultured monocytes derived from seronegative donors can be differentiated in vitro into multi-nucleated giant cells by exposure to allogeneic cells. The degree of differentiation was positively correlated with the level of CMV replication.[186] Latently infected monocytes and CD33+ bone marrow cells became permissive for CMV reactivation and viral replication after, respectively, exposure to T-cell–conditioned medium and hydrocortisone[187] and exposure to the combination of interferon-γ, tumor necrosis factor α, and interleukin-4[32] (see Fig. 40.1). When monocytes from healthy, seropositive donors were grown in a mitogen-stimulated culture system containing allogeneic adherent mononuclear cells, the resulting differentiated monocyte-derived macrophages initiated production of infectious CMV.[31] These studies demonstrated that naturally infected PBMNCs contain latent CMV and that exposure to allogeneic cells or to appropriate cytokine milieus, such as would be encountered in transfusion recipients, renders them permissive to viral reactivation with production of infectious CMV[32] (see Fig. 40.1).

There may be additional factors, including recipient-related mechanisms that modulate the incidence and severity of TT-CMV.[63] For example, compared with immunologically competent transfusion recipients, patients who are immunocompromised have higher rates of TT-CMV and CMV diseases such as retinitis, esophagitis, and interstitial pneumonitis.[67, 142] Even among immunocompromised patients, there are factors that can affect a recipient's susceptibility to CMV infection and disease. Among recipients of cadaveric renal transplants who were at risk for CMV infection, the immunosuppressive regimen employed significantly influenced survival.[188] The development of GVHD affects the incidence of CMV infection and disease in BMT recipients.[167, 168] In a study of 181 recipients of allogeneic BMT, CMV infections occurred in 34 of 81 patients who developed acute GVHD, compared with 20 of 100 patients who did not ($P < .001$). Of the 34 patients who developed both CMV infection and GVHD, diagnosis of GVHD preceded the onset of CMV infection by a mean of 33.7 days, suggesting that GVHD predisposed the patients to CMV infection.[170] A comparison of seronegative recipients of either autologous or seronegative allogeneic transplants showed that both groups had similar rates of TT-CMV, but the incidence of CMV interstitial pneumonitis was significantly greater after allogeneic transplantation, particularly if the allogeneic recipients developed GVHD.[159–161] Preiksaitis[63] recently suggested that the following factors may also predispose to TT-CMV: sequential transfusion over a long period (as opposed to large transfusion volumes given at one time), the use of HLA-matched donors, repetitive transfusions from the same donor, and the degree of immunosuppression and cytokine expression profile in the host.[63] However, the biologic variables potentially affecting TT-CMV are difficult to dissect in the clinical setting, and

probably are more amenable to investigation in experimental models. For example, a murine model of TT-CMV has been developed in which the incidence of TT-CMV is affected by viral load and by MHC mismatches between blood donor and recipient.[189, 190]

Prevention of TT-CMV

The incidence of TT-CMV, as well as other untoward effects of transfusion, can be reduced by limiting transfusions to appropriate, clinically indicated circumstances. However, if transfusions are necessary, the most common approach to decrease the risk of TT-CMV is the use of either CMV-seronegative or filtered components (see Table 40.4). Nonetheless, it is clear that there remains a small residual risk of TT-CMV associated with the use of either type of component.[185]

SERONEGATIVE BLOOD COMPONENTS

Multiple studies, including prospective, randomized, controlled trials, have demonstrated that exclusive use of CMV-seronegative units for transfusion can decrease the incidence of TT-CMV, compared with the use of unscreened units.[93, 150, 153, 155, 156, 191] In an early study, none of 90 seronegative newborns transfused with seronegative components contracted CMV infection, compared with 13.5% of seronegative newborns who received transfusions from seropositive donors.[93] The exclusive use of seronegative units in immunocompromised adult seronegative recipients of allogeneic seronegative BMT also decreased both the incidence of TT-CMV and the severity of resulting CMV disease, compared with the use of unscreened blood products.[155] However, the use of seronegative units was beneficial only in seronegative recipients of seronegative donor marrow. Seronegative recipients of seropositive BMT had a 46% incidence of CMV infection when transfused with unscreened blood, which was not significantly different from the 32% incidence when these patients received seronegative blood products.[155] The absence of a beneficial effect of seronegative transfusions for seronegative recipients of seropositive BMT was also observed in another study.[153] Among nonimmunosuppressed seronegative patients, transfusion of seronegative blood components can also prevent TT-CMV,[150] although there are few indications for the use of seronegative blood in this population. Based on these and other data, seronegative units remain the gold standard for the prevention of TT-CMV in susceptible transfusion recipients (see Table 40.4).

Despite exclusive use of seronegative units for transfusion, up to 4% of susceptible recipients have developed TT-CMV.[153, 155, 185] False-negative donor serology may have contributed to some of these cases of breakthrough TT-CMV, particularly in studies that used earlier-generation serology assays.[152, 191] Even sensitive and specific current EIA-based and particle agglutination assays, which detect anti-CMV antibodies of IgG, IgM, and in some cases IgA classes, can show significant disagreement when applied to samples from blood donors.[64] Alternatively, some of the donors may have been in the 6- to 8-week "window phase" after primary CMV infection, during which anti-CMV antibodies cannot be detected reliably[62] (see Fig. 40.2). During this period, there are high peripheral blood viral loads,[62] suggesting that transfusions from these apparently seronegative donors may be infectious. Detection of anti-CMV antibodies of the IgM class early during the course of infection appears to be important for prevention of TT-CMV.[192] In one study, patients who received components with detectable IgM anti-CMV antibodies had a TT-CMV rate of 8.4% (7 of 83 recipients), compared with a rate of 0.3% (1 of 280 patients) among those who received blood without IgM anti-CMV ($P<.001$).[193] In this same study, only 1 of 163 neonates who received seropositive but IgM-negative blood developed TT-CMV.[193] However, other investigators found that screening for IgM anti-CMV antibodies had poor sensitivity and specificity for identifying infectious blood components.[63]

FILTERED BLOOD COMPONENTS

The seroprevalence rate for CMV ranges from 40% to 80% in the United States.[4, 64, 67] The difficulties in maintaining a sufficient inventory of CMV-seronegative blood components motivated efforts to identify alternative strategies to provide CMV-safe components for susceptible patients. Because WBCs latently infected with CMV are the primary vector for TT-CMV, removal of WBCs from components was an obvious approach to mitigate TT-CMV. Current third-generation filtration technology can produce a 3- to 4-$\log_{10}$ reduction in monocytes and other leukocytes in blood components.[194] Alternatively, platelets can be prepared from donors by apheresis procedures, resulting in process-leukoreduced components with approximately 10^5 to 10^6 residual leukocytes, depending on instrumentation and separation technique.[195] This level of leukoreduction has been shown to significantly reduce the incidence of TT-CMV in multiple studies.[142, 154, 196–199]

In the largest prospective, randomized, controlled clinical trial to address this issue to date, 502 seronegative recipients of autologous or seronegative allogeneic BMT were randomly assigned to receive either unscreened blood products leukoreduced by filtration at the bedside or CMV-seronegative components.[185] Between 21 and 100 days after transplantation, the predefined window phase for identifying TT-CMV, the probabilities of developing CMV infection were similar in patients receiving filtered units and in those receiving seronegative components (2.4% versus 1.3%, respectively; $P=1.00$). The probabilities of developing CMV disease were also similar in these two groups (2.4% versus 0%, respectively; $P=1.00$). Based on an intention-to-treat analysis, the authors concluded that the seronegative and the filtered units carried equivalent risks of TT-CMV. The interpretation of this study was complicated by an analysis of all data from days 0 through 100 that showed a statistically greater progression to CMV disease in the group receiving filtered components (2.4%, compared with 0% among those receiving CMV-seronegative components; $P=.03$). In fact, five of six patients who contracted CMV from filtered units developed CMV disease that progressed to fatal CMV pneumonia, whereas none of four patients infected with CMV from seronegative components developed CMV disease ($P = .005$ by Fisher's exact test).[185, 200] The biologic basis for this difference remains unexplained,[200, 201] leaving open the possibility that there are differences between filtered and seronegative units with respect to the risk of TT-CMV. However, it should be noted that bedside filtration, as used in this study, is unlikely to produce the degree and reproducibility of leukoreduction achievable with prestorage filtration methods.

In a recent review, Preiksaitis[63] provided a detailed discussion of the theoretical and observed differences between CMV-seronegative units and filtered units. The current American Association of Blood Banks (AABB) guidelines state that a component with less than 5×10^6 residual leukocytes may be considered CMV-safe,[202] although it has been suggested that this guideline be revised downward to 1×10^6 leukocytes in the future.

OTHER COMMON COMPONENT-PROCESSING METHODOLOGIES

In seronegative neonates, the exclusive use of frozen deglycerolized RBCs markedly reduces the incidence of TT-CMV, providing a third option for patients at risk for TT-CMV.[142, 203, 204] However, given the labor-intensive nature of preparing frozen deglycerolized RBCs, this approach is rarely used.

In contrast, it is unclear whether washing of components can adequately decrease the incidence of TT-CMV. In one study of seronegative neonates, transfusion of washed RBCs from seropositive donors was associated with a 1.3% incidence of TT-CMV,[205] which was less than the historical incidence of 13% to 37%.[93, 153–155] However, in another study, transfusion of washed RBCs resulted in an 11.1% incidence of TT-CMV in seronegative neonates.[206] Given these conflicting data together with the logistics of washing blood components, this procedure cannot be recommended as a preparation of CMV-safe blood components.

Likewise, standard γ-irradiation protocols used to prevent transfusion-associated GVHD are not effective at abrogating TT-CMV.

IMMUNOGLOBULIN PREPARATIONS AND ANTIVIRAL DRUGS

The efficacy of passively acquired maternal anti-CMV antibodies to abrogate CMV infection and disease in neonates suggested that CMV immunoglobulin preparations may be useful in immunocompromised adults. In an early randomized trial of prophylactic hyperimmune CMV IVIG, BMT recipients receiving IVIG were protected against CMV infection ($P=.009$), interstitial pneumonia, and CMV mortality ($P=.014$), compared with the control group.[207] Other studies have produced similar findings.[208] A meta-analysis derived from 12 published clinical trials of prophylactic IVIG in BMT recipients confirmed that passive CMV antibodies can significantly reduce fatal CMV infection (95% confidence interval [CI], 0.23 to 0.99), CMV pneumonitis (95% CI, 0.42 to 0.89), non-CMV interstitial pneumonia (95% CI, 0.35 to 0.95), and total CMV mortality (95% CI, 0.55 to 0.99).[94] However, the efficacy of IVIG in preventing TT-CMV is more difficult to assess. For example, when seronegative study patients were transfused with seronegative blood (the current standard of care), there was no significant effect of IVIG on CMV infection and disease.[153] Furthermore, intramuscular CMV IVIG was ineffective at preventing TT-CMV in seronegative patients who received seropositive granulocyte infusions.[209]

In recipients of allogeneic BMT, ganciclovir can provide effective prophylaxis against CMV disease.[210, 211] However, ganciclovir can also cause untoward effects, including marrow suppression with neutropenia, delayed reconstitution of cellular immunity predisposing to opportunistic infections, and outgrowth of resistant viral mutants.[212–214] Even limited use of ganciclovir caused severe neutropenia in 33% (10 of 30) of treated patients, 7 of whom subsequently developed opportunistic infections.[215] Furthermore, despite adequate control of CMV infection in these patients, they experienced increased mortality from other infectious complications including *Aspergillus fumigatus*, *Streptococcus pneumoniae*, and *Pneumocystis carinii* pneumonia.[215] In a randomized, placebo-controlled trial of prophylactic ganciclovir in BMT recipients, use of ganciclovir led to delayed recovery of anti-CMV CTL activity, which might predispose patients to late-onset CMV disease.[101] Up to 15% of BMT recipients develop late CMV disease after discontinuation of ganciclovir prophylaxis,[210] and the mortality of late-onset disease approaches 70%.[101] Prolonged ganciclovir therapy can also lead to the selection of drug-resistant CMV mutants. In one study, 5 (38%) of 13 AIDS patients treated with ganciclovir for longer than 3 months shed resistant mutant virus.[216] Children receiving T-cell–depleted BMT also appear to be at increased risk for development of ganciclovir-resistant mutants, as well as strains resistant to the antiviral compounds foscarnet and cidofovir.[217] These concerns underscore the importance of preventing CMV transmission rather than treating resulting CMV infections and disease.[218] Furthermore, when compared with the proven efficacy of seronegative or filtered units to decrease the incidence of TT-CMV, the use of IVIG or antiviral agents (or both) would be more expensive and possibly not as effective; therefore, these interventions cannot be recommended as a means for abrogation of TT-CMV.

NAT-SCREENED COMPONENTS

With standard serologic assays, both uninfected donors and those in the window phase of a CMV infection test as seronegative. Some window-phase donors have high plasma- and WBC-associated viral loads; therefore, although their blood is seronegative, it may be infectious on transfusion.[62, 90] Blood components from most CMV-seropositive donors do not produce TT-CMV, but serologic testing is unable to distinguish these units from infectious seropositive units. Filter leukoreduction decreases the incidence of TT-CMV, but immunocompromised patients who acquire TT-CMV from filtered blood can develop significant CMV-associated disease.[185] Therefore, neither serologic screening nor leukoreduction produces a blood supply that is completely CMV-safe. In analogy with nucleic acid testing (NAT) screening for HIV and hepatitis C virus, NAT screening for CMV DNA may identify blood components that can produce TT-CMV and may serve as a useful adjunct to serology and filtration.

Because most seropositive donors are remotely infected (longer than 6 months before donation), they are likely to have peripheral blood viral loads near or below the limits of detection of even sensitive NAT assays. Assays sufficiently sensitive to detect these low viral loads may be subject to problems including nonspecific amplification of background DNA. For this reason, it is not surprising that several studies investigating the presence of CMV DNA in healthy blood donors have yielded conflicting results. Some investigators identified CMV DNA in WBCs or isolated monocytes from both seropositive and seronegative donors.[219–221] In a study of 270 healthy blood donors in Sweden, the use of a nested PCR technique demonstrated CMV DNA in PBMNCs from 14% of seronegative donors using both UL123 and UL32 PCR assays, although the CMV DNA detection rate increased to 55% when monocyte-enriched samples from seronegative

donors were assayed.[222] These investigators also identified CMV DNA in 100% of seropositive donors. In contrast, other investigators have been unable or only rarely able to identify CMV by PCR in peripheral blood from seropositive or seronegative donors.[79, 90, 121, 122, 124, 223–225] These latter findings appear more consistent with the clinical observations that seronegative blood components only rarely transmit CMV infection to transfusion recipients and that only 0.4% to 12% of seropositive blood units appear capable of CMV transmission.[150, 151, 175] The variability of the results in these prior studies demonstrate that technical hurdles remain before implementation of CMV NAT for testing of the blood supply.

In order to identify CMV PCR assays with appropriate performance characteristics for screening healthy blood donors, a multicenter trial was undertaken to determine the sensitivity, specificity, and reproducibility of seven previously described assays.[226] In practice, the DNA yield from 250,000 WBCs (approximately 2 μg of DNA) is the maximum tolerated input for most PCR assays. Based on estimates that 0.004% to 0.12% of PBMNCs are latently infected,[31, 34] it was predicted that an average of 4 to 120 latently infected cells would be present per 250,000 WBCs (PBMNCs typically comprise 40% of WBCs). Given the reported presence of 2 to 13 viral genomes per latently infected cell,[34] it was hypothesized that PCR assays used in donor screening should be sufficiently sensitive to detect 8 to 1560 CMV GE 250,000 WBCs. Five of the examined assays displayed sufficient sensitivity for donor screening based on consistent detection of a minimum of 25 CMV GE in analytical controls constructed to contain from 1 to 100 CMV GE in background DNA from 250,000 cells.[226] Of these five assays, two detected CMV DNA in a subset of 20 pedigreed CMV-seronegative samples. However, these results were found to be inconsistent when the seronegative samples were reanalyzed. The other three sensitive assays did not detect CMV DNA in the seronegative samples, and two of these tests were selected for further study. These assays, a nested PCR directed at the CMV UL93 ORF and the Roche Monitor assay, were used to screen 1000 blood samples from healthy donors.[64] Of the 416 seropositive donor samples, two (0.5%) tested positive for CMV DNA with both assays, whereas seven other samples tested positive on only one assay and did not confirm on retesting. When the two positive samples were subjected to limiting-dilution analysis they were found to have viral loads of 1 to 10 copies per 250,000 WBCs, demonstrating that CMV DNA loads in healthy blood donors are at or below the limits of detection of even sensitive PCR assays. Six of the seronegative samples tested positive on only one assay and were not confirmed on repeat testing. These results suggested that only a small percentage of seropositive samples from healthy blood donors have viral loads that are reproducibly detectable by extremely sensitive PCR assays, potentially limiting the use of PCR to prevent TT-CMV. The minimal viral load required for TT-CMV has not been determined, and it must be assumed at present that any CMV-seropositive or CMV DNA-positive unit is potentially infectious.

VIRAL INACTIVATION, CMV VACCINATION, AND ADOPTIVE IMMUNOTHERAPY TO DECREASE THE INCIDENCE OF TT-CMV

As opposed to current approaches such as the use of seronegative and filtered components, the application of pathogen inactivation technology to cellular blood components carries the potential for completely preventing TT-CMV, as well as eliminating the transmission of other infectious agents. The psoralen derivative 8-methoxypsoralen (8-MOP), when exposed to ultraviolet light, inactivates a spectrum of both gram-positive and gram-negative organisms that can contaminate platelet components, including *Staphylococcus aureus, Staphylococcus epidermidis, Escherichia coli, Yersinia enterocolitica, Salmonella choleraesuis, Serratia marcescens,* and *Pseudomonas aeruginosa.*[227] Bacterial concentrations of 10^4 to 10^7 colony-forming units (CFU) per milliliter can be inactivated, which compares favorably with estimated bacterial concentrations of 10 to 10^3 CFU/mL in naturally infected units.[228] In vitro platelet function was not adversely affected[227] by 8-MOP treatment. Similar results were recently reported with another psoralen derivative, S-59, which could efficiently inactivate more than 10^6 plaque-forming units per milliliter of HIV, duck hepatitis B virus, or bovine diarrhea virus (a model for hepatitis C virus) in experimentally infected platelet components.[229]

Viral inactivation technology has now entered clinical trials and has been the subject of several detailed reviews.[230–232] Given the limited risk of transfusion-associated CMV disease in seropositive recipients, vaccination of seronegative patients before immunosuppression may mitigate the risks of CMV in this population. Use of an attenuated Towne CMV strain as a live virus vaccine in 237 renal transplant recipients demonstrated that vaccinated seronegative recipients of seropositive grafts rates of infection similar to those of unvaccinated controls but experienced less severe disease. Furthermore, the survival of cadaveric renal grafts at 36 months was improved by vaccination ($P = 0.04$ compared with the control group).[233] Although there were no episodes of Towne CMV reactivation after latency among these immunosuppressed patients, this possibility must be considered when evaluating the safety of this approach. The use of recombinant CMV proteins as subunit vaccines represents a potentially safer method of vaccination. In experimental settings, recombinant gB protein can induce protective immunity,[96] and anti-gB antibodies in naturally infected donors comprise a large component of the CMV-neutralizing activity in seropositive donor serum.[11, 96]

Recovery of CMV-specific CTLs after BMT provides protection from CMV infection and disease.[97–99, 101] However, at 40 days after transplantation, 65% of BMT recipients had deficient CD8+ CTL responses in one study.[99] In immunocompromised patients who cannot mount an effective CTL response, passive transfer of CTLs is an attractive approach to augment cellular immunity. However, early attempts to restore cellular immunity through administration of unselected donor T cells to BMT recipients was associated with GVHD.[234–236] In an alternative approach, CD3+, CD8+, CD4–, CMV-specific CTLs were cloned from CMV-seropositive marrow donors, expanded in culture, and then infused into BMT recipients.[237] Each recipient received four infusions, 1 week apart, in escalating doses. Importantly, the CMV antigen-specific CTLs did not produce GVHD or other morbidity in recipients.[237] Further studies demonstrated that transferred clones could persist and retain anti-CMV cytotoxic activity for at least 12 weeks after infusion.[238] However, CTL activity declined if recipient anti-CMV CD4+ T cells were not generated. There was no evidence of CMV viremia or disease in any patient receiving CTL therapy.[238]

Although adoptive cellular immunotherapy is an attractive approach for prophylaxis in immunocompromised patients, the currently used methods for deriving and expanding donor CTL clones are lengthy, labor-intensive, and costly. However, as this technology improves and becomes more commonplace, transfusion medicine physicians will probably play a significant role in the procurement, processing, and administration of CTL components.

RECOMMENDATIONS

Based on the data presented here, the exclusive use of CMV-seronegative blood components remains the standard of care for the transfusion of seronegative, immunocompromised patients who are susceptible to TT-CMV (see Table 40.4). If seronegative units are not available, the evidence suggests that filtered, unscreened components are an acceptable substitute. Although the AABB guidelines state that seronegative and leukoreduced units are equivalent for prevention of TT-CMV,[239] other panels that have reviewed this issue are in disagreement. For example, Swiss clinical practice recommendations consider seronegative units to be the gold standard for prevention of TT-CMV and conclude that leukoreduced units have not yet been proven equivalent for this purpose.[240] A Canadian consensus conference reached similar conclusions when the majority of the panel agreed that seronegative blood components should continue to be provided to at-risk patients despite implementation of universal leukoreduction in Canada.[241] The use of frozen deglycerolized RBCs is also an acceptable alternative to the use of seronegative units, but their preparation is expensive and labor-intensive. In contrast, washed RBC and platelet components cannot be considered CMV-safe. The use of IVIG and ganciclovir, or other antiviral drugs, is unlikely to be clinically efficacious or cost-effective for the prevention of TT-CMV.

At the present time, there is no compelling scientific argument for the implementation of CMV NAT screening to prevent TT-CMV. Using the most sensitive and reproducible PCR tests currently available, only about 0.2% of blood donations are found to contain CMV DNA. Furthermore, there are no studies to correlate the risk of TT-CMV with the presence of CMV DNA, although such an association is theoretically attractive. Nonetheless, the potential of CMV NAT to detect seronegative window-phase donations, as well as components that retain a residual CMV load after filtration, remains an interesting possibility to be evaluated. However, implementation of CMV vaccination or virus-inactivated cellular blood components in the future is likely to render these issues moot.

■ Epstein-Barr Virus (HHV-4)

The genome of EBV, a gamma-herpesvirus, is 172 kb in length. Two genetically distinguishable types of EBV exist, EBV-1 and EBV-2, as well a number of variants resulting from genomic recombination. In immunocompetent patients, primary infection with EBV results in a spectrum of clinical sequelae ranging from asymptomatic infection to heterophile-positive infectious mononucleosis.[35, 242] EBV can also cause lymphomagenesis, as can the other human gamma-herpesvirus, HHV-8. EBV is an etiologic agent in endemic Burkitt's lymphoma, AIDS-related lymphoma, post-transplantation lymphoproliferative disease (PTLD), and nasopharyngeal carcinoma.[242]

After immune-mediated resolution of acute infection, EBV is not completely eliminated but rather achieves a lifelong latent state. The EBV genome is episomal in latently infected B cells, which probably represent the true EBV reservoir in the latently infected host. One in every 10^5 to 10^6 B cells is estimated to be latently infected after primary infection. Latent EBV in B cells may undergo sporadic reactivation with subsequent release of infectious progeny virus. Eleven viral gene products are known to be expressed during latent infection, including nuclear antigens (EBNA-1, -2, -3A, -3B, -3C, and -LP), membrane proteins (LMP-1, -2A, and -2B), and noncoding nuclear RNAs (EBER-1 and -2).[35] These latent gene products disrupt B-cell regulatory mechanisms, leading to the characteristic polyclonal B-cell lymphoproliferation seen in infectious mononucleosis.

EBV is transmitted by close contact, and the majority of the adult population (>95%) has been infected with EBV, based on serologic investigations. Seropositive individuals are at risk for reactivation of latent EBV infection if they become immunocompromised, for example in the setting of pharmacologic immunosuppression for organ or marrow transplantation.[242] However, the most significant EBV-associated risk is that of primary EBV infection occurring during immunosuppression for transplantation. Primary infection can be community acquired, or it can result from blood transfusion or transplantation from an EBV-seropositive donor.[242] An important clinical example is pediatric orthotopic liver transplantation, where EBV-associated PTLD has been identified in 10% to 20% of patients immunosuppressed with tacrolimus.[243-245] PTLD encompasses a range of disorders from benign polyclonal B-cell lymphoid hyperplasia to malignant high-grade non-Hodgkin's lymphoma. In pediatric orthopic liver transplantation, PTLD is a cause of significant morbidity, including graft loss,[246] as well as mortality rates of up to 20%.[247]

Transmission of EBV by blood transfusion can manifest in a similar manner to classic infectious mononucleosis. As with TT-CMV, viral genotyping has been used to document TT-EBV from a blood donor to a recipient, who subsequently developed EBV-driven PTLD.[248] In most cases of TT-EBV the blood donor was found to be in the incubation period for infectious mononucleosis, with high B-cell viral loads.[249] Although the use of EBV-seronegative blood components may reduce the incidence of TT-EBV, they are difficult to obtain given the high seroprevalence of EBV (Table 40.5). Because EBV is highly B-cell associated and B cells are efficiently removed by blood filtration,[194] exclusive use of leukoreduced cellular blood components for transfusion is likely to decrease the probability of TT-EBV infection in at-risk seronegative patients. However, this possibility has not been subject to controlled clinical trials.

■ Human Herpesvirus 6

HHV-6 was first identified in lymphocytes from AIDS patients with lymphoproliferative diseases, and it was originally named human B-cell lymphotropic virus.[250] However, the primary tropism of HHV-6 is now recognized to be CD4+ T lymphocytes, although it can also infect CD8+ T cells, NK cells, monocytes, macrophages, and megakaryocytes. The linear double-stranded DNA genome of HHV-6 consists of a 143-kb unique segment flanked by 8- to 13-kb terminal direct repeats. Overall, there is 66% sequence similarity between HHV-6 and CMV, the prototypical beta-herpesvirus,[251] and greater than 90% sequence similarity between the two HHV-6 variants, HHV-6A and HHV-6B.

HHV-6B is the principal etiologic agent of the childhood illness roseola infantum (sixth disease), which manifests with a fever of 2 to 5 days' duration followed by a maculopapular skin rash (exanthem subitum) and rapid defervescence.[252] Serologic investigations have demonstrated that HHV-6 is endemic, with at least 70% of children infected by 1 year of age[253] and more than 90% of the population displaying evidence of community-acquired infection during infancy. HHV-6, like other herpesviruses, can persist in a latent state, possibly within PBMNCs. In addition to roseola infantum, in immunocompetent individuals there is a weak association between HHV-6 infection and diseases including heterophile-negative mononucleosis, hepatitis, multiple sclerosis, chronic fatigue syndrome, hemophagocytic syndrome, encephalitis, Rosai-Dorfman disease, Kawasaki disease, Kikuchi disease, sarcoidosis, a variety of lymphoproliferative disorders, and rare cases of anemia and granulocytopenia.[254] However, significant problems are rare in immunocompetent individuals. In contrast, immunocompromised patients can experience HHV-6-related complications including fever, leukopenia, graft rejection, interstitial pneumonitis, encephalitis, and marrow suppression.[255-258] Fatal HHV-6 encephalitis has been documented after BMT.[259]

HHV-6 transmission by BMT and solid organ transplantation has been demonstrated.[256, 260] However, although PCR analysis of PBMNCs showed HHV-6 DNA in up to 90% of blood donors,[261] HHV-6 transmission by blood transfusion has not been definitively documented (see Table 40.5). In analogy

Table 40.5 Transfusion Transmission of Leukocyte-Associated Human Herpesviruses

Virus	% of Recipients Who Are Seronegative	Morbidity after Transfusion Transmission	Special Components for Susceptible Recipients	
			Seronegative Donor	Filtered
CMV	20%–60%	Yes	Acceptable	Acceptable
EBV	<5%	Rare	n/a	?
HHV-6	<5%	Not documented	n/a	?
HHV-7	<5%	Not documented	n/a	?
HHV-8	70%–95%	Not documented	n/a	?

n/a, not routinely available; ?, No clinical evidence for reduction in the risk of transfusion-transmission, but possibly effective since viruses are leukocyte-associated with EBV, another highly seroprevalent WBC-associated HHV, seronegative units are not generally available for transfusion of susceptible recipients. Although filtered components are hypothesized to reduce the risk of TT-HHV-6, clinical efficacy has not been shown.

Human Herpesvirus 7

Along with HHV-6A, HHV-7 is the only other HHV with primary tropism for T lymphocytes. HHV-6 and HHV-7 are closely related beta-herpesviruses, with an overall 40% sequence similarity. The HHV-7 genome consists of a long unique segment of 133 kb, flanked by single direct repeats of approximately 6 kb on each end.[262] HHV-7, which was originally isolated in 1990 from CD4+ T lymphocytes of a healthy individual,[263] displays much more restricted tropism than HHV-6 does. In culture, HHV-7 can infect only activated CD4+ T cells and the CD4+ cell line SupT1,[264] although in vivo HHV-7 also infects cells of the salivary glands.[265] Infections occur slightly later in life with HHV-7 than with HHV-6, but most children are seropositive by 5 years of age. Although a causative role for HHV-7 in pityriasis rosea and a minority of cases of exanthem subitum has been suggested,[266–268] the spectrum of diseases attributable to this virus is still unclear. Because HHV-7 infects CD4+ T cells and viral DNA was identified in WBCs from 66% of German blood donors,[269] HHV-7 may be transmissible by blood transfusion. The same considerations regarding TT-HHV-6 apply to this virus (see Table 40.5).

Human Herpesvirus 8

HHV-8, a gamma-herpesvirus also known as Kaposi sarcoma herpesvirus, was originally isolated from Kaposi sarcoma (KS) skin lesions using representational difference analysis.[270] The HHV-8 genome is approximately 170 kb in size and encodes an estimated 81 ORFs.[271, 272] Sequence analysis revealed that HHV-8 is closely related to herpesvirus saimiri and the other human gamma-herpesvirus, EBV.[270] As with EBV, HHV-8 can cause uncontrolled proliferation of infected cells. In addition to KS, HHV-8 is also associated with primary effusion lymphoma and multicentric Castleman disease in patients with POEMS syndrome (polyneuropathy, organomegaly, endocrinopathy, M protein, and skin changes).[273–275] There is still significant debate concerning the role of HHV-8 in the pathogenesis of multiple myeloma and monoclonal gammopathy of undetermined significance (MGUS).[276, 277] If HHV-8 is present in multiple myeloma lesions, it is generally agreed that it is not in the malignant plasma cells, but rather in a subset of surrounding stromal cells. The case has been made that HHV-8 has not yet fulfilled Koch's postulates or Hill's epidemiologic criteria for causality of multiple myeloma.[277]

HHV-8 is transmitted primarily through sexual contact, and infection is rare before puberty. The seroprevalence of HHV-8 has been intensely investigated. In most studies, 1% to 11% of the healthy adults in Western countries had detectable anti-HHV-8 antibodies.[278–281] However, when HHV-8 lytic antigens were used as serologic targets, up to 25% of the general population, 90% of HIV-infected homosexual men, and almost all patients with KS had detectable antibodies.[282] HHV-8 can be transmitted by infected renal allografts

transplanted into seronegative recipients.[283] However, the same study argued against frequent transmission by blood products, because no episodes of HHV-8 seroconversion were documented among seronegative recipients of seronegative transplants who received blood transfusions. Nonetheless, HHV-8 DNA was identified in PBMCs of 55% of patients with KS[284] and in the blood of some renal transplantation patients.[285] An HHV-8 seroprevalence of 35% to 82% has been reported in healthy non-HIV–infected individuals in Central Africa.[279, 280, 282] Approximately 22% of apparently healthy Central African blood donors had low levels of WBC-associated HHV-8 DNA, compared with 0% to 2% of healthy Europeans.[284, 286, 287] These studies raise the question of whether HHV-8 may be transmissible by transfusion, although TT-HHV-8 has not been demonstrated.[288, 289] Although the risk of transmitting HHV-8 by blood transfusion is currently unclear, the clinical issues associated with providing HHV-8 "safe" blood components are more similar to those associated with CMV than with EBV, HHV-6, or HHV-7 (see Table 40.5). For this reason, it may be possible to provide either HHV-8-seronegative units or filtered components to abrogate the risk of TT-HHV-8. Further investigations are necessary to validate the efficacy and usefulness of these approaches.

REFERENCES

1. Roizman B: Herpesviridae. In Fields BN, et al. (eds): Fields Virology. Philadelphia: Lippincott-Raven, 1996, pp 2221–2230.
2. Roizmann B, et al: The family Herpesviridae: An update. The Herpesvirus Study Group of the International Committee on Taxonomy of Viruses. Arch Virol 1992;123:425–449.
3. Mach M, Stamminger T, Jahn G: Human cytomegalovirus: Recent aspects from molecular biology. J Gen Virol 1989;70:3117–3146.
4. Mocarski ES: Cytomegalovirus and their replication. In Fields BN, et al. (eds): Fields Virology. Philadelphia: Lippincott-Raven, 1996, pp 2447–2492.
5. LaFemina RL, Hayward GS: Replicative forms of human cytomegalovirus DNA with joined termini are found in permissively infected human cells but not in non-permissive Balb/c-3T3 mouse cells. J Gen Virol 1983;64:373–389.
6. Bolovan-Fritts CA, Mocarski ES, Wiedeman JA: Peripheral blood CD14(+) cells from healthy subjects carry a circular conformation of latent cytomegalovirus genome. Blood 1999;93:394–398.
7. Wright HTJ, Goodheart CR, Lielausis A: Human cytomegalovirus: Morphology by negative staining. Virology 1964;23:419–424.
8. Bresnahan WA, Shenk T: A subset of viral transcripts packaged within human cytomegalovirus particles. Science 2000;288:2373–2376.
9. Fish KN, et al: Human cytomegalovirus persistently infects aortic endothelial cells. J Virol 1998;72:5661–5668.
10. Chee MS, et al: Analysis of the protein-coding content of the sequence of human cytomegalovirus strain AD169. Curr Top Microbiol Immunol 1990;154:125–169.
11. Marshall GS, et al: Antibodies to recombinant-derived glycoprotein B after natural human cytomegalovirus infection correlate with neutralizing activity. J Infect Dis 1992;165:381–384.
12. Pietropaolo RL, Compton T: Direct interaction between human cytomegalovirus glycoprotein B and cellular annexin II. J Virol 1997;71:9803–9807.
13. Wright JF, Kurosky A, Wasi S: An endothelial cell-surface form of annexin II binds human cytomegalovirus. Biochem Biophys Res Commun 1994;198:983–989.
14. Compton T, Nowlin DM, Cooper NR: Initiation of human cytomegalovirus infection requires initial interaction with cell surface heparan sulfate. Virology 1993;193:834–841.
15. Boyle KA, Compton T: Receptor-binding properties of a soluble form of human cytomegalovirus glycoprotein B. J Virol 1998;72:1826–1833.
16. Pietropaolo R, Compton T: Interference with annexin II has no effect on entry of human cytomegalovirus into fibroblast cells. J Gen Virol 1999;80:1807–1816.

17. Keay S, Baldwin B: Anti-idiotype antibodies that mimic gp86 of human cytomegalovirus inhibit viral fusion but not attachment. J Virol 1991;65:5124–5128.

18. Huber MT, Compton T: Characterization of a novel third member of the human cytomegalovirus glycoprotein H-glycoprotein L complex. J Virol 1997;71:5391–5398.

19. Keay S, Merigan TC, Rasmussen L: Identification of cell surface receptors for the 86-kilodalton glycoprotein of human cytomegalovirus. Proc Natl Acad Sci U S A 1989;86:10100–10103.

20. Keay S, Baldwin B: The human fibroblast receptor for gp86 of human cytomegalovirus is a phosphorylated glycoprotein. J Virol 1992;66:4834–4838.

21. Boyle KA, Pietropaolo RL, Compton T: Engagement of the cellular receptor for glycoprotein B of human cytomegalovirus activates the interferon-responsive pathway. Mol Cell Biol 1999;19:3607–3613.

22. Keay S, et al: Increases in (Ca2+) i mediated by the 92.5-kDa putative cell membrane receptor for HCMV gp86. Am J Physiol 1995;269:C11–C21.

23. Grundy JE, McKeating JA, Griffiths PD: Cytomegalovirus strain AD169 binds beta 2 microglobulin in vitro after release from cells. J Gen Virol 1987;68:777–784.

24. Pizzorno MC, et al: Trans-activation and autoregulation of gene expression by the immediate-early region 2 gene products of human cytomegalovirus. J Virol 1988;62:1167–1179.

25. Stenberg RM, et al: Regulated expression of early and late RNAs and proteins from the human cytomegalovirus immediate-early gene region. J Virol 1989;63:2699–2708.

26. Malone CL, Vesole DH, Stinski MF: Transactivation of a human cytomegalovirus early promoter by gene products from the immediate-early gene IE2 and augmentation by IE1: Mutational analysis of the viral proteins. J Virol 1990;64:1498–1506.

27. Kari B, Radeke R, Gehrz R: Processing of human cytomegalovirus envelope glycoproteins in and egress of cytomegalovirus from human astrocytoma cells. J Gen Virol 1992;73:253–260.

28. Kondo K, Kaneshima H, Mocarski ES: Human cytomegalovirus latent infection of granulocyte-macrophage progenitors. Proc Natl Acad Sci U S A 1994;91:11879–11883.

29. Mendelson M, et al: Detection of endogenous human cytomegalovirus in CD34+ bone marrow progenitors. J Gen Virol 1996;77:3099–3102.

30. Zhuravskaya T et al: Spread of human cytomegalovirus (HCMV) after infection of human hematopoietic progenitor cells: Model of HCMV latency. Blood 1997;90:2482–2491.

31. Soderberg-Naucler C, Fish KN, Nelson JA: Reactivation of latent human cytomegalovirus by allogeneic stimulation of blood cells from healthy donors. Cell 1997;91:119–126.

32. Hahn G, Jores R, Mocarski ES: Cytomegalovirus remains latent in a common precursor of dendritic and myeloid cells. Proc Natl Acad Sci U S A 1998;95:3937–3942.

33. Koffron AJ, et al: Cellular localization of latent murine cytomegalovirus. J Virol 1998;72:95–103.

34. Slobedman B, Mocarski ES: Quantitative analysis of latent human cytomegalovirus. J Virol 1999;73:4806–4812.

35. Rickinson AB, Kieff E: Epstein-Barr virus. In Fields BN, et al. (eds): Fields Virology. Philadelphia: Lippincott-Raven, 1996, pp 2397–2446.

36. Kondo K, Xu J, Mocarski ES: Human cytomegalovirus latent gene expression in granulocyte-macrophage progenitors in culture and in seropositive individuals. Proc Natl Acad Sci U S A 1996;93:11137–11142.

37. Kondo K, Mocarski ES: Cytomegalovirus latency and latency-specific transcription in hematopoietic progenitors. Scand J Infect Dis Suppl 1995;99:63–67.

38. Adams A, Lindahl T: Epstein-Barr virus genomes with properties of circular DNA molecules in carrier cells. Proc Natl Acad Sci U S A 1975;72:1477–1481.

39. Gardella T, et al: Detection of circular and linear herpesvirus DNA molecules in mammalian cells by gel electrophoresis. J Virol 1984;50:248–254.

40. Decker LL, et al: The Kaposi sarcoma-associated herpesvirus (KSHV) is present as an intact latent genome in KS tissue but replicates in the peripheral blood mononuclear cells of KS patients. J Exp Med 1996;184:283–288.

41. Garcia-Blanco MA, Cullen BR: Molecular basis of latency in pathogenic human viruses. Science 1991;254:815–820.

42. Yu Y, et al: Expression of a murine cytomegalovirus early-late protein in "latently" infected mice. J Infect Dis 1995;172:371–379.

43. Jault FM, et al: Cytomegalovirus infection induces high levels of cyclins, phosphorylated Rb, and p53, leading to cell cycle arrest. J Virol 1995;69:6697–6704.

44. Dittmer D, Mocarski ES: Human cytomegalovirus infection inhibits G1/S transition. J Virol 1997;71:1629–1634.

45. Salvant BS, Fortunato EA, Spector DH: Cell cycle dysregulation by human cytomegalovirus: Influence of the cell cycle phase at the time of infection and effects on cyclin transcription. J Virol 1998;72:3729–3741.

46. Bresnahan WA, et al: Inhibition of cellular Cdk2 activity blocks human cytomegalovirus replication. Virology 1997;231:239–247.

47. Poma EE, et al: The human cytomegalovirus IE1-72 protein interacts with the cellular p107 protein and relieves p107-mediated transcriptional repression of an E2F-responsive promoter. J Virol 1996;7:7867–7877.

48. Hengel H, Brune W, Koszinowski UH: Immune evasion by cytomegalovirus: Survival strategies of a highly adapted opportunist. Trends Microbiol 1998;6:190–197.

49. Goldmacher VS, et al: A cytomegalovirus-encoded mitochondria-localized inhibitor of apoptosis structurally unrelated to Bcl-2. Proc Natl Acad Sci U S A 1999;96:12536–12541.

50. Fish KN, Britt W, Nelson JA: A novel mechanism for persistence of human cytomegalovirus in macrophages. J Virol 1996;70:1855–1862.

51. Emery VC, et al: The dynamics of human cytomegalovirus replication in vivo. J Exp Med 1999;190:177–182.

52. Hengel H, et al: Macrophages escape inhibition of major histocompatibility complex class I-dependent antigen presentation by cytomegalovirus. J Virol 2000;74:7861–7868.

53. Beersma MF, Bijlmakers MJ, Ploegh HL: Human cytomegalovirus down-regulates HLA class I expression by reducing the stability of class I H chains. J Immunol 1993;151:4455–4464.

54. Wiertz EJ, Mukherjee S, Ploegh HL: Viruses use stealth technology to escape from the host immune system. Mol Med Today 1997;3:116–123.

55. Riddell SR, et al: Class I MHC-restricted cytotoxic T lymphocyte recognition of cells infected with human cytomegalovirus does not require endogenous viral gene expression. J Immunol 1991;146:2795–2804.

56. Riddell SR, et al: Selective reconstitution of CD8+ cytotoxic T lymphocyte responses in immunodeficient bone marrow transplant recipients by the adoptive transfer of T cell clones. Bone Marrow Transplant 1994;14(Suppl 4):S78–S84.

57. Heise MT, Connick M, Virgin HWT: Murine cytomegalovirus inhibits interferon gamma-induced antigen presentation to CD4 T cells by macrophages via regulation of expression of major histocompatibility complex class II-associated genes. J Exp Med 1998;187:1037–1046.

58. Hoglund P, et al: Host MHC class I gene control of NK-cell specificity in the mouse. Immunol Rev 1997;155:11–28.

59. Farrell HE, et al: Inhibition of natural killer cells by a cytomegalovirus MHC class I homologue in vivo. Nature 1997;386:510–514.

60. Dworsky ME, et al: Occupational risk for primary cytomegalovirus infection among pediatric health-care workers. N Engl J Med 1983;309:950–953.

61. Stagno S, Cloud GA: Working parents: The impact of day care and breast-feeding on cytomegalovirus infections in offspring. Proc Natl Acad Sci U S A 1994;91:2384–2389.

62. Zanghellini F, et al: Asymptomatic primary cytomegalovirus infection: Virologic and immunologic features. J Infect Dis 1999;180:702–707.

63. Preiksaitis JK: The cytomegalovirus—"safe" blood product: Is leukoreduction equivalent to antibody screening? Transfus Med Rev 2000;14:112–136.

64. Roback JD, et al: Cytomegalovirus (CMV) DNA is detected infrequently in healthy US blood donors: Results of a multicenter trial. Transfusion 2000;40:20S.

65. Adler SP: Transfusion-associated cytomegalovirus infections. Rev Infect Dis 1983;5:977–993.

66. Stagno S, et al: Primary cytomegalovirus infection in pregnancy: Incidence, transmission to fetus, and clinical outcome. JAMA 1986;256:1904–1908.

67. Britt WJ, Alford DA: Cytomegalovirus. In Fields BN, et al. (eds): Fields Virology. Philadelphia: Lippincott-Raven, 1996, pp 2493–2523.

68. Stagno S, et al: Congenital cytomegalovirus infection: The relative importance of primary and recurrent maternal infection. N Engl J Med 1982;306:945–949.

69. Alford CA, et al: Congenital and perinatal cytomegalovirus infections. Rev Infect Dis 1990;12(Suppl 7):S745–S753.

70. Reiser H, et al: Human cytomegalovirus replicates in primary human bone marrow cells. J Gen Virol 1986;67:2595–2604.

71. Maciejewski JP, et al: Infection of hematopoietic progenitor cells by human cytomegalovirus. Blood 1992;80:170–178.

72. von Laer D, et al: Detection of cytomegalovirus DNA in CD34+ cells from blood and bone marrow. Blood 1995:86:4086–4090.

73. Sindre H, et al: Human cytomegalovirus suppression of and latency in early hematopoietic progenitor cells. Blood 1996;88:4526–4533.

74. Soderberg-Naucler C, Fish KN, Nelson JA: Interferon-gamma and tumor necrosis factor-alpha specifically induce formation of cytomegalovirus-permissive monocyte-derived macrophages that are refractory to the antiviral activity of these cytokines. J Clin Invest 1997;100:3154–3163.

75. Gerna G, et al: Human cytomegalovirus infection of the major leukocyte subpopulations and evidence for initial viral replication in polymorphonuclear leukocytes from viremic patients. J Infect Dis 1992;166:1236–1244.

76. Revello MG, et al: In vitro generation of human cytomegalovirus pp65 antigenemia, viremia, and leukoDNAemia. J Clin Invest 1998;101:2686–2692.

77. Crapnell K, et al: In vitro infection of megakaryocytes and their precursors by human cytomegalovirus. Blood 2000;95:487–493.

78. Vonka V, Benyeshmelnick M: Thermoinactivation of human cytomegalovirus. J Bacteriol 1966;91:221–226.

79. Tegtmeier GE, et al: CMV DNA in plasma of seroconverting and anti-CMV seroprevalent blood donors [Abstract]. Transfusion 1999;39(Suppl 10):116s.

80. Schaade L, et al: Detection of cytomegalovirus DNA in human specimens by LightCycler PCR. J Clin Microbiol 2000;38:4006–4009.

81. Stagno S, et al: Comparative serial virologic and serologic studies of symptomatic and subclinical congenitally and natally acquired cytomegalovirus infections. J Infect Dis 1975;132:568–577.

82. Gerna G, et al: Monitoring of human cytomegalovirus infections and ganciclovir treatment in heart transplant recipients by determination of viremia, antigenemia, and DNAemia. J Infect Dis 1991;164:488–498.

83. Cope AN, et al: Interrelationships among quantity of human cytomegalovirus (HCMV) DNA in blood, donor-recipient serostatus, and administration of methylprednisolone as risk factors for HCMV disease following liver transplantation. J Infect Dis 1997;176:1484–1490.

84. Spector SA, et al: Plasma cytomegalovirus (CMV) DNA load predicts CMV disease and survival in AIDS patients. J Clin Invest 1998;101:497–502.

85. Gor D, et al: Longitudinal fluctuations in cytomegalovirus load in bone marrow transplant patients: Relationship between peak virus load, donor/recipient serostatus, acute GVHD and CMV disease. Bone Marrow Transplant 1998;21:597–605.

86. Hassan-Walker AF, et al: Quantity of human cytomegalovirus (CMV) DNAemia as a risk factor for CMV disease in renal allograft recipients: Relationship with donor/recipient CMV serostatus, receipt of augmented methylprednisolone and antithymocyte globulin (ATG). J Med Virol 1999;58:182–187.

87. Cox F, Hughes WT: Cytomegaloviremia in children with acute lymphocytic leukemia. J Pediatr 1975;87:190–194.

88. Diosi P, Moldovan E, Tomescu N: Latent cytomegalovirus infection in blood donors. Br Med J 1969;4:660–662.

89. Jordan MC: Latent infection and the elusive cytomegalovirus. Rev Infect Dis 1983;5:205–215.

90. Revello MG, et al: Human cytomegalovirus in blood of immunocompetent persons during primary infection: Prognostic implications for pregnancy. J Infect Dis 1998;177:1170–1175.

91. Tamura T, et al: Virus excretion and neutralizing antibody response in saliva in human cytomegalovirus infection. Infect Immun 1980;29:842–845.

92. Waner JL, et al: Cervical excretion cytomegalovirus: Correlation with secretory and humoral antibody. J Infect Dis 1977;136:805–809.

93. Yeager AS, et al: Prevention of transfusion: Acquired cytomegalovirus infections in newborn infants. J Pediatr 1981;98:281–287.

94. Bass EB, et al: Efficacy of immune globulin in preventing complications of bone marrow transplantation: A meta-analysis. Bone Marrow Transplant 1993;12:273–282.

95. Britt WJ, et al: Cell surface expression of human cytomegalovirus (HCMV) gp55-116 (gB): Use of HCMV-recombinant vaccinia virus-infected cells in analysis of the human neutralizing antibody response. J Virol 1990;64:1079–1085.

96. Gonczol E, et al: High expression of human cytomegalovirus (HCMV)-gB protein in cells infected with a vaccinia-gB recombinant: The importance of the gB protein in HCMV immunity. Vaccine 1991;9:631–637.

97. Quinnan GV, et al: Cytotoxic T cells in cytomegalovirus infection: HLA-restricted T-lymphocyte and non-T-lymphocyte cytotoxic responses correlate with recovery from cytomegalovirus infection in bone-marrow-transplant recipients. N Engl J Med 1982;307:7–13.

98. Quinnan GV, et al: HLA-restricted cytotoxic T lymphocytes are an early immune response and important defense mechanism in cytomegalovirus infections. Rev Infect Dis 1984;6:156–163.

99. Reusser P, et al: Cytotoxic T-lymphocyte response to cytomegalovirus after human allogeneic bone marrow transplantation: Pattern of recovery and correlation with cytomegalovirus infection and disease. Blood 1991;78:1373–1380.

100. Reusser P, et al: Cytomegalovirus-specific T-cell immunity in recipients of autologous peripheral blood stem cell or bone marrow transplants. Blood 1997;89:3873–3879.

101. Li CR, et al: Recovery of HLA-restricted cytomegalovirus (CMV)-specific T-cell responses after allogeneic bone marrow transplant: Correlation with CMV disease and effect of ganciclovir prophylaxis. Blood 1994;83:1971–1979.

102. Jonjic S, et al: Site-restricted persistent cytomegalovirus infection after selective long-term depletion of CD4+ T lymphocytes. J Exp Med 1989; 169(4): pp 1199–1212.

103. Steffens HP, et al: Preemptive CD8 T-cell immunotherapy of acute cytomegalovirus infection prevents lethal disease, limits the burden of latent viral genomes, and reduces the risk of virus recurrence. J Virol 1998;72:1797–1804.

104. Orange JS, et al: Requirement for natural killer cell-produced interferon gamma in defense against murine cytomegalovirus infection and enhancement of this defense pathway by interleukin 12 administration. J Exp Med 1995;182:1045–1056.

105. Welsh RM, et al: Natural killer (NK) cell response to virus infections in mice with severe combined immunodeficiency: The stimulation of NK cells and the NK cell-dependent control of virus infections occur independently of T and B cell function. J Exp Med 1991;173:1053–1063.

106. Presti RM, et al: Interferon gamma regulates acute and latent murine cytomegalovirus infection and chronic disease of the great vessels. J Exp Med 1998;188:577–588.

107. Fennie EH, et al: Reduced mortality in murine cytomegalovirus infected mice following prophylactic murine interferon-gamma treatment. Antiviral Res 1988;10:27–39.

108. Hengel H, et al: Restoration of cytomegalovirus antigen presentation by gamma interferon combats viral escape. J Virol 1994;68:289–297.

109. Orange JS, Biron CA: Characterization of early IL-12, IFN-alphabeta, and TNF effects on antiviral state and NK cell responses during murine cytomegalovirus infection. J Immunol 1996;156:4746–4756.

110. Riddell SR, Greenberg PD: Principles for adoptive T cell therapy of human viral diseases. Annu Rev Immunol 1995;13:545–586.

111. Phipps PH, et al: Comparison of five methods of cytomegalovirus antibody screening of blood donors. J Clin Microbiol 1983;18:1296–1300.

112. Adler SP, et al: Detection of cytomegalovirus antibody with latex agglutination. J Clin Microbiol 1985;22:68–70.

113. Beckwith DG, et al: Comparison of a latex agglutination test with five other methods for determining the presence of antibody against cytomegalovirus. J Clin Microbiol 1985;21:328–331.

114. McHugh TM, et al: Comparison of six methods for the detection of antibody to cytomegalovirus. J Clin Microbiol 1985;22:1014–1019.

115. Taswell HF, et al: Comparison of three methods for detecting antibody to cytomegalovirus. Transfusion 1986;26:285–289.

116. Gleaves CA, et al: Comparison of standard tube and shell vial cell culture techniques for the detection of cytomegalovirus in clinical specimens. J Clin Microbiol 1985;21:217–221.

117. Brumback BG, et al: Comparison of culture and the antigenemia assay for detection of cytomegalovirus in blood specimens submitted to a reference laboratory. J Clin Microbiol 1997;35:1819–1821.

118. van der Bij W, et al: Cytomegalovirus (CMV) antigenemia: Rapid diagnosis and relationship with CMV-associated clinical syndromes in renal allograft recipients. Transplant Proc 1989;21:2061–2064.

119. van der Bij W, et al: Comparison between viremia and antigenemia for detection of cytomegalovirus in blood. J Clin Microbiol 1988;26:2531–2535.

120. van der Bij W, et al: Rapid immunodiagnosis of active cytomegalovirus infection by monoclonal antibody staining of blood leucocytes. J Med Virol 1988;25:179–188.
121. Jiwa NM, et al: Rapid detection of human cytomegalovirus DNA in peripheral blood leukocytes of viremic transplant recipients by the polymerase chain reaction. Transplantation 1989;48:72–76.
122. Cassol SA, et al: Primer-mediated enzymatic amplification of cytomegalovirus (CMV) DNA: Application to the early diagnosis of CMV infection in marrow transplant recipients. J Clin Invest 1989;83:1109–1115.
123. Kidd IM, et al: Provision of prognostic information in immunocompromised patients by routine application of the polymerase chain reaction for cytomegalovirus. Transplantation 1993;56:867–871.
124. Nolte FS, et al: Early detection of human cytomegalovirus viremia in bone marrow transplant recipients by DNA amplification. J Clin Microbiol 1995;33:1263–1266.
125. Abecassis MM, et al: The role of PCR in the diagnosis and management of CMV in solid organ recipients: What is the predictive value for the development of disease and should PCR be used to guide antiviral therapy? Transplantation 1997;63:275–279.
126. Mazzulli T, et al: Cytomegalovirus antigenemia: Clinical correlations in transplant recipients and in persons with AIDS. J Clin Microbiol 1993;31:2824–2827.
127. Tanabe K, et al: Comparative study of cytomegalovirus (CMV) antigenemia assay, polymerase chain reaction, serology, and shell vial assay in the early diagnosis and monitoring of CMV infection after renal transplantation. Transplantation 1997;64:1721–1725.
128. Barber L, et al: Comparative study of three PCR assays with antigenaemia and serology for the diagnosis of HCMV infection in thoracic transplant recipients. J Med Virol 1996;49:137–144.
129. Ferreira-Gonzalez A, et al: Clinical utility of a quantitative polymerase chain reaction for diagnosis of cytomegalovirus disease in solid organ transplant patients. Transplantation 1999;68:991–996.
130. Caliendo AM, et al: Comparison of quantitative cytomegalovirus (CMV) PCR in plasma and CMV antigenemia assay: Clinical utility of the prototype AMPLICOR CMV MONITOR test in transplant recipients. J Clin Microbiol 2000;38:2122–2127.
131. Gerna G, et al: Human cytomegalovirus immediate-early mRNA detection by nucleic acid sequence-based amplification as a new parameter for preemptive therapy in bone marrow transplant recipients. J Clin Microbiol 2000;38:1845–1853.
132. Witt DJ, et al: Analytical performance and clinical utility of a nucleic acid sequence-based amplification assay for detection of cytomegalovirus infection. J Clin Microbiol 2000;38:3994–3999.
133. Kreel I, et al: A syndrome following total body perfusion. Surg Gynecol Obstet 1960;111:317–321.
134. Smith D: A syndrome resembling infectious mononucleosis after open-heart surgery. Br Med J 1964;1:945–948.
135. Klemola E, Kaariainen L: Cytomegalovirus as a possible cause of a disease resembling infectious mononucleosis. Br Med J 1965;5470:1099–1102.
136. Kaariainen L, Klemola E, Paloheimo J: Rise of cytomegalovirus antibodies in an infectious-mononucleosis-like syndrome after transfusion. Br Med J 1966;5498:1270–1272.
137. Lamb SG, Stern H: Cytomegalovirus mononucleosis with jaundice as presenting sign. Lancet 1966;2:1003–1006.
138. Nankervis GA, Kuman ML: Diseases produced by cytomegaloviruses. Med Clin North Am 1978;62:1021–1035.
139. Sandler SG, Grumet FC: Posttransfusion cytomegalovirus infections. Pediatrics 1982;69:650–653.
140. Tegtmeier GE: Transfusion-transmitted cytomegalovirus infections: Significance and control. Vox Sang 1986;51(Suppl 1):22–30.
141. Sayers MH, et al: Reducing the risk for transfusion-transmitted cytomegalovirus infection. Ann Intern Med 1992;116:55–62.
142. Hillyer CD, et al: Methods for the reduction of transfusion-transmitted cytomegalovirus infection: Filtration versus the use of seronegative donor units. Transfusion 1994;34:929–934.
143. Tolpin MD, et al: Transfusion transmission of cytomegalovirus confirmed by restriction endonuclease analysis. J Pediatr 1985;107:953–956.
144. Stevens DP, et al: Asymptomatic cytomegalovirus infection following blood transfusion in tumor surgery. JAMA 1970;211:1341–1344.
145. Adler SP, Baggett J, McVoy M: Transfusion-associated cytomegalovirus infections in seropositive cardiac surgery patients. Lancet 1985;2:743–747.
146. Huang ES, et al: Cytomegalovirus: Genetic variation of viral genomes. Ann N Y Acad Sci 1980;354:332–346.
147. Adler SP, McVoy MM: Cytomegalovirus infections in seropositive patients after transfusion: The effect of red cell storage and volume. Transfusion 1989;29:667–671.
148. Prince AM, et al: A serologic study of cytomegalovirus infections associated with blood transfusions. N Engl J Med 1971;284:1125–1131.
149. Winston DJ, et al: Cytomegalovirus infections associated with leukocyte transfusions. Ann Intern Med 1980;93:671–675.
150. Wilhelm JA, Matter L, Schopfer K: The risk of transmitting cytomegalovirus to patients receiving blood transfusions. J Infect Dis 1986;154:169–171.
151. Preiksaitis JK, Brown L, McKenzie M: The risk of cytomegalovirus infection in seronegative transfusion recipients not receiving exogenous immunosuppression. J Infect Dis 1988;157:523–529.
152. Preiksaitis JK, et al: Transfusion- and community-acquired cytomegalovirus infection in children with malignant disease: A prospective study. Transfusion 1997;37:941–946.
153. Bowden RA, et al: Cytomegalovirus immune globulin and seronegative blood products to prevent primary cytomegalovirus infection after marrow transplantation. N Engl J Med 1986;314:1006–1010.
154. Bowden RA, et al: Use of leukocyte-depleted platelets and cytomegalovirus-seronegative red blood cells for prevention of primary cytomegalovirus infection after marrow transplant. Blood 1991;78:246–250.
155. Miller WJ, et al: Prevention of cytomegalovirus infection following bone marrow transplantation: a randomized trial of blood product screening. Bone Marrow Transplant 1991;7:227–234.
156. Lee PI, et al: Transfusion-acquired cytomegalovirus infection in children in a hyperendemic area. J Med Virol 1992;36:49–53.
157. Hillyer CD, et al: Transfusion of the HIV seropositive patient: Immunomodulation, viral reactivation, and limiting exposure to EBV (HHV-4), CMV (HHV-5) and HHV-6, 7, and 8. Transfus Med Rev 1999;13:1–17.
158. Avery RK: Prevention and treatment of cytomegalovirus infection and disease in heart transplant recipients. Curr Opin Cardiol 1998;13:122–129.
159. Applebaum FR, et al: Nonbacterial nonfungal pneumonia following marrow transplantation in 100 identical twins. Transplantation 1982;33:265–268.
160. Santos GW, Hess AD, Vogelsang GB: Graft-versus-host reactions and disease. Immunol Rev 1985;88:169–192.
161. Wingard JR, et al: Cytomegalovirus infection after autologous bone marrow transplantation with comparison to infection after allogeneic bone marrow transplantation. Blood 1988;71:1432–1437.
162. Carlquist JF, et al: Accelerated rejection of murine cardiac allografts by murine cytomegalovirus-infected recipients: Lack of haplotype specificity. J Clin Invest 1993;91:2602–2608.
163. Evans PC, et al: An association between cytomegalovirus infection and chronic rejection after liver transplantation. Transplantation 2000;69:30–35.
164. George MJ, et al: The independent role of cytomegalovirus as a risk factor for invasive fungal disease in orthotopic liver transplant recipients. Boston Center for Liver Transplantation CMVIG-Study Group; Cytogam, MedImmune, Inc. Gaithersburg, Maryland. Am J Med 1997;103:106–113.
165. Preiksaitis JK: Indications for the use of cytomegalovirus-seronegative blood products. Transfus Med Rev 1991;5:1–17.
166. de Cates CR, Roberton NR, Walker JR: Fatal acquired cytomegalovirus infection in a neonate with maternal antibody. J Infect 1988;17:235–239.
167. Meyers JD, Flournoy N, Thomas ED: Risk factors for cytomegalovirus infection after human marrow transplantation. J Infect Dis 1986;153:478–488.
168. Wingard JR, et al: Cytomegalovirus infections in bone marrow transplant recipients given intensive cytoreductive therapy. Rev Infect Dis 1990;12(Suppl 7):S793–S804.
169. Pillay D, et al: Risk factors for viral reactivation following bone marrow transplantation. Ann Hematol 1992;64(Suppl):A148–A151.
170. Miller W, et al: Cytomegalovirus infection after bone marrow transplantation: An association with acute graft-v-host disease. Blood 1986;67:1162–1167.
171. Glenn J: Cytomegalovirus infections following renal transplantation. Rev Infect Dis 1981;3:1151–1178.

172. Chou SW: Acquisition of donor strains of cytomegalovirus by renal-transplant recipients. N Engl J Med 1986;314:1418–1423.

173. Chou S, Kim DY, Norman DJ: Transmission of cytomegalovirus by pretransplant leukocyte transfusions in renal transplant candidates. J Infect Dis 1987;155:565–567.

174. Grundy JE, et al: Symptomatic cytomegalovirus infection in seropositive kidney recipients: Reinfection with donor virus rather than reactivation of recipient virus. Lancet 1988;2:132–135.

175. Hillyer CD, Snydman DR, Berkman EM: The risk of cytomegalovirus infection in solid organ and bone marrow transplant recipients: Transfusion of blood products. Transfusion 1990;30:659–666.

176. Kurtz JB, et al: The problem of cytomegalovirus infection in renal allograft recipients. Q J Med 1984;53:341–349.

177. Tegtmeier GE: Cytomegalovirus infection as a complication of blood transfusion. Semin Liver Dis 1986;6:82–95.

178. Adler SP: Data that suggest that FFP does not transmit CMV [Letter]. Transfusion 1988;28:604.

179. Bowden R, Sayers M: The risk of transmitting cytomegalovirus infection by fresh frozen plasma. Transfusion 1990;30:762–763.

180. Hersman J, et al: The effect of granulocyte transfusions on the incidence of cytomegalovirus infection after allogeneic marrow transplantation. Ann Intern Med 1982;96:149–152.

181. Ho M: Epidemiology of cytomegalovirus infections. Rev Infect Dis 1990;12(Suppl 7):S701–S710.

182. Dworkin RJ, et al: Survival of cytomegalovirus in viremic blood under blood bank storage conditions. J Infect Dis 1990;161:1310–1311.

183. Tegtmeier GE: Posttransfusion cytomegalovirus infections. Arch Pathol Lab Med 1989;113:236–245.

184. Adler SP, et al: Cytomegalovirus infections in neonates acquired by blood transfusions. Pediatr Infect Dis 1983;2:114–118.

185. Bowden RA, et al: A comparison of filtered leukocyte-reduced and cytomegalovirus (CMV) seronegative blood products for the prevention of transfusion-associated CMV infection after marrow transplant. Blood 1995;86:3598–3603.

186. Ibanez CE, et al: Human cytomegalovirus productively infects primary differentiated macrophages. J Virol 1991;65:6581–6588.

187. Lathey JL, Spector SA: Unrestricted replication of human cytomegalovirus in hydrocortisone-treated macrophages. J Virol 1991;65:6371–6375.

188. Rubin RH, et al: Multicenter seroepidemiologic study of the impact of cytomegalovirus infection on renal transplantation. Transplantation 1985;40:243–249.

189. Cheung KS, Lang DJ: Transmission and activation of cytomegalovirus with blood transfusion: A mouse model. J Infect Dis 1977;135:841–845.

190. Roback JD, et al: Transfusion-transmitted cytomegalovirus infection (TT-CMV): Influence of leukoreduction (LR) and allogeneic interactions in a murine model. Transfusion 1999;39:2S.

191. Bowden RA, et al: Cytomegalovirus-seronegative blood components for the prevention of primary cytomegalovirus infection after marrow transplantation: Considerations for blood banks. Transfusion 1987;27:478–481.

192. Beneke JS, et al: Relation of titers of antibodies to CMV in blood donors to the transmission of cytomegalovirus infection. J Infect Dis 1984;150:883–888.

193. Lamberson HV, et al: Prevention of transfusion-associated cytomegalovirus (CMV) infection in neonates by screening blood donors for IgM to CMV. J Infect Dis 1988;157:820–823.

194. Roback JD, Bray RA, Hillyer CD: Longitudinal monitoring of WBC subsets in packed RBC units after filtration: Implications for transfusion transmission of infections. Transfusion 2000;40:500–506.

195. Sweeney JD, et al: In vitro and in vivo effects of prestorage filtration of apheresis platelets. Transfusion 1995;35:125–130.

196. Verdonck LF, et al: Cytomegalovirus seronegative platelets and leukocyte-poor red blood cells from random donors can prevent primary cytomegalovirus infection after bone marrow transplantation. Bone Marrow Transplant 1987;2:73–78.

197. Gilbert GL, et al: Prevention of transfusion-acquired cytomegalovirus infection in infants by blood filtration to remove leucocytes. Neonatal Cytomegalovirus Infection Study Group. [See comments.] Lancet 1989;1:1228–1231.

198. de Graan-Hentzen YC, et al: Prevention of primary cytomegalovirus infection in patients with hematologic malignancies by intensive white cell depletion of blood products. Transfusion 1989;29:757–760.

199. De Witte T, et al: Prevention of primary cytomegalovirus infection after allogeneic bone marrow transplantation by using leukocyte-poor random blood products from cytomegalovirus-unscreened blood-bank donors. Transplantation 1990;50:964–968.

200. Landaw EM, Kanter M, Petz LD: Safety of filtered leukocyte-reduced blood products for prevention of transfusion-associated cytomegalovirus infection [Letter]. Blood 1996;87:4910.

201. Bowden RA, Slichter S, Sayers M: Safety of filtered leukocyte-reduced blood products for prevention of transfusion-associated cytomegalovirus infection [Response]. Blood 1996;87:4910–4911.

202. Smith DMJ: Leukocyte Reduction for the Prevention of Transfusion-Transmitted Cytomegalovirus (TT-CMV). Bulletin 97-2. 1997: American Association of Blood Banks, Bethesda, MD 1997, pp 10–11.

203. Brady MT, et al: Use of deglycerolized red blood cells to prevent post-transfusion infection with cytomegalovirus in neonates. J Infect Dis 1984;150:334–339.

204. Taylor BJ, et al: Frozen deglycerolyzed blood prevents transfusion-acquired cytomegalovirus infections in neonates. Pediatr Infect Dis 1986;5:188–191.

205. Luban NL, et al: Low incidence of acquired cytomegalovirus infection in neonates transfused with washed red blood cells. Am J Dis Child 1987;141:416–419.

206. Demmler GJ, et al: Posttransfusion cytomegalovirus infection in neonates: Role of saline-washed red blood cells. J Pediatr 1986;108:762–765.

207. Condie RM, O'Reilly RJ: Prevention of cytomegalovirus infection by prophylaxis with an intravenous, hyperimmune, native, unmodified cytomegalovirus globulin: Randomized trial in bone marrow transplant recipients. Am J Med 1984;76:134–141.

208. Winston DJ, et al: Intravenous immune globulin for prevention of cytomegalovirus infection and interstitial pneumonia after bone marrow transplantation. Ann Intern Med 1987;106:12–18.

209. Meyers JD, et al: Prevention of cytomegalovirus infection by cytomegalovirus immune globulin after marrow transplantation. Ann Intern Med 1983;98:442–446.

210. Goodrich JM, et al: Early treatment with ganciclovir to prevent cytomegalovirus disease after allogeneic bone marrow transplantation. N Engl J Med 1991;325:1601–1607.

211. Boeckh M, Gooley TA, Bowden RA: Effect of high-dose acyclovir on survival in allogeneic marrow transplant recipients who received ganciclovir at engraftment or for cytomegalovirus pp65 antigenemia. J Infect Dis 1998;178:1153–1157.

212. Goodrich JM, et al: Ganciclovir prophylaxis to prevent cytomegalovirus disease after allogeneic marrow transplant. Ann Intern Med 1993;118:173–178.

213. Winston DJ, et al: Ganciclovir prophylaxis of cytomegalovirus infection and disease in allogeneic bone marrow transplant recipients: Results of a placebo-controlled, double-blind trial. Ann Intern Med 1993;118:179–184.

214. Prentice HG, Kho P: Clinical strategies for the management of cytomegalovirus infection and disease in allogeneic bone marrow transplant. Bone Marrow Transplant 1997;19:135–142.

215. Broers AE, et al: Increased transplant-related morbidity and mortality in CMV-seropositive patients despite highly effective prevention of CMV disease after allogeneic T-cell-depleted stem cell transplantation. Blood 2000;95:2240–2245.

216. Drew WL, et al: Prevalence of resistance in patients receiving ganciclovir for serious cytomegalovirus infection. J Infect Dis 1991;163:716–719.

217. Eckle T, et al: Drug-resistant human cytomegalovirus infection in children after allogeneic stem cell transplantation may have different clinical outcomes. Blood 2000;96:3286–3289.

218. Erice A, et al: Progressive disease due to ganciclovir-resistant cytomegalovirus in immunocompromised patients. N Engl J Med 1989;320:289–293.

219. Stanier P, et al: Persistence of cytomegalovirus in mononuclear cells in peripheral blood from blood donors. [See comments.] BMJ 1989;299:897–398.

220. Bevan IS, et al: Polymerase chain reaction for detection of human cytomegalovirus infection in a blood donor population. Br J Haematol 1991;78:94–99.

221. Taylor-Wiedeman J, et al: Monocytes are a major site of persistence of human cytomegalovirus in peripheral blood mononuclear cells. J Gen Virol 1991;72:2059–2064.

222. Larsson S, et al: Cytomegalovirus DNA can be detected in peripheral blood mononuclear cells from all seropositive and most seronegative healthy blood donors over time. Transfusion 1998;38:271–278.

223. Rowley AH, et al: Rapid detection of cytomegalovirus DNA and RNA in blood of renal transplant patients by in vitro enzymatic amplification. Transplantation 1991;51:1028–1033.

224. Bitsch A, et al: Failure to detect human cytomegalovirus DNA in peripheral blood leukocytes of healthy blood donors by the polymerase chain reaction. [See comments]. Transfusion 1992;32:612–617.

225. Smith KL, et al: Detection of cytomegalovirus in blood donors by the polymerase chain reaction. Transfusion 1993;33:497–503.

226. Roback JD, et al: Multicenter evaluation of PCR methodologies to detect cytomegalovirus DNA in blood donors. Transfusion 2001;41:1249–1257.

227. Lin L, et al: Photochemical inactivation of pathogenic bacteria in human platelet concentrates. Blood 1994;83:2698–2706.

228. Blajchman MA: Transfusion-associated bacterial sepsis: The phoenix rises yet again [Editorial; Comment]. Transfusion 1994;34:940–942.

229. Lin L, et al: Photochemical inactivation of viruses and bacteria in platelet concentrates by use of a novel psoralen and long-wavelength ultraviolet light. Transfusion 1997;37:423–435.

230. Corash L: Inactivation of viruses, bacteria, protozoa, and leukocytes in platelet concentrates: Current research perspectives. Transfus Med Rev 1999;13:18–30.

231. Corash L: Inactivation of viruses, bacteria, protozoa and leukocytes in platelet and red cell concentrates. Vox Sang 2000;78(Suppl 2):205–210.

232. Grass JA, et al: Inactivation of leukocytes in platelet concentrates by photochemical treatment with psoralen plus UVA. Blood 1998;91:2180–2188.

233. Plotkin SA, et al: Effect of Towne live virus vaccine on cytomegalovirus disease after renal transplant: A controlled trial. [See comments.] Ann Intern Med 1991;114:525–531.

234. Storb R, et al: Marrow transplantation with or without donor buffy coat cells for 65 transfused aplastic anemia patients. Blood 1982;59:236–246.

235. Kolb HJ, et al: Donor leukocyte transfusions for treatment of recurrent chronic myelogenous leukemia in marrow transplant patients. Blood 1990;76:2462–2465.

236. Papadopoulos EB, et al: Infusions of donor leukocytes to treat Epstein-Barr virus-associated lymphoproliferative disorders after allogeneic bone marrow transplantation. [See comments.] N Engl J Med 1994;330:1185–1191.

237. Riddell SR, et al: Restoration of viral immunity in immunodeficient humans by the adoptive transfer of T cell clones. [See comments.] Science 1992;257:238–241.

238. Walter EA, et al: Reconstitution of cellular immunity against cytomegalovirus in recipients of allogeneic bone marrow by transfer of T-cell clones from the donor. [See comments.] N Engl J Med 1995;333:1038–1044.

239. Smith DMJ: Leukocyte Reduction for the Prevention of Transfusion-Transmitted Cytomegalovirus (TT-CMV). Bulletin 97-2. Bethesda, MD: American Association of Blood Banks, 1997, pp 10–11.

240. Zwicky C, et al: [Prevention of post-transfusion cytomegalovirus infection: Recommendations for clinical practice.] Schweiz Med Wochenschr 1999;129:1061–1066.

241. Blajchman MA, et al: Proceedings of a consensus conference: Prevention of post-transfusion CMV in the era of universal leukoreduction. Transfus Med Rev 2001;15:1–20.

242. Griffin BE, Xue SA: Epstein-Barr virus infections and their association with human malignancies: Some key questions. Ann Med 1998;30:249–259.

243. Thomas JA, Crawford DH, Burke M: Clinicopathologic implications of Epstein-Barr virus related B cell lymphoma in immunocompromised patients. J Clin Pathol 1995;48:287–290.

244. Reding R, et al: Conversion from cyclosporine to FK506 for salvage of immunocompromised pediatric liver allografts: Efficacy, toxicity, and dose regimen in 23 children. Transplantation 1994;57:93–100.

245. Sokal EM, et al: Early signs and risk factors for the increased incidence of Epstein-Barr virus-related posttransplant lymphoproliferative diseases in pediatric liver transplant recipients treated with tacrolimus. Transplantation 1997;64:1438–1442.

246. Green M, et al: Serial measurement of Epstein-Barr viral load in peripheral blood in pediatric liver transplant recipients during treatment for posttransplant lymphoproliferative disease. Transplantation 1998;66:1641–1644.

247. McDiarmid S, et al: One hundred children treated with tacrolimus after primary orthotopic liver transplantation. Transplant Proc 1998;30:1397–1398.

248. Alfieri C, et al: Epstein-Barr virus transmission from a blood donor to an organ transplant recipient with recovery of the same virus strain from the recipient's blood and oropharynx. Blood 1996;87:812–817.

249. Walsh JH, Gerber P, Purcell RH: Viral etiology of the postperfusion syndrome. Am Heart J 1970;80:146.

250. Salahuddin SZ, et al: Isolation of a new virus, HBLV, in patients with lymphoproliferative disorders. Science 1986;234:596–601.

251. Lawrence GL, et al: Human herpesvirus 6 is closely related to human cytomegalovirus. J Virol 1990;64:287–299.

252. Yamanishi K, et al: Identification of human herpesvirus-6 as a causal agent for exanthem subitum. [See comments.] Lancet 1988;1:1065–1067.

253. Farr TJ, et al: The distribution of antibodies to HHV-6 compared with other herpesviruses in young children. Epidemiol Infect 1990;105:603–607.

254. Braun DK, Dominguez G, Pellett PE: Human herpesvirus 6. Clin Microbiol Rev 1997;10:521–567.

255. Kadakia MP, et al: Human herpesvirus 6: Infection and disease following autologous and allogeneic bone marrow transplantation. Blood 1996;87:5341–5354.

256. Lau YL, et al: Primary human herpes virus 6 infection transmitted from donor to recipient through bone marrow infusion. Bone Marrow Transplant 1998;21:1063–1066.

257. Singh N, Carrigan DR: Human herpesvirus-6 in transplantation: An emerging pathogen. Ann Intern Med 1996;124:1065–1071.

258. Wang FZ, et al: Lymphotropic herpesviruses in allogeneic bone marrow transplantation. Blood 1996;88:3615–3620.

259. Drobyski WR, et al: Brief report: Fatal encephalitis due to variant B human herpesvirus-6 infection in a bone marrow-transplant recipient. N Engl J Med 1994;330:1356–1360.

260. Ward KN, Gray JJ, Efstathiou S: Brief report: Primary human herpesvirus 6 infection in a patient following liver transplantation from a seropositive donor. J Med Virol 1989;28:69–72.

261. Cuende JI, et al: High prevalence of HHV-6 DNA in peripheral blood mononuclear cells of healthy individuals detected by nested-PCR. J Med Virol 1994;43:115–118.

262. Nicholas J: Determination and analysis of the complete nucleotide sequence of human herpesvirus. J Virol 1996;70:5975–5989.

263. Frenkel N, et al: Isolation of a new herpesvirus from human CD4+ T cells. [Published erratum appears in Proc Natl Acad Sci U S A 1990;87:7797.] Proc Natl Acad Sci U S A 1990;87:748–752.

264. Black JB, et al: Biologic properties of human herpesvirus 7 strain SB. Virus Res 1997;52:25–41.

265. Black JB, et al: Frequent isolation of human herpesvirus 7 from saliva. Virus Res 1993;29:91–98.

266. Tanaka K, et al: Human herpesvirus 7 another causal agent for roseola (exanthem subitum). J Pediatr 1994;125:1–5.

267. Drago F, et al: Human herpesvirus 7 in patients with pityriasis rosea: Electron microscopy investigations and polymerase chain reaction in mononuclear cells, plasma and skin; [See comments.] Dermatology 1997;195:374–378.

268. Drago F, et al: Human herpesvirus 7 in pityriasis rosea [Letter]. Lancet 1997;349:1367–1368.

269. Wilborn F, et al: Human herpesvirus type 7 in blood donors:Detection by the polymerase chain reaction. J Med Virol 1995;47:65–69.

270. Chang Y, et al: Identification of herpesvirus-like DNA sequences in AIDS-associated Kaposi's sarcoma. [See comments.] Science 1994;266:1865–1869.

271. Renne R, et al: The size and conformation of Kaposi's sarcoma-associated herpesvirus (human herpesvirus 8) DNA in infected cells and virions. J Virol 1996;70:8151–8154.

272. Russo JJ, et al: Nucleotide sequence of the Kaposi sarcoma-associated herpesvirus (HHV8). Proc Natl Acad Sci U S A 1996;93:14862–14867.

273. Cesarman E, et al: Kaposi's sarcoma-associated herpesvirus-like DNA sequences in AIDS-related body-cavity-based lymphomas. [See comments.] N Engl J Med 1995;332:1186–1191.

274. Knowles DM, Cesarman E: The Kaposi's sarcoma-associated herpesvirus (human herpesvirus-8) in Kaposi's sarcoma, malignant lymphoma, and other diseases. Ann Oncol 1997;8(Suppl 2):123–129.

275. Belec L, et al: Human herpesvirus 8 infection in patients with POEMS syndrome-associated multicentric Castleman's disease. Blood 1999;93:3643–3653.

276. Berenson JR, Vescio RA: HHV-8 is present in multiple myeloma patients. Blood 1999;93:3157–3159; discussion 3164–3166.

277. Tarte K, Chang Y, Klein B: Kaposi's sarcoma-associated herpesvirus and multiple myeloma: Lack of criteria for causality. Blood 1999;93:3159–3163; discussion 3163–3164.

278. Kedes DH, et al: The seroepidemiology of human herpesvirus 8 (Kaposi's sarcoma-associated herpesvirus): Distribution of infection in KS risk groups and evidence for sexual transmission. [See comments.] [Published erratum appears in Nat Med 1996;2:1041.] Nat Med 1996;2:918–924.

279. Gao SJ, et al: KSHV antibodies among Americans, Italians and Ugandans with and without Kaposi's sarcoma. [See comments.] Nat Med 1996;2:925–928.

280. Simpson GR, et al: Prevalence of Kaposi's sarcoma associated herpesvirus infection measured by antibodies to recombinant capsid protein and latent immunofluorescence antigen. Lancet 1996;348:1133–1138.

281. Chatlynne LG, et al: Detection and titration of human herpesvirus-8-specific antibodies in sera from blood donors, acquired immuno deficiency syndrome patients, and Kaposi's sarcoma patients using a whole virus enzyme-linked immunosorbent assay. Blood 1998;92:53–58.

282. Lennette ET, Blackbourn DJ, Levy JA: Antibodies to human herpesvirus type 8 in the general population and in Kaposi's sarcoma patients. [See comments.] Lancet 1996;348:858–861.

283. Regamey N, et al: Transmission of human herpesvirus 8 infection from renal-transplant donors to recipients. [See comments.] N Engl J Med 1998;339:1358–1363.

284. Whitby D, et al: Detection of Kaposi sarcoma associated herpesvirus in peripheral blood of HIV-infected individuals and progression to Kaposi's sarcoma. [See comments.] Lancet 1995;346:799–802.

285. Hudnall SD, et al: Serologic and molecular evidence of human herpesvirus 8 activation in renal transplant recipients. J Infect Dis 1998;178:1791–1794.

286. Belec L, et al: High prevalence in Central Africa of blood donors who are potentially infectious for human herpesvirus 8. Transfusion 1998;38:771–775.

287. De Milito A, et al: Lack of evidence of HHV-8 DNA in blood cells from heart transplant recipients. Blood 1997;89:1837–1838.

288. Operskalski EA, et al: Blood donations and viruses. Lancet 1997;349:1327.

289. LaDuca JR, et al: Detection of human herpesvirus 8 DNA sequences in tissues and bodily fluids. J Infect Dis 1998;178:1610–1615.

Chapter 41

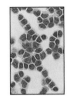

Bacterial Infections

Mindy Goldman
Morris A. Blajchman

Septic shock was one of the earliest recognized complications of blood transfusion,[1] and cases of life-threatening reactions resulting from bacterial contamination continue to be reported.[2–5] Prospective studies have indicated that the range of clinical severity is very wide and that mild reactions are often misidentified as febrile nonhemolytic transfusion reactions.[6–13] Indeed, although severe reactions are rare, data from surveillance cultures demonstrate that bacteria are the microorganisms most frequently present in cellular blood components. Because platelet concentrates are stored at room temperature, they offer the most favorable medium for bacterial growth, and bacterial contamination has been the limiting factor in the length of platelet storage that is permissible. Although they are most common with platelet components, reactions associated with contaminated red blood cells (RBCs), plasma, cryoprecipitate, and albumin have also been reported.[14–16] Moreover, bacterial contamination remains one of the residual complications of autologous transfusions.[17–20]

Methods suggested to detect bacteria in components range from simple visual inspection to sophisticated polymerase chain reaction (PCR) amplification of bacterial nucleic acid.[21] Changes in every step of blood component preparation, from donor screening to phlebotomy procedures, component production, and storage, have been proposed to decrease the frequency of contamination. In several countries, cultures are obtained routinely on platelets, in some cases to permit extended storage of up to 7 days before transfusion. Finally, methods of chemical inactivation of bacteria are under active development and may eliminate the problem of bacterial contamination in the future.[22]

■ Presentation and Prevalence

Red Blood Cell Concentrates

Transfusion reactions associated with contaminated RBC units are extremely severe, with a mortality rate of approximately 70%.[4, 5, 16] Temperatures higher than 38.5°C, rigors, and hypotension usually begin during the transfusion; nausea, vomiting, dyspnea, and diarrhea occur in a significant number of cases. Septic shock, oliguria, and disseminated intravascular coagulation are also frequent complications.[23] Anesthetized patients may present with hypotension, oliguria, and excessive bleeding. As discussed later, the majority of RBC-associated reactions are caused by gram-negative organisms, such as *Yersinia enterocolitica*, which possess endotoxin in their outer membrane.[4, 5, 16, 24]

The acute reactions are thought to be caused by infusion of endotoxin followed by massive release by the recipient of cytokines (i.e., tumor necrosis factor-α), that are important mediators in the pathogenesis of shock.[25, 26] In most of the reported reactions, the RBCs had been stored for longer than 21 days and therefore carried a high bacterial and endotoxin load.[23]

There have been four reports of septic shock related to the contamination of autologous RBC units; all four patients survived.[17–20] In retrospect, in the three cases involving *Y. enterocolitica* (which can cause enterocolitis), the donors had experienced gastrointestinal symptoms in the days preceding or following their autologous donation.[17, 18, 20] In the case involving *Serratia liquefaciens*, an infected toe ulcer may have been the source of a transient bacteremia at the time of autologous blood donation.[19]

There have been few prospective studies examining the frequency of bacterial contamination in patients receiving RBC transfusions. In two consecutive studies done at the Dana Farber Cancer Institute, cultures of RBCs and recipients involved in transfusion reactions demonstrated a possible contamination of 1 in 38,465 units transfused, for a rate of 2.6 per 100,000 transfusions.[8, 11]

Platelet Concentrates

In the reported cases of sepsis associated with platelet transfusion, patients presented with fever, hypotension, and chills

Table 41.1 Prevalence of Bacterial Contamination of Platelet Concentrates—Prospective Studies

Reference (year)	Apheresis Platelets		Random Donor Platelets	
	No. Contaminated/ No. Tested	Rate per 100,000 units	No. Contaminated/ No. Tested	Rate per 100,000 units
Morrow et al (1991)[6]	1/9519	5	6/74,598	8
Blajchman et al (1992)[7]	14/6055	230	—	—
Barrett et al (1993)[8]	5/17,928	28	1/4272	23
Yomtovian et al (1993)[9]	0/2476	0	6/15,705	38
Chiu et al (1994)[10]	—	—	10/21,503	46
Dzieczkowski et al (1995)[11]	1/5197	19	—	—
Blajchman et al (1994)[12]	—	—	16/31,610	51
Leiby et al (1997)[13]	—	—	4/4995	80
Blajchman et al (1997)[14]	—	—	7/10,065	70
Liu et al (1999)[15]	—	—	14/26,210	53

beginning during or shortly after transfusion.[23] More rarely, symptoms begin up to 2 weeks after transfusion. Half the patients develop shock requiring vasopressors, and the mortality rate is almost 25%. Most reactions occur with platelet concentrates that are more than 3 days old.[6] Because only the most severe reactions are likely to be recognized and reported, case reports represent the severe end of the clinical spectrum of transfusion reactions associated with bacterial contamination. Prospective studies demonstrate that the majority of recipients of contaminated platelet transfusions develop either no symptoms, or fever and chills with no clinical sequelae.[6, 8–11] These reactions may be clinically indistinguishable from febrile nonhemolytic transfusion reactions, and therefore the prevalence of bacterial contamination of platelets may be underestimated.[27, 28] In the prospective studies summarized in Table 41.1, the prevalence of bacterial contamination in apheresis platelets ranged from 0 to 230 per 100,000 platelet units, and the prevalence of contamination of random donor platelets ranged from 8 to 80 per 100,000 units.[6–15]

Fresh Frozen Plasma and Cryoprecipitate

Patients who receive contaminated plasma products have been reported to develop wound infections, endocarditis, or septicemia with unusual organisms several days after receiving cryoprecipitate or plasma thawed in a contaminated water bath.[29, 30]

Peripheral Blood Stem Cells

Although many studies have demonstrated that up to 4.5% of peripheral blood stem cell collections yield positive bacterial cultures, no adverse sequelae from the infusion of culture-positive collections have been reported. The recipients often are receiving prophylactic antibiotic treatment at the time of reinfusion.[31]

Determinants of Clinical Severity

As mentioned previously, the clinical consequences of the bacterial contamination of a blood component range from minimal or no reaction to fatal septic shock. Table 41.2 summarizes the bacterial and recipient characteristics known to influence clinical severity.[23]

Table 41.2 Determinants of Clinical Severity

Organism

Gram-negative organisms elaborating endotoxins
Virulence factors permitting bacterial growth

Bacterial load infused

Time of storage: >21 days for red blood cells, >3 days for platelets
Volume of component

Host characteristics

Concomitant administration of antibiotic
Degree of immunosuppression
Overall medical status
Age

■ Microorganisms Implicated

Red Blood Cell Concentrates

Because RBC concentrates are stored at 4°C, they provide an inhospitable environment for most organisms. The exceptions are *Y. enterocolitica*, other Enterobacteriaceae, and the psychrophilic pseudomonads.

Y. enterocolitica is responsible for half of the reported cases of RBC-associated sepsis, with a case-fatality rate of approximately 60%.[4, 5, 32–34] Frequency varies markedly in different geographic locations. For example, eight cases were reported in New Zealand from 1991 to 1995, for a transfusion incidence rate of 1 in 65,000; only 10 cases were reported in the United States in a similar time frame, for a transfusion incidence rate of 1 in 500,000.[4, 5] Almost 50 cases have been reported in the world literature. Differences in virulence have been reported among various strains. In addition, temperature-sensitive plasmid-encoded virulence factors appear to confer resistance to complement binding and phagocytosis.[35–37] Because *Y. enterocolitica* lacks siderophores, its growth is enhanced in an iron-rich environment such as stored RBCs. Data from inoculation experiments show that a lag phase of approximately 2 weeks is followed by exponential growth. A concentration of 10^9 organisms per millimeter is reached usually after 4 weeks of storage, with a parallel rise in endotoxin level.[38]

Pseudomonas species are gram-negative rods commonly found in soil and water. Certain species, such as *Pseudomonas putida* and *Pseudomonas fluorescens*, grow well at 4°C and are frequent contaminants in refrigerated environments.[39]

Platelet Concentrates

Because platelets are stored at 22°C, they provide a hospitable culture medium for a wide variety of bacteria. In both case reports and prospective studies, the majority of organisms isolated in platelet-associated bacteremic episodes are part of the normal skin flora.[6–15] Coagulase-negative staphylococci are the most frequently isolated organisms. Although the minimum inoculum size necessary for bacterial proliferation varies in different studies with different organisms, for many strains a very small inoculum, such as 1 colony-forming unit (CFU) per milliliter, may be sufficient for bacterial growth. In inoculation experiments, there is usually a lag phase, followed by exponential growth, to reach a maximum concentration of 10^8 to 10^9 organisms per milliliter on day 2 to day 5, depending on the organism.[40] Given the same initial inoculum, a larger volume of plasma, such as that found in an apheresis unit, may result in a larger bacterial load after several days of storage.[40]

Plasma and Cryoprecipitate

Pseudomonas cepacia and *Pseudomonas aeruginosa* are environmental organisms that grow optimally at 30°C. They have been isolated from cryoprecipitate and plasma thawed in contaminated water baths.[29, 30] *Borrelia burgdorferi*, the etiologic agent of Lyme disease, can survive in platelets, RBCs, and plasma under usual storage conditions.[41] Because spirochetemia has been documented in patients with early Lyme disease, the possibility for transmission by transfusion exists, although it has not yet been reported.[41–43]

■ Other Organisms

Tick-borne organisms, such as *Rickettsia rickettsii*, *Ehrlichia equi*, and *Ehrlichia chaffeensis*, the etiologic agents of Rocky Mountain spotted fever and ehrlichiosis, may theoretically be transmitted by transfusion. In July 1997, 700 blood components were recalled from donations made at a military base in Fort Chaffee, Arkansas because of the development of symptoms of tick-borne illnesses (e.g., fever, headache, rash) in some donors who may have been exposed to ticks during military exercises.[44] Twelve donors were found to have a confirmed or a probable case of Rocky Mountain spotted fever or ehrlichiosis; however, none of the 10 recipients who received units from the infected donors became ill.

Orientia tsutsugamuchi, the etiologic agent of scrub typhus, survived up to 10 days of refrigerated storage in inoculation experiments in RBCs.[45] Because bacteremia can occur before the development of clinical infection, the possibility for transmission by RBC transfusion exits.

■ Mechanisms of Contamination

Possible mechanisms of blood component contamination, listed in Table 41.3, involve the blood donor, the collection procedure, the collection pack, and blood processing procedures.

Donor Bacteremia

Obviously, most bacteremic people are symptomatic and would not be accepted as blood donors. In many countries, including Canada and the United States, donor temperature must be lower than 37.5°C. However, donors in an asymptomatic incubation period or in the recovery phase from an upper respiratory tract infection or gastroenteritis have been linked to episodes of bacterial contamination.[5, 16] In cases of transfusion-associated *Y. enterocolitica* septicemia reported to the U.S. Centers for Disease Control and Prevention (CDC),

Table 41.3 Sources of Bacterial Contamination

Mechanism (Ref. No.)	Examples of Implicated Organisms
Donor bacteremia	
Incubation or recovery period in a patient with gastroenteritis[5]	*Yersinia enterocolitica, Campylobacter jejuni*
Incubation period of an upper respiratory tract infection[6]	*Streptococcus pyogenes*
Incubation period of septicemia[46]	*Staphylococcus aureus*
Early Lyme disease[47]	*Borrelia burgdorferi*
Chronic low-grade infection	
Osteomyelitis[48]	*Salmonella choleraesuis*
Syphilis[16]	*Treponema pallidum*
Toe ulceration[19]	*Serratia liquefaciens*
After a dental or medical procedure[16]	*S. aureus*
Blood collection	
Inadequate skin disinfection	*Staphylococcus epidermidis, S. aureus, diphtheroids*
Scarred phlebotomy site[49]	*Enterococci, staphylococci*
Contaminated vacuum tubes[50]	*Serratia marcescens*
Contaminated apheresis solutions[51]	*Enterobacter cloacae*
Blood bag manufacture	
Bag exterior contaminated at manufacturing plant[52,53]	*S. marcescens*
Contamination during manufacture of fractionation products[54]	*Pseudomonas cepacia*
Container damage or defect	
Leaky seals[55,56]	*Serratia species*
Cracked vials[57]	*E. cloacae*
Blood processing	
Contamination during thawing[29]	*P. cepacia, Pseudomonas aeruginosa*

approximately 75% of donors recalled diarrhea in the days preceding or following their donation.[5] Gastrointestinal symptoms were also noted retrospectively in the *Y. enterocolitica* cases in autologous donors, discussed previously.[17, 18, 20] The following Canadian case illustrates *Staphylococcus aureus* septicemia in a recipient that was most likely of donor origin.[46]

A 76-year-old man with myelodysplasia was admitted to hospital for fever 3 days after transfusion of a pool of five units of prestorage filter-leukoreduced random donor platelet concentrates. He was not premedicated and did not have any symptoms during or after transfusion of the platelet pool. He developed septic shock and died 3 days after admission. Blood cultures were positive for *S. aureus*. One of the platelet units had been produced from a donation made 4 days before transfusion by a 36-year-old regular blood donor. The donor felt unwell 3 days after the donation, with dizziness, vomiting, and diarrhea, and presented to the emergency room, where he was kept for observation. The next day, he went into septic shock with blood cultures positive for *S. aureus*. He was subsequently found to have a new heart murmur, and echocardiography demonstrated rupture of the posterior leaflet of the mitral valve. He had a stormy hospital course but survived. Soon after the patient's admission to the hospital, a family member informed the attending physician that the patient had recently donated blood. This information was transmitted to the blood distributor, Canadian Blood Services, who attempted to recall the platelet component. The *S. aureus* isolates from both the donor and the recipient were found to be identical on antibiotic sensitivity testing profiles and gene mapping, indicating that they were probably from the same source. Had the blood donor not presented with a septic episode subsequent to donation, the link between fatal septicemia and the blood transfusion would not have been made in this recipient.

Lyme disease is caused by the tick-borne spirochete, *B. burgdorferi*, and is transmitted by ticks of the genus *Ixodes*. It is most common in coastal areas of New England and New York, although cases have been reported from most American states and parts of Canada.[59] A unique skin lesion, erythema migrans, often associated with a flu-like illness, develops in the 2-week period after a tick bite, and spirochetemia has been documented by PCR in this phase of the disease.[42] Because many people do not recall having a tick bite or primary illness, it is possible that spirochetemia can occur in relatively asymptomatic donors. However, six recipients of blood components from donors subsequently diagnosed as having Lyme disease were not infected, and a study done in Connecticut at the peak of the deer tick season demonstrated no clinical or laboratory evidence of disease transmission in multitransfused cardiothoracic surgery patients.[58, 60, 61]

Similarly, donors infected with *Treponema pallidum* can be asymptomatic and have a negative nonspecific serologic test for syphilis during periods of spirochetemia. The spirochete is inactivated after several days of storage at 4°C, but rare cases of transmission have been reported with blood stored for less than 24 hours.[16]

Isolated cases of bacterial contamination have been linked to donors with intermittent, low-grade bacteremia associated with chronic infection or transitory bacteremia after dental repair.[16, 48]

Blood Collection

The majority of organisms isolated from contaminated platelet concentrates are part of normal skin flora and are thought to enter into the needle during venipuncture.[62] Organisms such as *Staphylococcus epidermidis*, *S. aureus*, and *Bacillus* species are also frequent contaminants in blood culture studies. It is postulated that, despite adequate surface disinfection, viable bacteria remain in the deeper layers of the skin, especially with a scarred phlebotomy site.[49] The donor's skin may also be the source of unusual pathogens. A fatal platelet transfusion reaction due to *Clostridium perfringens* was linked to a donor who had frequently changed his children's diapers.[3] Arm swab cultures of this donor revealed the presence of *C. perfringens* and other bacteria that are normal components of fecal flora, such as *Escherichia coli* and *Streptococcus faecalis*.

Contaminated vacuum tubes used for specimen collection after donation and nonsterile intravenous solutions used during apheresis procedures were implicated in episodes of *Serratia marcescens* and *Enterobacter cloacae* sepsis, respectively.[50, 51]

Blood Bag Manufacture

In June 1991, six patients in Denmark and Sweden developed *S. marcescens* septicemia after transfusion of RBCs (five patients) or platelets (one patient). At least five more cases with milder symptoms were subsequently diagnosed.[52, 53] All of the episodes were related to blood bags produced in a plant in Belgium. The same ribotype of *S. marcescens* was isolated from each recipient, the implicated products, 0.3% to 1.5% of blood units collected during this time period, and the dust in the factory. It was hypothesized that *S. marcescens* had contaminated the exterior of the blood bags, which were put into a clean but not sterile outer plastic package. *S. marcescens* grows well at 4°C and 22°C, even under poor nutritional conditions, and may use the plasticizer leaking out of the blood bag as a carbon source. After massive contamination of the exterior of the blood bag, the bacteria probably entered the unit at the time of blood donation, either through suction into the needle or contamination of the phlebotomist's hands and subsequently of the donor's skin.[55]

In 1973, a cluster of cases of *P. cepacia* was traced to low-frequency contamination of a lot of albumin vials in the United States.[54]

Container Damage or Defect

Two episodes of bacterial contamination in Sweden were attributed to a leaky seal and tubing damaged by a clamp.[55] In 1995, the National Blood Authority in England withdrew 7000 blood bags because of faulty seals in some of the bags.[56] At least one case of post-transfusion *Serratia* septicemia may have been caused by the faulty bags.

In 1996, several cases of *E. cloacae* septicemia in the United States were related to damage to albumin vials during transport in the manufacturing facility, which resulted in cracks. This led to the recall of 10 lots of albumin and 1 lot of factor VIII by the manufacturer.[57]

Blood Processing

Contamination of plasma or cryoprecipitate on thawing in heavily contaminated water baths may lead to *P. cepacia* or

P. aeruginosa bacteremia, endocarditis, or mediastinal wound infection.[29, 30, 58] Contamination can occur as a result of microscopic cracks in the bags or entry of bath water into the packs at the time of pooling. Although bacterial contamination may theoretically occur during platelet pooling, in cases of sepsis associated with platelet pools contamination has always been traced to a constituent unit. A study of 1437 random donor platelet pools did not detect any contamination after pooling.[63] Because of the short time frame between pooling and transfusion in North America, the introduction of small numbers of bacteria most likely would be of little clinical consequence. However, if a sterile connecting device is used to weld tubing of platelet or RBC units before more lengthy storage, care must be taken to ensure that the connections are tight.

■ Bacteriologic Surveillance of Cellular Blood Products

Bacteriologic surveillance is part of hemovigilance in several countries. Surveillance may involve culturing of a certain number of products as part of quality assurance, culturing of recipients and of the remaining blood products of all recipients who experience transfusion reactions, and reporting of such transfusion reactions to a central registry.

French law requires reporting of all transfusion reactions to the Agence Française du Sang.[64] Designated personnel in each hospital are responsible for submitting standardized reports, and the reactions are graded according to severity and possible etiology. Of the 12,058 moderate and severe reactions reported in 1996 and 1997, 405 (1.3%) were thought to be caused by bacterial contamination, as were 5 (15%) of the 33 fatal reactions for which transfusion-related causality could be established clearly. From 1994 to mid-1997, the estimated frequency of a bacteria-associated transfusion reaction was 1 in 60,000 transfused components, with 1 in 185,000 components resulting in a severe reaction and 1 in 700,000 resulting in a lethal reaction. Four reactions occurred in association with autologous RBC transfusions, two of which were contaminated with *Y. enterocolitica*.[64, 65] The Bachthem (France) study is a national case-control study started in 1996 to determine risk factors and sources of contamination in cases of transfusion reactions caused by bacteria.[66] Perhaps because of increased awareness of the frequency of these reactions, some French transfusion services are performing routine cultures on all platelet concentrates before transfusion.[67]

In the United Kingdom, the Serious Hazards of Transfusion (SHOT) voluntary reporting system was started in late 1996 to compile reports of severe transfusion reactions.[68]

In the United States, the Bacterial Contamination (BaCon) study was initiated in 1998 by the American Association of Blood Banks (AABB), the American Red Cross, the CDC, and the Department of Defense. The aims of the American study are to increase awareness of and determine the frequency of bacterial contamination of blood products through standardized investigation and reporting of suspected septic reactions in hospitals in the United States.[71] From January 1, 1998, through June 30, 1999, there were 12 definite cases of post-transfusion sepsis reported, involving 5 platelet pools, 6 apheresis platelets, and 1 RBC concentrate. Eight cases

involved gram-positive organisms, and four involved gram-negative organisms. All three fatal reactions involved gram-negative organisms.[72]

Several countries, including Canada, Holland, and Germany, perform bacteriologic surveillance on randomly selected RBC and platelet components.[16, 69, 70] Because the rate of positive cultures is influenced by many factors, including the time, volume, and method of blood product sampling and the culture system used, uniform requirements have been instituted by the Paul Ehrlich Institute in Germany to permit comparisons among institutions and over time as modifications in procedures are introduced. Approximately 1% of platelet and RBC concentrates are cultured. Data from the surveillance cultures in various countries show a contamination rate of 0.3% to 0.5%.

■ Approaches to Reduce Transfusion-Associated Septic Reactions

Measures proposed to prevent transfusion-associated bacterial sepsis are listed in Table 41.4.

Extension of Donor Screening

Retrospective questioning of donors of RBC units contaminated with *Y. enterocolitica* often reveals symptoms of gastroenteritis, such as abdominal pain and diarrhea, that occurred during the month preceding donation. However, several studies have demonstrated that the addition of questions about such symptoms would lead to unacceptable donor loss and the exclusion of many healthy blood donors.[23, 73] Screening of blood donors for the presence of antibodies to *Y. enterocolitica* antigens was shown also to be of very little utility.[74]

Donors who develop diarrhea or a contagious disease in the week after donation may be asked to notify the transfusion service. In a study done in Montreal, Canada, components from 0.03% of donors were recalled owing to the development in the donor of diarrhea, vomiting, fever, or streptococcal pharyngitis during the week after donation. None of the transfused components was shown to be associated with transfusion reactions, and all components still in inventory were culture-negative.[75] Therefore, it is very likely that blood donors who develop these symptoms after donation are rarely infectious.

Table 41.4 Possible Methods to Prevent Transfusion-Associated Bacterial Sepsis

Extension of donor screening[23,73–77]

Improved donor skin disinfection[78–81]

Removal of first aliquot of donor blood[82,83]

Limitation of component storage time[23]

Pretransfusion detection[21]

Altered blood processing

    Leukocyte reduction[85,86]

    Reduced holding temperature and time prior to component preparation[87–89]

    Component storage temperature[90,91]

    Waterbath disinfection[58]

Chemical or photochemical decontamination
    Psoralens[22,109,110]

Donors may be asked about tick bites in areas of Lyme disease endemicity. However, because there have been no reported cases of Lyme disease transmission from asymptomatic donors, an AABB Advisory Group concluded that the addition of a specific question about tick bites was not necessary.[76]

Donors may be questioned about dental or medical procedures in the hours or days before donation. Although it has been demonstrated that many procedures can cause transient bacteremia, it is probably unnecessary to create long donor exclusion periods, which would lead to significant and probably inappropriate donor deferrals.[77]

Improved Skin Disinfection

Because the majority of the bacteria found in platelet concentrates are part of the normal skin flora, improvements in skin disinfection may lead to lower blood product contamination rates. Studies examining the effects of various disinfection techniques on blood culture contamination rates and vascular catheter infection rates suggest that significant differences may result from the use of improved disinfection protocols.[23]

In addition to the specific antiseptic, the mode of application used (scrub, sponge, swab, applicator) can influence efficacy. Two studies examining the rate of positive skin surface cultures after various protocols demonstrated greater efficacy of an isopropyl alcohol scrub followed by an ampule containing tincture of iodine, compared with povidone-iodine.[78, 79] Similar results were reported in a large U. K. study comparing 10 methods of skin disinfection.[80] For donors who are allergic to iodine, the tincture of iodine may be replaced by chlorhexidine; green soap, however, results in little microbial killing.[79] In the United Kingdom, skin surface cultures after donor arm disinfection are monitored as part of quality control.[81]

Removal of the First Aliquot of Donor Blood

Bacteria that are part of normal skin flora may be introduced into the blood bag in association with a skin core that enters the collection needle at the time of venisection.[62] The removal of the first few milliliters of donor blood therefore may decrease the bacterial load in the collection bag.[82]

In a French study,[83] 3440 units of blood were collected in special bags that allowed for the diversion of two separate 15-mL aliquots of blood at the beginning of the venipuncture. An automated blood culture system was then used to culture the two aliquots; if either of these cultures was positive, the RBC and plasma concentrates of the corresponding unit also were cultured. Two percent of bacterial cultures of the aliquots were positive for organisms that are part of the normal skin flora; in 73% of positive cultures, bacteria were detected only in the first aliquot. Seven of the 116 corresponding RBC and plasma units also had positive cultures.[83] Blood collection sets that divert the first few milliliters of blood to a satellite bag for donor testing are now in routine use in France.

Limitation of Component Storage

Most severe septic transfusion reactions occur with RBC concentrates stored for longer than 21 days and platelet concentrates stored for longer than 3 days. In 1986, the U.S. Food and Drug Administration reduced the platelet storage time from 7 to 5 days because of concern about case reports of

platelet-associated sepsis with concentrates transfused after 6 or 7 days of storage. However, reduction of RBC or platelet storage times may have a severe effect on blood product supply.[23] Another approach is to use pretransfusion detection methods for components stored for longer periods, as described in the next section.

Pretransfusion Detection

The ideal test for the detection of bacteria in blood components does not currently exist.[21] Because the initial inoculum of bacteria is probably very small (fewer than 10 organisms per milliliter), even a very sensitive technique, such as an automated culture system, will miss some contaminated units if the test is performed in the blood collection center shortly after collection. The number of bacteria in components associated with severe transfusion reactions is usually greater than 10^6 organisms per milliliter. Therefore, a less sensitive technique may be adequate to detect clinically significant contamination in the hospital transfusion service before transfusion. However, such a test would have to be rapid to avoid delaying product issue, and it should not require specialized equipment or personnel. In all cases, the technique should be specific, to avoid blood wastage or delays in product issuing. This is frequently problematic, particularly because the bacteria involved in contamination of platelets are often part of normal skin flora.

Studies done by Blajchman and associates[14] using the BacT/Alert automated blood culture system illustrate some of these issues. Over an 18-month period, 16,290 random donor platelet concentrates were cultured on day 1; 10,065 of these concentrates were also available for culture on day 3. Cultures were considered true positives if the organism isolated from the original platelet segment could also be detected in one of the blood components of the associated donation. There were seven true-positive cultures on day 3, for a prevalence of 70 per 100,000 units; only four of these had positive cultures detected on day 1 (prevalence, 25 per 100,000 units). All units that had true-positive cultures on day 1 remained positive on day 3. Most cultures were positive within a 24-hour incubation period. These data demonstrate that early sampling leads to false-negative results. In addition, there were cultures that were considered false-positives. Despite the limitations of this method, it is currently being used in some European centers on pooled buffy-coat platelet concentrates and apheresis platelets. Because of the greater volume of these products, a larger sample (usually 10 mL) can be cultured, improving sensitivity. In some cases this has permitted an extension of the platelet shelf life to 7 days, with decreased platelet unit outdating.[84]

In the prospective study by Liu and colleagues, 14 contaminated platelet concentrates were found to be associated with 9 contaminated RBC units and 4 contaminated fresh frozen plasma units from the same donations.[15] Therefore, culturing of platelet concentrates may also decrease transfusion of contaminated RBC and plasma units. Detection methods have been reviewed[21] and are summarized, along with some of their strengths and weaknesses, in Table 41.5.

Leukocyte Reduction

Phagocytes may be important in the elimination of viable bacteria present in blood components during the first few hours after venipuncture.[108] In the case of organisms such as

Table 41.5   Bacterial Detection Techniques

Method	Sensitivity (CFU/mL)		Strengths	Weaknesses	Current Applications
	Lower limit	Consistent detection			
Visual inspection of red cells, compare bag to segments[92,93]	10^5	10^8	Quick, easy, inexpensive	Insensitive, poor specificity	Mandatory in AABB Standards
Platelet swirling[94,98]	10^7	10^8	Quick, easy, inexpensive	Insensitive, poor specificity	Used in some countries as indicator of platelet viability
Microscopic examination Acridine orange[95]	10^3	10^5	Quick, inexpensive	Requires fluorescence microscope, some technical skill	Research
Gram stain[96]	10^5	10^7	Quick, inexpensive	Relatively insensitive, requires some technical skill	Routine use in some hospitals
Metabolic changes pH, glucose dipsticks for platelets[97,98]	10^3	10^7	Quick, easy, inexpensive	Poor sensitivity for certain organisms, results vary with collection kits and processing methods	Routine use in some hospitals
Blood gas analysis[99,100]	10^7	10^8	Quick, easy, inexpensive	Insensitive, results vary with bag permeability	Research
Endotoxin assay[38]	10^1	10^5	Relatively quick	Variable sensitivity, applicable only to gram-negative organisms	Research
Automated culture systems[14,83,101,102]	10^1	10^1	Very sensitive, partial automation	Lengthy incubation time, costly, specificity may be poor	Routine use in some European hospitals
Microvolume fluorimetry using an antibiotic probe[103]	10^3	10^3	Sensitivity, speed	Specialized equipment, preliminary results	Research
DNA/RNA assays Ribosomal RNA chemiluminescence assay[104–106]	10^2	10^5	Relativity quick and sensitive	Specialized equipment, labor-intensive, costly	Research
Polymerase chain reaction[107]	10^3	10^4	Relativity quick and sensitive	Species-specific, specialized equipment, labor-intensive, costly, false-positives	Research

Y. enterocolitica, the bacteria may already be present in the phagocytes in the donor's blood; with bacteria introduced from the donor's skin, phagocytosis may occur during initial storage, particularly if there is a room temperature hold before refrigeration. Bacteria may then be released back into the blood component as the leukocytes disintegrate during storage, or they may be eliminated by prestorage leukodepletion. Several spiking experiments have demonstrated reduced bacterial growth of *Y. enterocolitica* in contaminated RBC units that were leukoreduced in the hours after contamination.[85, 86] Data on the efficacy of leukoreduction in preventing growth of other bacterial strains in RBC or platelet concentrates have been less conclusive.[85]

Temperature and Time of Storage before Component Preparation

There is marked variability among countries in regard to the time and temperature of whole blood storage before component preparation. Time and temperature of storage may influence bacterial growth, phagocytosis, and complement-mediated killing. The few studies done on this subject have come to varying conclusions, possibly because of confounding variables such as differences in component preparation methods and leukoreduction.[87–89]

Lowering Component Storage Temperature

Platelet storage at 22°C is necessary to maintain platelet hemostatic efficacy, but this temperature provides a hospitable culture medium for many microorganisms. The development of storage solutions that permit retention of platelet function at 4°C would considerably decrease bacterial growth.[90] One study has indicated that proliferation of *Y. enterocolitica* in RBC concentrates may be decreased by storage at 0°C.[91] This interesting approach needs further study.

Water Bath Disinfection

Water baths should be emptied and disinfected weekly, to prevent heavy growth of organisms such as *P. cepacia* and *P. aeruginosa*. Plasma and cryoprecipitate units should be kept dry during thawing by use of a plastic overwrap.[58]

Photochemical Decontamination

A variety of photodynamic methods that inactivate viruses, bacteria, and protozoa are under development.[22] Psoralens bind to nucleic acids by intercalation and, on illumination with ultraviolet A (UVA) light, cause irreparable damage to the nucleic acids, inhibiting proliferation. Use of the novel psoralen S-59 followed by UVA light exposure has been shown to inactivate viruses and bacteria while preserving platelet function.[109] Clinical trials of apheresis platelets treated with this agent are underway currently in Europe and the United States. Other compounds are under development for use with RBC concentrates.[110]

■ Preferred Approach

Hospital Transfusion Service

A high index of suspicion is necessary to correctly diagnose a transfusion-associated septic reaction. The presence of a septic reaction should be considered if a blood product recipient develops a fever of 38°C or higher (or a 1°C rise in temperature), shaking chills, tachycardia, or hypotension during or shortly after transfusion. Nausea, vomiting, diarrhea, skin rash, and dyspnea also may be present. Patients under general anesthesia may present with hypotension, excessive bleeding, and oliguria.

If a septic reaction is suspected, the transfusion should be stopped and an intravenous line for venous access should be left in place. The blood bag should be returned to the blood bank and inspected for evidence of color change, hemolysis, clots, or bag defects. A Gram stain should be done on the remaining blood component, but this test may be negative in one third of cases. Aerobic and anaerobic cultures of the remaining product should be performed. Nutrient broth may be introduced into the blood bag if very little product remains for culture. Blood cultures also should be taken from the recipient. Symptoms are often nonspecific, so, in the case of a severe reaction, serologic investigation to rule out an acute hemolytic reaction due to an immunologic incompatibility should also be done.

For patients with a severe septic reaction, broad-spectrum antibiotic coverage (e.g., the combination of a β-lactam antibiotic with an aminoglycoside) should be initiated before culture results are obtained. Aggressive supportive care with intravenous fluids and vasopressors may be necessary if septic shock occurs.

Ideally, the diagnosis is firmly established when the same organism is isolated from the blood component and the patient. In some studies, microbial identity has been compared with the use of antibiotic susceptibility tests and PCR-based methods. Laboratory diagnosis can be difficult, because cultures from a recipient who is taking antibiotics may be negative, and cultures of the remaining blood component may be positive due to post-transfusion contamination.

Finally, the blood supplier should be informed as soon as possible about the suspected septic transfusion reaction.

The detection of an unusual pathogen such as *Y. enterocolitica* or *P. cepacia* in a transfusion recipient should prompt a search for a possible contaminated blood component. Clustering of cases of septicemia with unusual organisms such as *S. marcescens* should prompt a search for contaminated blood components or another iatrogenic cause (e.g., contaminated saline solutions).

Blood Supplier

When informed of a possible septic transfusion reaction, the transfusion service should recall and culture the other components from the same donation. If a defect is found in the bag or a cluster of cases has been reported, quarantine and investigation of other bags from the same lot may be necessary. In the case of an organism that is not part of normal skin flora, the donor should be contacted and asked about the development of infections before or shortly after blood donation.

Transfusion services should encourage the hospitals they supply to report septic transfusion reactions, and they in turn should report such reactions to national registries. This will permit the detection of small clusters of infections, such as the outbreak of *S. marcescens* in Scandinavia, that are related to blood bag contamination. Estimates of the frequency of such reactions are an important part of transfusion medicine hemovigilance, in order to continue to improve the safety of the blood supply.

Subsequent to the completion of this chapter many additional publications have appeared relevant to the topic of the bacterial contamination of blood products. Thus for up-to-date information relating to the topic of this chapter, the reader is referred to two recent publications by the authors.[23, 111]

REFERENCES

1. Borden CW, Hall WH: Fatal transfusion reactions from massive bacterial contamination of blood. N Engl J Med 1951;245:760–765.
2. Boulton FE, Chapman ST, Walsh TH: Fatal reaction to transfusion of red-cell concentrate contaminated with *Serratia liquefaciens*. Transfus Med 1998;8:15–18.
3. McDonald CP, Hartley S, Orchard K, et al: Fatal *Clostridium perfringens* sepsis from a pooled platelet transfusion. Transfus Med 1998;8:19–22.
4. Theakston EP, Morris AJ, Streat SJ, et al: Transfusion-transmitted *Yersinia enterocolitica* infection in New Zealand. Aust N Z J Med 1997;127:62–67.
5. Centers for Disease Control and Prevention. Red blood cell transfusions contaminated with *Yersinia enterocolitica*—United States, 1991–1996, and initiation of a national study to detect bacteria-associated transfusion reactions. MMWR Morb Mortal Wkly Rep 1997;46:553–555.
6. Morrow JF, Braine HG, Kickler TS, et al: Septic reactions to platelet transfusions. JAMA 1991;266:555–558.
7. Blajchman MA, Ali AM: Bacteria in the blood supply: an overlooked issue in transfusion medicine. *In* Nance, SJ (ed). Blood Safety: Current Challenges. Bethesda, MD: American Association of Blood Banks, 1992, pp 213–228.
8. Barrett BB, Anderson JW, Anderson KC: Strategies for the avoidance of bacterial contamination of blood components. Transfusion 1993;33:228–233.
9. Yomtovian R, Lazarus HM, Goodnough LT, et al: A prospective microbiologic surveillance program to detect and prevent the transfusion of bacterially contaminated platelets. Transfusion 1993;33:902–909.
10. Chiu EKW, Yuen KY, Lie AKW, et al: A prospective study on symptomatic bacteremia from platelet transfusion and its management. Transfusion 1994;34:950–965.
11. Dzieczkowski JS, Barrett BB, Nester D, et al: Characterization of reactions after exclusive transfusion of white cell-reduced cellular blood components. Transfusion 1995;35:20–25.
12. Blajchman MA, Ali A, Lyn P, et al: A prospective study to determine the frequency of bacterial contamination in random donor platelet concentrates [Abstract]. Blood 1994;84S:529a.
13. Leiby DA, Kerr KL, Compos JM, et al: A prospective analysis of microbial contaminants in outdated random-donor platelets from multiple sites. Transfusion 1997;37:259–263.
14. Blajchman MA, Ali A, Lyn P, et al: Bacterial surveillance of platelet concentrates: quantitation of bacterial load [Abstract]. Transfusion 1997;37(Suppl):74S.

15. Liu H, Yuen K, Cheng T, et al: Reduction of platelet transfusion-associated sepsis by short-term bacterial culture. Vox Sang 1999;77:1–5.

16. Goldman M, Blajchman MA: Blood product-associated bacterial sepsis. Transfus Med Rev 1991;5:73–83.

17. Richards C, Kolins J, Trindale CD: Autologous transfusion-transmitted *Yersinia enterocolitica* [Letter]. JAMA 1992;268:1541–1542.

18. Sire JM, Michelet C, Mesnard R, et al: Septic shock due to *Yersinia enterocolitica* after autologous transfusion [Letter]. Clin Infect Dis 1993;17:954–955.

19. Duncan KL, Ransley J, Elterman M: Transfusion-transmitted *Serratia liquefaciens* from an autologous blood unit [Letter]. Transfusion 1994;34:738–739.

20. Haditsch M, Binder L, Gabriel C, et al: *Yersinia enterocolitica* septicemia in autologous blood transfusion. Transfusion 1994;34:907–909.

21. Mitchell KMT, Brecher ME: Approaches to the detection of bacterial contamination in cellular blood products. Transfus Med Rev 1999;13:132–144.

22. Corash L: Inactivation of viruses, bacteria, protozoa, and leukocytes in platelet concentrates: current research perspectives. Transfus Med Rev 1999;13:18–30.

23. Goldman M, Blajchman MA: Bacterial contamination. *In* Popovsky M (ed). Transfusion Reactions (2nd edition). Bethesda, MD: American Association of Blood Banks, 2001, pp 129–154.

24. Tipple MA, Bland LA, Murphy MJ, et al: Sepsis associated with transfusion of red cells contaminated with *Yersinia enterocolitica*. Transfusion 1990;30:207–213.

25. McAllister SK, Bland LA, Arduino MJ, et al: Patient cytokine response in transfusion-associated sepsis. Infect Immun 1994;62:2126–2128.

26. Schwalbe B, Späth-Schwalbe E: Endotoxin concentrations and cytokine responses in a patient with fatal transfusion-associated sepsis [Letter]. Transfusion 1998;38:703–705.

27. Olsen KE, Sandler SG: Febrile neutropenia contributes to underreporting of potential septic platelet transfusion reactions [Letter]. Vox Sang 1996;70:118.

28. Zaza S, Tokars JI, Yomtovian R, et al: Bacterial contamination of platelets at a university hospital: increased identification due to intensified surveillance. Infect Control Hosp Epidemiol 1994;15:82–87.

29. Rhame FS, McCullough J: Follow-up on nosocomial *Pseudomonas cepacia* infection. MMWR Morb Mortal Wkly Rep 1979;28:409.

30. Casewell MW, Slater NGP, Cooper JE: Operating theatre water-baths as a cause of pseudomonas septicaemia. J Hosp Infect 1981;2:237–240.

31. Attarian H, Bensinger WI, Buckner CD, et al: Microbial contamination of peripheral blood stem cell collections. Bone Marrow Transplant 1996;17:699–702.

32. Aber RC: Transfusion-associated *Yersinia enterocolitica*. Transfusion 1990;30:193–195.

33. Mitchell R, Barr A: Transfusing *Yersinia enterocolitica* [Letter]. BMJ 1992;305:1095–1096.

34. Beresford AM: Transfusion reaction due to *Yersinia enterocolitica* and review of other reported cases. Pathology 1995;27:133–135.

35. Lian CJ, Hwang WS, Pai CH: Plasmid-mediated resistance to phagocytosis in *Yersinia enterocolitica*. Infect Immun 1987;55:1176–1183.

36. Gibb AP, Martin KM, Davidson GA, et al: Modeling the growth of *Yersinia enterocolitica* in donated blood. Transfusion 1994;34:304–310.

37. Högman CF, Engstrand L: Factors affecting growth of *Yersinia enterocolitica* in cellular blood products. Transfus Med Rev 1996;10:259–275.

38. Arduino MJ, Bland LA, Tipple MA, et al: Growth and endotoxin production of *Yersinia enterocolitica* and *Enterobacter agglomerans* in packed erythrocytes. J Clin Microbiol 1989;27:1483–1485.

39. Stevens AR, Legg JS, Henry BS, et al: Fatal transfusion reactions from contamination of stored blood by cold growing bacteria. Ann Intern Med 1953;39:1228–1239.

40. Wagner SJ, Moroff G, Katz AJ, Friedman LI: Comparison of bacteria growth in single and pooled platelet concentrates after deliberate inoculation and storage. Transfusion 1995;35:298–302.

41. Badon SJ, Fister RD, Cable RG: Survival of *Borrelia burgdorferi* in blood products. Transfusion 1989;29:581–583.

42. Goodman JL, Bradley JF, Ross AE, et al: Bloodstream invasion in early Lyme disease: results from a prospective, controlled, blinded study using the polymerase chain reaction. Am J Med 1995;99:6–12.

43. Aoki SK, Holland PV: Lyme disease: another transfusion risk? Transfusion 1989;29:646–650.

44. Arguin PM, Singleton J, Rotz LD et al: An investigation into the possibility of transmission of tick-borne pathogens via blood transfusion. Transfusion 1999;39:828–833.

45. Casleton BG, Salata K, Dasch GA, et al: Recovery and viability of *Orientia tsutsugamushi* from packed red cells and the danger of acquiring scrub typhus from blood transfusion. Transfusion 1998;38:680–689.

46. Alport T, Sher G: Personal communication. August 1999.

47. Burrascano JJ: Transmission of *Borrelia burgdorferi* by blood transfusion [Abstract]. International Conference on Lyme Borreliosis, 1992, p A44a.

48. Rhame FS, Root RK, MacLowry JD, et al: Salmonella septicemia from platelet transfusions: study of an outbreak traced to a hematogenous carrier of *Salmonella cholerae suis*. Ann Intern Med 1973;78:633–641.

49. Anderson KC, Lew MA, Gorgone BC, et al: Transfusion-related sepsis after prolonged platelet storage. Am J Med 1986;81:405–411.

50. Blajchman MA, Thornley JH, Richardson H, et al: Platelet transfusion-induced *Serratia marcescens* sepsis due to vacuum tube contamination. Transfusion 1979;19:39–44.

51. Kosmin M: Bacteremia during leukapheresis [Letter]. Transfusion 1980;20:115.

52. Heltberg O, Skov F, Gerner-Smidt P, et al: Nosocomial epidemic of *Serratia marcescens* septicemia ascribed to contaminated blood transfusion bags. Transfusion 1993;33:221–227.

53. Högman CF, Fritz H, Sandberg L: Posttransfusion *Serratia marcescens* septicemia [Editorial]. Transfusion 1993;33:189–191.

54. Steere AC, Terrey JH, Mackel DC, et al: *Pseudomonas* species bacteremia caused by contaminated normal human serum albumin. J Infect Dis 1977;135:729–735.

55. Högman CF, Engstrand L: Serious bacterial complications from blood components: how do they occur? Transfus Med 1998;8:1–3.

56. Dyer O: Blood authority investigates faulty blood bags. BMJ 1995;311:145.

57. AABB Weekly Report 1996(Oct. 11):6.

58. Halkier-Sorensen L, Kragballe K, Nedergaard St, et al: Lack of transmission of *Borrelia burgdorferi* by blood transfusion [Letter]. Lancet 1990;1:550.

59. Centers for Disease Control and Prevention. Lyme disease–United States, 1996. MMWR Morb Mortal Wkly Rep 1997;46:531–535.

60. Cable R, Krause P, Badon S, et al: Acute blood donor co-infection with *Babesia microti* [Abstract]. Transfusion 1993;33(Suppl):50S.

61. Gerber MA, Shapiro ED, Krause PJ, et al: The risk of acquiring Lyme disease or babesiosis from a blood transfusion. J Infect Dis 1994;170:231–234.

62. Gibson T, Norris W: Skin fragments removed by injection needles. Lancet 1958;2:983–985.

63. Morrissey AB, Jacobs MR, Lazarus H, Yomtovian R: Lack of contribution of the pooling and transfusion process to bacterial contamination of platelets [Abstract]. Transfusion 1992;32(Suppl):41S.

64. Noel L, Debeir J, Cosson A: The French haemovigilance system. Vox Sang 1998;74(Suppl 2):441–445.

65. Perez P, Ngombet R, Debeir J, et al: Les incidents transfusionnels par contamination bactérienne: synthèse de la littérature et des données d'hémovigilance. Transfus Clin Biol 1998;5:203–210.

66. Noël L, Audurier A: Contaminations bactériennes des produits sanguins labiles [Abstract]. Transfus Clin Biol 1998;5(Suppl 1):256S.

67. Girard M, Bombail Girard D, Meyer B, et al: Contrôle bactériologique systématique des concentrés de plaquettes d'aphérèse [Abstract]. Transfus Clin Biol 1998;5(Suppl 1):163S.

68. Williamson LM, Love EM: Reporting serious hazards of transfusion: the SHOT program. Transfus Med Rev 1998;12:28–35.

69. Walther-Wenke G: Contamination rates of blood components in Germany. International Symposium on New Aspects in Microbial Safety of Blood Components, Sept 7–8, Heidelberg, 1999.

70. Soeterboek AM, Welle FHW, Marcelis JH, et al: Sterility testing of blood products in 1994/1995 by three cooperating blood banks in The Netherlands. Vox Sang 1997;72:61–62.

71. AABB Weekly Report 1997(Nov. 21):4–5.

72. Kuehnert MJ, Roth VR, Haley NR, et al: Transfusion-transmitted bacterial infection in the United States, 1998 through 2000. Transfusion 2001;41:1493–1499.

73. Grossman BJ, Kollins P, Lau PM, et al: Screening blood donors for gastrointestinal illness: a strategy to eliminate carriers of *Yersinia enterocolitica*. Transfusion 1991;31:500–501.

74. Morris AJ, Woodfield DG: Antibody screening for recent *Yersinia enterocolitica* infection in blood donors [Letter]. Transfusion 1998;38:511–512.

75. Goldman M, Long A, Roy G, et al: Incidence of positive bacterial cultures after donor call-back [Letter]. Transfusion 1996;36:1035.

76. AABB News Briefs 1989;12:1–4.

77. Ness PM, Perkins HA: Transient bacteremia after dental procedures and other minor manipulations. Transfusion 1980;20:82–85.

78. Pleasant H, Marini J, Stehling L: Evaluation of three skin preps for use prior to phlebotomy [Abstract]. Transfusion 1994;34(Suppl):14S.

79. Goldman M, Roy G, Fréchette N, et al: Evaluation of donor skin disinfection methods. Transfusion 1997;37:309–312.

80. McDonald CP, Lowe P, Roy A, et al: Evaluation of donor arm disinfection techniques. Vox Sang 2001;80:135–141.

81. Kitchen AD, Howe PHJ: Donor arm swabbing: how clean is clean? [Abstract]. Transfus Med 1995;5(Suppl):50.

82. Olthuis H, Puylaert C, Verhagen C, Valk L: Method for removal of contamination bacteria during venipuncture [Abstract]. International Society for Blood Transfusion Regional Congress, Venice. 1995:77.

83. Vassort-Bruneau C, Perez P, Janus G, et al: New collection system to prevent contamination with skin bacteria [Abstract]. Vox Sang 1998;74(Suppl 1):1039.

84. Ollgaard M, Albjerg L, Georgsen J: Monitoring of bacterial growth in platelet concentrates: one year's experience with the BactAlert™ System [Abstract]. Vox Sang 1998;74(Suppl 1):1126.

85. Goldman M, Delage G: The role of leukodepletion in the control of transfusion-transmitted disease. Transfus Med Rev 1995;9:9–19.

86. Heal JM, Cohen HJ: Do white cells in stored blood component reduce the likelihood of posttransfusion bacterial sepsis? [Editorial]. Transfusion 1991;31:581–583.

87. Reesink HW, Hanfland P, Hertfelder H, et al: International forum: what is the optimal storage temperature for whole blood prior to preparation of blood components? Vox Sang 1993;65:320–327.

88. Pietersz RNI, Reesink HW, Dekker MA, et al: Elimination of *Yersinia enterocolitica* by a 20h hold of whole blood and removal of leukocytes by filtration [Abstract]. Transfusion 1992;32(Suppl):66S.

89. Wagner S, Moroff G, Katz A, Friedman L: Bacterial levels in components, prepared from deliberately inoculated whole blood held for 8 and 24 hours at room temperature [Abstract]. Transfusion 1994;34(Suppl):9S.

90. Currie LM, Harper JR, Allan H, et al: Inhibition of cytokine accumulation and bacterial growth during storage of platelet concentrates at 4°C with retention of in vitro functional activity. Transfusion 1997;37:18–24.

91. Bradley RM, Gander RM, Patel SK, et al: Inhibitory effect of 0°C storage on the proliferation of *Yersinia enterocolitica* in donated blood. Transfusion 1997;37:691–695.

92. Hoppe PA: Interim measures of detection of bacterially contaminated red cell components. Transfusion 1992;32:199–201.

93. Kim DM, Brecher ME, Bland LA, et al: Visual identification of bacterially contaminated red cells. Transfusion 1992;32:221–225.

94. Bertolini F, Murphy S: A multicenter inspection of the swirling phenomenon in platelet concentrates prepared in routine practice. Transfusion 1996;36:128–132.

95. McCarthy LR, Senne JE: Evaluation of acridine orange stain for detection of microorganisms in blood culture. J Clin Microbiol 1980;11:281–285.

96. Reik H, Rubin SJ: Evaluation of the buffy-coat smear for rapid detection of bacteria. JAMA 1981;245:357–359.

97. Burstain JM, Brecher ME, Workman K, et al: Rapid identification of bacterially contaminated platelets using reagent strips: glucose and pH analysis as markers of bacterial metabolism. Transfusion 1997;37:255–258.

98. Wagner SJ, Robinette D: Evaluation of swirling, pH, and glucose tests for the detection of bacterial contamination in platelet concentrates. Transfusion 1996;36:989–993.

99. Arpi M, Bremmelgaard A, Abel Y, et al: A novel screening method for the detection of microbial contamination of platelet concentrates [Letter]. Vox Sang 1993;65:335–336.

100. Hogman CF, Gong J: Studies of one invasive and two noninvasive methods for detection of bacterial contamination of platelet concentrates. Vox Sang 1994;67:351–355.

101. Wagner SJ, Robinette D: Evaluation of an automated microbiologic blood culture device for detection of bacteria in platelet components. Transfusion 1998;38:674–679.

102. Mertens G, Muylle L: False-positive and false-negative results of sterility testing of stored platelet concentrates [Letter]. Transfusion 1999;39:539–540.

103. Brecher ME, Wong ECC, Chen SE, et al: Vancomycin linked probes and microvolume fluorimetry for the rapid detection of gram positive bacterial contamination in platelet products [Abstract]. Transfusion 1998;38(Suppl):106S.

104. Brecher ME, Boothe G, Kerr A: The use of a chemiluminescence-linked universal bacterial ribosomal RNA gene probe and blood gas analysis for the rapid detection of bacterial contamination in white cell-reduced and nonreduced platelets. Transfusion 1993;33:450–457.

105. Brecher ME, Hogan JJ, Boothe G, et al: Platelet-bacterial contamination and the use of a chemiluminescence-linked universal bacterial ribosomal RNA gene probe. Transfusion 1994;34:1–6.

106. Chaney R, Rider J, Pamphilon D: Direct detection of bacteria in cellular blood products using bacterial ribosomal RNA-directed probes coupled to electrochemiluminescence. Transfus Med 1999;9:177–188.

107. Feng P, Keasler SP, Hill WE: Direct identification of Yersinia enterocolitica in blood by polymerase chain reaction amplification. Transfusion 1992;32:850–854.

108. Högman CF, Gong J, Eriksson L, et al: White cells protect donor blood against bacterial contamination. Transfusion 1991;31:620–626.

109. Lin L, Cook DN, Wiesehahn GP, et al: Photochemical inactivation of viruses and bacteria in platelet concentrates by use of a novel psoralen and long-wavelength ultraviolet light. Transfusion 1997;37:423–435.

110. Cook D, Stassinopoulos A, Wollowitz S, et al: In vivo analysis of packed red blood cells treated with S-303 to inactivate pathogens [Abstract]. Blood 1998;92(Suppl):503a.

111. Blajchman MA, Goldman M: Bacterial contamination of platelet concentrates: incidence, significance, and prevention. Semin Hemat 2001;38(4-Suppl 11):20–26.

Chapter 42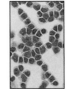

Additional Infectious Complications

Jay E. Menitove

Gary E. Tegtmeier

Additional infectious complications of blood transfusions include spirochete, protozoan, prion, parvovirus, and animal-to-human or zoonotic infections. Fortunately, these complications occur infrequently in the United States. However, changing global travel and emigration patterns and increasing use of xenotransplantation require ongoing awareness and surveillance for emerging infectious diseases.

This chapter describes agents endemic to the United States and those more prevalent in other parts of the world that have been transmitted or have a theoretical risk of transmission by transfusion, as well as measures to reduce the occurrence of this transfusion hazard.

■ Babesia

Babesiosis, a zoonosis caused by the rodent-borne piroplasm protozoan, *Babesia microti*, is transmitted by *Ixodes scapularis*, the deer or black-legged tick (Table 42.1).

I. scapularis also transmits the agents of Lyme disease and human granulocyte ehrlichiosis (discussed later).[1-4]

The white-footed mouse (*Peromyscus leucopus*) is the natural reservoir for *B. microti*; once infected, a mouse remains parasitemic indefinitely. *I. scapularis* transmits the piroplasm most frequently during the summer months. Endemic areas include coastal areas and islands of New England and New York as well as parts of California, Washington, Missouri, Wisconsin, and Minnesota.[2, 5, 6] Ticks coinfected with *B. microti* and *Borrelia burgdorferi* (the agent of Lyme disease) transmit *B. microti* less frequently than *B. burgdorferi* because the tick is a less competent host for *B. microti*. However, the intraerythrocytic site for *B. microti* favors transfusion transmission of this agent over *B. burgdorferi*, which is less frequently parasitemic.[6]

In humans, circulating *B. microti* DNA persists for an average of 82 days in asymptomatic patients and in those not given specific treatment. Coinfection with Lyme disease does

Table 42.1 Tick-borne Diseases

	Babesiosis	Lyme disease	HME	HGE	RMSF
Agent	*Babesia microti*	*Borrelia burgdorferi*	*Ehrlichia chaffeensis*	*Anaplasma phagocytophila*	*Rickettsia rickettsii*
Vector	*Ixodes scapularis*	*I. scapularis* *Ixodes pacificus*	*Ambylomma americanum*	*I. scapularis* *I. pacificus*	*Dermacentor variabilis*
Survival in blood component	Yes	Yes	Yes	Yes	Yes
Reported no. of transfusion-transmitted cases	>20	0	0	?1	1

HGE, human granulocytic ehrlichiosis; HME, human monocytic ehrlichiosis; RMSF, Rocky Mountain spotted fever.
Modified from McQuiston JH, Childs JE, Chamberland ME, Tabor E. Transmission of tick-borne agents of disease by blood transfusion: a review of known and potential risks in the United States. Transfusion 2000;40:274–284.

not alter the duration of parasitemia. Parasites circulate for only 16 days in persons who are treated with clindamycin and quinine. Patients with silent *Babesia* infections—approximately one third of infected individuals—are at risk for recrudescence spontaneously or after splenectomy or immunosuppression.[3] These persons also pose a risk through allogeneic blood donation, because the parasite retains infectivity in refrigerated or frozen stored red blood cell (RBC) components and in the residual RBCs contained in platelet concentrates stored at room temperature.[4, 7, 8]

To date, at least 24 cases of post-transfusion babesiosis have been reported.[2, 4, 5, 9–13] On the basis of these cases, the overall risk of acquiring transfusion-associated babesiosis is less than 1 in 1 million allogeneic blood donations, although the risk may vary regionally. A study conducted in Connecticut involving 155 cardiothoracic surgery patients given RBCs and platelet concentrates collected during the peak deer tick season identified 1 patient with babesiosis, representing a 0.17% risk per RBC unit transfused (95% confidence interval, 0.004% to 0.9%) and a 0% risk for platelet concentrates (95% confidence interval, 0% to 0.8%).[14]

The severity of clinical *B. microti* infections varies. Asplenia, older age, immunodeficiency syndromes, and liver disease increase the risk for severe illness. In acute, symptomatic cases, fatigue, malaise, weakness, and fever occur in more than 90% of the patients. Shaking chills, diaphoresis, nausea, anorexia, headaches, and myalgia occur frequently. Heart murmurs, hepatomegaly, and splenomegaly are found in 10% to 20% of patients; jaundice occurs less frequently. The average hemoglobin concentration was 11.3 g/dL in one report involving a review of hospitalized patients with community-acquired babesiosis.[1] In endemic areas, this diagnosis should be considered in patients with flu-like systemic symptoms during the summer.[3] More than one third of such patients reported a tick bite within 30 days before their hospitalization. Transfusion-acquired cases have an incubation period of 2 to 6.5 weeks.[2, 5, 10–13]

Examination of blood smears for piroplasms, antibabesial antibody assays, and polymerase chain reaction (PCR) assays for babesial DNA provide laboratory evidence of infection.[1, 3]

Blood collection agencies ask all prospective donors whether they have ever had babesiosis. Those answering affirmatively are deferred. However, donors are not asked about a recent history of tick bites or geographic residence because of the low predictive value associated with these questions.[4, 15] Serologic or PCR testing is impractical at this time. Hence, clinical awareness and suspicion leading to prompt intervention with antibiotic therapy are important for recognizing and treating this infrequent complication of transfusion therapy.

■ Lyme Disease

Lyme disease is a tick-borne zoonosis caused by infection with the *B. burgdorferi* spirochete (see Table 42.1). More than 12,000 cases occur annually in the United States, none of which have been reported to be associated with transfusion. Endemic areas include the northeastern, mid-Atlantic, and upper north-central regions of the United States, as well as several areas in northwestern California.[4, 16–18]

Infected *Ixodes* ticks (*I. scapularis* or *Ixodes pacificus*) serve as vectors. The ticks feed predominantly in the late spring and early summer during their nymphal stage. Lyme disease results predominantly from bites of infected nymphs. In endemic areas, 15% to 30% of *Ixodes* nymphs are infected with *B. burgdorferi*.

Patients with Lyme disease present with a characteristic erythema migrans rash accompanied by fever, malaise, headaches, myalgia, and arthralgia. The rash occurs over 7 to 14 days (range, 3 to 30 days) after a tick bite. *B. burgdorferi* spirochetes disseminate from the entry site via cutaneous, lymphatic, and blood-borne routes. Spirochetes have been isolated from the blood of patients with symptomatic Lyme disease.[19] Also, *B. burgdorferi* has been isolated from erythema migrans lesions. Treatment with antibiotics resolves the infection.

Serologic tests include enzyme-linked immunoassays and indirect fluorescent antibody tests. Western blot testing is used to confirm the results of reactive screening tests. PCR tests are available on a research basis. Currently, the diagnosis of Lyme disease is made primarily on a clinical basis.[18]

The possibility of transmission by blood transfusion requires consideration because the spirochete survives during routine storage of RBCs and frozen plasma storage.[20–23] However, there have been no confirmed reports of transfusion-associated Lyme disease.[24] Transfusion of RBCs or platelets collected from donors during peak deer tick activity to 155 patients undergoing cardiothoracic surgery resulted in no serologic or clinical evidence of Lyme disease.[4, 14] Presumably, the spirochetemic period occurs simultaneously with the onset of nonspecific symptoms for which potential donors would be deferred from blood donation. Individuals with a history of Lyme disease are accepted as blood donors provided they have been treated and are asymptomatic.

■ Transfusion Transmission of Other Tick-Borne Pathogens

Two emerging tick-borne zoonoses (see Table 42.1), human monocytic ehrlichiosis (HME) and human granulocytic ehrlichiosis (HGE), are reported with increasing frequency in the United States.[4, 24]

HME is caused by *Ehrlichia chaffeensis*. Most of the reported cases have occurred in the south-central and southeastern United States. HME is transmitted to humans through the bite of a Lone Star tick (*Amblyomma americanum*) previously infected by contact with deer or possibly dogs.

HGE is caused by *Anaplasma phagocytophila* which is related closely to species that infect horses (*Ehrlichia equi*) or ruminants (*Ehrlichia phagocytophila*). This illness occurs predominantly in the northeastern and upper midwestern areas of the United States and is transmitted to humans by *I. scapularis* or *I. pacificus* ticks.[4, 17, 24, 25] Fifty percent of ticks examined in one study in Connecticut were infected with the HGE agent, but none was infected with *E. chaffeensis*.[26] Another human ehrlichiosis, caused by *Ehrlichia ewingii*, also has been reported.[27]

Patients with HME and those with HGE present similarly, with fever, headache, myalgia, thrombocytopenia, leukopenia, and elevated liver enzyme concentrations. A rash occurs in one third of patients with HME. Membrane-bound intracytoplasmic ehrlichia aggregates or morulae are present in monocytes. Complications include respiratory distress, renal failure, neurologic disorders, and disseminated intravascular coagulation.

Septicemia, vasculitis, and thrombotic thrombocytopenic purpura should be considered in the differential diagnosis.[4, 24, 25] Doxycycline is the treatment of choice.

Because ehrlichia are present in blood, transfusion transmission must be considered. One case of transfusion-associated HGE occurred 9 days after an RBC transfusion donated by an asymptomatic donor who had been exposed to extensive deer ticks 2 months previously. The infected RBCs were stored for 30 days before transfusion.[28] An extensive epidemiologic study in Arkansas involving military trainee blood donors who had been exposed to tick bites and unknowingly infected with the agents of ehrlichiosis and Rocky Mountain spotted fever (RMSF) found no clinical illness among the recipients of RBCs and platelets donated by these soldiers.[29] However, possible seroconversion to RMSF occurred in one of the recipients.[29]

There is a single case report of clinical illness associated with transfusion-transmitted RMSF infection[30] (see Table 42.1). The donor developed symptoms of RMSF 3 days after donation. The recipient developed fever and headache 6 days after receiving the implicated *Rickettsia rickettsii*–infected transfusion.

Although the risk of transfusion transmission of these agents is low, clinical suspicion is important because appropriate antibiotic intervention is effective.

■ Malaria

Malaria is a protozoan disease caused by four species of the genus *Plasmodium*: *P. falciparum*, *P. vivax*, *P. ovale*, and *P. malariae* (Table 42.2). These protozoa are transmitted to humans by the bite of an infected female mosquito of the genus *Anopheles*. Infection of the human host, absent treatment, results in a chronic intraerythrocytic infection that can be transmitted by blood transfusion.

Malaria is a huge global public health problem, with an estimated annual incidence of 300 to 500 million cases and 3 million deaths per year.[31] Malarial endemic areas include parts of Africa, Asia, Central America, Hispaniola, North America, Oceania, and South America.

During the early part of the 20th century, specifically 1914, an estimated 600,000 cases of malaria occurred in the continental United States, but since the 1940s improved socioeconomic conditions, water management, vector control, and case management have prevented endemic malaria transmission.[32] Ongoing malaria surveillance in the United States continues to recognize cases in immigrants and in residents and travelers to areas of the world where malaria transmission still occurs. Each year, a few cases are reported that might represent local mosquito-borne transmission.[33] Congenital infections and transfusion-acquired infections round out the sources of malaria cases diagnosed each year in the United States.

Although the signs and symptoms of malaria are variable, most patients are febrile, and many also manifest headache, chills, sweating, nausea, vomiting, diarrhea, back pain, myalgia, and cough. A diagnosis of malaria should be considered for any patient with symptoms who has a history of travel to a malaria-endemic area or recent blood transfusion. Malaria also should be considered in the differential diagnosis of patients who have fever of unknown origin regardless of their travel history.

Of 1167 cases of malaria in the United States with onset of symptoms in 1995, one was acquired by organ transplantation and one by blood transfusion.[34] Of 1014 reported cases in 1994, two were transfusion-acquired.[35] The overwhelming majority of cases are imported, with roughly half occurring among immigrants or refugees and half among U.S. travelers, both civilian and military. About 85% of the cases among travelers occur in persons who failed to take prophylactic drugs or who were given ineffective drugs.

Mosquitos of the genus *Anopheles*, with few exceptions, feed between dusk and dawn. The exceptions are daytime feedings in densely shaded woodlands or dark interiors of houses or shelters. Therefore, travelers who visit malarial areas during bright daylight hours are at little or no risk for acquiring malaria if they return to a nonmalarial area before dusk.

Transfusion-transmitted malaria occurs at an estimated rate of 0.25 cases per 1 million blood units collected.[36] Because of this low incidence and the lack of a laboratory test approved by the U.S. Food and Drug Administration (FDA), prevention of transfusion-transmitted malaria continues to depend solely on the donor deferral guidelines established by the FDA and most recently updated in 1994.[37] Currently, prospective donors who are residents of countries where malaria is not endemic but who have traveled to a malaria-endemic area are temporarily deferred until 1 year after their departure from the endemic area if they have remained free of symptoms suggestive of malaria. Immigrants, refugees, citizens, and residents of malaria-endemic areas are deferred for 3 years after their departure from the endemic area if they have remained free of symptoms suggestive of malaria. Prospective donors with a history of malaria are deferred for 3 years after becoming asymptomatic.

The three cases of post-transfusion malaria due to *P. falciparum* that occurred between 1996 and 1998, two of which were fatal,[38] prompted a review by the Centers for

Table 42.2 Transfusion-Transmitted Malaria in the United States 1963–1999*

	Plasmodium falciparum	Plasmodium vivax	Plasmodium ovale	Plasmodium malariae
Transfusion-associated cases, 1963–1998 (% of total)	33 (36%)	25 (27%)	5 (5%)	25 (27%)
Average incubation period (days)	17 (range, 8–36)	20 (range, 11–42)	24 (range, 18–30)	51 (range, 8–90)
Relapse	No (manifests clinically within 1 year	Yes (usually within 3 years	Yes (usually within 3 years	Yes (prolonged)

*3 cases were due to mixed infections. The etiology of two cases was unknown.

Disease Control and Prevention (CDC) of all cases of trans-fusion-transmitted malaria reported to CDC between 1963 and 1999[39] (see Table 42.2). A total of 93 cases (2.5 per year) were reported during this interval. Thirty-three cases (36%) were caused by *P. falciparum*, 25 (27%) by *P. vivax*, 25 (27%) by *P. malariae*, 5 (5%) by *P. ovale*, 3 (3%) by mixed species, and 2 (2%) by an undetermined species. *P. falciparum* cases increased in frequency over the period 1990 to 1999, account-ing for 10 (71%) of 13 cases during that interval, compared with 15 (24%) of 45 cases reported between 1970 and 1989. Of 10 (11%) fatal cases overall, 6 were associated with *P. falciparum*, 2 with *P. vivax*, and 2 with *P. malariae*.

The incubation period of cases ranged from 8 to 90 days, with *P. falciparum* having the shortest time (mean, 17 days; range, 8 to 36 days) and *P. malariae* having the longest (mean, 51 days, range, 8 to 90 days). The period between onset of symptoms and the time of diagnosis ranged from 1 to 180 days, with a median of 10 days. Ninety-four percent of the cases were associated with transfusion of whole blood or RBCs; 6% were platelet-associated.

Implicated donors were defined as having met one or more of the following criteria: (1) a blood smear that demonstrated malaria parasites, (2) a positive result on malaria serology, and (3) being the only donor. Ninety-one donors were impli-cated in the 93 cases. Two blood products each from two implicated donors were transfused to four different patients. The median number of donors per case was seven (range, 1 to 192). Donors were overwhelmingly male (90%) and ranged in age from 19 to 59 years (median, 27 years). Foreign-born donors accounted for 59% (63% of those from Africa); 41% were born in the United States.

Of 58 donors implicated in the cases for which epidemio-logic follow-up was complete, serology was the most effective tool for identifying transmitting donors (72%); only 10% were identified by a positive blood smear. Serology and blood smear were both positive in 15%, and 3% were implicated as the only donor to a case.

Analysis of all cases using current donor deferral guide-lines revealed that 23 cases occurred despite proper applica-tion of the guidelines. When reviewed against the guidelines in place at the time they occurred, 3 cases could not be evaluated because their dates of onset were before 1970, when guidelines were vague; 18 of the remaining 20 cases would still have occurred but 2 would have been prevented if then-current guidelines had been applied properly. Not surprisingly, most (65%) of the cases that occurred where guidelines were followed were caused by *P. malariae*.

The continued occurrence of cases despite proper adminis-tration of the history questions highlights the reality that malaria risk from transfusion, although low, cannot be fully prevented by questioning of donors. Though the deferral guidelines currently in place are based on the biology of the four species of *Plasmodia* that cause malaria, they represent a balance struck between maximizing safety and minimizing donor loss. *P. vivax* and *P. ovale*, species that give rise to relapsing infections, rarely persist longer than 3 years.[40] However, some infections do persist, and individuals with these prolonged infections will transmit malaria if their blood is transfused. Likewise, disease caused by *P. falciparum*, a nonrelapsing species, manifests within 1 year after departure from a malarious area 99% of the time,[34] but a report of *falciparum* malaria occurring 13 years after departure from a malarious area has been published.[41] The well-known ability

of *P. malariae* to persist asymptomatically for decades in some individuals further highlights the difficulty of eradicat-ing the risk of post-transfusion malaria through questioning of donors.[42]

From time to time, proposals to screen donors for evidence of malaria have been advanced, but no FDA-approved tests or policies for screening donors are currently in place. Selective screening of high-risk donors has been suggested as an alter-native to universal screening.[43] Blood smear diagnosis is both impractical and insensitive as a donor screening technique. The indirect fluorescent antibody test (IFA) is useful diag-nostically but is unsuitable for large-scale donor screening, although it could be used to test high-risk donors and to determine their suitability.[43] Although antibody assays detect most individuals with parasitemia, they also are positive in persons who are no longer parasitemic.[44] Hence, noninfec-tious donors would be deferred if selective antibody screening were implemented. PCR is another promising test option that has sensitivity and specificity, but it is currently unstandard-ized and unavailable outside research laboratories.[45]

In roughly two thirds of the cases of post-transfusion malaria reported in the CDC review,[39] the donor screening process failed. These failures highlight the difficulties of obtaining accurate travel and immigration histories from donors. The American Association of Blood Banks has advocated the use of uniform donor screening questions to elicit malaria risk from prospective donors, including ques-tions that inquire about a history of malaria and about the prospective donor's travel history within the past 3 years. A "yes" answer to travel outside the United States and Canada triggers further inquiry to pinpoint travel destinations in malarious areas.

The FDA is currently revising its guidelines for deferral of blood donors because of a risk of malaria. The agency will issue the new guidelines sometime in the year 2002 or 2003. The proposed guidelines were discussed at the FDA's Blood Products Advisory Committee meeting in June 1999.[46] In addition to retaining the provisions for donor deferral outlined in the FDA memo of July 26, 1994,[37] the revised guideline recommends adding the following question sequence to the donor history form: (1) "Were you born in the United States?" (2) If yes, ask: "In the past 3 years have you been outside the United States or Canada?" (3) If the answer to (1) is no, ask: "When did you arrive in the United States and, since your arrival, have you traveled outside the United States or Canada?" If the answer to question (2) or the second question in (3) is yes, follow up questions will be asked of the donor to determine when and which country or countries were visited.

The impetus for revision of the guidelines includes the increased number of imported malaria cases in the United States, the large number of postdonation events related to malaria reported to the FDA, and the recognition that eliciting an accurate donor history is the only currently available defense against transfusion-transmitted malaria.

■ Chagas Disease

American trypanosomiasis, or Chagas disease, is a zoonosis caused by the hemoflagellate protozoan parasite *Trypanosoma cruzi* (Table 42.3). The life cycle of *T. cruzi* involves transmission from insect vectors to mammalian hosts includ-ing humans. *T. cruzi* infects humans when triatomid

Table 42.3 Transfusion-Associated Chagas Disease

Agent	*Trypanosoma cruzi*
Vector	Triatomid (reduviid) bugs
No. of transfusion-associated cases in United States and Canada	6 (platelet concentrates involved in at least 4 cases)
Implicated donors	Born in Chagas-endemic geographic region 16 to 33 years before implicated transfusion

(reduviid) or kissing bugs ingest a blood meal and deposit infected feces into the wound or when contaminated feces contact the mucosal surface of the eye or mouth. Hematogenous spread occurs subsequently. In addition *T. cruzi* crosses the placenta.

Acute Chagas disease is associated with fever, facial edema, generalized lymphadenopathy, and hepatosplenomegaly. Symptomatic myocarditis and meningoencephalitis can occur. Fulminant illness can occur in grown children or immunocompromised persons. In more than 95% of patients the illness is mild and symptoms resolve in 4 to 6 weeks. If untreated, patients enter an indeterminate phase. The low-grade parasitemia that is present in this phase presents a risk of transfusion transmission and of vertical transmission to infants. Between 12% and 48% of recipients of parasitemic blood become infected. Ten percent to 30% of patients progress from the indeterminate asymptomatic phase to a chronic symptomatic phase associated with cardiac enlargement, apical aneurysms, mural thrombi, megaesophagus, or megacolon appearing years to decades after infection.[42, 47–51]

An estimated 16 to 18 million people are infected in South America, Central America, and Mexico, where Chagas disease is endemic and triatomid insects reside in cracks of rural and suburban houses with adobe walls. There have been only five case reports of autochthonous transmission in the United States.[52]

Since 1989, five cases of transfusion-associated Chagas disease have been reported in the United States and Canada.[53–56] A sixth case involving a multiple myeloma patient without symptoms of Chagas disease was detected as part of a research study.[56] All six cases involved patients with malignancies, and in at least four of the cases platelets were the implicated blood component. Centrifugation may sediment *T. cruzi* into platelets during platelet concentrate preparation from whole blood, or storage at room temperature may favor parasite survival. *T. cruzi* has been shown to survive in refrigerated RBCs and whole blood.[51] Symptoms developed approximately 2 to 3 months after transfusion. In five of the reported cases, a donor emigrating from a *T. cruzi* endemic region (Bolivia, Mexico, Paraguay, Chile) was identified. Three of the donors emigrated between 16 and 33 years before the implicated transfusion.

Estimates of risk for transfusion-associated Chagas disease have evolved from studies conducted among immigrants from endemic regions. During the mid-1980s, 4.9% of 205 Nicaraguan and Salvadorian immigrants living in Washington, D.C., had serologic evidence of *T. cruzi* infection, and parasites were isolated from half of them.[57] In California, 0.06% to 0.33% of donors had geographic risk factors or serologic evidence of *T. cruzi* risk.[58–63] In Miami, 0.1% had *T. cruzi* antibodies.[63] Although a correlation exists between the percentage of immigrants from endemic areas and the percentage of donors with serologic evidence of *T. cruzi* infection, investigators have identified seropositive donors who were born in the United States.[64] Congenital transmission may have occurred in these individuals.

Approximately 2.5% of U.S. blood donors have a geographic risk of *T. cruzi* exposure, 0.003% to 0.14% are seropositive, and approximately 50% of infected donors have lifelong parasitemia.[51, 63, 64] Interventions to reduce the risk of transfusion-transmitted Chagas disease include questioning donors about geographic location of birth, extended stay or transfusion in areas endemic for Chagas disease, or serologic testing.[51, 58, 61] Currently, no tests are licensed by the FDA for blood screening, although highly specific confirmatory tests are available.[65] Donor history questions may be only 75% effective.[51] Leukocyte reduction by filtration appears to be effective in reducing *T. cruzi* transmission.[66]

The impact of transfusion-associated Chagas disease in the United States remains undefined. In only 1 case, of approximately 20 investigated, was a previous recipient of blood from a seropositive transfusion recipient found to be infected with *T. cruzi*.[56, 60, 63, 64] This may reflect a relative paucity of platelet transfusion recipients in the study cohort or fewer immuno-compromised patients. Ongoing monitoring is needed to define the risk of transfusion-transmitted Chagas disease in the United States.

■ Syphilis

Serologic testing of blood donations for syphilis was instituted in 1938 and required by regulation beginning in 1958. No cases of transfusion-associated syphilis have been reported in the United States since 1969.[67] An FDA advisory panel proposed eliminating the requirement for serologic syphilis testing in 1985, but changes were not made because of a potential benefit of such testing in preventing transmission of human immunodeficiency virus (HIV). Subsequently, observational data did not support this assumption. A National Institutes of Health Consensus Statement, issued in January 1995, recommended continuation of syphilis testing because its role in preventing transfusion-transmitted syphilis was not "understood."[68] Multiple factors—improved donor selection, uniform serologic testing, and lack of spirochete viability in blood stored at refrigerated temperatures—apparently contribute to the current lack of transfusion-transmitted syphilis cases.[67, 68]

There is no single optimal laboratory test for syphilis, and the infective agent, *Treponema pallidum*, cannot be cultured in vitro. During treponema infection, nontreponemal and treponemal antibodies are produced. The nontreponemal antibodies (reagin antibodies) react against phospholipid isolated from beef heart or cardiolipin. These antibodies are detected by the Venereal Disease Research Laboratory (VDRL), rapid plasma reagin (RPR), and other tests and are produced in response to the interaction of infected host tissue with *T. pallidum*. They parallel the pathologic course but have no relation to immunity. Treponema-specific antibodies have a higher serologic sensitivity in the early stages of syphilis but are less effective indicators of disease activity. During the first 3 weeks after primary infection, the VDRL is positive in 30% of cases and the fluorescent treponemal antibody-absorption (FTA-ABS) test is positive in 50%. Other treponemal antibody tests, often used to confirm nontreponemal tests, include *T. pallidum* particle aggregation (TP-PA) and recombinant antigen tests. An automated test for treponemal antibodies, PK $^{+M}$treponema pallidum (PK-TP), using the olympus PK 7200, is in wide use currently.[69]

The typical first sign of syphilis, a chancre, appears 3 to 90 days (average, 21 days) after exposure. The exact timing of spirochetemia and *T. pallidum* dissemination from the chancre and of seroconversion is not known. Secondary syphilis, characterized by a disseminated rash and spirochetemia, occurs 6 to 8 weeks after infection. Serologic tests are almost universally positive. If patients remain untreated, recurrent fulminant secondary syphilis recurs within 2 years in approximately 20%. Subsequently, patients become immune to reinfection and become noninfectious. VDRL titers decrease over time. Treponemal antibodies remain indefinitely in both treated and untreated patients, unless patients are treated in the primary stage.

Tertiary syphilis develops after a variable length of time. Reactivation is clinically and serologically noticeable via anticardiolipin and treponemal antibody detection.[69, 70, 71]

Reaction patterns characterized by positive RPR or PK-TP tests and negative FTA-ABS reactions (so-called false-positive reactions) may be caused by hepatitis, mononucleosis, viral pneumonia, chickenpox, measles, immunizations, pregnancy, or laboratory error. Persistent false-positive reactions have been reported in patients with rheumatoid arthritis, cirrhosis, ulcerative colitis, vasculitis, and older age.[69, 71]

Another factor mitigating transfusion-associated syphilis are the loss of *T. pallidum* viability during storage. Spirochetes survive 96 to 120 hours at refrigerated temperatures.[70, 72, 73] However, viability at room temperature (e.g., in platelet concentrates) has not been studied. By implication, loss of viability during storage is an incomplete protection mechanism, favoring retention of serologic testing.

Currently, blood from donations with reactive syphilis tests is discarded. If the confirmatory test is positive, donors are deferred for 1 year; they are then allowed to donate again, provided that they have undergone adequate treatment for syphilis and the serologic screening tests are negative.

■ Human Parvovirus

Human parvovirus B19 (Table 42.4) was discovered serendipitously in human plasma during blood donor screening for hepatitis B surface antigen in 1975.[74] For 6 years it was a virus in search of a disease. It was then found to be the cause of the transient aplastic crisis in patients with sickle cell anemia[75] and subsequently in patients with other inherited hemolytic diseases,[76] in whom it can result in severe reticulocytopenia and anemia.

B19 was later found to be the etiologic agent of fifth disease or erythema infectiosum, a common childhood illness that manifests as an erythematous rash.[77] Arthropathy is a frequent complication of adult-acquired B19 infection, particularly in women.[78, 79] Encephalitis and meningitis are infrequent but potentially severe complications of B19 infection in both children and adults.[80, 81]

B19 can infect the fetus via transplacental transmission, resulting in hydrops fetalis and fetal death in approximately 10% of cases.[82] Adverse outcomes are most often associated with first- and second-trimester infections. However, most women infected with B19 during pregnancy deliver unaffected infants.[83]

Table 42.4   Parvovirus

Agent	Human parvovirus B19 (a nonenveloped DNA virus)
Associated illnesses	Fifth disease (erythema infection), red cell aplasia
Transmission	Respiratory Transplacental (fetal death in 10%) Organ transplantation
Tropism	Blood group P antigen
At-risk transfusion recipients	Patients with inherited hemolytic disorders Pregnant women Solid and marrow transplant recipients AIDS patients

Although B19 infections in immunocompetent individuals are usually self-limited, persistent infections often occur in immunocompromised patients, with resultant RBC aplasia. Persistent B19 infections of transplant recipients,[84] leukemia patients,[85] and patients with acquired immunodeficiency syndrome (AIDS)[86, 87] have been documented.

B19 infects only humans and is highly tropic for erythroid progenitor cells, gaining access to cells through the blood group P antigen, which has been identified as the virus receptor.[88] Viral replication is dependent on cellular functions expressed only during the S phase of the cell cycle. Hence, only dividing cells with the P receptor can be productively infected. Cells with the P receptor that are not in S phase may be infected and "killed" because of the toxic effect of a nonstructural viral protein expressed by the B19 genome.[89]

B19 infection is ubiquitous in human populations and is already prevalent in pediatric age groups. Seroprevalence studies show antibody frequencies of 50% in high school age children and up to 90% in older adults.[89] Epidemics and sporadic infections may occur at any time of year, with major outbreaks of erythema infectiosum occurring every 3 to 6 years.

The respiratory route is the most common avenue for B19 transmission. Vertical transmission is much less common. Because of the transient, high-titer viremia that accompanies acute asymptomatic B19 infection, virus transmission by blood,[90–92] blood derivatives,[93] and organ transplantation[84] has been well documented.

The difficulty of adapting B19 to cell culture impeded the development of serologic tests for diagnosis and epidemiologic studies. Before the availability of recombinant and synthetic antigens, the only source of viral antigens was the blood of B19-infected patients or blood donors. Now, both immunoglobulin G (IgG)–specific and IgM-specific immunoassays based on recombinant or synthetic antigens are commercially available, as are supplemental Western blot and immunofluorescence assays.[93]

Direct detection of B19 was originally accomplished by counterimmunoelectrophoresis or immune electron microscopy. More recently, sophisticated molecular methods to detect the virus have become available in the form of dot-blot hybridization assays, in situ hybridization, and PCR. PCR has become the method of choice for direct detection of B19 and is especially useful in the identification of persistent infections among immunocompromised patients and asymptomatic blood and plasma donors.

Although early B19 antigen prevalence studies of blood donors using counterimmunoelectrophoresis agar gel diffusion showed relatively low rates of infection, ranging from 0.005% to 0.002%, PCR-based investigations have found rates in the range of 0.03% to 0.6%, emphasizing the insensitivity of the gel-based methods.[93]

Despite the documented transmission of B19 to blood recipients, the incidence of such infections is thought to be low because of the high prevalence of B19 antibody in adults and the possible mitigating effect of B19 antibody in antigen-positive donors. However, no large-scale, prospective studies of recipients of blood components have been published to assess the risk of B19 infection in this population. By contrast, recipients of plasma derivatives have been recognized to be at risk for B19 for some time.[93] Despite the application of viral inactivation steps to pooled plasma products beginning in the mid-1980s, the risk of B19 infection is still high in heavily transfused patients (58% to 98%).[93] This situation prevails because B19 is a small, nonenveloped, DNA virus that is highly resistant to chemical and physical agents. The relatively high prevalence of B19-positive donors detected by PCR ensures that practically every plasma pool will contain B19.

Prospective studies involving small numbers of previously untreated hemophiliacs for evidence of B19 transmission have verified the conclusions from the cross-sectional studies mentioned previously. Seroconversion rates ranging from 17% to 71% were observed with concentrates inactivated by a variety of methods. Although these studies were uncontrolled, the proximity of seroconversion and PCR positivity in recipients in relation to the first infusion of concentrate makes it highly unlikely that the observed infections were community acquired and confirms the ongoing risk of infection from virally inactivated concentrates.[93]

The highly resistant nature of B19 is illustrated in reports of B19 detection by PCR in lots of recombinant factor VIII. Anecdotal reports of seroconversion in recipients of recombinant factor VIII have yet to be documented. The suspected source of contamination is the albumin used to stabilize the recombinant factor VIII. One study showed 3 of 12 albumin samples to be positive for B19 DNA, whereas a second study failed to detect B19 in 29 different lots. Whether the presence of B19 sequences detectable by PCR predicts infectivity awaits the development of a suitable in vitro assay for infectivity. Second-generation recombinant products omit albumin as a stabilizer and therefore should not pose a risk of B19 infection to hemophilia patients.

Postmarketing studies of a solvent detergent–treated fresh frozen plasma have shown evidence for B19 infection in volunteers infused with this product. This has prompted the manufacturer to introduce PCR testing of minipools for B19 DNA as an in-process step to reduce the viral load in pools to less than 10^4 genome equivalents per milliliter. Fresh frozen plasma derived from such pools carries a greatly reduced risk for B19 transmission.[94] Plasma fractionators in the United States and Europe have implemented, or are in the process of implementing, B19 testing of minipools by nucleic acid amplification testing as an in-process step, a development that may have implications for blood centers providing recovered plasma to commercial fractionators.[95]

Evolving policy vis á vis B19 and recipients of blood and blood components may emulate that already in place for cytomegalovirus. Vulnerable target populations may receive blood products screened with nucleic acid amplification tests to reduce the risk of B19 infection. At-risk populations identified to date include patients with inherited hemolytic abnormalities, pregnant women, recipients of solid organ and marrow transplants, and AIDS patients. Provision of blood products with reduced risk to these vulnerable patients awaits the commercial availability of nucleic acid amplification assays and the development of standards for these products.

■ Creutzfeldt-Jakob Disease (CJD) and New Variant CJD

Transmissible spongiform encephalopathies (TSEs) occurring in humans include kuru, Creutzfeldt-Jakob disease (CJD), Gerstmann-Sträussler-Scheinker disease, fatal familial insomnia, and variant CJD (vCJD). TSEs occurring in animals include scrapie, wasting disease of deer and elk, and bovine spongiform encephalopathy.[96–100]

The presumed TSE infectious agents are classified as prions, or proteinaceous infectious particles, and lack nucleic acid.[97] These agents resist treatments that inactivate viruses or nucleic acids, such as alcohol, formalin, ionizing irradiation, proteases, and nucleases, but are disrupted by autoclaving, phenols, detergents, and extremes in pH that affect proteins. All prion disease involves modification of a constituent of mammalian cells, prion protein (PrP). Normal, cellular PrP is designated PrP^c, and the protease-resistant protein associated with disease, a conformationally altered isoform of PrP, is designated PrP^{sc}. The conversion of PrP^c to PrP^{sc} results in refolding of a portion of the α-helical and coil structure of PrP^c into β-sheets. PrP^c is soluble in nondenaturing detergents and is digested by protease, whereas PrP^{sc} is insoluble and resistant, respectively.

CJD occurs at an incidence of 0.5 to 1.5 cases per 1 million population worldwide. This rate has been stable. Between 1979 and 1996, 4468 cases of CJD were reported in the United States.[96, 99] Sporadic CJD, causing 80% of CJD cases, occurs in persons 50 to 70 years of age and is manifested by dementia, myoclonus, and pyramidal tract and cerebellar signs. The mean survival time is 5 months. Approximately 10% to 15% of CJD cases occur in patients with a family history of CJD, suggesting an autosomal dominant inheritance pattern. More than 20 mutations for the genes on the short arm of chromosome 20 that encode PrP have been identified.

The remaining CJD cases involve iatrogenic transmission. CJD was transmitted by a corneal transplant from a patient with undiagnosed CJD, and stereotactic electroencephalographic silver electrodes previously implanted in a patient with CJD resulted in two iatrogenic CJD cases.[96, 99] At least 21 U.S. and 55 French recipients of intramuscular human growth hormone injections prepared from cadaveric pituitary glands from donors with unsuspected CJD have died.[100–103] The mean incubation period was 9 to 20 years, with some cases occurring 30 years after exposure. Cadaveric dura mater grafting with a commercial product prepared by batch processing resulted in at least 61 CJD cases worldwide, some occurring 16 years after graft placement.[104]

In sporadic and iatrogenic cases of CJD, a polymorphism involving codon 129 in the PrP gene sequence located on chromosome 20 appears to affect susceptibility. Normally 37% of the population are methionine/methionine homozygous and 11% are valine/valine homozygous at codon 129. The remaining 52% are heterozygous. Homozygous individuals represent almost 90% of sporadic and iatrogenic CJD cases.[96, 100]

Intracerebral inoculation with human prions from a CJD case resulted in transmission of CJD in transgenic mice expressing human PrP.[105] Other animal studies demonstrated transmission of a mouse-adapted human TSE strain by buffy coats, plasma, cryoprecipitate, and Cohn fractions I + II + III via intracerebral and intravenous inoculation.[106, 107] Studies involving immune-deficient mice suggested that differentiated B cells are needed for transporting intraperitonally inoculated TSE agents to nervous tissue.[108]

In contrast, no evidence of transfusion-associated CJD was documented in case-control studies involving more than 600 patients with CJD or in recipients of blood from persons who subsequently developed CJD.[109–116] Examination of brain tissue from deceased hemophilia patients showed no evidence of CJD.[117, 118] Nonetheless, the iatrogenic cases and the theoretical risk of CJD transmission by blood led the FDA to issue a recommendation to defer donors if they have one or more blood relatives with CJD or if they have received human pituitary–derived growth hormone injections or a dura mater transplant. All in-date products from donors with these risk factors must be quarantined and destroyed, and the previous recipients of blood from implicated donors, with the exception of those who have only one family member with CJD, must be notified.[119]

In the spring of 1985, several dairy cows in the United Kingdom displayed aggressive behavior, ataxia, and falling. These "mad cows" were found to have spongiform lesions in brain tissue resembling scrapie that was subsequently termed bovine spongiform encephalopathy (BSE). More than 160,000 cattle succumbed to BSE, but almost 1 million may have been infected. Because the mean incubation period for BSE is 5 years and most cows were slaughtered between 2 and 3 years of age, most cattle did not manifest disease.[96, 97, 100] Approximately 50,000 BSE-infected cattle entered the food chain before the first BSE case was recognized in 1986. Subsequently, the onset of the BSE epidemic was traced to feeding cattle a meat and bone meal made from sheep, cattle, and pig offal; the rendering process presumably resulted in the feeding of scrapie-infected material to cows. Use of sheep offal was banned in 1989. After March 1996, only animals younger than 30 months were allowed to be used for foodstuffs.[100]

Surveillance of human CJD cases was reinstated in the United Kingdom after recognition of the BSE epidemic. Ten of 207 CJD patients in 1994 and 1995 had unusual neuropathologic changes.[120–122] They presented predominately with psychiatric and sensory symptoms, ataxia, dementia, and myoclonus. All were younger than 45 years of age, a distinctly unusual characteristic for CJD. Electroencephalographic features were not typical of CJD, and florid PrP plaques were seen on neuropathologic examination. Median survival time was 14 months, in contrast to 4 months for CJD. These cases were considered to represent a new variant of CJD (vCJD). As of February 2000, 52 fatal cases of vCJD had been reported in the United Kingdom, 2 in France, and 1 in Ireland.[123] All patients tested were homozygous for methionine at PrP codon 129. Because a long incubation period is likely, the extent of the epidemic remains unknown.

Table 42.5   Donor Deferral Requirements for Variant Creutzfeldt-Jakob Disease (vCJD)

Permanent deferral
   Donors diagnosed with vCJD or CJD

Indefinite deferral
   Recipients of dura mater transplant; human pituitary-derived growth hormone; or bovine insulin since 1980
   One or more blood relatives with CJD
   Donors who spent 3 months or more cumulatively in the United Kingdom (England, Scotland, Wales, Northern Ireland, Isle of Man, Channel Islands, Gibraltar, and the Falkland Islands) from 1980 through 1996
Military personnel (current and former) and their dependents who spent time on military bases in northern Europe (1980–1990), or elsewhere in Europe (1980–1996), for 6 months or more
Donors who received a transfusion in the United Kingdom between 1980 and the present
Donors who lived in Europe for 5 years or more between 1980 and the present

Extensive investigations using animal models provided evidence that the same prion strain causes BSE and vCJD; the new variant therefore is distinct from classic CJD.[124–126] Ingestion of British beef appears to be a risk factor for BSE in nonhuman primates.[127]

Concern about transfusion transmission of vCJD arises because PrP^{sc} is found consistently in the lymphoreticular system of vCJD patients, because B lymphocytes appear to play a role in transporting TSEs, and because of findings in animal studies.[106, 108, 128] Universal blood component leukocyte reduction has been instituted in the United Kingdom and in other European countries in an effort to interdict lymphocytes from transmitting vCJD during transfusion.[98] However, evidence supporting the effectiveness of this intervention is uncertain.[129]

In light of the theoretical risk of transmitting vCJD by transfusion, the FDA revised its recommendation about CJD in November 1999 and January 2002.[99] In addition to previous CJD recommendations, donors who visited or resided in the United Kingdom for a cumulative period of 3 months or longer between 1980 and 1996 are deferred indefinitely. In addition, donors who injected bovine insulin after 1980 are indefinitely deferred. Prior notification of recipients of blood from these donors is not recommended by the FDA. In-date blood components and plasma intended for derivative production, however, must be recalled, quarantined, and destroyed. Ongoing surveillance of vCJD cases is being conducted, including a recommendation to notify the CDC about all patients younger than 55 years of age who are diagnosed with CJD (Table 42.5).

■ Leishmaniasis

Visceral forms of leishmaniasis result from infection with *Leishmania donovani* or *Leishmania infantum*. Cutaneous lesions occur in persons infected with *Leishmania braziliensis* or *Leishmania tropica*, the cause of Old World cutaneous leishmaniasis. However, at least eight soldiers returning from eastern Saudi Arabia after Operation Desert Storm developed visceral leishmaniasis that was attributed to *L. tropica*.[130, 131] The leishmania organisms, transmitted primarily by bites from infected sand flies, infect approximately 12 million persons in the tropical and subtropical regions of the Sudan, Eastern India, Bangladesh, Nepal, Brazil, and the Mediterranean.[132]

In the most severe manifestation of visceral leishmaniasis, kala-azar, patients have marked hepatosplenomegaly, pancytopenia, hypergammaglobulinemia, and cachexia. The incubation period is approximately 6 months.[132]

At least six transfusion-associated cases of leishmaniasis due to *L. donovani* have been reported.[133] Four of the patients were newborns, and two were young children. The latter two were infected from blood donated in China by their mother, who developed kala-azar 1 month after donation. Both children developed kala-azar. Two newborns received blood from a traveler to Spain, who developed skin lesions and lymphadenopathy 2 months after the donation. Biopsies from the donor revealed leishmania parasites. One of the transfused infants developed anemia, failure to thrive, and kala-azar. In the other cases, reported from Sweden and Belgium, the implicated donor was asymptomatic or not determined.

After being transmitted by a sand fly bite, parasites became intracellular in monocytes, which circulate for an undefined period until they localize in internal organs. Anti-*L. donovani* antibodies form shortly after infection. In Brazil,[134] 9% of blood donors and 7% of multitransfused dialysis patients in a low-incidence kala-azar region had antibodies against *L. donovani*. In comparison, antibodies were not detected in patients undergoing continuous ambulatory peritoneal dialysis—suggesting, but not proving, transfusion transmission. On follow-up, some of the blood donors had clinical symptoms, but this information was not available for transfusion recipients.[134] In a French study,[131] 76 of 565 blood donors had antibodies to *L. infantum*, and 16 had evidence of parasitemia by PCR or culture. Low-level or transient parasitemia was suspected.

Veterans of Operation Desert Storm were deferred from blood donation through 1993, after a report of *L. tropica*–related viscerotropic leishmaniasis in eight soldiers. The patients had nonspecific clinical manifestations, including prolonged fever, malaise, abdominal pain, and intermittent diarrhea, that occurred up to 7 months after they returned to the United States.[130] *L. tropica* was found in the bone marrow of seven patients and in a lymph node in one patient. Intracellular amastigotes were seen in the peripheral blood of the one patient in whom this was studied.[133] *L. tropica* within human monocytes survives in blood stored at 1° to 6°C, in frozen RBCs, and in platelet concentrates stored at room temperature. However, *L. tropica* has not been detected in relatively cell-free fresh frozen plasma. Animal studies demonstrate transmission by contaminated blood.[133]

No cases of transfusion-transmitted leishmaniasis have been reported in the United States to date. For this reason, surveillance rather than active measures (including donor deferral or testing) appears to be appropriate.

Toxoplasmosis

Toxoplasma gondii is a ubiquitous parasite whose usual host is the domestic cat. Infection sometimes results in lymphadenopathy, malaise, fever, headache, sore throat, splenomegaly, hepatomegaly, and rash. Retinopathy and lethal infections occur in immunocompromised hosts.

Transfusion transmission was reported in 1971. However, the cases occurred among leukemia patients given granulocyte transfusions obtained from other leukemic patients.[42] More recently, a case report suggested that a patient undergoing chemotherapy for a leukemic relapse 3 years after receiving an allogeneic marrow transplant developed toxoplasma pneumonitis. A person with serologic evidence of recent toxoplasma infection donated one of the units of blood transfused to the patient.[135] Previously, a 52-year-old woman with drug-induced thrombocytopenia developed toxoplasmic retinochoroiditis presumably related to a platelet transfusion.[136]

The paucity of reported cases indicates that this infection represents a remote risk to transfusion recipients.

Xenogeneic Infections

Xenotransplantation of pig and nonhuman primate organs and tissues has emerged as a result of the unavailability of such tissues from humans for transplantation and as therapy for Parkinson and Huntington diseases. Infectious outbreaks traced to animal sources (e.g., hantavirus, Ebola, HIV, BSE) raise concern that xenotransplantation might lead to other zoonoses.

Additionally, integrated proviruses, or endogenous animal viruses, are incorporated into vertebrate genomes and are inherited in mendelian fashion. Although these endogenous retroviruses may not be expressed in the natural host, they can infect cells in another species. Such xenotropic viruses therefore pose a risk to human xenotransplant recipients that cannot be prevented by raising the animals in sterile or pathogen-free environments. Although agents causing acute illness are detected promptly, infectious agents with long latent periods may pose a greater risk, because dissemination could be widespread before clinical awareness occurs.[137, 138]

Two different porcine endogenous retrovirus (PERV) proviruses capable of infecting human cells have been identified.[139–141] Several studies found no evidence for PERV infection among recipients of pig pancreatic islet cell transplants; dialysis patients whose blood was perfused through pig kidneys, spleens, and livers; or recipients of pig skin grafts.[142–144] Of possible concern, porcine cells persisted intravascularly in a microchimeric state for up to 8.5 years in 23 of 100 patients whose blood was perfused through pig spleens.[144]

Because of the theoretical risk of zoonosis transmission by blood and blood products from xenotransplant recipients, the FDA recommended in December 1999 that persons exposed to xenotransplantation products (live cells, tissues, or organs used in xenotransplantation), close contacts of such persons, and health care and laboratory workers exposed to blood and body fluids of xenotransplant product recipients should be deferred indefinitely from donating blood and blood components.[145]

REFERENCES

1. White DJ, Talarico J, Chang HG, et al: Human babesiosis in New York State: review of 139 hospitalized cases and analysis of prognostic factors. Arch Intern Med 1998;158:2149–2154.
2. Dobroszycki J, Herwaldt BL, Boctor F, et al: A cluster of transfusion-associated babesiosis cases traced to a asymptomatic donor. JAMA 1999;281:927–930.
3. Krause PJ, Spielman A, Telford SR, et al: Persistent parasitemia after acute babesiosis. N Engl J Med 1998;339:160–165.

4. McQuiston JH, Childs JE, Chamberland ME, Tabor E: Transmission of tick-borne agents of disease by blood transfusion: a review of known and potential risks in the United States. Transfusion 2000;40:274–284.

5. Linden JV, Wong SJ, Chu FK, et al: Transfusion-associated transmission of babesiosis in New York State. Transfusion 2000;40:285–289.

6. Krause PJ, Telford SR, Ryan R, et al: Geographical and temporal distribution of babesial infection in Connecticut. J Clin Microbiol 1991;29:1–4.

7. Popovsky MA: Transfusion-transmitted babesiosis. Transfusion 1991;31:296–298.

8. Grabowski EF, Giardina PJV, Goldberg D, et al: Babesiosis transmitted by a transfusion of frozen-thawed blood. Ann Intern Med 1982;96:466–467.

9. Smith RP, Evans AT, Popovsky M, et al: Transfusion-acquired babesiosis and failure of antibiotic treatment. JAMA 1986;256:2726–2727.

10. Mintz ED, Anderson JF, Cable RG, Hadler JL: Transfusion-transmitted babesiosis: a case report from a new endemic area. Transfusion 1991;31:365–368.

11. Wittner M, Rowin KS, Tanowitz HB, et al: Successful chemotherapy of transfusion babesiosis. Ann Intern Med 1982;96:601–604.

12. Herwaldt BL, Kjemtrup AM, Conrad PA, et al: Transfusion-transmitted babesiosis in Washington state: first reported case caused by WA1-type parasite. J Infect Dis 1997;175:1259–1262.

13. Marcus LC, Valigorsky JM, Fanning WL, et al: A case report of transfusion-induced babesiosis. JAMA 1982;248:465–467.

14. Gerber MA, Shapiro ED, Krause PJ, et al: The risk of acquiring Lyme disease or babesiosis from a blood transfusion. J Infect Dis 1994;170:231–234.

15. Popovsky MA, Lindberg LE, Syrek AL, Page PL: Prevalence of *Babesia* antibody in a selected blood donor population. Transfusion 1988;28:59–61.

16. Aoki SK, Holland PV: Lyme disease: another transfusion risk? Transfusion 1989;29:646–650.

17. Spach DH, Liles WC, Cambell GL, et al: Tick-borne diseases in the United States. N Engl J Med 1993;329:936–946.

18. Centers for Disease Control and Prevention. Recommendations for the use of Lyme disease vaccine. Recommendations of the Advisory Committee on Immunization Practices (ACIP). MMWR Morb Mortal Wkly Rep 1999;48:RR-7.

19. Nadelman RB, Pavia CS, Magnarelli LA, Wormser GP: Isolation of *Borrelia burgdorferi* from the blood of seven patients with Lyme disease. Am J Med 1990;88:21–26.

20. Baranton G, Saint-Girons I: *Borrelia burgdorferi* survival in human blood samples. Ann N Y Acad Sci 1988;539:444–445.

21. Badon SJ, Fister RD, Cable RD: Survival of *Borrelia burgdorferi* in blood products. Transfusion 1989;29:581–583.

22. Nadelman RB, Sherer C, Mack L, et al: Survival of *Borrelia burgdorferi* in human blood stored under blood banking conditions. Transfusion 1990;30:298–301.

23. Johnson SE, Swaminathan B, Moore P, et al: *Borrelia burgdorferi*: survival in experimentally infected human blood processed for transfusion. J Infect Dis 1990;162:557–559.

24. McQuiston JH, Paddock CD, Holman RC, Childs JE: The human ehrlichioses in the United States. Emerg Infect Dis 1999;5:635–642.

25. Goodman JL: Ehrlichiosis: ticks, dogs, and doxycycline. N Engl J Med 1999;341:195–197.

26. Magnarelli L, Ijdo J, Anderson J, et al: Human exposure to a granulocytic *Ehrlichia* and other tick-borne agents in Connecticut. J Clin Microbiol 1998;36:2823–2827.

27. Buller RS, Arens M, Hmiel SP, et al: *Ehrlichia ewingii*, a newly recognized agent of human ehrlichiosis. N Engl J Med 1999;341:148–155.

28. Eastlund T, Persing D, Mathieson D, et al: Human granulocyte ehrlichiosis after red cell transfusion. Transfusion 1999;93:117S.

29. Arguin PM, Singleton J, Rotz LD, et al: An investigation into the possibility of transmission of tick-borne pathogens via blood transfusion. Transfusion 1999;39:828–833.

30. Wells GM, Woodward TE, Fiset P, Hornick RB: Rocky Mountain spotted fever caused by blood transfusion. JAMA 1978;239:2763–2765.

31. World Health Organization. World malaria situation in 1993. Wkly Epidemiol Rec 1996;71:17–24.

32. Pan American Health Organization. Report for Registration of Malaria Eradication from the United States of America. Washington, DC: Pan American Health Organization, 1969.

33. Zucker JR: Changing patterns of autochthonous malaria transmission in the United States: a review of recent outbreaks. Emerging Infect Dis 1996;2:37–43.

34. Williams HA, Roberts J, Kachur SP, et al: Malaria surveillance—United States, 1995. MMWR Morb Mortal Wkly Rep 1999;48:SS-1.

35. Kachur SP, Reller ME, Barber AM, et al: Malaria surveillance—United States, 1994. MMWR Morb Mortal Wkly Rep 1997;46:SS-5.

36. Guerrero IC, Weniger BC, Schultz MG: Transfusion malaria in the United States, 1972–1981. Ann Intern Med 1983;99:221–226.

37. Zoon K: Recommendations for Deferral of Donors for Malaria Risk. Letter to all registered blood establishments. Rockville, MD, U.S. Department of Health and Human Services, Food and Drug Administration, July 24, 1994.

38. Transfusion-transmitted malaria—Missouri and Pennsylvania, 1996–1998. MMWR Morb Mortal Wkly Rep 1999;48:253–556.

39. Mungai M, Tegtmeier G, Chamberland M, Parise M: Transfusion-transmitted malaria in the U. S., 1963–1998. N Engl J Med 2001;344:1973–1978.

40. Vu Thi TH, Tran VB, Phan NT et al: Screening donor blood for malaria by polymerase chain reaction. Trans R Soc Trop Med Hyg 1995;89:44–47.

41. Besson PP, Robert JF, Reviron J, et al: Á propos de deux observations du paludisme transfusionnel. [Two cases of transfusional malaria.] Revue Française de Transfusion et d'Immunohématologie 1976;19:369–373.

42. Shulman IA: Parasitic infections and their impact on blood donor selection and testing. Arch Pathol Lab Med 1994;118:366–370.

43. Brasseur P, Bonneau J-C: Le paludisme transfusionnel: risque, prévention et coût. Revue Française de Transfusion et Hématologie 1981;24:597–608.

44. Sulzer AJ, Wilson M: The indirect fluorescent antibody test for the detection of occult malaria in blood donors. Bull World Health Organ 1971;45:375–379.

45. Kachur SP, Bloland PB: Malaria. In Wallace RB (ed.) Maxcy-Rosenau-Last Textbook of Public Health and Preventive Medicine, 14th ed. Norwalk: Appleton & Lange, 1998, pp 313–326.

46. U.S. Department of Health and Human Services, Food and Drug Administration, Center for Biologics Evaluation and Research. Proceedings of the Blood Products Advisory Committee, 63rd meeting, Washington, DC, June 18, 1999.

47. Kirchhoff LV: American trypanosomiasis (Chagas' disease): a tropical disease now in the United States. N Engl J Med 1993;329:639–644.

48. Schmunis GA: *Trypanosoma cruzi*, the etiologic agent of Chagas' disease: status in the blood supply in endemic and nonendemic countries. Transfusion 1991;31:547–557.

49. Wendel S, Gonzaga AL: Chagas' disease and blood transfusion: a new world problem? Vox Sang 1993;64:1–12.

50. Moraes-Souza H, Bordin JO: Strategies for prevention of transfusion-associated Chagas' disease. Transfus Med Rev 1996;10:161–170.

51. Shulman IR: Intervention strategies to reduce the risk of transfusion-transmitted *Trypanosoma cruzi* infection in the United States. Transfus Med Rev 1999;13:227–234.

52. Herwaldt BL, Grijalva MJ, Newsome AL, et al: Use of polymerase chain reaction to diagnose the fifth reported US case of autochthonous transmission of *Trypanosoma cruzi*, in Tennessee, 1998. J Infect Dis 2000;181:395–399.

53. Nickerson P, Orr P, Schroeder ML, et al: Transfusion-associated *Trypanosoma cruzi* infection in a non-endemic area. Ann Intern Med 1989;111:851–853.

54. Grant IH, Gold JWM, Wittner M, et al: Transfusion-associated acute Chagas' disease acquired in the United States. Ann Intern Med 1989;111:849–851.

55. Cimo PL, Luper WE, Scouros MA: Transfusion-associated Chagas' disease in Texas: report of case. J Tex Med 1993;89:48–50.

56. Leiby DA, Lenes BA, Tibbals MA, Tames-Olmedo MT: Prospective evaluation of a patient with *Trypanosoma cruzi* infection transmitted by transfusion. N Engl J Med 1999;341:1237–1239.

57. Kirchhoff LV, Gam AA, Gilliam FC: American trypanosomiasis (Chagas' disease) in Central American immigrants. Am J Med 1987;82:915–920.

58. Appleman MD, Shulman IA, Saxena S, Kirchhoff LV: Use of a questionnaire to identify potential blood donors at risk for infection with *Trypanosoma cruzi*. Transfusion 1993;33:61–64.

59. Brashear RJ, Winkler MA, Schur JD, et al: Detection of antibodies to *Trypanosoma cruzi* among blood donors in the southwestern and western United States: I. Evaluation of the sensitivity and specificity of an enzyme immunoassay for detecting antibodies to *T. cruzi*. Transfusion 1995;35:213–218.

60. Kerndt PR, Waskin HA, Kishhoff LV, et al: Prevalence of antibody to *Trypanosoma cruzi* among blood donors in Los Angeles, California. Transfusion 1991;31:814–818.

61. Galel SA, Kirchhoff LV: Risk factors for *Trypanosoma cruzi* infection in California blood donors. Transfusion 1996;36:227–231.

62. Shulman IA, Appleman MD, Saxena S, et al: Specific antibodies to *Trypanosoma cruzi* among blood donors in Los Angeles, California. Transfusion 1997;37:727–731.

63. Leiby DA, Read EJ, Lenes BA, et al: Seroepidemiology of *Trypanosoma cruzi*, etiologic agent of Chagas' disease, in US blood donors. J Infect Dis 1997;176:1047–1052.

64. Leiby DA, Fucci MH, Stumpf RJ: *Trypanosoma cruzi* in low-to moderate- risk blood donor population: seroprevalence and possible congenital transmission. Transfusion 1999;39:310–315.

65. Leiby DA, Wendel S, Takaoka DT, et al: Serologic testing for *Trypanosoma cruzi*: comparison of radioimmunoprecipitation assay with commercially available indirect immunofluorescence assay, indirect hemagglutination assay, and enzyme-linked immunosorbent assay kits. J Clin Microbiol 2000;38:639–642.

66. Moraes-Souza H, Bordin JO, Bardossy L, MacPherson DW: Prevention of transfusion-associated Chagas' disease: efficacy of white cell-reduction filters in removing *Trypanosoma cruzi* from infected blood. Transfusion 1995;35:723–726.

67. Herrera GA, Lackritz RS, Janssen VP, et al: Serologic test for syphilis as a surrogate marker for human immunodeficiency virus infection among United States blood donors. Transfusion 1997;37:836–840.

68. Infectious Disease Testing for Blood Transfusions. NIH Consensus Statement 1995;13:1–27.

69. Aberle J, Grasse SL, Notari OE, et al: Predictive value of past and current screening tests for syphilis in blood donors: changing from a rapid plasma reagin test to an automated specific treponemal test for screening. Transfusion 1999;39:206–211.

70. Cable RG: Evaluation of syphilis testing of blood donors. Transfus Med Rev 1996;10:296–302.

71. Wicher K, Horowitz H, Wicher V: Laboratory methods of diagnosis of syphilis for the beginning of the third millennium. Microbe Infect 1999;1:1035–1049.

72. Van der Slais JJ, Onvlee PC, Kothe FCHA, et al: Transfusion syphilis: survival of *Treponema pallidum* in donor blood. Vox Sang 1984;47:197–204.

73. Van der Sluis JJ, Ten Kate FJW, Vuzevski VD, et al: Transfusion syphilis: survival of *Treponema pallidum* in stored donor blood. Vox Sang 1985;49:390–399.

74. Cossart YE, Field AM, Cant B, et al: Parvovirus-like particles in human sera. Lancet 1975;2:72–73.

75. Pattison HR, Jones SE, Hodgson J, et al: Parvovirus infections and hypoplastic crisis in sickle-cell anemia. Lancet 1981;1:664–665.

76. Young N: Hematologic and hematopoietic consequences of parvovirus B19 infection. Semin Hematol 1988;25:159–172.

77. Anderson MJ, Lewis E, Kidd IM, et al: An outbreak of erythema infectiosum associated with human parvovirus infection. J Hyg 1984;93:85–93.

78. Reid DM, Reid TMS, Brown T, et al: Human parvovirus-associated arthritis: a clinical and laboratory description. Lancet 1985;1:422–425.

79. Woolf AD, Campion GV, Chishick A, et al: Clinical manifestations of human parvovirus B19 in adults. Arch Intern Med 1989;149:1153–1156.

80. Cassinotti P, Schultze D, Schlageter P, et al: Persistent human parvovirus B19 infection following an acute infection with meningitis in an immunocompetent patient. Eur J Clin Microbiol Infect Dis 1993;12:701–704.

81. Watanabe T, Satoh M, Oda Y: Human parvovirus B19 encephalopathy. Arch Dis Child 1994;70:71.

82. Knott PD, Wepley GAC, Anderson MJ: Serologically proved intrauterine infection with parvovirus. Br Med J 1984;289:1660.

83. Public Health Laboratory Service Working Party on Fifth Disease. Prospective study of human parvovirus (B19) infection in pregnancy. Br Med J 1990;316:1166–1170.

84. Azzi A, Zakrzewska K, Bertoni E, et al: Persistent parvovirus B19 infections with different clinical outcome in renal transplant recipients: diagnostic relevance of PCR and of quantification of B19 DNA in sera. Clin Microbiol Infect 1996;2:105–108.

85. Azzi A, Macchia PA, Favre C, et al: Aplastic crisis caused by B19 virus in a child during induction therapy for acute lymphoblastic leukemia. Haematologica 1989;74:191–194.

86. Frickofen N, Abkowitz JL, Safford M, et al: Persistent parvovirus infection in patients infected with human immunodeficiency virus type 1 (HIV-1): a treatable cause of anemia in AIDS. Ann Intern Med 1990;113:926–933.

87. Musiani M, Zerbini M, Gentilomi G, et al: Persistent B19 parvovirus infections in hemophilic HIV-1 infected patients. J Med Virol 1995;46:103–108.

88. Brown KE, Anderson SM, Young NS: Erythrocyte P antigen-cellular receptor for B19 virus. Science 1993;262:114–117.

89. Brown KE, Young NS, Liu JM: Molecular, cellular and clinical aspects of parvovirus B19 infection. Clin Rev Oncol Hematol 1994;16:1–31.

90. Zanella A, Rossi F, Cesana C, et al: Transfusion-transmitted human parvovirus B19 infection in a thalassemic patient. Transfusion 1995;35:769–772.

91. Cohen BJ, Beard S, Knowles WA, et al: Chronic anemia due to parvovirus infection in a bone marrow transplant patient after platelet transfusion. Transfusion 1997;37:947–952.

92. Jordan J, Tiangco B, Kiss J, et al: Human parvovirus B19: prevalence of viral DNA in volunteer blood donors and clinical outcomes of transfusion recipients. Vox Sang 1998;75:97–102.

93. Azzi, A, Morfini M, Mannucci PM: The transfusion-associated transmission of parvovirus B19. Transfus Med Rev 1999;13:194–204.

94. U.S. Food and Drug Administration, Center for Biologics Evaluation and Research. Workshop on Implementation of Nucleic Acid Testing. Bethesda, MD: U.S. Department of Health and Human Services, December 1999.

95. National Institutes of Health, National Heart, Lung and Blood Institute. Parvovirus B19 Workshop: Implications for Transfusion Medicine. Bethesda, MD: U.S. Department of Health and Human Services, December 1999.

96. Johnson RT, Gibbs CJ: Creutzfeldt-Jacob disease and related transmissible spongiform encephalopathies. N Engl J Med 1998;339:1994–2004.

97. Prusiner SB: Prions. Proc Natl Acad Sci U S A 1998;95:13363–13383.

98. Murphy MF: New variant Creutzfeldt-Jacob disease (nvCJD): the risk of transmission by blood transfusion and the potential benefit of leukocyte-reduction of blood components. Transfus Med Rev 1999;13:75–83.

99. FDA Guidance: Revised Precautionary Measures to Reduce the Possible Risk of Transmission of Creutzfeldt-Jakob disease (CJD) and New Variant Creutzfeldt-Jakob Disease (nvCJD) by Blood and Blood Products. Rockville, MD U.S. Department of Health and Human Services, revised January 2002.

100. Collinge J: Variant Creutzfeldt-Jacob disease. Lancet 1999;354:317–323.

101. Brown P: Donor pool size and the risk of blood-borne Creutzfeldt-Jacob disease. Transfusion 1998;38:312–315.

102. Huillard d'Aignaux J, Costagliola D, Maccario J, et al: Incubation period of Creutzfeldt-Jacob disease in human growth hormone recipients in France. Neurology 1999;53:1197–1201.

103. Fradkin JE, Schonberger LB, Mills JL, et al: Creutzfeldt-Jacob disease in pituitary growth hormone recipients in the United States. JAMA 1991;265:880–884.

104. Centers for Disease Control and Prevention. Creutzfeldt-Jacob disease associated with cadaveric dura mater grafts—Japan, January 1979–May 1996. MMWR Morb Mortal Wkly Rep 1997;46:1066–1069.

105. Collinge J, Palmer MS, Sidle KC, et al: Unaltered susceptibility to BSE in transgenic mice expressing human prion protein. Nature 1995;378:779–783.

106. Brown P, Rohwer RG, Dunston BC, et al: The distribution of infectivity in blood components and plasma derivatives in experimental models of transmissible spongiform encephalopathy. Transfusion 1998;38:810–816.

107. Brown P, Cervenakova L, McShane LM, et al: Further studies of blood infectivity in an experimental model of transmissible spongiform encephalopathy, with an explanation of why blood components do not transmit Creutzfeldt-Jacob disease in humans. Transfusion 1999;39:1169–1178.

108. Klein MA, Frigg R, Flechsig, et al: A crucial role for B cells in neuroinvasive scrapie. Nature 1997;390:387–390.

109. Sullivan MT, Schonberger LB, Kessler D, et al: Creutzfeldt-Jakob Disease (CJD) investigational lookback study. Transfusion 1997;37:2S.

110. Heye N, Hensen S, Müller N: Creutzfeldt-Jakob disease and blood transfusion. Lancet 1994;343:298–299.

111. Esmonde TFG, Will RG, Slattery JM, et al: Creutzfeldt-Jacob disease and blood transfusion. Lancet 1993;341:205–207.

112. van Duijn CM, Delasnerie-Laupretre N, Masullo C, et al: Case-control study of risk factors of Creutzfeldt-Jacob disease in Europe during 1993–1995. Lancet 1998;351:1081–1085.

113. Collins S, Law MG, Fletcher A, et al: Surgical treatment and risk of sporadic Creutzfeldt-Jacob disease: a case-control study. Lancet 1999;353:693–697.

114. Will RG, Kimberlin RH: Creutzfeldt-Jacob disease and the risk from blood or blood products. Vox Sang 1998;75:178–180.

115. Turner M: The impact of new variant Creutzfeldt-Jacob disease in blood transfusion practice. Br J Haematol 1999;106:842–850.

116. Wientjens DPWM, Davanipour Z, Hofman A, et al: Risk factors for Creutzfeldt-Jacob disease: a reanalysis of case-control studies. Neurology 1996;46:1287–1291.

117. Evatt B, Austin H, Barnhart E, et al: Surveillance for Creutzfeldt-Jacob disease among persons with hemophilia. Transfusion 1998;38:817–820.

118. Lee CA, Ironside JW, Bell JE, et al: Retrospective neuropathological review of prion disease in UK haemophilic patients. Thromb Haemost 1998;80:909–911.

119. U.S. Food and Drug Administration, Center for Biologics Evaluation and Research. Revised Precautionary Measures to Reduce the Possible Risk of Transmission of Creutzfeldt-Jakob Disease (CJD) by Blood and Blood Products. Rockville, MD, U.S. Department of Health and Human Services, 1996.

120. Will RG, Ironside JW, Zeidler M, et al: A new variant of Creutzfeldt-Jacob disease in the UK. Lancet 1996;347:921–925.

121. Zeidler M, Stewart GE, Barraclogh CR, et al: New variant Creutzfeldt-Jacob disease: neurological features and diagnostic tests. Lancet 1997;350:903–907.

122. Zeidler M, Johnstone EC, Bamber RWK, et al: New variant Creutzfeldt-Jacob disease: psychiatric features. Lancet 1997;350:908–910.

123. ABC Newsletter. 2000;March 24:9.

124. Bruce ME, Will RG, Ironside JW, et al: Transmissions to mice indicate that 'new variant' CJD is caused by the BSE agent. Nature 1997;389:498–501.

125. Hill AF, Desbruslais M, Joiner S, et al: The same prion strain causes vCJD and BSE. Nature 1997;389:448–450.

126. Scott MR, Will R, Ironside J, et al: Compelling transgenetic evidence for transmission of bovine spongiform encephalopathy prions to humans. Proc Natl Acad Sci 1999;96:15137–15142.

127. Bons N, Mestre-Frances N, Belli P, et al: Natural and experimental oral infection of nonhuman primates by bovine spongiform encephalopathy agents. Proc Natl Acad Sci U S A 1999;96:4046–4051.

128. Hill AF, Butterworth RJ, Joiner S, et al: Investigation of variant Creutzfeldt-Jacob disease and other human prion diseases with tonsil biopsy samples. Lancet 1999;353:183–189.

129. Kleinman S: New variant Creutzfeldt-Jacob disease and white cell reduction: risk assessment and decision making in the absence of data. Transfusion 1999;39:920–924.

130. Magaill AJ, Grögal M, Gasser RA, et al: Visceral infection caused by Leishmania tropica in veterans of Operations Desert Storm. N Engl J Med 1993;328:1383–1387.

131. Fichoux YL, Quaranta JF, Aufeuvre JP, et al: Occurrence of Leishmania infantum parasitemia in asymptomatic blood donors living in an area endemicity in Southern France. J Clin Microbiol 1999;37:1953–1957.

132. CDC. Viscerotropic leishmaniasis in persons returning from Operation Desert Storm 1990–1991. MMWR Morb Mortal Wkly Rep 1992;41:63–65.

133. Grogl M, Daugirda JL, Hoover DL, et al: Survivability and infectivity of viscerotropic Leishmania tropica from Operation Desert Storm participants in human blood products maintained under blood bank conditions. Am J Trop Med Hyg 1993;49:308–315.

134. Luz KG, Da Silva VO, Gomes EM, et al: Prevalence of anti-Leishmania donovani antibody among Brazilian blood donors and multiply transfused hemodialysis patients. Am J Trop Med Hyg 1997;57:168–171.

135. Saad R, Vincent JF, Cimon B, et al: Pulmonary toxoplasmosis after allogeneic bone marrow transplantation: case report and review. Bone Marrow Transplant 1996;18:211–212.

136. Nelson JC, Kauffmann JH, Ciavarella D, Senisi WJ: Acquired toxoplasmic retinochoroiditis after platelet transfusions. Ann Ophthalmol 1989;21:253–254.

137. Chapman LE, Folks TM, Saloman DR, et al: Xenotransplantation and xenogeneic infections. N Engl J Med 1995;333:1498–1501.

138. Stoye JP, Le Tissier P, Takeuchi Y, et al: Endogenous retroviruses: a potential problem for xenotransplantation? Ann N Y Acad Sci 1998;862:67–74.

139. Le Tissier P, Stoye JP: Two sets of human-tropic pig retrovirus. Nature 1997;389:681–682.

140. Wilson CA, Wong S, Muller J, et al: Type C retrovirus released from porcine primary peripheral blood mononuclear cells infects human cells. J Virol 1998;72:3082–3087.

141. Weiss RA: Zenografts and retroviruses. Science 1999;285:1221–1222.

142. Patience C, Patton GS, Takeuchi Y, et al: No evidence of pig DNA or retroviral infection in patients with short-term extracorporeal connection to pig kidneys. Lancet 1998;352:699–701.

143. Heneine W, Tibell A, Switzer WM, et al: No evidence of infection with porcine endogenous retrovirus in recipients of porcine islet-cell xenografts. Lancet 1998;352:695–699.

144. Paradis K, Langford G, Long Z, et al: Search for cross-species transmission of porcine endogenous retrovirus in patients treated with living pig tissue. Science 1999;285:1236–1241.

145. FDA Guidance: Precautionary Measures to Reduce the Possible Risk of Transmission of Zoonoses by Blood and Blood Products from Xenotransplantation Product Recipients and Their Contacts. Rockville MD U. S. Department of Health and Human Services, December 1999.

i. Practical Considerations

Chapter **43**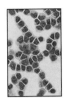

Practical and Technical Issues and Adverse Reactions in Therapeutic Apheresis

Mark E. Brecher

Helen G. Jones

M. Joleen Randels

Nicholas A. Bandarenko

The age-old notion of "bad blood," which was the basis of blood letting, ultimately evolved to the more sophisticated blood separation techniques of today. Apheresis, a word of Latin derivation (from the word *aphairesis*),[1] emerged in the early 20th century. In 1914 at Johns Hopkins Hospital, Rowntree, Abel, and Turner used "plasmapheresis" to mitigate symptoms after bilateral nephrectomy in dogs. Although these experiments were associated with deaths (due to apparent overbleeding and hemorrhage), the improvement in the clinical condition of those animals successfully treated was "marked." The term *apheresis* has since been generalized to refer to the separation of blood into its components, removal of one component, and return of the remainder. Thus, *leukapheresis* means the removal of leukocytes, and *erythrocytapheresis* means the removal of erythrocytes. Alternative terms such as plasma exchange and erythrocyte exchange are frequently used interchangeably for plasmapheresis and erythrocytapheresis, respectively. Some authors have suggested that the term *plasma exchange* be reserved for low-volume procedures involving no more than 500 to 600 mL of plasma and *plasmapheresis* for large-volume procedures, but these terms are frequently used interchangeably.

In the 1950s, therapeutic application of these techniques emerged for the treatment of patients with hyperviscosity syndromes.[2-6] An acceleration in the interest and development of apheresis applications had to await the arrival of automated cell separators in the 1970s.[7, 8] The past 3 decades are testimony to major advances in apheresis, including equipment, automation, plastics, microprocessors, and separation techniques. Today, apheresis has become a standard of care for a variety of diseases. These are summarized in Table 43.1. The relative fraction of therapeutic apheresis procedures by type is illustrated in Figure 43.1.

It is intriguing that, even today, requests for therapeutic apheresis inevitably arise out of desperation or ignorance in diseases and conditions for which therapeutic options have been exhausted. However, apheresis procedures are not without risk or cost. One must be judicious in its application and strive to do no harm. Objective evidence provided by published clinical and basic research provides the rationale for therapeutic apheresis. Nevertheless, clinical situations do arise in which there exists little or no literature to provide guidance. Under such circumstances, a reasoned collegial approach, weighing the potential risks and benefits for the patient, is mandatory, and a full informed consent is essential.

■ Modeling of Apheresis Kinetics

Kinetic modeling of apheresis exchange is generally based on an isolated one-compartment intravascular model. This model assumes that the component removed is neither synthesized nor degraded substantially during the procedure, that it remains within the intravascular compartment, and that there is instantaneous mixing. In the short term, these assumptions work relatively well when applied to solutes that are located predominantly in the intravascular compartment, such as immunoglobulin M (IgM) and red blood cells (RBCs); they work less well for proteins such as IgG, which are predominantly extravascular in distribution. The intravascular distributions of IgG, IgA, IgM, albumin, and fibrinogen are approximately 45%, 42%, 76%, 40%, and 80%, respectively.[9]

Table 43.1   Role of Apheresis and Treatment Categories by AABB and ASFA Guidelines

Disorder	Procedure	AABB Category	ASFA Category
ABO-incompatible organ or marrow transplant	TPE	III	II
AIDS (symptoms of immunodeficiency)	TPE	IV	NR
Amyotrophic lateral sclerosis	TPE	IV	IV
Aplastic anemia	TPE	IV	III
Bullous pemphigoid	TPE	NR	II
Burn shock, refractory	TPE	III	NR
Cancer (nonhematologic)	TPE/staph protein A	NR	III/III
Chronic inflammatory demyelinating polyneuropathy (CIDP)	TPE	I	I
Coagulation factor inhibitors	TPE	III	II
Cold agglutinin disease	TPE	II	NR
Cryoglobulinemia	TPE	I	I
Cutaneous T-cell lymphoma	Photopheresis/cytapheresis	II/II	I/III
Drug overdose and poisoning (protein bound)	TPE	II	II
Eaton-Lambert syndrome	TPE	II	I
Fabry disease (glycosphingolipids)	TPE	NR	III
Focal segmental glomerulonephritis	TPE	III	NR
Goodpasture syndrome	TPE	I	I
Guillian-Barré syndrome	TPE	I	I
Hemolytic transfusion reaction (life-threatening)	Rec cell exchange	III	NR
Hemolytic uremic syndrome	TPE	II	II
Hepatic failure (fulminant/acute)	TPE	IV	III
Homozygous familial hypercholesterolemia	TPE/selective removal	I/NR	II/I
Hypereosinophilia	Cytapheresis	IV	NR
Hyperparasitemia (malaria)	RBC exchange	II	NR
Hyperviscosity	TPE	I	I
Idiopathic thrombocytopenia purpura (ITP)	TPE/staph protein A	IV/III	III/III
Leukemia with hyperleukocytosis syndrome	Cytoreduction	I	I
Leukemia without hyperleukocytosis syndrome	Cytoreduction	IV	NR
Lupus nephritis	TPE	IV	NR
Maternal treatment for hemolytic disease of the newborn (HDN)	TPE	III	III
Multiple sclerosis	TPE/cytapheresis	III	III
Myasthenia gravis	TPE	I	I
Organ transplant rejection	TPE/photopheresis/cytapheresis	NR/III/III	IV/III/NR
Paraneoplastic syndromes	TPE	NR	III
Paraproteinemic peripheral neuropathy	TPE	NR	II
Pemphigus vulgaris	TPE/photopheresis	II/NR	II/III
Peripheral Blood Stem Cell progenitor cells for hematopoietic reconstitution	Cytapheresis	I	NR
Polymyositis/dermatomyositis	TPE/cytapheresis	IV/IV	III–IV*/NR
Post-transfusion purpura	TPE	I	I
Systemic sclerosis	TPE/photopheresis/lympho-cytaplasmapheresis	III/III/NR	III/III/III
Psoriasis	TPE	IV	IV
Quinine/quinidine thrombocytopenia	TPE	II	NR
Rapidly progressive glomerulonephritis	TPE	II	II
Rasmussen encephalitis	TPE	III	NR
Raynaud disease	TPE	NR	II
RBC aplasia	TPE	III	NR
Refsum disease (phytanic acid)	TPE	I	I
Renal transplant rejection	TPE	IV	IV
Rheumatoid arthritis (RA)	TPE/cytapheresis	IV/III	IV/III
Schizophrenia	TPE	IV	IV
Sickle cell syndromes (prophylactic use in pregnancy)	RBC exchange	I(III)	I(NR)
Systemic lupus erythematosus (SLE)	TPE	NR	II
Systemic vasculitis (primary or secondary to RA or SLE)	TPE	II	II
Thrombocytosis, symptomatic	Cytoreduction	I	I
Thrombotic thrombocytopenic purpura	TPE	I	I
Thyroid storm	TPE	III	III
Transfusion refractoriness due to alloantibodies	TPE/staph protein A	III/NR	III/III
Warm autoimmune hemolytic anemia	TPE	III	III

*Consensus not reached. NR, disorder not ranked; ABBB, American Association of Blood Banks; ASFA, American Society for Apheresis; RBC, red blood cell; TPE, therapeutic plasma exchange; I, standard acceptable therapy; II, sufficient evidence to suggest efficacy usually as adjunctive therapy; III, inconclusive evidence of efficacy or uncertain risk/benefit ratio; IV, lack of efficacy in controlled trials.

Reproduced with permission from Abel J, Rountree LG, Turner BB. Plasma removal with return of corpuscles (plasmapheresis). Pharmacol Exp Ther 1914;5:62–91.

Figure 43.1 Relative frequency of therapeutic procedures by type, based on data from 18 institutions in the United States encompassing 3421 procedures. PE, plasma exchange; PBSC, peripheral blood stem cells. (Data from McLeod BC, Sniecinski I, Ciavarella D, et al. Frequency of immediate adverse effects associated with therapeutic apheresis. Transfusion 1999;39:282–288.)

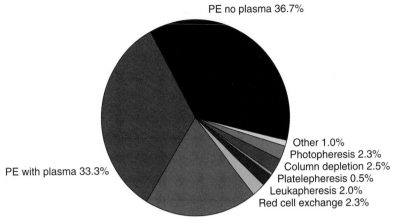

PE no plasma 36.7%

Other 1.0%
Photopheresis 2.3%
Column depletion 2.5%
Platelepheresis 0.5%
Leukapheresis 2.0%
Red cell exchange 2.3%

PE with plasma 33.3%

Autologous PBSC 19.4%

For continuous-flow plasma exchange, the removal of plasma or solute can be described by the same differential equation that applies to isovolemic hemodilution:

$$\frac{dS}{dV_{ex}} = \frac{-S}{PV}$$

where S is the solute concentration, V_{ex} is the volume exchanged, and PV is the plasma volume.

This equation can be integrated to yield

$$V_{ex} = PV \times \ln(S_i / S_f)$$

where S_i is the initial solute concentration and S_f is the final solute concentration.

This equation can be modified to yield

$$\text{Fraction remaining} = S_f S_i = e^{-V_{ex}/PV}$$

For intermittent flow, if the replacement is given after removal of the plasma, after N repetitions of plasma removal the remaining fraction of the plasma (and the analyte in question) is given by the following equation:

$$\text{Fraction remaining} = \{(PV - \text{volume removed}) \div PV\}^N$$

If the replacement is given before removal of the plasma, after N repetitions of plasma removal, the remaining fraction of the plasma (and the analyte in question) is given by the equation

$$\text{Fraction remaining} = \{PV \div (PV + \text{volume removed})\}^N$$

Because of the initial hemodilution that occurs if the replacement is given before removal of the plasma, for each cycle of plasma removal, the fraction remaining is less than if the replacement had been given only after each repetition of plasma removal. A comparison of continuous-versus intermittent-flow plasma exchange is illustrated in Figure 43.2.

Calculations for RBC exchanges, although somewhat more complicated, can be achieved in a similar manner. In this case, total blood volume (TBV) is substituted for PV and the solute of interest is either the hemoglobin concentration or the hematocrit. For example, continuous-flow apheresis can be used for a patient with sickle cell disease who has a TBV of 5 L and a hematocrit of 32%. If it is assumed that the patient has 100% hemoglobin S and the therapeutic goal is to decrease the percentage of hemoglobin S to 30% while maintaining the patient's hematocrit at 32%, the amount of blood that must be processed is given by the following equation:

$$V_{ex} = 5000 \text{ mL} \times \ln(100\% \div 30\%) = 6020 \text{ mL}$$

The volume of RBCs needed for replacement in order to maintain the patient's hematocrit at 32% throughout the procedure would be

$$6020 \text{ mL} \times 0.32 = 1926 \text{ mL}$$

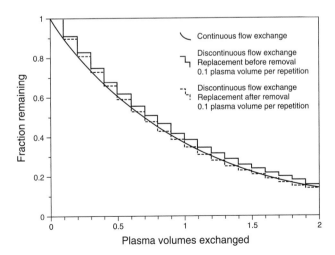

Figure 43.2 Theoretical fraction of solute remaining after plasma exchange for continuous- and discontinuous-flow separation.

Table 43.2 Summary of Current Apheresis Technology

Manufacturer	Instrument	Type	Flow	Access	D/I	Procedure/Products
Haemonetics	V-50	C, bowl	I		D, T	PL, PLT, Gran
	PCS/PCS-2	C, bowl	I		D	PL
	MCS/MCS Plus	C, bowl	I		D, T	PL, PLT, Gran, RBCs, PBSCs
COBE (Gambro BCT)	Spectra	C, channel	C	1, 2	D, T	PL, PLT, Gran, PBSC, TPE, RBCEx, cytoreduction
	Trima	C, channel	C	1, 2	D	PLT, PL, RBCs
Fenwal	CS3000 Plus	C, bags	C	1, 2	D, T	PL, PLT, Gran (mononuclear cells, PBSCs, TPE), RBCEx
	Amicus	C, bags	C	1, 2	D	PL, PLT (future PBSCs and possibly RBCs)
	Autopheresis-C	SM	I	1	D	PL
Fresenius	AS104	C, channel	C	1, 2	D, T	PL, PLT, Gran, PBSCs
Therakos (Johnson & Johnson)	UVAR Photopheresis Machine	C, bowl	I	1, 2	T	Photopheresis

C, centrifuge; SM, spinning membrane; I, intermittent; C, continuous; 1, single needle; 2, dual needle; D, donor; T, therapeutic; PL, plasma; PLT, platelets; Gran, granulocytes; RBC, red blood cells; PBSCs, peripheral blood stem cells; TPE, therapeutic plasma exchange; RBCEx, red blood cell exchange.

If it is assumed that a typical allogeneic unit contains 200 mL of RBCs, then 10 units (1926 mL ÷ 200 mL/unit = 9.6 units) would be needed.

■ Overview of Technology

Current apheresis instrumentation involves the separation of blood components, segregation of the component being targeted using on-line automated technology, and delivery of the remaining components back to the individual donor or patient. The use of temporary anticoagulation (with citrate alone or in combination with heparin) and disposable sterile plastic tubing sets enables these basic steps to be accomplished by a variety of instruments, which typically accommodate flow rates of 30 to 150 mL/min from either central or peripheral venous access.[10] Variations in the design of apheresis separators affect their efficiency of collection and removal and influence their suitability for specific donor or therapeutic applications. Currently licensed automated apheresis equipment separates blood components by either centrifugation or filtration and can operate with either continuous or intermittent flow. Table 43.2 summarizes the current technology.

Differential Centrifugation

Because of differences in density, anticoagulated whole blood separates into components when centrifuged. Mature RBCs have the greatest relative density, followed by neocytes, granulocytes, mononuclear cells (including lymphocytes, peripheral blood progenitor cells), then platelets, and finally plasma. Whole blood pumped into the apheresis separator enters a rotating bowl or chamber, tubular rotor, or belt-shaped channel. Once equilibrium is reached, the desired fraction can be selectively removed. An optical sensor may aid in maintaining the interface between components, and all systems have a mechanism to prevent twisting of the tubing that feeds the separation chamber.

With intermittent flow (discontinuous flow), whole blood is processed in batches (Fig. 43.3). With each cycle the centrifuge device is filled; separation occurs until the dense component fills the separation container. Then processing is interrupted to empty the device. Haemonetics Inc. (Braintree, MA) manufactures the most widely used, currently licensed intermittent-flow centrifugation devices. These separators are useful for the collection of plasma, platelets, leukocytes, or RBCs by a single or double venous access.

The Latham bowl is the centrifuge chamber in Haemonetics models V50, MCS, and MCS Plus. This conical-shaped chamber has a stationary stem joined to the rotating bowl by a rotating seal. Blood enters the bottom (stationary stem) and rises between two conical surfaces. The centrifugal forces cause a vertical interface between RBCs (outside layer) and plasma (inside layer). Plasma, being of lower density, eventually exits the top of the bowl as the RBC layer widens. Ultimately the RBCs fill the entire bowl, necessitating interruption of processing to empty the bowl (see Fig. 43.2). The development of a surge technique has enabled greater purity of platelet and mononuclear cell products. This process involves blocking the flow of whole blood into the Latham bowl when an optical sensor detects the buffy coat. Then, plasma from a reservoir bag is flushed rapidly into the still rotating bowl. The plasma flows through the cellular layers, floating off platelets initially, followed by lymphocytes.

The plasmapheresis bowl used with Haemonetics models V50 and PCS-2 is designed exclusively for the collection of plasma. A cylindrical modification of the Latham bowl, it operates on the same principle.

Continuous-flow separators enable removal of components of different densities without interruption of processing. Equipment presently licensed includes apheresis separators manufactured by Gambro BCT (Lakewood, CO), Fenwal (Baxter Biotech, Deerfield, IL), and Fresenius AG (Bad Hamburg, Germany).

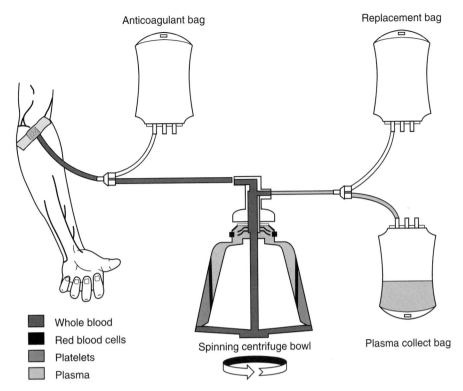

Anticoagulant bag

Replacement bag

Whole blood

Red blood cells

Platelets

Plasma

Spinning centrifuge bowl

Plasma collect bag

Figure 43.3 Example of an intermittent-flow apheresis procedure. Depicted is a simplified representation of a plasma exchange. Whole blood enters the Latham bowl through a central channel and is dispersed at the bottom of the bowl. The blood is then forced to the periphery of the bowl and rises between two concentric conical surfaces. The centrifugal force causes the plasma, platelet-rich plasma, and red blood cells (RBCs) to form vertical layers. As more whole blood enters the bowl, the lighter plasma is forced up through an effluent tube and directed to the plasma collect bag. When the bowl is filled with RBCs, the centrifuge is stopped and the pumps are reversed, permitting the RBCs to be reinfused to the patient.

The COBE Spectra uses continuous-flow technology and is capable of double- or single-needle plateletpheresis (converts to intermittent flow for single-needle procedures) and double-needle leukapheresis as well as therapeutic procedures. The separation chamber is a belt-shaped channel with a lariat-like configuration to prevent twisting of the afferent and efferent lines. This system lacks a rotating seal. The plasma/buffy coat/RBC interface is automatically controlled by a microprocessor. Different software is used depending on the type of procedure (e.g., plasma exchange, granulocyte collection, plateletpheresis). For plateletpheresis, a dual-stage channel is employed that maximizes product quality, including minimal contamination with leukocytes.

Like the COBE Spectra, the Fenwal CS3000 Plus is a sealless system that relies on continuous-flow technology and is largely automated with numerous preprogrammed procedures. A closed system of plastic bags serve as the collection and separation chambers. Pressure plates, which are specific to the procedure being performed, affect the shape of these chambers, allowing a single tubing set to accommodate several different procedures. The addition of a novel platelet chamber, the TNX-6 separation chamber, has decreased the leukocyte content of platelet products collected with this system.

Fenwal's more recent continuous-flow cell separator, the Amicus, is a more portable, efficient, operator-friendly device. Its novel features include ease of loading the disposable tubing kit and a unique drive mechanism for its centrifuge.

The separation and collection containers resemble a belt around a spool and are uniquely configured to promote collection of small- to large-sized platelets, to concentrate RBCs, and to minimize mononuclear cell contamination of platelet products.

The Fresenius AS104 blood separator is another continuous-flow device that uses a sealless centrifugation. It offers multiple preprogrammed options as well as customized programming. For plateletpheresis, a dual-stage channel is used. A single-stage channel is used for granulocyte collections. The device is also capable of therapeutic plasmapheresis. Plasma collection as a by-product of plateletpheresis is a practical option; however, two-unit plasmapheresis collections are limited by the cost of disposable software. The AS104 does have the advantage of very low extracorporeal volume with two-needle procedures.

Filtration

Membrane-based blood separators rely on differences in the actual size of particles rather than their density. In order of increasing size are platelets (3 μm), RBCs (7 μm), lymphocytes (10 μm), and granulocytes (13 μm). Separation of plasma from cellular elements becomes very practical because of the smaller size of instrumentation, the lower extracorporeal volume, and the removal of all cellular debris, compared with centrifugal systems.

There are two basic types of filtration separators. The hollow-fiber systems consist of a bundle of narrow, hollow fibers with perforations along their surfaces. These are contained within a larger cylinder. As whole blood enters, the plasma passes through the pores along the fibers, leaving a more concentrated cell suspension to exit the fibers; plasma can be collected via a side port. In the flat-plate membrane system, whole blood passes between two membranes and plasma escapes through pores, to be collected separately from the cellular elements.

Filtration and centrifugation may be combined. Centrifugation can force plasma to separate from cellular elements via pores. Central placement of the filtration device moves the cellular elements away from the filter pores for improved efficiency. An example of this technology is the Fenwal Autopheresis-C. Originally used for plasma collection, this device, with an increased pore size, can also be used to harvest platelets, albeit with limited efficacy. This is a discontinuous device that requires a single needle to access the donor.

Filtration techniques have been developed to attempt selective removal of a plasma constituent. If the undesirable or pathologic component is of large size, filtration of the separated plasma may afford reasonable removal. Addition of a second column with smaller pore sizes can be used. The arrangement of two or more columns in series is known as *cascade filtration*. Removal of low-density lipoproteins in familial hypercholesterolemia is an example of this application.[11]

Affinity Adsorption Apheresis

Affinity adsorption apheresis involves the selective extraction of immunologic or nonimmunologic substances from the circulation by means of a column, with the benefit of returning nonextracted proteins (e.g., clotting factors) to the patient. The column contains a sorbent or ligand attached to a carrier to which patient plasma is exposed while in the extracorporeal circuit. The most commonly used column is the staphylococcus protein A column, in which staph protein A as the ligand is attached to silica as the carrier (e.g., Prosorba column, Cypres Inc., Seattle, WA). These columns adsorb immune complexes and immunoglobulins via their Fc portion (with greatest affinity for IgG subclasses 1, 2, and 4 and lower affinity for IgG subclass 3, IgM, and IgA).[12] The majority of patients tolerate affinity apheresis without complications, although several reports have associated significant toxicity and at least one fatality with use of the staph protein A column.[13–17] It is approved for clinical use in the United States for the treatment of idiopathic thrombocytopenia purpura and, more recently, for refractory rheumatoid arthritis.

Photopheresis

An alternative approach to immunomodulation and tumor cell therapy is the use of extracorporeal photopheresis. After oral ingestion of 8-methoxypsoralen, leukapheresis is performed, and the buffy coat is exposed to ultraviolet radiation and subsequently reinfused into the patient.[18–20] Possible mechanisms for the beneficial effects include activation of treated macrophages with subsequent release of cytokines (e.g., tumor necrosis factor) and possibly anticlonotypic immune attack toward the malignant cell populations.[21]

■ Hemapheresis "Dose" or Goal

The required volume of blood that must be processed to achieve a treatment goal is based on the patient's TBV, PV, or RBC volume. Because the efficacy of collection of the component being removed decreases with increasing volume processed (see earlier discussion), it may be necessary to process several TBVs to reach a specific therapeutic goal. Patients being treated with plasma exchange typically have one PV removed per exchange. In contrast, with cytapheresis, multiple blood volumes may have to be processed to achieve a therapeutic endpoint. For example, patients requiring RBC exchange for sickle cell disease or malaria may require exchange of 1 to 2.5 times their TBV to reach a therapeutic goal of 90% hemoglobin A or to reduce the parasitic load to less than 5%. Similarly, leukocytoreduction, used to treat patients with hyperleukocytosis, may require the processing of 1.5 to 2 times the TBV to reduce the leukocyte count by 50%.

Extracorporeal Blood Volume Assessment and Treatment Dose Calculation

To assess the patient's ability to tolerate the extracorporeal circuit and to determine the "treatment dose," the patient's TBV, RBC volume, and PV must first be calculated. In general, two methods are commonly used to calculate TBV. One approach employs gender and weight, and the second uses the additional variable of height. Although both methods overestimate the TBV in obese patients and underestimate it in very muscular patients, they do provide a reasonable approximation of the TBV (Table 43.3).

The patient's RBC volume and PV are calculated based on the TBV and the patient's current hematocrit.

The total extracorporeal volume is the amount of cells and plasma that is needed to displace the saline used for priming the lines (manufacturers usually provide this volume). The RBC extracorporeal volume is the RBC volume required to fill the bowl or channel and all the tubing, which

Table 43.3 Calculation of Total Blood Volume (TBV)

Patient Habitus	TBV (mL/kg of body weight)			
	Obese	Thin	Normal	Muscular
Rule of Fives[22]				
Male	60	65	70	75
Female	55	60	65	70
Infant/child	—	—	80/70	—
Nadler's Formula (for adults)[23]				
Male	(0.006012 × Height in inches³)/(14.6 × Weight in pounds) + 604			
Female	(0.005835 × Height in inches³)/(15 × Weight in pounds) + 183			

is proportional to the patient's hematocrit. The lower the hematocrit, the more whole blood must be processed before RBCs are returned to the patient. Therefore, the fraction of RBCs that is extracorporeal can greatly exceed the fraction of extracorporeal "blood." For example, the total volume of the extracorporeal circuit may be 10% of the TBV, but more than 10% of the packed RBC volume may be contained in the extracorporeal circuit. The extracorporeal volume also varies depending on the system (continuous versus intermittent flow), type of procedure, and ancillary equipment such as blood warmers or single-needle devices.

Management of Extracorporeal Volume

The general standard of care is for neither the total extracorporeal blood volume nor the extracorporeal RBC volume to exceed 15%. If the total extracorporeal volume is 15% to 20% but the extracorporeal RBC volume is less than 15% (i.e., in a patient with a high hematocrit), a saline bolus or colloid prime may be needed to prevent hypotension secondary to intravascular hypovolemia.

If the extracorporeal total volume is less than 15% but the patient has a low hematocrit, the extracorporeal RBC volume may exceed 15%. The patient should be carefully monitored for signs of hypoxia. If the patient has a history of cardiac or pulmonary problems or becomes symptomatic (short of breath, tachycardic, or requiring oxygen), priming of the extracorporeal circuit with RBCs should be considered. For asymptomatic patients, both adults and children, one approach is to calculate the intraprocedure hematocrit:

Intraprocedure hematocrit
= [(Initial RBC volume − extracorporeal RBC volume)
÷ TBV] × 100

This formula assumes that the patient is maintained in an isovolemic state during the procedure. If the intraprocedure hematocrit is equal to or greater than 24% in an asymptomatic patient, the patient typically will not require transfusion. Asymptomatic patients with chronic anemia may be able to tolerate even lower hematocrits.

■ Choice of Replacement Solutions for Plasma Exchange

In the 1970s, following the introduction of cell separators for plasma exchange, it was common practice to replace plasma removed with stored allogeneic plasma. Complications with viral contamination (particularly hepatitis) and citrate toxicity led to the search for a safer alternative. Because large amounts of plasma protein that provided colloidal osmotic pressure were being removed, it seemed reasonable to replace the removed human plasma protein with human-derived plasma protein in the form of 5% albumin (which is ≥96% pure albumin) or plasma protein fraction (≥83% pure albumin). These replacement solutions largely resolved the problems of disease transmission and citrate toxicity. Subsequently, partial saline replacement was integrated into replacement regimens.[24, 25]

In recent years, market recalls (due to Creutzfeldt-Jakob disease or bacterial contamination) and increased demand have compromised the availability of albumin and purified protein fraction. Decreased availability, rising costs, recognition of drug interactions with albumin (i.e., angiotensin-converting enzyme [ACE] inhibitors), and a fear of disease transmission led several groups to the use of colloidal starches (hydroxyethyl starches, also known as HES) as partial or full replacement for plasma during plasma exchange.[26–31] One regimen currently in use includes 3% Hespan (6% Hespan diluted 1:1 with normal saline) at 110% replacement initially, followed by a final liter of replacement with 5% albumin at 100% replacement.[29] An alternative approach employs 10% pentastarch for the first half of the colloid replacement, followed by 5% albumin.[31] In some cases, 25% albumin is diluted to 5% albumin for use as replacement. Hemolysis has occurred when hypotonic solutions were used as a diluent; 25% albumin should be diluted with normal saline.[32–34]

In specific clinical settings, patients may require replacement of a specific plasma protein (such as von Willebrand factor metalloprotease in thrombocytopenic thrombotic purpura) or clotting factors in patients at increased risk for bleeding (e.g., Goodpasture syndrome with pulmonary hemorrhage). In such cases, plasma or modified plasma (e.g., solvent detergent–treated plasma, cryoreduced plasma supernatant) may be indicated as full or partial replacement.

Supplementation of replacement solutions (saline, colloidal starches, and albumin) with calcium can reduce the incidence of hypocalcemia secondary to citrate toxicity. In one study, the incidence of citrate toxicity was reduced from 35.6% to 8.6% with a constant calcium gluconate infusion.[35] Possible regimens include addition of 10% calcium gluconate (10 mL per liter of return fluid) or addition of calcium chloride (CaCl$_2$, 200 mg per liter of return fluid).[7, 34] Most patients tolerate hypocalcemia without major adverse effects. However, patients with fulminant liver failure require close monitoring of ionized calcium levels to avoid severe hypocalcemia.

■ Vascular Access

Apheresis procedures require high blood flow rates. Such rates can typically be achieved via peripheral venous access with one or two large-bore needles (16 to 18 gauge). However, the absence of peripheral access or an inability to augment venous return by fist clenching (in patients who are unconscious, confused, or uncooperative and in those who have significant muscle weakness or are easily fatigued) often necessitates the placement of a central catheter.[10] Routine central catheters are flexible and are designed for positive pressure; such "soft-walled" catheters collapse under the negative pressure exerted by the cell separators during blood withdrawal. Therefore, more rigid, specifically designed apheresis or dialysis catheters are required for apheresis procedures. Central catheters are not without risk, and much of the morbidity associated with apheresis procedures is catheter-related. Catheters can be associated with infection (line or catheter sepsis), bleeding, pneumothorax or hemothorax (if placed in the chest), and air emboli. Before the placement of a central catheter, decisions must be made regarding the optimal location of the catheter for a given patient. For example, femoral catheters are relatively easy to place but are associated with increased risk of infection. Such placement may be appropriate for a patient who requires a catheter for a brief period, whereas a subclavian or tunneled catheter may be more appropriate for prolonged access.

■ Anticoagulants

Citrate, heparin, or a combination of citrate and heparin is used during apheresis to prevent coagulation in the extracorporeal circuit. To determine the anticoagulant of choice, the patient should be carefully evaluated for the ability to tolerate citrate versus heparin anticoagulation. Other considerations include an assessment of how the patient will tolerate an increased intravascular volume, the type and length of the procedure, the type and volume of replacement fluid, the type of vascular access, and the inlet blood flow.

Citrate prevents coagulation by binding ionized calcium, which is required for multiple steps in the coagulation cascade. A healthy liver metabolizes citrate as quickly as it is infused at typical rates. If the infusion rate exceeds hepatic metabolism, transient hypocalcemia can occur. Low calcium levels may induce mild paresthesias (perioral, distal extremities) or progress to gastrointestinal symptoms, hypotension, and, in the most extreme situations, cardiac dysrhythmias or seizures. The patient with liver failure is at greatest risk. In such clinical settings, management requires frequent monitoring of ionized calcium and the possible addition of a calcium drip, a decreased citrate infusion rate, or both.

Citrate is available in three forms: ACD-A, ACD-B, and a concentrate of trisodium citrate. ACD-A is the most widely used form; it is a 3% citrate solution that may be administered at a ratio of whole blood to anticoagulant (WB:ACD ratio) of 9:1 to 14:1. ACD-B is a 2% citrate solution that is usually administered at a ratio of 6:1 to 9:1. ACD-B is used primarily with systems that have a fixed WB:ACD ratio to reduce the risk of citrate toxicity. Trisodium citrate is used with leukopheresis. Between 30 and 40 mL of trisodium citrate concentrate (46.7%) is mixed with 500 mL of a sedimenting agent (HES or Pentastarch) during leukopheresis, permitting the anticoagulant pump to titrate the sedimenting agent as well as the anticoagulant. Trisodium citrate may also be diluted with normal saline to make a solution similar to ACD. Trisodium citrate should never be administered undiluted.

Heparin, unlike citrate, is not rapidly metabolized (approximate half-life, 90 minutes) and results in systemic anticoagulation. This anticoagulant can be particularly problematic during plasmapheresis with non-plasma replacement (e.g., 5% albumin, HES) because of the removal of plasma-associated clotting factors. Heparin may be used alone or in combination with ACD-A or ACD-B. When a combination is used, less heparin and a lower volume of ACD-A are required for effective anticoagulation. Such combinations therefore decrease the incidence of citrate toxicity, minimize the systemic anticoagulation caused by heparin alone, and reduce the total fluid volume of the procedure. Use of heparin alone may result in platelet aggregation during cytapheresis procedures.

■ Drug Clearance

On rare occasions, plasma exchange is used to assist in the treatment of acute drug toxicity when other modalities such as gastric lavage, dialysis, hemoperfusion, and forced diuresis have been ineffective. Drugs that are lipophilic and highly protein bound, with long half-lives and small volumes of distribution, are most effectively removed. Plasma exchange has been used to improve clearance of barbiturates, theophylline, vincristine, cisplatin, digoxin-antidigoxin antibody complexes (in the presence of renal failure), paraquat, quinidine, tricyclic antidepressants, acetaminophen, and phenytoin.

More commonly, one encounters the question of the effect of plasma exchange on therapeutic drug dosing. In general, drugs that are most affected have a small volume of distribution and are extensively protein bound (similar to drugs that are treated with plasma exchange in acute toxicity). Drug kinetics in the context of plasma exchange has not been extensively studied. The limited data suggest that supplemental dosing of prednisone, digoxin, cyclosporine, ceftriaxone, ceftazidime, valproic acid, and phenobarbital after plasma exchange is not necessary.[36, 37] In contrast, dosing of certain drugs such as salicylates and tobramycin should be supplemented, and phenytoin, for which there are conflicting reports of clearance, requires careful patient monitoring. In general, removal of a drug is likely to be increased during the distribution phase after administration. Therefore, it would seem prudent, when possible, to administer drug doses after a plasma exchange and not immediately before an exchange.

■ Effect of Plasma Exchange on Clotting

Therapeutic plasma exchange is generally associated with the rapid (and repeated) removal of large quantities of plasma and its associated coagulant proteins.[9, 28, 29, 38, 42, 43] When coagulant protein-deficient replacement fluids such as albumin, saline, or colloidal starches are used, an acute fall in clotting factor activity, varying from 40% to 70% of baseline, can be observed immediately after the exchange. This depletion is usually associated with a small prolongation in measured prothrombin time (PT) and activated partial thromboplastin time (aPTT), although such values frequently remain within the normal range. Fibrinogen, having a volume of distribution that is almost exclusively intravascular, is the clotting factor most depleted. Levels of clotting factors usually return to normal within 1 to 2 days after an exchange. The consensus is that, in the absence of an underlying hemostatic defect or liver disease, use of clotting factor–free replacement solutions is appropriate.

An unintentional consequence of plasma removal is a reduction in circulating platelets. Mean reduction of platelets after a plasma exchange has been variably reported to range from 9.4% to 52.6%.[7, 29, 39–41] This wide range probably reflects differences in the amount of PV processed, the cell separator used, and the settings employed. Larger volumes processed and low speed settings (decreased centrifugal force) are associated with greater platelet loss.[44] Despite mean decreases in platelet counts of 52.6% after 1.6 PVs exchanged, Sultan and colleagues[38] found that the platelets [as well as all clotting factors measured, with the exception of antithrombin III (AT III)] had almost reached or even exceeded their initial values after 48 to 96 hours (just before the next plasma exchange).[38] We have also observed normal platelet counts 48 hours after exchange of 1 PV (just before the next plasma exchange).

In a hemostatically compromised patient or if large-volume daily exchanges are performed, hemostatic parameters should be monitored, and the replacement fluid should be supplemented with plasma or platelets as clinically indicated.

■ Adverse Reactions

Adverse reactions associated with therapeutic apheresis are uncommon. A 1995 survey conducted by the American Association of Blood Banks Hemapheresis Committee, involving 18 centers and 3429 procedures, reported 242 adverse invents in 163 procedures (4.75% of all procedures, 6.87% of first-time procedures, and 4.28% of repeat procedures).[8] Mild reactions were not reported in this study. The types of reactions reported were as follows: transfusion reactions, 1.6%; citrate-related nausea and vomiting, 1.2%; hypotension, 1.0%; vasovagal nausea and vomiting, 0.5%; diaphoresis, 0.5%; tachycardia, 0.4%; respiratory distress, 0.3%; tetany or seizure, 0.2% (associated with fresh frozen plasma replacement); and chills or rigors, 0.2%. Three deaths, attributed to primary disease, were reported in this study. Although deaths have occurred in patients being treated with therapeutic apheresis, most have occurred in critically ill patients and were not thought to be secondary to the apheresis procedures. Mortality rates are largely a function of the patient population treated. For example, it is known that 10% to 20% of patients with thrombotic thrombocytopenic purpura will die while receiving therapy.[45, 46] Overall, estimated mortality rates ranging from 1 per 1000 to 3 per 10,000 procedures more accurately reflect the underlying disease state than the risk of the procedure.[8, 47]

Adverse reactions or complications that occur in the setting of therapeutic apheresis may be caused by the procedure (anticoagulant, replacement fluids), by an underlying condition (anemia; renal, cardiac, or hepatic disease; sepsis; dehydration), or by adjunctive therapy (vasopressors, antihypertensives, diuretics). Before therapy is initiated, the patient should be carefully evaluated for risk factors and a care plan should be developed to minimize risk.

Although the following reactions may occur outside the setting of apheresis, the use of citrate anticoagulation and the large volume and rapid infusion of a variety of replacement solutions predispose the apheresis subject to adverse events. Mild hypocalcemia or citrate reaction (characterized by tingling, oral paresthesias, or chest discomfort) is the most commonly encountered adverse reaction. Such reactions are usually mild and easily managed by slowing the infusion rate, changing the WB:ACD ratio, or giving oral calcium. More severe reactions may be treated or prevented by administering intravenous calcium. Calcium chloride may be added to the replacement fluid (200 mg per liter of 5% albumin or of 3% to 6% HES) or given at a very slow rate intravenously (200 mg, diluted to at least 20 mg/mL, infused over 2 minutes) when replacing with fresh frozen plasma.

Allergic-type reactions, ranging from mild urticaria to anaphylaxis, are associated with the use of replacement fluids including plasma, HES, and albumin. Premedication with antihistamines may prevent allergic reactions in most patients, but some patients develop mild to severe reactions even with premedication. In this group of patients, multiple strategies may be required. In addition to premedication with antihistamines such as histamine[1] antagonists (e.g., diphenhydramine), use of a histamine[2] blocker (e.g., hydroxyzine, cimetidine) and a continuous antihistamine drip may be effective in preventing breakthrough reactions.

Atypical allergic or anaphylactoid reactions have been described, respectively, with ethylene oxide gas sterilization of tubing sets and with drug interactions between ACE inhibitors and albumin. Ethylene oxide reactions are usually characterized by periorbital edema with chemosis and tearing.[48] Double priming of the tubing is useful to prevent the recurrence of such a reaction. ACE inhibitor reactions are associated with albumin infusion during therapeutic plasma exchange.[26] It is thought that the symptoms are caused by rapid infusion of low levels of prekallikrein activator (a metabolite of clotting factor XII) found in the albumin product, which activates prekallikrein to bradykinin, a naturally occurring vasoactive peptide. Metabolism of bradykinin is inhibited by the ACE inhibitor, leading to an accumulation of bradykinin. The patient may experience mild to severe facial flushing, hypotension, and a feeling of doom. ACE inhibitor therapy should be discontinued 24 to 48 hours before the start of therapeutic plasma exchange. If the patient's condition is such that the procedure cannot be delayed for 24 to 48 hours, a colloidal starch such as HES may be used for replacement.

■ Conclusion

The field of apheresis continues to evolve in both the technology and the understanding of how the pathophysiology of disease can be affected by apheresis. Careful assessment of the patient and expertise in therapeutic apheresis are essential to optimize therapy and minimize adverse consequences. Chapters 44 and 45 explore in depth the use of therapeutic apheresis for both cellular and plasma therapy.

REFERENCES

1. Abel J, Rowntree LG, Turner BB: Plasma removal with return of corpuscles (plasmaphaeresis). J Pharmacol Exp Ther 1914;5:625–627.
2. Adams WS, Bland WH, Bassett SH. A method of human plasmapheresis. Proc Soc Exp Biol Med 1952;80:377–379.
3. Skoog WA, Adams WA. Plasmapheresis in a case of Waldenström's macroglobulinemia. Clin Res 1959;7:96.
4. Schwab PJ, Fahey JL. Treatment of Waldenström's macroglobulinaemia by plasmapheresis. N Engl J Med 1969;263:574–579.
5. Solomon A, Fahey JL. Plasmapheresis therapy in macroglobulinaemia. Ann Intern Med 1963;58:789–800.
6. Reynolds WA. Late report of the first case of plasmapheresis for Waldenström's macroglobulinemia. JAMA 1981;245:606–607.
7. Owen HG, Brecher ME: Management of the therapeutic apheresis patient. In McLeod BC, Price TH, Drew MJ (eds): Apheresis: Principles and Practice. Bethesda, MD, American Association of Blood Banks, 1997, pp 223–249.
8. McLeod BC, Sniecinski I, Ciavarella D, et al. Frequency of immediate adverse effects associated with therapeutic apheresis. Transfusion 1999;39:282–288.
9. McCullough J, Chopek M. Therapeutic plasma exchange. Lab Med 1981;12:745–753.
10. Hodgson WJB, Mercan S. Hemapheresis listening post: Optimal venous access. Transfus Sci 1991;12:274.
11. Leitman SF, Smith JW, Gregg RE. Homozygous hypercholesterolemia: Selective removal of low density lipoproteins by secondary membrane filtration. Transfusion 1989;29:341.
12. Pineda AA: Immunoaffinity apheresis columns: Clinical application and therapeutic mechanisms of action. In Sacher RA, Brubaker DB, Kasprisin DO, McCarthy LJ (eds): Cellular and Humoral Immunotherapy and Apheresis. Arlington, VA, American Association of Blood Banks, 1991, p 31.
13. Belak M, Widder RA, Brunner R, et al. Immunoadsorption with protein A Sepharose or silica. Lancet 1994;343:792–793.
14. Garey DC, Perry E, Jackson B. Fatal pulmonary reaction with staph protein A immune adsorption for pure red cell aplasia. Transfusion 1988;28:245a.
15. Snyder HW Jr, Cochran SK, Balint JP Jr, et al. Experience with protein A-immunoadsorption in treatment-resistant adult immune thrombocytopenic purpura. Blood 1992;79:2237–2245.

16. Smith RE, Gottschall JL, Pisciotta AV. Life-threatening reaction to staphylococcal protein A immunomodulation. J Clin Apheresis 1992;7:4–5.

17. Young JB, Ayus JC, Miller LK, et al. Cardiopulmonary toxicity in patients with breast carcinoma during plasma perfusion over immobilized protein A. Am J Med 1983;75:278–288.

18. Edelson R, Berger C, Gasparro F, et al. Treatment of cutaneous T-cell lymphoma by extracorporeal photochemotherapy: Preliminary results. N Engl J Med 1987;316:297–303.

19. Gollnick HP, Owsianowski M, Ramaker J, et al. Extracorporeal photopheresis: A new approach for the treatment of cutaneous T cell lymphomas. Recent Results Cancer Res 1995;139:409–415.

20. Armus S, Keyes B, Cahill C, et al. Photopheresis for the treatment of cutaneous T-cell lymphoma. J Am Acad Dermatol 1990;23:898–902.

21. Zic J, Arzubiaga C, Salhany KE, et al. Extracorporeal photopheresis for the treatment of cutaneous T-cell lymphoma. J Am Acad Dermatol 1992;27:729–736.

22. Gilcher RO: Apheresis: principles and practices. In Rossi EC, Simon TL, Moss GS, Gould SA (eds): Principles of Transfusion Medicine, 2nd ed. Baltimore, MD, Williams & Wilkins, 1996, pp 537–545.

23. Nadler SB, Hidalgo JU, Bloch T. Prediction of blood volume in normal human adults. Surgery 1962;51:224.

24. Lasky LC, Finnerty EP, Glenis L, Polesky HF. Protein and colloid osmotic pressure changes with albumin and/or saline replacement during plasma exchange. Transfusion 1984;24:256–259.

25. McLeod BC, Sassetti RJ, Stefoski D, Davis FA. Partial plasma protein replacement in therapeutic plasma exchange. J Clin Apheresis 1983;1:115–118.

26. Owen, HG, Brecher ME. Atypical reactions associated with ACE inhibitors and apheresis. Transfusion 1994;34:891–894.

27. Brecher ME, Owen HG. Washout kinetics of colloidal starch as a partial or full replacement for plasma exchange. J Clin Apheresis 1996;11:123–126.

28. Owen HG, Brecher ME, Partial colloid replacement for therapeutic plasma exchange. J Clin Apheresis 1997;12:87–92.

29. Brecher ME, Owen HG, Bandarenko N. Alternatives to albumin: starch replacement for plasma exchange. J Clin Apheresis 1997;12:146–153.

30. Owen HG, Brecher ME, Howard JF, Bandarenko N. Minimizing hypovolemic reactions with 3% hetastarch replacement during therapeutic plasma exchange [Abstract]. J Clin Apheresis 1999;14:91.

31. Gross AG, Weinstein R. Pentastarch as partial replacement fluid for therapeutic plasma exchange: Effect on plasma proteins, adverse events during treatment, and serum ionized calcium. J Clin Apheresis 1999;14:114–121.

32. Steinmuller DR. A dangerous error in the dilution of 25 percent albumin [Letter]. N Engl J Med 1998;338:1226–1227.

33. Pierce LR, Gaines A, Varricchio F, Epstein J. Hemolysis and renal failure associated with the inappropriate use of sterile water to dilute human albumin 25%. N Engl J Med 1998;338:1226–1227.

34. Pierce LR, Gaines A, Finlayson JS, et al. Hemolysis and acute renal failure due to the administration of albumin diluted in sterile water [Letter]. Transfusion 1999;39:110–111.

35. Weinstein R. Prevention of citrate reactions during therapeutic plasma exchange by constant infusion of calcium gluconate with the return fluid. J Clin Apheresis 1996;11:204–210.

36. Pramodini B K-B, Woo MW. A review of the effects of plasmapheresis on drug clearance. Pharmacotherapy 1997;17:684–695.

37. Stigelman WH, Henry DH, Talbert RL, Townsend RJ. Removal of prednisone and prednisolone by plasma exchange. Clinical Pharmacy 1984;3:402–407.

38. Sultan Y, Bussel A, Maisonneuve P, et al. Potential danger of thrombosis after plasma exchange in the treatment of patients with immune disease. Transfusion 1979;19:558–593.

39. Orlin JB, Berkman EM. Partial plasma exchange using albumin replacement: Removal and recovery of normal plasma constituents. Blood 1980;56:1055–1059.

40. Wood L, Jacobs P. The effect of serial therapeutic plasmapheresis on platelet count, coagulation factors, plasma immunoglobulin and complement levels. J Clin Apheresis 1986;3:124–128.

41. Flaum MA, Cueo RA, Appelbaum FR, et al. The hemostatic imbalance of plasma-exchange transfusion. Blood 1979;54:694–702.

42. Simon TL. Coagulation disorders with plasma exchange. Plasma Ther Transfus Technol 1982;3:147–153.

43. Domen RE, Kennedy MS, Jones LL, Senhauser DA. Hemostatic imbalances produced by plasma exchange. Transfusion 1984;24:336–339.

44. Owen HG, Koo A, McAteer M, Brecher ME. Evaluation of platelet loss during TPE on the COBE SPECTRA. J Clin Apheresis 1997;12:28.

45. Bandarenko N, Brecher ME. United States Thrombotic Thrombo-cytopenic Purpura Apheresis Study Group (US TTP ASG): multicenter survey and retrospective analysis of current efficacy of therapeutic plasma exchange. J Clin Apheresis 1998;13:133–141.

46. Brailey L, Brecher ME, Bandarenko N. Thrombotic thrombocytopenia purpura. Ther Apheresis 1999;3:20–24.

47. Huestis DW: Complications of therapeutic apheresis. In Valbonesi M, Pineda AA, Bigs JC (eds): Therapeutic Hemapheresis. Milan, Wichtig Editore, 1986, pp 179–186.

48. Leitman SF, Boltansky H, Alter HJ, et al. Allergic reactions in healthy plateletpheresis donors caused by sensitization to ethylene oxide gas. N Engl J Med 1986;315:1192–1196.

Chapter **44**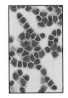

Therapeutic Plasma Exchange

Bruce C. McLeod

Like many true stories, the history of therapeutic plasma exchange (TPE) is sprinkled with serendipity. TPE arose from the ideas and efforts of a number of people who had no intention of treating patients and was helped along by others who were not interested in a device for exchanging plasma. After a long period of inadvertent stage setting, TPE emerged over a fairly short interval as a credible therapy and has become an important treatment for a number of diseases.

Seminal credit is usually given to Abel and Rowntree,[1] who, in pursuing higher yields of antisera for serotherapy, devised manual plasmapheresis in 1914 to obtain more plasma from immunized horses without exsanguinating them. Skoog and Adams[2] and Schwab and Fahey[3] later applied this technique to patients with the hyperviscosity syndrome. Recognition should also be extended to Dr. Edwin Cohn and his associates[4] (especially his engineering consultant Alan Latham[5]), who, in the 1950s, adapted for blood component donation the concept of continuous flow centrifugation invented 60-odd years earlier for the dairy industry by Carl Gustav Patrick De Laval.[6] Nor should one forget to mention Dr. Emil Freireich, George Judson, and others at the National Cancer Institute, who, in the 1960s, constructed a centrifugal blood cell separator to remove white blood cells from patients with chronic myelogenous leukemia.[7] Further refinement of concepts originating with these workers led eventually to the commercial availability of several semiautomated blood separator instruments for clinical use.

■ Rationale for Therapeutic Plasma Exchange

In the 1960s and early 1970s, the notion of treating a patient with a large-scale plasma exchange carried out with such an instrument began to take hold, first in Rh-sensitized women[8–10] and patients with systemic lupus erythematosus (SLE)[11, 12] and then in other illnesses. The common threads linking these disorders were the beliefs that a circulating macromolecule was a crucial pathogenetic factor and that meaningful clinical improvement could be brought about by removing the material.

TPE has often been likened to the practice of bloodletting to remove evil humors. The notion of therapeutic removal is a sound one that has changed little since medieval times; however, the concept of an evil humor has been refined. There are three subtypes of molecules that are candidates for therapeutic removal: (1) molecules that are troublesome because of their binding specificity—these are always antibodies and usually autoantibodies; (2) molecules that confer troublesome physical properties on the plasma and hence on the blood, such as hyperviscosity or cold insolubility—these are also usually antibodies although they are often in immune complexes; and (3) molecules that have a nonimmune toxicity, such as low-density lipoproteins (LDLs). An important therapeutic effect arising from removal is more easily envisioned for large molecules having a relatively long half-life in the circulation and a corresponding low synthetic rate. In fact, the majority of successfully treated disorders are due to pathogenic immunoglobulin G (IgG), which has these properties. It has been hypothesized at various times that removal of complement or coagulation proteins, or both, or mediators of inflammation derived from them or secreted by inflammatory cells might contribute to a therapeutic effect. Such mechanisms are unlikely to be of clinical importance because the candidate molecules have relatively short half-lives or rapid synthetic rates, and in fact no such effect has been proved.

TPE can also be used in a fourth way, not foreseen by medieval barbers or 19th century physicians, and that is to achieve relatively high levels of a normal plasma constituent

Table 44.1 Rationales for Therapeutic Plasma Exchange

Goal of TPE Therapy	Example
Remove antibody with harmful specificity	Autoantibody
Remove protein (usually antibody) with harmful physical property	Hyperviscosity
Remove nonantibody toxin	Low-density lipoprotein
Correct deficiency of plasma factor	Thrombotic thrombocytopenic purpura

that is not available in a concentrated form. These four distinct rationales for TPE are summarized in Table 44.1.

■ General Principles of Therapeutic Plasma Exchange

Mathematical Principles

Patients sometimes liken TPE to an oil change, and it is instructive to consider why this analogy is misleading. A 5-L oil exchange that is nearly 100% efficient can be performed on an automobile engine in 10 minutes because the engine is not running during the exchange. By contrast, limitations are imposed on the rate and efficiency of TPE by the need to keep the heart pumping and the blood stream nearly full throughout the procedure. These requirements dictate that only a small proportion of the total blood volume be extracorporeal at any given moment. TPE must therefore proceed gradually, either continuously or in small increments. Consequently, as an exchange progresses, an increasing proportion of the material removed is not the patient's plasma but replacement fluid infused earlier in the procedure.

In such a process, the behavior of an entirely intravascular substance that is absent in the replacement medium is described by the formula

$$y_x = y_0 e^{-x}$$

where y_0 is the starting concentration of the substance, e is the base natural logarithm, and y_x is the concentration of the substance after x patient plasma volumes have been exchanged. If y_0 is assigned a normalized value of 1.0, a plot of the function yields the smooth asymptotic middle curve in Figure 44.1, which describes a continuous exchange. The flanking curves, which describe small incremental discontinuous exchanges, are similar.[13] Experimental work has shown that this formula is also predictive of exchange outcomes for macromolecules such as LDL[14] and IgG[15] that have a substantial extravascular reservoir, if equilibration between the intravascular and extravascular compartments is slow relative to the rate of removal.

As noted earlier, the molecule targeted for removal in many patients is an IgG antibody. Because slightly more than half of IgG is extravascular[13] and removal of intravascular IgG becomes progressively less efficient with larger exchange volumes, most practitioners choose to limit an exchange to 1 to 1.5 patient plasma volumes, which removes 60% to 75% of intravascular material and limits side effects associated with depletion of normal plasma components. Equilibration with extravascular sources over 1 to 2 days raises the intravascular IgG level, and further removal by exchange can then be undertaken more advantageously. The effects of a series of TPEs on intravascular, extravascular, and total IgG are shown schematically in Figure 44.2.

For reasons given subsequently, human serum albumin is the most common replacement fluid in TPE. In these cases, all plasma constituents except albumin are removed but not replaced, and removal in an individual exchange is almost completely nonselective.[15] However, because most other plasma constituents are resynthesized much more rapidly than IgG, a series of such exchanges results in fairly selective lowering of IgG levels over a course of exchanges,[16] as shown in Figure 44.3.

Regulation of IgG Metabolism

Because reduction of IgG levels is a frequent goal of TPE, it is worthwhile to consider certain details of IgG metabolism. The catabolic rates for IgG1, IgG2, and IgG4, which

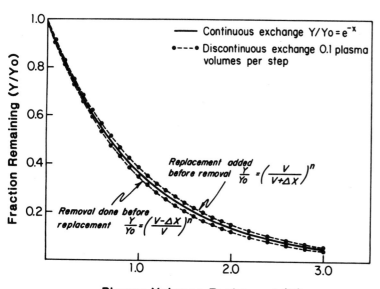

Figure 44.1 Calculated fraction of intravascular substance remaining during a plasma exchange, assuming no equilibration with extravascular material. (From Chopek M, McCullough J: Protein and biochemical changes during plasma exchange. In Berkman EM, Umlas J [eds]: Therapeutic Hemapheresis. Washington DC, American Association of Blood Banks, 1980, p 17.)

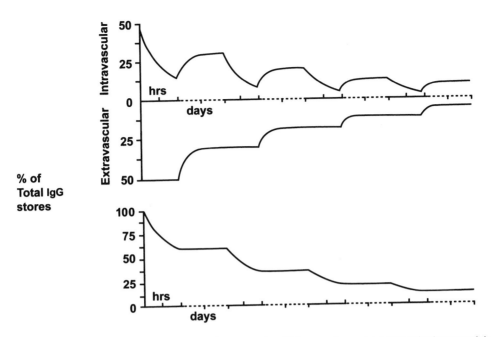

% of Total IgG stores

Figure 44.2 Computer-generated curve estimating amounts of intravascular and extravascular immunoglobulin G (IgG) (upper curves) and total IgG (lower curve) during a course of 4 one-plasma-volume TPEs with an IgG-free replacement medium. Published formulas were used for rates of removal during exchanges and reequilibration after exchanges.[13] No correction was made for continuing synthesis.

constitute about 90% of total IgG, are proportional to total IgG level. Accordingly, their half-lives are inversely proportional to concentration.[17–20] This observation has long been attributed to the existence of a saturable receptor that protects IgG from catabolic pathways.[21] This receptor has been characterized and shown to be identical to the FcRn receptor in neonatal intestinal epithelium.[22]

Synthetic rates for IgG are difficult to measure in humans. Certain animal experiments concerning levels of specific antibody fostered the belief that the synthetic rate for IgG is variable and exhibits negative feedback, such that synthesis increases when IgG or specific antibody levels, or both, are lower.[23] By contrast, Junghans[24] has shown that knockout mice genetically deficient for the FcRn receptor, which rapidly catabolize IgG, have the same IgG synthetic rate as normal mice despite maintaining very low IgG levels. This observation argues against any feedback regulation of IgG synthesis and suggests that the generalized hypogammaglobulinemia induced by TPE would not produce any rebound increase in IgG synthesis.

Intravenous immunoglobulin (IVIG) therapy has been reported effective in a number of antibody-mediated diseases in which TPE has also been used. Yu and Lennon[25] have proposed that the beneficial action of IVIG is to compete with endogenous IgG antibodies for FcRn receptors and thereby promote increased catabolism of the latter, including pathogenic antibodies. In this view, the therapeutic effects of IVIG and TPE are essentially the same; that is, both lower harmful autoantibody levels. TPE lowers levels quickly but may be followed by slower catabolism, whereas IVIG presumably has a slower onset of action but promotes rapid catabolism.

Figure 44.3 Total protein, albumin, and immunoglobulin G (IgG) levels before and after TPE with albumin/saline replacement. Exchanges were carried out three times per week for 3 weeks on seven patients. Points and ranges represent means and standard deviations. Note the disproportionate decrease in IgG levels. (From McLeod BC, Sassetti RJ, Stefoski D, Davis FA. Partial plasma protein replacement in therapeutic plasma exchange. J Clin Apheresis 1983;1:117.)

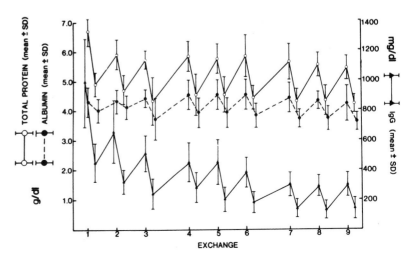

Table 44.2 Colloid Replacement Fluids for Therapeutic Plasma Exchange

Fluid	Advantages	Disadvantages
5% Albumin	Viral safety Convenience Reactions rare	High cost Most proteins not replaced
Single-donor plasma*	All proteins replaced	High cost Inconvenient† Citrate reactions Urticaria Infection possible
Solvent/detergent plasma	All proteins partially replaced‡ Lipid-coated viruses inactivated	Very high cost Inconvenient† Citrate reactions Urticaria Pooled product
6% Hetastarch	Low cost Viral safety Convenience	No proteins replaced Hypotensive reactions Dosage limit Slow catabolism

*Fresh frozen plasma or cryoprecipitate-poor plasma.
†Must be thawed prior to use; must match patient's ABO type.
‡Coagulation factors ≥80% of normal levels.

Replacement Fluids

Saline replacement alone can suffice when only 500 to 1000 mL of plasma is removed in a manual plasmapheresis, but colloid must be given in a multiliter plasma exchange. Available colloid replacement fluids are listed in Table 44.2, which also summarizes their relative advantages and disadvantages. The standard replacement medium for most indications is 5% human serum albumin in normal saline; however, substitution of 25% to 50% of the volume removed with saline is well tolerated in certain groups of patients.[16, 26] Although it is a pooled product, albumin is considered preferable to plasma as a source of replacement colloid because (1) it can be pasteurized under conditions that inactivate known blood-borne infectious agents, (2) it can be given without regard to blood type, and (3) it does not require thawing or other preparation prior to use. Adverse reactions to albumin are infrequent.[27] Albumin exchanges produce temporary deficiencies of other plasma proteins, such as coagulation factors; however, these are usually subclinical and are rapidly corrected by reequilibration and resynthesis.[15, 28] Reports have suggested that there is increased mortality among trauma and sepsis patients resuscitated or supplemented with albumin as opposed to crystalloid alone.[29, 30] Although further developments in this area will bear watching, no corresponding trend has been apparent in decades of albumin use in TPE.

There are a few circumstances in which replacement with donor plasma is deemed preferable. Prominent among these is the treatment of thrombotic microangiopathies.[31] Affected patients are customarily exchanged with fresh frozen plasma (FFP) or cryoprecipitate-poor plasma because of abundant evidence that thrombotic thrombocytopenic purpura responds better to plasma than albumin. In addition, plasma is often given to patients with preexisting thrombocytopenia or humoral coagulopathy, who may have bleeding complications when the dilutional coagulopathy of an albumin exchange is superimposed. Use of plasma is associated with a higher incidence of immediate adverse effects, however, most notably urticarial and hypocalcemic reactions.[32]

One group has tried infusing a solution of hydroxyethyl starch (HES), a less costly volume expander, in the early part of an exchange. They reasoned that recommended dosage limitations for HES would not actually be exceeded because much of the infused HES would be removed in exchange for albumin infused later. This group has reported successes, albeit with a higher incidence of side effects.[33]

Selective Extraction of Plasma Components

Practitioners of TPE have long recognized the apparent wastefulness inherent in removing and discarding *all* plasma components in an effort to deplete just *one*. The concept of selective extraction of the pathogenic component from separated plasma, with recovery and reinfusion of the rest, was recognized early as an attractive goal. Experience with off-line separation of cryoglobulins[34] provided early evidence of practicality and efficacy; however, although a number of methods and applications for on-line separation have been explored,[35] commercial availability and widespread acceptance have been slow to be realized.

Prominent obstacles to commercially practical devices have included the high cost and limited capacity of sorbents that are biocompatible and truly selective and the high extracorporeal volume associated with on-line sorbent modules that have a depletion capacity equivalent to that of TPE. In the past decade, two devices have become available that utilize pairs of small, low-capacity sorbent modules. Flow cycles are alternated, with one module absorbing material from patient's plasma while the absorbent capacity of the other is regenerated by elution. This approach to selective extraction requires an additional instrument to manage the cycling-elution-regeneration process. A semiselective system of this type that utilizes staphylococcal protein A to deplete IgG is in use in Europe,[36] and a Japanese device for selection extraction of LDL from patients with familial hypercholesterolemia is also approved in the United States.[37]

Indication Categories

Subsequent sections of this chapter deal with specific indications for TPE. To help practitioners assess the potential utility of apheresis therapy in specific circumstances, two organizations, the American Society for Apheresis (ASFA) and the American Association of Blood Banks (AABB), have described indication categories for therapeutic apheresis.[38, 39] The definitions used by the two organizations are similar and can be summarized as follows. Category I denotes diseases for which apheresis therapy is a standard and acceptable first-line therapy, although not always mandatory. Category II includes diseases in which it is a valuable second-line therapy, to be offered when first-line measures fail or are poorly tolerated. Category III indicates either uncertainty related to a paucity of data or controversy because of conflicting reports. Category IV implies negative data from controlled trials or anecdotal reports. The indication categories assigned by both organizations are given in tabular form for the diseases in each of the following sections.

■ Therapeutic Plasma Exchange in Neurologic Disorders

Immune processes, especially those that produce circulating antibody to structures in the nervous system, have been implicated in a number of neurological diseases, and TPE

Table 44.3 Indication Categories for Therapeutic Plasma Exchange in Neurological Disorders

Disorder	Indication Categories* ASFA	Indication Categories* AABB
Guillain-Barré syndrome	I	I
Chronic inflammatory demyelinating polyneuropathy	I	I
Peripheral neuropathy with monoclonal gammopathy	I/II	NR
Myasthenia gravis	I	I
Lambert-Eaton myasthenic syndrome	II	I
Paraneoplastic neurologic syndromes	III	NR
Rasmussen encephalitis	III	III
Sydenham chorea	II	NR
PANDAS	III	NR
Multiple sclerosis	III	III

*I, standard first-line therapy; II, second-line therapy; III, controversial; IV, no efficacy; NR, not rated.
AABB, American Association of Blood Banks; ASFA, American Society for Apheresis; PANDAS, pediatric antoimmune neuropsychiatric disorders associated with streptococcal infection.

has become an important therapeutic modality for many of them.[40] The diseases to be considered in this section are listed in Table 44.3, along with their ASFA-AABB indication categories.

Guillain-Barré Syndrome

The Guillain-Barré syndrome (GBS) is a disease of the peripheral nervous system. It is the most common cause of acute paralysis with areflexia in the Western world, having an incidence of 1 to 2 cases per 100,000 population per year. It typically begins with symmetrical distal paresthesias, followed by leg and arm weakness. Symptoms progress proximally and reach a nadir by 14 to 30 days after onset. About a quarter of those affected have a mild illness and remain ambulatory throughout. The remaining patients are disabled by more serious paralysis and may have oropharyngeal and respiratory weakness as well. About one quarter require ventilatory assistance at some point, and the worst cases are marked by quadriplegia, ophthalmoplegia, and prolonged ventilator dependence. Variant presentations, with arm weakness predominating or with symptoms limited to ophthalmoplegia, ataxia, and areflexia (Fisher syndrome), are also possible. Spinal tap usually reveals few cells and only a moderately elevated protein concentration. A conduction block indicative of demyelination is usually found in electrophysiological studies, although inexcitability may be seen in the axonal form of GBS.[41–43]

Several lines of evidence suggest that the demyelination observed histopathologically is due to circulating antineuronal antibodies. Early experiments showed that sera from GBS patients produced demyelination in experimental animals.[44, 45] Other studies have identified antimyelin antibodies in the serum of many patients with GBS.[46–48] There is a clinical association of GBS with a history of recent infection,[41] especially *Campylobacter jejuni* infection,[49–51] and studies have suggested a specific link to the Penner strain 19 of *C. jejuni* in 30% to 40% of GBS cases,[52] with antibodies formed to a strain-specific lipopolysaccharide that may be

antigenically similar to the myelin ganglioside GM1.[53] Epidemic Chinese acute motor neuropathy, an illness of rural Chinese children, is clinically similar to GBS and is also associated with *C. jejuni* infection and anti-GM1 antibodies.[54]

Spontaneous recovery is the rule in GBS and is perhaps associated with the decline in antibody levels expected after recovery from infection. Patients with mild illness require no therapy, but more severely affected patients need careful observation so that appropriate intervention with supportive therapies, such as mechanical ventilation, can be accomplished in a timely fashion.[41–43] Neither oral nor pulse intravenous steroids are beneficial in GBS.[55] Several small series and case reports suggested that TPE could favorably alter the course of the disease.[56–60] This evidence of benefit was confirmed by sizable randomized controlled trials that documented its effectiveness in shortening recovery time and reducing disability.[61–66]

The North American trial enrolled 245 disabled patients, 142 of whom received TPE.[63] At 4 weeks after entry, 59% of the treated patients had improved one clinical grade versus 39% of control subjects, with the mean improvements being 1.1 and 0.4 grades, respectively. The median time to improve one grade was only 19 days in treated patients versus 40 days in control patients, and median times to walk unassisted were 53 and 85 days, respectively. For ventilated patients, the median times to weaning were 24 and 48 days, respectively, and the median times to walk unassisted were 97 and 169 days. Similar hastening of recovery in severely affected patients was shown in the trial by the French Cooperative Group involving 220 patients.[64] In another study that enrolled 556 patients, the French group showed that benefit from TPE accrued even to mildly affected patients.[65] The typical treatment schedule in these trials included five or six exchanges of 1 to 1.5 plasma volumes over 7 to 14 days. Albumin replacement and FFP were specifically compared in the French trial. FFP caused more side effects[67] but offered no therapeutic advantage.[64] GBS patients may need careful monitoring, perhaps in an intensive care unit, because they may have autonomic neuropathy and are more likely to experience hemodynamic instability during TPE.[68]

Later evidence suggested that IVIG is also beneficial in GBS. The Dutch group reported that 53% of IVIG-treated GBS patients improved by one grade at 4 weeks after treatment, versus only 34% of TPE-treated patients.[69] The median time to improve one grade in this trial was 27 days with IVIG and 41 days with TPE. This trial was controversial, in part because the TPE patients did so poorly (comparable to untreated control patients in the North American trial). A later large multi-institutional trial compared IVIG, TPE, and TPE followed by IVIG, with 121 to 130 patients in each treatment group.[70] The mean disability grade improvements at 4 weeks were 0.8, 0.9, and 1.1, respectively, and the median times to walk unassisted were 51, 49, and 40 days, respectively. Although the trends favored TPE plus IVIG, none of the differences was statistically significant.

Chronic Inflammatory Demyelinating Polyneuropathy

Chronic inflammatory demyelinating polyneuropathy (CIDP) is an acquired neuropathy that has either a continuously progressive or an intermittent, relapsing course. Both sensory loss and weakness are typically present, with both proximal and distal sites usually affected. Proximal weakness helps to distinguish CIDP from other chronic neuropathies, and progression for more than 2 months differentiates it from GBS. Nerve conduction studies should reveal evidence of demyelination, as should nerve biopsies. Nerve root biopsies may show patchy inflammatory infiltrates. The cerebrospinal fluid protein is moderately elevated but the cell count is usually less than $10/\mu L$. Assuming certain exclusionary criteria are met, CIDP is deemed "possible" on the basis of clinical and electrophysiological findings, "probable" if cerebrospinal fluid is also examined and found consistent, and "definite" if compatible nerve pathology is also demonstrated. Treatment is recommended for all these groups, and responsiveness to treatment is similar for all three. CIDP may be idiopathic or may arise in the context of an associated disease, such as inflammatory bowel disease, chronic active hepatitis, connective tissue disease, Hodgkin disease, human immunodeficiency virus (HIV) infection, or monoclonal gammopathy.[71–73]

The etiology of CIDP remains unclear; however, the disease associations, the similarities to GBS, and the histopathology all support an immune process. The fact that some cases are associated with a monoclonal protein suggests an antibody-mediated disorder, as does the finding that experimental allergic neuritis, an animal model of CIDP, can be transferred with serum.[74] Later studies have shown antibody to myelin components such as GM1,[75] P_0 and P_2 proteins,[76] and β tubulin[77] in the sera of patients with CIDP, although no cause-and-effect relationship has been established.

Most patients with CIDP respond to corticosteroids in moderately high doses. Standard therapy consists of a course of prednisone at perhaps 100 mg/day for an adult, followed by gradual tapering to alternate-day therapy when a functional plateau is reached.[72]

The successful application of TPE in GBS, along with evidence for a circulating factor in CIDP, provided the rationale for early trials of TPE in CIDP patients who had not responded to steroids or were unable to tolerate them. A double-blind, sham-controlled crossover trial of 3 weeks of TPE reported by Dyck and colleagues[78] in 1986 showed improvement in 5 of 15 treated patients, with a similar proportion responding after crossover in the group randomly assigned to sham. Many patients worsened after TPE was stopped, however. A similar study was reported by Hahn and coworkers[79] in 1996 with 18 previously untreated patients. Twelve of 15 patients who completed the trial improved during the TPE portion. Improvement began after a shorter delay than is usually seen with steroid therapy, and its rate was more rapid. These patients were given prednisone for 6 months after completing TPE, and many maintained good function after recovery from a brief relapse when TPE was stopped.

An effect of IVIG on CIDP has also been sought. Early controlled trials comparing IVIG with a control infusion of albumin were not conclusive but suggested a superior effect for IVIG.[80–83] Hahn and colleagues[84] have published a double-blind, placebo-controlled trial with crossover in 30 patients. Study patients were permitted to take low stable doses of prednisone. Overall, 19 patients, or 63%, responded to IVIG and 5 (17%) responded to placebo. Two studies comparing IVIG with TPE in CIDP have been published. In an uncontrolled retrospective study by Choudhary and Hughes,[85] 21 of 33 patients (64%) had major improvement after TPE treatment while, at the same institution, 14 of 21 patients (67%)

responded to IVIG. In a prospective observer-blinded crossover study of 20 patients at the Mayo Clinic, both therapies were adjudged to produce rapid and statistically significant improvement and the authors concluded that either therapy was appropriate as a primary treatment.[86] TPE protocols in the preceding studies have tended to specify relatively long courses of treatment. A proposed schedule is 3 one-plasma-volume exchanges per week for 2 weeks, followed by 2 exchanges per week for another 4 weeks.[72]

Peripheral Neuropathy and Monoclonal Gammopathy

About 10% of patients with polyneuropathy have a circulating monoclonal immunoglobulin. The background incidence of such proteins is only 1% in adults older than 50 and rises to only 3% in adults older than 70.[87, 88] Thus, the epidemiology suggests a causal relationship. This idea has been strengthened by studies showing that antimyelin antibody activity is expressed by the monoclonal proteins of many patients with neuropathy. Antibody to a carbohydrate epitope on myelin-associated glycoprotein (MAG) is found in a majority of IgM-associated neuropathies.[89] The same epitope occurs in myelin glycoprotein P_0 and on other gangliosides in nerve cell membranes.[90, 91] Anti-MAG injection is known to produce demyelination in experimental animals.[92] Other patients have antibodies to myelin sheath sulfatides, to membrane-associated chondroitin sulfate C moieties, or to the GM1 ganglioside.[90, 91]

Clinical features of monoclonal gammopathy–associated neuropathy are mostly similar to those of CIDP[72]; however, sensory features tend to be more prominent and, although progression tends to be slower, it is also more relentless, and spontaneous improvement is uncommon.[93, 94] Neuropathy is more prevalent in patients with IgM paraproteins than in those with IgG or IgA[95] except in osteosclerotic myeloma, in which the prevalence of neuropathy with IgG or IgA proteins is quite high, sometimes as a part of the POEMS syndrome (polyneuropathy, organomegaly, endocrinopathy, monoclonal protein, skin changes).[96] Nerve biopsies show demyelination, axonal degeneration, and fiber loss, and immunofluorescence may demonstrate IgM and complement in IgM-associated cases.[88]

Patients with B-cell malignancies such as myeloma or Waldenström macroglobulinemia should be treated with chemotherapy protocols appropriate for their diagnosis and may experience improvement in the neuropathy. Many patients have neuropathy in the context of a monoclonal gammopathy of undetermined significance (MGUS) and are treated with immunosuppressive regimens similar to those used in CIDP.[88]

TPE has been shown to be effective in MGUS-associated neuropathy. In a sham-controlled trial in 39 patients, twice-weekly exchange led to improvement in disability scores, weakness scores, and electrodiagnostic parameters in the blinded portion of the trial. Similar improvement occurred subsequently in sham-treated patients who received true TPE in an open follow-up.[97] Response was more frequent in patients with IgG and IgA paraproteins than in those with IgM. This trend was also noted in other studies.[98–100]

Myasthenia Gravis

Myasthenia gravis (MG) is a disease of the neuromuscular junction characterized by weakness or undue fatigability, or both, in skeletal muscle. Ocular myasthenia, with diplopia and ptosis, is a frequent presentation, but other muscles are eventually affected in most patients. Involvement of muscles innervated by other cranial nerves leads to the most serious symptoms, including inability to swallow secretions and respiratory insufficiency.[101]

Most patients with myasthenia have circulating antibodies to a portion of the α subunit of the acetylcholine receptor molecule (AChR) on the muscle cell motor end plate.[102, 103] There are at least three mechanisms by which such antibodies can cause weakness.

1. They can block receptors competitively so that acetylcholine released from the nerve ending cannot gain access.

2. They can increase turnover of receptors in a manner that requires cross-linking and leads to a decreased number of receptors available to receive signals.

3. They can mediate target cell damage by complement or inflammatory cell attack, or both.[104]

The third mechanism probably leads to the most common histopathological findings, which are simplification of the normally convoluted junctional folds that bear the receptors and occasional inflammatory cell infiltrates in these areas.[105]

There are two approaches to drug therapy of myasthenia. Agents such as neostigmine and pyridostigmine inhibit degradation of acetylcholine at the neuromuscular junction and thereby enhance its action on remaining receptors.[105, 106] Immunosuppressive drugs, such as prednisone and azathioprine, are also used to reduce damage to receptors through either general anti-inflammatory properties or decreased antibody levels.[107]

Surgical treatment is also used. The incidence of malignant thymoma is increased among patients with myasthenia. Some of these patients improve after surgical resection of the thymus. This observation stimulated trials of thymectomy in patients not known to have tumors, and these patients may experience disease remission as well.[105–107]

Given the relationship between circulating antibody, pathology, and symptoms in myasthenia, TPE has seemed a reasonable approach to therapy.[108] A controlled trial has never been published, but numerous open trials have suggested that the therapy can bring about rapid symptomatic improvement in concert with lower levels of circulating anti-AChR antibody. TPE has also been effective in patients who test negative for antibody, perhaps suggesting that not all pathogenic antibodies are detected by available assays.[105–107, 109–111]

As a result of this universally favorable experience, TPE is widely accepted as a therapy for myasthenia. It is not, however, recommended for all patients. Rather, it is reserved for those with severe disease and those who either do not respond to other therapies or cannot tolerate them. Patients whose respiration, deglutition, or locomotion is inadequate are good candidates for the rapid improvement brought by TPE, even at initial treatment.[105] TPE can also be useful to optimize muscle function before surgery, especially thymectomy.[112] Occasional patients do best with regular TPE at 2- to 4-week intervals in addition to maintenance drug therapy.[113] Semiselective adsorption of IgG with protein A–Sepharose has been tried in myasthenia, also with favorable results.[114–118]

Myasthenia may also respond to IVIG.[119] Although no randomized trials have been done to prove efficacy, a controlled study compared IVIG with TPE in 87 patients. Either three or five infusions of IVIG at 0.4 g/kg were found equivalent to three TPE treatments. A shorter median time to response for TPE-treated patients (9 days vs. 15 days) did not achieve statistical significance ($p = .14$).[120] A multicenter retrospective chart review found significantly better ventilatory status at 2 weeks and functional status at 1 month in patients treated with TPE.[121]

Lambert-Eaton Myasthenic Syndrome

Lambert-Eaton myasthenic syndrome (LEMS) is characterized clinically by fatigue and weakness. It differs from MG in that oculomotor and bulbar symptoms are rarely prominent but signs of dysautonomia, such as dry mucous membranes and orthostatic hypotension, are common. LEMS most often occurs as a paraneoplastic syndrome. About 60% of cases are associated with small cell lung cancer, and associations with other tumors are also known. In many cases, the neuromuscular symptoms antedate any other sign of tumor.[105, 122–124]

LEMS is also a disease of the neuromuscular junction, but the defect is in the nerve cell ending instead of the muscle cell. LEMS is caused by circulating antibody directed against the "active zones" of the nerve terminus, which are thought to be the site of the voltage-gated calcium channels (VGCCs) that mediate electrical events in neuromuscular impulse transmission. The physiological result is a reduction in the amount of acetylcholine released by depolarization events, with consequent weakness in affected skeletal muscles as well as dysfunction at some autonomic nerve endings.[125, 126] The LEMS antibodies appear to be restricted to a subset of VGCCs that share the ability to bind one of the ω-conotoxins.[127]

Curiously, cholinesterase inhibitors are less effective in LEMS than in MG.[128] Agents that prolong nerve action potentials by blocking voltage-gated potassium channels may improve muscle strength in LEMS patients, presumably by enhancing acetylcholine release; 3,4-diaminopyridine is currently considered the most promising of these.[129, 130]

Immunosuppressive drugs such as cortisone and azathioprine may be helpful in LEMS, and paraneoplastic cases may respond to specific antitumor therapy.[131, 132]

TPE has been helpful in LEMS. Responses are often slower and more modest than those seen in MG, suggesting that more time is required to heal a damaged nerve ending.[11, 128, 133] IVIG has also been reported to be effective in trials in both the short and long term.[134]

Other Paraneoplastic Neurological Syndromes

A number of distinct neurological syndromes have been defined that are associated with malignant tumors and are characterized by circulating antibody to structures in the nervous system. Paraneoplastic encephalomyelitis is characterized by seizures, mental changes, and cerebellar and autonomic dysfunction. It is often associated with anti-Hu (also called ANNA-1), an antibody to a 38- to 40-kD antigen found in the nuclei of neurons and of small cell lung cancer cells. Paraneoplastic cerebellar degeneration produces ataxia, dysarthria, and down-beating nystagmus. It may arise in association with ovarian, breast, and small cell lung cancers as well as with Hodgkin disease. About 40% of patients have circulating anti-Yo, an antibody to 34- and 62-kD antigens in Purkinje cells. Paraneoplastic opsoclonus-myoclonus syndrome is characterized by both vertical and horizontal dysrhythmic conjugated eye movements. It may occur in children with neuroblastoma and in adults with lung, breast, or other tumors. Cases seen with breast or gynecological cancers may have circulating anti-Ri (also called ANNA-2), an antibody to 55- and 80-kD antigens in neuronal nuclei. Paraneoplastic stiff-man syndrome is characterized by stiffness and spasm in axial muscles and is associated with antibody to amphiphysin, a 128-kD synaptic vesicle protein. Cancer-associated retinopathy causes photosensitivity and gradual visual loss. It is associated with anti-CAR, an antibody to antigens shared by retinal neurons and small cell lung cancer cells.[135, 136]

Treatment of these syndromes is difficult. They seldom respond well to antitumor measures, even when these are otherwise effective, or to pharmacological immunosuppression. TPE has been used in a number of these cases, usually with disappointing results.[135, 136]

Non-neoplastic Disorders with Anti-CNS Antibodies

Rasmussen encephalitis is a rare, acquired disorder that begins in childhood, often after a viral infection. Seizures are a prominent clinical feature but, unlike patients with idiopathic epilepsy, patients with Rasmussen encephalitis develop progressive, usually unilateral neurological deficits including hemiparesis and mental retardation. Histopathological studies show inflammation and atrophy of brain tissue, usually confined to one hemisphere.[137]

Studies have revealed circulating IgG antibody to the Glu R3 receptor for the central nervous system (CNS) neurotransmitter glutamate.[138] It is hypothesized that these autoantibodies arise in response to a cross-reactive microbial antigen.[139, 140] Treatment with either TPE[140, 141] or IVIG[142] has been reported to bring temporary clinical improvement.

Sydenham chorea is an acquired movement disorder of children that follows group A streptococcal infection.[143] Many children with typical chorea also exhibit obsessive-compulsive symptoms,[144] and some children who have obsessive-compulsive disorder, tics, and other neurological symptoms without chorea have evidence of streptococcal infection (pediatric autoimmune neuropsychiatric disorders associated with streptococcal infection [PANDAS]).[145]

There is evidence to suggest that a cross-reactive antibody response to streptococcal antigens could mediate symptoms in some patients,[146, 147] although this is not universally accepted.[148] Small controlled trials have indicated that TPE and IVIG may both be beneficial in Sydenham chorea[149] and in PANDAS.[150]

Multiple Sclerosis

Multiple sclerosis (MS) is a demyelinating disease of the CNS that results in localized neurologic dysfunction. Two clinical patterns can be distinguished. About 70% of patients have acute attacks that resolve partially or fully over time (relapsing-remitting). The other 30% have gradual but continual progression of disease (chronic progressive). Attack frequency in relapsing-remitting MS tends to decrease with disease duration, and some patients may change to a chronic progressive pattern.[151]

Discrete plaques of demyelination in white matter are the pathological hallmarks of MS. These areas, which are easily visualized on magnetic resonance imaging (MRI), are initially inflammatory but progress to fibrosis.[151] The mechanism of their appearance remains a mystery, but most experts in the field suspect involvement of the immune system. An animal model of MS (experimental allergic encephalomyelitis [EAE]) can be induced by immunization with myelin basic protein or other myelin proteins. EAE appears to be mediated by T cells and can be passively transferred with T cells from immunized animals.[152, 153] Most evidence points to a disordered cellular immune response in MS as well, and it has been difficult to implicate circulating antibody in the pathogenesis of MS.[154]

Treatment of MS is problematic. Studies are complicated by the natural tendencies for acute attacks to subside and for attack frequency to decline, as well as other spontaneous fluctuations in disease activity. Clinical measurement tools such as the Expanded Disability Status Scale have been devised to quantify improvement or progressive disability, or both. These bring some objectivity to clinical studies but are arithmetically arbitrary and subject to interrater variability.[151, 155]

Immunosuppressive and immunomodulatory drugs have been the mainstay of pharmacological treatment in MS. Resolution of acute attacks is thought to be promoted by short courses of either corticosteroids or adrenocorticotropic hormone. These agents may promote faster return of normal nerve conduction by lessening edema and inflammation around new plaques.[151] It is doubtful whether the relentless progression of disability is halted by these measures, although vigorous use of intravenous steroids for optic neuritis may delay the onset of frank MS that it often portends.[156] Cyclosporin, total lymphoid irradiation, and cytotoxic immunosuppressants such as azathioprine and cyclophosphamide provide only modest benefits that may not warrant their attendant risks.[157] Mitoxantrone[158] and low-dose methotrexate[156] have also been tried. Interferon-β has shown promise,[159–164] as has glatiramer acetate, a mixture of synthetic polypeptides that may modulate immune responses to myelin basic protein.[165–167] These agents reduce the frequency of acute attacks and the appearance of new lesions on MRI.

IVIG has also been tried in MS. Prophylactic administration was reported to reduce the frequency of attacks in open trials. In three controlled trials there has been a decrease in the frequency of attacks.[168–170] MRI was not monitored in one study[168]; in another, fewer gadolinium-enhancing lesions were found in IVIG-treated patients[169]; in the third, the number of lesions seen without enhancement was the same after 2 years in both treatment and control groups.[170] A review advises that IVIG should still be regarded as experimental.[171]

The rationale for use of TPE in MS is unclear because there is so little evidence to implicate any circulating factor in the etiology of acute attacks or chronic progression. TPE has been used, however, and uncontrolled studies have reported encouraging results.[172–174] In controlled studies it has been more difficult to discern benefit, even with vigorous TPE regimens.[175, 176] The first randomized, double-blind sham-controlled study in chronic progressive MS was reported to show significant benefit for patients receiving TPE in addition to cyclophosphamide and prednisone.[177] The study was subsequently questioned because of anomalies in statistical analysis and because extraordinary recoveries in several of the TPE patients have not been reproduced in subsequent trials, suggesting that some patients with the relapsing-remitting form were inadvertently misclassified and entered into the trial.[154, 157, 178] Two later sham-controlled trials have not shown convincing benefit.[179, 180] Although TPE may yet be found useful in some subset of MS patients, such as those with prolonged severe demyelination,[181] most neurologists view it as controversial at best. The American Academy of Neurology classified TPE as "possibly useful" in MS.[182]

■ Therapeutic Plasma Exchange in Hematological and Oncological Disorders

Blood is the organ that can be most directly manipulated by therapeutic apheresis, and TPE has been tried in a variety of hematological and oncological conditions. These are listed in Table 44.4 along with their assigned indication categories.

Monoclonal Proteins

In addition to peripheral neuropathy, four other syndromes associated with monoclonal immunoglobulins are regarded as clinical indications for TPE. All five are listed in Table 44.5. The three syndromes that almost always occur in the setting of a malignant B-cell disorder are discussed here, and cryoglobulinemia is discussed in a later section.

The hyperviscosity syndrome was the first condition to be treated successfully with manual plasmapheresis, the precursor to TPE.[2, 3] The full-blown syndrome includes neurological symptoms, a bleeding diathesis, a distinctive retinopathy characterized by alternating dilated and constricted segments in retinal veins (link sausage veins), and hypervolemia related to an expanded plasma volume. Symptoms seldom occur if the relative serum viscosity is less than 4 and become more likely when it exceeds 6. The syndrome is most often seen in patients with IgM paraproteins in the context of Waldenström

Table 44.4 Indication Categories for Therapeutic Plasma Exchange in Hematological-Oncological Disorders

Disorder	Indication Categories*	
	ASFA	AABB
Hyperviscosity syndrome	I	I
Hemolytic disease of the newborn	III	NR
ABO-incompatible marrow transplant	II	III
Platelet alloimmunization and refractoriness	III	III
Thrombotic thrombocytopenic purpura	I	I
Hemolytic-uremic syndrome	III	II
Post-transfusion purpura	I	I
Idiopathic thrombocytopenic purpura	III	IV
Autoimmune hemolytic anemia	III	III
Aplastic anemia	III	IV
Pure red blood cell aplasia	III	III
Coagulation factor inhibitors	II	III

*I, standard first-line therapy; II, second-line therapy; III, controversial; IV, no efficacy; NR, not rated.
AABB, American Association of Blood Banks; ASFA, American Society for Apheresis.

Table 44.5 Paraprotein-Related Indications for Therapeutic Plasma Exchange

Indication	Implicated Ig Classes
Hyperviscosity	IgM > IgG/IgA
Coagulopathy	IgM > IgA > IgG
Myeloma kidney	Light chains
Neuropathy	IgM > IgG/IgA
Cryoglobulinemia	
Type I	IgM/IgG/IgA
Type II	IgM >> IgG/IgA

Ig, immunoglobulin.

macroglobulinemia but may occur in multiple myeloma as well.[183–185]

At higher paraprotein levels, the relationship between viscosity and paraprotein concentration is nonlinear and a relatively large change in viscosity may follow a relatively small change in concentration. As a consequence, the two-unit manual plasmapheresis technique available in the 1950s could lower an elevated viscosity enough to relieve symptoms. When combined with the fact that most affected patients have IgM paraproteins that are roughly 80% intravascular, this nonlinear relationship also predicts that a one-plasma-volume automated exchange will provide a wide margin of safety and can be done less often in the hyperviscosity syndrome than is necessary in many other conditions.[183, 186] Viscosity measurements should guide therapy, of course, but treatment every 1 to 2 weeks is often adequate.

Interference by paraprotein molecules in platelet and clotting factor interactions may occur even in the absence of hyperviscosity. Coagulopathies are found in 60% of patients with macroglobulinemia, 40% of patients with IgA myeloma, and 15% of patients with IgG myeloma.[187] Should they prove clinically significant, TPE therapy can help to restore adequate hemostasis.

Renal failure occurs in 3% to 9% of myeloma patients and carries a poor prognosis. In many such cases, renal biopsy demonstrates accumulation of free light chains in renal tubules. With normal renal function, urinary excretion of light chains far exceeds the amounts that could be removed by TPE, but in renal failure the reverse may be true.[188–190] Two controlled studies have shown higher rates of recovery of renal function in patients who received TPE therapy. In one study, three of seven dialysis-dependent patients who received TPE recovered renal function while none of five control patients did.[191] In the other, 13 of 15 patients in the treatment group recovered renal function compared with only 2 of 14 control subjects.[192]

Alloantibodies to Blood Cells

Alloantibodies to red blood cells and platelets may contribute to a disease process in a number of situations. Antibody removal has been used as a treatment in several of these pathologic states.

Hemolytic disease of the newborn was one of the first conditions to be approached with automated apheresis instruments.[8–10, 193] Efforts were made to lower anti-D titers by TPE in sensitized D-negative mothers carrying a D-positive fetus in the hope of ameliorating fetal red blood cell destruction.

The incidence of this condition has dropped dramatically as prophylaxis with Rh immune globulin has become more widespread, and intrauterine transfusion with D-negative red blood cells has proved to be a more effective treatment for an affected fetus.[194] TPE is seldom used in this circumstance now, but it may still be helpful in pregnancies with early evidence of fetal involvement because intrauterine transfusion is not feasible before about 18 weeks of gestation.[195, 196] Early institution of TPE was associated with successful delivery after multiple prior abortions in compelling case reports involving anti-M[197] and anti-P.[198]

TPE has also been used to remove isoagglutinins in the context of transplantation. Allogeneic stem cell transplantation across a major ABO barrier (e.g., group A donor into group O recipient) is feasible if a hemolytic transfusion reaction to red blood cells in the transplant can be avoided. For bone marrow transplants this was first accomplished by exhaustive pretransplantation TPE of the recipient to lower the relevant isoagglutinin titer.[199] Immunoadsorption columns containing A or B substance have subsequently been used.[200] Ultimately, however, it has proved preferable simply to remove most of the red blood cells from the bone marrow graft before transplantation.[201] Peripheral blood stem cell grafts contain smaller quantities of red blood cells and can usually be infused safely without any manipulation. Red blood cell engraftment is sometimes delayed in this setting, however, and TPE has been tried, both before transplantation to avoid delayed engraftment and after transplantation to correct it, with uncertain results in both cases.[202]

Solid-organ transplantation across a major ABO barrier can result in hyperacute rejection and is usually avoided for this reason. In desperate circumstances, however, considerations of organ availability have sometimes dictated use of an ABO-incompatible liver after pretransplantation TPE of the recipient, often with a satisfactory outcome.[203–205]

Organ transplantation across a minor ABO barrier (e.g., group O donor into group A recipient) does not increase the risk of rejection; however, it is sometimes followed, within 1 to 3 weeks after transplantation, by a hemolytic anemia related to isoagglutinin secretion by B lymphocytes carried in the transplanted organ. Hemolysis mediated by these "passenger lymphocytes" is most often seen in heart-lung or liver transplantation, where the volume of lymphoid tissue transplanted is relatively high.[206] Severe hemolysis in this setting may be partially ameliorated by TPE in combination with compatible red blood cell transfusion.[207]

Alloimmunization to platelets can cause clinical refractoriness to platelet transfusions.[208] Removal of antibody has been attempted, both with TPE[209] and with a protein A–silica column.[210, 211] IVIG has also been tried.[212–214] However, the results have been inconclusive and transfusion of compatible platelets is still the best option.

Thrombotic Thrombocytopenic Purpura and Hemolytic-Uremic Syndrome

Thrombotic Thrombocytopenic Purpura

Thrombotic thrombocytopenic purpura (TTP) is characterized by microangiopathic hemolytic anemia and thrombocytopenia, often severe. Fever, CNS changes, and renal abnormalities may be seen in advanced cases, although frank renal failure is uncommon.[215] A rare relapsing form usually begins in childhood, but most cases are sporadic and occur in adults.[216] Women are predominantly affected, accounting for 70% of cases.[217] TTP is usually idiopathic but the syndrome may be seen in association with other illnesses, such as SLE[218] and HIV infection.[219] Idiopathic TTP was formerly associated with a mortality rate of 95%, but empirical studies in the 1970s and 1980s demonstrated much better survival in patients who received TPE with plasma replacement. Some patients, including children with the relapsing form of the disease, respond to simple plasma infusion.[216]

A convincing account of the pathogenesis of TTP has been offered. It involves a plasma enzyme (a metalloproteinase designated as ADA MTS 13) that cleaves the ultralarge von Willebrand factor (ULvWF) multimers secreted by endothelial cells, yielding the smaller polymers found in normal plasma. Children with relapsing TTP have an inherited deficiency of this enzyme,[220] and in idiopathic adult cases there is an acquired deficiency related to the presence of an autoantibody that inhibits the enzyme.[221, 222] In either instance, persistence of ULvWF in the circulation apparently promotes inappropriate adherence of platelets to endothelial cells and to each other, leading to consumptive thrombocytopenia and microvascular obstructions. The latter cause mechanical trauma to red blood cells and varying degrees of end-organ ischemia. Periodic plasma infusion may abort or prevent attacks in congenitally deficient patients.[220] Idiopathic cases respond better to TPE (78% response rate vs. 63% for plasma infusion in a Canadian study),[223] presumably because exchange removes inhibitory antibody as well as supplying the deficient proteinases. Exchanges are usually carried out daily until the platelet count and lactate dehydrogenase (as a marker of hemolysis) have normalized.

Various immunosuppressive measures, such as glucocorticoid therapy,[224] vincristine,[225] and splenectomy,[226] have been advocated as adjunctive treatments. Discovery of an autoimmune etiology provides support for their use in idiopathic but not in congenital cases. Further work may clarify whether SLE- and HIV- associated cases are due to a similar autoantibody.

A syndrome similar to TTP has been identified in some patients taking the antiplatelet drug ticlopidine. Autoantibody-induced deficiency of the metalloproteinase has been demonstrated in patients with this syndrome,[227] and plasma exchange therapy has been reported to improve survival (76% survival vs. 50% for patients without exchange in a retrospective study).[228]

Hemolytic-Uremic Syndrome

The hemolytic-uremic syndrome (HUS) is characterized by microangiopathic hemolysis, renal insufficiency, and mild to moderate thrombocytopenia.[229] In children it may occur in a self-limited form that follows infection with a verotoxin-producing *Escherichia coli* (diarrhea + or D+); however, some pediatric cases lack this association (D–).[230, 231] Familial and nonfamilial forms affect adults.[221] Nonfamilial cases may be idiopathic or may be associated with prior chemotherapy or stem cell transplantation.[232]

Because of overlapping clinical manifestations, it has long been supposed that the pathogenesis of HUS was similar to that of TTP. Largely on this basis, TPE and protein A column therapy have been recommended for D– childhood HUS and for adult HUS. Responses have generally been less favorable than in TTP, particularly in HUS associated with chemotherapy and transplantation.[233, 234]

Levels of the vWF-cleaving metalloproteinase have now been studied in adult patients with both familial and nonfamilial forms of HUS. Neither severe deficiency nor inhibitory activity has been found.[221] Thus, the prior supposition of a pathogenic mechanism shared with TTP would seem to be in error. Deficiency of complement factor H has been identified in some patients with familial HUS.[235–237] This might provide some rationale for plasma therapy; however, for most cases the role of TPE is unclear at this time. Similar comments apply to the HELLP syndrome of hemolysis, elevated liver enzymes, and low platelets in pregnant women,[238] which shares clinical features with TTP, HUS, and preeclampsia.

Post-Transfusion Purpura

Post-transfusion purpura (PTP) is a rare syndrome in which the platelet count drops abruptly to dangerously low levels about 1 week after an allogeneic transfusion. Patients who develop the syndrome lack the common allele for one of the platelet-specific glycoprotein antigens, most often the human platelet-specific antigen 1a (HPA-1a) on glycoprotein (GP) IIIa. Most affected patients have had multiple pregnancies or prior transfusions and have been immunized thereby to the platelet-specific antigen coded by the prevalent allele. The transfusion that precipitates the illness appears to stimulate an anamnestic response with an increasing IgG antibody titer, most often anti–HPA-1a. PTP is self-limited and usually resolves without treatment in several weeks; however, bleeding complications, including fatal CNS hemorrhage, may occur.[239–241]

Although PTP is linked to a platelet-specific alloantibody response, the mechanism of extensive destruction of antigen-negative autologous platelets remains obscure. The following four possibilities have been proposed: (1) platelet antigen–antiplatelet antibody immune complexes bind to autologous platelets and mediate their destruction; (2) autologous platelets adsorb soluble alloantigen derived from the transfusion; (3) a simultaneous platelet autoantibody response occurs; (4) a broad alloimmune response produces antibodies that cross-react with autologous platelets.[242]

Treatment of PTP is advisable because many patients have bleeding complications. High-dose corticosteroids are usually given empirically, and pulse methylprednisolone at 1 g/day has been reported effective. Platelet transfusions, even those from antigen-negative donors, do not raise the platelet count and may cause severe reactions. Daily TPE usually promotes a rise in platelet count within a few days and is considered an effective treatment for this reason, even though controlled trials have not been done.[243] Exchanges usually include FFP replacement to avoid a superimposed humoral coagulopathy. IVIG leads to similarly prompt increases in platelet count and has become the favored treatment modality for this group of patients.[244]

Idiopathic Thrombocytopenic Purpura

Idiopathic thrombocytopenic purpura (ITP) is an autoimmune illness affecting platelets. Most patients have an IgG autoantibody directed against a platelet membrane glycoprotein antigen. ITP sometimes accompanies warm autoimmune hemolytic anemia (Evans syndrome). A pediatric form of ITP is acute and self-limited; recovery is the rule with or without treatment. Adult cases, most of which occur in women, seldom remit without therapy, and most progress to the chronic form of the disease. An ITP-like syndrome also occurs in association with SLE and HIV.[245]

The goal of treatment in ITP is prevention of bleeding. Because most platelets circulating in ITP patients are relatively young and more hemostatically active, avoidance of hemorrhage can be accomplished without normalization of the platelet count. Corticosteroids, splenectomy, and IVIG are the mainstays of therapy.[245] Some favorable anecdotal reports of TPE in ITP appeared in the 1970s.[246, 247] One small controlled trial suggested a lower rate of splenectomy in patients receiving exchange.[248] In the absence of confirmatory trials, however, enthusiasm for this approach has waned, and TPE is seldom used in ITP.

Favorable responses to protein A–silica column treatment have been reported, first in ITP associated with HIV infection[249] and later in patients with chronic ITP without HIV.[250] The mechanism of action of protein A in this disease is uncertain. A subtractive mechanism involving antiplatelet antibody is unlikely because responses have been reported with treatment of as little as 250 mL of plasma per week. Bearing this uncertainty in mind, the protein A–silica column remains an option for chronic ITP refractory to more standard therapies.

Autoimmune Hemolytic Anemia

Autoimmune hemolytic anemia (AHA) is caused by autoantibodies to red blood cells. Such antibodies are either cold or warm agglutinins. Cold agglutinins are usually IgM antibodies directed against the I/i antigens; they bind preferentially at low temperatures and produce the syndrome of complement-mediated intravascular hemolysis known as cold agglutinin disease (CAD). Warm agglutinins are usually IgG and are often directed against an antigen that is not expressed on Rh_{null} cells. They bind better at body temperature and produce a predominantly extravascular hemolytic syndrome (warm autoimmune hemolytic anemia [WAHA]). AHA can be idiopathic but may also be associated with an infection, a lymphoproliferative disorder, or another autoimmune disease.[251, 252]

Most cases require treatment. Standard therapy is aimed at inhibiting antibody production or reducing destruction of sensitized cells, or both. Corticosteroids, IVIG, and splenectomy are often effective in WAHA, and other immunosuppressive drugs may be tried if these measures fail.[251] All approaches are less successful in CAD.[252]

TPE to deplete circulating antibody has been tried in both WAHA and CAD when conventional treatments have failed.[253–259] IgM antibodies in CAD are predominantly intravascular and only loosely bound to cells. Thus, their removal by TPE should be relatively efficient. Such therapy, when added to conventional drug treatment, has been reported to transiently lower antibody titers and transfusion requirements in CAD. In WAHA much of the circulating antibody is bound to red blood cells; TPE has also been tried in this disorder, but it is less likely to be helpful.

Aplastic Anemia and Pure Red Blood Cell Aphasia

Aplastic anemia and pure red blood cell aplasia are bone marrow disorders. The former leads to pancytopenia, whereas in the latter there is only reticulocytopenic anemia. At least some cases of both conditions are likely to be immunologically mediated. Allogeneic bone marrow transplantation is the preferred treatment for aplastic anemia if a suitable donor is available, but immunosuppressive therapies, such as corticosteroids, cytotoxic drugs, cyclosporin, and antithymocyte globulin, are effective in some cases.[260–262]

In a minority of patients it is possible to demonstrate a serum factor, probably antibody, that is inhibitory to the growth of relevant marrow-derived precursor cells in culture.[263] These observations provided an explicit rationale for TPE, and this therapy has been reported in a handful of cases in both disorders. Results in aplastic anemia have been mixed, with responses more likely in patients demonstrating serum inhibitory activity.[263–265] In pure red blood cell aplasia, all reported instances of TPE treatment have led to improvement, which is sometimes quite dramatic in patients with serum inhibitory activity.[266–269] Thus, although TPE is not a primary therapy for either disorder, it is an option for patients who have not responded to more conventional treatment, especially those who have serum inhibitory factors.

Coagulation Factor Inhibitors

Coagulation factor inhibitors are IgG antibodies directed against components of the humoral clotting cascade. They inactivate the targeted factor and interfere with clotting. They may be autoantibodies that arise in individuals with no prior bleeding disorder. Alternatively, they may be alloantibodies arising in genetically deficient patients as a result of exposure to a "foreign protein" in the course of factor replacement therapy.[270, 271] Factor VIII is the clotting protein most often affected by antibodies of either type.

The goals of treatment for patients with inhibitors are, first, control of individual bleeding episodes and, eventually, suppression of inhibitor synthesis.[272, 273] Depending on the inhibitor titer, the first goal can usually be achieved by infusion of high doses of human factor VIII, porcine factor VIII (which is usually only partially cross-reactive with anti–human factor VIII antibodies),[274] or, for patients with the highest titers, factor VIII–bypassing products, including recombinant factor VIIa.[275] TPE with plasma replacement may be employed during a bleeding episode to reduce inhibitor titers enough to allow infused human or porcine factor VIII to circulate and bring about hemostasis.[276–278] Suppression of inhibitor synthesis is approached with immunosuppressive measures, including high-dose corticosteroids, cytotoxic agents,[279] cyclosporin,[280] and IVIG.[281] Tolerance-inducing protocols have been devised for congenitally deficient patients with alloimmune inhibitors.[282, 283] These involve regular infusion of exogenous factor VIII. In the so-called Malmö protocol, extensive TPE or IgG depletion with protein A–Sepharose column procedures is used to lower the inhibitor titer at the onset of treatment so that infused factor can circulate.[284] Patients with inhibitors usually need frequent, large (two or three plasma volumes) exchanges with FFP replacement. Central venous access is frequently required; catheter placement in the context of a refractory bleeding disorder is challenging to all concerned and often mandates use of a factor VIII–bypassing product for wound hemostasis.[285]

TPE has also been reported for treatment of patients with antiphospholipid antibodies.[286] These may interfere with in vitro assays of coagulation, such as the partial thromboplastin time. However, unlike the inhibitory antibodies described above, they usually promote inappropriate coagulation in vivo and cause thrombotic events.

■ Therapeutic Plasma Exchange in Other Immunological Disorders

TPE has been tried in a number of rheumatic diseases and other diseases that are considered to have an immune or autoimmune etiology. These are listed in Table 44.6 along with the indication categories assigned by ASFA and AABB.

Cryoglobulinemia

Cryoglobulins are defined as serum proteins that precipitate reversibly at 4°C, although some precipitate at higher temperatures. The precipitates always contain immunoglobulins, and immunoelectrophoretic or immunofixation analysis allows distinction of three types.[287]

Type I cryoglobulins consist of a single species of monoclonal immunoglobulin. These are usually found in myeloma, Waldenström macroglobulinemia, or other lymphoproliferative disorders (see Table 44.5). Cryoglobulin levels are often quite high (>500 mg/dL) and may cause Raynaud phenomenon or acral necrosis related to microvascular obstruction, as well as other symptoms. Type II cryoglobulins have both a monoclonal and a polyclonal component. The former is usually an IgMk with anti-IgG activity that binds polyclonal IgG in an immune complex. These typically produce a lower extremity cutaneous vasculitis and may cause other, more serious visceral manifestations of immune complex disease. Many cases occur in association with chronic hepatitis C infection.[288] Type III cryoglobulins are mixed polyclonal, often with IgM anti-IgG binding IgG in immune complexes. These may arise in acute infections, such as hepatitis B, and in severe rheumatoid arthritis or other chronic inflammatory states. Clinical manifestations resemble those of serum sickness.[287, 289]

If there is an associated condition, cryoglobulin levels and related symptoms may decrease with treatment of the primary disorder, for example, chemotherapy for myeloma or

Table 44.6 Indication Categories for Therapeutic Plasma Exchange in Rheumatic and Other Immune Disorders

Disorder	Indication Categories[*]	
	ASFA	AABB
Cryoglobulinemia	II	I
Rheumatoid arthritis	III, (II for IA[†])	NR
Systemic lupus erythematosus	IV	IV
Systemic vasculitis	III	II
Polymyositis and dermatomyositis	IV	IV
Goodpasture syndrome	I	I
Rapidly progressive glomerulonephritis	II	II
Renal transplantation		
Rejection	IV	IV
Presensitization	III	NR
Recurrent focal glomerulosclerosis	III	NR
Heart transplant rejection	III	NR

[*]I, standard first-line therapy; II, second-line therapy; III, controversial; IV, no efficacy; NR, not rated.
[†]IA, protein A-silica immunoadsorption;
AABB, American Association of Blood Banks; ASFA, American Society for Apheresis.

interferon for hepatitis C virus infection. For idiopathic and secondary cases of mixed cryoglobulinemia, prednisone therapy may be effective in relieving symptoms, and alkylating agents may be useful for patients with severe symptoms resistant to prednisone.[289]

TPE reduces cryoglobulin levels and controls symptoms,[290] even in the absence of other treatments,[34] but expense and inconvenience usually preclude such use. Plasma exchange therapy should be started promptly for patients who present with severe acral ischemia or visceral manifestations of vasculitis.[291] In such patients it can help gain and maintain control of symptoms until aggressive drug therapy takes hold. Patients with chronic ulcers in the setting of cutaneous vasculitis may also benefit.[292] Care should be taken to warm replacement fluids to body temperature before reinfusion.

Rheumatoid Arthritis

Rheumatoid arthritis (RA) is a disease of unknown etiology that is more prevalent in women. It is the most common chronic inflammatory joint disease and a leading cause of disability. Most patients have rheumatoid factor, an IgM autoantibody to IgG; however, because this finding is absent in many otherwise typical cases and because it occurs in other patients who do not have arthritis, it is not thought to be directly involved in pathogenesis.[293]

Conservative treatment of RA includes nonsteroidal anti-inflammatory agents, low-dose oral corticosteroids, and intra-articular steroids. More severely affected patients eventually receive slow-acting antirheumatic agents that are probably immunomodulatory, such as antimalarials, gold compounds, and methotrexate.[294] Tumor necrosis factor inhibitors have been approved for use in RA.[295]

TPE was tried in RA in the 1970s and 1980s, but controlled trials did not show benefit.[296, 297] There were subsequent reports of lymphapheresis, with or without TPE in addition. Some controlled trials showed significant but short-lived benefit,[298] whereas others did not.[299] In practice, the prospect of no more than a modest chance of only modest benefit from a costly and inconvenient therapy has discouraged treatment with therapeutic apheresis.

A sham-controlled trial of 12 weekly protein A–silica column treatments produced improvement in 33% of 48 treated patients versus only 9% of 43 control subjects. Benefit persisted for about 8 months on average, and a subsequent course was again beneficial in seven of nine initial responders.[300] Despite the fact that its mechanism of action is unclear, this device has gained Food and Drug Administration (FDA) approval for use in RA, and postmarketing clinical experience is beginning to accumulate.

Systemic Lupus Erythematosus

SLE has been viewed as the prototypical autoimmune disease. The occurrence of antibodies to DNA, especially those specific for double-stranded DNA (anti–ds-DNA), identifies a group of patients who may have autoantibodies to a variety of other determinants. Their clinical syndromes comprise a disparate mixture in which skin disease, joint disease, cytopenias, or nephritis may be the sole or dominant manifestation.[301]

Immunosuppressive measures are the cornerstone of therapy for SLE. Most patients receive prednisone in varying doses, and those with severe disease may also be given azathioprine or cyclophosphamide.[302] The plethora of autoantibodies that

seem relevant to clinical signs made SLE an obvious target for plasma exchange therapy, and it was one of the first illnesses to be treated with automated TPE in the early 1970s. A number of case reports and uncontrolled series suggested a favorable effect.[11, 12, 303, 304]

Lupus nephritis is a particularly devastating expression of SLE in which glomerular deposition of anti–ds-DNA and immune complexes is believed to play a prominent pathogenic role. It thus seemed an attractive context for randomized trials. A controlled trial with only eight patients suggested benefit.[305] However a multi-institutional randomized controlled trial comparing oral cyclophosphamide plus TPE with oral cyclophosphamide alone failed to show any advantage for the patients receiving TPE.[26] A later international trial included patients with a variety of severe manifestations. It was structured to take advantage of an enhanced sensitivity to a properly timed pulse dose of intravenous cyclophosphamide that was believed to follow removal of pathogenic antibody by TPE.[306] As mentioned earlier, subsequent work with knockout mice deficient for the FcRn receptor suggested that enhanced susceptibility would not occur.[24] In any case, this trial also failed to show any benefit associated with TPE, either in all patients[307] or in a subgroup with nephritis.[308] Thus, several large controlled studies have failed to reveal any worthwhile effect of TPE in SLE.

Systemic Vasculitis

Systemic vasculitis is an inclusive term applied to a group of disorders that cause inflammation in blood vessel walls with resultant ischemic tissue damage. Vasculitis syndromes are conveniently classified on the basis of the size of vessels typically involved, as shown in Table 44.7. Most are of unknown etiology. The presence of immune complexes in some syndromes and of autoantibodies, such as antineutrophil cytoplasmic antibodies (ANCAs) found in Wegener granulomatosis (c-ANCA) and polyarteritis (p-ANCA), in others has lent credence to the notion that humoral immune factors are somehow involved.[309]

Prednisone is the first-line therapy for most vasculitic syndromes. Cyclophosphamide is often added in more severe cases.[310] Randomized controlled trials in renal vasculitis,[311] as well as in a group of patients with polyarteritis or Churg-Strauss angiitis,[312] have shown little evidence that long-term benefit is conferred by addition of TPE to drug therapy. Nevertheless, it may be requested for patients who are not responding to maximal drug therapy.

Table 44.7 Classification of Systemic Vasculitis

Large vessel vasculitis
   Giant cell (temporal) arteritis
   Takayasu arteritis

Medium-sized vessel vasculitis
   Polyarteritis nodosa
   Kawasaki syndrome

Small vessel vasculitis
   Wegener granulomatosis
   Churg-Strauss syndrome
   Microscopic polyangiitis
   Henoch-Schönlein purpura
   Essential cryoglobulinemic vasculitis
   Cutaneous leukocytoclastic angiitis

Polymyositis and Dermatomyositis

Polymyositis and dermatomyositis are inflammatory diseases of skeletal muscle. A characteristic dermatitis, typically involving the eyelids, knuckles, neck, and shoulders, is also found in the latter condition. Proximal weakness with biochemical evidence of muscle cell enzyme leakage is the usual presentation. The diagnosis is confirmed by characteristic inflammatory histology in a biopsy specimen from an affected muscle. The natural history is progressive fiber loss, eventually leading to profound, irreversible weakness. An autoimmune etiology is suspected, but an antibody specific for skeletal muscle has not yet been implicated.[313]

Initial treatment is high-dose prednisone, which can often be tapered to levels that are tolerable in the long term. Resistant disease is treated with azathioprine, methotrexate, or an alkylating agent, or a combination thereof.[314] Controlled trials have also shown that IVIG infusion reduces muscle enzyme levels and improves strength temporarily.[315]

Several uncontrolled series have been interpreted to show that TPE was beneficial, but these were confounded by concurrent escalations in immunosuppressive drug therapy.[316–318] A randomized, controlled trial was reported in which 12 patients received TPE, 12 received lymphapheresis, and 12 received sham apheresis, with no changes in drug therapy.[319] There was no difference in the response rate among the three groups. Thus, despite the successes with IVIG there appears to be no role for TPE in the treatment of polymyositis.

Goodpasture Syndrome

Goodpasture syndrome (GPS) is an illness characterized clinically by rapidly progressive glomerulonephritis and pulmonary hemorrhage. Renal biopsy shows crescent formation in many glomeruli on light microscopy and linear subendothelial immune deposits on immunofluorescence and electron microscopy. Lung biopsy may show similar subendothelial deposits.[320, 321] In 95% of cases the syndrome is associated with circulating antibody that binds to glomerular basement membrane (anti-GBM).[322] These antibodies are directed against a noncollagenous sequence near the carboxyl terminus of the α-3 chain of a type of collagen (type IV) that is found in appreciable quantities only in renal and pulmonary basement membranes.[323] Untreated GPS progresses quickly and relentlessly, and most patients die of uremia or of complications of lung hemorrhage.[322]

Since the classical report by Lockwood and colleagues in 1975,[324] the recommended treatment for GPS has been aggressive TPE combined with high-dose prednisone and cyclophosphamide.[325, 326] TPE reduces anti-GBM levels quickly to minimize progression of tissue damage.[327] Exchanges are usually carried out daily and may be continued for 2 weeks.[328] It is therefore prudent to give some FFP replacement in the latter part of each exchange to replete coagulation factors and avoid exacerbations of lung bleeding related to dilutional coagulopathy.

The only controlled trial on record failed to show an advantage for GPS patients who received TPE; however, this study has been largely discounted because the TPE schedule (every 3 days) was not sufficiently aggressive and because, despite randomization, the extent of renal damage at entry was not comparable in the TPE and control groups.[329] Early

treatment is preferred because it has been noted that patients with dialysis-dependent renal failure at the onset of treatment are not likely to recover renal function.[328, 330] A corollary is that patients whose renal biopsies show an irreversible lesion and who do not have pulmonary hemorrhage are unlikely to benefit from TPE.

Other Rapidly Progressive Glomerulonephritis

In addition to GPS, there are two other categories of rapidly progressive glomerulonephritis (RPGN) as shown in Table 44.8. In both of these, the light microscopic findings are similar to those in GPS with severe glomerular inflammation and crescent formation. Some cases may even have associated lung hemorrhage. The distinction among RPGN subcategories rests on immunofluorescence microscopy and electron microscopy, which show granular (vs. linear in GPS) subendothelial immune deposits, usually taken to be immune complexes, in one group of patients and absence or relative scarcity of immune deposits in the other (pauci-immune RPGN).[331] Patients in each group may have isolated, idiopathic renal disease or may have accompanying features that suggest a diagnosis of systemic vasculitis, for example, mixed cryoglobulinemia or Henoch-Schönlein purpura for granular–immune complex RPGN and microscopic polyangiitis or Wegener granulomatosis for patients with pauci-immune RPGN, many of whom test positive for ANCA.[332, 333]

Because treatments for the two categories are similar, some trials and series have included patients with both types of RPGN.[334, 335] Virtually all patients receive prednisone and most receive cyclophosphamide, either orally or intravenously. TPE has been used extensively in patients with both types of disease, and early uncontrolled series tended to credit it with a beneficial effect. Two controlled trials, one published in 1988[336] and the other in 1992,[337] showed no advantage overall for patients who received TPE in addition to immunosuppressive drugs. However, a separate analysis of the small subgroup in the second study who presented with dialysis-dependent renal failure suggested that such patients have a better chance of recovering renal function if they receive TPE.[337] A comparable trend was not noticed in the trial conducted by Guillevin and colleagues.[338] A more recent prospective, randomized trial by Stegmayr and coworkers[330] compared TPE with immunoadsorption. Among 38 patients with non-GPS RPGN, 87% of whom had ANCA, 70% avoided long-term dialysis. TPE and immunoadsorption were equally effective. Thus, TPE continues to be controversial in non-GPS RPGN. It is probably not justified as a first-line therapy, except (paradoxically) in patients who present with dialysis dependence,[339] but it may be offered to patients who progress despite immunosuppressive drug therapy.

Table 44.8 Subtypes of Rapidly Progressive Glomerulonephritis (RPGN)

Nomenclature	Quality of Subendothelial Immune Deposits
Goodpasture syndrome	Linear
Immune complex RPGN	Granular
Pauci-immune RPGN	Scant or none

Solid-Organ Transplantation

TPE has been used in the organ transplant setting both to treat and to prevent rejection as well as to treat recurrence of certain diseases in a transplanted organ. Photopheresis has also been tried for the same purposes, mostly in heart transplantation.

Rejection

Cellular immunity is thought to mediate rejection of most organ allografts; however, rapid antibody-mediated rejection may occur in patients who have preexisting antibodies to ABO or human leukocyte antigen (HLA) antigens expressed by the graft.[340] Histologically, such hyperacute rejection is characterized by fibrin deposition, endothelial damage, and neutrophil infiltration in small blood vessels; damage to the graft parenchyma is mainly ischemic.[341] All treatments, including TPE, have been futile in hyperacute rejection. Vascular changes reminiscent of hyperacute rejection may be seen in later rejection episodes. These are sometimes taken to indicate antibody-mediated rejection, even when immuno-fluorescence microscopy and tests for circulating antibody are negative.[341]

Prophylactic immunosuppression with corticosteroids and either cyclosporin or tacrolimus is standard post-transplantation management for kidney and liver transplantation.[342] Heart recipients may also receive azathioprine or mycophenolate mofetil.[343] Rejection episodes occurring in spite of these measures are treated with pulse steroids or anti–T-cell antibody preparations, or both.[344]

TPE was used extensively in the late 1970s and early 1980s to treat renal transplant rejection after a number of case reports and uncontrolled series suggested it was beneficial.[345–350] In the middle and late 1980s, however, five controlled trials were reported. Four showed no significant benefit for patients receiving TPE in addition to standard drug therapy, even in the subgroups with vascular histology in transplant biopsies.[351–354] In the single study suggesting benefit, the mean time of treatment was 10 to 11 months after transplantation, when antibody-mediated rejection is unlikely.[355] The last and largest study was reported by Blake and colleagues,[354] who concluded that TPE therapy could no longer be recommended for this purpose. Despite this, use of TPE in this context continues to be reported.[356–360]

Notwithstanding its ineffectiveness in renal transplantation, preliminary experience with TPE has also been reported in the context of cardiac allograft rejection. Favorable courses have been seen in individual patients who were also receiving other therapies, but no controlled trials have been reported.[361, 362] Vascular rejection is more difficult to detect or exclude in the endomyocardial biopsies done to monitor cardiac allografts because few blood vessels are found in this part of the heart muscle. Immunofluorescence microscopy positive for IgG is the usual criterion for humoral rejection; however, one group has suggested that this diagnosis be made, and TPE employed, in patients who have relatively normal biopsies in the context of deteriorating cardiac function.[363, 364] Controlled data to support this assertion are lacking.

TPE has been used prior to transplantation in patients presensitized to HLA antigens. Patients whose sera react with lymphocytes from a large proportion of the population have a diminished chance of a compatible crossmatch with an available donor and hence a low likelihood of receiving a transplant. Prospective immunosuppression, combined with removal of antibody by TPE or protein A–Sepharose immunoadsorption, has been tried as a means to obtain a compatible crossmatch and prevent hyperacute rejection. Several groups have reported that patients prepared in this way who receive kidney transplants have quite respectable graft survival rates.[365–372] Similar protocols have facilitated successful transplantation of ABO-incompatible kidneys and livers.[373–378]

In summary, the preponderance of evidence from controlled trials shows that TPE is not effective in reversing established rejection of renal allografts. Nonetheless, pre-transplantation antibody removal can allow transplantation for otherwise ineligible candidates, especially those with high-titer antibodies to one or two HLA antigens whose titer-sensitive cross-reactions can be suppressed.

Recurrence of Disease

Focal glomerulosclerosis (FGS) is a disease that causes nephrosis and renal failure, predominantly in children. It recurs in about 30% of patients with allografts, suggesting that a humoral factor may play a role in the pathogenesis.[379] There is evidence to implicate a 50-kD plasma factor that binds to protein A but has not been further characterized.[380, 381] Several reports describe reductions in proteinuria and improved renal function when recurrence of FGS is treated with stepped-up immunosuppression and TPE.[379, 382–384]

GPS may occasionally recur in an allograft,[385] although this can usually be avoided by delaying renal transplantation until anti-GBM titers have dropped spontaneously. If it recurs, it should be treated promptly with TPE and cyclophosphamide.

A diffuse coronary artery disease, termed allograft vasculopathy, sometimes develops in transplanted hearts. It is the leading cause of morbidity and mortality in allograft recipients who survive beyond 1 year.[343] It may be related to continuing hyperlipidemia[386] or to chronic rejection.[387] Selective depletion of LDLs, discussed in more detail in the following section on hypercholesterolemia, has been thought helpful in a few transplant patients with persistent lipoprotein abnormalities.[388] Photopheresis has also been used as an anti-rejection measure in this setting.[389]

■ Therapeutic Plasma Exchange in Toxic and Metabolic Disorders

This section covers several conditions in which removal of nonantibody substances present in plasma has been deemed therapeutically attractive or advisable. These are listed in Table 44.9 along with the indication categories assigned to them by ASFA and AABB.

Hypercholesterolemia

Familial hypercholesterolemia (FH) is an inherited disorder characterized by highly elevated levels of circulating LDL, cholesterol (650 to 1000 mg/dL), and lipoprotein (a) (Lpa). In homozygotes, cholesterol deposits in the form of skin xanthomas and coronary atheromas develop in the first decade of life, and death from myocardial infarction prior to age 20 is common. Heterozygotes also have elevated LDL, cholesterol (350 to 500 mg/dL), and Lpa levels; xanthomas may develop

Table 44.9   Indication Categories for Therapeutic Plasma Exchange in Metabolic Disorders

Disease	Indication Categories*	
	ASFA	AABB
Homozygous familial hypercholesterolemia	II, (I for LDL-P[†])	I
Refsum disease	I	I
Overdose or poisoning	III	II
Acute hepatic failure	III	IV

*I, standard first-line therapy; II, second-line therapy; III, controversial; IV, no efficacy.
[†]LDL-P, low-density lipoprotein apheresis (i.e., selective depletion of LDL). AABB, American Association of Blood Banks; ASFA, American Society For Apheresis.

by age 20 and coronary atherosclerosis by age 30. A genetically determined deficiency of cell surface LDL receptors in these patients interferes with cholesterol off-loading from LDL into cells and with the normal negative feedback regulation of LDL synthesis, leading to the elevations in LDL and cholesterol.[390]

Less severe forms of hypercholesterolemia can be influenced by dietary modifications and are amenable to therapy with several categories of drugs, including 3-hydroxy-3-methylglutaryl coenzyme A (HMG-CoA) reductase inhibitors, bile acid binding resins, and nicotinic acid. However, FH homozygotes and some FH heterozygotes respond poorly to these measures and are at high risk for premature death. Drastic surgical therapies such as ileal bypass, portacaval shunt, and liver transplantation may be offered to such patients if they have evidence of coronary artery disease.[390] Alternatively, repeated physical removal of LDL and its associated cholesterol can be accomplished by various modalities of therapeutic apheresis.

A one-plasma-volume TPE lowers LDL and cholesterol levels by 50% or more, and long-term treatment every 1 to 2 weeks can bring about shrinkage of cutaneous xanthomas and regression of coronary deposits.[391–394] TPE removes both LDL and Lpa but it also depletes high-density lipoproteins (HDLs), which are felt to have a salutary antiatherogenic action. This apparent disadvantage has engendered efforts to remove LDL semiselectively and on line from patient's plasma separated by an apheresis device and then return the LDL-depleted plasma to the patient.

Several systems that have been designed to accomplish this goal are listed in Table 44.10. Secondary filtration systems employ a plasma filter with a pore size that retains the very large LDL molecule while sieving smaller ones such as albumin[395]; however, these systems typically remove about half of plasma HDL.[396] In a heparin extracorporeal LDL precipitation (HELP) system, LDL precipitated by heparin at acid pH is removed by filtration from patient's plasma that is then dialyzed on line to restore a physiological pH.[397] Lpa is also depleted, and HDL levels fall by 15%.[396] LDL immunoadsorption columns contain an LDL-specific antibody linked to Sepharose particles.[398, 399] The need to reuse columns to achieve cost-effectiveness is an awkward feature of this technology.[396] A final system, the Kaneka Liposorber, uses a pair of regenerable dextran sulfate columns that absorb LDL but not HDL or Lpa.[37, 400] All these systems remove LDL

Table 44.10   Selective Extraction Methods for Lipoproteins

Immunoadsorption with anti-LDL antibody
Secondary membrane filtration
Heparin precipitation (HELP system)
Chemical adsorption to dextran sulfate

HELP, heparin extracorporeal low-density lipoprotein precipitation; LDL, low-density lipoprotein.

effectively, but only the dextran sulfate system is FDA approved and commercially available in the United States. Although this system lowers HDL considerably less than TPE for a given decrement in LDL, it has no application other than the treatment of hypercholesterolemia. Consequently, a center acquiring it must use it regularly on multiple patients to make it economically feasible.

Refsum Disease

Refsum disease is an inherited disorder caused by deficiency of the peroxisomal enzyme phytanoyl-CoA hydroxylase, which participates in the normal degradation of phytanic acid by α-oxidation. Symptoms usually begin in the third decade of life as a result of accumulation of diet-derived phytanic acid in plasma lipoproteins and in tissue lipid stores. Peripheral neuropathy, cerebellar ataxia, and retinitis pigmentosa are found in almost all cases. Anosmia, deafness, ichthyosis, renal failure, and arrhythmias may also occur. Slow progression is the usual course, but abrupt deterioration, including sudden death, may follow a marked increase in plasma phytanic acid levels.[401]

Early diagnosis is important so that dietary intake of phytanic acid through dairy products, meats, and ruminant fats can be curtailed. Diet is the mainstay of treatment, leading to gradual clearing of phytanate stores by slow ω-oxidation and gradual symptomatic improvement in most patients. Adequate nutrition must be maintained, however, because overly rapid catabolism of endogenous fat can raise plasma phytanic acid levels acutely and cause clinical exacerbations.[401]

TPE has been reported in a number of cases of Refsum disease and removes large quantities of phytanic acid incorporated into plasma lipids.[402] Selective lipoprotein depletion is also effective.[403] Apheresis is probably most appropriate for patients who have very high plasma phytanate levels, particularly those with exacerbation of symptoms. Skin disease, neuropathic symptoms, and ataxia usually improve as plasma levels drop. Cranial nerve defects usually do not.[401]

Drug Overdose and Poisoning

Toxic effects may arise from intentional or inadvertent exposure to excessive doses of pharmacological agents as well as from harmful agents encountered in the environment. Management techniques are similar for both types of events and include attempts to remove toxin still in the gastrointestinal tract, efforts to promote or enhance renal elimination, and direct removal from the blood by hemodialysis, hemoperfusion (e.g., over charcoal columns), or TPE.[404] If available, specific antidotes may also be given.[405] Most patients are treated with more than one modality.

TPE has been tried in a number of patients with drug overdose or poisoning. It has been reported to be beneficial, when used along with other therapies, in cases involving substances that bind tightly to plasma proteins.[406] Examples include methylparathion,[407] vincristine,[408] and cisplatin.[409] It has also been reported for severe hyperthyroidism, either endogenous or exogenous, although its effectiveness is limited by extensive binding of L-thyroxine to tissue proteins.[410] TPE has been used in several cases of poisoning caused by ingestion of the *Amanita phalloides* mushroom[411, 412]; however, diuresis has been shown to clear far more *Amanita* toxin.[413]

The literature on this topic is older and is entirely anecdotal. Furthermore, TPE has always been used in combination with other, presumably effective therapies, making it difficult to formulate firm, rational guidelines. Nevertheless, it seems reasonable to offer TPE to severely affected patients with poisoning or overdose who have high blood levels of an agent known to bind to plasma proteins. On the other hand, TPE has shown minimal or no beneficial effect in overdosage of drugs known to bind to tissue proteins and lipids, including barbiturates,[414] chlordecone,[415] aluminum,[416] tricyclic antidepressants,[417] benzodiazepines,[414] quinine,[418] phenytoin,[419] digoxin, digitoxin,[420] prednisone, prednisolone,[421] tobramycin,[422] and propranol.[423]

Acute Hepatic Failure

Acute hepatic failure (AHF) is an uncommon condition that arises from a severe liver insult. Hepatitis B and acetaminophen overdosage are important causes. Additional cases are due to drug reactions, Wilson disease, vascular anomalies, acute fatty liver of pregnancy, and a variety of toxins. AHF results in a myriad of metabolic imbalances and synthetic defects. Clinical symptoms include jaundice, coagulopathy, renal failure, and encephalopathy. Liver transplantation is the treatment of choice, leading to 60% to 80% long-term survival versus greater than 60% mortality for patients without transplantation. Many fatal outcomes are due to complications of cerebral edema.[424–426]

Conservative therapy is essentially supportive. Fluid, electrolyte, and nutritional supplements are adjusted to correct metabolic abnormalities. Bowel sterilization with enteral antibiotics is recommended to minimize ammonia production by intestinal flora. Pressors are given as needed for hemodynamic support, and plasma products are infused to combat coagulopathy. Osmotic diuretics, sedatives, hyperventilation, and proper positioning are all employed to reduce intracranial pressure.[424–426]

TPE with plasma replacement has inherent appeal as a strategy to restore metabolic homeostasis, remove toxic metabolites that may cause cerebral edema, and supply deficient plasma proteins, such as coagulation factors, in quantity without inducing volume overload. However, evaluations of the effectiveness of this approach have been mixed.[425] Some investigators have felt that TPE was helpful in stabilizing patients and maintaining them until an organ became available for transplantation.[427] Improvements in neurologic status, blood pressure, and cerebral blood flow were attributed to exchanges in one study[428]; however, intracranial pressure, which is a key prognostic indicator, did not fall. Hemoperfusion over activated charcoal, which lowers plasma ammonia levels, has also shown no advantage over intensive supportive care alone.[426]

Potential problems with extensive TPE arise from the diminished ability of patients with AHF to metabolize the citrate in infused plasma. Citrate accumulation leads to ionized hypocalcemia and to alterations in arterial ketone body ratios that may interfere with regeneration of hepatocytes.[429] Thus, although TPE can partially reverse coagulopathy and other synthetic deficits in these patients, a favorable net impact on outcome has been difficult to demonstrate.

The Bioartificial Liver being tested by the Circe Corporation is a promising new development. It contains a suspension of pig liver cells in the exterior space surrounding the fibers in a hollow fiber filter cartridge. Patient's plasma, separated by an apheresis device and passed through a charcoal column to remove ammonia, is then brought into "metabolic contact" with the porcine hepatocytes as it flows through the hollow fibers. A nonrandomized study showed decreases in both ammonia levels and intracranial pressure readings in patients treated for 6 to 8 hours per day with the device, which is intended as a bridge to liver transplantation.[430]

■ Conclusion

It can be seen from the foregoing that TPE is an effective therapy for a number of disorders, especially those mediated by autoreactive antibodies or paraproteins. Refinements in instrumentation that are outside the scope of this chapter have made it a safe therapy as well. Thus, it should play an important role in the treatment of selected diseases for the foreseeable future.

REFERENCES

1. Abel JJ, Rowntree LG, Turner BB: Plasma removal with return of corpuscles (plasmapheresis). J Pharmacol Exp Ther 1914;5:625.
2. Skoog WA, Adams WS: Plasmapheresis in a case of Waldenström's macroglobulinemia. Clin Res 1959;7:96.
3. Schwab PJ, Fahey JL: Treatment of Waldenström's macroglobulinemia by plasmapheresis. N Engl J Med 1960;263:574.
4. Cohn EJ, Tullis JL, Surgenor DM, et al: Biochemistry and biomechanics of blood collection, processing and analysis. Abstract of paper presented at the National Academy of Science, New Haven, CT, Nov 5–7, 1951. Science 1951;114:479.
5. Latham A: Early developments in blood cell separation technology. Vox Sang 1986;51:249.
6. De Laval CGP: U.S. Patent 247,804, 1881.
7. Freireich EJ, Judson G, Levin RH: Separation and collection of leukocytes. Cancer Res 1965;25:1516.
8. Powell L: Intense plasmapheresis in the pregnant Rh sensitized woman. Am J Obstet Gynecol 1968;101:153.
9. Bowman JM, Peddle LJ, Anderson C: Plasmapheresis in severe Rh iso-immunization. Vox Sang 1968;15:272.
10. Clarke CA, Elson CJ, Bradley J, et al: Intensive plasmapheresis as a therapeutic measure in Rhesus-immunised women. Lancet 1970;2:793.
11. Verrier Jones J, Cumming RH, Bucknall RC, et al: Plasmapheresis in the management of acute systemic lupus erythematosus. Lancet 1976;1:709.
12. Verrier Jones J, Cumming RH, Bacon PA, et al: Evidence for a therapeutic effect of plasmapheresis in patients with systemic lupus erythematosus. Q J Med 1979;448:555.
13. Chopek M, McCullough J: Protein and biochemical changes during plasma exchange. In Berkman EM, Umlas J (eds): Therapeutic Hemapheresis: A Technical Workshop. Washington, DC, American Association of Blood Banks, 1980, p 13.
14. Kellogg RM, Hester JP: Kinetics modeling of plasma exchange: intra- and post-plasma exchange. J Clin Apheresis 1988;4:183.
15. Orlin JB, Berkman EM: Partial plasma exchange using albumin replacement: removal and recovery of normal plasma constituents. Blood 1980;56:1055.
16. McLeod BC, Sassetti RJ, Stefoski D, Davis FA: Partial plasma protein replacement in therapeutic plasma exchange. J Clin Apheresis 1983;1:115.

17. Waldmann TA, Strober W: Metabolism of immunoglobulins. Prog Allergy 1969;13:1.

18. Strober W, Wochner RD, Barlow MH, et al: Immunoglobulin metabolism in ataxia telangiectasia. J Clin Invest 1968;47:1905.

19. Wells JV, Fudenberg HH: Metabolism of radio-iodinated IgG in patients with abnormal serum IgG levels. 1. Hypergamma-globulinaemia. Clin Exp Immunol 1971;9:761.

20. Wells JV, Fudenberg HH: Metabolism of radio-iodinated IgG in patients with abnormal serum IgG levels. II. Hypogamma-globulinaemia. Clin Exp Immunol 1971;9:775.

21. Brambell, FWR, Hemmings WA, Morris IG: A theoretical model of γ-globulin catabolism. Nature 1964;203:1352.

22. Junghans RP, Anderson CL: The protection receptor for IgG catabolism is the β_2-microglobulin–containing neonatal intestinal transport receptor. Proc Natl Acad Sci USA 1996;93:5512.

23. Dau PC: Immunologic rebound. J Clin Apheresis 1995;10:210.

24. Junghans RP: IgG Biosynthesis: no "immunoregulatory feedback." Blood 1997;90:3815.

25. Yu Z, Lennon VA: Mechanism of intravenous immune globulin therapy in antibody-mediated autoimmune diseases. N Engl J Med 1999;340:227.

26. Lewis EJ, Hunsicker LG, Lan SP, et al: A controlled trial of plasmapheresis therapy in severe lupus nephritis. N Engl J Med 1992;326:1371.

27. Pool M, McLeod BC: Pyrogen reactions to human serum albumin in plasma exchange. J Clin Apheresis 1995;10:81.

28. Keller AJ, Urbaniak SJ: Intensive plasma exchange on the cell separator: effects on serum immunoglobulins and complement components. Br J Haematol 1978;38:531.

29. Cochrane Injuries Group Albumin Reviewers: Human albumin administration in critically ill patients: systematic review of randomized controlled trials. Br Med J 1998;317:235.

30. Tjoeng MM, Bartelink AK, Thijs LG: Exploding the albumin myth. Pharm World Sci 1999;21:17.

31. Rossi EC: Plasma exchange in the thrombotic microangiopathies. In Rossi EC, Simon TL, Moss GS, Gould SA (eds): Principles of Transfusion Medicine, 2nd ed. Baltimore, Williams & Wilkins, 1996, p 577.

32. McLeod BC, Price TH, Owen H, et al: Frequency of immediate adverse effects associated with therapeutic apheresis. Transfusion 1999;39:282.

33. Owen HG, Brecher ME: Partial colloid replacement for therapeutic plasma exchange. J Clin Apheresis 1997;12:146.

34. McLeod B, Sassetti R: Plasmapheresis with return of cryoglobulin depleted autologous plasma (cryoglobulinpheresis) in cryoglobulinemia. Blood 1980;55:866.

35. Vamvakas EC, Pineda AA: Selective extraction of plasma constituents. In McLeod BC, Price TH, Drew MJ (eds): Apheresis: Principles and Practice. Bethesda, Md, AABB Press, 1997, p 378.

36. Gjöstrup P, Watt RM: Therapeutic protein A immunoadsorption: a review. Transfus Sci 1990;281.

37. Gordon BR, Kelsy SF, Dau PC, et al: Long-term effects of low-density lipoprotein apheresis using an automated dextran sulfate cellulose adsorption system. Liposorber Study Group. Am J Cardiol 1998;81:407.

38. McLeod BC: Introduction to the third special issue on clinical applications of therapeutic apheresis. J Clin Apheresis 2000;15:1.

39. McLeod B, Ciavarella D, Owen H, et al: Guidelines for Therapeutic Hemapheresis. AABB Hemapheresis Committee document. Bethesda, Md, AABB, revised October 1995.

40. Consensus Conference: The utility of therapeutic plasmapheresis for neurological disorders. JAMA 1986;256:1333.

41. Ropper AH: The Guillain-Barré syndrome. N Engl J Med 1992;326:1130.

42. van der Meché FGA: The Guillain-Barré syndrome. Baillieres Clin Neurol 1994;3:73.

43. Hughes RA, Rees JH: Guillain-Barré syndrome. Curr Opin Neurol 1994;7:386.

44. Cook SD, Dowling PC, Murray MR, Whitaker JN: Circulating demyelinating factors in acute idiopathic polyneuropathy. Arch Neurol 1971;24:136.

45. Feasby TE, Hahn AF, Gilbert JJ: Passive transfer studies in Guillain-Barré polyneuropathy. Neurology 1982;32:1159.

46. Koski CI, Gratz E, Sutherland J, et al: Clinical correlation with anti–peripheral myelin antibodies in Guillain-Barré syndrome. Ann Neurol 1986;19:573.

47. McFarlin DE: Immunological parameters in Guillain-Barré syndrome. Ann Neurol 1990;27(Suppl 1):525.

48. Vriesendorp FJ, Mayer RF, Koski CL: Kinetics of anti–peripheral nerve myelin antibody in patients with Guillain-Barré syndrome treated and not treated with plasmapheresis. Arch Neurol 1991;48:858.

49. Vriesendorp FJ, Mishu B, Blaser MJ, Koski CL: Serum antibodies to GM1, GD16, peripheral nerve myelin, and *Campylobacter jejuni* in patients with Guillain-Barré syndrome and controls. Ann Neurol 1993;34:130.

50. Rees JH, Gregson NA, Hughes RA: Anti–ganglioside GM1 antibodies in Guillain-Barré syndrome and their relationship to *Campylobacter jejuni* infection. Ann Neurol 1995;38:809.

51. Rees JH, Soudain SE, Gregson NA, Hughes RAC: *Campylobacter jejuni* infection and Guillain-Barré syndrome. N Engl J Med 1995;333:1374.

52. Willison HJ, Kennedy PGE: Gangliosides and bacterial toxins in Guillain-Barré syndrome. J Neuroimmunol 1993;46:105.

53. Yuki N, Taki T, Inagaki F, et al: A bacterium lipopolysaccharide that elicits Guillain Barré syndrome has a GM_1, ganglioside-like structure. J Exp Med 1993;178:1771.

54. McKhann GM, Cornblath DR, Griffen JW, et al: Acute motor axonal neuropathy: a frequent cause of flaccid paralysis in China. Ann Neurol 1993;33:333.

55. Guillain-Barré Syndrome Steroid Trial Group: Double-blind trial of intravenous methylprednisone in Guillain-Barré syndrome. Lancet 1993;341:586.

56. Brettle RP, Gross MLP, Legg NJ, et al: Treatment of acute polyneuropathy by plasma exchange. Lancet 1978;2:1100.

57. Schooneman F, Janot C, Streiff F, et al: Plasma exchange in Guillain-Barré syndrome: ten cases. Plasma Ther 1981;2:117.

58. Valbonesi M, Garelli S, Mosconi L, et al: Plasma exchange as a therapy for Guillain-Barré syndrome with immune complexes. Vox Sang 1981;41:74.

59. de Jager AEJ, The TH, Smit Sibinga CTS, Das PC: Plasma exchange in the Guillain Barré syndrome. Br Med J 1981;283:794.

60. Rumpl E, Mayr U, Gerstenbrand F, et al: Treatment of Guillain-Barré syndrome by plasma exchange. J Neurol 1981;225:207.

61. Greenwood RJ, Newsom-Davis J, Hughes RA, et al: Controlled trial of plasma exchange in acute inflammatory polyradiculoneuropathy. Lancet 1984;1:877.

62. Osterman PG, Lundemo G, Pirskanen R, et al: Beneficial effects of plasma exchange in acute inflammatory polyradiculoneuropathy. Lancet 1984;2:1296.

63. The Guillain-Barré Syndrome Study Group: Plasmapheresis and acute Guillain-Barré syndrome. Neurology 1985;35:1096.

64. French Cooperative Group on Plasma Exchange and Guillain-Barré Syndrome: Efficiency of plasma exchange in Guillain-Barré syndrome: role of replacement fluids. Ann Neurol 1987;22:753.

65. French Cooperative Group on Plasma Exchange in Guillain-Barré Syndrome: Plasma exchange in Guillain-Barré syndrome: one-year follow-up. Ann Neurol 1992;32:94.

66. Jansen PW, Perkin RM, Ashwal S: The Guillain-Barré syndrome in childhood: natural course and efficacy of plasmapheresis. Pediatr Neurol 1993;9:16.

67. Bouget J, Chevret S, Chastang C, Raphael J-C, and The French Cooperative Group: Plasma exchange in Guillain-Barré syndrome: results from the French prospective, double-blind, randomized, multicenter study. Crit Care Med 1993;21:651.

68. McLeod BC: The technique of therapeutic apheresis. J Crit Illness 1991;6:487.

69. van der Meché FGA, Schmitz PIM, The Dutch Guillain-Barré Study Group: A randomized trial comparing intravenous immune globulin and plasma exchange in Guillain-Barré syndrome. N Engl J Med 1992;326:1123.

70. Plasma Exchange/Sandoglobulin Guillain-Barré Syndrome Trial Group: Randomised trial of plasma exchange, intravenous immunoglobulin, and combined treatments in Guillain-Barré syndrome. Lancet 1997;349:225.

71. Barohn RJ, Kissel JT, Warmolts JR, Mendell JR: Chronic inflammatory demyelinating polyradiculopathy. Arch Neurol 1989;46:878.

72. Mendell JR: Chronic inflammatory demyelinating polyradiculopathy. Annu Rev Med 1993;44:211.

73. Glass JD, Cornblath DR: Chronic inflammatory demyelinating polyneuropathy and paraproteinemic neuropathies. Curr Opin Neurol 1994;7:393.
74. Saida K, Sumner AJ, Saida T, et al: Antiserum-mediated demyelination: relationship between remyelination and functional recovery. Ann Neurol 1980;8:12.
75. Simone IL, Annunziata P, Maimone D, et al: Serum and CSF anti-GM1 antibodies in patients with Guillain-Barré syndrome and chronic inflammatory demyelinating polyneuropathy. J Neurol Sci 1993;114:49.
76. Khalili-Shirazi A, Atkinson P, Gregson N, Hughes RAC: Antibody response to P_0 and P_2 myelin proteins in Guillain-Barré syndrome and chronic inflammatory demyelinating polyradiculoneuropathy. J Neuroimmunol 1993;46:245.
77. Connolly AM, Pestronk A, Trotter JL, et al: High-titer selective anti–beta-tubulin antibodies in chronic demyelinating polyneuropathy. Neurology 1993;43:557.
78. Dyck PJ, Daube J, O'Brien P, et al: Plasma exchange in chronic inflammatory demyelinating polyradiculoneuropathy. N Engl J Med 1986;314:461.
79. Hahn AF, Bolton CF, Pillay N, et al: Plasma-exchange therapy in chronic inflammatory demyelinating polyneuropathy. A double-blind, sham-controlled, cross-over study. Brain 1996;119:1055.
80. van Doom PA, Vermeulen M, Brand A, et al: Intravenous immunoglobulin treatment in patients with chronic inflammatory demyelinating polyneuropathy. Arch Neurol 1991;48:217.
81. Faed JM, Day B, Pollack M, et al: High-dose intravenous human immunoglobulin in chronic inflammatory demyelinating polyneuropathy. Neurology 1989;39:422.
82. van Doom PA, Brand A, Strengers PFW, et al: High-dose intravenous immunoglobulin treatment in chronic inflammatory demyelinating polyneuropathy. Neurology 1990;40:209.
83. Vermeulen M, van Doom PA, Brand A, et al: Intravenous immunoglobulin treatment in patients with chronic inflammatory demyelinating polyneuropathy: a double blind, placebo controlled study. J Neurol Neurosurg Psychiatry 1993;56:36.
84. Hahn AF, Bolton CF, Zochodne D, Feasby TE: Intravenous immunoglobulin treatment in chronic inflammatory demyelinating polyneuropathy. A double-blind, placebo-controlled, cross-over study. Brain 1996;119:1067.
85. Choudhary PP, Hughes RAC: Long-term treatment of chronic inflammatory demyelinating polyradiculoneuropathy with plasma exchange or intravenous immunoglobulin. Q J Med 1995;88:493.
86. Dyck PJ, Litchy WJ, Kratz KM, et al: A plasma exchange versus immune globulin infusion trial in chronic inflammatory demyelinating polyradiculoneuropathy. Ann Neurol 1994;36:838.
87. Kyle RA: Monoclonal proteins in neuropathy. Neurol Clin 1992;10:713.
88. Bosch EP, Smith BE: Peripheral neuropathies associated with monoclonal proteins. Med Clin North Am 1993;77:125.
89. Baldini L, Nobile-Orazio E, Guffanti A, et al: Peripheral neuropathy in IgM monoclonal gammopathy and Waldenström's macroglobulinemia: a frequent complication in elderly males with low MAG-reactive serum monoclonal component. Am J Hematol 1994;45:25.
90. Nemni R, Gerosa E, Piccolo G, Merlini G: Neuropathies associated with monoclonal gammopathies. Haematologica 1994;79:557.
91. Gabriel JM, Erne B, Miescher GC, et al: Expression patterns of human PNS myelin proteins in neuropathies associated with anti-myelin antibodies. Schweiz Arch Neurol Psychiatr 1994;145:22.
92. Tatum AH: Experimental paraprotein neuropathy: demyelination by passive transfer of human IgM anti-myelin–associated glycoprotein. Ann Neurol 1993;33:502.
93. Smith IS: The natural history of chronic demyelinating neuropathy associated with benign IgM paraproteinemia: a clinical and neurophysiological study. Brain 1994;117:949.
94. Simmons Z, Albers JW, Bromberg MB, Feldman EL: Long-term follow-up of patients with chronic inflammatory demyelinating polyradiculoneuropathy, without and with monoclonal gammopathy. Brain 1995;118:359.
95. Nobile-Orazio E, Barbieri S, Baldini L, et al: Peripheral neuropathy in monoclonal gammopathy of undetermined significance: prevalence and immunopathogenetic studies. Acta Neurol Scand 1992;85:383.
96. Miralles GD, O'Fallon JR, Talley NJ: Plasma-cell dyscrasia with polyneuropathy: the spectrum of POEMS syndrome. N Engl J Med 1992;327:1919.

97. Dyck PJ, Low PA, Windebank AJ, et al: Plasma exchange in polyneuropathy associated with monoclonal gammopathy of undetermined significance. N Engl J Med 1991;325:1482.
98. Siciliano G, Moriconi L, Gianni G, Richieri E: Selective techniques of apheresis in polyneuropathy associated with monoclonal gammopathy of undetermined significance. Acta Neurol Scand 1994;89:117.
99. Oksenhendler E, Chevret S, Leger JM, et al: Plasma exchange and chlorambucil in polyneuropathy associated with monoclonal IgM gammopathy. J Neurol Neurosurg Psychiatry 1995;59:243.
100. Bleasel AF, Hawke SH, Pollard JD, McLeod JG: IgG monoclonal paraproteinemia and peripheral neuropathy. J Neurol Neurosurg Psychiatry 1993;56:52.
101. Hopkins LC: Clinical features of myasthenia gravis. Neurol Clin North Am 1994;12:243.
102. Lindstrom JM, Seybold ME, Lennon VA, et al: Antibody to acetylcholine receptor in myasthenia gravis. Neurology 1976;26:1054.
103. Masselli, RA: Pathophysiology of myasthenia gravis and Lambert-Eaton syndrome. Neurol Clin 1994;12:285.
104. Richman DP, Wollman RL, Maselli RA, et al: Effector mechanisms of myasthenic antibodies. Ann NY Acad Sci 1993;681:264.
105. Sanders DB, Scoppetta C: The treatment of patients with myasthenia gravis. Neurol Clin 1994;12:343.
106. Genkins G, Sivak M, Tartter PI: Treatment strategies in myasthenia gravis. Ann NY Acad Sci 1993;681:603.
107. Cornelio F, Antozzi C, Mantegazza R, et al: Immunosuppressive treatments. Their efficacy on myasthenia gravis patients' outcome and on the natural course of the disease. Ann NY Acad Sci 1993;681:594.
108. Dau PC, Lindstrom JM, Cassel CK, et al: Plasmapheresis and immunosuppressive drug therapy in myasthenia gravis. N Engl J Med 1977;297:1134.
109. Dau PC: Plasmapheresis therapy in myasthenia gravis. Muscle Nerve 1980;3:468.
110. Pollard JD, Basten A, Hassall JE, et al: Current trends in the management of myasthenia gravis: plasmapheresis and immunosuppressive therapy. Aust NZ J Med 1989;10:212.
111. Seybold ME: Plasmapheresis in myasthenia gravis. Ann NY Acad Sci 1987;505:584.
112. d'Empaire G, Hoaglin DC, Perlo VP, Pontoppidan H: Effect of pre-thymectomy plasma exchange on postoperative respiratory function in myasthenia gravis. J Thorac Cardiovasc Surg 1985;89:592.
113. Rodnitzy RL, Bosch EP: Chronic long-interval plasma exchange in myasthenia gravis. Arch Neurol 1984;41:715.
114. Splendiani G, Passlacqua S, Barbera G, et al: Semi-selective immunoadsorption treatment in myasthenia gravis. Biomater Artif Cells Immobilization Biotechnol 1992;20:1145.
115. Ichikawa M, Koh CS, Hata Y, et al: Immunoadsorption plasmapheresis for severe generalized myasthenia gravis. Arch Dis Child 1993;69:236.
116. Sawada K, Malchesky PS, Koo AP: Myasthenia gravis therapy: immunoadsorbent may eliminate need for plasma products. Cleve Clin J Med 1993;60:60.
117. Berta E, Confalonieri P, Simoncini O, et al: Removal of antiacetylcholine receptor antibodies by protein-A immunoadsorption in myasthenia gravis. Int J Artif Organs 1994;17:603.
118. Benny WB, Sutton DMC, Oger J, et al: Clinical evaluation of a staphylococcal protein A immunoadsorption system in the treatment of myasthenia gravis patients. Transfusion 1999;39:682.
119. Gajdos P: Intravenous immune globulin in myasthenia gravis. Clin Exp Immunol 1994;97(Suppl 1):49.
120. Gajdos P, Chevret S, Clair B, et al: Clinical trial of plasma exchange and high-dose intravenous immunoglobulin in myasthenia gravis. Ann Neurol 1997;41:789.
121. Qureshi AI, Choudry MA, Akber MS, et al: Plasma exchange vs. intravenous immunoglobulin treatment in myasthenic crisis. Neurology 1999;52:629.
122. Newsom-Davis J: Lambert-Eaton myasthenic syndrome. Springer Semin Immunopathol 1985;8:129.
123. Jablecki C: Lambert-Eaton myasthenic syndrome. Muscle Nerve 1984;7:250.
124. O'Neill JH, Murray NM, Newsom-Davis J: The Lambert-Eaton myasthenic syndrome: a review of 50 cases. Brain 1988;11:577.
125. Hewett SJ, Atchison WD: Specificity of Lambert-Eaton myasthenic syndrome immunoglobulin for nerve terminal calcium channels. Brain Res 1992;599:324.

126. Rosenfield MR, Wong E, Dalmace J, et al: Cloning and characterization of a Lambert-Eaton myasthenic syndrome antigen. Ann Neurol 1993;33:113.

127. Sher E, Carbone E, Clementi F: Neuronal calcium channels as target for Lambert-Eaton myasthenic syndrome autoantibodies. Ann NY Acad Sci 1993;681:373.

128. Dau PC, Denys EH: Plasmapheresis and immunosuppressive drug therapy in the Eaton-Lambert syndrome. Ann Neurol 1982;11:570.

129. Lundh H, Nilsson O, Rosen I: Treatment of Lambert-Eaton syndrome: 3,4-diaminopyridine and pyridostigmine. Neurology 1984;34:1324.

130. Cooke JD, Hefter H, Brown SH, et al: Lambert-Eaton syndrome: evaluation of movement performance following drug therapy. Clin Neurophysiol 1994;34:87.

131. Jenkyn LR, Brooks PL, Forcier RJ, et al: Remission of the Lambert-Eaton syndrome and small cell anaplastic carcinoma of the lung induced by chemotherapy and radiotherapy. Cancer 1980,46:1123.

132. Chalk CH, Murray NM, Newsom-Davis J, et al: Response of the Lambert-Eaton myasthenic syndrome to treatment of associated small-cell lung carcinoma. Neurology 1990;40:1552.

133. Lisak RP: Plasma exchange in neurologic disease. Arch Neurol 1984;41:654.

134. Takano H, Tanaka M, Koike R, et al: Effect of intravenous immunoglobulin in Lambert-Eaton myasthenic syndrome with small-cell lung cancer: correlation with the titer of anti–voltage-gated calcium channel antibody. Muscle Nerve 1994;17:1123.

135. Moll JWB, Vecht CJ: Immune diagnoses of paraneoplastic neurological disease. Clin Neurol Neurosurg 1995;97:71.

136. Graus F, Rene R: Clinical and pathological advances on central nervous system paraneoplastic syndromes. Rev Neurol (Paris) 1992;148:496.

137. Oguni H, Andermann F, Rasmussen TB: The natural history of the syndrome of chronic encephalitis and epilepsy: a study of the MNI series of forty-eight cases. In Andermann F (ed): Chronic Encephalitis and Epilepsy: Rasmussen's Syndrome. Boston, Butterworth-Heinemann, 1991, p 7.

138. Rodgers SW, Andrews PI, Gahring LC, et al: Autoantibodies to glutamate receptor Glu R3 in Rasmussen's encephalitis. Science 1994;265:648.

139. Andrews PI, McNamara JO: Rasmussen's encephalitis: an autoimmune disorder? Curr Opinion Neurobiol 1996;6:673.

140. Rogers SW, Andrews PI, Gahring LC, et al: Autoantibodies to glutamate receptor GluR3 in Rasmussen's encephalitis. Science 1994;265:648.

141. Andrews PI, Dichter MA, Berkovic SF, et al: Plasmapheresis in Rasmussen's encephalitis. Neurology 1996;46:242.

142. Hart YM, Cortez M, Andermann F, et al: Medical treatment of Rasmussen's syndrome (chronic encephalitis and epilepsy): effect of high dose steroids or immunoglobulins in 19 patients. Neurology 1994;44:1030.

143. Swedo SE, Leonard HL, Schapiro MB, et al: Sydenham's chorea: physical and psychological symptoms of St. Vitus' dance. Pediatrics 1993;91:706.

144. Swedo SE, Rapoport JL, Cheslow DL, et al: High prevalence of obsessive-compulsive symptoms in patients with Sydenham's chorea. Am J Psychiatry 1989;146:246.

145. Swedo SE, Leonard HL, Garvey M, et al: Pediatric autoimmune neuropsychiatric disorders associated with streptococcal infections: clinical description of the first 50 cases. Am J Psychiatry 1998;155:264.

146. Husby G, van de Rijn I, Zabriskie JB, et al: Antibodies reacting with cytoplasm of subthalamic and caudate nuclei neurons in chorea and acute rheumatic fever. J Exp Med 1976;144:1094.

147. Zabriskie JB: Rheumatic fever: a model for the pathological consequences of microbial-host mimicry. Clin Exp Rheumatol 1986;4:65.

148. Singer HS: PANDAS and immunomodulatory therapy. Lancet 1999;354:1137.

149. Garvey MA, Swedo SW, Shapiro MB, et al: Intravenous immunoglobulin and plasmapheresis as effective treatments in Sydenham's chorea. Neurology 1996;46:A147.

150. Perlmutter SJ, Leitman SF, Garvey MA, et al: Therapeutic plasma exchange and intravenous immunoglobulin for obsessive-compulsive disorder and tic disorders in childhood. Lancet 1999;354:1153.

151. Weinshenker BG, Sibley WA: Natural history and treatment of multiple sclerosis. Curr Opin Neurol Neurosurg 1992;5:203.

152. Owens T, Sriram S: The immunology of multiple sclerosis and its animal model, experimental allergic encephalomyelitis. Neuro Clin 1995;13:51.

153. Hafler DA, Weiner HL: Immunologic mechanisms and therapy in multiple sclerosis. Immunol Rev 1995;144:75.

154. Goodin DS: The use of immunosuppressive agents in the treatment of multiple sclerosis: a critical review. Neurology 1991;41:980.

155. Noseworthy JH, Ebers GC, Vandervoort MK, et al: The impact of blinding on the results of a randomized, placebo-controlled multiple sclerosis clinical trial. Neurology 1994;44:16.

156. Jacobs L, Goodkin DE, Rudick RA, Herndon R: Advances in specific therapy for multiple sclerosis. Curr Opin Neurol 1994;7:250.

157. Goodkin DE, Ransohoff RM, Rudick RA: Experimental therapies for multiple sclerosis: current status. Cleve Clin J Med 1992;59:63.

158. van Oosten BW, Truyen L, Barkhof F, Polman CH: Multiple sclerosis therapy. A practical guide. Drugs 1995;49:200.

159. Jacobs LD, Cookfair DL, Rudick RA, et al: Intramuscular interferon beta-1a for disease progression in relapsing multiple sclerosis. The Multiple Sclerosis Collaborative Research Group. Ann Neurol 1996;39:285.

160. Rudick RA, Goodkin DE, Jacobs LD, et al: Impact of interferon beta-1a on neurologic disability in relapsing multiple sclerosis. The Multiple Sclerosis Collaborative Group (MSCRG). Neurology 1997;49:358.

161. Simon JH, Jacobs LD, Campion M, et al: Magnetic resonance studies of intramuscular interferon beta-1a for relapsing multiple sclerosis. The Multiple Sclerosis Collaborative Research Group. Ann Neurol 1998;43:79.

162. Jacobs L, Johnson KP: A brief history of the use of interferons as treatment of multiple sclerosis. Arch Neurol 1994;51:1245.

163. IFNB Multiple Sclerosis Study Group: Interferon beta-1b is effective in relapsing remitting multiple sclerosis. I. Clinical results of a multicenter, randomized, double-blind, placebo-controlled trial. Neurology 1993;43:655.

164. Paty DW, Li DKB, UBC MS/MRI Study Group, IFNB Multiple Sclerosis Study Group: Interferon beta-1b is effective in relapsing-remitting multiple sclerosis. II. MRI analysis results of a multicenter randomized, double-blind, placebo-controlled trial. Neurology 1993;43:662.

165. Johnson KP: Experimental therapy of relapsing-remitting multiple sclerosis with copolymer-1. Ann Neurol 1994;36(Suppl):S115.

166. Wolinsky J: Copolymer 1: a most reasonable alternative therapy for early relapsing-remitting multiple sclerosis with mild disability. Neurology 1995;45:1245.

167. Johnson KP, Brooks BR, Cohen JA, et al and the Copolymer I Multiple Sclerosis Study Group: Extended use of glatiramer acetate (Copaxone) is well tolerated and maintains its clinical effect on multiple sclerosis relapse rate and degree of disability. Neurology 1998;50:701.

168. Fazekas F, Deisenhammer F, Strasser-Fuchs S, et al: Randomised placebo-controlled trial of monthly intravenous immunoglobulin therapy in relapsing-remitting multiple sclerosis. Austrian Immunoglobulin in Multiple Sclerosis Study Group. Lancet 1997;349:589.

169. Sorensen PS, Wanscher B, Jensen CV, et al: Intravenous immunoglobulin G reduces MRI activity in relapsing multiple sclerosis. Neurology 1998;50:1273.

170. Achiron A, Gabbay U, Gilad R, et al: Intravenous immunoglobulin treatment in multiple sclerosis. Effect on relapses. Neurology 1998;50:398.

171. Arnason BGW: Immunologic therapy of multiple sclerosis. Annu Rev Med 1999;50:291.

172. Dau PC, Petajan JM, Johnson KP, et al: Plasmapheresis and immunosuppressive drug therapy in multiple sclerosis. Neurology 1980;30:1023.

173. Weiner HL, Dawson DM: Plasmapheresis in multiple sclerosis: preliminary study. Neurology 1980;30:1029.

174. Khatri BO, McQuillen MP, Hoffman RG, et al: Plasma exchange in chronic progressive multiple sclerosis: a long term study. Neurology 1991;41:409.

175. Hauser SL, Dawson DM, Lehrich JR, et al: Intensive immunosuppression in progressive multiple sclerosis: a randomized three-arm study of high dose intravenous cyclophosphamide, plasma exchange, and ACTH. N Engl J Med 1983;308:173.

176. Tindall RSA, Walker JE, Ehle AL, et al: Plasmapheresis in multiple sclerosis: prospective trial of pheresis and immunosuppression versus immunosuppression alone. Neurology 1982;32:739.

177. Khatri BO, McQuillen MP, Harrington GJ, et al: Chronic progressive multiple sclerosis: double-blind controlled study of plasmapheresis in patients taking immunosuppressive drugs. Neurology 1985;35:312.

178. Weiner HL: An assessment of plasma exchange in progressive multiple sclerosis. Neurology 1985;35:320.
179. Weiner HL, Dau P, Khatri BO, et al: Double-blind study of true versus sham plasma exchange in patients being treated with immunosuppression for acute attacks of multiple sclerosis. Neurology 1989;39:1143.
180. The Canadian Cooperative Multiple Sclerosis Study Group: The Canadian cooperative trial of cyclophosphamide and plasma exchange in progressive multiple sclerosis. Lancet 1991;337:441.
181. Rodriguez M, Karnes WE, Bartleson JD, Pineda AA: Plasmapheresis in acute episodes of fulminant CNS inflammatory demyelination. Neurology 1993;43:1100.
182. Assessment of plasmapheresis. Report of the Therapeutics and Technology Assessment Subcommittee of the American Academy of Neurology. Neurology 1996;47:840.
183. McGrath MA, Penny R: Paraproteinemias. Blood hyperviscosity and clinical manifestations. J Clin Invest 1976;58:1155.
184. Salmon SE, Cassady RJ: Plasma cell neoplasms. In DeVita VT, Hellman S, Rosenberg SA (eds): Cancer: Principles and Practice of Oncology. New York, Lippincott-Raven, 1997, p 2344.
185. Kyle RA: Multiple myeloma and other plasma cell disorders. In Hoffman R, Benz EJ, Shattil SJ, Furie B (eds): Hematology, Basic Principles and Practice. New York, Churchill Livingstone, 1995, p 1354.
186. Kipps TJ: Macroglobulinemia. In Beutler E, Lichtman M, Coller BS, Kipps TJ (eds): Hematology, 5th ed. New York, McGraw-Hill, 1995, p 1127.
187. Glaspy JA: Hemostatic abnormalities in multiple myeloma and related disorders. Hematol Oncol Clin North Am 1992;6:1301.
188. Bear RA, Cole EH, Slang A, et al: Treatment of acute renal failure due to myeloma kidney. Can Med Assoc J 1980;123:750.
189. Misiani R, Tiraboschi G, Mingardi G, Mecca G: Management of myeloma kidney: an anti-light chain approach. Am J Kidney Dis 1987;10:28.
190. Solling K, Solling J: Clearance of Bence-Jones proteins during peritoneal dialysis or plasmapheresis in myelomatosis associated with renal failure. Contrib Nephrol 1988;68:259.
191. Johnson WJ, Kyle RA, Pineda AA, et al: Treatment of renal failure associated with multiple myeloma. Plasmapheresis, hemodialysis, and chemotherapy. Arch Intern Med 1990;150:863.
192. Zucchelli P, Pasquali S, Cagnoli L, Ferrari G: Controlled plasma exchange trial in acute renal failure due to multiple myeloma. Kidney Int 1988;33:1175.
193. Fraser ID, Bothamley JE, Bennett MO, et al: Intensive antenatal plasmapheresis in severe Rhesus isoimmunisation. Lancet 1976;1:6.
194. Mollison PL, Engelfriet CP, Contreras M: Haemolytic disease of the fetus and newborn. In Blood Transfusion in Clinical Medicine. London, Blackwell Science, 1997, p 390.
195. Filbey D, Berseus O, Lindeberg S, Wesstrom G: A management programme for Rh alloimmunization during pregnancy. Early Hum Dev 1987;15:11.
196. Watson WJ, Katz VL, Bowes WA: Plasmapheresis during pregnancy. Obstet Gynecol 1990;76:451.
197. Furukawa K, Nakajima T, Kogure T, et al: Example of a woman with multiple intrauterine deaths due to anti-M who delivered a live child after plasmapheresis. Exp Clin Immunogenet 1993;10:161.
198. Shirey R, Ness P, Kickler T, et al: The association of anti-P and early abortion. Transfusion 1987;27:189.
199. Gale RP, Feig S, Ho W, et al: ABO blood group system and bone marrow transplantation. Blood 1977;50:185.
200. Bensinger WI, Baker DA, Buckner DD, et al: Immunoadsorption for removal of A and B blood group antibodies. N Engl J Med 1981;301:160.
201. Braine HG, Sensenbrenner LL, Wright SK, et al: Bone marrow transplantation with major ABO incompatibility using erythrocyte depletion of marrow prior to infusion. Blood 1982;60:420.
202. Gmur JP, Burger J, Schaffner A, et al: Pure red cell aplasia of long duration complicating major ABO incompatible bone marrow transplantation. Blood 1990;75:290.
203. Fischel RJ, Ascher NL, Payne WD, et al: Pediatric liver transplantation across ABO blood group barriers. Transplant Proc 1989;21:2221.
204. Renard TH, Shimaoka S, Le Bherz D, et al: ABO incompatible liver transplantation in children: a prospective approach. Transplant Proc 1993;25:1953.
205. Mor E, Skerrett D, Manzarbeitia C, et al: Successful use of an enhanced immunosuppressive protocol with plasmapheresis for ABO-incompatible mismatched grafts in liver transplant recipients. Transplantation 1995;59:986.
206. Ramsey G: Red cell antibodies arising from solid organ transplants. Transfusion 1991;31:76.
207. Lundgren G, Asaba H, Bergstrom J, et al: Fulminating anti-A autoimmune hemolysis with anuria in a renal transplant recipient: a therapeutic role of plasma exchange. Clin Nephrol 1981;16:211.
208. Kickler TS: The challenge of platelet alloimmunization: management and prevention. Transfusion 1990;30:8.
209. Bensinger WI, Buckner CD, Clift RA, et al: Plasma exchange for platelet alloimmunization. Transplantation 1986;41:602.
210. Christie DJ, Howe RB, Lennon SS, Sauro SC: Treatment of refractoriness to platelet transfusion by protein A column therapy. Transfusion 1993;33:234.
211. Lopez-Plaza I, Miller K, Leitman SF: Ineffectiveness of protein A adsorption in the treatment of platelet refractoriness. J Clin Apheresis 1992;7:33.
212. Lee EJ, Norris D, Schiffer CA: Intravenous immune globulin for patients alloimmunized to random donor platelet transfusions. Transfusion 1987;27:245.
213. Kickler T, Braine HG, Piantadosi S, et al: A randomized, placebo-controlled trial of intravenous gammaglobulin in alloimmunized thrombocytopenic patients. Blood 1987;70:313.
214. Ziegler ZR, Shadduck RK, Rosenfeld CS, et al: High-dose intravenous gamma globulin improves responses to single-donor platelets in patients refractory to platelet transfusion. Blood 1987;70:1433.
215. Amorosi EL, Ultmann JE: Thrombotic thrombocytopenic purpura: report of 16 cases and review of the literature. Medicine (Baltimore) 1966;45:139.
216. Moake JL: Thrombotic thrombocytopenic purpura. Thromb Haemost 1995;74:240.
217. Torok TJ, Holman RC, Chorba TL: Increasing mortality from thrombotic thrombocytopenic purpura in the United States–analysis of national mortality data, 1968–1991. Am J Hematol 1995;50:84.
218. Porta C, Caporali R, Montecucco C: Thrombotic thrombocytopenic purpura and autoimmunity: a tale of shadows and suspects. Haematologia 1999;84:260.
219. Rarick MU, Espina B, Mocharnuk R, et al: Thrombotic thrombocytopenic purpura in patients with human immunodeficiency virus infection: a report of three cases and review of the literature. Am J Hematol 1992;40:103.
220. Furlan M, Robles R, Solenthaler M, et al: Deficient activity of von Willebrand factor–cleaving protease in chronic relapsing thrombotic thrombocytopenic purpura. Blood 1997;89:3097.
221. Furlan M, Robles R, Galbusera M, et al: Von Willebrand factor–cleaving protease in thrombotic thrombocytopenic purpura and the hemolytic-uremic syndrome. N Engl J Med 1998;339:1578.
222. Tsai H-M, Lian EC-Y: Antibodies to von Willebrand factor–cleaving protease in acute thrombotic thrombocytopenic purpura. N Engl J Med 1998;339:1585.
223. Rock GA, Shumak KH, Buskard NA, et al: The Canadian Apheresis Study Group. Comparison of plasma exchange with plasma infusion in the treatment of thrombotic thrombocytopenic purpura. N Engl J Med 1991;325:393.
224. Bell WR, Braine HG, Ness PM, Kickler TS: Improved survival in thrombotic thrombocytopenic purpura–hemolytic uremic syndrome. Clinical experience in 108 patients. N Engl J Med 1991;325:398.
225. O Connor NTJ, Bruce-Jones P, Hill LF: Vincristine therapy for thrombotic thrombocytopenic purpura. Am J Hematol 1992;39:234.
226. Onundarson PT, Rowe JM, Heal JM, Francis CW: Response to plasma exchange and splenectomy in thrombotic thrombocytopenic purpura. Arch Intern Med 1992;152:791.
227. Tsai H-M, Rue L, Sarode R, et al: Antibody inhibitors to von Willebrand factor metalloproteinase and increased binding of von Willebrand factor to platelets in ticlopidine associated thrombotic thrombocytopenic purpura. Ann Intern Med 2000;132:794.
228. Bennett CL, Weinberg PD, Rozenberg-Ben-Dor K, et al: Thrombotic thrombocytopenic purpura associated with ticlopidine. A review of 60 cases. Ann Intern Med 1998;128:541.
229. Gasser C, Gautier E, Steck A, et al: Hämolytisch-urämische Syndrome: bilaterale Nierenrinden-nekrosen bei akuten erworbenen hämolytischen Anämien. Schweiz Med Wochenschr 1955;85:905.
230. Robson WL, Leung AKC, Kaplan BS: Hemolytic-uremic syndrome. Curr Probl Pediatr 1993;23:16.

231. Loirat C, Baudouin V, Sonsino E, et al: Hemolytic-uremic syndrome in the child. Adv Nephrol 1993;22:141.
232. George JN, Gilcher RO, Smith JW, et al: Thrombotic thrombocytopenic purpura-hemolytic uremic syndrome: diagnosis and management. J Clin Apheresis 1998;13:120.
233. Snyder HW, Mittelman A, Oral A, et al: Treatment of cancer chemotherapy–associated thrombotic thrombocytopenic purpura/hemolytic uremic syndrome by protein A immunoadsorption of plasma. Cancer 1993;71:1882.
234. Sarade R, McFarland JG, Flomenberg N, et al: Therapeutic plasma exchange does not appear to be effective in the management of thrombotic thrombocytopenic purpura/hemolytic uremic syndrome following bone marrow transplantation. Bone Marrow Transplant 1995;16:271.
235. Rougier N, Kazatachkine MD, Rougier J-P, et al: Human complement factor H deficiency associated with hemolytic uremic syndrome. J Am Soc Nephrol 1998;9:2318.
236. Warwicker P, Donne RL, Goalship JA, et al: Familial relapsing haemolytic uraemic syndrome and complement factor H deficiency. Nephrol Dial Transplant 1999;14:1229.
237. Zipfel PF, Hellwage J, Friese MA, et al: Factor H and disease: a complement regulator affects vital bodily functions. Mol Immunol 1999;36:241.
238. Martin JN, Files JC, Blake PG, et al: Plasma exchange for preeclampsia. I. Postpartum use for persistently severe preeclampsia-eclampsia with HELLP syndrome. Am J Obstet Gynecol 1990;162:126.
239. Mueller-Eckhardt C: Post-transfusion purpura. Br J Haematol 1986;64:419.
240. Shulman NR, Reid DM: Platelet immunology. In Colman RW, Hirsh J, Marder VJ, Salzman EW (eds): Hemostasis and Thrombosis. Philadelphia, JB Lippincott, 1994, p 414.
241. McCrae KR, Herman JH: Posttransfusion purpura: two unusual cases and a literature review. Am J Hematol 1996;52:205.
242. Newman PJ, McFarland JG, Aster RH: Alloimmune thrombocytopenias. In Loscalzo J, Schafer AI (eds): Thrombosis and Hemorrhage. Boston, Blackwell Scientific, 1994, p 429.
243. Laursen B, Morling N, Rosenkvist J, et al: Post-transfusion purpura treated with plasma exchange by Haemonetics cell separator. Acta Med Scand 1978;203:539.
244. Mueller-Eckhardt C, Kiefel V: High dose IgG for post-transfusion purpura—revisited. Blut 1988;57:163.
245. George JN, El-Harake MA, Aster RH: Thrombocytopenia due to enhanced platelet destruction by immunologic mechanisms. In Beutler E, Lichtman MA, Coller BS, Kipps TJ (eds): Williams Hematology, 5th ed. New York, McGraw-Hill, 1995, p 1315.
246. Branda RF, Tate DY, McCullough JJ, et al: Plasma exchange in the treatment of fulminant idiopathic (autoimmune) thrombocytopenic purpura. Lancet 1978;1:688.
247. Isbister JP, Biggs JC, Penny R: Experience with large volume plasmapheresis in malignant paraproteinemia and immune disorders. Aust NZ J Med 1978;8:154.
248. Marder VJ, Nusbacher J, Anderson FW: One-year follow-up of plasma exchange therapy in 14 patients with idiopathic thrombocytopenic purpura. Transfusion 1981;21:291.
249. Mittelman A, Bertram J, Henry DH, et al: Treatment of patients with HIV thrombocytopenia and hemolytic uremic syndrome with protein A (proSorba) immunoadsorption. Semin Hematol 1989;26(Suppl 11):15.
250. Snyder HW Jr, Cochran SK, Balint JP, et al: Experience with protein A-immunoadsorption in treatment resistant immune thrombocytopenic purpura. Blood 1992;79:2237.
251. Packman CH, Leddy JP: Acquired hemolytic anemia due to warm-reacting autoantibodies. In Beutler E, Lichtman MA, Coller BS, Kipps TJ (eds): Williams Hematology, 5th ed. New York, McGraw-Hill, 1995, p 677.
252. Packman CH, Leddy JP: Cryopathic hemolytic syndromes. In Beutler E, Lichtman MA, Coller BS, Kipps TJ (eds): Williams Hematology, 5th ed. New York, McGraw-Hill, 1995, p 685.
253. Silberstein LE, Berkman EM: Plasma exchange in autoimmune hemolytic anemia (AIHA). J Clin Apheresis 1983;1:238.
254. Valbonesi M, Guzzini D, Zerbi D, et al: Successful plasma exchange for a patient with chronic demyelinating polyneuropathy and cold agglutinin disease due to anti-Pr_a. J Clin Apheresis 1986;3:109.
255. Kutti J, Wadenvik H, Safai-Kutti S, et al: Successful treatment of refractory autoimmune hemolytic anemia by plasmapheresis. Scand J Hematol 1984;32:149.
256. Andersen O, Taaning E, Rosenkvist J, et al: Autoimmune hemolytic anemia treated with multiple transfusions, immunosuppressive therapy, plasma exchange and desferrioxamine. Acta Paediatr Scand 1984;73:145.
257. McConnell ME, Atchison JA, Kohaut E, Castleberry RP: Successful use of plasma exchange in a child with refractory autoimmune hemolytic anemia. Am J Pediatr Hematol Oncol 1987;9:158.
258. von Keyserlingk H, Meyer-Sabellek W, Arntz R, Hiller H: Plasma exchange treatment in autoimmune hemolytic anemia of the wane antibody type with renal failure. Vox Sang 1987;52:298.
259. Geurs F, Ritter K, Mast A, Van Maele V: Successful plasmapheresis in corticosteroid-resistant hemolysis in infectious mononucleosis: role of autoantibodies against triosephosphate isomerase. Acta Haematol 1992;88:142.
260. Shadduck RK: Aplastic anemia. In Beutler E, Lichtman MA, Coller BS, Kipps TJ (eds): Williams Hematology, 5th ed. New York, McGraw-Hill, 1995, p 238.
261. Erslev AJ: Pure red cell aplasia. In Beutler E, Lichtman MA, Coller BS, Kipps TJ (eds): Williams Hematology, 5th ed. New York, McGraw-Hill, 1995, p 448.
262. Young NS, Barrett AJ: The treatment of severe acquired aplastic anemia. Blood 1995;85:3367.
263. Fitchen JJ, Cline MJ, Saxon A, et al: Serum inhibitors of hematopoiesis in a patient with aplastic anemia and systemic lupus erythematosus. Am J Med 1979;6:537.
264. Abdou NI: Plasma exchange in the treatment of aplastic anemia. In Tindall RSA (ed): Therapeutic Apheresis and Plasma Perfusion. New York, Alan R Liss, 1982, p 337.
265. Young NS, Klein HG, Griffith P, et al: Therapeutic plasma exchange and lymphocyte depletion in aplastic anemia and pure red cell aplasia. In Nose Y, Malchesky PS, Smith JW, et al (eds): Plasmapheresis. New York, Raven Press, 1983, p 339.
266. Messner HA, Fause AA, Curtis JE, et al: Control of antibody-mediated pure red cell aplasia by plasmapheresis. N Engl J Med 1981;304:1334.
267. Freund LG, Hippe E, Strandgaard S, et al: Complete remission in pure red cell aplasia after plasmapheresis. Scand J Hematol 1985;35:351.
268. Khelif A, Van HV, Tremisi JP, et al: Remission of acquired pure red cell aplasia following plasma exchanges. Scand J Hematol 1985;35:13.
269. Berlin G, Lieden G: Long-term remission of pure red cell aplasia after plasma exchange and lymphocytapheresis. Scand J Haematol 1986;36:121.
270. Ludlam CA, Morrison AE, Kessler C: Treatment of acquired hemophilia. Semin Hematol 1994;31(Suppl 4):16.
271. Ewenstein BM: Factor VIII and other coagulation factor inhibitors. In Loscalzo J, Schafer AI (eds): Thrombosis and Hemorrhage. Boston, Blackwell Scientific, 1994, p 729.
272. Garvey MB: Incidence and management of patients with acquired factor VIII inhibitors: the practical experience of a tertiary care hospital. In Kessler CM (ed): Acquired Hemophilia. Princeton, NJ, Excerpta Medica, 1995, p 91.
273. Kessler CM: Factor VIII inhibitors—an algorithmic approach to treatment. Semin Hematol 1994;31(Suppl 4):33.
274. Kessler CM: The treatment of acquired factor VIII inhibitors: worldwide experience with porcine factor VIII. In Kessler CM (ed): Acquired Hemophilia. Princeton, NJ, Excerpta Medica, 1995, p 71.
275. Lusher J, Ingerslev S, Roberts H, Hedner U: Clinical experience with recombinant factor VIIa. Blood Coagul Fibrinolysis 1998;9:119.
276. Wensley RT, Stevens RF, Burn AM, et al: The role of intensive plasma exchange in the prevention and management of haemorrhage in patients with inhibitors to factor VIII. Br Med J 1980;281:1388.
277. Slocombe GW, Newland AC, Colvin MP, et al: The role of intensive plasma exchange in the management of hemophilia patients with inhibitors. Br J Haematol 1981;47:577.
278. Bona RD, Pasquale DN, Kalish RI, et al: Porcine factor VIII and plasmapheresis in the management of hemophilia patients with inhibitors. Am J Hematol 1986;21:201.
279. Lusher JM: Management of patients with factor VIII inhibitors. Transfus Med Rev 1987;1:123.
280. Pflieger G, Boda Z, H'arsfalvi J, et al: Cyclosporin treatment of a woman with acquired hemophilia due to factor VIII:C inhibitor. Postgrad Med J 1989;65:400.
281. Schwartz RS, Gabriel DA, Aledort LM, et al: A prospective study of treatment of acquired (autoimmune) factor VIII inhibitors with high-dose intravenous gammaglobulin. Blood 1995;86:797.
282. Ewing NP, Sanders NL, Dietrich SL, Kaspar CK: Induction of immune tolerance to factor VIII in hemophiliacs with inhibitors. JAMA 1988;259:65.

283. Gruppo RA, Valdez LP, Stout RD: Induction of immune tolerance in patients with hemophilia A and inhibitors. Am J Pediatr Hematol Oncol 1992;4:82.

284. Nilsson IM, Berntorp E, Zettervoll O: Induction of immune tolerance in patients with hemophilia and antibodies to factor VIII by combined treatment with intravenous IgG, cyclophosphamide, and factor VIII. N Engl J Med 1988;318:947.

285. Smith OP, Hann IM: rVIIa therapy to secure haemostasis during central line insertion in children with high-responding FVIII inhibitors. Br J Haematol 1996;92:1002.

286. Nakamura Y, Yoshida K, Itoh S, et al: Immunoadsorption plasmapheresis as a treatment for pregnancy complicated by systemic lupus erythematosus with positive antiphospholipid antibodies. Am J Reprod Immunol 1999;41:307.

287. Brouet JC, Clauvel JP, Danon F, et al: Biologic and clinical significance of cryoglobulins: a report of 86 cases. Am J Med 1974;57:775.

288. Bloch KJ: Cryoglobulinemia and hepatic C Virus. N Engl J Med 1992;327:1521.

289. Foerster J: Cryoglobulins and cryoglobulinemia. In Lee GR, Bithell TC, Foerster J, et al (eds): Wintrobe's Clinical Hematology. Philadelphia, Lea & Febiger, 1993, p 2284.

290. Berkman EM, Orlin JB: Use of plasmapheresis and partial plasma exchange in the management of patients with cryoglobulinemia. Transfusion 1980;20:171.

291. Bombardieri S, Maggiore Q, L Abbate A, et al: Plasma exchange in essential mixed cryoglobulinemia. Plasma Ther Transfus Technol 1981;2:101.

292. McGovern TW, Enzenauer RJ, Fitzpatrick JE: Treatment of recalcitrant leg ulcers in cryoglobulinemia types I and II with plasmapheresis. Arch Dermatol 1996;132:498.

293. Goronzy J, Weyland C: Rheumatoid arthritis. In Klippel (ed):Primer on the Rheumatic Diseases. Atlanta, Arthritis Foundation, 1997, p 155.

294. Paget S: Rheumatoid arthritis, treatment. In Klippel (ed): Primer on the Rheumatic Diseases. Atlanta, Arthritis Foundation, 1997, p 168.

295. Moreland LW: Inhibitors of tremor necrosis factor for rheumatoid arthritis. J Rheumatol 1999;26(Suppl 57):7.

296. Rothwell R, Davis P, Gordon P, et al: A controlled study of plasma exchange in the treatment of severe rheumatoid arthritis. Arthritis Rheum 1980;23:785.

297. Dwosh I, Giles A, Ford P: Plasmapheresis therapy in rheumatoid arthritis. A controlled, double-blind, crossover trial. N Engl J Med 1983;308:1124.

298. Wallace D, Goldfinger D, Lowe C, et al: A double-blind, controlled study of lymphoplasmapheresis versus sham apheresis in rheumatoid arthritis. N Engl J Med 1982;306:1406.

299. Karch J, Klippel J, Plotz P, et al.: Lymphapheresis in rheumatoid arthritis. A randomized trial. Arthritis Rheum 1981;24:867.

300. Hester J, Felson D, Gendreau M: Phase III trial of ProSorba column for severe rheumatoid arthritis. J Clin Apheresis 1998;13:90.

301. Pisesky D: Systemic lupus erythematosus. In Klippel (ed): Primer on the Rheumatic Diseases. Atlanta, Arthritis Foundation, 1997, p 246.

302. Klippel J: Systemic lupus erythematosus: treatment. In Klippel J (ed): Primer on the Rheumatic Diseases. Atlanta, Arthritis Foundation, 1997, p 258.

303. Parry HF, Moran CJ, Snaith ML, et al: Plasma exchange in systemic lupus erythematosus. Ann Rheum Dis 1981;40:224.

304. Jones JV: Plasmapheresis in SLE. Clin Rheum Dis 1982;8:243.

305. Huston DP, White MJ, Maltiolo C, et al: A controlled trial of plasmapheresis and cyclophosphamide therapy of lupus nephritis. Arthritis Rheum 1983;26(Suppl):S33.

306. Euler HH, Schwab UM, Schroeder JO, Hasford J: The Lupus Plasmapheresis Study Group: rationale and updated interim report. Artif Organs 1996;20:356.

307. Schroeder JO, Schwab U, Zennet R, et al: Plasmapheresis and subsequent pulse cyclophosphamide in severe systemic lupus erythematosus. Preliminary results of the LPSG Trial. Arthritis Rheum 40:S325, 1997.

308. Wallace DJ, Goldfinger D, Pepkowitz S, et al: Randomized control of pulse/synchronization cyclophosphamide/apheresis for proliferative lupus nephritis. J Clin Apheresis 1998;13:163.

309. Cupps T: Vasculitis: epidemiology, pathology and pathogenesis. In Klippel J (ed): Primer on the Rheumatic Diseases. Atlanta, Arthritis Foundation, 1997, p 289.

310. Hoffman G: Vasculitis: treatment. In Klippel J (ed): Primer on the Rheumatic Diseases. Atlanta, Arthritis Foundation, 1997, p 301.

311. Pusey CD, Rees AJ, Evans DJ, et al: Plasma exchange in focal necrotizing glomerulonephritis without anti-GBM antibodies. Kidney Int 1991;40:757.

312. Guillevin L, Fain O, Lhote F, et al: Lack of superiority of steroids plus plasma exchange to steroids alone in the treatment of polyarteritis nodosa and Churg-Strauss syndrome. A prospective, randomized trial in 78 patients. Arthritis Rheum 1992;35:208.

313. Olsen NJ, Wortmarm RL: Inflammatory and metabolic diseases of muscle. In Klippel JH, Weyand CM, Wortmann RL (eds): Primer on the Rheumatic Diseases. Atlanta, Arthritis Foundation, 1997, p 276.

314. Kaye SA, Isenberg DA: Treatment of polymyositis and dermatomyositis. Br J Hosp Med 1994;52:463.

315. Dalakas MC: Controlled studies with high-dose intravenous immunoglobulin in the treatment of dermatomyositis, inclusion body myositis and polymyositis. Neurology 1998;51:537.

316. Dau PC: Plasmapheresis in idiopathic inflammatory myopathy. Arch Neurol 1981;38:544.

317. Khatri BO, Luprecht G, Weiss SA: Plasmapheresis and immunosuppressive drug therapy in polymyositis. Muscle Nerve 1982;5:568.

318. Cecere FA, Spiva DA: Combination plasmapheresis/leukocytapheresis for the treatment of dermatomyositis/polymyositis. Plasma Ther Transfus Technol 1982;3:401.

319. Miller FW, Leitman SF, Cronin ME, et al: Controlled trial of plasma exchange and leukapheresis in polymyositis and dermatomyositis. N Engl J Med 1992;326:1380.

320. Meguid El Nahas A, Wilkie M: Rapidly progressive glomerulonephritis. In Jamison RL, Wilkinson R (eds): Nephrology. London, Chapman & Hall, 1997, p 586.

321. Glassock RJ, Cohen AH, Adler SG: Primary glomerular diseases. In Brenner BM (ed): The Kidney. Philadelphia, WB Saunders, 1996, p 1392.

322. Wiseman KC: New insights on Goodpasture's syndrome. ANNA J 1993;20:17.

323. Kalluri R, Gunwar S, Reeders ST, et al: Goodpasture syndrome: localization of the epitope for the autoantibodies to the carboxy-terminal region of the alpha 3(IV) chain of basement membrane collagen. J Biol Chem 1991;266:24018.

324. Lockwood CM, Boulton-Jones JM, Lowenthal RM, et al: Recovery from Goodpasture's syndrome after immunosuppressive treatment and plasmapheresis. Br Med J 1975;2:252.

325. Pusey CD, Lockwood CM, Peters DK: Plasma exchange and immunosuppressive drugs in the treatment of glomerulonephritis due to antibodies to the glomerular basement membrane. Int J Artif Organs 1983;6:15.

326. Glassock RJ: Intensive plasma exchange in crescentic glomerulonephritis: help or no help? Am J Kidney Dis 1992;20:270.

327. Madore F, Lazarus JM, Brady HR: Therapeutic plasma exchange in renal diseases. J Am Soc Nephrol 1997;7:367.

328. Bolton WK: Goodpasture's syndrome. Kidney Int 1996;50:1753.

329. Johnson JP, Moore J, Austin HA, et al: Therapy of anti–glomerular basement membrane antibody disease: analysis on the prognostic significance of clinical, pathologic, and treatment factors. Medicine (Baltimore) 1985;64:219.

330. Stegmayr BG, Almroth G, Berlin G, et al: Plasma exchange or immuno-adsorption in patients with rapidly progressive glomerulonephritis. A Swedish multicenter study. Int J Artif Organs 1999;22:81.

331. Lewis EJ, Schwartz MN: Idiopathic crescentic glomerulonephritis. Semin Nephrol 1982;2:193.

332. Glassock RJ, Cohen AH, Adler SG: Primary glomerular diseases. In Brenner BM (ed): The Kidney. Philadelphia, WB Saunders, 1996, p 1392.

333. Jayne DRW, Marshall PD, Jones SJ, Lockwood CM: Autoantibodies to GBM and neutrophil cytoplasm in rapidly progressive glomerulonephritis. Kidney Int 1990;37:965.

334. Burran WP, Avasthi P, Smith KJ, et al: Efficacy of plasma exchange in severe idiopathic rapidly progressive glomerulonephritis. Transfusion 1986;26:382.

335. Sakellariou G: Plasmapheresis as a therapy in specific forms of acute renal failure. Nephrol Dial Transplant 1994;9:210.

336. Glöckner WM, Sieberth HG, Wichmann HE, et al: Plasma exchange and immunosuppression in rapidly progressive glomerulonephritis: a controlled, multi-center study. Clin Nephrol 1988;29:1.

337. Cole E, Cattran D, Magil A, et al: A prospective randomized trial of plasma exchange as additive therapy in idiopathic crescentic glomerulonephritis. Am J Kidney Dis 1992;20:261.

338. Guillevin L, Fain O, Lhote F, et al: Lack of superiority of steroids plus plasma exchange to steroids alone in the treatment of polyarteritis nodosa and Churg-Strauss syndrome. A prospective, randomized trial in 78 patients. Arthritis Rheum 1992;35:208.

339. Levy JB, Pusey CD: Still a role for plasma exchange in rapidly progressive glomerulonephritis? J Nephrol 1997;10:7.

340. Milford EL, Hancock W, Carpenter CB: Immunopathogenetic mechanisms of allograft rejection. In Tishler CC, Brenner BM (eds): Renal Pathology: With Clinical and Functional Correlations. Philadelphia, JB Lippincott, 1994, p 1581.

341. Croker BP, Ramos EL: Pathology of the renal allograft. In Tishler CC, Brenner BM (eds): Renal Pathology: With Clinical and Functional Correlations. Philadelphia, JB Lippincott, 1994, p 1591.

342. McCarthy SA, Zeevi A, Thomson AW, et al: Prevention and management of rejection. In Shapiro R, Simmons RL, Starzl TE (eds): Renal Transplantation. Stamford, CT, Appleton & Lange, 1997, p 149.

343. Winkel E, DiSesa VJ, Costanzo MR: Advances in heart transplantation. Dis Mon 1999;45:63.

344. Kirlin JK, Bourge RC, McGiffin DC: Recurrent or persistent allograft rejection: therapeutic options and recommendations. Transplant Proc 1997;29(Suppl 8a):40S.

345. Cardella CJ, Sutton D, Uldall PR, de Veber GA: Intensive plasma exchange and renal transplant rejection. Lancet 1977;1:264.

346. Rifle G, Chalopin JM, Ture JM, et al: Plasmapheresis in the treatment of renal allograft rejections. Transplant Proc 1979;11:20.

347. Adams MB, Kauffman HM, Hussey CV, et al: Plasmapheresis in the treatment of refractory renal allograft rejection. Transplant Proc 1981;13:491.

348. Vangelista A, Frasca GM, Nanni Costa A, et al: Value of plasma exchange in renal transplant rejection induced by specific HLA antibodies. Trans Am Soc Artif Intern Organs 1982;28:599.

349. Cardella CJ, Sutton D, Falk JA, et al: Effect of intense plasma exchange on renal transplant rejection and serum cytotoxic antibody. Transplant Proc 1978;10:617.

350. Bankowski LHW, Corteste J, Lutton JL, Saunders PH: Plasmapheresis—adjunctive treatment for steroid-resistant rejection in renal transplantation. J Urol 1984;131:14.

351. Soulillou JP, Guyot C, Guimbretiere J, et al: Plasma exchange in early kidney graft rejection associated with anti-donor antibodies. Nephron 1983;35:158.

352. Allen NH, Ayer P, Geoghegan T, et al: Plasma exchange in acute renal allograft rejection: a controlled trial. Transplantation 1983;35:425.

353. Kirubakaran MG, Disney APS, Norman J, et al: A controlled trial of plasmapheresis in the treatment of renal allograft rejection. Transplantation 1981;32:164.

354. Blake P, Sutton D, Cardella C: Plasma exchange in acute renal transplant rejection. Prog Clin Biol Res 1990;337:249.

355. Bonomini V, Vangelista A, Frasca GM, et al: Effects of plasmapheresis in renal transplant rejection: a controlled study. Trans Am Soc Artif Intern Organs 1985;31:698.

356. Gannedahl G, Ohlman S, Persson U, et al: Rejection associated with early appearance of donor-reactive antibodies after kidney transplantation treated with plasmapheresis and administration of 15-deoxyspergualin. A report of two cases. Transpl Int 1992;5:189.

357. Grandtnerova B, Javorsky P, Kolacny J, et al: Treatment of acute humoral rejection in kidney transplantation with plasmapheresis. Transplant Proc 1995;27:934.

358. Loss GE Jr, Grewal HP, Siegel CT, et al: Reversal of delayed hyperacute renal allograft rejection with a tacrolimus-based therapeutic regimen. Transplant Proc 1998;30:1249.

359. Aichberger C, Nussbaumer W, Rosmanith P, et al: Plasmapheresis for the treatment of acute vascular reaction in renal transplantation. Transplant Proc 1997;29:169.

360. Abe M, Sannomiya A, Koike T, et al: Removal of anti-donor antibody by double-filtration plasmapheresis to prevent chronic rejection in kidney transplantation. Transplant Proc 1998;30:3108.

361. Partanen J, Nieminen MS, Krogerus L, et al: Heart transplant rejection treated with plasmapheresis. J Heart Lung Transplant 1992;11:301.

362. Malafa M, Mancini MC, Myles JL, et al: Successful treatment of acute humoral rejection in a heart transplant patient. J Heart Lung Transplant 1992;11:486.

363. Costanzo-Nordin MR, Heroux AL, Radvany R, et al: Role of humoral immunity in acute cardiac allograft rejection. J Heart Lung Transplant 1993;12:S143.

364. Heroux AL, Costanzo-Nordin MR, Radvany R, et al: The enigma of acute allograft dysfunction without cellular rejection: role of humoral immunity. J Heart Lung Transplant 1993;12:S91.

365. Taube D, Palmer A, Welsh K, et al: Removal of anti-HLA antibodies prior to transplantation: an effective and successful strategy for highly sensitized renal allograft recipients. Transplant Proc 1989;21:694.

366. Backman U, Fellstrom B, Frodin L, et al: Successful transplantation in highly sensitized patients. Transplant Proc 1989;21:762.

367. Alarabi A, Backman U, Wikstrom B, et al: Plasmapheresis in HLA-immunosensitized patients prior to kidney transplantation. Int J Artif Organs 1997;20:51.

368. Hodge EE, Klingman LL, Koo AP, et al: Pretransplant removal of anti-HLA antibodies by plasmapheresis and continued suppression on cyclosporine-based therapy after heart-kidney transplant. Transplant Proc 1994;26:2750.

369. Hakim R, Milford E, Himmelfarb J, et al: Extracorporeal removal of anti-HLA antibodies in transplant candidates. Am J Kidney Dis 1990;16:423.

370. Kupin WL, Venkat KK, Hayashi H, et al: Removal of lymphocytotoxic antibodies by pretransplant immunoadsorption therapy in highly sensitized renal transplant recipients. Transplantation 1991;51:324.

371. Miura S, Okazaki H, Sato T, et al: Beneficial effects of double-filtration plasmapheresis on living related donor renal transplantation in presensitized recipients. Transplant Proc 1995;27:1040.

372. Miura S, Okazaki H, Sato T, et al: Successful renal transplantation in presensitized recipients with double-filtration plasmapheresis and 15-deoxyspergualin. Transplant Proc 1997;29:350.

373. Ishikawa A, Itoh M, Ushlyama T, et al: Experience of ABO-incompatible living kidney transplantation after double filtration plasmapheresis. Clin Transplant 1998;12:80.

374. Renard TH, Andrews WS: An approach to ABO-incompatible liver transplantation in children. Transplantation 1992;53:116.

375. Takahashi K, Yogisawa T, Sonda K, et al: ABO-incompatible kidney transplantation in a single center trial. Transplant Proc 1993;25:271.

376. Boudreaux JP, Hayes DH, Mizrahi S, et al: Successful liver/kidney transplantation across ABO incompatibility. Transplant Proc 1993;25:1874.

377. Aswad S, Mendez R, Mendez RG, et al: Crossing the ABO blood barrier in renal transplantation. Transplant Proc 1993;25:267.

378. Mor E, Skerrett D, Manzarbeitia C, et al: Successful use of an enhanced immunosuppressive protocol with plasmapheresis for ABO-incompatible mismatched grafts in liver transplant recipients. Transplantation 1995;59:986.

379. Artero M, Biava C, Amend W, et al: Recurrent focal glomerulosclerosis: natural history and response to therapy. Am J Med 1992;92:375.

380. Artero ML, Sharma R, Savin VJ, Vincenti F: Plasmapheresis reduces proteinuria and serum capacity to injure glomeruli in patients with recurrent focal glomerulosclerosis. Am J Kidney Dis 1994;23:574.

381. Savin VJ, Sharma R, Sharma M, et al: Circulating factor associated with increased glomerular permeability to albumin in recurrent focal segment of glomerulosclerosis. N Engl J Med 1996;334:878.

382. Cochat P, Kassir A, Colon S, et al: Recurrent nephrotic syndrome after transplantation: early treatment with plasmapheresis and cyclophosphamide. Pediatr Nephrol 1993;7:50.

383. Oetliker OH, Zimmerman A, Bianchetti MG: Treatment of recurrent idiopathic nephrotic syndrome after transplantation using plasmapheresis and intensified immunosuppression over 2 months [letter]. Pediatr Nephrol 1993;7:508.

384. Delucchi A, Cano F, Rodriguez E, Wolff E: Focal segmental glomerulosclerosis relapse after transplantation: treatment with high cyclosporine doses and a short plasmapheresis course [letter]. Pediatr Nephrol 1994;8:786.

385. Dixon FJ, McPhaul JJ, Lemer RA: The contribution of transplantation to the study of glomerulonephritis—the recurrence of glomerulonephritis in renal transplants. Transplant Proc 1969;1:194.

386. Kobashigawa JA: Transplant coronary artery disease: targeting nonalloimmune-dependent causes. Transplant Proc 1997;29 (Suppl 8A):47S.

387. Crisp SJ, Dunn MJ, Rose JS, et al: Antiendothelial antibodies after heart transplantation: the accelerating factor in transplant-associated coronary artery disease? J Heart Lung Transplant 1994;13:81.

388. Thiery J, Meiser B, Wenke K, et al: Heparin-induced extracorporeal low-density-lipoprotein plasmapheresis (HELP) and its use in heart transplant patients with severe hypercholesterolemia. Transplant Proc 1995;27:1950.

389. Barr ML, McLaughlin SN, Murphy MP, et al: Prophylactic photopheresis and effect on graft atherosclerosis in cardiac transplantation. Transplant Proc 1995;27:1993.

390. Goldstein JL, Hobbs HH, Brown MS: Familial hypercholesterolemia. In Scriver CR, Beuadet AL, Sly WS, Valle D (eds): The Metabolic and Molecular Basis of Inherited Disease. New York, McGraw-Hill, 1995, p 1981.

391. Thompson GR, Miller JP, Breslow JL: Improved survival of patients with homozygous familial hypercholesterolaemia treated with plasma exchange. Br Med J 1985;291:1671.

392. Kamanabroo D, Ulrich K, Grobe H, Assman G: Plasma exchange in type II hypercholesterolemia. Prog Clin Biol Res 1988;255:347.

393. Leren TP, Fagerhol MK, Leren P: Sixteen years of plasma exchange in a homozygote for familial hypercholesterolemia. J Intern Med 1993;233:195.

394. Beigel Y, Bar J, Cohen M, Hod M: Pregnancy outcome in familial homozygous hypercholesterolemic females treated with long-term plasma exchange. Acta Obstet Gynecol Scand 1998;77:603.

395. Leitman SF, Smith JW, Gregg RE: Homozygous familial hypercholesterolemia: selective removal of low-density lipoproteins by secondary membrane filtration. Transfusion 1989;9:341.

396. Matsuda Y, Malchesky PS, Nose Y: Assessment of currently available low-density lipoprotein apheresis systems. Artif Organs 1994;18:93.

397. Armstrong VW, Eisenhauer T, Noll D, et al: Extracorporeal plasma therapy: the HELP system for the treatment of hyperlipoproteinemia. In Widhalm K, Maito HK (eds): Recent Aspects of Diagnosis and Treatment of Lipoprotein Disorders: Impact on Prevention of Atherosclerotic Diseases. New York, Alan R Liss, 1988, p 327.

398. Stoffel W, Borberg H, Greve V: Application of specific extracorporeal removal of low density lipoprotein in familial hypercholesterolaemia. Lancet 1981;2:1005.

399. Saal SD, Parker TS, Gordon BR, et al: Removal of low-density lipoproteins in patients by extracorporeal immunoadsorption. Am J Med 1986;80:583.

400. Yamamoto A, Kojima S, Shiba-Harada M, et al: Assessment of the biocompatibility and long-term effect of LDL-apheresis by dextran sulfate–cellulose column. Artif Organs 1992;16:177.

401. Steinberg D: Refsum's disease. In Scriver CR, Beuadet AL, Sly WS, Valle D (eds): The Metabolic and Molecular Basis of Inherited Disease. New York, McGraw-Hill, 1995, p 2351.

402. Gibberd FB: Plasma exchange for Refsum's disease. Transfus Sci 1993;14:23.

403. Gutsche H-U, Siegmund JB, Hoppmann I: Lipapheresis: an immunoglobulin-sparing treatment for Refsum's disease. Acta Neurol Scand 1996;94:190.

404. Giorgi DF, Jagoda A: Poisoning and overdose. Mt Sinai J Med 1997;64:283.

405. Trujillo MH, Guerrero J, Fragachan C, Fernandez MA: Pharmacologic antidotes in critical care medicine: a practical guide for drug administration. Crit Care Med 1998;26:377.

406. Jones JS, Dougherty J: Current status of plasmapheresis in toxicology. Ann Emerg Med 1986;15:474.

407. Luzhnikov EA, Yaroslavsky AA, Molodenkov MN, et al: Plasma perfusion through charcoal in methylparathion poisoning. Lancet 1977;1:38.

408. Pierga JY, Beuzeboc P, Dorval T, et al: Favorable outcome after plasmapheresis for vincristine overdose. Lancet 1992;1:185.

409. Chu G, Mantin R, Shen YM, et al: Massive cisplatin overdose by accidental substitution for carboplatin. Toxicity and management. Cancer 1993;72:3707.

410. Ligtenberg J, Tulleken J, Zijlstra J: Plasmapheresis in thyrotoxicosis. Ann Intern Med 1999;131:71.

411. Mercuriali F, Sichia G: Plasma exchange for mushroom poisoning. Transfusion 1977;17:644.

412. Ponikvar R, Drinovec J, Kandus A, et al: Plasma exchange in management of severe acute poisoning with *Amanita phalloides*. In Rock G (ed): Apheresis. New York, Wiley-Liss, 1990, p 327.

413. Piqueras J, Duran-Suarez JR, Massuet L, Hernandez-Sanchez JM: Mushroom poisoning: therapeutic apheresis or forced diuresis. Transfusion 1987;27:116.

414. Seyffart G: Plasmapheresis in treatment of acute intoxications. Trans Am Soc Artif Organs 1982;28:673.

415. Guzelian PS: New approaches for treatment of humans exposed to a slowly excreted environmental chemical (chlordecone). Z Gastroenterol 1984;22:16.

416. Elliott HL, MacDougall AI, Haase G, et al: Plasmapheresis in the treatment of dialysis encephalopathy. Lancet 1978;2:940.

417. Tilz GP, Teubl I, Kopplhuber C, et al: Therapeutic plasmapheresis: a new form of adjuvant treatment. Med Klin 1976;71:1952.

418. Sabato JK, Pierce RM, West RH, Gurr FW: Hemodialysis, peritoneal dialysis, plasmapheresis and forced diuresis for the treatment of quinine overdose. Clin Nephrol 1981;16:264.

419. Larsen LS, Sterrett JR, Whitehead B, Marcus SM: Adjunctive therapy of phenytoin overdose—a case report using plasmapheresis. J Toxicol Clin Toxicol 1986;24:37.

420. Keller F, Hauff A, Schultze G, et al: Effect of repeated plasma exchange on steady state kinetics of digoxin and digitoxin. Arzneimittelforschung 1984;34:83.

421. Stigelman WH, Henry DH, Talbert RL, Townsend RJ: Removal of prednisone and prednisolone by plasma exchange. Clin Pharm 1984;3:402.

422. Appelgate R, Schwartz D, Bennett WM: Removal of tobramycin during plasma exchange therapy. Ann Intern Med 1981;94:820.

423. Talbert RL, Wong YY, Duncan DB: Propranolol plasma concentrations and plasmapheresis. Drug Intell Clin Pharm 1981;15:993.

424. Lee WM: Acute liver failure. Am J Med 1994;96(Suppl 1A):3S.

425. Lee WM: Acute liver failure. N Engl J Med 1993;329:1862.

426. Caraceni P, van Thiel DH: Acute liver failure. Lancet 1995;345:163.

427. Kondrup J, Almdal T, Vilstrup H, et al: High volume plasma exchange in fulminant hepatic failure. Int J Artif Organs 1992;15:669.

428. Larsen FS, Hansen BA, Ejlersen L, et al: Cerebral blood flow, oxygen metabolism and transcranial Doppler sonography during high-volume plasmapheresis in fulminant hepatic failure. Eur J Gastroenterol Hepatol 1995;8:261.

429. Saibara T, Maeda T, Onishi S, Yamamoto Y: Plasma exchange and the arterial blood ketone body ratio in patients with acute hepatic failure. J Hepatol 1994;20:617.

430. Chen SS, Hewitt WR, Watanabe FD, et al: Clinical experience with a porcine hepatocyte-based liver support system. Int J Artif Organs 1996;19:664.

Chapter 45

Therapeutic Cytapheresis

Edahn Isaak

Cytapheresis is a term composed of two parts: *Cyto-* is a prefix that translates as "cell," and *apheresis* means "to take away" or "to remove." The term *cytapheresis* therefore refers to the medical practice of removing cells, either those primary to the disease process or those associated with it. One of the earliest forms of cytapheresis was blood-letting, a therapy that dates back to the Middle Ages in Europe. At that time, people believed that the health of an individual depended on the balance of four bodily "humours," that disease was caused by an imbalance of these humours, and that health would be improved by restoring the balance through blood-letting. Today, advances in the understanding of pathobiology and in the equipment available for cytapheresis have resulted in renewed interest among medical professionals. Disease states that are characterized by the presence of abnormal cell populations may be mitigated by removal of these populations, and cytapheresis has become a mainstay of medical treatment for several disease states, including malignancies, inflammatory conditions, and infections. Indeed, there is a growing list of disease entities for which cytapheresis is considered appropriate therapy (Table 45.1).

Despite the growing number of indications for which cytapheresis may be used, much of the literature over the past 30 years points to three limitations. First, there are many anecdotal descriptions in the form of single case reports or small case series. Second, there is a perception in the community of medical professionals who perform cytapheresis that a reporting bias may exist, so that individual researchers who achieve successful outcomes may be more inclined to publish their results than are those individuals achieving less successful outcomes. Finally, there are few sham-controlled, double-blinded studies that can validate the true effectiveness of cytapheresis as a therapy. Some investigators who have published their results

Table 45.1 Indications for Cytapheresis

Malignancies

Acute myelogenous leukemia
Chronic myelogenous leukemia
Acute lymphocytic leukemia
Chronic lymphocytic leukemia
Hairy cell leukemia
Sezary syndrome
Neuroblastoma
Polycythemia vera
Essential thrombocythemia

Inflammatory conditions

Rheumatoid arthritis
Ulcerative colitis
Crohn disease
Porphyria cutanea tarda
Chronic iron overload

Infections

Malaria
Babesiosis

Miscellaneous

Methemoglobinemia
Reactive thrombocytosis

point out that the concept of a "sham" trial not only entails a dedication of expensive resources but also may be unethical. Although practicing professionals should be cognizant of the limitations inherent in a procedure that may not have been rigorously proven to be effective for a given disease state, they should also consider the increasing body of evidence attesting to the usefulness of cytapheresis in those conditions.

■ Definitions

Cytapheresis is traditionally divided into three entities, depending on which fraction of the cellular population has been targeted for removal: leukocytes, erythrocytes, and thrombocytes. Although treatment of some disease entities involves therapy aimed at removing more than one fraction, this basic three-part division serves as a useful format from which an understanding can be garnered. Based on etymology, *leukocytapheresis* means removal of white blood cells (WBCs), *erythrocytapheresis* means removal of red blood cells (RBCs), and *thrombocytapheresis* means removal of thrombocytes. When cytapheresis is performed with the use of density centrifugation, the fraction of the cellular population that is removed in the greatest percentage is the one for which the procedure is named. However, recent innovations in technology, such as the G-1 column and the Asahi filter, are used to remove overlapping populations of cells. Because procedures involving these innovations are often mentioned without specific enumeration of the exact cellular elements targeted and removed, terms have been employed without being rigorously defined. This lack of specificity in the terminology has resulted in some confusion. In addition to the terms already mentioned, some investigators have proposed the additional terms *lymphocytapheresis* and *granulocytapheresis*.[1]

■ Leukocytapheresis

Ten years ago, the two most common indications for leukocytapheresis were the prevention of leukostasis and the prevention of tumor lysis syndrome, conditions found in patients with certain forms of leukemia. In addition, leukocytapheresis was used to treat infiltrative hematologic tumors such as mycosis fungoides. Over the past decade, the list of potential indications has expanded to include several systemic inflammatory conditions and some solid tumors. The literature describing leukocytapheresis as therapy for systemic inflammatory conditions such as rheumatoid arthritis and inflammatory bowel disease, and for solid tumors such as neuroblastoma, is predominantly anecdotal and consists of several case reports and several small case series. The applications of leukocytapheresis are described here by disease category, including hematologic malignancies, solid tumors, and systemic inflammatory diseases.

Hematologic Malignancies

As previously mentioned, the primary indications for leukocytapheresis in the context of hematologic malignancies are the prevention and treatment of leukostasis and of tumor lysis syndrome. Leukostasis is a complication that is primarily associated with primitive blastic cells in various types of acute myelogenous leukemia (AML).[2] These blasts can be myelocytic, myelomonocytic, or monocytic. In the literature these cells are described as "sticky," and it is now appreciated that this characterization results from an abnormal overexpression of adhesion molecules.[3] When the number of these cells exceeds 100,000/mL, blood viscosity increases.[4] This affects the microcirculation in the lungs and other vital organs by forming white thrombi that then obstruct microvascular channels. These thrombi compete with the local cells for oxygen, and the resulting hypoxia causes the release of toxic cytokines, which results in further invasion and damage to the endothelium. Patients with leukostasis thus experience neurologic and pulmonary symptoms leading to death.

When the WBC count is markedly elevated, the patient is also at risk for tumor lysis syndrome. High rates of cell proliferation and death result in hyperuricemia, hyperkalemia, hypocalcemia, and hyperphosphatemia, which may result in renal failure. In addition, the effects of these complications can be augmented by chemotherapy. Standard therapy for the treatment of tumor lysis syndrome includes hydration, alkalinization of the urine, administration of allopurinol, and correction of electrolyte imbalances. Leukocytapheresis can be used as a supplement to this chemotherapy and functions by decreasing the tumor load.

In addition to the prevention of leuokostasis and tumor lysis syndrome, some authorities have suggested that leukocytapheresis contributes to therapy by making the malignant cells more susceptible to chemotherapy via effects on cell cycle distribution.[5] As leukocytapheresis proceeds, the tumor burden is decreased, and the remaining tumor cells may be stimulated to divide, thus increasing the number of cells in S phase of the cell cycle. Because chemotherapeutic agents such as cytarabine target cells in S phase, the potential efficacy of the chemotherapeutic agent may be increased.

Myeloid Leukemias

The adhesive properties of the primitive blasts in AML are more significant than those in other forms of leukemia. Consequently, leukostasis and tumor lysis syndrome are potentially more problematic in the myeloid leukemias,[6] in which vascular sludging due to high numbers of blasts represents a true emergency. If untreated, leukostasis can result in cerebral ischemia,[7] pulmonary infarction, and myocardial ischemia. Even early reports showed that leukocytapheresis could alleviate the symptoms of leukostasis in leukemia,[8] and it was shown that leukocytapheresis was most valuable because of the rapid cytoreduction associated with its use.

In one of the larger published case series examining hematologic malignancies and response to leukocytapheresis, Steeper and associates[9] evaluated 20 patients, 6 of whom had AML. A total of nine procedures were done on these six patients, with an average of 1.8 blood volumes processed. The mean WBC count before leukocytapheresis was 213,000/mL, and after the procedure it was 65,000/mL. The procedures resulted in potentially significant decreases in hemoglobin and platelet count—23% and 53%, respectively. In addition, four patients with chronic myelogenous leukemia (CML) underwent a total of six procedures, with 2 blood volumes processed in each procedure. The WBC count decreased from a mean of 180,000 to 76,000/mL. Leukocytapheresis resulted in a 12% overall decrease in hemoglobin and a 41% overall decrease in platelet count. Although leukocytapheresis is clearly helpful in lowering the WBC count, this effect does not translate into any long-term benefit. Patients with CML who are treated solely with leukocytapheresis do not achieve remission, and the occurrence of blast crisis is neither prevented nor delayed.[10]

AML and CML share some important pathophysiologic features. In the series reported by Steeper and colleagues,[9] leukemic cellular aggregates and white thrombi were found in 40% of patients. The thrombi were believed to be the immediate cause of death in 24% of the patients with AML and 65% of those with CML. All patients with WBC counts greater than 200,000/mL and more than half of those with counts between 50,000 and 200,000/mL who died had cellular aggregates and white thrombi in histologic sections from their tissues. Although leukocytapheresis should not be used as sole therapy in either AML or CML, most investigators suggest that there is clear benefit in the use of cytapheresis for the purpose of cytoreduction.[11]

CML in chronic phase in pregnant patients represents a unique situation in which leukocytapheresis can be beneficial. Standard therapy for CML can include busulfan, hydroxyurea, interferon-α, and bone marrow transplantation, all of which have the potential to produce teratogenic effects in a fetus. Caplan and coworkers[12] reported the first attempt to use leukocytapheresis as therapy for CML in a pregnant patient, requiring toxic agents during the second half of her gestation. Fitzgerald and associates[13] reported the first successful case in 1986, followed by Strobl and colleagues[14] in 1999. In the report by Strobl, leukocytapheresis was initiated during the 13th week of gestation and continued over the next 8 weeks. At week 21, the WBC count was less than 50,000/mL. Although therapy was discontinued, the WBC count remained stable, and the patient had an uneventful delivery 17 weeks later.

Lymphoid Leukemia

Chronic lymphocytic leukemia is predominantly a disease of the elderly population. Individuals with this disorder usually develop lymphocytosis, followed by organomegaly and ultimately by anemia and thrombocytopenia. Leukocytapheresis can be used to reduce the organomegaly.[15] However, chronic lymphocytic leukemia is an indolent disorder, and there is little benefit in performing leukocytapheresis, compared with standard therapy.[16]

The treatment of acute lymphocytic leukemia generally involves chemotherapy and stem cell transplantation. In contrast to the myeloid leukemias, leukostasis and tumor lysis syndrome are not common in acute lymphocytic leukemia, even with blast counts in excess of 100,000/mL. Therefore, these are not clear indications for leukocytapheresis.[9] Nevertheless, Woloskie and colleagues[17] described the case of a 3-week-old infant who was treated with leukocytapheresis followed by bone marrow transplantation. The WBC count was reduced from 567,900 to 116,000/mL. The long-term outcome of this intervention was not reported.

Mycosis Fungoides

Mycosis fungoides is a CD4-positive T-cell tumor that infiltrates the upper dermis in an interstitial pattern and the epidermis in small collections called Pautrier microabscesses. This skin involvement manifests as erythematous lesions varying from patches to generalized erythroderma. These lesions can be intensely pruritic. When the neoplastic cells circulate either in the lymphatics or in the blood vessels, the disorder is called Sezary syndrome.

Edelson and associates[18] reported the use of leukocytapheresis in a patient with advanced Sezary syndrome. The patient had a WBC count greater than 200,000/mL and had undergone splenomegaly and lymphadenopathy. Leukocytapheresis lowered the number of the circulating neoplastic cells and resulted in decreased infiltration of the skin. Pineda and Winkelman[19] reported on five patients; leukocytapheresis was performed a total of 17 times, and an

average of 2.54×10^9 Sezary cells were removed. In 1984, Decaro and colleagues[20] published a case report describing the use of leukocytapheresis in a patient who was refractory to chemotherapy and to phototherapy, a standard treatment for this entity in which the skin lesions are exposed to ultraviolet light. Five procedures were performed over a 15-day period, and a total of 6.94×10^9 leukocytes were removed. After five treatments, the skin lesions were completely resolved, and a biopsy showed a marked decrease in the number of lymphocytes in the skin.

Although there can be short-term benefit with leukocytapheresis, this does not translate to long-term cures. Three patients[21] received two to three procedures every week over a course of months. Six to seven liters were processed each time, and the procedures resulted in an average reduction of 35% to 56% of the circulating Sezary cells. Although the patients responded favorably for a period of time, the authors suggested that leukocytapheresis as a sole, long-term, therapeutic modality was ineffective.

PHOTOPHERESIS

Although leukocytapheresis can be used to treat Sezary syndrome, the therapy of choice is *photopheresis.*[22] Patients are given an oral dose of 8-methoxypsoralen; this agent intercalates within the DNA of the leukocytes. Two hours later, the patients undergo a modified form of leukocytapheresis in which the leukocytes are passed through a specialized column and exposed to ultraviolet A light. This irradiation cross-links the DNA of photosensitized leukocytes and ultimately causes the leukocytes to undergo apoptosis. Edelson and coworkers[23] were the first to report the use of this therapy. They treated 37 patients and achieved a 73% response rate. Most of the patients who responded had generalized erythroderma, as opposed to the more localized forms of the disease. Evans and associates[22] evaluated 23 patients to determine whether any clinical parameter could be used to predict a positive response to photopheresis. Their results indicated that only a higher tumor burden was predictive of a positive response. They hypothesized that there may be a minimum tumor burden that is critical to the mode of action of photopheresis.

Hairy Cell Leukemia

Hairy cell leukemia is a B-cell neoplastic disorder with a variable course.[24] In the pancytopenic phase, treatment options are limited, although leukocytapheresis has been used with some success in several cases.[25] Theoretically, these favorable effects resulted from the removal of humoral factors, which can inhibit normal hematopoiesis. Although the treatment was not curative, leukocytapheresis could be repeated each time the disease progressed. Choudhury and colleagues[26] treated a patient with three successive courses of leukocytapheresis over a period of 2 years. A total of 26 procedures were performed. An average of 312 mL of buffy coat was removed at each procedure, and the leukocyte concentrate contained an average of 4.56×10^9 WBCs. Seventy-five percent of these cells were shown to be T cells, and 15% were B cells. Only 2% to 4% were leukemic cells. Nevertheless, the patient improved, with a hemoglobin concentration of 15.5 g/dL and a platelet count of 110,000/mL after the final leukocytapheresis procedure. The skin lesions of the patient resolved, and he remained asymptomatic 2 years later.

Solid Tumors

Granulocytosis occurs in association with certain advanced solid tumors.[27] Solid tumors may produce cytokines, such as granulocyte colony-stimulating factor (G-CSF) and granulocyte-macrophage colony-stimulating factor (GM-CSF), which stimulate marrow production of granulocytes. It is believed that these granulocytes interact with the T cells of the immune system of the host, and that this interaction has a suppressive effect on the ability of the host to mount an effective immunologic response against the malignancy. Tabuchi and associates[28] described the use of the G-1 column (Japan Immuno Research Co., Ltd., Takasaki, Japan) in the treatment of two patients with solid tumors. The G-1 column has a capacity of 300 mL and is packed with 220 mg of cellulose acetate beads. The flow rate was set at 30 mL/min, and each procedure lasted 60 minutes. The first patient had metastatic breast carcinoma and underwent 26 procedures; the lesions resolved, and the patient survived for 3 years without further cancer therapy. The second patient had metastatic rectal carcinoma and showed radiologic evidence of improvement after 88 treatments. Despite these anecdotal successes, further studies involving a large number of patients and proper control cohorts are necessary to evaluate the role of the G-1 column in the treatment of solid tumors.

Systemic Inflammatory Diseases

Rheumatoid Arthritis

Rheumatoid arthritis is a chronic, inflammatory disease that affects multiple joints in a symmetrical distribution and also can affect multiple extra-articular sites.[29] In addition to the classic inflammatory tissue, known as pannus, synovial histology is characterized by the presence of chronic inflammatory cells.[30] Although there is no known cure, medical therapy consists of several options. Pharmacotherapy is the first line of treatment. Once the pharmacologic agents have been tried, other options include plasmapheresis and leukocytapheresis. Plasmapheresis was first reported in 1963.[31] Multiple studies later showed that leukocytapheresis was a viable and clinically effective alternative.[32–36] Karsh and colleagues[35] described this clinical efficacy in a randomized, double-blind study. Morning stiffness decreased from 170 to 80 minutes in the treatment group, whereas this clinical parameter actually increased from 155 to 210 minutes in the control group. The treated cohort showed an 18% decrease in joint count, compared with no change in the control group.

Leukocytapheresis as therapy for rheumatoid arthritis is performed in three different ways. The initial studies involved the use of centrifugation as a means to effect a separation of the leukocytic population. The second method was introduced in the late 1980s and involves the use of a technologically innovative filter.[37] The filter is composed of polyester fibers, which trap leukocytes and platelets. The filter is cylindrical in shape and is interposed within an extracorporeal circuit.[38] The third option is the G-1 column, which was originally designed to remove activated neutrophils from the blood of patients with from extensive carcinomatosis.[39]

In a study comparing plamapheresis and leukocytapheresis, the latter proved to be the more efficacious mode of therapy in terms of clinical improvement[40]: those patients treated with lymphocytapheresis had lower levels of rheumatoid factor and higher levels of grasping power than did the patients treated with plasmapheresis. The reason for the clinical efficacy remains unclear, but the hypothesis is that leukocytapheresis removes cells associated with humoral factors, inflammatory cytokines, and other soluble mediators, thus exerting an immunomodulatory effect. Because leukocytapheresis can be performed by three different methods, controversy has centered on which of the three modalities is superior.

Hidaka and Suzuki[41] published a study in 1997 on filter leukocytapheresis in a population of 22 patients. An average of 96% of the leukocytes, 93% of the neutrophils, and 100% of the lymphocytes entering the filter were removed. Circulating neutrophils and lymphocytes decreased during the procedure and then began to rise. After three procedures performed over a 3-week period, the number of circulating activated T-cell subsets had increased. However, the number of activated T cells in the synovial fluid had decreased. The authors concluded that leukocytapheresis with a filter is an effective mode of therapy and that the efficacy may be related to a redistribution of activated T cells from the synovial space to the circulation. Wallace[42] challenged these assertions and stated that filtration leukocytapheresis removed only 1.9×10^9 lymphocytes per procedure, whereas centrifugation removed more than twice that amount. He also argued that circulating lymphopenia correlated with clinical improvement, and that Hidaka's group had not achieved this. Additionally, Wallace argued that there was no rationale for removing granulocytes. Hidaka and associates countered by asserting that Japanese patients are smaller than Americans and that the decreased number of removed lymphocytes could be attributed to this observation. They also pointed out that the role of granulocytes and of monocytes in the pathogenesis of rheumatoid arthritis has not been fully elucidated.[43, 44]

As the controversy over centrifugation versus filtration developed, a third form of leukocytapheresis using the G-1 column was employed in a clinical trial on 40 patients.[45] The authors reported 61% effectiveness and no side effects. Subsequent trials continued to produce promising and consistent results.[39] Basic science research on the column revealed that there were multiple changes in the phenotypic expression of adhesion molecules on the surface of granulocytes that passed through the column and there were also changes in the expression of various inflammatory mediators. Despite the published successful results with the G-1 column, delineation of its place and that of the other forms of leukocytapheresis in the treatment of rheumatoid arthritis awaits further study and clarification.

Inflammatory Bowel Disease

Inflammatory bowel disease includes both ulcerative colitis and Crohn disease. In ulcerative colitis, acute and chronic inflammatory cells are present within the colonic mucosa. These infiltrating leukocytes release multiple proteases and inflammatory mediators, which ultimately are responsible for extensive mucosal damage.[46] Injury to the epithelium from the proinflammatory cytokines results in the clinical manifestations. In Crohn disease, the inflammation within the bowel is discontinuous and transmural and can result in granulomas. Similar to the situation with rheumatoid arthritis, the primary mode of medical therapy for both forms of inflammatory bowel disease is pharmacologic. However, initial studies with leukocytapheresis have demonstrated its usefulness as adjunctive therapy.

All three forms of leukocytapheresis, which were previously discussed in the context of the treatment of rheumatoid arthritis, have been applied in the management of refractory inflammatory bowel disease. Leukocytapheresis performed with a centrifuge has been successful in inducing remission in inflammatory bowel disease refractory to glucocorticoids.[47] Four treatments were performed over a period of 4 weeks; at the end of the fourth week, a remission rate of 68% was reported. Kawamura and coworkers[48] used filtration leukocytapheresis to treat 16 patients with inflammatory bowel disease. After three or four treatments, 11 of the 12 patients with ulcerative colitis achieved remission, with two relapses among them. All four of the patients with Crohn disease improved, and there were no relapses. Shimoyama and colleagues[49] treated 53 patients with weekly leukocytapheresis for five weeks, using the G-1 column. During the 60-minute treatments, the column adsorbed an average of 26% of the granulocytes, 20% of the monocytes, and 2% of the lymphocytes. Fifty-nine percent of the patients achieved a remission.

■ Erythrocytapheresis

Erythrocytapheresis is a term that may be translated, "to take away red blood cells." There are currently three general categories of disease for which erythrocytapheresis is used. The first group consists of those entities in which pathology is caused by an abnormality in iron metabolism. These disorders include hereditary hemochromatosis, transfusion-associated iron overload, methemoglobinemia, and miscellaneous disorders such as porphyria cutanea tarda. The second category of diseases includes those entities in which there is an increase in RBC mass. These can be primary, such as polycythemia vera, or secondary, such as chronic disorders associated with a state of generalized hypoxia. The third category of diseases comprises those entities in which various infectious agents target the RBC, including malaria and babesiosis.

Disorders of Iron Metabolism

Hereditary Hemochromatosis

Hereditary hemochromatosis is a genetic disorder that results, over time, in a progressive increase in body iron stores. This increase in iron stores causes pathologic changes in several organ systems, including the liver, pancreas, heart, and skeletal system.[50–53] Patients ultimately develop liver cirrhosis, diabetes, cardiomyopathy, and arthropathy. Standard therapy for hereditary hemochromatosis consists of periodic phlebotomy or chelation with deferoxamine.[54] If patients are properly treated before permanent organ damage occurs, there is a good possibility that they will live to reach their normal life expectancy. The only component of the disease process that does not respond well to therapy is the arthropathy.

In addition to phlebotomy and chelation, erythrocytapheresis may be used in the treatment of hereditary hemochromatosis, as was first reported in 1983.[55] Kellner and Zoller[56] subsequently performed a prospective study of eight patients with hereditary hemochromatosis. Procedures were carried out every 4 weeks until serum ferritin levels dropped to less than 300 μg/L. This goal was achieved in all eight patients within a mean of 8.5 months. Serum iron levels and transferrin saturations followed the trend of the serum ferritins. Clinical re-examination revealed normal liver iron stores; however, there was no improvement in liver histology. Maintenance therapy then consisted of repeated erythrocytapheresis every 5 to 6 months. Because plasma protein levels and platelet counts were unaffected by the therapy, the investigators recommended that erythrocytapheresis should be considered as a therapeutic option in patients with hypoproteinemia and low platelet counts.

Transfusion-Associated Iron Overload

Several of the chronic anemias, most commonly sickle cell anemia, are treated with periodic simple transfusion therapy. Pediatric patients with sickle cell anemia are at risk for cerebrovascular complications, especially in the latter part of the first decade of life.[57] Although chronic transfusion therapy is efficacious, a therapeutic end point has not been clearly established, so the transfusion therapy is continued indefinitely.[58] The most significant consequence is iron overload.[59]

The traditional treatment for iron overload is chelation with deferoxamine. However, its effectiveness is limited by several factors, including expense and poor compliance. An alternative to treatment is erythrocytapheresis, which was first reported as an option in 1994.[60] The initial study showed that erythrocytapheresis was safe and effective and that, although total blood use was increased by 73% compared with simple transfusion, iron load decreased by 87% and some patients were able to discontinue chelation therapy.

Hillard and associates[61] studied 11 patients with a history of sickle cell anemia complicated by stroke. The patients were initially treated with simple transfusion and then converted to erythrocytapheresis. Hemoglobin levels remained relatively constant. Erythrocytapheresis was performed on average every 35 days, in contrast to transfusion, which was performed every 30 days. There was a mild increase in the fraction of hemoglobin S while the patients were being treated with erythrocytapheresis, but there were no clinical sequelae associated with the increase. Consistent with previous reports in the literature, there was a significant increase in RBC usage (53%); however, none of the patients developed an alloantibody or an infectious complication. The results of therapy with erythrocytapheresis in the 11 patients depended on the pretreatment serum ferritin level and on chelation status. Patients receiving chelation therapy who had a serum ferritin concentration greater than 5000 ng/mL remained stable. One patient receiving chelation therapy with a serum ferritin concentration of 4000 ng/mL experienced a decline in iron load. The best result occurred in a patient whose ferritin level was less than 500 ng/mL when he began erythrocytapheresis. This patient was able to maintain a low serum ferritin concentration without the need for chelation therapy. The investigators concluded that erythrocytapheresis is a safe alternative to standard therapy and that erythrocytapheresis is most effectively used as initial therapy, before there is an advanced degree of iron overload.[61]

Methemoglobinemia

Methemoglobinemia results from the oxidation of hemoglobin to the ferric state, which prevents the iron moiety from binding oxygen.[62] This disorder may be congenital or acquired. Congenital forms are caused by rare defects in the pathways involved in the reduction of hemoglobin. The acquired form results when oxidative stress is applied to hemoglobin. Standard therapy for the acquired form of methemoglobinemia is methylene blue. However, individuals who are glucose-6-phosphate dehydrogenase-deficient or who have severe refractory methemoglobinemia do not respond to standard therapy. The major option for such patients is RBC exchange.

Exchange transfusion has been used successfully in the past.[63] It can be performed manually as a whole blood exchange, or it can be performed as an automated exchange. Golden and Weinstein[64] reported the case of a 26-month-old boy with glucose-6-phosphate dehydrogenase deficiency and severe, acquired methemoglobinemia. The patient was cyanotic and in respiratory failure. After there was no response to treatment with methylene blue or to manual exchange, the patient underwent an automated RBC exchange. A single procedure, in which a 1.3 RBC volume exchange was performed, lowered the methemoglobin level from 32% to 7%. The patient was uneventfully discharged from the hospital 2 days later.

Porphyria Cutanea Tarda

Porphyria cutanea tarda is a disorder characterized by a photosensitive dermatosis and hepatic siderosis.[65] The expression of the disease is determined by several contributing factors, among which is the degree of hepatic iron accumulation. This accumulation is usually treated with phlebotomy. Although erythrocytapheresis can be used to treat the hepatic iron accumulation, it usually is not necessary.

Increases in Red Blood Cell Mass

Polycythemia Vera

Polycythemia vera is a myeloproliferative disorder that results in an abnormal increase in the number of RBCs.[66] Both the hematocrit and the blood volume increase, which leads to the development of a hyperviscosity syndrome. Patients with polycythemia vera who experience this syndrome complain of headache, dizziness, and visual disturbances, and they are at increased risk for thrombosis. Because the increase in RBC mass is pathologic, patients benefit from therapy aimed at reducing the RBC mass to physiologic levels. Standard treatment consists of therapeutic phlebotomy and chemotherapy. Erythrocytapheresis can be considered as an alternative to standard therapy in three circumstances.

The first circumstance involves the need to rapidly decrease the hematocrit in a symptomatic patient when the degree of decrease in RBC mass that the patient requires exceeds the level that can be achieved through phlebotomy. In the second circumstance, the patient has not only erythrocytosis but also a concomitant thrombocytosis. Finally, some patients require frequent phlebotomy to maintain their hematocrit near a normal level of 45%. For such patients, erythrocytapheresis can be used to increase the interval between treatments. Centurioni and colleagues[67] treated three patients with polycythemia vera, each of whom had required two or three phlebotomies every month to maintain a proper hematocrit. With erythrocytapheresis, the interval between treatments was extended to approximately 3 months in each case.

Secondary Erythrocytosis

Secondary erythrocytosis occurs in individuals with cyanotic congenital cardiac disease, chronic pulmonary insufficiency, and other conditions associated with chronic hypoxemia.[68] In contrast to polycythemia vera, in which the increase in RBC mass is pathologic and maladaptive, the increase associated with secondary erythrocytosis is adaptive. These patients can tolerate hematocrit levels in the range of 55% to 65% without symptoms of hyperviscosity, and many do not require therapy for the elevated hematocrit. When therapy is required owing to symptoms of hyperviscosity, phlebotomy is considered to be standard treatment.[69] Although erythrocytapheresis remains an option, it is usually unnecessary.

Infections

Malaria

Malaria is caused by infection with species of the blood parasite, *Plasmodium*. The manifestations of malaria differ, depending on which plasmodial organism is involved. The most aggressive form, also known as malignant tertian malaria, is caused by *Plasmodium falciparum*. The presentation of this disease depends not only on the infecting organism but also on the immune status of the host.[70] *P. falciparum* is transferred to a human host through the bite of the female *Anopheles* mosquito. After an initial phase of replication in the liver, the merozoites are released into the blood stream, where each merozoite is capable of infecting an RBC. Replicative cycles occur at intervals of 48 hours and produce paroxysms of fever and chills. Infected RBCs develop an altered membrane structure that results in an increased tendency of the RBC to adhere in the microvasculature and to cause thrombosis. Individuals with no immunity to the parasite are most susceptible to serious complications and death. Individuals with some degree of immunity can tolerate higher parasitic loads (>5%) with less risk.[71]

Malaria caused by *Plasmodium falciparum* is initially treated with chloroquine. Because *P. falciparum* is chloroquine-resistant, parenteral quinidine gluconate is used. Apheresis, in the form of plasmapheresis or erythrocytapheresis, can be useful as ancillary therapy. Plasmapheresis can remove free hemoglobin and toxic cytokines[72]; however, it is of limited value and is not generally recommended.

Erythrocytapheresis should be considered in several instances. First, infected individuals with greater than 10% parasitemia and complications such as renal failure or cerebral malaria may be good candidates.[73] Patients with parasitemia in the range of 5% to 10% with metabolic complications such as shock and acidosis should also be considered. Zhang and colleagues[74] treated three patients who had parasitemia ranging from 20% to 40% with symptoms of cerebral involvement. The desired end points of therapy, including hematocrit and fraction of cells remaining, were entered into a COBE Spectra, (COBE Laboratories, Lakewood, CO) and the instrument performed the necessary calculations. In all cases parasitemia was decreased by more than 80%, and all three patients recovered uneventfully. Weir and associates[75] also treated three patients with parasitemia ranging from 30% to 60% and symptoms of cerebral malaria. The patients received loading doses of quinidine, followed by RBC exchange. Two patients required a second exchange. Parasitemia levels were less than 1% within 24 hours after the last exchange, and all three patients were uneventfully discharged within 18 days after admission. Although erythrocytapheresis may be useful in additional circumstances, there are no controlled trials to definitively validate its use.

Babesiosis

Babesiosis is caused by infection with a protozoal parasite. The disease is transmitted from animals to humans by *Ixodes dammini* and is most commonly caused by infection with *Babesia microti*. Most of these infections are subclinical.[76] However, asplenic patients and patients with acquired immune deficiency syndrome may have more serious manifestations, including renal failure, disseminated intravascular coagulation, and pulmonary edema.[77] Although pharmacotherapy is the standard treatment, erythrocytapheresis is used when the level of parasitemia is elevated. Evenson and colleagues[77] treated two patients with babesiosis. The first had a parasitemia of 30% and underwent two RBC exchanges; despite a successful treatment outcome, with parasitemia less than 1%, the patient died from medical complications of pancreatitis. The second patient underwent three RBC exchanges and one plasma exchange; he received pharmacotherapy concurrently and was apparently free from infection at last follow-up.

There are no controlled studies on the role of erythrocytapheresis in the management of babesiosis, and Evenson's group was the first to report a case suggesting a possible role for plasma exchange. Because no consensus exists on the exact level of parasitemia at which erythrocytapheresis is indicated, a level of 5% (as for malaria) has been suggested by Evenson and colleagues.[77]

■ Thrombocytapheresis

Thrombocytapheresis is a term that translates as "to take away platelets." There are two general categories of disease for which thrombocytapheresis can be used: primary causes and secondary (or reactive) causes of thrombocytosis. The term *thrombocytosis* describes platelet counts that are greater than the accepted upper limit of the reference range for platelets in peripheral blood. Extreme thrombocytosis refers by convention to peripheral blood platelet counts greater than 1,000,000/mL.[78] Primary causes of thrombocytosis belong to a category of disease entities known as myeloproliferative disorders and include essential thrombocythemia, polycythemia vera, CML, and myeloid metaplasia. Secondary causes of thrombocytosis include many diverse disease entities (Table 45.2), and their incidence varies among populations of different ages. Secondary thrombocytosis in children is generally a result of infection; in teenagers, it is usually caused by trauma; and in those age 40 years or older, it is most commonly caused by malignancy or infection.

Patients who present with extreme thrombocytosis may be prone to either thrombosis or hemorrhage; however, the platelet count alone is not a reliable indicator of the risk of these complications.[79–81] It is more important to differentiate between primary and secondary causes of thrombocytosis,

because thrombotic and hemorrhagic events are much more common in primary thrombocytosis, and reactive thrombocytosis usually does not require intervention. In one study of 280 patients, 56% of those with primary thrombocytosis experienced thrombotic or hemorrhagic complications. In contrast, only 4% of the patients with reactive thrombocytosis experienced similar complications, and the thrombotic episodes could be explained by atherosclerosis or other concomitant disease processes.

Primary causes of thrombocytosis share some overlapping features. Clinical presentation and prognostic implications vary, so criteria to differentiate among the primary causes of thrombocytosis have been published by the Polycythemia Vera Study Group.[82] When thrombocytosis is a component of the patient's presentation, standard therapy involves the use of single agents such as hydroxyurea,[83] anegrilide,[84] and interferon-α.[85] As an adjunct to chemotherapy, thrombocytapheresis can be used to rapidly lower the peripheral platelet count. This application was first performed in 1966.[86] Patients who should be considered as candidates for thrombocytapheresis include those with evidence of thrombosis or hemorrhage, those who are either elderly or pregnant, and with cardiovascular disease.

Table 45.2 Diseases Causing Reactive Thrombocytosis

Acute blood loss
Iron deficiency
Cobalamin deficiency
Nonhematologic malignancies
Infectious diseases
Connective tissue diseases
Inflammatory bowel disease
Vasculitis
Splenectomy
Exercise
Medications

REFERENCES

1. Sawada K, Shimoyama T: Therapeutic cytapheresis for inflammatory bowel disease. Ther Apheresis 1998;2:90–92.
2. Grima K: Therapeutic apheresis in hematological and oncological diseases. J Clin Apheresis 2000;15:28–52.
3. Cartron JP, Bailly P, Le Van Kim C, et al: Insights into the structure and function of membrane polypeptides carrying blood group antigens. Vox Sang 1998;74(Suppl 2):29–64.
4. Thiebaut A, Thomas X, Belhabri A, et al: Impact of pre-induction therapy leukapheresis on treatment outcome in adult acute myelogenous leukemia presenting with hyperleukocytosis. Ann Hematol 2000;79:501–506.
5. Powell BL, Gregory BW, Evans JK, et al: Leukapheresis induced changes in cell cycle distribution and nucleoside transporters in patients with untreated acute myeloid leukemia. Leukemia 1991;5:1037–1042.
6. Lichtman MA: Rheology of leukocytes, leukocyte suspensions and blood in leukemia: Possible relationship to clinical manifestations. J Clin Invest 1973;52:350–358.
7. Fritz RD, Forkner CE, Freireich EJ, et al: The association of fatal intracerebral hemorrhage and blastic crisis in patients with acute leukemia. N Engl J Med 1959;261:59–64.
8. Eisenstaedt RS, Berkman EM: Rapid cytoreduction in acute leukemia: Management of cerebral leukostasis by cell pheresis. Transfusion 1978;18:113–115.
9. Steeper TA, Smith JA, McCullough J: Therapeutic cytapheresis using Fenwal CS-3000 blood cell separator. Vox Sang 1985;48:193–200.
10. Vallejos CS, McCredie KB, Briten GM: Biological effects of repeated leukapheresis of patients with acute myelogenous leukemia. Blood 1973;42:925–933.
11. Lowenthal RM, Buskard NA, Park J, et al: Intensive leukapheresis as initial therapy for chronic granulocytic leukemia. Blood 1975;46:835–844.
12. Caplan SN, Coco FV, Berkman EM: Management of chronic myelocytic leukemia in pregnancy by cell pheresis. Transfusion 1978;18:120–124.
13. Fitzgerald D, Rowe JM, Heal J: Leukapheresis for the control of chronic myelogenous leukemia during pregnancy. Am J Hematol 1986;22:213–218.
14. Strobl FJ, Voelkerding KV, Smith EP: Management of chronic myeloid leukemia during pregnancy with leukapheresis. J Clin Apheresis 1999;14:42–44.
15. Silvergleid AJ: Applications and limitations of hemapheresis. Annu Rev Med 1983;34:69–89.
16. Curtis JE, Hersch EM, Freireich EJ: Leukapheresis of chronic lymphocytic leukemia. Blood 1973;39:163–175.

17. Woloskie S, Armelagos H, Meade JM, et al: Leukodepletion for acute lymphocytic leukemia in a three-week old infant. J Clin Apheresis 2001;16:31–32.

18. Edelson RM, Facktor M, Andrews A, et al: Successful management of the Sezary syndrome: Mobilization and removal of neoplastic T cells by leukapheresis. N Engl J Med 1974;291:293–294.

19. Pineda AA, Winkelman RK: Leukapheresis in the treatment of Sezary syndrome. J Am Acad Dermatol 1981;5:544–549.

20. Decaro JH, Novoa JE, de Anda D, et al: Leukapheresis in a patient with Sezary syndrome. Vox Sang 1984;47:276–279.

21. Muller N, Lange CE: Long-term cytapheresis in the treatment of Sezary syndrome. Int J Artif Organs 1984;7:143–146.

22. Evans AV, Wood BP, Scarisbrick JJ, et al: Extracorporeal photopheresis in Sezary syndrome: Hematologic parameters as predictors of response. Blood 2001;98:1298–1301.

23. Edelson R, Berger C, Gasparro F, et al: Treatment of cutaneous T-cell lymphoma by extracorporeal photochemotherapy: Preliminary results. N Engl J Med 1987;316:297–303.

24. Katayama I, Finkel HE: Leukemic reticuloendotheliosis: A clinicopathologic study with review of the literature. Am J Med 1974;57:115–126.

25. Worsley A, Cuttner J, Gordon R, et al: Therapeutic leukocytapheresis in a patient with hairy cell leukemia presenting with a white cell count greater than 500,000/microliter. Transfusion 1982;22:308–310.

26. Choudhary AM, Bhoopalam NB, Hoffstadter LK: Effect of intense leukocytapheresis in pancytopenic phase of hairy cell leukemia. Transfusion 1983;23:526–529.

27. Robinson AW: Granulocytosis in neoplasia. Ann N Y Acad Sci 1974;230:212–218.

28. Tabuchi T, Hideyuki U, Saniabadi AR, et al: Granulocyte apheresis as a possible new approach in cancer therapy: A pilot study involving two cases. Cancer Detect Prev 1999;23:417–421.

29. Zvaifler NJ: The immunopathology of joint inflammation in rheumatoid arthritis. Adv Immunol 1973;16:265–336.

30. Ziff M: Role of the endothelium in chronic inflammatory synovitis. Arthritis Rheum 1991;34:1345–1352.

31. Jaffe IA: Comparison of the effect of plasmapheresis and penicillamine on the level of circulating rheumatoid factor. Ann Rheum Dis 1963;22:71–76.

32. Karsh J, Wright DJ, Klippel JH, et al. Lymphocyte depletion by continuous flow cell centrifugation in rheumatoid arthritis: Clinical effects. Arthritis Rheum 1979;22:1055–1059.

33. Wallace DJ, Goldfinger D, Gatti R, et al. Plasmapheresis and lymphoplasmapheresis in the management of rheumatoid arthritis. Arthritis Rheum 1979;22:703–709.

34. Wright DJ, Karsh J, Fauci AS, et al: Lymphocyte depletion and immunosuppression with repeated leukapheresis by continuous flow centrifugation. Blood 1981;58:451–458.

35. Karsh J, Klippel JH, Plotz PH, et al: Lymphapheresis in rheumatoid arthritis: A randomized trial. Arthritis Rheum 1981;24:867–873.

36. Wallace DJ, Goldfinger D, Lowe C, et al: A double-blind controlled study of lymphoplasmapheresis versus sham apheresis in rheumatoid arthritis. N Engl J Med 1982;306:1406–1410.

37. Kondoh T, Hidaka Y, Katoh H, et al: Evaluation of a filtration lymphocytapheresis (LCP) device for use in the treatment of patients with rheumatoid arthritis. Artif Organs 1991;15:180–188.

38. Sirchia G, Rebulla P, Parravicini A, et al: Leukocyte depletion of red cell units at the bedside by transfusion through a new filter. Transfusion 1987;27:402–405.

39. Kyogoku M, Kasukawa R: Clinical and basic studies on the G-1 column, a new extracorporeal therapeutic device effective in controlling rheumatoid arthritis. Inflamm Res 1998;47(Suppl):166–176.

40. Ogawa H, Matsumoto Y: The efficacy of plasmapheresis or leuko-cytapheresis. Ther Apheresis 1997;1:330–335.

41. Hidaka T, Suzuki K: The mechanism of the efficiency of leukocytapheresis on rheumatoid arthritis. Ther Apheresis 1997;1:215–218.

42. Wallace D: Leukocytapheresis and rheumatoid arthritis: Comment on the article by Hidaka et al. Arthritis Rheum 1999;42:2255.

43. Ohara M, Saniabadi AR, Kokuma S, et al: Granulocytapheresis in the treatment of patients with rheumatoid arthritis. Artif Organs 1997;21:989–994.

44. Hahn G, Stuhlmuller B, Hain N, et al: Modulation of monocyte activation in patients with rheumatoid arthritis by leukapheresis therapy. J Clin Invest 1993;91:862–870.

45. Kasukawa R, Yoshima S, Ohara M, et al: Extracorporeal granulocyte adsorption treatment of patients with rheumatoid arthritis using cellulose acetate beads. Inflammation 1994;14:239–254.

46. Weissman G: Lysosomal mechanism of tissue injury in arthritis. N Engl J Med 1972;286:141–147.

47. Kohgo Y: Recent advances in therapy for patients with inflammatory bowel disease. Intern Med 2000;39:342–345.

48. Kawamura A, Saitoh M, Yonekawa M, et al: New technique of leukocytapheresis by the use of nonwoven polyester fiber filter for inflammatory bowel disease. Ther Apheresis 1999;3:334–337.

49. Shimoyama T, Sawadi K, Hiwatashi N, et al: Safety and efficacy of granulocyte and monocyte adsorption apheresis in patients with active ulcerative colitis: A multicenter study. J Clin Apheresis 2001;16:1–9.

50. Adams PC, Kertesz AE, Valberg LS: Clinical presentation of hemochromatosis: A changing scene. Am J Med 1991;90:445–449.

51. Adams PC, Speechly M, Kertesz AE: Long-term survival analysis in hereditary hemochromatosis. Gastroenterology 1991;101:368–372.

52. Adams PC, Halliday JW, Powell LW: Early diagnosis and treatment of hemochromatosis. Adv Intern Med 1989;34:111–126.

53. Askari AD, Muir WA, Rosner TA: Arthritis of hemochromatosis: Clinical spectrum, relation to histocompatibility antigens, and effectiveness of early phlebotomy. Am J Med 1983;75:957–965.

54. Cohen A, Witzleben C, Schwartz E: Treatment of iron overload. Semin Liver Dis 1984;4:228–238.

55. Conte D, Brunelli L, Bozzani A, et al: Erythrocytapheresis in idiopathic haemochromatosis. Br Med J 1983;286:939.

56. Kellner H, Zoller WG: Repeated isovolumic large-volume erythrocytapheresis in the treatment of idiopathic hemochromatosis. Z Gastroenterol 1992;30:779–783.

57. Frepong KO: Stroke in sickle-cell disease: Demographic, clinical and therapeutic considerations. Semin Hematol 1991;28:213–219.

58. Wang WC, Kovnar EH, Tonkin IL, et al: High risk of recurrent stroke after discontinuance of five to twelve years of transfusion therapy in patients with sickle-cell disease. J Pediatr 1991;118:377–382.

59. Cohen A, Kron E, Brittenham G: Toxicity of transfusional iron overload in sickle-cell anemia. Blood 1984;64(Suppl 1):47.

60. Kim HC, Dugan NP, Silber JH, et al: Erythrocytapheresis therapy to reduce iron overload in chronically transfused patients with sickle-cell disease. Blood 1994;83:1136–1142.

61. Hillard LM, Williams BF, Lounsbury AE, et al: Erythrocytapheresis limits iron accumulation in chronically transfused sickle-cell patients. Am J Hematol 1998;59:28–35.

62. Mansouri A, Lurie AA: Concise review: Methemoglobinemia. Am J Hematol 1992;42:7–12.

63. Mier RJ: Treatment of aniline poisoning with exchange transfusion. Clin Toxicol 1988;26:357–364.

64. Golden PJ, Weinstein R: Treatment of high-risk, refractory acquired methemoglobinemia with automated red blood cell exchange. J Clin Apheresis 1988;13:28–31.

65. Bulaj Z, Phillips JD, Ajioka RS, et al: Hemochromatosis genes and other factors contributing to the pathogenesis of porphyria cutanea tarda. Blood 2000;95:1565–1571.

66. Conley CL: Polycythemia vera. JAMA 1990;263:2481–2483.

67. Centurioni R, Leoni P, Candela M, et al: Neocytapheresis in the treatment of polycythemia vera. Recent Prog Med 1996;87:161–163.

68. Pollari G, Antonini V, Izzo A, et al: The role of erythrocytapheresis in secondary erythrocytosis therapy. Clin Hemorheol Microcirc 1999;21:353–355.

69. Perloff JK, Rosove MH, Child JS, et al: Adults with cyanotic congenital heart disease: Hematologic management. Ann Intern Med 1998;109:406–413.

70. Glenister FK, Coppel RL, Cowman AF, et al: Contribution of parasite proteins to altered mechanical properties of malaria-infected red cells. Blood 2002;99:1060–1063.

71. Vachon F, Wolff M, Lebras J: Exchange transfusion as an adjunct to the treatment of severe falciparum malaria. Infect Dis Clin North Am 1992;14:1269–1270.

72. Phillips P, Nantel S, Benny WB: Exchange transfusion as an adjunct to the treatment of severe falciparum malaria: A case report and review. Rev Infect Dis 1990;12:1100–1108.

73. White NJ: The treatment of malaria. N Engl J Med 1996;335:800–806.

74. Zhang Y, Telleria JM, Vinetz JM, et al: Erythrocytapheresis for *Plasmodium falciparum* infection complicated by cerebral malaria and hyperparasitemia. J Clin Apheresis 2001;16:15–18.

75. Weir EG, King KE, Ness PM, et al: Automated RBC exchange transfusion: Treatment for cerebral malaria. Transfusion 2000;40:702–707.

76. Ruebush TK, Cassidy PB, March HJ, et al: Human babesiosis on Nantucket Island: Clinical features. Ann Intern Med 1977;86:6–9.

77. Evenson DA, Perry E, Kloster B, et al: Therapeutic apheresis for babesiosis. J Clin Apheresis 1998;13:32–36.

78. Buss DH, Cashell AW, O'Connor ML, et al: Occurrence, etiology and clinical significance of extreme thrombocytosis: A study of 280 cases. Am J Med 1994;96:247–253.

79. Barbui T, Cortelazzo S, Viero P: Thrombohemorrhagic complication in 101 cases of myeloproliferative disorders: Relationship to platelet numbers and function. Eur J Cancer Clin Oncol 1983:19:1593–1599.

80. Kessler CM, Klein HG, Havlik RJ: Uncontrolled thrombocytosis in chronic myeloproliferative disorders. Br J Haematol 1982;50:157–167.

81. Buss DH, Stuart JJ, Lipscomb GE: The incidence of thrombotic and hemorrhagic disorders in association with extreme thrombocytosis: An analysis of 129 cases. Am J Hematol 1985;20:365–372.

82. Kutti J, Wadenvik H: Diagnostic and differential criteria of essential thrombocythemia and reactive thrombocytosis. Leuk Lymphoma 1996;22(Suppl 1):41–45.

83. Schafer AI: Essential thrombocythemia. Prog Hemost Thrombosis 1991;10:69–96.

84. Mughal TI: Primary thrombocythemia: A current perspective. Stem Cells 1995;13:355–359.

85. Carlo-Stella C, Cazzola M, Gasner A, et al: Effects of recombinant alpha and gamma interferons on the in-vitro growth of circulating hematpoietic progenitor cells (CFU-GEMM, CFU-Mk, BFU-E, and CFU-GM) from patients with myelofibrosis with myeloid metaplasia. Blood 1987;70:1014–1019.

86. Colman RW, Sievers CA, Pugh RP: Thrombocytopheresis: A rapid and effective approach to symptomatic thrombocytosis. J Clin Lab Med 1966;68:389–399.

Chapter 46

Bone Marrow and Peripheral Blood Stem Cell Transplantation

Avichai Shimoni
Richard Champlin

Hematopoietic cellular transplantation (HCT) involves engraftment of stem cells and progenitor cells that can be collected from the bone marrow, peripheral blood, or umbilical cord blood. *Autologous* transplants use a patient's own hematopoietic cells, usually after cryopreservation. *Syngeneic* transplants involve a genetically identical twin donor. *Allogeneic* transplants are donated by another person.

Bone marrow transplantation (BMT) has been studied in animal models since the late 1940s as a means to rescue recipients exposed to lethal radiation. Allogeneic transplantation from a human leukocyte antigen (HLA)-identical donor was first successfully used in 1968 in three children with congenital immune deficiency.[1] In 1977, Thomas and colleagues reported the first large series of 100 patients with end-stage leukemia treated with allogeneic transplantation; a few patients achieved long-term remissions.[2] Autologous transplants have been widely employed since the mid 1980s. Since then, thousands of patients with a variety of diseases have received HCT, with continuous growth of this approach each year. The indications for HCT have become better defined, and much progress has been achieved in improving supportive care and prevention of transplant-related complications. This chapter focuses on the principles of clinical HCT, the indications and results of HCT in specific diseases, specific transplant-related complications, and methods for the prevention and treatment of these complications.

■ Rationale for Hematopoietic Transplantation

HCT is an effective treatment for a range of hematologic, immunologic, metabolic, and neoplastic diseases (Table 46.1).[3, 4] Allogeneic transplants may be used for treatment of bone marrow failure states, immune deficiencies,

or inborn errors of metabolism involving hematopoietic tissues, by establishing a new, normally functioning hematopoietic system. Autologous transplants have also been used as treatment of autoimmune diseases,[5–8] as a vehicle for gene therapy using genetically modified stem/progenitor cells or lymphocytes,[9, 10] for correction of metabolic defects, and for immunotherapy.[11–13]

The most common application of HCT is for treatment of malignant diseases.[14] Dose-intensive therapy in association with HCT is an effective treatment for a wide range of hematologic malignant diseases and selected solid tumors. Many chemotherapy drugs and radiation produce a dose-dependent antitumor response. Higher doses produce greater cytoreduction and may overcome low-level drug resistance. Myelosuppression is the dose-limiting toxicity of many chemotherapeutic agents and total-body radiation (TBI). Doses of some agents can be markedly escalated, to three- to fivefold higher than conventional maximally tolerated doses, if administration of these drugs is followed by autologous or allogeneic transplantation to restore hematopoiesis. Treatment doses are limited by nonhematologic toxicity to normal tissues.

Allogeneic transplants may also confer an immune-mediated graft-versus-malignancy (GVM) effect that may eradicate tumor cells surviving high-dose cytotoxic therapy.[15–18] Extensive experimental data support the presence of a graft-versus-leukemia (GVL) or GVM effect. The risk of relapse of the malignant disease after HCT is increased in syngeneic transplants,[17, 19, 20] or when T cells are depleted from an allograft as a means to prevent graft-versus-host disease (GVHD).[21] Patients with acute and chronic GVHD have a reduced risk of relapse, a finding suggesting a relationship between the GVL effect and GVHD.[22, 23] Withdrawal of immunosuppressive treatment given for prevention of GVHD

Table 46.1 Diseases Treated with Hematopoietic Transplantation

Malignant
    Leukemia
        Acute myeloid leukemia
        Myelodysplastic syndromes
        Acute lymphoblastic leukemia
        Chronic myeloid leukemia and related myeloproliferative disorders
        Chronic lymphocytic leukemia
    Non-Hodgkin's and Hodgkin's lymphoma
    Multiple myeloma and related plasma cell dyscrasias
    Solid tumors: breast, testicular, ovarian, small cell lung cancer; pediatric solid tumors: neuroblastoma,
        Ewing sarcoma, medulloblastoma, renal cell cancer, melanoma

Nonmalignant
    Aplastic anemia and related bone marrow failure states
    Paroxysmal noctural hemoglobinuria
    Hemoglobinopathies: thalassemia, sickle cell anemia
    Congenital disorders of hematopoiesis: Fanconi anemia and related syndromes
    Congenital immune deficiencies: serve combined immune deficiency, Wiskott-Aldrich syndrome,
        chronic granulomatous disease, and related syndromes
    Inborn errors of metabolism
    Autoimmune disorders: rheumatoid arthritis, systemic lupus erythematosus, multiple sclerosis and related syndromes

can occasionally lead to restoration of remission in patients having a relapse of their disease after HCT.[24] The most direct evidence of the GVL effect comes from the observation that infusion of donor lymphocytes (DLI) can reinduce remission in patients who have a relapse after HCT.[25, 26]

GVL effects have been best studied in patients with chronic myelogenous leukemia, a disease in which the Philadelphia chromosome and the resulting bcr-abl rearrangement can be used to detect residual leukemia cells. Minimal residual disease can frequently be detected by sensitive techniques early after allogeneic HCT.[27] In patients receiving syngeneic or T-cell–depleted transplants, these cells generally produce relapse.[21] In patients receiving unmodified (T-cell–replete) allografts, malignant cells are generally eliminated within 6 to 12 months, presumably related to an ongoing GVL effect. GVL effects have also been shown in acute myeloid leukemia (AML), myelodysplastic syndromes (MDSs), and chronic lymphocytic leukemia (CLL). GVM has been documented in multiple myeloma, indolent lymphomas, and Hodgkin disease.[28–31] GVM effects may also affect some solid tumors, particularly renal cell carcinoma[32] and breast cancer.[33]

GVL effects may be directed against certain potential target antigens. This process may involve immune reactivity against broadly expressed major or minor histocompatibility antigens, targets that overlap with those of GVHD. With DLIs, patients may achieve an antileukemic immune effect without developing clinical evidence of GVHD. In responding patients, host-derived normal hematopoietic cells are eliminated concomitantly with the malignant disease. These observations suggest that the GVL effect may result from reactivity against minor histocompatibility antigens restricted to the hematopoietic system and shared by normal and malignant hematopoietic cells *(antihematopoietic effect)*. Malignancy-specific antigens, such as the products of mutated or rearranged genes or overexpressed cellular antigens, may also be involved. Alternatively, a different threshold for GVL and GVHD may explain this phenomenon; malignant cells may be more sensitive than normal cells to a common immunologic mechanism. Development of

methods to separate GVL effects and GVHD, and to generate antigen-specific antitumor responses, is a major goal of ongoing research. In all, allogeneic HCT is a means to deliver dose-intensive chemoradiotherapy as well as a adoptive cellular immunotherapy for the treatment of malignant disease.

■ Donor Selection

For autologous HCT, the patient's own hematopoietic stem cells are used. Autologous transplants are most commonly used as a means to support dose-intensive cytotoxic therapy for treatment of malignant diseases. Autotransplants have the advantage that the hematopoietic cells will not be rejected or produce GVHD. However, autologous transplants may be contaminated by malignant cells and do not confer a GVL effect. Unmodified autologous transplants cannot be used for genetic or acquired diseases in which the hematopoietic cells are injured or defective, although autologous hematopoietic cells can potentially be used as vehicles for gene therapy designed to correct deficiency states.

Allogeneic transplants are collected from a related or an unrelated donor. The human leukocyte antigen (HLA) system is the major histocompatibility complex (MHC) in humans, and the results of allogeneic transplantation depend on the histocompatibility between donor and recipient. The HLA system is encoded by genes present in several closely linked loci on the short arm of chromosome 6.[34] Class I loci include HLA-A, HLA-B, and HLA-C alleles. The class II region includes HLA-DR, HLA-DQ, and HLA-DP loci. Compatibility was initially defined by serologic assays. The serologic groups were further divided into specific alleles by molecular oligonucleotide typing. Most transplants are performed from an HLA genotypically identical sibling donor; in this situation, each sibling has inherited the same pair of sixth chromosomes and the identical class I and II genes.

Most patients lack an HLA-identical sibling donor. Related donor-recipient pairs that are mismatched for only one A, B, or D HLA locus have a higher incidence of GVHD and graft failure, but survival similar to that in patients who receive transplants from HLA-identical siblings. Registries of potential unrelated donors have been established to provide HCT to patients lacking a histocompatible relative. HLA gene frequencies vary considerably among racial groups, and a patient is likely to find a match among potential donors of their own racial and ethnic group. Linkage disequilibrium occurs such that some common haplotypes occur, but approximately 50% of people have rare haplotypes. More than 4 million potential unrelated bone marrow donors are accessible in registries worldwide, and approximately half of patients can access an HLA-A–, HLA-B–, and HLA-DR–dentical donor. Unrelated donor transplants have been successful, although the incidence and severity of GVHD is increased compared with transplants from HLA-genotypically identical siblings.[35, 36] This phenomenon is presumably related to greater genetic disparity; these pairs are more likely to be mismatched for HLA variants and minor histocompatibility loci than related donors. Serologic HLA typing does not detect many clinically important molecular alleles, and molecular allele typing is now routinely performed for selection of donors.[37] Studies in which unrelated donors were selected using molecular allele typing methods have had a reduced risk of GVHD, and results are approaching those seen with transplants from HLA-identical siblings.[38, 39]

Recipients of related transplants mismatched for two or more loci have poorer results, with a high risk of graft rejection, GVHD, and other complications.[40, 41] Haploidentical donors are readily available for most patients. Aggressive T-cell depletion (4- to 5-log reduction) of the donor hematopoietic cells can prevent GVHD, but it results in a higher rate of graft failure. Results have been improved with the use of high "megadoses" of T-depleted peripheral blood progenitor cells (PBPCs) and with intensive myeloablative and immunosuppressive conditioning.[42, 43] Delayed immune reconstitution and opportunistic infections remain the major complications.

■ Preparative Regimen and Engraftment

The intensive pretransplant treatment is generally termed a *preparative regimen* or *conditioning*. This regimen provides intensive immunosuppression that is required to prevent rejection of an allogeneic hematopoietic transplant and to allow sustained engraftment. More intensive pretransplant immunosuppression is required for HCT than is necessary to prevent rejection of solid organ allografts such as kidney, liver, or heart. The immunosuppressive preparative treatment administered before transplantation must severely suppress the recipient's immunity, including T-lymphocyte and natural killer (NK) cell function. In addition, engraftment is enhanced by myelosuppressive preparative therapy, possibly by providing "space" in the bone marrow microenvironment to allow engraftment of hematopoietic stem cells.[44, 45] The intensity of immunosuppressive therapy required for engraftment varies, depending on the immunocompetence of the recipient and the composition of the transplanted cells. High doses of donor stem cells enhance engraftment, and T cells present in the allograft also enhance engraftment by an alloreactive antihematopoietic or graft-versus-host effect.[43, 46, 47]

For the treatment of malignant diseases, the preparative regimen is also directed at eradication of tumor or abnormal hematopoietic tissue. The preparative regimen generally involves chemotherapeutic drugs alone or in combination

with TBI. The classical ablative regimens used in the treatment of leukemia involve the combination of high-dose cyclophosphamide with either TBI[48, 49] or high-dose busulfan.[50, 51] Most studies did not find a survival advantage for one of the regimens. These regimens are sufficient to produce engraftment of more than 98% of allogeneic transplants from HLA-identical siblings. More intensive immunosuppression is necessary for HLA-nonidentical transplants or if T cells are depleted from the allograft, to prevent GVHD. The addition of other myeloablative drugs (e.g., thiotepa) or immunosuppressive drugs (e.g., antithymocyte globulin [ATG]) has been employed to enhance engraftment in these settings.

The use of myeloablative transplantation is limited to younger patients in good medical condition (see later). The discovery of the curative potential of the immune-mediated GVL effect led to a novel approach using lower-dose, relatively nontoxic preparative regimens. These nonmyeloablative conditioning regimens have been designed not to eradicate the malignant disease, but rather to provide sufficient immunosuppression to achieve engraftment and to allow induction of the GVL effect.[52–54] Further immune manipulations, such as early withdrawal of immunosuppressive therapy or DLI, may be required. These regimens were originally designed to extend the use of allogeneic transplants to older patients and to those with comorbidities who were not eligible to receive an ablative preparative regimen. Nonablative regimens are being investigated as an alternative strategy to reduce transplant-related morbidity in a variety of settings.[55–58] Most regimens include purine analogues as the immunosuppressive agents, but low-dose TBI has also been investigated for this purpose.[59, 60] Engraftment has been achieved in most patients, with favorable outcomes in patients with chemosensitive, low-burden disease.

■ Cell Sources for Hematopoietic Transplantation

HCT requires collection of sufficient numbers of hematopoietic stem cells for reconstitution of hematopoiesis and immunity in the recipient.[61, 62] A major area of ongoing research is characterization of the phenotype and of the function of hematopoietic stem cells. Human repopulating stem and progenitor cells express the CD34 cell-surface antigen, which comprises approximately 1% of the bone marrow.[63, 64] Highly enriched CD34 positively selected cells have been used for autologous or allogeneic HCT, with resulting rapid hematologic recovery.[65] Repopulating cells also express c-kit,[66] thy-1,[67] and AC133.[68] More primitive CD34– stem cells have been described that can differentiate into CD34+ progenitors.[69, 70] CD34 expression is reversibly expressed by activated stem cells.[71]

Hematopoietic stem cells primarily reside in the bone marrow, and, initially, the procedure involved collection and transplantation of bone marrow cells. Donors require general or regional anesthesia. One to 1.5 L of marrow is harvested by multiple aspirations, usually from the posterior superior iliac crests.[72] Adequate collections include 2 to 5×10^8 nucleated cells/kg and 0.5 to 3×10^6 CD34+ cells/kg. The procedure is generally safe for the donor. Rare complications may occur, primarily relating to general anesthesia and to infection or injury at the site of marrow aspirations.[73–78]

PBPCs have been used as an alternative source of hematopoietic cells for transplantation.[79, 80] Hematopoietic stem cells are present in low frequency in the peripheral blood, but they can be "mobilized" from the marrow during recovery from myelosuppressive chemotherapy and by treatment with various cytokines.[81, 82] Treatment with granulocyte colony-stimulating factor (G-CSF) increases the frequency of CD34+ cells 25-fold and allows collection of an adequate dose for transplantation by apheresis.[83] Stem cell factor,[84] thrombopoietin,[85] and flt-3 ligand[86] also mobilize progenitors, particularly in combination with G-CSF.

The rate of hematopoietic recovery after HCT depends on the number of CD34+ cells/kg infused. The minimum number of cells necessary for transplantation is not well defined, but optimal hematopoietic recovery requires $\geq 5 \times 10^6$ CD34+ cells/kg.[87] PBPCs produce more rapid hematologic recovery than bone marrow and are now used for most autologous transplants. PBPCs contain approximately 1 log more T cells than a bone marrow harvest, and this influences the immunologic effects after allogeneic HCT.[88] The rate of acute GVHD is unchanged with PBPCs compared with bone marrow,[89, 90] but chronic GVHD has been increased in several studies.[91, 92] Two studies reported improved early survival after allogeneic transplantation of PBPCs compared with bone marrow in high-risk patients.[92, 93] PBPCs have been used for unrelated allogeneic transplants.

Umbilical cord blood has been proposed as an alternative source of hematopoietic stem cells for transplantation from related or unrelated donors. Umbilical cord blood is relatively enriched for hematopoietic stem and progenitor cells.[94, 95] The major limitation is the small number of hematopoietic cells, less than 10% of the cell dose administered in typical BMT. Many unrelated cord blood registries and collection centers have been established.[96, 97] Transplant results have been related to the cell dose transplanted per kilogram of the recipient's body weight, with the best results if more than 3×10^8 nucleated cells/kg are infused.[98, 99] The time to engraftment and hematologic recovery after cord blood transplantation depend on the cell dose administered and may be prolonged to more than 6 weeks in some patients. Because of the size of the units, cord blood transplants have been most successful in children, but they are also under investigation in adults. Umbilical cord blood transplants have been associated with a relatively low rate of GVHD, and this feature has allowed the use of partially mismatched unrelated donors.[98–100]

Once the conditioning therapy is completed, the hematopoietic cells are infused intravenously. The cells circulate transiently, and sufficient numbers of stem cells home to the bone marrow to restore hematopoiesis. Peripheral blood counts are profoundly suppressed after high-dose chemotherapy but generally recover within 3 to 4 weeks after BMT. The date of engraftment is generally defined as the first of three consecutive white blood counts with an absolute neutrophil count greater than 0.5×10^9/L. The hematopoietic growth factors G-CSF and granulocyte-macrophage CSF (GM-CSF) accelerate recovery of granulocyte counts, but they have no effect on erythrocytes or platelets. Transplantation of PBPCs generally produces more rapid hematopoietic recovery than BMT and accelerates recovery of platelets as well as granulocytes.

Allogeneic engraftment of donor cells can be documented by acquisition of donor type cell-surface antigens, isoenzymes, chromosome markers, or DNA restriction fragment length polymorphisms.[101–105] After successful transplantation, cells of the hematologic and immunologic systems are primarily derived from the bone marrow donor, although in some cases, mixed chimerism occurs in which both donor- and recipient-derived cells are present. Mixed chimerism has been more frequent after T-cell depletion of the donor graft and after nonmyeloablative conditioning.[59] Most parenchymal cells of visceral organs and mesenchymal cells remain host in origin, although a small fraction are donor-derived.[106, 107]

■ Autologous Transplantation, Tumor Cell Contamination, and Purging

For autologous transplantation, the patient must first undergo collection of hematopoietic stem cells and cryopreservation.[108–110] Cryopreservation can be reliably performed, and the stored cells remain viable for more than 5 years.

Hematopoietic cell collection should ideally occur at a time when the bone marrow is normally cellular and the blood and marrow do not contain malignant cells. Malignant cells may contaminate autologous stem cell products; the likelihood varies by the diagnosis and disease stage. Mobilized PBPCs tend to have a lower frequency of tumor cell contamination than do bone marrow harvests.[111] PBPC transplants can be performed in patients in which marrow harvesting is not feasible, such as those with prior pelvic radiotherapy.

Tumor cells can be identified in histologically normal product by a variety of techniques including cell culture, flow cytometry, immunohistochemistry, and polymerase chain reaction (PCR) for amplification of clone specific markers, such as a typical translocation or immunoglobulin gene rearrangement. Gene marking studies using retroviral gene vectors have shown that tumor cells contained in the graft can contribute to relapse in patients with leukemia, neuroblastoma, and presumably other diagnoses.[112–114] Numerous clinical studies have shown that tumor cell contamination of the autograft is associated with shortened disease-free survival.[115–117] Purging methods have been developed to deplete tumor cells from the autograft in an attempt to improve outcomes.[118] Purging methods most often use monoclonal antibodies combined with complement, immunomagnetic beads or conjugated toxins.[115] Positive selection of CD34+ cells is another widely used approach,[119–121] and combined methods are investigated as a potentially better purging strategy. Pharmacologic purging include ex vivo treatment of the autograft with chemotherapeutic agents such as 4-hydroxycyclophosphamide and are mostly applied to autografts of patients with AML.[122, 123]

The clinical benefit of purging is not well documented. Successful purging of marrow harvests of patients with follicular lymphoma or with breast cancer were associated with superior outcome.[115–117] However, the presence of tumor cells in the autograft may correlate with the extent of systemic residual disease, and this is not a direct evidence that reinfused tumor cells caused relapse. Most patients relapse in sites of prior disease, and inadequate systemic cytoreduction is believed to be the major cause of relapse. An alternative explanation is that tumor cells in the graft home preferentially to sites of prior disease where the microenvironment supports their growth. There are no randomized studies documenting reduced relapse rates using purged versus unpurged autologous transplants, and the role of purging remains controversial.

■ Selection of Autologous or Allogeneic Transplantation

Selection of the type of transplantation for a patient, autologous or allogeneic, depends on the type of malignant disease, age, availability of a suitable donor, ability to collect a tumor-free autograft, stage and status of disease (e.g., bone marrow involvement, bulk of disease, and chemosensitivity to conventional chemotherapy), and the susceptibility of the disease to GVM effects. The advantages and disadvantages of autologous versus allogeneic transplants are outlined in Table 46.2.

Autologous transplantation is readily available, and no need exists to identify a donor. The patient has no risk of GVHD and no need for immunosuppressive therapy to prevent GVHD and graft rejection. Immune reconstitution after autologous HCT is faster than after allogeneic transplants and the risk of opportunistic infections is low. Graft failure occurs rarely. Treatment-related mortality is lower than 5% in most studies, and elderly patients can tolerate treatment relatively well.[124, 125] However, autologous transplants have several drawbacks. The autograft may be contaminated with clonogenic tumor cells that can contribute to relapse of disease. Autologous transplantation relies solely on the effect of high-dose cytoreductive treatment, and it lacks the allogeneic immune-mediated GVM effect. In most malignant diseases, relapse rates are higher after autologous HCT than with allogeneic HCT, although this difference is offset in some settings by a lower rate of treatment-related mortality. Prior therapy, especially with multiple courses of alkylating agents or purine analogues, may deplete the stem cell pool and may result in poor stem cell collection and persistent pancytopenia after HCT.[126] Patients with extensive prior therapy are also at high risk of developing myelodysplasia and secondary acute leukemia after autologous HCT.[127, 128]

Allogeneic HCT has the advantage that the graft is free of contaminating tumor cells. In addition, the graft contains donor-immunocompetent cells that may produce an immune GVM effect. This situation generally leads to a lower risk of disease recurrence than with autologous HCT. However, allogeneic transplants may be associated with certain potentially fatal complications such as graft rejection and GVHD. Immune reconstitution is slower after allogeneic HCT, and opportunistic infections are more frequent. Treatment-related mortality is significantly higher after allografts than with autologous transplants. Only 20% to 30% of patients have an HLA-identical related donor available. Treatment-related mortality is increased with mismatched or unrelated allogeneic transplants.

Allogeneic HCT has usually been limited to younger patients in good general condition because of the increased risk of regimen-related toxicity and GVHD with advanced age. Improvement in supportive care, infection control, and GVHD prophylaxis and treatment have enabled many centers to treat older patients, but only a few centers consider patients older than 55 to 60 years. Most malignant diseases that are effectively treated by allogeneic HCT are more common in elderly patients. Nonmyeloablative conditioning regimens are under evaluation to reduce the risk of allogeneic transplantation in elderly patients, with induction of the GVM effect as the primary goal of treatment.[52, 55, 59]

In general, allogeneic transplants have been used predominantly in the treatment of leukemia—AML, chronic myeloid leukemia (CML), and acute lymphoblastic leukemia (ALL)—and myelodysplasia. Autologous transplants have been used more often in solid tumors, lymphoma, and myeloma. Understanding of the role of the GVM effect in certain diseases, as well as the ability to collect a tumor-free autograft and to employ better cytoreductive treatments, may change the trend in certain diseases.

The outcome of HCT relates to the selection of patients and the timing of transplantation during the natural history of the malignant disease. The best results occur when HCT is performed early in the disease course, when the malignancy is still sensitive to chemoradiotherapy treatment and the tumor burden is low. Conversely, HCT done as last resort is associated with high rates of both relapse and treatment-related toxicity. The patient with a malignant disease may also develop infection, organ toxicity, or poor performance status over time, which markedly increases the risk of transplant-related complications. In general, transplantation should be offered early to patients with diseases that are at high risk of relapse or transformation to a more aggressive form, as well as to patients with early disease recurrence. Patients with high cure rates with conventional chemotherapy, such as AML with favorable cytogenetics or standard-risk ALL, are generally not

Table 46.2 Advantages and Disadvantages of Autologous and Allogeneic Transplantation

	Autologous	Allogeneic
Availability	Readily available	Need for a histocompatible donor
Graft rejection	None	2%–20% (depending on HLA matching)
Graft-versus-host disease	None, no need for immunosuppressive treatment	20%–>50% depending on HLA match and donor type; immunosuppressive treatment required
Immune reconstitution	Rapid, infections less frequent	Slow, infections more frequent
Treatment-related mortality	< 5%	20%–40% depends on patient and disease factors (lower for nonablative (regimens)
Patient eligibility	< 70 yr, normal organ function	<55 yr, normal organ function (older patients and with comorbidities may be eligible for nonablative regimens)
Graft-versus-leukemia effect	None	Operative in certain malignant diseases
Tumor cell contamination of graft	Frequent	None
Post-transplant relapse rate	Higher	Lower

offered HCT during the first remission. The possibility of future HCT should be considered early in the course of appropriate malignant diseases, and early identification of a potential donor is advisable so that a transplant procedure can be promptly performed should the disease recur. The specific indications for allogeneic and autologous transplantation are further discussed for each specific diagnosis.

Response to conventional chemotherapy generally determines the likelihood of response to transplant. Demonstration of chemosensitivity is usually required before one attempts autologous HCT. The best results have been achieved in patients with chemosensitive disease relapse or when HCT is performed in high-risk patients as consolidation of response, particularly in patients with minimal disease at the time of the transplant procedure. Patients with partial response to initial chemotherapy are also good candidates. Primary resistance can sometimes be overcome by dose-intensive treatment, such as in patients with primary refractory acute leukemia, Hodgkin disease, or multiple myeloma, early in the course. However, patients with bulky disease, refractory relapse, or multiple relapses of malignant disease generally have poor results.

■ Complications of Hematopoietic Cell Transplantation

Intensive chemoradiotherapy and HCT may be associated with certain serious complications, as listed in Table 46.3. These include the following: toxicities resulting from the pretransplant conditioning regimen; infections resulting from neutropenia; and post-transplant immunodeficiency and

Table 46.3   Complications of Hematopoietic Transplantation

Regimen-related toxicity
    Mucositis and gastroenteritis
    Veno-occlusive disease of the liver
    Interstitial pneumonitis
    Diffuse alveolar hemorrhage
    Hemorrhagic cystitis
    Cytokine release syndrome (engraftment syndrome)
    Thrombotic thrombocytopenic purpura and hemolytic disorders
    Encephalopathy
    Cyclophosphamide- or radiation-induced myocarditis or pericarditis
    Renal failure

Immune-mediated disorders
    Graft failure
    Acute graft-versus-host disease
    Chronic graft-versus-host disease

Infections and immunodeficiency
    Bacterial
    Fungal: *Candida* species, *Aspergillus* species, others
    Viral: cytomegalovirus, herpesviruses, respiratory viruses, adenoviruses, hepatitis viruses, others
    Epstein-Barr virus–associated lymphoproliferative disease
    Parasitic: *Pneumocystis carinii*

Recurrent disease

Late complications
    Growth disturbances
    Poor dentition
    Hypothyroidism
    Sterility and hypogonadism
    Cataracts
    Avascular necrosis of bone
    Hypertension
    Secondary malignant diseases

immune-mediated processes, such as graft rejection and GVHD. Relapse of the original malignant disease is one of the major causes of treatment failure. Some of these complications are specific clinicopathologic syndromes unique to HCT. Several processes may coexist. Clinical assessment and histopathologic evaluation are necessary for accurate diagnosis and treatment.

Graft Failure and Graft-versus-Host Disease

Graft failure is defined as the failure to establish hematopoietic engraftment (primary graft failure) or loss of an established graft (secondary graft failure). Operationally, this entity is defined when granulocytes fail to recover to more than $0.5 \times 10^9/L$ or fall to less than this level for more than 3 days after initial recovery. Graft failure after autologous HCT occurs rarely and is most often related to infusion of an inadequate stem cell number or ex vivo manipulations of the autograft. Purging techniques that may injure or reduce the numbers of hematopoietic stem cells increase the risk of graft failure, and it is recommended that autologous untreated, backup marrow or PBPCs be stored when one plans high-risk graft manipulations; this backup collection can be infused to rescue patients if graft failure occurs.

Graft failure after allogeneic HCT is most commonly the result of immunologic rejection. *Graft rejection* is caused by host-derived cytotoxic T lymphocytes or NK cells directed against donor hematopoietic cells.[129, 130] Rejection occurs in fewer than 2% of transplants from an HLA-identical sibling. The risk is increased up to 10% to 20% in recipients of HLA-mismatched or matched unrelated donor transplants.[41, 131, 132] CD8+ T lymphocytes posses a graft facilitating effect, and T-lymphocyte depletion from the allogeneic graft increases the risk of graft failure.[133, 134] Other accessory cells with graft-facilitating activity also exist.[135] The barrier for engraftment can be overcome by infusion of a larger number of stem cells[43] and by intensifying the myeloablative and immunosuppressive intensity of the preparative regimen.[42]

Graft failure or poor graft function may be caused by various drugs, by GVHD, and by infections that occur in the early post-transplant period. Ganciclovir, given for prevention or treatment of cytomegalovirus (CMV) infections, is the most common drug producing graft failure; this failure is generally reversible when the drug is discontinued. Trimethoprim-sulfamethoxazole, given to prevent *Pneumocystis carinii* infections, is modestly myelosuppressive, and it only rarely produces graft failure. CMV,[136] parvovirus,[137] human herpesvirus 6,[138] and mycobacterial and fungal infections may also compromise the graft. Occasionally, poor engraftment results from microenvironment or marrow stroma dysfunction related to prior therapy.

Graft failure that is not the result of rejection can often be successfully treated with the growth factors G-CSF or GM-CSF.[139, 140] A second stem cell infusion from the same donor or an alternative donor, after further immunosuppression with ATG, corticosteroids, or other agents, may result in successful engraftment. Autologous backup stem cells stored before HCT can rescue a patient with graft failure.

Acute Graft-versus-Host Disease

GVHD is a major, potentially life-threatening complication of allogeneic transplantation. GVHD is divided into two clinical syndromes, depending on the time of onset. Acute GVHD typically develops within the first 100 days after HCT, whereas chronic GVHD develops later, although the classic manifestations of chronic GVHD may occur as early as 50 days after transplantation.

Acute GVHD results from reactivity of donor T lymphocytes directed against disparate major or minor histocompatibility antigens of the recipient. The current understanding of the pathogenesis of acute GVHD suggests three phases.[141] The first involves conditioning regimen–related tissue injury resulting in cytokine release, upregulation of HLA molecules, activation of macrophages, and generation of a proinflammatory state. During the second phase, alloreactive T cells recognize antigen disparities presented on host dendritic cells, are activated, and are expanded. The third phase includes generation of effector cells and cytokines that cause tissue injury and inflammation. Acute GVHD requires the presence of donor T lymphocytes and recipient antigen-presenting cells.[142]

Clinically, acute GVHD involves the skin, the gastrointestinal (GI) tract, and the liver. The hematopoietic and immune systems are also targets. Patients with acute GVHD have more severe immunodeficiency and are at high risk of infection. It is unclear why other tissues are not directly affected by GVHD. A maculopapular rash, which is typically pruritic and confluent, is usually the first presentation. When the condition is severe, generalized erythroderma, bullae, and desquamation may occur. Acute GVHD of the liver targets the biliary epithelium and produces cholestatic hepatitis, with marked elevation of bilirubin and alkaline phosphatase. Synthetic function is usually preserved early in the course of the disease. GVHD can affect the entire GI tract, by targeting epithelial cells. GI GVHD characteristically produces secretory diarrhea, abdominal pain, and, on rare occasions, ileus. Upper GI GVHD produces nausea, vomiting, and anorexia, which may occur without lower GI or other tissue involvement.[143] Conjunctivitis and other ocular manifestations, anemia, and thrombocytopenia may also occur.

Acute GVHD is a clinical syndrome, and its diagnosis should be based on clinical assessment, supported by biopsies of involved tissues.[144, 145] The staging and grading of acute GVHD are based on the severity of involvement of the various tissues and are outlined in Table 46.4. In general, grade I is mild and does not require treatment. Grade II is moderate and requires systemic treatment, and grades III and IV are severe and life-threatening. Severe GVHD is associated with a poor prognosis because of direct tissue damage, debilitation, and severe immunodeficiency caused by both the GVHD process itself and its treatment with immunosuppressive drugs.

The most important factor in predicting the risk of occurrence of GVHD is HLA disparity between the donor and the recipient.[39, 146] With current immunosuppressive prophylaxis, the incidence of GVHD in recipients of hematopoietic transplants from an HLA-identical sibling is 25% to 50% and is directed against minor histocompatibility antigens. A higher incidence, up to 70% to 90%, has been reported after

Table 46.4 Clinical Staging and Grading of Graft-versus-Host Disease

Acute			
Stage	Skin*	Liver[†]	Gut[†]
1	Maculopapular rash < 25%	Bilirubin 2–3 mg/dL	Diarrhea 500–1000 mL or persistent nausea[‡]
2	Maculopapular rash 25%–50%	Bilirubin 3–6 mg/dL	Diarrhea 1000–1500 mL
3	Generalized erythroderma	Bilirubin 6–15 mg/dL	Diarrhea > 1500 mL
4	Desquamation and bullae	Bilirubin > 15 mg/dL	Severe abdominal pain or ileus

Overall Grade[§]	Severity	Skin		Liver		Gut
0	None	0		0		0
I	Mild	1–2		0		0
II	Moderate	3	or	1	or	1
III	Severe			2–3	or	2–3
IV"	Life-threatening	4	or	4	or	4

Chronic[¶]	
Limited	Localized skin involvement and/or hepatic dysfunction
Extensive	1. Generalized skin involvement or 2. Localized skin involvement and/or hepatic dysfunction, plus any of the following: a. liver histology showing chronic aggressive hepatitis, bridging necrosis or cirrhosis b. eye involvement (Schirmer test < 5 mm wetting) c. involvement of mucosalivary glands or oral mucosa d. involvement of any other target organ

*Extents determined by rule of nines or burn chart.
[†]Downgrade one stage for additional causes of elevated bilirubin or diarrhea.
[‡]Requires histologic evidence of GVHD in the stomach or duodenum.
[§]Minimal organ stage required to determined grade.
"Grade IV may also be determined with lower organ involvement with extreme decrease in performance status.
[¶]Data from reference 551.
Data from gluclesberg H, Storb R, Fefer A: Clinical manifestations of graft-versus-host disease in human recipients of marrow from HLA-identical sibling donors. Transplantation 1974;18:295–304; and Przepiorlea D, Weisdorf D, Martin P, et al: Consensus conference on acute GVHD grading. Bone marrow Transplant 1995;15:825–828.

receipt of transplants from mismatched and unrelated donors. Allelic molecular matching for class I and II HLA molecules has reduced this incidence toward the rates observed in matched siblings, although greater disparity for minor histocompatibility antigens in unrelated donors will likely continue to produce a higher risk of GVHD.[147] Older age is associated with an increased incidence of GVHD. Increased donor age has also been shown to be associated with a higher incidence of GVHD in unrelated donor transplants. Male-related minor histocompatibility antigens, H-Y, are potential targets of GVHD.[148] Sex-mismatched grafts (female donor→male recipient) have a higher rate of associated acute GVHD, particularly if the female donor is sensitized to male antigens by pregnancy or prior blood transfusions.[149, 150] Despite infusion of greater numbers of lymphocytes, PBPC transplants are not associated with increased rates of acute GVHD compared with BMT, although chronic GVHD may be increased.[92] Umbilical cord blood transplants are associated with a lower incidence of GVHD than bone marrow allografts.[151]

Less intensive, nonmyeloablative conditioning regimens may also limit the severity of GVHD, presumably by reducing toxicities and generation of inflammatory cytokines that facilitates development of GVHD.[54] Some studies show a role of host and donor infection with herpesviruses that increases the risk of GVHD.[152]

The most effective method for prevention of GVHD is depletion of T lymphocytes from the graft by various techniques.[21, 153–157] However, this method has not resulted in better survival because of the increased risk of graft failure, relapse, and opportunistic infections caused by loss of graft facilitation, the GVM effect, and anti-infection immunity effects of T cells, respectively. Pharmacologic immunosuppression, administered immediately before HCT and in the first several months afterward, is the alternative method of prevention of GVHD. Corticosteroids, methotrexate, ATG, cyclosporine, and tacrolimus (FK506) have been used for GVHD prevention. The standard regimen currently combines cyclosporine or FK506 with three or four doses of methotrexate administered in the first 11 days after HCT[158–160] Cyclosporine and FK506 prevent activation of T cells, whereas methotrexate targets T cells that were activated at the early post-transplant phase by host antigens. The addition of corticosteroids is the first line of therapy in patients who develop acute GVHD. These drugs may be administered topically for limited GVHD of the skin, but they are usually administered intravenously at a starting dose of methylprednisolone 2 mg/kg for other manifestations. Approximately half of patients have a sustained response,[161] and the steroid dose can be tapered gradually. Steroid-resistant GVHD has an unfavorable prognosis. Although 30% to 40% of the patients respond to second-line therapy such as ATG,[162] most patients succumb to infections or direct manifestations of GVHD. The prognosis is best for GVHD limited to the skin. Acute GVHD involving the liver or multiple organs has a poorer prognosis; only 30% of patients respond to immunosuppressive therapy. Newer investigational agents for treatment of acute GVHD include monoclonal antibodies against activated T cells, such as anti-CD25,[163] sirolimus, and cytokine inhibitors. Successful treatment requires meticulous supportive care with special attention to prevention of opportunistic infections. Octreotide (a somatostatin analogue) has been useful in controlling secretory diarrhea associated with GVHD.[164]

Chronic Graft-versus-Host Disease

Chronic GVHD is a related syndrome affecting 25% to 40% of recipients of allogeneic transplantation who survive more than 3 months after the procedure.[165] It most often occurs between 90 and 200 days after transplantation, but the onset may be delayed to the second year. Chronic GVHD is more common in older patients and in patients with prior acute GVHD, although approximately one third of affected patients have a de novo presentation without prior acute GVHD.[165, 166] Chronic GVHD may be more prevalent after HCT with PBPCs than after BMT.[92]

Chronic GVHD has protean clinical manifestation similar to those seen in several autoimmune disorders, such as progressive systemic sclerosis, Sjögren syndrome, and primary biliary cirrhosis.[167, 168] It is a syndrome of immune dysregulation with generation of autoreactive T cells directed against shared MHC determinants and production of autoantibodies. Chronic GVHD is associated with thymic dysfunction and failure of the thymus to delete autoreactive cells and induce tolerance. Chronic GVHD is also associated with profound immunosuppression, and the major risk to these patients relates to the high incidence of opportunistic infections.

Chronic GVHD most often involves the skin, liver, oral cavity, and eyes. Skin involvement may be acute, with erythema, hyperkeratosis, and desquamation, or it may be more insidious, with gradual thickening and tightness of the skin and limitation of joint flexibility. Additional symptoms include a sicca syndrome with dry eyes, dry mouth, and lichenoid changes in the oral cavity. Liver involvement produces cholestatic changes. Bronchiolitis obliterans is a life-threatening complication that may occur without other major manifestations of chronic GVHD and may result in pulmonary failure.[169] Intestinal involvement with anorexia, dysphagia, malabsorption, and wasting is now rare. Serositis and autoimmune manifestations also occur rarely. Secondary infections are common causes of morbidity and mortality. Chronic GVHD may become a chronic debilitating disease affecting quality of life, and it remains the major determinant of late transplant-related morbidity.[170, 171]

Chronic GVHD is classified as *limited* when it involves certain regions of the skin and or liver (see Table 46.4). It is considered *extensive* when it involves multiple organs, when skin involvement is extensive, or when the liver histology indicates advanced changes. The prognosis of chronic GVHD is worse when it is extensive and in the progressive form. Thrombocytopenia has been associated with a poor outcome.[171]

Corticosteroids are the first line of therapy for chronic GVHD.[172] The chronic nature of this syndrome requires long-term therapy for at least 6 to 9 months, and therefore reduced doses and, if possible, alternate-day doses are preferable, to minimize the complications resulting from long-term steroid therapy. Cyclosporine and FK506 are used in combination with steroids in high-risk patients, as defined earlier, or in patients with poor response to steroids.[173, 174] Mycophenolate mofetil has some efficacy and is useful as a steroid-sparing agent, to allow reduction of the corticosteroid dose.[175] Thalidomide is an effective agent for salvage therapy in some patients.[176] Psoralen plus ultraviolet A light[177] or extracorporeal photopheresis is also studied as an effective treatment modality.[178, 179] Aggressive antimicrobial prophylaxis and early treatment of infections are essential.

■ Organ Toxicity from High-Dose Chemotherapy

Pretransplant cytoreductive treatment approaches the limit of tolerance for several tissues. The lungs and liver are the most susceptible to toxic damage, but severe toxicity may also involve the GI tract, heart, bladder, nervous system, and, rarely other tissues. The actual risk of toxicity results from a complex interrelationship of predisposing, preexisting factors, the preparative regimen, and other post-transplant complications. Investigators continuously search for more effective and less toxic conditioning regimens to improve the outcome after HCT.

Oral Mucositis and Gastroenteritis

In patients receiving HCT, the dose-limiting toxicity of TBI and many chemotherapy drugs is in the GI tract. *Oral mucositis* and chemoradiotherapy-related *gastroenteritis* frequently occur during the initial several weeks after HCT.[180] The severity depends on the intensity of the conditioning regimen. This results in dysphagia, pain, nausea, and diarrhea. Extremely severe mucositis may result in upper airway obstruction and aspiration pneumonitis, and gastroenteritis may be complicated by GI bleeding. Treatment is supportive and includes continuous intravenous narcotics for pain relief, intravenous fluids, and, if necessary, parenteral hyperalimentation. Mucositis and GI toxicity usually resolve after engraftment.

Veno-occlusive Disease

Veno-occlusive disease (VOD) of the liver is defined clinically by the combination of direct hyperbilirubinemia, painful hepatomegaly, and fluid retention with ascites and weight gain. It is the result of hepatic toxicity of chemotherapy and radiation and complicates 10% to 60% of HCT cases.[181–183] The onset of VOD is usually before day 30 after transplantation. The severity of VOD is classified as mild (when it requires no treatment and resolves completely), moderate (when it requires treatment but resolves completely by day 100), or severe (when it does not resolve completely or results in death). Severe VOD may result in multiorgan failure, renal or pulmonary failure, and encephalopathy, and it is usually fatal.

VOD is more common in patients with pretransplant active hepatitis, hepatic fibrosis or cirrhosis, iron overload, or abnormal liver function tests.[184] It is more common in patients with prior transplantation or prior radiation to the liver, with more intensive conditioning regimens using increased total-dose or single-dose radiation, and with the use of busulfan, especially associated with higher plasma levels. VOD may also be more frequent in recipients of mismatched and unrelated allogeneic transplants.

VOD is a hepatotoxic process with endothelial damage, obstruction of small intrahepatic venules, and damage to the centrilobular hepatocytes and sinusoids. The clinical diagnosis requires two of three criteria—jaundice, hepatomegaly, and ascites—occurring within 20 days after transplantation. VOD resulting from the preparative regimen should be differentiated from other drug toxicity (especially that caused by cyclosporine, methotrexate, or trimethoprim-sulfamethoxazole), GVHD, sepsis, and congestive heart failure. Ultrasound scanning of the abdomen may show hepatomegaly, ascites, and reversal of portal flow. The definite diagnosis relies on histologic evaluation. Transjugular liver biopsy can be performed, even in thrombocytopenic patients, and the hepatic wedge pressure can be determined (greater than 10 mm Hg is suggestive of VOD).[185]

Treatment of VOD is primarily supportive and includes restriction of sodium and water, use of diuretics, and control of pain. Heparin has been reported as potentially useful prophylactically to prevent VOD,[186, 187] but this agent is not widely used because of concern regarding bleeding. Ursodiol has been shown to be useful in prevention of VOD and may be considered in patients at high risk of developing VOD.[188] As treatment, thrombolytic therapy has resulted in contradictory outcomes and is limited by the high risk of bleeding.[189, 190] Transjugular intrahepatic portal-systemic shunting has been used to control ascites.[191] Defibrotide, a drug with fibrinolytic activity, has had encouraging results.[192] Liver transplantation have been successful in rare patients.[193] Dialysis and mechanical ventilation have been used in patients with severe multiorgan failure, albeit with little impact on survival.

Pulmonary Toxicity

Regimen-related *pulmonary toxicity* occurs in up to 10% of recipients of HCT.[194, 195] The *idiopathic pneumonia syndrome* relates to a syndrome of diffuse pulmonary inflammation in the absence of identifiable infectious pathogens.[196] This syndrome occurs more frequently in recipients of allogeneic transplants and may be more common after receipt of transplants from an unrelated donor. It has been associate with TBI-containing cytoreductive regimens, and the risks increases with a larger total dose and dose rate. Cyclophosphamide, busulfan, and carmustine (BCNU) are also associated with pulmonary toxicity. Advanced age, prior radiation therapy to the chest, acute GVHD, and the use of methotrexate are other risk factors for the idiopathic pneumonia syndrome.

Patients with the idiopathic pneumonia syndrome may present with fever, nonproductive cough, tachypnea, hypoxemia, and diffuse interstitial or alveolar infiltrates on chest radiography. Idiopathic pneumonia usually occurs early in the course within a few weeks of HCT. The presentation is nonspecific and cannot be differentiated easily from an infection. Bronchoalveolar lavage (BAL) is essential for the diagnosis of infectious process but is often nondiagnostic. Open lung biopsy may be needed for definite diagnosis. Rapid deterioration with development of hypoxemic respiratory failure is common, and mortality exceeds 60%. Treatment is predominantly supportive. High-dose corticosteroids are of unproven efficacy, except in certain instances.

Pneumonitis is particularly common in patients receiving BCNU at high doses as a preparative regimen for autologous HCT.[197] The onset may be delayed until a few months after the transplant procedure. Early recognition of the condition and administration of high-dose corticosteroids are essential to avoid a fatal outcome.

Diffuse alveolar hemorrhage occurs among recipients of autologous and allogeneic transplants. It is defined by hypoxemia, rapid onset of diffuse alveolar opacities, and progressively bloody return from BAL. Overt hemoptysis is rare. The condition usually occurs early in the course and coincides with engraftment. It seems likely that, like idiopathic pneumonia, this disorder is related to lung injury by the preparative regimen, cytokine release, acute GVHD, or infection in the presence of thrombocytopenia. Late-onset diffuse alveolar hemorrhage is most often associated with underlying infection. Treatment includes high-dose corticosteroids and correction of thrombocytopenia or underlying coagulopathy.[198] Pulmonary infiltrates may occur as part of the *engraftment syndrome*.[199] This is a poorly defined syndrome of fever, skin rash, capillary leak, and transient pulmonary infiltrates, and it relates to cytokine release at the time of engraftment. A short course of high-dose corticosteroids is the appropriate treatment.

Approximately 10% of allogeneic transplant recipients with chronic GVHD develop progressive airflow obstruction consistent with *bronchiolitis obliterans*.[200] It occurs late in the course and may lead to respiratory failure. It is usually treated with immunosuppressive treatment and aggressive infection prevention and control. Pulmonary VOD is another rare cause of late-onset respiratory failure in the absence of pulmonary infiltrates.

Hemorrhagic Cystitis

Hemorrhagic cystitis is a common occurrence after high-dose cyclophosphamide, but it may also occur after other chemotherapy or radiation treatments.[201] The damage to the bladder wall is mediated by acrolein, a metabolite of cyclophosphamide that is toxic to transitional epithelium.[202] Hemorrhagic cystitis may be associated with viral infection of the bladder, most commonly with polyoma virus, adenovirus, and CMV.[203, 204] Hemorrhagic cystitis may develop acutely or as delayed complication weeks to months after HCT. Patients may present with suprapubic pain, dysuria, hematuria, urinary frequency, and obstruction of urinary flow by clots. The course may be protracted and resistant to therapy, with recurrent flares of symptoms. Mesna is a uroprotective agent that binds to acrolein and, together with hyperhydration, may reduce the risk of bladder toxicity.[205] Some centers advocate prophylactic bladder irrigation.[206] Initial treatment of hemorrhagic cystitis includes hydration and correction of thrombocytopenia. Bladder irrigation and aggressive pain control are frequently required. When these measures fail, cauterization or fulguration with formalin may control symptoms. On rare occasions, superpubic cystotomy or cystectomy needs to be performed.[207]

Hemolytic Complications

Hemolytic reactions may result from ABO incompatibility between the donor and the recipient. The incompatibility may be major when the recipient plasma contains isohemagglutinins against donor RBC or minor when the donor plasma contains isohemagglutinins against recipient RBC. ABO incompatibility is not a contraindication for allogeneic transplant. Red blood cells should be removed from the donor graft to prevent acute hemolytic reaction with major ABO incompatibility, and plasma should be removed in pairs with minor ABO incompatibility. Delayed hemolysis, delayed erythropoiesis, and even pure red blood cell aplasia can complicate ABO incompatibility.

Thrombotic microangiopathy may occur after transplantation, with a range of symptoms from asymptomatic laboratory evidence of microangiopathy to full-blown thrombotic thrombocytopenic purpura. Factors implicated in initiating endothelial injury include chemotherapeutic agents, radiation, cyclosporine and FK506, CMV and fungal infections, and cytokine-release syndromes. Treatment with plasma exchange

results in response in some patients. Early onset of thrombotic thrombocytopenic purpura, association with cyclosporine and FK506, and neurologic manifestations have been associated with poor outcome, with a mortality rate of 85% when two or three of these risk factors are present.

Other Organ Toxicities

Cardiac toxicity is most often related to high-dose cyclophosphamide.[208] Abnormalities range from asymptomatic electrocardiographic abnormalities and pericarditis to hemorrhagic myocardial necrosis resulting in fatal heart failure. Corticosteroids have been employed in the treatment of these complications, with variable success.

Renal toxicity is common and multifactorial and most often results from the use of nephrotoxic drugs such as cyclosporine, FK506, amphotericin, foscarnet, and nephrotoxic antibiotics.[209] Renal failure may complicate sepsis or VOD as part of a multiorgan failure state.

Metabolic encephalopathy may complicate sepsis, renal, hepatic, or respiratory failure, or the use of sedative-hypnotic drugs. Cyclosporine and FK506 used for prevention of GVHD may be associated with a variety of neurologic complications including tremor, headaches, seizures, and encephalopathy, with more pronounced involvement of the occipital lobes.[210, 211] Magnetic resonance imaging typically shows multifocal T2-weighted hyperintense white matter lesions. Treatment requires discontinuing the medication or decreasing the dose.

Late Complications

Late complications include cataracts, dental abnormalities, hypothyroidism and hypogonadism, permanent sterility in most but not all patients, growth retardation, osteoporosis, and avascular necrosis of the hip or other bones.[165, 212, 213]

Patients have an increased risk of solid and hematologic secondary tumors after HCT.[214, 215] Solid tumors, mostly head and neck cancers, squamous cell carcinomas, melanomas, and brain and thyroid cancers, are more common in recipients of TBI-containing regimens, and the cumulative incidence is up to 7% at 15 years. Myelodysplasia and secondary leukemia occur more commonly after autologous HCT, in 4% to 18% of patients within 2.5 to 8.5 years of the transplantation procedure.[216, 217] Data suggest that myelodysplasia is associated more with extensive prior therapy, rather than with the high-dose chemotherapy given before the transplant per se.

■ Immunodeficiency and Infections

Recipients of hematopoietic transplants have a severe *immunodeficiency* state involving both T and B cells. Intensive preparative regimens ablate the host immune system. Myeloid cells, macrophages and monocytes, and lymphocytes are subsequently produced from precursor cells present in the graft. The most profound abnormalities occur within the first 6 months, followed by slow recovery over the first year. Patients with HLA-mismatched or unrelated donor transplants have more severe immunodeficiency and risk of *opportunistic infections*, particularly if T-cell depletion is used to prevent GVHD.[218] Recipients of autologous and syngeneic transplants also have a period of immunodeficiency, but their recovery may be more rapid, and post-transplant infections are less frequent and severe than after allogeneic HCT.

Patients with chronic GVHD have a profound immunodeficiency state for prolonged periods and are highly susceptible to unusual infections. Recipients of hematopoietic transplants may be susceptible to unusual opportunistic infections and also to acute overwhelming infections. Prophylactic strategies against an array of potential infections and rapid recognition and treatment of infections are essential parts of successful management of transplant recipients.[219] Immunoglobulin repletion should be considered in patients with documented immunoglobulin deficiency. Revaccinations should be performed on immune recovery. Isolation measurements, especially meticulous hand washing, are important in prevention of nosocomial acquisition of infections.

Bacterial Infections

Bacterial infections are common in the early post-transplantation period because of neutropenia, disruption of normal mucosal barriers, and the nearly universal use of indwelling intravenous catheters. The most common bacterial pathogens during this period are gram-positive aerobic bacteria such as coagulase-negative staphylococci and α-hemolytic streptococci. Gram-negative enteric bacteria are also common pathogens. Vancomycin is an effective prophylactic treatment against gram-positive bacteria; it should be used conservatively, given the emergence of vancomycin-resistant enterococci.[220, 221] Penicillin is often used as an alternative for infection prophylaxis. Quinolones (such as norfloxacin or ciprofloxacin) are used for prevention of enteric gram-negative infections during the time of neutropenia.[222] Treatment of fever in the neutropenic transplant recipient requires early initiation of broad-spectrum intravenous antibiotics.[223, 224]

B-cell function recovery may be delayed, and transplant recipients, especially those with chronic GVHD, may suffer from hypogammaglobulinemia, opsonization defect, and functional hyposplenia. These patients are more prone to infections with encapsulated bacteria, such as pneumococci and *Haemophilus*, as late as 1 year after HCT. Continuous antibacterial prophylaxis should be considered for these patients, and vaccinations against pneumococci and *Haemophilus* are recommended early during the second year after HCT.[225]

Fungal Infections

Invasive *fungal infections* remain a significant hazard for transplant recipients. Fungal infection may occur during the neutropenic phase or later, during the first few months after transplant until immune recovery, and especially in patients immunocompromised by GVHD and corticosteroid therapy.[226] *Candida albicans* infections have become much less frequent since the introduction of fluconazole as prophylaxis against systemic candidiasis.[227, 228] Fluconazole is usually given for the first 100 days or for the duration of immunosuppression. Resistant fungal species such as *Torulopsis glabrata* and *Candida krusei* have emerged as major pathogens.[229] Molds, especially *Aspergillus* species, but also *Fusarium*, Mucorales, and other pathogens, have become the major hazard to transplant recipients.[230–232] The most common manifestation of invasive *Aspergillus* infection is fungal pneumonia, with nodular or interstitial infiltrates on chest radiography. Sinusitis, brain abscesses, and, rarely, disseminated disease are other manifestations. The diagnosis is frequently difficult to obtain because BAL cultures are often negative. The radiologic appearance on the chest radiograph and chest computed tomography scan and a persistent fever despite antibiotic treatment are often presumed to represent fungal infection. Prolonged empiric therapy with high-dose amphotericin or its liposomal formulations and, rarely, surgical intervention for removal of focal lesions are indicated, but the mortality rate remain high.[233] Measures to prevent aspergillosis include air filtration. Low-dose systemic or inhaled amphotericin is under study as prophylaxis.

Viral Infections

Cytomegalovirus Infection and Disease

CMV is one of the most common pathogens infecting recipients of allogeneic hematopoietic transplants. CMV infections occur, but they are less common after autologous transplantation. CMV pneumonitis was the major cause of infectious mortality before the availability of effective antiviral therapy, ganciclovir and foscarnet.[234] Patients who are seronegative for CMV may acquire the infection through blood product transfusions or donor marrow, if the donor is seropositive. Infections can be prevented by using filtered or seronegative blood products.[235, 236] However, in most seropositive patients, CMV infection results from reactivation of latent virus infection acquired before HCT.[237]

CMV infection is defined as active CMV replication and isolation of CMV from the blood or other tissues. *CMV disease* is defined when organ-related syndromes and tissue damage occur, and CMV is isolated from the affected tissue. CMV viremia, antigenemia, and recovery of CMV from BAL in an otherwise asymptomatic patient are highly predictive of development of CMV disease.[238] CMV pneumonia may follow in 60% of these patients within 14 days. Shedding of the virus in the throat or urine is not predictive of subsequent CMV disease. The risk of CMV disease increases with age, receipt of a mismatched or unrelated transplant, presence of GVHD, and treatment with high-dose corticosteroids.[239, 240]

CMV pneumonitis is the most common manifestation of CMV disease, and it is responsible for more than half of the cases of post-transplantation interstitial pneumonitis. Before the introduction of monitoring and prevention methods against CMV disease, 15% to 30% of marrow recipients developed pneumonitis, and the mortality rate was high. Historically, CMV disease occurred most often in the first 3 months after HCT, with a median time of 50 to 60 days after HCT. The natural pattern of CMV disease has changed with the introduction of prophylactic treatment;[241, 242] the time to onset has been delayed to more than 100 days, and CMV disease can occur late in the first year, especially in patients with chronic GVHD. CMV may also cause enteritis, with ulcerative lesions that may involve the esophagus, stomach, and small and large intestine, and it may cause diarrhea, abdominal pain, and vomiting. Prolonged fever and a mononucleosis-like syndrome, hepatitis, and encephalitis are other manifestations. CMV disease may also be associated with graft failure and thrombotic thrombocytopenic purpura. Myelosuppression may occur.[243]

CMV infection in seronegative patients can be prevented by the selection of seronegative donors, if possible, and by transfusion of CMV-negative or leukocyte-depleted blood products. CMV disease in seropositive patients can be prevented before reactivation of the virus (prophylactic treatment) or at the first signs of CMV infection and before CMV disease occurs (preemptive treatment). Rapid methods for detection of CMV are needed to allow good monitoring of CMV after HCT. The most common method is the CMV antigenemia test, which uses immunofluorescence of peripheral blood leukocytes with antibodies directed against the CMV pp65 antigen.[238] The shell vial method is commonly used for rapid detection of CMV in culture, and the PCR test has also been developed for rapid detection of CMV DNA.

Ganciclovir is an effective treatment to prevent CMV infection and disease;[242, 244, 245] however, its use may be complicated with adverse effects, most notably neutropenia. Prophylactic treatment with ganciclovir has not improved overall survival rates after HCT, presumably because of increased rates of other infections resulting from neutropenia.[241, 242] The alternative method is to treat CMV preemptively, by administering antiviral therapy only for those patients in whom the virus is reactivated, before CMV disease occurs. This method requires close monitoring but has been shown to have a significant positive effect on mortality. Some patients may develop CMV disease simultaneously with the first detection of CMV infection. Prophylactic treatment of patients at high risk of developing CMV disease is commonly employed.

CMV infection is usually treated with ganciclovir,[246] initially with an intensive induction phase of 2 weeks' duration, and then followed by a maintenance phase. Foscarnet is an alternative for patients with poor graft function.[247] The treatment of CMV pneumonia requires the combination of ganciclovir and intravenous immunoglobulin.[244] Ganciclovir alone has not resulted in improved outcome. Combination treatment with foscarnet may be needed in patients with resistant strains. Cidofovir is considered third-line therapy.[248] CMV infections are controlled by T cells. Adoptive transfer of T-cell clones has been effective for immunotherapy to prevent CMV disease, and approaches for cellular immunotherapy are under investigation.[249]

Hepatitis Viruses

Infection with *hepatitis B and C viruses* before HCT is common and is not considered a contraindication for transplantation unless the infection is accompanied by liver cirrhosis or severe abnormalities in liver function tests.[256, 257] Virus replication may increase during the period of immunosuppression and may lead to chronic infection.[258] Some patients with hepatitis B or C may develop fulminant hepatitis at the time of immune recovery as a result of an immune response against infected hepatocytes. Patients with hepatitis B should be followed-up with serial hepatitis B virus DNA levels, and antiviral therapy with lamivudine or famciclovir is recommended for patients with rising levels, to suppress hepatitis B virus replication. Hepatitis C usually does not require treatment during the immunosuppression period, but it may flare at the time of immune recovery, and it can be treated at that time. Long-term HCT survivors with hepatitis C have an increased risk of chronic hepatitis and cirrhosis.

Other Viral Infections

Mucosal *herpes simplex infections* are common during the first month after HCT, and prophylactic treatment with acyclovir may decrease their occurrence. *Respiratory viruses* such as respiratory syncytial virus (RSV), parainfluenza, and influenza viruses may cause severe, occasionally fatal, lower respiratory infection with high mortality rates in the first few months after HCT.[250] Diagnosis of RSV may be made by rapid antigen test on nasal washing or BAL. Inhaled ribavirin and RSV-specific immunoglobulin have resulted in clinical responses.[251] Neuroaminidase inhibitors are used successfully for the treatment of influenza infections, but no proven treatment exists for parainfluenza.

Adenovirus infection may result in pneumonia, enteritis, hepatitis, hemorrhagic cystitis, and nephritis.[252, 253] No proven treatment exists. Intravenous ribavirin results in inconsistent outcomes.

Varicella-zoster virus infections are common late posttransplant infections.[254] Localized herpes zoster is the most common clinical presentation; however, the risk of multidermatome disseminated infection and visceral dissemination is increased. Visceral dissemination rarely occurs in the absence of cutaneous disease. Abdominal zoster may present with upper abdominal pain, fever, and GI symptoms. Viral pneumonia, fulminant hepatitis, pancreatitis, and encephalitis are other rare manifestations of disseminated disease. Patients with cutaneous zoster should be treated early with high-dose intravenous acyclovir to prevent dissemination. Varicella-zoster immune globulin may prevent infections in patients exposed to the virus. Acyclovir and valacyclovir are used routinely for prevention of infection with herpesviruses during the first 3 months.

Human herpesvirus 6 infections also occur in immunocompromised transplant recipients; patients infected with this virus may present with pneumonitis, encephalitis, or marrow failure.[255] A PCR test is useful in the diagnosis. The virus is resistant to acyclovir but may respond to foscarnet.

Post-transplant Lymphoproliferative Disease

Post-transplant lymphoproliferative disease (PTLD) is a life-threatening complication of allogeneic transplantation.[259] It is more prevalent in recipients of T-cell–depleted marrow grafts, in recipients of transplants from unrelated donors, in patients with GVHD, and especially in those treated with aggressive immunosuppressive treatment including ATG. PTLD in hematopoietic transplant recipients arises from transformation of donor-derived B lymphocytes by Epstein-Barr virus (EBV) infection. Patients who are seronegative to EBV before HCT may develop PTLD early in the course because of primary EBV infection, and the disease may be rapidly progressive. Seropositive patients may develop a more indolent form as a late complication of prolonged immunosuppression. PTLD presents with systemic symptoms, adenopathy, and, frequently, extranodular lesions in the GI tract, liver, and central nervous system. Treatment includes withdrawal of immunosuppression and administration of the anti-CD20 monoclonal antibody, rituximab. Cellular therapy with DLI, at a relatively low cell number, has had dramatic results in controlling PTLD.[260] Methods have been developed to generate EBV-specific cytotoxic lymphocytes for the treatment of this complication.[261] Patients with increasing levels of EBV DNA are at the highest risk of PTLD and are candidates for preemptive immunotherapy.[262]

Pneumocystis carinii Infection

Pneumocystis carinii is an opportunistic parasite that may cause bilateral interstitial pneumonia in up to 15% of patients who are not receiving prophylactic treatment to prevent it.[263] The onset is usually delayed toward the later post-transplant phase. Patients with *Pneumocystis carinii* pneumonia usually present with gradual onset of dyspnea, cough, fever, hypoxemia, and diffuse pulmonary infiltrates. The diagnosis of *Pneumocystis carinii* pneumonia is made by cytologic evaluation of silver-stained preparations of BAL. Treatment includes trimethoprim-sulfamethoxazole or intravenous pentamidine. Supplementation of corticosteroids may be beneficial in patients with hypoxemia. Prophylactic treatment with trimethoprim-sulfamethoxazole almost eliminated the occurrence of this infection. Pentamidine, administered intravenously or by inhalation, and dapsone are the alternative medications for patients with allergy to sulfa drugs or marrow suppression, but they do not completely eliminate the risk of this complication.[264, 265] *Pneumocystis carinii* pneumonia prophylaxis should be continued for at least 6 to 12 months after HCT and for as long as immunosuppressive drugs are administered.

■ Treatment of Relapse after Hematopoietic Transplantation

Relapse after HCT is generally associated with a poor outcome.[266] In recipients of allogeneic transplants, withdrawal of immunosuppressive therapy may occasionally be sufficient to allow a GVL effect and to restore remission, often in association with GVHD.[24] Standard chemotherapy can control rapidly proliferating malignant diseases for variable durations, especially if relapse occurs after a long prior remission. Cytokines have been used in patients with disease relapses. Treatment with G-CSF has achieved transient remission in a few patients with AML with smoldering relapse.[267] Interleukin-2 has some effect, but it has been investigated more commonly in combination with cellular therapy. Interferon may achieve hematologic and cytogenetic responses in patients with CML and relapses in the chronic phase.[268]

Donor lymphocyte infusions (DLIs) are an effective treatment for relapse of CML in cytogenetic and chronic phases. DLI has a less striking effect in patients with more advanced disease.[25, 26] Complete remission can be achieved with DLI in up to 80% of patients with CML relapsing in an early phase. Patients with advanced CML are less likely to respond. Response in CML are usually durable. DLIs in relapse of AML or MDS result in response in about one third of the patients, and responses are often transient. The less favorable outcome in AML is partially related to a rapid proliferation of the leukemia cells before an effective GVL response is generated. Some groups have advocated administration of chemotherapy, before DLI, in an attempt to achieve transient control of the disease, and the outcome with this approach may be better. Patients with ALL rarely respond to DLI. DLIs have reinduced remissions in patients with multiple myeloma, CLL, and, rarely, other malignant diseases.

The major complications after DLI are marrow aplasia and GVHD. Marrow aplasia occurs in 20% to 40% of patients and is related to elimination of host leukemic hematopoiesis

before reconstitution of donor-derived hematopoiesis. This complication occurs more often when the percentage of donor cells in the marrow before DLI is low, and it is rare in patients with low-grade cytogenetic relapse.[269] Aplasia is often reversible, but a few patients require infusion of additional donor stem cells. GVHD, acute or chronic, may occur in 60% of DLI recipients. It is often responsive to immunosuppressive therapy. GVHD is associated with response, but in CML, responses can occur in the absence of clinically overt GVHD. Overall, DLI-related mortality is approximately 20%, and it is most often related to infection associated with aplasia or immunosuppressive therapy for GVHD.

A few strategies have been developed to reduce the risk of GVHD while retaining the beneficial GVL effect. Depletion of CD8+ cells has been shown to reduce the risk of GVHD, with no compromise of remission rate.[270, 271] Another approach is to use escalating number of lymphocytes.[272] The rate of GVHD and the leukemia response in CML depend on the dose of cells administered. Approximately 20% of patients with CML respond to a low dose of lymphocytes of 1×10^7 CD3 cells/kg, a dose that is rarely associated with GVHD. Escalating doses may then be given as needed to achieve response, with ultimately a lower risk of GVHD than that associated with a large initial dose.[273] Donor lymphocytes can be transduced in vitro with a suicide gene, herpes simplex virus thymidine kinase, which renders them susceptible to ganciclovir. If GVHD occurs, ganciclovir can be used to eliminate the process.[274] An intensive effort is directed at developing strategies to generate specific targeted immunotherapy[16, 275] directed against host hematopoietic minor histocompatibility antigens[276] or tumor-specific or overexpressed antigens.[277] This approach may potentially enhance the efficiency and safety of cellular immunotherapy.

Second transplants have been performed in a limited number of patients.[278–280] A second allogeneic transplant may salvage a patient who has a relapse after an autologous transplant. The outcome depends on the length of the prior remission, the stage and aggressiveness of the disease, and the age and performance status of the recipient. Second transplants within 1 year of the first in adults are associated with a high risk of transplant-related mortality because of cumulative toxicity. Patients who have a relapse within 100 days of HCT have a minimal chance of responding. Nonmyeloablative regimens have been used to reduce the toxicity associated with a second transplant and may provide a platform for effective immunotherapy.[281]

■ Hematopoietic Transplantation in the Treatment of Specific Diseases

Acute Myeloid Leukemia

HCT has been extensively used for the treatment of patients with AML.[282] The objective of HCT is to administer high-dose chemoradiotherapy to eradicate the malignant cells, followed by transplantation of normal marrow to rescue the patient from severe myelosuppression. Allogeneic HCT also provides an immune GVL effect against AML.

AML is more common with advanced age, but about 30% of patients are younger than 55 years. With current induction chemotherapy, 60% to 80% of adult patients achieve complete remission, and with modern consolidation regimens, incorporating high-dose cytarabine, 20% to 40% of patients are long-term survivors. Patients who do not respond to initial treatment or who subsequently have a relapse have a poor outcome with conventional chemotherapy.

Most patients have received high-dose cyclophosphamide and TBI or the combination of busulfan and cyclophosphamide[50, 283] as a preparative regimen before HCT. Most studies showed no difference in outcome between the two regimens; only one randomized study showing an advantage for TBI, with concerns about busulfan bioavailability in that study.[284] Most patients achieve complete remission after HCT. The major causes of treatment failure are GVHD, regimen-related toxicity, infections, and recurrent leukemia. More intensive regimens designed to have greater antileukemic activity by increasing TBI dose or by adding additional chemotherapeutic agents to the conditioning regimen have been associated with a lower relapse rate, but also with a higher rate of complications resulting from toxicity, and overall survival has not improved.[285] T-lymphocyte depletion reduces treatment toxicity by preventing GVHD; however, overall survival in most studies remained unchanged because of increased risk of relapse, graft failure, and infections. More recently, improved results were reported with T-cell–depleted allogeneic transplants in AML in first remission.[286–288]

Nonmyeloablative regimens have been investigated as a means to decrease regimen-related toxicity, but they may also be associated with higher relapse rate in patients who are not in remission at the time of HCT.[53] Other novel approach include the use of antimyeloid monoclonal antibodies that are radiolabeled or conjugated to toxins that can target the malignant cells or marrow with little systemic toxicity.[289, 290]

The outcome after allogeneic transplantation primarily depends on the disease status (remission vs. relapse), the cytogenetic abnormality of the leukemia, the patient's age, and the histocompatibility between donor and recipient.[291]

The best results are achieved when HCT is performed in patients in first remission.[292, 293] Long-term disease-free survival is 40% to 60% in this setting, and fewer than 30% of patients have a relapse after transplant. Allogeneic HCT can result in long-term disease-free survival in 20% to 30% of patients who fail to achieve first remission[294] or with first relapse of AML.[295] Results are similar when employing allogeneic HCT as the initial treatment of early leukemic relapse or after reinduction of a second remission.[296] Patients in early relapse who have a readily available donor should therefore proceed directly to HCT; otherwise, reinduction chemotherapy is required. Patients in advanced AML, in second or subsequent relapse, have an unfavorable outcome, with only 10% to 20% long-term survivors, predominantly because of the high relapse rate. Approximately 10% of patients with chemotherapy-refractory relapse achieve long-term survival after allogeneic BMT.

It remains an unresolved question whether patients with a sibling donor should receive allogeneic transplant while they are in first remission or at the time of disease relapse. The rationale for early HCT includes treatment of the patients with a relatively low burden of malignant cells, before the development of resistant leukemia. In addition, patients in remission are generally in better medical condition than patients with advanced leukemia and can better tolerate the intensive preparative regimen. However, about 25% of patients in first remission are already cured, and they will be unnecessarily exposed to the potential toxicity of HCT. Because about 30% of patients in early first relapse can still be cured with HCT, the overall cure rate may not be different if HCT is delayed to early first relapse.

Numerous studies have compared allogeneic HCT with autologous HCT and consolidation chemotherapy in patients with AML in first remission.[297–300] Results have been conflicting, in part because of various regimens used and the different type, intensity, and number of consolidation cycles before HCT and because only a portion of patients received the assigned treatment in each study. In general, most studies have shown a significantly lower relapse rate in patients receiving allogeneic HCT. Relapse rates after autologous transplantation are higher, but they are still superior to chemotherapy in most studies. A few studies also showed survival advantage of patients with allogeneic HCT. No study showed survival advantage of the other modalities.

The most important predictor of outcome with chemotherapy or with transplantation treatments is the cytogenetic abnormality of the leukemia.[301, 302] The t(15;17), y(8;21), and inv16 cytogenetic abnormalities are favorable, and patients with these abnormalities should initially be treated with standard chemotherapy using high-dose cytarabine consolidation, with allogeneic HCT reserved for patients who have a relapse.[303] Diploid cytogenetics are intermediate, and all the others such as trisomy 8, monosomy 5 and 7, complicated cytogenetics, and others confer poor prognosis. Patients with poor-risk cytogenetics should be offered allogeneic HCT.[301, 304]

Other prognostic factors have been reported that predict for shortened duration of remission, such as high initial white blood cell count, histologic subtype (monocytoid morphology being adverse), a prior preleukemic syndrome, and a slow response to initial induction chemotherapy or the need for more than one induction course.[305, 306] Patients with these characteristics should also be considered for early HCT. The patient's age appears to be an important prognostic factor, and the best results have been reported in patients less than 20 years of age. Age is another major prognostic factor with allogeneic BMT; it is reasonable to offer allogeneic transplantation to all young patients with AML in first remission who have a matched sibling donor.[307]

Elderly patients have a higher rate of regimen-related toxicity and GVHD. Most centers have limited transplantation to patients less than 55 to 60 years of age who have an HLA-identical sibling donor. However, AML is more common in advanced age. Elderly patients are more likely to have adverse cytogenetics and antecedent hematologic disorders and thus an unfavorable outcome. The use of nonmyeloablative regimens for induction of GVL as the main goal of treatment has opened the option of allogeneic transplantation to patients up to 75 years of age who have chemotherapy-sensitive disease.[53, 55, 308]

The risks of allogeneic transplantation are increased in patients without an HLA-identical sibling donor. Transplants from a matched unrelated donor or a related mismatched donor should be considered in patients after relapse, in those with poor-risk cytogenetic abnormalities, or in patients with an antecedent hematologic disorder.[309, 310] Assays to detect minimal numbers of leukemia cells may allow selection of patients at high risk of relapse and may possibly guide the selection of therapy.

Autologous BMT has also been evaluated as treatment for AML.[123, 311-313] Patients undergo procurement and cryopreservation of bone marrow cells while they are in remission. These patients may then receive similar marrow ablative chemoradiotherapy followed by reinfusion of the cryopreserved hematopoietic cells to restore hematopoiesis. The major limitation is the high likelihood that the "remission" bone marrow may be contaminated by small numbers of leukemic cells, which would be cryopreserved and reinfused with the autologous marrow. For patients with a cytogenetic marker, cytogenetic studies should be performed immediately before cryopreservation of hematopoietic cells. The autologous marrow would not be likely to mediate the favorable GVL effect, as described for allogeneic transplantation.

Numerous techniques have been explored to deplete occult leukemic cells from the harvested bone marrow in vitro before cryopreservation. Immunologic approaches using anti-AML monoclonal antibodies[314] or pharmacologic agents, such as 4-hydroperoxycyclophosphamide[123] or mafosphamide,[122] have been studied. Although some of the best results are reported in series using purged marrow, no controlled studies have been done, and the efficacy of purging remains to be determined.

For patients receiving autologous marrow transplants while the disease is in relapse, the major problem has been rapid relapse of leukemia; the median duration of remission has been 3 to 5 months, and fewer than 10% of patients have survived for 1 year. Better results have occurred with autologous marrow transplantation in patients in first or second remission.[122, 123] Approximately 20% to 40% of patients who received transplants while they were in second remission achieve prolonged disease-free survival. These data indicate that this approach can be successful, and relapse of leukemia may not invariably occur.

For patients with relapsed AML who lack a sibling or syngeneic donor, whether to pursue an unrelated donor transplant, a haploidentical transplant, or an autologous transplant depends on circumstances. Autologous transplantation should be considered only when the patient is in a well-established remission and the harvested cells were collected in remission with cytogenetics and molecular markers also indicating remission at the time of collection. Because the search for an unrelated donor often takes 2 to 6 months to identify a donor and to procure marrow, the patient's disease status must allow this lead time. One study reported similar survival with autologous and unrelated donor marrow transplantation; there were fewer relapses, but higher treatment-related mortality with the unrelated transplants.[315] Unrelated umbilical cord blood transplants may also be effective, but the rates of delayed engraftment and treatment-related mortality in adults are high.[96] Aggressively, T-cell–depleted haploidentical BMT can salvage 20% to 30% of patients with relapsed AML.[316] To have a successful outcome with haploidentical BMT, the cell-processing laboratory needs to have technology available to reduce T cells by 4 to 5 logs and to infuse more than 6×10^6 CD34+ cells/kg.

Relapse after allogeneic HCT is associated with a grim outcome. Early relapse is most often fatal. A few patients who have a relapse more than 1 year after HCT achieved durable remission with a second transplant, especially when they could be reinduced into remission with chemotherapy. DLIs have resulted in only short-lived responses. Better results may

be achieved with induction chemotherapy followed by DLI. Allogeneic HCT may be an appropriate salvage approach for patients who have a relapse after an autologous HCT, and a nonmyeloablative regimen may be considered to reduce toxicity, especially if the relapse is early.

Myelodysplastic Syndromes

MDSs are a group of clonal hematologic disorders, manifested by peripheral cytopenias and a high risk of transformation to AML. They may occur de novo or secondary to prior chemotherapy, such as with alkylating agents and etoposide, or after autologous transplantation for another malignant disease. MDS most often occurs in elderly patients, but about 10% of patients are young.

The outcome is determined by the French-American-British (FAB) morphologic classification. Patients with refractory anemia or refractory anemia with ringed sideroblasts (early MDS) have longer survival than patients with refractory anemia with excess myeloblasts or chronic myelomonocytic leukemia (advanced MDS). Low-, intermediate-, and high-risk groups have been defined based on marrow blast percentage, cytopenias, and karyotype.[317] The median survival of patients with low-risk IPPS scores is 5.7 years, but only 0.4 years for high-risk patients.

Allogeneic HCT is a potentially curative treatment for MDS.[318-320] The timing of transplantation is controversial. Patients with high-risk disease, excess blasts, severe neutropenia, transfusion dependency, and high-risk cytogenetic abnormalities are considered candidates. Patients with low-risk disease should not be offered HCT, unless they are extremely young or have life-threatening cytopenias. The conditioning regimens used are similar to those used for AML. Patients with hypocellular MDS who were treated with a protocol similar to that used for aplastic anemia fared worse because of the high incidence of relapse, a finding supporting the importance of ablative therapy.[321] However, the GVL effect has been documented for MDS. Nonmyeloablative transplants have been successful in some patients, and DLIs can restore remission in some patients with post-transplantation relapse. Little evidence indicates that pretransplant induction chemotherapy improves outcome. Patients with a readily available donor can proceed to allogeneic HCT as front-line treatment.[322]

The outcome is related to the MDS morphology and related prognostic factors.[318] The relapse rate after HCT for early MDS is less than 10%, and long-term disease-free survival is 50% to 60%. The risk of relapse for patients with refractory anemia with excess blasts is approximately 30%, with 30% to 40% long-term survival. Survival is better for young patients and when HCT is performed early after diagnosis, and it is worse after receipt of transplants from an unrelated donor. The relapse rate after HCT for therapy-related MDS is similar to that in de novo MDS, but treatment-related complications occur more often, probably because these patients are usually heavily pretreated for their primary malignant disease.[323]

Anecdotal reports of the use of autologous transplants for MDS have been published.[324] Some patients have normal stem cells that coexist with the abnormal clone, such as patients with de novo AML. These patients can achieve nonclonal remission with intensive chemotherapy and, theoretically, normal stem cells can be collected at recovery from chemotherapy. Detection of residual disease in the autograft may be difficult. Too few autologous transplants have been performed to allow conclusions.

Acute Lymphoblastic Leukemia

HCT is an effective treatment for ALL.[325–327] Intensive chemotherapy regimens have resulted in cure of approximately 70% of children with ALL. Substantial improvement has also been reported in the treatment of adult ALL with similar regimens; 80% to 90% achieve complete remission with induction regimens, and 30% to 35% can be cured.[328] Consequently, HCT has generally been reserved for patients after relapse, for patients who fail to achieve remission with initial chemotherapy, and for a subset of patients in first remission with a high-risk of recurrence of the disease.

HCT in first remission is controversial.[329, 330] Most studies have shown no survival advantage for patients having HCT because a reduced relapse rate is offset by treatment-related mortality. Patients may be selected for transplant based on prognostic features at diagnosis that predict for subsequent relapse. Advanced age, high leukocyte count at diagnosis (more than 30×10^9/L), poor prognostic cytogenetic abnormalities such as t(9;22) and t(4;11), non–T-cell phenotype, and longer time to achieve complete remission have been identified as adverse prognostic factors.[294, 327, 331] A study of the French Group on Therapy for Adult ALL reported improved outcome of patients with high-risk ALL having allogeneic HCT in first remission, in comparison with those having autologous HCT or continuous chemotherapy.[332] Patients with Philadelphia chromosome–positive ALL have an extremely poor prognosis, with only 5% achieving long-term disease-free survival. Allogeneic HCT in first remission can cure 30% to 40% and can be considered standard treatment for these patients.[331, 333] The use of other adverse prognostic factors to select patients for HCT in first remission is more controversial.

HCT offers the only chance for cure for most patients with refractory or relapsing disease.[294, 334, 335] Children with relapse occurring more than 36 months after first remission, or more than 12 months after completion of maintenance chemotherapy, may still be cured with chemotherapy.[336] However, the outcome of most adults with relapsing disease is dismal, and they should be considered for HCT.[327, 337] About 20% to 30% of patients with primary refractory ALL can be salvaged with allogeneic HCT. The International Bone Marrow Transplant Registry (IBMTR) analysis showed leukemia-free survival of 53%, 40%, and 21% among patients in first remission, second or subsequent remission, or in relapse at the time of transplantation, respectively.

Although transplants from an unrelated donor are associated with higher risks compared with transplants from an HLA-identical sibling, they are indicated in the same situations. Encouraging results have been reported for unrelated donor transplants in patients with Philadelphia chromosome–positive ALL in first remission.[338] ALL in relapse is often a rapidly progressive disease, and many patients die or become ineligible for HCT during the time it takes to identify and collect marrow from an unrelated donor. Transplants from a haploidentical related donor have also been generally unsuccessful.[42]

The most common preparative regimen used for HCT in ALL includes TBI and high-dose cyclophosphamide plus or minus other chemotherapeutic agents. TBI-containing regimens have been associated with improved disease-free survival, in comparison with regimens that do not contain TBI.[339] Intensification of radiation or addition of other agents has generally not improved overall outcome.

Patients with active leptomeningeal leukemia should have the central nervous system disease treated before HCT and then should receive monthly intrathecal methotrexate for up to 18 months.[340] Intrathecal methotrexate prophylaxis is also recommended for patients without leptomeningeal disease. Prior intrathecal treatment or prophylactic cranial radiation does not necessarily preclude the use of TBI.

Recurrent leukemia is a major problem in patients with ALL after HCT. The GVL effect is less striking in ALL than in AML and CML.[17] Patients with GVHD have a lower risk of relapse, but relapse after receipt of T-cell–depleted transplants or syngeneic transplants is not markedly increased.[20] DLIs are only rarely successful in restoring remission in post-transplant relapse.[25]

Autologous HCT has also been evaluated in patients with ALL, mostly in children.[341–343] Certain monoclonal antibodies to leukemia-associated antigens are available in ALL that are nonreactive with normal hematopoietic progenitors. These include antibodies to the common ALL antigen (CALLA) or certain T-cell antigens. Some patients have received autologous transplants using bone marrow that was treated ex vivo with one or more of these antibodies and complement. Limitations to this technique include probable antigenic heterogeneity among neoplastic cells, and it is unclear whether leukemic stem cells express these cell-surface antigens. Although selected patients with ALL in second remission have achieved prolonged remissions after receiving intensive chemotherapy, TBI, and autologous transplantation using anti-CALLA antibody and complement-treated marrow, the most autologous transplants have resulted in long-term survival rates of 20% or less. These data are difficult to interpret because many of the successful cases involved patients with a relatively good prognosis with conventional treatment, such as patients who have a relapse after a long first remission and in whom maintenance therapy has been discontinued. Results in patients with average or poor prognostic features have been much less encouraging.

Chronic Myeloid Leukemia

CML is a hematologic malignant disease characterized by excessive clonal proliferation of myeloid cells and their progenitors. In more than 90% of cases, the Philadelphia chromosome, t(9;22), is a marker of the malignant clone, and in most of the others, the translocation can be identified by a PCR test. CML is more common with advanced age, and the median age of onset is 60 years.

The disease can be divided into two phases: an initial chronic phase, in which cell maturation is normal, followed by transformation to an acute phase (blast crisis), characterized by maturation arrest at the level of the myeloblast or lymphoblast. The blast crisis phase resembles acute leukemia and is most often fatal. Some patients develop a transient accelerated phase before the development of overt blast crisis.

CML can be treated with chemotherapy, interferon-based therapies, and HCT. Hydroxyurea is the standard chemotherapeutic agent used in chronic-phase CML and is able to control the disease symptomatically. Interferon, with or without cytarabine, achieves hematologic control in most patients. Unlike with hydroxyurea, approximately 30% of patients may achieve a major cytogenetic response, some a complete response and, rarely, complete molecular remission.[344, 345] Interferon-based therapy may prolong life; the median survival of responders exceeds 8 years. However, in most patients, interferon is not curative, and blastic crises ultimately occur. Interferon therapy may also be associated with side effects and intolerance in some patients. An inhibitor of the abl tyrosine kinase (STI 571) involved in the Philadelphia chromosome translocation is a novel promising agent.[346, 347] It has entered clinical trials and may also achieve cytogenetic responses, but the long-term outcome is unknown.

Allogeneic HCT is an effective treatment for CML that can cure the disease.[348–350] Most patients have received busulfan and cyclophosphamide, or cyclophosphamide and TBI, as the preparative regimen. Both regimens appear equally effective.[351] The oral busulfan formulation is erratically absorbed, and relapse rates depend on the levels of busulfan achieved.[352, 353] Intravenous busulfan has more reliable pharmacokinetics and appears to have less toxicity[354]; this formulation appears preferable to the oral preparation; however, no comparative trials have been conducted. It has not been possible to improve the antileukemic effect of the preparative regimen with additional chemotherapy or higher doses of radiation without a concomitant increase in toxicity.[352]

The major determinants of transplant outcome are the stage of the disease at the time of HCT, the patient's age, the type of donor, and the interval from diagnosis to transplantation. The best results have been reported for patients receiving transplant during the chronic phase, with a disease-free survival of approximately 50% to 80% at 5 years. If HCT is performed within the first 1 to 2 years of diagnosis, and from a HLA-genotypically identical sibling, survival may be 80% to 90%.[350, 355] However, allogeneic transplantation is associated with a risk of early treatment-related mortality, and the survival advantage of HCT in patients with standard-risk CML may not become apparent until after more than 4 years after HCT.[356] Survival advantage becomes apparent earlier in patients with CML in the late chronic phase and with risk factors such as marked splenomegaly and increased numbers of peripheral and bone marrow blasts or basophils. HCT is the only treatment that potentially allows long-term survival in advanced CML. However, the outcome is much less favorable. For patients undergoing HCT during a blast crisis, only approximately 10% to 20% become long-term survivors and remain in continuous remission. Patients who are in an accelerated phase have a 35% chance of prolonged survival. The major cause of treatment failure in advanced CML is disease relapse. Patients who receive transplants during a blast crisis have a 60% relapse rate, in comparison with 10% to 20% for those who receive transplants during the chronic phase.

Younger patients fare better than older ones because of better tolerance to myeloablative treatment and lower rates of GVHD. More recently, nonmyeloablative regimens have allowed treatment of elderly patients as well, with promising results. Transplants from an unrelated donor are associated with a higher rate of treatment-related complications and an inferior outcome. The best results occur in younger patients who undergo HCT within 1 year of diagnosis,[350] with overall survival up to 85%.[38, 355] Improving HLA typing by allelic typing of class I and II antigens may improve the results with unrelated donor transplants to approach those achieved with a matched sibling donor. The chronic nature of chronic-phase CML allows time for a prolonged search for the optimal donor. Syngeneic transplants are safe, but the risk of relapse is approximately 50% because of lack of a GVL effect.[20] Overall, the best results have been achieved in patients who receive a transplant within 1 year of diagnosis.

The effect of prior treatment with interferon on the outcome of subsequent HCT is controversial. Interferon may upregulate HLA expression on selected tissues and theoretically may increase the risk of GVHD. In addition, interferon treatment may be associated with decreased performance status, which theoretically may increase the risk of transplant-related complications. Analysis at the M.D. Anderson Cancer Center in Houston, Texas, showed that prior interferon treatment was not associated with increased risk of complications in patients receiving transplants from HLA-matched siblings.[357] The Seattle group showed worse results because of increased GVHD in unrelated donor transplant recipients who were given more than 6 months of interferon treatment.[358] No adverse effects were observed in matched sibling transplants analyzed by the IBMTR.[359] The effects of interferon appear to be reversible, although it may take several months. The risks of adverse outcome may lessen if interferon is discontinued at least 3 months before HCT.[360]

The major limitation of allogeneic HCT is the risk of transplant-related complications, associated with an overall mortality rate of approximately 20% within the first 6 months of HCT. Acute GVHD may occur in 20% to 35% of patients. Strategies have been developed to deplete T lymphocytes from the graft at the initial HCT procedure. This approach reduces GVHD, but the risks of rejection and relapse are substantially increased, resulting in inferior disease-free survival rates.[361] T-cell depletion has been combined with DLIs either prophylactically or at the time of early relapse.[362–364] Overall, survival and GVHD rates have not changed with these strategies.

The timing of HCT remains an issue of continuing debate.[365, 366] The risks of early HCT must be balanced against the risks of delaying the treatment, risks that include transformation to blast crisis and a less favorable outcome of HCT when it is performed beyond 1 year of diagnosis or after disease acceleration. No reliable tests are available to detect imminent transformation to blast crisis. Patients' values and preferences are crucial for treatment planning. Our approach to patients with CML in chronic phase is to offer early allogeneic HCT for patients younger than 40 years with an HLA-matched sibling donor. Older patients or those with no sibling donor are offered a trial of interferon-based therapy. Patients who do not achieve hematologic remission within 3 to 6 months or who have no cytogenetic response within 6 to 12 months are offered a transplant from an HLA-matched related or unrelated donor. Extremely young patients may be offered an unrelated donor transplant initially. Elderly patients, more than 55 to 60 years of age, are eligible for HCT with a nonmyeloablative regimen after interferon-based therapies have failed. Patients with advanced CML should have HCT as soon as possible.

The high-dose preparative regimen may not completely eliminate all malignant cells, and a GVL effect is necessary to prevent relapse. Many patients may still have small numbers of Philadelphia chromosome–positive cells identified by cytogenetics or PCR for up to 6 to 12 months,[27] and these cells are gradually eliminated, presumably by the GVL effect. Relapse after HCT can be clinically overt, or it may be diagnosed only by cytogenetic or molecular analysis. Patients with subclinical recurrence of Philadelphia chromosome–positive cells may have spontaneous disappearance of these in a later analysis, especially if immunosuppressive treatment is withdrawn. In recipients of T-cell–depleted transplants, almost all patients with cytogenetic or molecular recurrence will progress to a clinically overt relapse. Infusion of donor T lymphocytes can ultimately salvage 80% to 90% of patients who have a relapse in a subclinical or chronic phase.[25, 273, 367] Most remissions achieved after DLI are durable, and they may be longer than those achieved after HCT. Patients who have a relapse in advanced phase is far less likely to respond to DLI. A response may take 3 to 4 months to 12 months, and sometimes multiple infusions are required. Patients may become pancytopenic at the time of response because of an antihost hematopoietic effect. This may be more common in patients with a higher percentage of host-derived hematopoiesis at the time of DLI.[269] Recovery of donor hematopoiesis usually follows, but some patients require infusion of more donor stem cells to support hematopoiesis. GVHD is the major risk, and it may occur in 60% of patients. Treatment-related mortality is about 20%. Strategies to separate the GVL effect from GVHD have been investigated (see earlier). Interferon and second transplants have been other modalities used for disease relapse after HCT.[268]

Autologous transplants have also been investigated for the treatment of CML.[368–370] Initial studies used bone marrow or stem cells collected during the chronic phase of the disease. When the patients later progressed to blastic phase, they received intensive chemotherapy, followed by reinfusion of cryopreserved autologous cells,[223, 224] with the objective to restore the early chronic phase. However, the blast crisis phase was often chemoresistant, and remission was short-lived. Another approach has been to attempt to collect autologous marrow or blood progenitor cells when they contain predominantly diploid cells. Marrow is harvested from patients in partial or complete cytogenetic remission after treatment with interferon or after recovery from intensive chemotherapy. The cells may be further treated in vitro to separate normal from leukemic cells by a variety of developmental approaches, including separation on the basis of HLA-DR expression, treatment with chemotherapeutic agents, or treatment in long-term culture.[371] Autologous transplants with this approach are of limited efficacy when HCT is performed after disease progression. When HCT is performed during chronic phase, these transplants may prolong the duration of the chronic phase, but they cannot be considered curative.

HCT has been used for the treatment of other myeloproliferative disorders such as agnogenic myeloid metaplasia and other syndromes.[372–374] The appropriate timing of HCT is not well defined. Most researchers have used transfusion requirement and other prognostic scoring systems to select patients for transplant.[375]

Chronic Lymphocytic Leukemia

CLL is a lymphoid malignant disease that typically has an indolent natural history and median survival exceeding 10 years.[376, 377] CLL is a clonal disorder of B cells characterized by the accumulation of small, mature-appearing lymphocytes, although rare T-cell variants also occur. The Rai system and the Binet system separate patients with CLL into prognostic groups.[378–380] The National Cancer Institute Working Group recommends the "three-risk group" modification of the original five-stage Rai staging system.[381] The median survival of the low-risk group is more than 14 years, that of the intermediate-risk group is 8 years, and that of the high-risk group is 4 years. Expression of CD38 and the serum level of β_2-microglobulin have major prognostic importance.[382, 383]

Chemotherapy is generally recommended if the disease causes symptoms or impaired performance status.[381] Chemotherapy has been palliative and is generally used for control of disease symptoms. Chlorambucil has been the standard of care since the 1970s and is useful to control leukocytosis and lymphadenopathy.[381] Fludarabine has been demonstrated to be a highly active agent,[384, 385] producing complete and partial remissions in most previously untreated patients. These remissions are transient, however, and overall survival has not been substantially improved; this disease is considered incurable. The prognosis is poorer once disease progression occurs after initial chemotherapy. Results depend on the response to salvage chemotherapy. The overall survival is approximately 2.5 to 4 years. This provides justification for evaluation of innovative strategies for these patients.

The bone marrow is extensively involved with malignant cells at diagnosis, and until the advent of fludarabine treatment, it was rare to achieve a bone marrow remission, a problem largely precluding consideration for autologous transplantation. Fludarabine alone, or in combination with other agents, has been established as effective cytoreductive treatment for CLL. Patients responding to treatment may achieve a prolonged remission, but the disease uniformly recurs, and overall survival has not been changed.[386, 387] Campath-1H, a monoclonal anti-CD52 antibody, also has activity against CLL,[388] and this agent allows collection of remission bone marrow or blood stem cells. Several studies of high-dose chemoradiotherapy with autologous HCT have been reported.[389–391] The autograft can be purged by monoclonal antibodies directed against B lymphocytes, and elimination of detectable systemic malignant cells is associated with improved survival.[392]

The role and optimal timing of autologous transplantation are controversial. The results of autologous transplants have been best when HCT is performed early in the disease. Investigators from the Dana Farber Cancer Center in Boston have treated patients as part of primary therapy and have achieved prolonged remissions.[392] The impact on survival in this selected group of lower-risk patients is unknown. The M.D. Anderson group has treated heavily pretreated patients with advanced disease, and only transient remissions have been achieved;[390] allogeneic transplantation was associated with a longer survival in this group. Thus, autologous transplantation is not a good option for advanced disease after failure of first-line therapy, but it is promising and deserves further study for consolidation of an initial response.

Allogeneic HCT has been studied predominantly in younger patients with advanced disease and poor prognosis.[391, 393, 394] Patients with chemosensitive disease have better outcome after HCT, but long-term survival has also been achieved in patients with refractory disease. An IBMTR analysis showed a 3-year survival of 46%, but also a high risk of transplant-related mortality.[395] A GVL effect has been shown in this disease,[396] and this has opened the way for studies using nonmyeloablative conditioning, to reduce toxicity and to extend the use of allogeneic transplantation options to the treatment of elderly patients up to age 75 years.[54] Encouraging preliminary results have been reported by many groups using this strategy.

The optimal timing of allogeneic transplantation is also controversial. Given the indolent course of this disease in newly diagnosed patients, it is generally recommended to delay allogeneic HCT until after failure of initial therapy. Patients showing no response or who have recurrent disease after fludarabine treatment have a poorer prognosis, a finding justifying the risk of allogeneic transplantation from an HLA-identical sibling. Delaying HCT until later in the course compromises the chance of long-term survival. Patients with multiply relapsed or chemotherapy-refractory disease have a much poorer outcome.[54, 395] Relatively few unrelated donor or mismatched transplants have been given to CLL patients. The risk of GVHD and treatment-related mortality is higher, and the role of transplants from alternative donors is uncertain.

Non-Hodgkin Lymphoma

Non-Hodgkin lymphomas are a heterogeneous group of lymphoid malignant diseases with a different natural history and prognosis. The treatment approach with both standard and high-dose chemotherapy predominantly relies on the histologic subtype. Lymphoid malignant diseases encompass a range of neoplasms with indolent to highly aggressive natural histories. Several classification systems have been proposed. A revised European-American (REAL) classification is widely used that incorporates immunophenotypical as well as morphologic criteria,[397] and a new World Health Organization classification has been proposed.[398] Lymphoid malignant diseases have been grouped into major categories: low-grade (including CLL), intermediate-grade, and high-grade diseases. These disorders result from malignant transformation and clonal proliferation of lymphoid cells and their progenitors. Each subtype is associated with characteristic cytogenetic and molecular abnormalities.[399–401] Clonal genetic abnormalities or immunoglobulin or T-cell receptor rearrangements can be detected by sensitive PCR-based techniques for identification of minimal residual disease or early relapse.[402, 403] Considerations of the role and timing of autologous or allogeneic transplants depend on their efficacy and on the effectiveness of treatment alternatives at different times in the natural history of each disorder.

Low-Grade Lymphoma

The low-grade lymphomas (small lymphocytic lymphoma, follicular small cleaved cell lymphoma, and follicular mixed cell lymphoma) are indolent diseases, but they are incurable with standard forms of chemotherapy. Follicular small cleaved cell lymphoma and follicular mixed cell lymphoma are the most common categories included among low-grade lymphomas; these diseases are associated with the t(14;18) resulting in rearrangement of the bcl-2 gene.[404]

Patients with low-grade lymphomas also have a median survival of 7 to 9 years.[405] The major factors influencing prognosis include stage, lactate dehydrogenase level, and β_2-microglobin level.[406–409] Patients may remain stable for years, and a policy of delaying chemotherapy until disease progression has produced long-term survival similar to that seen with initiating chemotherapy at diagnosis.[410] Initial chemotherapy using intensive combination chemotherapy regimens, such as cyclophosphamide, doxorubicin, vincristine, and prednisone (CHOP), results in complete and partial response rates of 50% to 70%, but no consistent improvement in survival over the use of a single alkylating agent or other conservative approaches. When the disease progresses after the initial chemotherapy, the prognosis worsens.[406, 411] Active chemotherapy regimens include ESHAP (etoposide, cytarabine, cisplatin, and corticosteroids), MINE (methotrexate, ifosfamide, mitoxantrone, and etoposide),[412] and FND (fludarabine, mitoxantrone, and dexamethasone).[413]

High-dose chemotherapy with autologous HCT has been extensively evaluated for low-grade lymphoma and has produced rates of complete remission of more than 80%. Patients receiving marrow or blood stem cell autografts effectively depleted of malignant cells using anti-B cell monoclonal antibodies may achieve prolonged remissions.[414–416] Controversy exists, however, regarding the role of autologous transplantation in this disease. Long-term survival is similar when high-dose therapy with autologous transplantation is compared with conservative forms of standard-dose chemotherapy.[417, 418] The use of autologous HCT is limited by involvement of the blood and bone marrow as a part of the natural history of these diseases, as well as by the inability of even high-dose chemoradiotherapy to eradicate systemic disease in most patients. In addition, patients have a high risk of secondary myelodysplasia and acute leukemia after autologous HCT in this disease.[127, 419, 420]

Allogeneic BMT has generally been reserved for patients with far-advanced low-grade lymphoma. High-dose cyclophosphamide and TBI, with or without other agents, or the combination of BCNU, etoposide, cytarabine, and melphalan (BEAM), have been the standard conditioning regimens. Several groups have reported extended disease-free survival in heavily pretreated patients.[421, 422] Other groups have also reported a high fraction of long-term remissions. Relapse rates after allogeneic HCT have been substantially lower than with HCT of purged autologous cells, most likely because of the graft-versus-lymphoma effect.[423, 424] Verdonck and associates published a study of 28 patients with advanced low-grade lymphoma and compared results with allogeneic versus autologous transplants.[424] The probability of disease progression among patients receiving allogeneic transplants was 0% versus 83% for autologous transplant recipients ($P = .002$), and progression-free survival at 2 years was 68% and 22%, respectively ($P = .049$). Van Besien and colleagues, for the IBMTR, analyzed results of allogeneic BMT from HLA-identical sibling donors in 113 patients with low-grade lymphoma.[425] Three-year probability of disease-free survival was 49% (95% confidence interval [CI], 39 to 59) and the probability of disease recurrence was 16% (95% CI, 9 to 27). The probability of treatment-related mortality was 28% (95% CI, 19 to 39). In multivariate analysis, a decreased Karnofsky score, the presence of chemotherapy resistant disease, and the use of a non-TBI regimen were independent predictors of survival.

Attal and colleagues performed a retrospective case-control analysis of 216 patients reported to the French Bone Marrow Transplant Group Registry from 1986 to 1996.[426] Seventy-two allogeneic transplants were matched with

144 autologous cases. Patients with allogeneic transplants had a significantly lower relapse rate, 12% at 60 months, with a plateau after 15 months, in contrast to 55% with autologous transplantation without an apparent plateau ($P < .001$). Transplant-related mortality was higher after allogeneic BMT (30% versus 4% with autotransplantation) ($P < .001$). The 4-year event-free survival was not significantly different, 53% for allogeneic BMT and 45% for autologous transplantation. The benefit of improved control of the malignant disease was largely offset by a higher rate of treatment-related mortality.

These studies indicate that high-dose chemoradiotherapy and allogeneic BMT are potentially curative for patients with advanced low-grade lymphoma. Unlike the case with autologous HCT, few relapses occurred after 2 years from transplantation, presumably because of a graft-versus-lymphoma effect or the lack of malignant cells in an allograft. The potential efficacy of allogeneic HCT must be balanced against its risks and the long natural history using conservative therapy. Given these considerations, no clear consensus exists regarding the timing of HCT. Nonmyeloablative preparative regimens for allogeneic HCT, the results of which have been encouraging, may reduce the risk of treatment-related mortality.[54, 427] This option should be considered for patients after failure of initial chemotherapy.

Mantle Cell Lymphoma

The diffuse forms of *mantle cell lymphoma* are associated with a poor prognosis.[428–430] Autologous HCT may be effective in chemoresponsive patients in first remission, but patients with resistant or recurrent disease have a high rate of treatment failure.[431, 432] Some small series or case reports have indicated success with allogeneic HCT in this disease.[433–436] Khouri and associates reported a series of 16 patients treated with allogeneic blood or marrow transplantation for diffuse type mantle cell lymphoma, 3 with blastic features;[433] 15 of these patients had stage 4 disease, and 11 had failed to respond or had suffered a relapse after previous chemotherapy. Disease-free survival was 55% at 3 years. These preliminary data indicate that allogeneic HCT using an ablative or nonmyeloablative regimen can induce durable remission in patients with mantle cell lymphoma. Allogeneic HCT appears promising in patients who fail to respond to initial chemotherapy or who have recurrent disease; its role in patients with newly diagnosed disease needs to be determined. Further clinical trials are needed.

Intermediate-Grade and High-Grade Lymphomas

Intermediate-grade and high-grade lymphomas are aggressive malignant diseases with a short natural history in the absence of effective therapy. These disorders are responsive to combination chemotherapy, and some patients achieve durable remissions. Chemotherapy for large cell lymphoma with the CHOP combination or with comparable regimens results in cure in approximately 40% for patients with diffuse large cell lymphoma.[437–442] The International Index has been the most widely accepted system.[443]

High-dose chemotherapy and autologous HCT improve cure rates for patients with recurrent large cell lymphoma who respond to salvage chemotherapy.[444, 445] The Parma study randomized patients younger than 60 years, with chemosensitive relapse, and no marrow or central nervous system involvement to continued salvage chemotherapy or to high-dose chemotherapy and autologous HCT.[446, 447] The 5-year event-free survival rates were 46% in the transplant group and 12% in the standard chemotherapy group; overall survival was also improved. Autologous HCT can therefore be considered standard treatment for that group of patients, although the foregoing inclusion criteria may apply to fewer than 50% of the patients with recurrent disease. Patients with refractory relapse have a minimal cure rate with autologous HCT.

Patients with chemotherapy-resistant disease and those with multiple relapses also have poor results; fewer than 20% have durable remissions. Patients achieving only a partial response to initial chemotherapy are rarely cured with chemotherapy and are appropriate candidates for autologous HCT; however, patients who continue to have disease progression through initial treatment only rarely achieve prolonged remission if autologous HCT is attempted at that time.[448] One study showed that patients with a slow antitumor response may do as well with continuing induction chemotherapy as with early HCT.[449]

Whether high-dose chemotherapy also contributes to improved survival when it is used in first remission for patients with aggressive non-Hodgkin lymphoma remains unsettled. Prospective studies failed to show a benefit of early HCT in low-risk patients. Two studies reported that high-dose chemotherapy with autologous HCT improves event-free survival of patients with intermediate-risk or high-risk disease,[450, 451] but other, smaller studies failed to confirm this benefit.[452] Ongoing clinical trials are addressing this issue. The rationale is to administer high-dose chemotherapy early, before the emergence of tumor resistance. High-dose chemotherapy appears most effective at a minimal disease state, and those studies that showed advantage of early HCT performed it after completion of a full chemotherapy course, rather than in the middle of the regimen.

The most common regimens used for conditioning include combinations BEAM (the most common regimen), CBV (cyclophosphamide, BCNU, and etoposide), or BEAC (BCNU, etoposide, cytarabine, and cyclophosphamide), accordingly. The role of allogeneic transplantation for aggressive lymphomas is controversial. Unlike the case for low-grade lymphomas, high-dose chemotherapy with autologous HCT is effective and potentially curative in patients with partial responses to induction chemotherapy, patients with chemotherapy-sensitive first relapse,[446, 447, 453] and high-risk patients in first remission.[415] Patients with recurrent large cell lymphoma with elevated lactate dehydrogenase levels, multiple relapses, and chemotherapy-insensitive disease have a poor prognosis with autologous HCT.[444]

High-dose therapy with allogeneic HCT has been examined in phase I and phase II studies in patients with intermediate-grade or high-grade lymphoma.[454] Most of these studies were in young patients with advanced disease. Some studies examined allografts for Burkitt lymphoma or lymphoblastic lymphoma in first remission.[455, 456] Results are difficult to interpret without concurrent controls, given the impact of eligibility criteria and patient selection on outcome. A prospective study by Ratanatharathorn and colleagues compared allogeneic BMT with autologous BMT and reported a significantly decreased recurrence rate and a trend toward improved disease-free survival with allogeneic transplantation.[457] Similar results were reported by Jones and associates.[458] Other studies have confirmed the relatively low relapse rate with allogeneic transplantation but found the benefit offset by higher rates of treatment-related mortality.[459, 460] A subsequent retrospective study by the European Bone Marrow Transplant Group compared allogeneic and autologous transplants.[460] They also reported a lower risk of relapse by allogeneic transplantation but, in general, inferior event-free survival and overall survival resulting from excessive treatment-related mortality. This study has been criticized for not accounting for potentially important prognostic differences between the allogeneic and autologous transplant groups; many physicians reserve allogeneic transplants for patients with a relatively poor response to chemotherapy or for patients in whom autologous transplants are not feasible.

A major problem with allogeneic HCT for recurrent intermediate-grade and high-grade lymphomas is the relatively high rate of treatment-related mortality in these heavily pretreated patients. The use of PBPC transplantation has been studied as an alternative approach for allogeneic transplantation. Preliminary studies indicate accelerated hematopoietic recovery,[461, 462] as well as potentially reduced early treatment-related morbidity.[463, 464] Preliminary studies at the M.D. Anderson Cancer Center demonstrated encouraging results in 21 patients with recurrent or resistant large cell lymphoma; 42% survived free of disease beyond 1 year.[465] Further study of allogeneic HCT is warranted.

Hodgkin's Disease

Remarkable progress has been made in the treatment of *Hodgkin's disease* since the 1980s, and many patients, even those presenting with advanced disease, can now be cured with combination chemotherapy or radiation treatment.[466] However, 20% to 30% of patients with advanced disease may fail to achieve complete remission with initial treatment, and approximately one third of those in remission may subsequently have a relapse. Although some of these patients may respond to additional chemotherapy, most ultimately die of the disease. High-dose chemotherapy and autologous HCT comprise an effective treatment capable of producing sustained remissions, and this approach is considered the treatment of choice for those who fail to achieve durable remission with standard-dose therapy.[467]

For patients with recurrent Hodgkin's disease, HCT results in a complete remission rate greater than 50% to 80% and a 40% to 60% disease-free survival rate at 3 to 5 years after transplantation.[467, 468] Numerous phase II studies have suggested that high-dose chemotherapy improves disease-free survival and possibly overall survival in comparison with standard chemotherapy in this setting. Only one randomized study showed improved disease-free survival with BEAM compared with miniBEAM.[469] The study was terminated early; the trend was for improved overall survival, but this was not statistically significant. Results in patients with an initial remission that is shorter than 1 year appear superior to those reported with standard salvage chemotherapy, and most researchers recommend high-dose therapy for these patients. Controversy remains regarding patients with a long first remission. Little evidence indicates that chemotherapy can cure patients in second or subsequent relapse, and these patients should proceed to HCT. Ongoing studies are evaluating the role of high-dose therapy with autologous HCT in patients with high-risk features as part of their initial therapy.[470]

The optimal roles and interactions of salvage chemotherapy and high-dose chemotherapy are uncertain. Some centers

have performed HCT as the first treatment in patients with disease relapse.[471] Others have instituted several courses of salvage chemotherapy with collection of the autograft between courses and institution of dose-intensive chemotherapy after achieving maximal cytoreduction. This latter approach has the appeal of providing treatment immediately after relapse and employing high-dose treatment at the time of minimal disease. Patients with bulky disease at the time of HCT are unlikely to achieve a prolonged remission.

Patients who fail to achieve complete remission with initial chemotherapy have a poor outcome; however, 20% to 40% can be salvaged by HCT.[472] Patients with a partial response fare better than patients with bulky progressive disease. It is unclear whether the latter group of patients should proceed to HCT or whether further attempts for debulking with chemotherapy should be attempted.

A few models for predicting the response and survival after HCT have been developed.[468, 473, 474] Prognostic factors include age, performance status, disease stage at HCT, number of extranodal sites involved, lactate dehydrogenase level, systemic symptoms at relapse, number of prior treatments, length of first remission, response to salvage treatment, and volume of disease at the time of HCT (minimal vs. bulky). These factors are similar to those for patients receiving standard salvage treatment. Patients with all favorable prognostic features have a greater than 70% disease-free survival at 4 years compared with approximately 20% for patients with multiple adverse features. These patient- and disease-related factors have such a major impact on outcome that it is difficult to compare treatment regimens among centers or in different subsets of patients in which prognostic features vary or are not defined.

Late relapses and a high incidence of secondary myelodysplasia (approximately 15%) continue to be major problems among long-term survivors.[475–477] Late infections and cardiac and pulmonary toxicity may also occur.

The most commonly employed regimens include alkylating agents and etoposide. The CBV regimen (see earlier) has been the most frequently used.[478, 479] TBI-containing regimens have also been investigated. The use of prior radiation therapy precludes TBI in many patients. No evidence suggests superior results with any of these regimens. TBI and high-dose carmustine should be used with caution in patients with prior chest irradiation or pulmonary disease, owing to the increased risk of pulmonary toxicity. Radiation therapy may be employed after high-dose chemotherapy for patients achieving only a partial response with HCT or to areas of prior bulky disease.[480]

Relatively few allogeneic transplants have been performed in patients with Hodgkin's disease.[481] Allogeneic HCT has the potential advantage of providing tumor-free graft and may be the only option for patients with extensive bone marrow involvement or those unable to collect a sufficient number of stem cells for transplantation. The donor-derived lymphoid cells may also have an immunotherapeutic effect analogous to that of the GVL effect. Allogeneic HCT is not associated with the same high risk of therapy-related myelodysplasia and may be a reasonable option for patients who already harbor cytogenetic abnormalities. However, allogeneic HCT is associated with a high treatment-related mortality in patients with Hodgkin's disease that exceeded 50% in some studies. This may be the result of the selection of patients with extremely advanced disease for allogeneic HCT. A European Bone Marrow Transplant Group analysis concluded that the risks of high-dose chemotherapy with allogeneic HCT outweighed the benefits compared with autologous HCT.[482] Studies in patients with advanced disease who were not suitable for autologous HCT showed a 15% to 20% salvage rate with HLA-matched sibling transplants.[483] Use of nonmyeloablative regimens to reduce treatment-related mortality is currently being investigated, and the preliminary results are encouraging. Clinical trials of allogeneic HCT should be considered only in patients who have a poor prognosis with autologous HCT or who have had a relapse after an autologous transplant.

Multiple Myeloma

Multiple myeloma is a common hematologic malignant disease that occurs in increasing frequently with advancing age. Standard chemotherapy can control the disease for variable periods, but only 5% of patients achieve complete remission, the median survival is 30 to 36 months, and fewer than 5% of all patients survive beyond 10 years of diagnosis.[484] Numerous phase II studies have suggested that high-dose chemotherapy improves the response rate and survival.[485–487] In a randomized study of patients with newly diagnosed multiple myeloma, high-dose chemoradiotherapy with autologous HCT was superior to standard chemotherapy;[488] 52% of the patients randomized to HCT were alive and 28% had no disease progression at 5 years, in comparison with 12% and 10%, respectively. High-dose chemotherapy with autologous HCT is now considered standard treatment for patients with multiple myeloma with an intermediate or high tumor mass.[489]

Chemosensitivity of the tumor is a major determinant of HCT outcome. Patients with chemosensitive disease who undergo HCT within the first year have a more favorable outcome, and 40% to 50% may achieve complete remission. Encouraging results have also been achieved in patients with primary refractory disease if HCT is performed early in the course of disease,[485, 490] but treatment is of only limited value in advanced resistant disease, especially in patients with refractory relapse.[491] Advanced age, high β_2-microglobulin level, and cytogenetic abnormalities involving chromosome 13 are the most prominent adverse prognostic factors.[492, 493]

With the introduction of PBPC transplants and better supportive care, autologous hematopoietic transplants have become considerably safer. Treatment-related mortality is typically less than 5%, even for elderly patients up to age 70 years. The most common regimen used includes high-dose melphalan with or without TBI. Others have used other combinations of alkylating agents.[494, 495] No evidence indicates the superiority of any of the regimens. TBI may increase toxicity, but it has not been shown to improve outcome. A randomized trial failed to demonstrate any advantage with the addition of TBI to high-dose melphalan. High-dose melphalan should be considered the present standard of care.

The timing of autologous HCT remains controversial. A few studies have suggested a better outcome when HCT is performed early, within 1 year of starting treatment. Others have advocated early collection of stem cells, but delaying high-dose chemotherapy itself to subsequent progression. A randomized French study of early versus late HCT did not show any survival difference, but patients randomized to early

HCT enjoyed longer periods without the need for chemotherapy.[496] High-dose chemotherapy increases progression-free survival, but relapse ultimately occurs in most patients. Various strategies have been investigated as ways to improve outcome. The Arkansas group has advocated the use of timely administered tandem transplants.[497] With this more aggressive approach, these investigators reported a median survival of 68 months and median progression-free survival of 43 months for patients with newly diagnosed disease who entered the program. Interim results from two European studies showed a trend for better survival with double versus single HCT that was not statistically significant.[498, 499] The difference may be more prominent in low-risk patients.

Another approach is to try to deplete the autograft of contaminating myeloma cells. One technique is positively to select CD34+ stem/progenitor cells, a procedure capable of depleting tumor cells by more than 3 log (99.9%). Although this approach can eliminate detectable cells in the autologous transplant in most patients, it has not been shown to improve remission duration or survival rates.[121] Most patients have a relapse resulting from residual resistant systemic disease. Improved treatments for cytoreduction are needed to increase the complete remission rate and to prolong the remission duration. Novel approaches include investigation of tumor vaccines,[500] post-transplant maintenance chemotherapy or interferon treatment,[501] and the use of bisphosphonates,[502] to address minimal residual disease with the goal of prolonging progression-free survival.

Relatively few allogeneic transplants have been performed in multiple myeloma. Most have been studies in young patients who have a relapse or disease progression during standard chemotherapy.[503] Patients have generally received high-dose melphalan and TBI or busulfan-cyclophosphamide–based conditioning regimens. Allogeneic HCT provides a tumor-free graft and also an immune graft-versus-myeloma effect. Relapse occurs almost invariably after autologous HCT, but it may be less common after allogeneic HCT. DLIs have reinduced remission in a few patients who had a relapse after allogeneic HCT, a finding consistent with the presence of a graft-versus-myeloma effect.[30, 31] However, the reduced relapse rate is offset by a high treatment-related mortality rate approaching 50% in heavily pretreated patients with multiple myeloma. Three-year progression-free survival is approximately 30% to 40%. Most comparative studies have shown that patients with autologous transplants have a better overall survival than do those with allografts, at least during the first few years after HCT.[504, 505] Results of allogeneic HCT may improve if patients undergo the procedure early instead of at advanced refractory stage, or if less toxic nonmyeloablative preparative regimens prove effective. A subset of patients with high-risk features, such as patients with chromosome 13 abnormalities, should be considered for allogeneic HCT early in their treatment plan. Allogeneic HCT has also been shown to rescue patients who have a relapse after autologous HCT.

Other plasma cell dyscrasias have also been effectively treated with high-dose melphalan and autologous HCT. This approach has become the treatment of choice for *primary amyloidosis*, a related, invariably fatal disease.[506, 507]

Solid Tumors

Breast cancer has been the most common disease treated by high-dose chemotherapy and autologous HCT. However, considerable controversy remains regarding the efficacy of high-dose therapy in this disease and the role of HCT-based therapies.[508] The most effective high-dose chemotherapy regimens used include combinations of alkylating agents and related drugs, including cyclophosphamide, melphalan, thiotepa, carmustine, cisplatin, or carboplatin.[509, 510] Taxanes are also being studied in preparative regimens.[511] Studies in patients with chemotherapy-responsive metastatic breast cancer have documented that this approach significantly increases the complete remission rate to more than 50%, with long-term disease-free survival in approximately 20%.[512] This result is better than expected with standard chemotherapy, although selection bias cannot be excluded.[513] The patients most likely to benefit are those with chemosensitive disease in minimal disease state (preferentially in complete remission) at the time of transplantation, no liver metastasis, and good performance status.[514, 515]

These same prognostic factors also apply to conventional-dose chemotherapy, and randomized trials are necessary to assess critically the efficacy of this form of therapy. A few randomized studies have been performed, with disparate results. Two studies showed an advantage in event-free survival with HCT,[516] but another randomized trial showed no benefit.[517] Autologous HCT has also been used as adjuvant therapy in patients with local regional breast cancer who are at high risk of disease relapse. This has generally been defined as stage II disease with 10 or more positive axillary nodes, stage III, particularly in failures of neoadjuvant therapy, and inflammatory breast cancer. In phase II studies, approximately 50% to 85% of these high-risk patients survived free of relapse at 5 years. Studies comparing HCT with standard chemotherapy in this setting did not show a survival advantage for HCT but did show a reduction in survival;[518, 519] however, studies have either had inadequate power or too short a follow-up period to have definitive results.

Relapse remains a major problem, and the use of biologic or immunologic therapies for minimal residual breast cancer after autologous HCT needs to be evaluated. Clinical studies using allogeneic HCT are exploring the potential of a GVM effect in this disease.[33]

A similar approach with autologous HCT has been used for the treatment of other chemotherapy-responsive solid tumors in adults, including ovarian cancer, testicular/germ cell carcinomas, and small cell carcinoma of the lung. *Testicular carcinoma* is a chemotherapy-responsive tumor that is frequently cured using standard chemotherapy. Patients in whom first-line and second-line chemotherapy regimens fail have received high-dose chemotherapy and autologous transplants. Response rates are high, and a few patients have achieved long-term remissions.[520]

Dose-intensive chemotherapy is being increasingly used for treating *ovarian cancer*.[521, 522] Like breast cancer, this tumor is sensitive to alkylating agents, platinum-based chemotherapy agents, taxanes, and topoisomerase I inhibitors. Transplants have not been used commonly in the adjuvant setting, but they have a role for patients with low-bulk disease after a second-look laparotomy and for patients with relapses of chemotherapy-sensitive low-bulk diseased.

Autologous transplants have been extensively studied in *small cell lung cancer*.[523] Patients with extensive disease or relapsed carcinoma have generally had only brief responses and modest clinical benefit. Better results have been obtained

as consolidation therapy for patients with limited small cell lung cancer, with prolongation of remission duration in some studies. Few patients are long-term survivors, and the efficacy of this approach remains to be established.

Autologous transplants have been studied in a range of *pediatric solid tumors* such as neuroblastoma and Ewing sarcoma, which are highly sensitive to chemotherapy and radiation, yet have a poor prognosis in patients with advanced disease.[524, 525]

Certain malignant diseases that are poorly responsive to conventional treatment have also been treated with high-dose chemotherapy and HCT, including melanoma, colon and other GI carcinomas, and non–small cell lung cancer. These patients have generally received escalated doses of single agents, such as melphalan or carmustine, or combinations of alkylating agents. This high-dose treatment has increased response rates, but these responses are usually brief, and it is unclear whether overall survival is improved.

More recently, allogeneic transplants using nonablative regimens achieved promising results in metastatic renal cell cancer.[32] A GVM effect was documented in some of these patients.

Aplastic Anemia

Aplastic anemia is a uncommon disease of primary bone marrow failure presenting with pancytopenia and bone marrow hypocellularity, either congenital or acquired. Severe aplastic anemia is defined as marrow cellularity of less than 25%, with a neutrophil count $<0.5 \times 10^9$/L, a platelet count $<20 \times 10^9$/L, or a total reticulocyte count $<40 \times 10^9$/L.[526] More than 50% of patients with severe aplastic anemia may die within 6 months of diagnosis. Effective treatments for aplastic anemia include immunosuppressive therapy (such as cyclosporine and ATG)[527, 528] and HCT.[529]

Syngeneic transplantation has been successful without conditioning in 50% of the recipients, a finding suggesting an intrinsic stem cell abnormality in some patients. Those who do not recover most often respond to a second infusion with immunosuppressive conditioning.[530] These and other data suggest an autoimmune pathophysiology in many patients.[531] Most allogeneic transplants for aplastic anemia have been from an HLA-matched sibling. The conditioning regimen is aimed to provide immunosuppression for prevention of graft rejection. Most studies use high-dose cyclophosphamide (200 mg/kg) with or without ATG, but many appear to have immune-mediated suppression of hematopoiesis.[532, 533]

Historically, graft rejection was a major complication of allogeneic transplantation for aplastic anemia, and it occurred in up to 30% of recipients.[532] Multiple blood transfusions may sensitize the recipient against the donor and may increase the risk of rejection. The more judicious use of transfusions and leukocyte depletion of the transfused blood products have reduced the risk of rejection. Intensification of immunosuppressive therapy with the addition of ATG may also reduce the risk.[533] The combination of cyclophosphamide with TBI or total nodal radiation can reduce the risk of graft rejection, but it is associated with increased toxicity and has not improved survival;[534] the addition of radiation adds toxicity and has not improved survival. The infusion of bone marrow with additional buffy coat cells was proposed as a means to reduce rejection rates,[535] but it was also associated with a higher incidence of chronic GVHD, and it is now discouraged.

Late graft rejection may occur when post-transplant immunosuppression administered for prevention of GVHD is withdrawn. With current regimens, with early HCT and a judicious transfusion policy, and with improved supportive care systems, fewer than 10% of patients reject the grafts, and long-term survival can be achieved in 80% to 90% of recipients of marrow from an HLA-matched sibling donor.

HCT from a partially matched related donor or a phenotypically matched unrelated donor requires additional immunosuppression for prevention of rejection, but the mode and dose are unknown.[555, 536] The results have been markedly inferior to those achieved with genotypically matched transplants, and fewer than 50% of these patients are long-term survivors.[537, 538]

Several studies have compared the effectiveness of allogeneic HCT and immunosuppressive therapy. Most studies have shown a survival advantage for patients younger than 40 years who undergo allogeneic HCT from an HLA-matched sibling. Immunosuppressive therapy has a higher risk of late complications such as relapse or development of myelodysplasia or AML. However, patients more than 40 to 50 years old have a higher risk of complications with allogeneic HCT, and this approach should be reserved for patients in whom immunosuppressive therapy has failed. Patients lacking an HLA-identical related donor should receive a trial of immunosuppressive therapy; alternative donor transplants should be considered only in those who fail to respond to this treatment.

Other Nonmalignant Disorders

Allogeneic HCT is a potentially curative treatment in a number of *congenital disorders* of the hematopoietic and immune systems. *Thalassemia*[539] and *sickle cell anemia*[540] are among the most common nonmalignant hematologic disorders curable with HCT. Results in patients with thalassemia have been more favorable when performed early and in patients who are not heavily transfused and who have no sign of severe hepatic iron overload or portal fibrosis. Most patients receive busulfan and cyclophosphamide to avoid the undesirable effects of TBI in young children. *Fanconi anemia* has been treated similarly to aplastic anemia, but with an extremely low-dose conditioning regimen because of the known sensitivity of these patients to the effects of radiation and alkylating agents.[541, 542] Patients are not cured of the nonhematologic manifestations of the disease, and many develop secondary solid tumors.

Allogeneic HCT has been the treatment of choice for infants with severe combined immunodeficiency.[543] Engraftment can be achieved in many patients even without conditioning in this disorder. Allogeneic HCT has been able to reverse the bone sclerosis in osteopetrosis.[544] The results in storage diseases have been inconsistent.[545] T-cell depletion may be useful in preventing GVHD. For patients without a matched sibling, both unrelated donor transplants or mismatched related transplants have been successful.[546, 547] In most disorders outcomes were better when transplants were given early, and promising results have been reported for transplants in utero.[548] In the future, gene modification of autologous cells may be a curative approach for some of these disorders.[549]

Interest in autologous HCT, with or without T-cell depletion of the graft, for the treatment of autoimmune disorders has increased.[7] Encouraging results have been reported in a limited number of patients with rheumatoid arthritis, systemic lupus erythematosus, multiple sclerosis, myasthenia gravis, and other disorders.[8, 550]

■ Future Directions

Since the early 1990s, HCT has become a much safer procedure, applicable to a larger patient population in a variety of disease processes. Most hematopoietic transplants are performed for treatment of malignant diseases. With the introduction of PBPC transplants and better supportive care, autologous HCT has been used safely in patients up to 70 years old. Relapse of the malignant disease remains the major cause of treatment failure; innovative strategies are required to eradicate minimal residual disease that survives high-dose therapy or contaminates an autograft. Targeted radiation therapy, such as monoclonal antibody–radionuclide immunoconjugates and bone-seeking isotopes such as holmium, are under active evaluation as a means to target radiotherapy to the tumor; this approach has little systemic toxicity other than myelosuppression. It may be possible to improve results further by using strategies to overcome drug-resistance mechanisms, such as administration of inhibitors to P glycoprotein or other mechanisms of drug resistance.

The immune GVM effect associated with allogeneic transplants illustrates the capability of the immune system to eliminate residual disease. Strategies to enhance immune antitumor mechanisms with both allogeneic HCT and autologous HCT are necessary. Tumor vaccines have been generated by ex vivo transfection of tumors with genes to improve presentation of antigens, costimulatory molecules, and various cytokines to enhance the immune response directed against the tumor. Autologous antigen-presenting cells, pulsed with tumor antigens, or by themselves when they originate from the malignant clone, have also been used to stimulate and expand, in vitro or in vivo, cytotoxic T lymphocytes and other effectors for cellular immunotherapy. Ongoing research efforts seek to generate antigen-specific immune cells directed against tumors and major pathogens, but with sparing of normal donor tissues. Once these processes are better understood, it will be possible to engineer the graft to provide specific immunotherapy without the undesirable complication of GVHD.

The collection of bone marrow or PBPCs offers the potential for ex vivo genetic therapy to improve treatment results. Transfection of genes for drug resistance such as the multiple drug resistance gene (mdr-1) into normal marrow cells or transfer of genes into lymphocytes to modify the immune response may improve patient outcomes.

In the allogeneic transplant setting, efforts are directed at expansion of the donor pool, reducing the toxicity of the procedure, and improving the methods to deliver immunotherapy. Most patients who are candidates for allogeneic HCT do not have an HLA-matched sibling donor. Further development of international unrelated donor registries for bone marrow, blood stem cells, and umbilical cord blood registries will increase the likelihood of finding a donor. Special attention is given to representation of ethnic minorities in these registries. New molecular methods to improve the precision of histocompatibility matching may decrease the risk of rejection and GVHD. Another approach is to use related partially matched donors. The risk of graft failure and GVHD can been minimized by infusions of large numbers of stem cells and aggressive T-cell depletion, but this type of transplantation is still limited by delayed immune reconstitution after transplant and by the high risk of infections. Strategies are being investigated to find ways to delete alloreactive T-cell subsets but retain subsets that contribute to graft facilitation, GVL effect, and infection control.

Considerable progress has been achieved in supportive care to prevent GVHD, CMV and other infections, and other transplant-related complications and to make allogeneic transplants increasingly safe over time. The finding that the GVL effect is responsible for much of the therapeutic potential of allogeneic transplants has opened the way for the use of nonmyeloablative regimens as means to allow engraftment of donor cells with reduced toxicity and to providing GVL as the primary treatment. Carefully planned prospective clinical trials will be required to define the role of this strategy, as well as the diseases and patient populations for which it will be useful.

REFERENCES

1. Gatti RA, Meuwissen HJ, Allen HD, et al: Immunological reconstitution of sex-linked lymphopenic immunological deficiency. Lancet 1968;2:1366–1369.
2. Thomas ED, Buckner CD, Banaji M, et al: One hundred patients with acute leukemia treated by chemotherapy, total body irradiation, and allogeneic marrow transplantation. Blood 1977;49:511–533.
3. Thomas ED, Storb R, Clift RA, et al: Bone-marrow transplantation. N Engl J Med 1975;292:832–843.
4. Forman S, Blume K, Thomas ED: Bone Marrow Transplantation. Boston, Blackwell Scientific, 1994.
5. Gratwohl A, Tyndall A: From autoimmunity to stem cell transplantation. Crit Rev Oncol Hematol 1999;30:159–172.
6. Snowden JA, Brooks PM, Biggs JC: Haemopoietic stem cell transplantation for autoimmune diseases. Br J Haematol 1997;99:9–22.
7. van Bekkum DW: Autologous stem cell therapy for treatment of autoimmune diseases. Exp Hematol 1998;26:831–834.
8. Burt RK, Traynor AE, Pope R, et al: Treatment of autoimmune disease by intense immunosuppressive conditioning and autologous hematopoietic stem cell transplantation. Blood 1998;92:3505–3514.
9. Brenner MK: Gene transfer to hematopoietic cells. N Engl J Med 1996;335:337–339.
10. Dunbar CE: Gene transfer to hematopoietic stem cells: Implications for gene therapy of human disease. Annu Rev Med 1996;47:11–20.
11. Hanania EG, Kavanagh J, Hortobagyi G, et al: Recent advances in the application of gene therapy to human disease. Am J Med 1995;99:537–552.
12. Donahue RE, Byrne ER, Thomas TE, et al: Transplantation and gene transfer of the human glucocerebrosidase gene into immunoselected primate CD34+Thy- 1+ cells. Blood 1996;88:4166–4172.
13. Kohn DB, Bauer G, Rice CR, et al: A clinical trial of retroviral-mediated transfer of a rev-responsive element decoy gene into CD34⁺ cells from the bone marrow of human immunodeficiency virus-1-infected children. Blood 1999;94:368–371.
14. Thomas ED: Bone marrow transplantation for malignant disease. J Clin Oncol 1983;1:517.
15. Barrett AJ, Malkovska V: Graft-versus-leukaemia: Understanding and using the alloimmune response to treat haematological malignancies. Br J Haematol 1996;93:754–761.
16. Champlin R, Khouri I, Kornblau S, et al: Allogeneic hematopoietic transplantation as adoptive immunotherapy: Induction of graft-vs-malignancy as primary therapy. Hematol Oncol Clin North Am 1999;13:1041–1057.
17. Horowitz MM, Gale RP, Sondel PM, et al: Graft-versus-leukemia reactions after bone marrow transplantation. Blood 1990;75:555–562.
18. Slavin S, Ackerstein A, Naparstek E, et al: The graft-versus-leukemia (GVL) phenomenon: Is GVL separable from GVHD? Bone Marrow Transplant 1990;6:155–161.
19. Gale RP, Champlin RE: How does bone marrow transplantation cure leukemia? Lancet 1984;2:28–30.
20. Gale RP, Horowitz MM, Ash RC, et al: Identical-twin bone marrow transplants for leukemia. Ann Intern Med 1994;120:646–652.
21. Marmont AM, Horowitz MM, Gale RP, et al: T-cell depletion of HLA-identical transplants in leukemia. Blood 1991;78:2120–2130.
22. Sullivan KM, Weiden PL, Storb R, et al: Influence of acute and chronic graft-versus-host disease on relapse and survival after bone marrow transplantation from HLA-identical siblings as treatment of acute and chronic leukemia. Blood 1989;73:1720–1728.
23. Weiden PL, Sullivan KM, Flournoy N, et al: Antileukemic effect of chronic graft-versus-host disease: Contribution to improved survival after allogeneic marrow transplantation. N Engl J Med 1981;304:1529–1532.
24. Collins RH Jr, Rogers ZR, Bennett M, et al: Hematologic relapse of chronic myelogenous leukemia following allogeneic bone marrow transplantation: Apparent graft-versus-leukemia effect following abrupt discontinuation of immunosuppression. Bone Marrow Transplant 1992;10:391–395.
25. Collins RH Jr, Shpilberg O, Drobyski WR, et al: Donor leukocyte infusions in 140 patients with relapsed malignancy after allogeneic bone marrow transplantation. J Clin Oncol 1997;15:433–444.
26. Kolb HJ, Schattenberg A, Goldman JM, et al: Graft-vs-leukemia effect of donor lymphocyte transfusions in marrow grafted patients. Blood 1995;86:2041–2050.
27. Radich JP, Gehly G, Gooley T, et al: Polymerase chain reaction detection of the *BCR-ABL* fusion transcript after allogeneic marrow transplantation for chronic myeloid leukemia: Results and implications in 346 patients. Blood 1995;85:2632–2638.
28. Kwak LW, Pennington R, Longo DL: Active immunization of murine allogeneic bone marrow transplant donors with B-cell tumor-derived idiotype: A strategy for enhancing the specific antitumor effect of marrow grafts. Blood 1996;87:3053–3060.
29. Van Besien KW, De Lima M, Giralt SA, et al: Management of lymphoma recurrence after allogeneic transplantation: The relevance of graft-versus-lymphoma effect. Bone Marrow Transplant 1997;19:977–982.
30. Verdonck LF, Lokhorst HM, Dekker AW, et al: Graft-versus-myeloma effect in two cases. Lancet 1996;347:800–801.
31. Tricot G, Vesole DH, Jagannath S, et al: Graft-versus-myeloma effect: Proof of principle. Blood 1996;87:1196–1198.
32. Childs RW, Clave E, Tisdale J, et al: Successful treatment of metastatic renal cell carcinoma with a nonmyeloablative allogeneic peripheral-blood progenitor-cell transplant: Evidence for a graft-versus-tumor effect. J Clin Oncol 1999;17:2044–2049.
33. Ueno NT, Rondón G, Mirza NQ, et al: Allogeneic peripheral-blood progenitor-cell transplantation for poor-risk patients with metastatic breast cancer. J Clin Oncol 1998;16:986–993.
34. Hansen JA, Choo SY, Geraghty DE, et al: The HLA system in clinical marrow transplantation. Hematol Oncol Clin North Am 1990;4:507–515.
35. Kernan NA, Bartsch G, Ash RC, et al: Analysis of 462 transplantations from unrelated donors facilitated by the National Marrow Donor Program. N Engl J Med 1993;328:593–602.
36. McGlave PB, Shu XO, Wen WQ, et al: Unrelated donor marrow transplantation for chronic myelogenous leukemia: 9 years' experience of the National Marrow Donor Program. Blood 2000;95:2219–2225.
37. Madrigal JA, Arguello R, Scott I, et al: Molecular histocompatibility typing in unrelated donor bone marrow transplantation. Blood Rev 1997;11:105–117.
38. Hansen JA, Gooley TA, Martin PJ, et al: Bone marrow transplants from unrelated donors for patients with chronic myeloid leukemia. N Engl J Med 1998;338:962–968.
39. Petersdorf EW, Mickelson EM, Anasetti C, et al: Effect of HLA mismatches on the outcome of hematopoietic transplants. Curr Opin Immunol 1999;11:521–526.
40. Beatty PG, Clift RA, Mickelson EM, et al: Marrow transplantation from related donors other than HLA-identical siblings. N Engl J Med 1985;313:765.
41. Anasetti C, Amos D, Beatty PG, et al: Effect of HLA compatibility on engraftment of bone marrow transplants in patients with leukemia or lymphoma. N Engl J Med 1989;320:197–204.
42. Aversa F, Tabilio A, Terenzi A, et al: Successful engraftment of T-cell-depleted haploidentical "three-loci" incompatible transplants in leukemia patients by addition of recombinant human granulocyte colony-stimulating factor–mobilized peripheral blood progenitor cells to bone marrow inoculum. Blood 1994;84:3948–3955.

43. Bachar-Lustig E, Rachamim N, Li HW, et al: Megadose of T cell–depleted bone marrow overcomes MHC barriers in sublethally irradiated mice. Nat Med 1995;1:1268–1273.

44. Terenzi A, Lubin I, Lapidot T, et al: Enhancement of T cell-depleted bone marrow allografts in mice by thiotepa. Transplantation 1990;50:717–720.

45. Lapidot T, Terenzi A, Singer TS, et al: Enhancement by dimethyl myleran of donor type chimerism in murine recipients of bone marrow allografts. Blood 1989;73:2025–2032.

46. Lapidot T, Lubin I, Terenzi A, et al: Enhancement of bone marrow allografts from nude mice into mismatched recipients by T cells void of graft-versus-host activity. Proc Natl Acad Sci U S A 1990;87:4595–4599.

47. Lapidot T, Faktorowich Y, Lubin I, et al: Enhancement of T-cell-depleted bone marrow allografts in the absence of graft-versus-host disease is mediated by CD8$^+$ CD4$^-$ and not by CD8$^-$ CD4$^+$ thymocytes. Blood 1992;80:2406–2411.

48. Thomas ED: Total body irradiation regimens for marrow grafting. Int J Radiat Oncol Biol Phys 1990;19:1285–1288.

49. Shank B: Total body irradiation for marrow or stem-cell transplantation. Cancer Invest 1998;16:397–404.

50. Santos GW, Tutschka PJ, Brookmeyer R, et al: Marrow transplantation for acute nonlymphocytic leukemia after treatment with busulfan and cyclophosphamide. N Engl J Med 1983;309:1347.

51. Tutschka PJ, Copelan EA, Klein JP: Bone marrow transplantation for leukemia following a new busulfan and cyclophosphamide regimen. Blood 1987;70:1382–1388.

52. Champlin RE, Khouri I, Kornblau S, et al: Reinventing bone marrow transplantation: Nonmyeloablative preparative regimens and induction of graft-vs-malignancy effects. Oncology 1999;3:621–628.

53. Giralt S, Estey E, Albitar M, et al: Engraftment of allogeneic hematopoietic progenitor cells with purine analog-containing chemotherapy: Harnessing graft-versus-leukemia without myeloablative therapy. Blood 1997;89:4531–4536.

54. Khouri I, Keating M, Korbling M, et al: Transplant Lite: Induction of graft-versus-leukemia using fludarabine-based nonablative chemotherpy and allogeneic blood progenitor cell transplantation as treatment for lymphoid malignancies. J Clin Oncol 1998;16:2817–2824.

55. Slavin S, Nagler A, Naparstek E, et al: Nonmyeloablative stem cell transplantation and cell therapy as an alternative to conventional bone marrow transplantation with lethal cytoreduction for the treatment of malignant and nonmalignant hematologic diseases. Blood 1998;91:756–763.

56. Sykes M, Preffer F, McAfee S, et al: Mixed lymphohaemopoietic chimerism and graft-versus-lymphoma effects after non-myeloablative therapy and HLA-mismatched bone-marrow transplantation. Lancet 1999;353:1755–1759.

57. Carella AM, Lerma E, Dejana A, et al: Engraftment of HLA-matched sibling hematopoietic stem cells after immunosuppressive conditioning regimen in patients with hematologic neoplasias. Haematologica 1998;83:904–909.

58. Childs R, Clave E, Contentin N, et al: Engraftment kinetics after nonmyeloablative allogeneic peripheral blood stem cell transplantation: Full donor T-cell chimerism precedes alloimmune responses. Blood 1999;94:3234–3241.

59. McSweeney PA, Storb R: Mixed chimerism: Preclinical studies and clinical applications. Biol Blood Marrow Transplant 1999;5:192–203.

60. Storb R, Yu C, Sandmaier BM, et al: Mixed hematopoietic chimerism after marrow allografts: Transplantation in the ambulatory care setting. Ann N Y Acad Sci 1999;872:372–376.

61. Spangrude GJ: Biological and clinical aspects of hematopoietic stem cells. Annu Rev Med 1994;45:93–104.

62. Weissman I, Spangrude G, Heimfeld S, et al: Stem cells. Nature 1991;353:26–26.

63. Civin CI, Almeida-Porada G, Lee MJ, et al: Sustained, retransplantable, multilineage engraftment of highly purified adult human bone marrow stem cells in vivo. Blood 1996;88:4102–4109.

64. Andrews RG, Bryant EM, Bartelmez SH, et al: CD34$^+$ marrow cells, devoid of T and B lymphocytes, reconstitute stable lymphopoiesis and myelopoiesis in lethally irradiated allogeneic baboons. Blood 1992;80:1693–1701.

65. Berenson RJ, Bensinger WI, Hill RS, et al: Engraftment after infusion of CD34$^+$ marrow cells in patients with breast cancer or neuroblastoma. Blood 1991;77:1717–1722.

66. Kawashima I, Zanjani ED, Almaida-Porada G, et al: CD34$^+$ human marrow cells that express low levels of Kit protein are enriched for long-term marrow-engrafting cells. Blood 1996;87:4136–4142.

67. Baum CM, Weissman IL, Tsukamoto AS, et al: Isolation of a candidate human hematopoietic stem-cell population. Proc Natl Acad Sci U S A 1992;89:2804–2808.

68. Yin AH, Miraglia S, Zanjani ED, et al: AC133, a novel marker for human hematopoietic stem and progenitor cells. Blood 1997;90:5002–5012.

69. Osawa M, Hanada K, Hamada H, et al: Long-term lymphohematopoietic reconstitution by a single CD34$^-$ low/negative hematopoietic stem cell. Science 1996;273:242–245.

70. Zanjani ED, Almeida-Porada G, Livingston AG, et al: Human bone marrow CD34$^-$ cells engraft in vivo and undergo multilineage expression that includes giving rise to CD34$^+$ cells. Exp Hematol 1998;26:353–360.

71. Sato T, Laver JH, Ogawa M: Reversible expression of CD34 by murine hematopoietic stem cells. Blood 1999;94:2548–2554.

72. Thomas ED, Storb R: Technique for human marrow grafting. Blood 1970;36:507–515.

73. Bortin MM, Buckner CD: Major complications from marrow harvesting for transplantation. Exp Hematol 1983;11:916.

74. Buckner CD, Clift RA, Sanders JE, et al: Marrow harvesting from normal donors. Blood 1984;64:630–634.

75. Baselga J, Reich L, Doherty M, Gulati S: Fat embolism syndrome following bone marrow harvesting. Bone Marrow Transplant 1991;7:485–486.

76. Klumpp TR, Mangan KF, Macdonald JS, Mesgarzadeh M: Fracture of the ilium: An unusual complication of bone marrow harvesting. Bone Marrow Transplant 1992;9:503–504.

77. Stroncek D, Strand R, Scott E, et al: Attitudes and physical condition of unrelated bone marrow donors immediately after donation. Transfusion 1989;29:317–322.

78. Stroncek DF, Holland PV, Bartch G, et al: Experiences of the first 493 unrelated marrow donors in the National Marrow Donor Program. Blood 1993;81:1940–1946.

79. Champlin RE: Peripheral blood progenitor cells: A replacement for marrow transplantation? Semin Oncol 1996;23:15–21.

80. Hartmann O, Le Corroller AG, Blaise D, et al: Peripheral blood stem cell and bone marrow transplantation for solid tumors and lymphomas: Hematologic recovery and costs—a randomized, controlled trial. Ann Intern Med 1997;126:600–607.

81. Socinski MA, Elias A, Schnipper L, et al: Granulocyte-macrophage colony stimulating factor expands the circulating haemopoietic progenitor cell compartment in man. Lancet 1988;1:1194–1197.

82. Sheridan WP, Begley CG, Juttner CA, et al: Effect of peripheral-blood progenitor cells mobilised by filgrastim (G-CSF) on platelet recovery after high-dose chemotherapy. Lancet 1992;339:640–644.

83. Anderlini P, Körbling M, Dale D, et al: Allogeneic blood stem cell transplantation: Considerations for donors. Blood 1997;90:903–908.

84. Glaspy JA, Shpall EJ, LeMaistre CF, et al: Peripheral blood progenitor cell mobilization using stem cell factor in combination with filgrastim in breast cancer patients. Blood 1997;90:2939–2951.

85. Somlo G, Sniecinski I, Ter Veer A, et al: Recombinant human thrombopoietin in combination with granulocyte colony-stimulating factor enhances mobilization of peripheral blood progenitor cells, increases peripheral blood platelet concentration, and accelerates hematopoietic recovery following high-dose chemotherapy. Blood 1999;93:2798–2806.

86. Sudo Y, Shimazaki C, Ashihara E, et al: Synergistic effect of FLT-3 ligand on the granulocyte colony-stimulating factor-induced mobilization of hematopoietic stem cells and progenitor cells into blood in mice. Blood 1997;89:3186–3191.

87. Shpall EJ, Champlin RE, Glaspy J: The effect of CD34+ peripheral blood progenitor cell dose on hematopoietic recovery. Biol Blood Marrow Transplant 1998;4:84–92.

88. Korbling M, Huh YO, Durett A, et al: Allogeneic blood stem cell transplantation: Peripheralization and yield of donor-derived primitive hematopoietic progenitor cells (CD34$^+$ Thy-1^{dim}) and lymphoid subsets, and possible predictors of engraftment and graft-versus-host disease. Blood 1995;86:2842–2848.

89. Przepiorka D, Smith TL, Folloder J, et al: Risk factors for acute graft-versus-host disease after allogeneic blood stem cell transplantation. Blood 1999;94:1465–1470.

90. Bensinger WI, Clift R, Martin P, et al: Allogeneic peripheral blood stem cell transplantation in patients with advanced hematologic malignancies: A retrospective comparison with marrow transplantation. Blood 1996;88:2794–2800.

91. Storek J, Gooley T, Siadak M, et al: Allogeneic peripheral blood stem cell transplantation may be associated with a high risk of chronic graft-versus-host disease. Blood 1997;90:4705–4709.

92. Champlin R, Schmitz N, Horowitz MM, et al: Blood stem cells versus bone marrow as a source of hematopoietic cells for allogeneic transplantation. Blood 2000;95:3701–3709.

93. Bensinger W, Martin P, Clift R, et al: A prospective randomized trial of peripheral blood stem cells or marrow for patients undergoing allogeneic transplantation for hematologic malignancies. Blood 1999;94(Suppl 1):368A.

94. Broxmeyer HE: Questions to be answered regarding umbilical cord blood hematopoietic stem and progenitor cells and their use in transplantation. Transfusion 1995;35:694–702.

95. Cairo MS, Wagner JE: Placental and/or umbilical cord blood: An alternative source of hematopoietic stem cells for transplantation. Blood 1997;90:4665–4678.

96. Rubinstein P, Carrier C, Scaradavou A, et al: Outcomes among 562 recipients of placental-blood transplants from unrelated donors. N Engl J Med 1998;339:1565–1577.

97. Silberstein LE, Jefferies LC: Placental-blood banking: A new frontier in transfusion medicine. N Engl J Med 1996;335:199–201.

98. Gluckman E, Rocha V, Boyer-Chammard A, et al: Outcome of cord-blood transplantation from related and unrelated donors. N Engl J Med 1997;337:373–381.

99. Kurtzberg J, Laughlin M, Graham ML, et al: Placental blood as a source of hematopoietic stem cells for transplantation into unrelated recipients. N Engl J Med 1996;335:157–166.

100. Wagner JE, Rosenthal J, Sweetman R, et al: Successful transplantation of HLA-matched and HLA-mismatched umbilical cord blood from unrelated donors: Analysis of engraftment and acute graft-versus-host disease. Blood 1996;88:795–802.

101. Carter AS, Bunce M, Cerundolo L, et al: Detection of microchimerism after allogeneic blood transfusion using nested polymerase chain reaction amplification with sequence-specific primers (PCR-SSP): A cautionary tale. Blood 1998;92:683–689.

102. Casarino L, Carbone C, Capucci MA, et al: Analysis of chimerism after bone marrow transplantation using specific oligonucleotide probes. Bone Marrow Transplant 1992;10:165–170.

103. Durnam DM, Anders KR, Fisher L, et al: Analysis of the origin of marrow cells in bone marrow transplant recipients using a Y-chromosome-specific in situ hybridization assay. Blood 1989;74:2220–2226.

104. Leclair B, Frégeau CJ, Aye MT, Fourney RM: DNA typing for bone marrow engraftment follow-up after allogeneic transplant: A comparative study of current technologies. Bone Marrow Transplant 1995;16:43–55.

105. McCann SR, Lawler M: Mixed chimaerism: Detection and significance following BMT. Bone Marrow Transplant 1993;11:91–94.

106. Gerson SL: Mesenchymal stem cells: No longer second class marrow citizens. Nat Med 1999;5:262–264.

107. Pittenger MF, Mackay AM, Beck SC, et al: Multilineage potential of adult human mesenchymal stem cells. Science 1999;284:143–147.

108. Aird W, Labopin M, Gorin NC, Antin JH: Long-term cryopreservation of human stem cells. Bone Marrow Transplant 1992;9:487–490.

109. Attarian H, Feng Z, Buckner CD, et al: Long-term cryopreservation of bone marrow for autologous transplantation. Bone Marrow Transplant 1996;17:425–430.

110. Rowley SD, Bensinger WI, Gooley TA, Buckner CD: Effect of cell concentration on bone marrow and peripheral blood stem cell cryopreservation. Blood 1994;83:2731–2736.

111. Ross AA, Cooper BW, Lazarus HM, et al: Detection and viability of tumor cells in peripheral blood stem cell collections from breast cancer patients using immunocytochemical and clonogenic assay techniques. Blood 1993;82:2605–2610.

112. Brenner MK, Rill DR, Moen RC, et al: Gene-marking to trace origin of relapse after autologous bone-marrow transplantation. Lancet 1993;341:85–86.

113. Deisseroth AB, Zu Z, Claxton D, et al: Genetic marking shows that Ph$^+$ cells present in autologous transplants of chronic myelogenous leukemia (CML) contribute to relapse after autologous bone marrow in CML. Blood 1994;83:3068–3076.

114. Rill DR, Santana VM, Roberts WM, et al: Direct demonstration that autologous bone marrow transplantation for solid tumors can return a multiplicity of tumorigenic cells. Blood 1994;84:380–383.

115. Gribben JG, Freedman AS, Neuberg D, et al: Immunologic purging of marrow assessed by PCR before autologous bone marrow transplantation for B-cell lymphoma. N Engl J Med 1991;325:1525–1533.

116. Vredenburgh JJ, Peters WP, Rosner G, et al: Detection of tumor cells in the bone marrow of stage IV breast cancer patients receiving high-dose chemotherapy: The role of induction chemotherapy. Bone Marrow Transplant 1995;16:815–821.

117. Sharp JG, Kessinger A, Mann S, et al: Outcome of high-dose therapy and autologous transplantation in non-Hodgkin's lymphoma based the presence of tumor in the marrow or infused hematopoietic harvest. J Clin Oncol 1996;14:214–219.

118. Champlin RE: Purging: The separation of normal from malignant cells for autologous transplantation. Transfusion 1996;36:910–918.

119. Shpall EJ, LeMaistre CF, Holland K, et al: A prospective randomized trial of buffy coat versus CD34$^-$ selected autologous bone marrow support in high-risk breast cancer patients receiving high-dose chemotherapy. Blood 1997;90:4313–4320.

120. Rowley SD, Loken M, Radich J, et al: Isolation of CD34$^+$ cells from blood stem cell components using the Baxter Isolex system. Bone Marrow Transplant 1998;21:1253–1262.

121. Vescio R, Schiller G, Stewart AK, et al: Multicenter phase III trial to evaluate CD34$^+$ selected versus unselected autologous peripheral blood progenitor cell transplantation in multiple myeloma. Blood 1999;93:1858–1868.

122. Gorin NC, Aegerter P, Auvert B, et al: Autologous bone marrow transplantation for acute myelocytic leukemia in first remission: A European survey of the role of marrow purging. Blood 1990;75:1606–1614.

123. Yeager AM, Kaizer H, Santos GW, et al: Autologous bone marrow transplantation in patients with acute nonlymphocytic leukemia, using ex vivo marrow treatment with 4-hydroperoxycyclophosphamide. N Engl J Med 1986;315:141–147.

124. Kusnierz-Glaz CR, Schlegel PG, Wong RM, et al: Influence of age on the outcome of 500 autologous bone marrow transplant procedures for hematologic malignancies. J Clin Oncol 1997;15:18–25.

125. Miller CB, Piantadosi S, Vogelsang GB, et al: Impact of age on outcome of patients with cancer undergoing autologous bone marrow transplant. J Clin Oncol 1996;14:1327–1332.

126. Bensinger W, Appelbaum F, Rowley S, et al: Factors that influence collection and engraftment of autologous peripheral-blood stem cells. J Clin Oncol 1995;13:2547–2555.

127. Friedberg JW, Neuberg D, Stone RM, et al: Outcome in patients with myelodysplastic syndrome after autologous bone marrow transplantation for non-Hodgkin's lymphoma. J Clin Oncol 1999;17:3128–3135.

128. Marolleau JP, Brice P, Morel P, Gisselbrecht C: Secondary acute myeloid leukemia after autologous bone marrow transplantation for malignant lymphomas. J Clin Oncol 1993;11:590–591.

129. Bordignon C, Keever CA, Small TN, et al: Graft failure after T-cell-depleted human leukocyte antigen identical marrow transplants for leukemia. II. In vitro analyses of host effector mechanisms. Blood 1989;74:2237–2243.

130. Fleischhauer K, Kernan NA, O'Reilly RJ, et al: Bone marrow-allograft rejection by T lymphocytes recognizing a single amino acid difference in HLA-B44. N Engl J Med 1990;323:1818–1822.

131. Petersdorf EW, Longton GM, Anasetti C, et al: Association of HLA-C disparity with graft failure after marrow transplantation from unrelated donors. Blood 1997;89:1818–1823.

132. Davies SM, Ramsay NKC, Haake RJ, et al: Comparison of engraftment in recipients of matched sibling or unrelated donor marrow allografts. Bone Marrow Transplant 1994;13:51–57.

133. Martin PJ: Donor CD8 cells prevent allogeneic marrow graft rejection in mice: Potential implications for marrow transplantation in humans. J Exp Med 1993;178:703–712.

134. Martin PJ, Hansen JA, Torok-Storb B, et al: Graft failure in patients receiving T cell-depleted HLA-identical allogeneic marrow transplants. Bone Marrow Transplant 1989;3:445.

135. Kaufman CL, Colson YL, Wren SM, et al: Phenotypic characterization of a novel bone marrow-derived cell that facilitates engraftment of allogeneic bone marrow stem cells. Blood 1994;84:2436–2446.

136. Simmons P, Kaushansky K, Torok-Storb B: Mechanisms of cytomegalovirus-mediated myelosuppression: Perturbation of stromal cell function versus direct infection of myeloid cells. Proc Natl Acad Sci U S A 1990;87:1386–1390.

137. Schleuning M, Jäger G, Holler E, et al: Human parvovirus B19-associated disease in bone marrow transplantation. Infection 1999;27:114–117.

138. Carrigan DR, Knox KK: Human herpesvirus 6 (HHV-6) isolation from bone marrow: HHV-6-associated bone marrow suppression in bone marrow transplant patients. Blood 1994;84:3307–3310.

139. Nemunaitis J, Singer JW, Buckner CD, et al: Use of recombinant human granulocyte-macrophage colony-stimulating factor in graft failure after bone marrow transplantation. Blood 1990;76:245–253.

140. Weisdorf DJ, Verfaillie CM, Davies SM, et al: Hematopoietic growth factors for graft failure after bone marrow transplantation: A randomized trial of granulocyte-macrophage colony-stimulating factor (GM-CSF) versus sequential GM-CSF plus granulocyte-CSF. Blood 1995;85:3452–3456.

141. Ferrara JLM, Deeg HJ: Mechanisms of disease: Graft-versus-host disease. N Engl J Med 1991;324:667–674.

142. Shlomchik WD, Couzens MS, Tang CB, et al: Prevention of graft versus host disease by inactivation of host antigen-presenting cells. Science 1999;285:412–415.

143. Weisdorf DJ, Snover DC, Haake R, et al: Acute upper gastrointestinal graft-versus-host disease: Clinical significance and response to immunosuppressive therapy. Blood 1990;76:624–629.

144. Glucksberg H, Storb R, Fefer A: Clinical manifestations of graft-versus-host disease in human recipients of marrow from HLA-identical sibling donors. Transplantation 1974;18:295–304.

145. Przepiorka D, Weisdorf D, Martin P, et al: Consensus conference on acute GVHD grading. Bone Marrow Transplant 1995;15:825–828.

146. Gajewski J, Gjertson D, Cecka M, et al: Impact of molecular subtype of HLA DR and DQ alleles on acute graft-vs.-host disease and relapse free survival in HLA serologically identical unrelated donor bone marrow transplants: Effect of T-cell depletion. Biol Blood Marrow Transplant 1997;3:76–82.

147. Martin PJ: Increased disparity for minor histocompatibility antigens as a potential cause of increased GVHD risk in marrow transplantation from unrelated donors compared with related donors. Bone Marrow Transplant 1991;8:217–223.

148. Rufer N, Wolpert E, Helg C, et al: HA-1 and the SMCY-derived peptide FIDSYICQV (H-Y) are immunodominant minor histocompatibility antigens after bone marrow transplantation. Transplantation 1998;66:910–916.

149. Flowers MED, Pepe MS, Longton G, et al: Previous donor pregnancy as a risk factor for acute graft-versus-host disease in patients with aplastic anaemia treated by allogeneic marrow transplantation. Br J Haematol 1990;74:492–496.

150. Gale RP, Bortin MM, vanBekkum DW, et al: Risk factors for acute graft-versus-host disease. Br J.Haematol 1987;67:397–406.

151. Wagner JE, Kernan NA, Steinbuch M, et al: Allogeneic sibling umbilical-cord-blood transplantation in children with malignant and non-malignant disease. Lancet 1995;346:214–219.

152. Boström L, Ringdén O, Jacobsen N, et al: A European multicenter study of chronic graft-versus-host disease: The role of cytomegalovirus serology in recipients and donors, acute graft-versus-host disease, and splenectomy. Transplantation 1990;49:1100–1105.

153. Champlin RE: T-cell depletion for allogeneic bone marrow transplantation: Impact on graft-versus-host disease, engraftment, and graft-versus-leukemia. J Hematother 1993;2:27–42.

154. Mitsuyasu R, Champlin RE, Gale RP, et al: Depletion of T-lymphocytes from donor bone marrow for the prevention of graft-versus-host disease following bone marrow transplantation. Ann Intern Med 1986;105:20–26.

155. Ash RC, Casper JT, Chitambar CR, et al: Successful allogeneic transplantation of T-cell-depleted bone marrow from closely HLA-matched unrelated donors. N Engl J Med 1990;322:485–494.

156. O'Reilly RJ: T-cell depletion and allogeneic bone marrow transplantation. Semin Hematol 1992;29(Suppl 1):20–26.

157. Reisner Y, Kapoor RJ, Kirkpatrick N, et al: Allogeneic bone marrow transplantation for acute leukemia with HLA-A and -B nonidentical parental marrow cells fractionated with soybean agglutinin and sheep red blood cells. Lancet 1981;2:327–331.

158. Nash RA, Piñeiro LA, Storb R, et al: FK506 in combination with methotrexate for the prevention of graft-versus-host disease after marrow transplantation from matched unrelated donors. Blood 1996;88:3634–3641.

159. Przepiorka D, Ippoliti C, Khouri I, et al: Tacrolimus and minidose methotrexate for prevention of acute graft-vs-host disease after matched unrelated donor marrow transplantation. Blood 1996;88:4383–4389.

160. Storb R, Pepe M, Deeg HJ, et al: Long-term follow-up of a controlled trial comparing a combination of methotrexate plus cyclosporine with cyclosporine alone for prophylaxis of graft-versus-host disease in patients administered HLA-identical marrow grafts for leukemia. Blood 1992;80:560–561.

161. Martin PJ, Schoch G, Fisher L, et al: A retrospective analysis of therapy for acute graft-versus-host disease: Initial treatment. Blood 1990;76:1464–1472.

162. Martin PJ, Schoch G, Fisher L, et al: A retrospective analysis of therapy for acute graft-versus-host disease: Secondary treatment. Blood 1991;77:1821–1828.

163. Przepiorka D, Kernan NA, Ippoliti C, et al: Daclizumab, a humanized anti-interleukin-2 receptor alpha chain antibody, for treatment of acute graft-versus-host disease. Blood 2000;95:83–89.

164. Ippoliti C, Champlin R, Bugazia N, et al: Use of octreotide in the symptomatic management of diarrhea induced by graft-versus-host disease in patients with hematologic malignancies. J Clin Oncol 1997;15:3350–3354.

165. Sullivan KM, Agura E, Anasetti C, et al: Chronic graft-versus-host disease and other late complications of bone marrow transplantation. Semin Hematol 1991;28:250–259.

166. Atkinson K, Horowitz MM, Gale RP, et al: Risk factors for chronic graft-versus-host disease after HLA-identical sibling bone marrow transplantation. Blood 1990;75:2459–2464.

167. Shulman HM, Sullivan KM, Weiden PL: Chronic graft-versus-host syndrome in man: A long-term clinicopathologic study of 20 Seattle patients. Am J Med 1980;69:204–217.

168. Parkman R: Is chronic graft versus host disease an autoimmune disease. Curr Opin Immunol 1993;5:800–803.

169. Holland HK, Wingard JR, Beschorner WE, et al: Bronchiolitis obliterans in bone marrow transplantation and its relationship to chronic graft-v-host disease and low serum IgG. Blood 1988;72:621–627.

170. Wingard JR, Piantadosi S, Vogelsang GB, et al: Predictors of death from chronic graft-versus-host disease after bone marrow transplantation. Blood 1989;74:1428–1435.

171. Pepe MS, Longton G, Pettinger M, et al: Summarizing data on survival, relapse, and chronic graft-versus-host disease after bone marrow transplantation: Motivation for a description of new methods. Br J Haematol 1993;83:602–607.

172. Siadak M, Sullivan KM: The management of chronic graft-versus-host disease. Blood Rev 1994;8:154–160.

173. Sullivan KM, Witherspoon RP, Storb R, et al: Alternating-day cyclosporine and prednisone for treatment of high-risk chronic graft-v-host disease. Blood 1988;72:555–561.

174. Tzakis AG, Abu-Elmagd K, Fung JJ, et al: FK 506 rescue in chronic graft-versus-host disease after bone marrow transplantation. Transplant Proc 1991;23:3225–3227.

175. Basara N, Blau WI, Kiehl MG, et al: Efficacy and safety of mycophenolate mofetil for the treatment of acute and chronic GVHD in bone marrow transplant recipient. Transplant Proc 1998;30:4087–4089.

176. Vogelsang GB, Farmer ER, Hess AD, et al: Thalidomide for the treatment of chronic graft-versus-host disease. N Engl J Med 1992;326:1055–1058.

177. Kapoor N, Pelligrini AE, Copelan EA, et al: Psoralen plus ultraviolet A (PUVA) in the treatment of chronic graft versus host disease: Preliminary experience in standard treatment resistant patients. Semin Hematol 1992;29:108–112.

178. Rossetti F, Zulian F, Dall'Amico R, et al: Extracorporeal photochemotherapy as single therapy for extensive, cutaneous, chronic graft-versus-host disease. Transplantation 1995;59:149–151.

179. Besnier DP, Chabannes D, Mahé B, et al: Treatment of graft-versus-host disease by extracorporeal photochemotherapy. Transplantation 1997;64:49–54.

180. Garfunkel AA, Tager N, Chausu S, et al: Oral complications in bone marrow transplantation patients: Recent advances. Isr J Med Sci 1994;30:120–124.

181. Bearman SI: The syndrome of hepatic veno-occlusive disease after marrow transplantation. Blood 1995;85:3005–3020.

182. McDonald GB, Hinds MS, Fisher LD, et al: Veno-occlusive disease of the liver and multiorgan failure after bone marrow transplantation: A cohort study of 355 patients. Ann Intern Med 1993;118:255–267.

183. Carreras E, Bertz H, Arcese W, et al: Incidence and outcome of hepatic veno-occlusive disease after blood or marrow transplantation: A prospective cohort study of the European group for blood and marrow transplantation. Blood 1998;92:3599–3604.

184. Frickhofen N, Wiesneth M, Jainta C, et al: Hepatitis C virus infection is a risk factor for liver failure from veno-occlusive disease after bone marrow transplantation. Blood 1994;83:1998–2004.

185. Carreras E, Grañena A, Navasa M, et al: Transjugular liver biopsy in BMT. Bone Marrow Transplant 1993;11:21–26.

186. Bearman SI, Hinds MS, Wolford JL, et al: A pilot study of continuous infusion heparin for the prevention of hepatic veno-occlusive disease after bone marrow transplantation. Bone Marrow Transplant 1990;5:407–411.

187. Attal M, Huguet F, Rubie H, et al: Prevention of hepatic veno-occlusive disease after bone marrow transplantation by continuous infusion of low-dose heparin: A prospective, randomized trial. Blood 1992;79:2834–2840.

188. Essell JH, Schroeder MT, Harman GS, et al: Ursodiol prophylaxis against hepatic complications of allogeneic bone marrow transplantation: A randomized, double-blind, placebo-controlled trial. Ann Intern Med 1998;128:975–981.

189. Bearman SI, Lee JL, Barón AE, McDonald GB: Treatment of hepatic venoocclusive disease with recombinant human tissue plasminogen activator and heparin in 42 marrow transplant patients. Blood 1997;89:1501–1506.

190. Baglin TP, Harper P, Marcus RE: Veno-occlusive disease of the liver complicating ABMT successfully treated with recombinant tissue plasminogen activator (rt-PA). Bone Marrow Transplant 1990;5:439–441.

191. Levy V, Azoulay D, Rio B, et al: Successful treatment of severe hepatic veno-occlusive disease after allogeneic bone marrow transplantation by transjugular intrahepatic portosystemic stent-shunt (TIPS). Bone Marrow Transplant 1996;18:443–445.

192. Abecasis MM, Silva JPC, Ferreira I, et al: Defibrotide as salvage therapy for refractory veno-occlusive disease of the liver complicating allogeneic bone marrow transplantation. Bone Marrow Transplant 1999;23:843–846.

193. Nimer SD, Milewicz AL, Champlin RE, Busuttil RW: Successful treatment of hepatic venoocclusive disease in a bone marrow transplant patient with orthotopic liver transplantation. Transplantation 1990;49:819–821.

194. Crawford SW, Hackman RC: Clinical course of idiopathic pneumonia after bone marrow transplantation. Am Rev Respir Dis 1993;147:1393–1400.

195. Weiner RS, Bortin MM, Gale RP, et al: Interstitial pneumonitis after bone marrow transplantation. Ann Intern Med 1986;104:168–175.

196. Springmeyer SC, Silvestri RC, Flournoy N, et al: Pulmonary function of marrow transplant patients. I. Effects of marrow infusion, acute graft-versus-host disease, and interstitial pneumonitis. Transplantation 1984;12:805–810.

197. Jones RB, Matthes S, Shpall EJ, et al: Acute lung injury following treatment with high-dose cyclophosphamide, cisplatin, and carmustine: Pharmacodynamic evaluation of carmustine. J Natl Cancer Inst 1993;85:640–647.

198. Raptis A, Mavroudis D, Suffredini AF, et al: High-dose corticosteroid therapy for diffuse alveolar hemorrhage in allogeneic bone marrow stem cell transplant recipients. Bone Marrow Transplant 1999;24:879–883.

199. Lee C-K, Gingrich RD, Hohl RJ, Ajram KA: Engraftment syndrome in autologous bone marrow and peripheral stem cell transplantation. Bone Marrow Transplant 1995;16:175–182.

200. Palmas A, Tefferi A, Myers TL, et al: Late-onset noninfectious pulmonary complications after allogeneic bone marrow transplantation. Br J Haematol 1998;100:680–687.

201. Sencer SF, Haake RJ, Weisdorf DJ: Hemorrhagic cystitis after bone marrow transplantation: Risk factors and complications. Transplantation 1993;56:875–879.

202. Al-Rawithi S, El-Yazigi A, Ernst P, et al: Urinary excretion and pharmacokinetics of acrolein and its parent drug cyclophosphamide in bone marrow transplant patients. Bone Marrow Transplant 1998;22:485–490.

203. Bedi A, Miller CB, Hanson JL, et al: Association of BK virus with failure of prophylaxis against hemorrhagic cystitis following bone marrow transplantation. J Clin Oncol 1995;13:1103–1109.

204. Chen FE, Liang RHS, Lo JY, et al: Treatment of adenovirus-associated haemorrhagic cystitis with ganciclovir. Bone Marrow Transplant 1997;20:997–999.

205. Shepherd JD, Pringle LE, Barnett MJ, et al: Mesna versus hyperhydration for the prevention of cyclophosphamide-induced hemorrhagic cystitis in bone marrow transplantation. J Clin Oncol 1991;9:2016–2020.

206. Turkeri LN, Lum LG, Uberti JP, et al: Prevention of hemorrhagic cystitis following allogeneic bone marrow transplant preparative regimens with cyclophosphamide and busulfan: Role of continuous bladder irrigation. J Urol 1995;153:637–640.

207. Baronciani D, Montesi M, Angelucci E, et al: Suprapubic cystotomy as treatment for severe hemorrhagic cystitis after bone marrow transplantation. Bone Marrow Transplant 1995;16:267–270.

208. Lee CK, Harman GS, Hohl RJ, Gingrich RD: Fatal cyclophosphamide cardiomyopathy: Its clinical course and treatment. Bone Marrow Transplant 1996;18:573–577.

209. Miralbell R, Bieri S, Mermillod B, et al: Renal toxicity after allogeneic bone marrow transplantation: The combined effects of total-body irradiation and graft-versus-host disease. J Clin Oncol 1996;14:579–585.

210. Devine SM, Newman NJ, Siegel JL, et al: Tacrolimus (FK506)-induced cerebral blindness following bone marrow transplantation. Bone Marrow Transplant 1996;18:569–572.

211. Reece DE, Frei-Lahr DA, Shepherd JD, et al: Neurologic complications in allogeneic bone marrow transplant patients receiving cyclosporin. Bone Marrow Transplant 1991;8:393–401.

212. Locatelli F, Giorgiani G, Pession A, Bozzola M: Late effects in children after bone marrow transplantation: A review. Haematologica 1993;78:319–328.

213. Sanders JE, Hawley J, Levy W, et al: Pregnancies following high-dose cyclophosphamide with or without high-dose busulfan or total-body irradiation and bone marrow transplantation. Blood 1996;87:3045–3052.

214. Curtis RE, Rowlings PA, Deeg HJ, et al: Solid cancers after bone marrow transplantation. N Engl J Med 1997;336:897–904.

215. Socie G, Henry-Amar M, Cosset JM, et al: Increased incidence of solid malignant tumors after bone marrow transplantation for severe aplastic anemia. Blood 1991;78:277–279.

216. Abruzzese E, Radford JE, Miller JS, et al: Detection of abnormal pretransplant clones in progenitor cells of patients who developed myelodysplasia after autologous transplantation. Blood 1999;94:1814–1819.

217. Armitage JO: Myelodysplasia and acute leukemia after autologous bone marrow transplantation. J Clin Oncol 2000;18:945–946.

218. Bacigalupo A, Mordini N, Pitto A, et al: Transplantation of HLA-mismatched CD34$^+$ selected cells in patients with advanced malignancies: Severe immunodeficiency and related complications. Br J Haematol 1997;98:760–766.

219. Powles R, Singhal S, Treleaven J, et al: Identification of patients who may benefit from prophylactic immunotherapy after bone marrow transplantation for acute myeloid leukemia on the basis of lymphocyte recovery early after transplantation. Blood 1998;91:3481–3486.

220. Edmond MB, Ober JF, Dawson JD, et al: Vancomycin-resistant enterococcal bacteremia: Natural history and attributable mortality. Clin Infect Dis 1996;23:1234–1239.

221. Kirkpatrick BD, Harrington SM, Smith D, et al: An outbreak of vancomycin-dependent *Enterococcus faecium* in a bone marrow transplant unit. Clin Infect Dis 1999;29:1268–1273.

222. Lew MA, Kehoe K, Ritz J, et al: Ciprofloxacin versus trimethoprim/sulfamethoxazole for prophylaxis of bacterial infections in bone marrow transplant recipients: A randomized, controlled trial. J Clin Oncol 1995;13:239–250.

223. Anaissie EJ, Vadhan-Raj S: Is it time to redefine the management of febrile neutropenia in cancer patients. Am J Med 1995;98:221–223.

224. Pizzo PA: Drug therapy: Management of fever in patients with cancer and treatment-induced neutropenia. N Engl J Med 1993;328:1323–1332.

225. Winston DJ, Ho WG, Schiffman G, et al: Pneumococcal vaccination of recipients of bone marrow transplants. Arch Intern Med 1983;143:1735–1737.

226. De Bock R: Epidemiology of invasive fungal infections in bone marrow transplantation. Bone Marrow Transplant 1994;14(Suppl 5):S1–S2.

227. Goodman JL, Winston DJ, Greenfield RA, et al: A controlled trial of fluconazole to prevent fungal infections in patients undergoing bone marrow transplantation. N Engl J Med 1992;326:845–851.

228. Van Burik JAH, Leisenring W, Myerson D, et al: The effect of prophylactic fluconazole on the clinical spectrum of fungal diseases in bone marrow transplant recipients with special attention to hepatic candidiasis: An autopsy study of 355 patients. Medicine (Baltimore) 1998;77:246–254.

229. Wingard JR, Merz WG, Rinaldi MG, et al: Increase in *Candida krusei* infection among patients with bone marrow transplantation and neutropenia treated prophylactically with fluconazole. N Engl J Med 1991;325:1274–1277.

230. Morrison VA, Haake RJ, Weisdorf DJ: Non-*Candida* fungal infections after bone marrow transplantation: Risk factors and outcome. Am J Med 1994;96:497–503.

231. Gamis AS, Gudnason T, Giebink GS, Ramsay NKC: Disseminated infection with *Fusarium* in recipients of bone marrow transplants. Rev Infect Dis 1991;13:1077–1088.

232. McWhinney PHM, Kibbler CC, Hamon MD, et al: Progress in the diagnosis and management of aspergillosis in bone marrow transplantation: 13 years' experience. Clin Infect Dis 1993;17:397–404.

233. Ribaud P, Chastang C, Latgé JP, et al: Survival and prognostic factors of invasive aspergillosis after allogeneic bone marrow transplantation. Clin Infect Dis 1999;28:322–330.

234. Meyers JD: Prevention of cytomegalovirus infection after marrow transplantation. Rev Infect Dis 1989;11(Suppl 7):S1691–S1705.

235. Bowden RA, Slichter SJ, Sayers M, et al: A comparison of filtered leukocyte-reduced and cytomegalovirus (CMV)-seronegative blood products for the prevention of transfusion-associated CMV infection after marrow transplant. Blood 1995;86:3598–3603.

236. Bowden RA, Sayers M, Flournoy N, et al: Cytomegalovirus immune globulin and seronegative blood products to prevent primary cytomegalovirus infection after marrow transplant. N Engl J Med 1986;314:1006–1010.

237. Winston DJ, Huang E-S, Miller MJ, et al: Molecular epidemiology of cytomegalovirus infections associated with bone marrow transplantation. Ann Intern Med 1985;102:16–20.

238. Boeckh M, Gooley TA, Myerson D, et al: Cytomegalovirus pp65 antigenemia–guided early treatment with ganciclovir versus ganciclovir at engraftment after allogeneic marrow transplantation: A randomized double-blind study. Blood 1996;88:4063–4071.

239. Boeckh M: Management of cytomegalovirus infections in blood and marrow transplant recipients. Adv Exp Med Biol 1999;458:89–109.

240. Enright H, Haake R, Weisdorf D, et al: Cytomegalovirus pneumonia after bone marrow transplantation: Risk factors and response to therapy. Transplantation 1993;55:1339–1346.

241. Goodrich JM, Bowden RA, Fisher L, et al: Ganciclovir prophylaxis to prevent cytomegalovirus disease after allogeneic marrow transplant. Ann Intern Med 1993;118:173–178.

242. Winston DJ, Ho WG, Bartoni K, et al: Ganciclovir prophylaxis of cytomegalovirus infection and disease in allogeneic bone marrow transplant recipients: Results of a placebo-controlled, double-blind trial. Ann Intern Med 1993;118:179–184.

243. Torok-Storb B, Boeckh M, Hoy C, et al: Association of specific cytomegalovirus genotypes with death from myelosuppression after marrow transplantation. Blood 1997;90:2097–2102.

244. Emanuel D, Cunningham I, Jules-Elysee K, et al: Cytomegalovirus pneumonia after bone marrow transplantation successfully treated with the combination of ganciclovir and high dose intravenous immune globulin. Ann Intern Med 1991;109:777–782.

245. Goodrich JM, Mori M, Gleaves CA, et al: Early treatment with ganciclovir to prevent cytomegalovirus disease after allogeneic bone marrow transplantation. N Engl J Med 1991;325:1601–1607.

246. Forman SJ, Zaia JA: Treatment and prevention of cytomegalovirus pneumonia after bone marrow transplantation: Where do we stand? Blood 1994;83:2392–2398.

247. Ippoliti C, Morgan A, Warkentin D, et al: Foscarnet for prevention of cytomegalovirus infection in allogeneic marrow transplant recipients unable to receive ganciclovir. Bone Marrow Transplant 1997;20:491–495.

248. Lalezari JP, Stagg RJ, Kuppermann BD, et al: Intravenous cidofovir for peripheral cytomegalovirus retinitis in patients with AIDS: A randomized, controlled trial. Ann Intern Med 1997;126:257–263.

249. Riddell S, Watanabe K, Goodrich J, et al: Restoration of viral immunity in immunodeficient humans by the adoptive transfer of T cell clones. Science 1992;257:238.

250. Whimbey E, Champlin RE, Couch RB, et al: Community respiratory virus infections among hospitalized adult bone marrow transplant recipients. Clin Infect Dis 1996;22:778–782.

251. Whimbey E, Champlin RE, Englund JA, et al: Combination therapy with aerosolized ribavirin and intravenous immunoglobulin for respiratory syncytial virus disease in adult bone marrow transplant recipients. Bone Marrow Transplant 1995;16:393–399.

252. Flomenberg P, Babbitt J, Drobyski WR, et al: Increasing incidence of adenovirus disease in bone marrow transplant recipients. J Infect Dis 1994;169:775–781.

253. Howard DS, Phillips GL II, Reece DE, et al: Adenovirus infections in hematopoietic stem cell transplant recipients. Clin Infect Dis 1999;29:1494–1501.

254. Han CS, Miller W, Haake R, Weisdorf D: Varicella zoster infection after bone marrow transplantation: Incidence, risk factors and complications. Bone Marrow Transplant 1994;13:277–283.

255. Carrigan DR: Human herpesvirus-6 and bone marrow transplantation. Blood 1995;85:294–295.

256. Strasser SI, McDonald GB: Hepatitis viruses and hematopoietic cell transplantation: A guide to patient and donor management. Blood 1999;93:1127–1136.

257. Liang R, Lau GKK, Kwong YL: Chemotherapy and bone marrow transplantation for cancer patients who are also chronic hepatitis B carriers: A review of the problem. J Clin Oncol 1999;17:394–398.

258. Ljungman P, Johansson N, Aschan J, et al: Long-term effects of hepatitis C virus infection in allogeneic bone marrow transplant recipients. Blood 1995;86:1614–1618.

259. Curtis RE, Travis LB, Rowlings PA, et al: Risk of lymphoproliferative disorders after bone marrow transplantation: A multi-institutional study. Blood 1999;94:2208–2216.

260. Papadopoulos EB, Ladanyi M, Emanuel D, et al: Infusions of donor leukocytes to treat Epstein-Barr virus–associated lymphoproliferative disorders after allogeneic bone marrow transplantation. N Engl J Med 1994;330:1185–1191.

261. Heslop H, Ng C, Li C, et al: Long-term restoration of immunity against Epstein-Barr virus infection by adoptive transfer of gene-modified virus-specific T lymphocytes. Nat Med 1996;2:551.

262. Gustafsson Å, Levitsky V, Zou JZ, et al: Epstein-Barr virus (EBV) load in bone marrow transplant recipients at risk to develop posttransplant lymphoproliferative disease: Prophylactic infusion of EBV-specific cytotoxic T cells. Blood 2000;95:807–814.

263. Masur H: Drug therapy: Prevention and treatment of *Pneumocystis* pneumonia. N Engl J Med 1992;327:1853–1860.

264. Przepiorka D, Selvaggi K, Rosenzweig PQ, et al: Aerosolized pentamidine for prevention of *Pneumocystis* pneumonia after allogeneic marrow transplantation. Bone Marrow Transplant 1991;7:324–325.

265. Souza JP, Boeckh M, Gooley TA, et al: High rates of *Pneumocystis carinii* pneumonia in allogeneic blood and marrow transplant recipients receiving dapsone prophylaxis. Clin Infect Dis 1999;29:1467–1471.

266. Giralt SA, Champlin RE: Leukemia relapse after allogeneic bone marrow transplantation: A review. Blood 1994;84:3603–3612.

267. Giralt S, Escudier S, Kantarjian H, et al: Preliminary results of treatment with filgrastim for relapse of leukemia and myelodysplasia after allogeneic bone marrow transplantation. N Engl J Med 1993;329:757–761.

268. Arcese W, Goldman JM, D'Arcangelo E, et al: Outcome for patients who relapse after allogeneic bone marrow transplantation for chronic myeloid leukemia. Blood 1993;82:3211–3219.

269. Van Rhee F, Lin F, Cullis JO, et al: Relapse of chronic myeloid leukemia after allogeneic bone marrow transplant: The case for giving donor leukocyte transfusions before the onset of hematologic relapse. Blood 1994;83:3377–3383.

270. Giralt S, Hester J, Huh Y, et al: CD8+ depleted donor lymphocyte infusion as treatment for relapsed chronic myelogenous leukemia after

allogeneic bone marrow transplantation: graft vs leukemia without graft vs. host disease. Blood 1995;86:4337–4343.

271. Alyea EP, Soiffer RJ, Canning C, et al: Toxicity and efficacy of defined doses of CD4+ donor lymphocytes for treatment of relapse after allogeneic bone marrow transplant. Blood 1998;91:3671–3680.

272. Mackinnon S, Papadopoulos EB, Carabasi MH, et al: Adoptive immunotherapy evaluating escalating doses of donor leukocytes for relapse of chronic myeloid leukemia after bone marrow transplantation: Separation of graft-versus-leukemia responses from graft-versus-host disease. Blood 1995;86:1261–1268.

273. Dazzi F, Szydlo RM, Craddock C, et al: Comparison of single-dose and escalating-dose regimens of donor lymphocyte infusion for relapse after allografting for chronic myeloid leukemia. Blood 2000;95:67–71.

274. Bonini C, Ferrari G, Verzeletti S, et al: HSV-TK gene transfer into donor lymphocytes for control of allogeneic graft-versus-leukemia. Science 1997;276:1719–1724.

275. Falkenburg JHF, Wafelman AR, Joosten P, et al: Complete remission of accelerated phase chronic myeloid leukemia by treatment with leukemia-reactive cytotoxic T lymphocytes. Blood 1999;94:1201–1208.

276. Mutis T, Verdijk R, Schrama E, et al: Feasibility of immunotherapy of relapsed leukemia with ex vivo–generated cytotoxic T lymphocytes specific for hematopoietic system–restricted minor histocompatibility antigens. Blood 1999;93:2336–2341.

277. Molldrem J, Lee PP, Wang CQ, et al: A PR1-human leukocyte antigen-A2 tetramer can be used to isolate low-frequency cytotoxic T lymphocytes from healthy donors that selectively lyse chronic myelogenous leukemia. Cancer Res 1999;56:2675–2681.

278. Barrett AJ, Locatelli F, Treleaven JG, et al: Second transplants for leukaemic relapse after bone marrow transplantation: High early mortality but favourable effect of chronic GVHD on continued remission. A report by the EBMT Leukaemia working party. Br J Haematol 1991;79:567–574.

279. Mrsíc M, Horowitz MM, Atkinson K, et al: Second HLA-identical sibling transplants for leukemia recurrence. Bone Marrow Transplant 1992;9:269–275.

280. Sanders JE, Buckner CD, Clift RA, et al: Second marrow transplants in patients with leukemia who relapse after allogeneic marrow transplants. Bone Marrow Transplant 1989;3:11.

281. Locatelli F: The role of repeat transplantation of haemopoietic stem cells and adoptive immunotherapy in treatment of leukaemia relapsing following allogeneic transplantation. Br J Haematol 1998;102:633–638.

282. Clift RA, Buckner CD: Marrow transplantation for acute myeloid leukemia. Cancer Invest 1998;16:53–61.

283. Copelan EA, Deeg HJ: Conditioning for allogeneic marrow transplantation in patients with lymphohematopoietic malignancies without the use of total body irradiation. Blood 1992;80:1648–1658.

284. Blaise D, Maraninchi D, Archimbaud E, et al: Allogeneic bone marrow transplantation for acute myeloid leukemia in first remission: A randomized trial of a busulfan-Cytoxan versus Cytoxan-total body irradiation as preparative regimen: A report from the Groupe d'Etudes de la Greffe de Moelle Osseuse. Blood 1992;79:2578–2582.

285. Clift RA, Buckner CD, Appelbaum FR, et al: Long-term follow-up of a randomized trial of two irradiation regimens for patients receiving allogeneic marrow transplants during first remission of acute myeloid leukemia. Blood 1998;92:1455–1456.

286. Aversa F, Terenzi A, Carotti A, et al: Improved outcome with T-cell–depleted bone marrow transplantation for acute leukemia. J Clin Oncol 1999;17:1545–1550.

287. Papadopoulos EB, Carabasi MH, Castro-Malaspina H, et al: T-cell–depleted allogeneic bone marrow transplantation as postremission therapy for acute myelogenous leukemia: Freedom from relapse in the absence of graft-versus-host disease. Blood 1998;91:1083–1090.

288. Soiffer RJ, Fairclough D, Robertson M, et al: CD6-depleted allogeneic bone marrow transplantation for acute leukemia in first complete remission. Blood 1997;89:3039–3047.

289. Matthews DC, Appelbaum FR, Eary JF, et al: Phase I study of 131I-anti-CD45 antibody plus cyclophosphamide and total body irradiation for advanced acute leukemia and myelodysplastic syndrome. Blood 1999;94:1237–1247.

290. Scheinberg DA, Lovett D, Divgi CR, et al: A phase I trial of monoclonal antibody M195 in acute myelogenous leukemia: Specific

bone marrow targeting and internalization of radionuclide. J Clin Oncol 1991;9:478–490.

291. Champlin RE, Gale RP: Acute myelogenous leukemia: Recent advances in therapy. Blood 1987;69:1551–1562, 1987

292. Applebaum FR, Fisher LD, Thomas ED: Chemotherapy vs marrow transplantation for adults with acute nonlymphocytic leukemia: A five year follow-up. Blood 1988;72:179–184.

293. Champlin RE, Ho WG, Gale RP, et al: Treatment of acute myelogenous leukemia: A prospective controlled trial of bone marrow transplantation versus consolidation chemotherapy. Ann Intern Med 1985;102:285–291.

294. Forman SJ, Schmidt GM, Nademanee AP, et al: Allogeneic bone marrow transplantation as therapy for primary induction failure for patients with acute leukemia. J Clin Oncol 1991;9:1570–1574.

295. Appelbaum FR, Clift RA, Buckner CD, et al: Allogeneic bone marrow transplantation for non-lymphoblastic leukemia after first relapse. Blood 1983;61:949–953.

296. Clift RA, Buckner CD, Appelbaum FR, et al: Allogeneic marrow transplantation during untreated first relapse of acute myeloid leukemia. J Clin Oncol 1992;10:1723–1729.

297. Burnett AK: Transplantation in first remission of acute myeloid leukemia. N Engl J Med 1998;339:1698–1700.

298. Cassileth PA, Harrington DP, Appelbaum FR, et al: Chemotherapy compared with autologous or allogeneic bone marrow transplantation in the management of acute myeloid leukemia in first remission. N Engl J Med 1998;339:1649–1656.

299. Reiffers J, Stoppa AM, Attal M, et al: Allogeneic vs autologous stem cell transplantation vs chemotherapy in patients with acute myeloid leukemia in first remission: The BGMT 87 study. Leukemia 1996;10:1874–1882.

300. Zittoun RA, Mandelli F, Willemze R, et al: Autologous or allogeneic bone marrow transplantation compared with intensive chemotherapy in acute myelogenous leukemia. N Engl J Med 1995;332:217–223.

301. Gale RP, Horowitz MM, Weiner RS, et al: Impact of cytogenetic abnormalities on outcome of bone marrow transplants in acute myelogenous leukemia in first remission. Bone Marrow Transplant 1995;16:203–208.

302. Bloomfield CD, Lawrence D, Byrd JC, et al: Frequency of prolonged remission duration after high-dose cytarabine intensification in acute myeloid leukemia varies by cytogenetic subtype. Cancer Res 1998;58:4173–4179.

303. Mayer RJ, Davis RB, Schiffer CA, et al: Intensive postremission chemotherapy in adults with acute myeloid leukemia. N Engl J Med 1994;331:896–903.

304. Schouten HC, Van Putten WLJ, Hagemeijer A, et al: The prognostic significance of chromosomal findings in patients with acute myeloid leukemia in a study comparing the efficacy of autologous and allogeneic bone marrow transplantation. Bone Marrow Transplant 1991;8:377–381.

305. Slovak ML, Kopecky KJ, Wolman SR, et al: Cytogenetic correlation with disease status and treatment outcome in advanced stage leukemia post bone marrow transplantation: A Southwest Oncology Group study (SWOG-8612). Leuk Res 1995;19:381–388.

306. Tallman MS, Kopecky KJ, Amos D, et al: Analysis of prognostic factors for the outcome of marrow transplantation or further chemotherapy for patients with acute nonlymphocytic leukemia in first remission. J Clin Oncol 1989;7:326–337.

307. Nesbit ME Jr, Buckley JD, Feig SA, et al: Chemotherapy for induction of remission of childhood acute myeloid leukemia followed by marrow transplantation or multiagent chemotherapy: A report from the Children's Cancer Group. J Clin Oncol 1994;12:127–135.

308. McSweeney P, Niederwieser D, Shizuru J, et al: Outpatient allografting with minimally myelosuppressive immunosuppressive conditioning of low-dose TBI and postgrafting cyclosporine and mycophenolate mofetil. Blood 1999;94(Suppl 1):393A.

309. Anasetti C: Transplantation of hematopoietic stem cells from alternate donors in acute myelogenous leukemia. Leukemia 2000;14:502–504.

310. Champlin R: Bone marrow transplantation for leukemia utilizing HLA-matched unrelated donors. Bone Marrow Transplant 1993;11(Suppl 1):74–77.

311. Burnett AK, Goldstone AH, Stevens RMF, et al: Randomised comparison of addition of autologous bone-marrow transplantation to intensive chemotherapy for acute myeloid leukaemia in first remission: Results of MRC AML 10 trial. Lancet 1998;351:700–708.

312. Cassileth PA, Andersen J, Lazarus HM, et al: Autologous bone marrow transplant in acute myeloid leukemia in first remission. J Clin Oncol 1993;11:314–319.

313. Ravindranath Y, Yeager AM, Chang MN, et al: Autologous bone marrow transplantation versus intensive consolidation chemotherapy for acute myeloid leukemia in childhood. N Engl J Med 1996;334:1428–1434.

314. Ball ED, Rybka WB: Autologous bone marrow transplantation for adult acute leukemia. Hematol Oncol Clin North Am 1993;7:201–231.

315. Busca A, Anasetti C, Anderson G, et al: Unrelated donor or autologous marrow transplantation for treatment of acute leukemia. Blood 1994;83:3077–3084.

316. Aversa F, Tabilio A, Velardi A, et al: Treatment of high-risk acute leukemia with T-cell–depleted stem cells from related donors with one fully mismatched HLA haplotype. N Engl J Med 1998;339:1186–1193.

317. Greenberg PL: Risk factors and their relationship to prognosis in myelodysplastic syndromes. Leukemia Res 1998;22(Suppl):S3–S6.

318. Appelbaum FR, Anderson J: Allogeneic bone marrow transplantation for myelodysplastic syndrome: Outcomes analysis according to IPSS score. Leukemia 1998;12(Suppl):S25–S29.

319. de Witte T, Gratwohl A: Bone marrow transplantation for myelodysplastic syndrome and secondary leukaemias. Br J Haematol 1993;84:361–364.

320. Deeg HJ, Shulman HM, Anderson JE, et al: Allogeneic and syngeneic marrow transplantation for myelodysplastic syndrome in patients 55 to 66 years of age. Blood 2000;95:1188–1194.

321. Appelbaum FR, Barrall J, Storb R, et al: Bone marrow transplantation for patients with myelodysplasia: Pretreatment variables and outcome. Ann Intern Med 1990;112:590–597.

322. Anderson JE, Gooley TA, Schoch G, et al: Stem cell transplantation for secondary acute myeloid leukemia: Evaluation of transplantation as initial therapy or following induction chemotherapy. Blood 1997;89:2578–2585.

323. Yakoub-Agha I, De la Salmonière P, Ribaud P, et al: Allogeneic bone marrow transplantation for therapy-related myelodysplastic syndrome and acute myeloid leukemia: A long-term study of 70 patients. Report of the French Society of Bone Marrow Transplant. J Clin Oncol 2000;18:963–971.

324. de Witte T, Van Biezen A, Hermans J, et al: Autologous bone marrow transplantation for patients with myelodysplastic syndrome (MDS) or acute myeloid leukemia following MDS. Blood 1997;90:3853–3857.

325. Borgmann A, Schmid H, Hartmann R, et al: Autologous bone-marrow transplants compared with chemotherapy for children with acute lymphoblastic leukaemia in a second remission: A matched-pair analysis. Lancet 1995;346:873–876.

326. Ritz J, Sallan SE, Bast RC, et al: Autologous bone marrow transplantation in CALLA positive acute lymphoblastic leukemia after in vitro treatment with J5 monoclonal antibody and complement. Lancet 1982;2:60–63.

327. Barrett AJ, Horowitz MM, Gale RP, et al: Marrow transplantation for acute lymphoblastic leukemia: Factors affecting relapse and survival. Blood 1989;74:862–871.

328. Kantarjian HM, O'Brien S, Smith TL, et al: Results of treatment with Hyper-CVAD, a dose-intensive regimen, in adult acute lymphocytic leukemia. J Clin Oncol 2000;18:547–561.

329. Zhang MJ, Hoelzer D, Horowitz MM, et al: Long-term follow up of adults with acute lymphoblastic leukemia in first remission treated with chemotherapy of bone marrow transplantation: The acute lymphoblastic leukemia working committee. Ann Intern Med 1995;15:428–431.

330. Forman SJ, Blume KG: Allogeneic bone marrow transplantation for acute leukemia. Hematol Oncol Clin North Am 1990;4:517–534.

331. Forman SJ, O'Donnell MR, Nademanee AP, et al: Bone marrow transplantation for patients with Philadelphia chromosome positive acute lymphoblastic leukemia. Blood 1987;70:587–588.

332. Sebban C, Lepage E, Vernant J-P, et al: Allogeneic bone marrow transplantation in adult acute lymphoblastic leukemia in first complete remission: A comparative study. J Clin Oncol 1994;12:2580–2587.

333. Barrett AJ, Horowitz MM, Ash RC, et al: Bone marrow transplantation for Philadelphia chromosome–positive acute lymphoblastic leukemia. Blood 1992;79:3067–3070.

334. Johnson FL, Thomas ED, Clark BS, et al: A comparison of marrow transplantation with chemotherapy for children with acute

335. Kersey JH, Weisdorf D, Nesbit ME, et al: Comparison of autologous and allogeneic bone marrow transplantation for treatment of high risk refractory acute lymphoblastic leukemia in second remission. N Engl J Med 1987;317:461–467.

336. Herzig R, Bortin MM, Gluckman E, et al: Optimal timing of bone marrow transplantation in patients with high risk acute lymphoblastic leukemia. Lancet 1987;1:786–788.

337. Champlin RE, Gale RP: Acute lymphoblastic leukemia: Recent advances in biology and therapy. Blood 1989;73:2051–2066.

338. Sierra J, Radich J, Hansen JA, et al: Marrow transplants from unrelated donors for treatment of Philadelphia chromosome–positive acute lymphoblastic leukemia. Blood 1997;90:1410–1414.

339. Davies SM, Ramsay NK, Klein JP, et al: Comparison of preparative regimens in transplants for children with acute lymphoblastic leukemia. J Clin Oncol 2000;18:340–347.

340. Thompson CB, Sanders JE, Flournoy N, et al: The risks of central nervous system relapse and leukoencephalopathy in patients receiving marrow transplants for acute leukemia. Blood 1986;67:195–199.

341. Brenner MK: Autologous bone-marrow transplantation in childhood acute lymphoblastic leukaemia. Lancet 1995;346:856–857.

342. Doney K, Buckner CD, Fisher L, et al: Autologous bone marrow transplantation for acute lymphoblastic leukemia. Bone Marrow Transplant 1993;12:315–321.

343. Sallan SE, Niemeyer CM, Billett AL, et al: Autologous bone marrow transplantation for acute lymphoblastic leukemia. J Clin Oncol 1989;7:1594–1601.

344. Kantarjian HM, O'Brien S, Smith TL, et al: Treatment of Philadelphia chromosome–positive early chronic phase chronic myelogenous leukemia with daily doses of interferon alpha and low-dose cytarabine. J Clin Oncol 1999;17:284–292.

345. Guilhot F, Chastang C, Michallet M, et al: Interferon alfa-2b combined with cytarabine versus interferon alone in chronic myelogenous leukemia. N Engl J Med 1997;337:223–229.

346. Druker B, Talpaz M, Resta D, et al: Clinical efficacy and safety of an abl specific tyrosine kinase inhibitor as targeted therapy for chronic myelogenous leukemia. Blood 1999;94(Suppl 1):368A.

347. Druker BJ, Tamure S, Buchdunger E, et al: Effects of a selective inhibitor of the abl tryosine kinase on the growth of bcr-abl positive cells. Nat Med 1996;2:561.

348. Champlin R, McGlave P: Allogeneic bone marrow transplantation for chronic myelogenous leukemia. In Forman SJ, Blume KG, Thomas ED (eds): Bone Marrow Transplantation. Boston, Blackwell Scientific Publications, pp 595–606.

349. Goldman JM, Szydlo R, Horowitz MM, et al: Choice of pretransplant treatment and timing of transplants for chronic myelogenous leukemia in chronic phase. Blood 1993;82:2235–2238.

350. Thomas ED, Clift RA: Indications for marrow transplantation in chronic myelogenous leukemia. Blood 1989;73:861–864.

351. Clift RA, Radich J, Appelbaum FR, et al: Long-term follow-up of a randomized study comparing cyclophosphamide and total body irradiation with busulfan and cyclophosphamide for patients receiving allogeneic marrow transplants during chronic phase of chronic myeloid leukemia. Blood 1999;94:3960–3962.

352. Clift RA, Buckner CD, Appelbaum FR, et al: Allogeneic marrow transplantation in patients with chronic myeloid leukemia in the chronic phase: A randomized trial of two irradiation regimens. Blood 1991;77:1660–1665.

353. Slattery JT, Clift RA, Buckner CD, et al: Marrow transplantation for chronic myelogenous leukemia: The influence of plasma busulfan levels on the outcome of transplantation. Blood 1997;89:3055–3060.

354. Andersson BS, Kashyap A, Gian V, et al: Conditioning therapy with intravenous busulfan and cyclophosphamide (IV BuCy2) for hematologic malignancies prior to allogeneic stem cell transplantation: a phase II study. Biol Blood Marrow Transplant 2002;8(3):145–154.

355. Goldman J, McGlave P, Szydlo R, et al: Impact of disease duration and prior treatment on outcome of bone marrow transplantation for chronic myelogenous leukemia. Exp Hematol 1992;62:830.

356. Gale RP, Hehlmann R, Zhang MJ, et al: Survival with bone marrow transplantation versus hydroxyurea or interferon for chronic myelogenous leukemia. Blood 1998;91:1810–1819.

357. Giralt SA, Kantarjian HM, Talpaz M, et al: Effect of prior interferon alfa therapy on the outcome of allogeneic bone marrow

transplantation for chronic myelogenous leukemia. J Clin Oncol 1993;11:1055–1061.

358. Morton AJ, Gooley T, Hansen JA, et al: Association between pretransplant interferon-α and outcome after unrelated donor marrow transplantation for chronic myelogenous leukemia in chronic phase. Blood 1998;92:394–401.

359. Giralt S, Szydlo R, Goldman JM, et al: Effect of short-term interferon therapy on the outcome of subsequent HLA-identical sibling bone marrow transplantation for chronic myelogenous leukemia: An analysis from the International Bone Marrow Transplant Registry. Blood 2000;95:410–415.

360. Hehlmann R, Hochhaus A, Kolb HJ, et al: Interferon-α before allogeneic bone marrow transplantation in chronic myelogenous leukemia does not affect outcome adversely, provided it is discontinued at least 90 days before the procedure. Blood 1999;94:3668–3677.

361. Goldman JM, Gale RP, Bortin MM, et al: Bone marrow transplantation for chronic myelogenous leukemia in chronic phase: increased risk of relapse associated with T-cell depletion. Ann Intern Med 1988;108:806–814.

362. Barrett AJ, Mavroudis D, Tisdale J, et al: T cell–depleted bone marrow transplantation and delayed T cell add-back to control acute GVHD and conserve a graft-versus-leukemia effect. Bone Marrow Transplant 1998;21:543–551.

363. Drobyski WR, Hessner MJ, Klein JP, et al: T-cell depletion plus salvage immunotherapy with donor leukocyte infusions as a strategy to treat chronic-phase chronic myelogenous leukemia patients undergoing HLA-identical sibling marrow transplantation. Blood 1999;94:434–441.

364. Sehn LH, Alyea EP, Weller E, et al: Comparative outcomes of T-cell–depleted and non–T-cell–depleted allogeneic bone marrow transplantation for chronic myelogenous leukemia: Impact of donor lymphocyte infusion. J Clin Oncol 1999;17:561–568.

365. Silver RT, Woolf SH, Hehlmann R, et al: An evidence-based analysis of the effect of busulfan, hydroxyurea, interferon, and allogeneic bone marrow transplantation in treating the chronic phase of chronic myeloid leukemia: Developed for the American Society of Hematology. Blood 1999;94:1517–1536.

366. Lee SJ, Kuntz KM, Horowitz MM, et al: Unrelated donor bone marrow transplantation for chronic myelogenous leukemia: A decision analysis. Ann Intern Med 1997;127:1080–1088.

367. Kolb HJ, Mittermüller J, Clemm C, et al: Donor leukocyte transfusions for treatment of recurrent chronic myelogenous leukemia in marrow transplant patients. Blood 1990;76:2462–2465.

368. Carella AM, Lerma E, Corsetti MT, et al: Autografting with Philadelphia chromosome–negative mobilized hematopoietic progenitor cells in chronic myelogenous leukemia. Blood 1999;93:1534–1539.

369. McGlave PB, De Fabritiis P, Deisseroth A, et al: Autologous transplants for chronic myelogenous leukaemia: Results from eight transplant groups. Lancet 1994;343:1486–1488.

370. Talpaz M, Kantarjian H, Liang J, et al: Percentage of Philadelphia chromosome (Ph)–negative and Ph-positive cells found after autologous transplantation for chronic myelogenous leukemia depends on percentage of diploid cells induced by conventional-dose chemotherapy before collection of autologous cells. Blood 1995;85:3257–3263.

371. Barnett MJ, Eaves CJ, Phillips GL, et al: Autografting with cultured marrow in chronic myeloid leukemia: Results of a pilot study. Blood 1994;84:724–732.

372. Guardiola P, Esperou H, Cazals-Hatem D, et al: Allogeneic bone marrow transplantation for agnogenic myeloid metaplasia. Br J Haematol 1997;98:1004–1009.

373. Anderson JE, Sale G, Appelbaum FR, et al: Allogeneic marrow transplantation for primary myelofibrosis and myelofibrosis secondary to polycythaemia vera or essential thrombocytosis. Br J Haematol 1997;98:1010–1016.

374. Przepiorka D, Giralt S, Khouri I, et al: Allogeneic marrow transplantation for myeloproliferative disorders other than chronic myelogenous leukemia: Review of forty cases. Am J Hematol 1998;57:24–28.

375. Barosi G: Myelofibrosis with myeloid metaplasia: Diagnostic definition and prognostic classification for clinical studies and treatment guidelines. J Clin Oncol 1999;17:2954–2970.

376. O'Brien S, Del Giglio A, Keating M: Advances in the biology and treatment of B-cell chronic lymphocytic leukemia. Blood 1995;85:307–318.

377. Foon KA, Rai KR, Gale RP: Chronic lymphocytic leukemia: New insights into biology and therapy. Ann Intern Med 1990;113:525–539.

378. Binet JL, Catovsky D, Chandra P, et al: Chronic lymphocytic leukemia: Proposals for a revised prognostic staging system. Br J Haematol 1981;48:365–367.

379. Rai KR, Sawitsky A, Cronkite EP, et al: Clinical staging of chronic lymphocytic leukemia. Blood 1975;46:219–234.

380. Rai KR, Han T: Prognostic factors and clinical staging in chronic lymphocytic leukemia. Hematol Oncol Clin North Am 1990;4:447–456.

381. Cheson BD, Bennett JM, Grever M, et al: National Cancer Institute–sponsored Working Group guidelines for chronic lymphocytic leukemia: Revised guidelines for diagnosis and treatment. Blood 1996;87:4990–4997.

382. Damle RN, Wasil T, Fais F, et al: Ig V gene mutation status and CD38 expression as novel prognostic indicators in chronic lymphocytic leukemia. Blood 1999;94:1840–1847.

383. Keating MJ, Lerner S, Kantarjian H: The serum β2-microglobulin level is more powerful than stage in predicting resonse and survival in chronic lymphocytic leukemia. Blood 1995;86(Suppl 1):606A.

384. Keating MJ, O'Brien S, Kantarjian H, et al: Long-term follow-up of patients with chronic lymphocytic leukemia treated with fludarabine as a single agent. Blood 1993;81:2878–2884.

385. O'Brien S, Kantarjian H, Beran M, et al: Results of fludarabine and prednisone therapy in 264 patients with chronic lymphocytic leukemia with multivariate analysis–derived prognostic model for response to treatment. Blood 1993;82:1695–1700.

386. Keating MJ, O'Brien S, Kantarjian H, et al: Long-term follow-up of patients with chronic lymphocytic leukemia treated with fludarabine as a single agent. Blood 1993;81:2878–2884.

387. Keating MJ, O'Brien S, Lerner S, et al: Long-term follow-up of patients with chronic lymphocytic leukemia (CLL) receiving fludarabine regimens as initial therapy. Blood 1998;92:1165–1171.

388. Bowen AL, Zomas A, Emmett E, et al: Subcutaneous CAMPATH-1H in fludarabine-resistant/relapsed chronic lymphocytic and B-prolymphocytic leukaemia. Br J Haematol 1997;96:617–619.

389. Dreger P, Von Neuhoff N, Kuse R, et al: Early stem cell transplantation for chronic lymphocytic leukaemia: A chance for cure? Br J Cancer 1998;77:2291–2297.

390. Khouri IF, Keating MJ, Vriesendorp HM, et al: Autologous and allogeneic bone marrow transplantation for chronic lymphocytic leukemia: Preliminary results. J Clin Oncol 1994;12:748–758.

391. Rabinowe SN, Soiffer RJ, Gribben JG, et al: Autologous and allogeneic bone marrow transplantation for poor prognosis patients with B-cell chronic lymphocytic leukemia. Blood 1993;82:1366–1376.

392. Provan D, Bartlett-Pandite L, Zwicky C, et al: Eradication of polymerase chain reaction-detectable chronic lymphocytic leukemia cells is associated with improved outcome after bone marrow transplantation. Blood 1996;88:2228–2235.

393. Khouri I, Champlin R: Allogeneic bone marrow transplantation in chronic lymphocytic leukemia. Ann Intern Med 1996;125:780–780.

394. Khouri IF, Przepiorka D, Van Besien K, et al: Allogeneic blood or marrow transplantation for chronic lymphocytic leukaemia: Timing of transplantation and potential effect of fludarabine on acute graft-versus-host disease. Br J Haematol 1997;97:466–473.

395. Michallet M, Archimbaud E, Bandini G, et al: HLA-identical sibling bone marrow transplantation in younger patients with chronic lymphocytic leukemia. Ann Intern Med 1996;124:311–315.

396. Rondón G, Giralt S, Huh Y, et al: Graft-versus-leukemia effect after allogeneic bone marrow transplantation for chronic lymphocytic leukemia. Bone Marrow Transplant 1996;18:669–672.

397. Harris NL, Jaffe ES, Stein H, et al: A revised European-American classification of lymphoid neoplasms: A proposal from the International Lymphoma Study Group. Blood 1994;84:1361–1392.

398. Harris NL, Jaffe ES, Diebold J, et al: World Health Organization classification of neoplastic diseases of the hematopoietic and lymphoid tissues: Report of the Clinical Advisory Committee Meeting—Airlie House, Virginia, November 1997. J Clin Oncol 1999;17:3835–3849.

399. Dierlamm J, Michaux L, Criel A, et al: Genetic abnormalities in chronic lymphocytic leukemia and their clinical and prognostic implications. Cancer Genet Cytogenet 1997;94:27–35.

400. Matutes E, Oscier D, Garcia-Marco J, et al: Trisomy 12 defines a group of CLL with atypical morphology: Correlation between cytogenetic, clinical and laboratory features in 544 patients. Br J Haematol 1996;92:382–388.

401. Juliusson G, Oscier DG, Fitchett M, et al: Prognostic subgroups in B-cell chronic lymphocytic leukemia defined by specific chromosomal abnormalities. N Engl J Med 1990;323:720–724.

402. Billadeau D, Blackstadt M, Greipp P, et al: Analysis of B-lymphoid malignancies using allele-specific polymerase chain reaction: A technique for sequential quantitation of residual disease. Blood 1991;78:3021–3029.

403. Provan D, Bartlett-Pandite L, Zwicky C, et al: Eradication of polymerase chain reaction-detectable chronic lymphocytic leukemia cells is associated with improved outcome after bone marrow transplantation. Blood 1996;88:2228–2235.

404. Croce CM: Molecular biology of lymphomas. Semin Oncol 1993;20(Suppl 5):31–46.

405. Horning SJ: Natural history of and therapy for the indolent non-Hodgkin's lymphomas. Semin Oncol 1993;20(Suppl 5):75–88.

406. Romaguera JE, McLaughlin P, North L, et al: Multivariate analysis of prognostic factors in stage IV follicular low-grade lymphoma: A risk model. J Clin Oncol 1991;9:762–769.

407. Coiffier B, Bastion Y, Berger F, et al: Prognostic factors in follicular lymphomas. Semin Oncol 1993;20(Suppl 5):89–95.

408. Decaudin D, Lepage E, Brousse N, et al: Low-grade stage III–IV follicular lymphoma: Multivariate analysis of prognostic factors in 484 patients: A study of the Groupe d'Etude des Lymphomes de l'Adulte. J Clin Oncol 1999;17:2499–2505.

409. López-Guillermo A, Montserrat E, Bosch F, et al: Applicability of the International Index for aggressive lymphomas to patients with low-grade lymphoma. J Clin Oncol 1994;12:1343–1348.

410. Portlock CS: Management of the low-grade non-Hodgkin's lymphomas. Semin Oncol 1990;17:51–59.

411. Weisdorf DJ, Andersen JW, Glick JH, Oken MM: Survival after relapse of low-grade non-Hodgkin's lymphoma: Implications for marrow transplantation. J Clin Oncol 1992;10:942–947.

412. Rodriguez MA, Cabanillas FC, Velasquez W, et al: Results of a salvage treatment program for relapsing lymphoma: MINE consolidated with ESHAP. J Clin Oncol 1995;13:1734–1741.

413. McLaughlin P, Hagemeister FB, Romaguera JE, et al: Fludarabine, mitoxantrone, and dexamethasone: An effective new regimen for indolent lymphoma. J Clin Oncol 1996;14:1262–1268.

414. Gribben JG, Freedman AS, Neuberg D, et al: Immunologic purging of marrow assessed by PCR before autologous bone marrow transplantation for B-cell lymphoma. N Engl J Med 1991;325:1525–1533.

415. Rohatiner AZS, Johnson PWM, Price CGA, et al: Myeloablative therapy with autologous bone marrow transplantation as consolidation therapy for recurrent follicular lymphoma. J Clin Oncol 1994;12:1177–1184.

416. Negrin RS, Kusnierz-Glaz CR, Still BJ, et al: Transplantation of enriched and purged peripheral blood progenitor cells from a single apheresis product in patients with non-Hodgkin's lymphoma. Blood 1995;85:3334–3341.

417. Freedman AS, Neuberg D, Gribben JG, et al: High-dose chemoradiotherapy and anti-B-cell monoclonal antibody purged autologous bone marrow transplantation in mantle-cell lymphoma: No evidence for long-term remission. J Clin Oncol 1998;16:13–18.

418. Johnson PWM, Rohatiner AZS, Whelan JS, et al: Patterns of survival in patients with recurrent follicular lymphoma: A 20-year study from a single center. J Clin Oncol 1995;13:140–147.

419. Krishnan A, Bhatia S, Slovak ML, et al: Predictors of therapy-related leukemia and myelodysplasia following autologous transplantation for lymphoma: An assessment of risk factors. Blood 2000;95:1588–1593.

420. Milligan DW, De Elvira MCR, Kolb HJ, et al: Secondary leukaemia and myelodysplasia after autografting for lymphoma: Results from the EBMT. Br J Haematol 1999;106:1020–1026.

421. Van Besien KW, Khouri IF, Giralt SA, et al: Allogeneic bone marrow transplantation for refractory and recurrent low-grade lymphoma: The case for aggressive management. J Clin Oncol 1995;13:1096–1102.

422. Van Besien KW, Mehra RC, Giralt SA, et al: Allogeneic bone marrow transplantation for poor-prognosis lymphoma: Response, toxicity, and survival depend on disease histology. Am J Med 1996;100:299–307.

423. Van Besien K, Thall P, Korbling M, et al: Allogeneic transplantation for recurrent or refractory non-Hodgkin's lymphoma with poor prognostic features after conditioning with thiotepa, busulfan and cyclophosphamide: Experience in 44 consecutive patients. Biol Blood Marrow Transplant 1997;3:150–156.

424. Verdonck LF, Dekker AW, Lokhorst HM, et al: Allogeneic versus autologous bone marrow transplantation for refractory and recurrent low-grade non-Hodgkin's lymphoma. Blood 1997;90:4201–4205.

425. Van Besien K, Sobocinski K, Rowlings PA, et al: Allogeneic bone marrow transplantation for low-grade lymphoma. Blood 1998;92:1832–1836.

426. Attal M, Socié G, Molina L, et al: Allogeneic bone marrow transplantation for refractory and recurrent follicular lymphoma: A case-matched analysis with autologous transplantation from the French Bone Marrow Transplant Group Registry data. Blood 1997;93(Suppl):1120A.

427. Khouri I, Lee M-S, Palmer L, et al: Transplant-lite using fludarabine-cyclophosphamide and allogeneic stem cell transplantation for low grade lymphoma. Blood 1999;94(Suppl):1553A.

428. Argatoff LH, Connors JM, Klasa RJ, et al: Mantle cell lymphoma: A clinicopathologic study of 80 cases. Blood 1997;89:2067–2078.

429. Hiddemann W, Unterhalt M, Hermann R, et al: Mantle-cell lymphomas have more widespread disease and a slower response to chemotherapy compared with follicle-center lymphomas: Results of a prospective comparative analysis of the German low-grade lymphoma study group. J Clin Oncol 1998;16:1922–1930.

430. Majlis A, Pugh WC, Rodriguez MA, et al: Mantle cell lymphoma: Correlation of clinical outcome and biologic features with three histologic variants. J Clin Oncol 1997;15:1664–1671.

431. Freedman AS, Neuberg D, Gribben JG, et al: High-dose chemoradiotherapy and anti–B-cell monoclonal antibody purged autologous bone marrow transplantation in mantle-cell lymphoma: No evidence for long-term remission. J Clin Oncol 1998;16:13–18.

432. Khouri IF, Romaguera J, Kantarjian H, et al: Hyper-CVAD and high-dose methotrexate/cytarabine followed by stem-cell transplantation: An active regimen for aggressive mantle-cell lymphoma. J Clin Oncol 1998;16:3803–3809.

433. Khouri I, Lee M-S, Romaguera J, et al: Allogeneic hematopoietic transplantation for mantle-cell lymphoma: Molecular remissions and evidence of graft-versus-malignancy. Ann Oncol 1999;10:1293–1299.

434. Adkins D, Brown R, Goodnough LT, et al: Treatment of resistant mantle cell lymphoma with allogeneic bone marrow transplantation. Bone Marrow Transplant 1998;21:97–99.

435. Corradini P, Ladetto M, Astolfi M, et al: Clinical and molecular remission after allogeneic blood cell transplantation in a patient with mantle-cell lymphoma. Br J Haematol 1996;94:376–378.

436. Khouri I, Romaguera J, Kantarjian H, et al: Mantle cell lymphoma: Improved outcome with hyper-CVAD/high-dose methotrexate-cytarabine (MTX-Ara-C) followed by autologous or allogeneic stem cell transplantation. Blood 1997;90(Suppl):2642A.

437. Coiffier B: Treatment of aggressive non-Hodgkin's lymphoma. Semin Oncol 1999;26:12–20.

438. Armitage JO: Drug therapy: Treatment of non-Hodgkin's lymphoma. N Engl J Med 1993;328:1023–1030.

439. Fisher RI, Gaynor ER, Dahlberg S, et al: Comparison of a standard regimen (CHOP) with three intensive chemotherapy regimens for advanced non-Hodgkin's lymphoma. N Engl J Med 1993;328:1002–1006.

440. Engelhard M, Brittinger G, Huhn D, et al: Subclassification of diffuse large B-cell lymphomas according to the Kiel classification: Distinction of centroblastic and immunoblastic lymphomas is a significant prognostic risk factor. Blood 1997;89:2291–2297.

441. Shipp MA: Prognostic factors in aggressive non-Hodgkin's lymphoma: Who has "high-risk" disease? Blood 1994;83:1165–1173.

442. Rodriguez J, Cabanillas F, McLaughlin P, et al: A proposal for a simple staging system for intermediate grade lymphoma and immunoblastic lymphoma based on the "tumor score." Ann Oncol 1992;3:711.

443. International Non-Hodgkin's Lymphoma Prognostic Factors Project: A predictive model for aggressive non-Hodgkin's lymphoma. N Engl J Med 1993;329:987–995.

444. Van Besien K, Tabocoff J, Rodriguez M, et al: High-dose chemotherapy with BEAC regimen and autologous bone marrow transplantation for intermediate grade and immunoblastic lymphoma: Durable complete remissions, but a high rate of regimen-related toxicity. Bone Marrow Transplant 1995;15:549–555.

445. Bosly A, Coiffier B, Gisselbrecht C, et al: Bone marrow transplantation prolongs survival after relapse in aggressive-

lymphoma patients treated with the LNH-84 regimen. J Clin Oncol 1992;10:1615–1623.

446. Philip T, Guglielmi C, Hagenbeek A, et al: Autologous bone marrow transplantation as compared with salvage chemotherapy in relapses of chemotherapy-sensitive non Hodgkin's lymphoma. N Engl J Med 1995;333:1540–1545.

447. Philip T, Armitage JO, Spitzer G, et al: High-dose therapy and autologous bone marrow transplantation after failure of conventional chemotherapy in adults with intermediate grade or high-grade non-Hodgkin's lymphoma. N Engl J Med 1987;316:1493–1498.

448. Philip T, Hartman O, Brian P, et al: High dose therapy and autologous bone marrow transplantation in partial remission after first line induction therapy for diffuse non-Hodgkin's lymphoma. J Clin Oncol 1988;8:784–791.

449. Martelli M, Vignetti M, Zinzani PL, et al: High-dose chemotherapy followed by autologous bone marrow transplantation versus dexamethasone, cisplatin, and cytarabine in aggressive non-Hodgkin's lymphoma with partial response to front-line chemotherapy: A prospective randomized Italian multicenter study. J Clin Oncol 1996;14:534–542.

450. Haioun C, Lepage E, Gisselbrecht C, et al: Benefit of autologous bone marrow transplantation over sequential chemotherapy in poor-risk aggressive non-Hodgkin's lymphoma: Updated results of the prospective study LNH87-2. J Clin Oncol 1997;15:1131–1137.

451. Gianni AM, Bregni M, Siena S, et al: High-dose chemotherapy and autologous bone marrow transplantation compared with MACOP-B in aggressive B-cell lymphoma. N Engl J Med 1997;336:1290–1297.

452. Verdonck LF, Van Putten WLJ, Hagenbeek A, et al: Comparison of CHOP chemotherapy with autologous bone marrow transplantation for slowly responding patients with aggressive non-Hodgkin's lymphoma. N Engl J Med 1995;332:1045–1051.

453. Philip T, Hartman O, Brian P, et al: High dose therapy and autologous bone marrow transplantation in partial remission after first line induction therapy for diffuse non-Hodgkins lymphoma. J Clin Oncol 1988;8:784–791.

454. VanBesien K, Champlin RE: Non-Hodgkins lymphoma: Allogeneic and autologous blood and marrow transplantation. Adv Oncol 2000;16:3–16.

455. de Witte T, Awwad B, Boezeman J, et al: Role of allogeneic bone marrow transplantation in adolescent or adult patients with acute lymphoblastic leukaemia or lymphoblastic lymphoma in first remission. Bone Marrow Transplant 1994;14:767–774.

456. Troussard X, Leblond V, Kuentz M, et al: Allogeneic bone marrow transplantation in adults with Burkitt's lymphoma or acute lymphoblastic leukemia in first complete remission. J Clin Oncol 1990;8:809–812.

457. Ratanatharathorn V, Uberti J, Karanes C, et al: Prospective comparative trial of autologous versus allogeneic bone marrow transplantation in patients with non-Hodgkin's lymphoma. Blood 1994;84:1050–1055.

458. Jones RJ, Ambinder RF, Piantadosi S, Santos GW: Evidence of a graft-versus-lymphoma effect associated with allogeneic bone marrow transplantation. Blood 1991;77:649–653.

459. Chopra R, Goldstone AH, Pearce R, et al: Autologous versus allogeneic bone marrow transplantation for non-Hodgkin's lymphoma: A case-controlled analysis of the European Bone Marrow Transplant Group registry data. J Clin Oncol 1992;10:1690–1695.

460. Peniket AJ, Ruiz de Elvira MC, Taghipour G, et al: Allogeneic transplantation for lymphoma produces a lower relapse rate than autologous transplantation but survival has not risen because of higher treatment-related mortality: A report of 764 cases from the EBMT lymphoma registry. Blood 1997;90(Suppl 1):1124A.

461. Bensinger WI, Weaver CH, Appelbaum FR, et al: Transplantation of allogeneic peripheral blood stem cells mobilized by recombinant human granulocyte colony-stimulating factor. Blood 1995;85:1655–1658.

462. Korbling M, Przepiorka D, Huh YO, et al: Allogeneic blood stem cell transplantation for refractory leukemia and lymphoma: Potential advantage of blood over marrow allografts. Blood 1995;85:1659–1665.

463. Przepiorka D, Anderlini P, Ippoliti C, et al: Allogeneic blood stem cell transplantation in advanced hematologic cancers. Bone Marrow Transplant 1997;19:455–460.

464. Przepiorka D, Ippolitti C, Khouri I, et al: Allogeneic transplantation for advanced leukemia: Improved short-term outcome with

blood stem cell grafts and tacrolimus. Transplantation 1996;62:1806–1810.

465. Przepiorka D, Van Besian K, Khouri I, et al: Carmustine, etoposide, cytarabine and melphalan as a preparative regimen for allogeneic transplantation for high-risk malignant lymphoma. Ann Oncol 1999;10:527–532.

466. Loeffler M, Brosteanu O, Hasenclever D, et al: Meta-analysis of chemotherapy versus combined modality treatment trials in Hodgkin's disease. J Clin Oncol 1998;16:818–829.

467. Bierman PJ, Vose JM, Armitage JO: Autologous transplantation for Hodgkin's disease: Coming of age. Blood 1994;83:1161–1164.

468. Jagannath S, Armitage JO, Dicke KA, et al: Prognostic factors for response and survival after high-dose cyclophosphamide, carmustine, and etoposide with autologous bone marrow transplantation for relapsed Hodgkin's disease. J Clin Oncol 1989;7:179–185.

469. Linch DC, Winfield D, Goldstone AH, et al: Dose intensification with autologous bone-marrow transplantation in relapsed and resistant Hodgkin's disease: Results of a BNLI randomised trial. Lancet 1993;341:1051–1054.

470. Federico M, Clo V, Carella AM: Preliminary analysis of clinical characteristics of patients enrolled in the HD01 protocol: A randomised trial of high dose therapy and autologous stem cell transplantation versus conventional therapy for patients with advanced Hodgkin's disease responding to first line therapy. Leuk Lymphoma 1995;15(Suppl 1):63–66.

471. Reece DE, Connors JM, Spinelli JJ, et al: Intensive therapy with cyclophosphamide, carmustine, etoposide ± cisplatin, and autologous bone marrow transplantation for Hodgkin's disease in first relapse after combination chemotherapy. Blood 1994;83:1193–1199.

472. Lazarus HM, Rowlings PA, Zhang MJ, et al: Autotransplants for Hodgkin's disease in patients never achieving remission: A report from the autologous blood and marrow transplant registry. J Clin Oncol 1999;17:534–545.

473. Burns LJ, Daniels KA, McGlave PB, et al: Autologous stem cell transplantation for refractory and relapsed Hodgkin's disease: Factors predictive of prolonged survival. Bone Marrow Transplant 1995;16:13–18.

474. O'Brien MER, Milan S, Cunningham D, et al: High-dose chemotherapy and autologous bone marrow transplant in relapsed Hodgkin's disease: A pragmatic prognostic index. Br J Cancer 1996;73:1272–1277.

475. André M, Henry-Amar M, Blaise D, et al: Treatment-related deaths and second cancer risk after autologous stem-cell transplantation for Hodgkin's disease. Blood 1998;92:1933–1940.

476. Harrison CN, Gregory W, Hudson GV, et al: High-dose BEAM chemotherapy with autologous haemopoietic stem cell transplantation for Hodgkin's disease is unlikely to be associated with a major increased risk of secondary MDS/AML. Br J Cancer 1999;81:476–483.

477. Traweek ST, Slovak ML, Nademanee AP, et al: Clonal karyotypic hematopoietic cell abnormalities occurring after autologous bone marrow transplantation for Hodgkin's disease and non-Hodgkin's lymphoma. Blood 1999;484:957–963.

478. Kessinger A, Bierman PJ, Vose JM, Armitage JO: High-dose cyclophosphamide, carmustine, and etoposide followed by autologous peripheral stem cell transplantation for patients with relapsed Hodgkin's disease. Blood 1991;77:2322–2325.

479. Reece DE, Nevill TJ, Sayegh A, et al: Regimen-related toxicity and non-relapse mortality with high-dose cyclophosphamide, carmustine (BCNU) and etoposide (VP16-213) (CBV) and CBV plus cisplatin (CBVP) followed by autologous stem cell transplantation in patients with Hodgkin's disease. Bone Marrow Transplant 1999;23:1131–1138.

480. Constine LS, Rapoport AP: Hodgkin's disease, bone marrow transplantation, and involved field radiation therapy: Coming full circle from 1902 to 1996. Int J Radiat Oncol Biol Phys 1996;36:253–255.

481. Gajewski JL, Phillips GL, Sobocinski KA, et al: Bone marrow transplants from HLA-identical siblings in advanced Hodgkin's disease. J Clin Oncol 1996;14:572–578.

482. Milpied N, Fielding AK, Pearce RM, et al: Allogeneic bone marrow transplant is not better than autologous transplant for patients with relapsed Hodgkin's disease. J Clin Oncol 1996;14:1291–1296.

483. Appelbaum FR, Sullivan K, Thomas ED, et al: Allogeneic marrow transplantation in the treatment of MOPP-resistant Hodgkin's disease. J Clin Oncol 1985;3:1490–1494.

484. Gore ME, Selby PJ, Viner C, et al: Intensive treatment of multiple myeloma and criteria for complete remission. Lancet 1989;2:879–882.

485. Alexanian R, Dimopoulos MA, Hester J, et al: Early myeloablative therapy for multiple myeloma. Blood 1994;84:4278–4282.

486. Barlogie B, Jagannath S, Vesole D, Tricot G: Autologous and allogeneic transplants for multiple myeloma. Semin Hematol 1995;32:31–44.

487. Fermand J-P, Chevret S, Ravaud P, et al: High-dose chemoradiotherapy and autologous blood stem cell transplantation in multiple myeloma: Results of a phase II trial involving 63 patients. Blood 1993;82:2005–2009.

488. Attal M, Harousseau JL, Stoppa AM, et al: A prospective, randomized trial of autologous bone marrow transplantation and chemotherapy in multiple myeloma. N Engl J Med 1996;335:91–97.

489. Gale RP, Park RE, Dubois RW, et al: Delphi-panel analysis of appropriateness of high-dose therapy and bone marrow autotransplants in newly diagnosed multiple myeloma. Leuk Lymphoma 1999;33:511–517.

490. Alexanian R, Dimopoulos MA, Delasalle KB, et al: Myeloablative therapy for primary resistant multiple myeloma. Stem Cells 1995;13:118–121.

491. Alexanian R, Dimopoulos M, Smith T, et al: Limited value of myeloablative therapy for late multiple myeloma. Blood 1994;83:512–516.

492. Jagannath S, Barlogie B, Dicke K, et al: Autologous bone marrow transplantation in multiple myeloma: Identification of prognostic factors. Blood 1990;76:1860–1866.

493. Tricot G, Sawyer JR, Jagannath S, et al: Unique role of cytogenetics in the prognosis of patients with myeloma receiving high-dose therapy and autotransplants. J Clin Oncol 1997;15:2659–2666.

494. Bensinger WI, Rowley SD, Demirer T, et al: High-dose therapy followed by autologous hematopoietic stem-cell infusion for patients with multiple myeloma. J Clin Oncol 1996;14:1447–1456.

495. Dimopoulos MA, Alexanian R, Przepiorka D, et al: Thiotepa, busulfan, and cyclophosphamide: A new preparative regimen for autologous marrow or blood stem cell transplantation in high-risk multiple myeloma. Blood 1993;82:2324–2328.

496. Fermand JP, Ravaud P, Chevret S, et al: High-dose therapy and autologous peripheral blood stem cell transplantation in multiple myeloma: Up-front or rescue treatment? Results of a multicenter sequential randomized clinical trial. Blood 1998;92:3131–3136.

497. Vesole DH, Barlogie B, Jagannath S, et al: High-dose therapy for refractory multiple myeloma: Improved prognosis with better supportive care and double transplants. Blood 1994;84:950–956.

498. Björkstrand B, Ljungman P, Bird JM, et al: Double high-dose chemoradiotherapy with autologous stem cell transplantation can induce molecular remissions in multiple myeloma. Bone Marrow Transplant 1995;15:367–371.

499. Harousseau JL, Milpied N, Laporte JP, et al: Double-intensive therapy in high-risk multiple myeloma. Blood 1992;79:2827–2833.

500. Kwak LW, Thielemans K, Massaia M: Idiotypic vaccination as therapy for multiple myeloma. Semin Hematol 1999;36:34–37.

501. Cunningham D, Powles R, Malpas J, et al: A randomized trial of maintenance interferon following a high-dose chemotherapy in multiple myeloma: Long-term follow-up results. Br J Haematol 1998;102:495–502.

502. Dhodapkar MV, Singh J, Mehta J, et al: Anti-myeloma activity of pamidronate in vivo. Br J Haematol 1998;103:530–532.

503. Gahrton G, Tura S, Ljungman P, et al: Allogeneic bone marrow transplantation in multiple myeloma. N Engl J Med 1991;325:1267–1273.

504. Björkstrand B, Ljungman P, Svensson H, et al: Allogeneic bone marrow transplantation versus autologous stem cell transplantation in multiple myeloma: A retrospective case-matched study from the European group for blood and marrow transplantation. Blood 1996;88:4711–4718.

505. Gahrton G, Svensson H, Björkstrand B, et al: Syngeneic transplantation in multiple myeloma: A case-matched comparison with autologous and allogeneic transplantation. Bone Marrow Transplant 1999;24:741–745.

506. Gertz MA, Lacy MQ, Dispenzieri A: Myeloablative chemotherapy with stem cell rescue for the treatment of primary systemic amyloidosis: A status report. Bone Marrow Transplant 2000;25:465–470.

507. Moreau P, Leblond V, Bourquelot P, et al: Prognostic factors for survival and response after high-dose therapy and autologous stem cell transplantation in systemic AL amyloidosis: A report on 21 patients. Br J Haematol 1998;101:766–769.

508. Anonymous: Chaos surrounds high-dose chemotherapy for breast cancer. Lancet 1999;353:1633–1633.

509. Antman K, Ayash L, Elias A, et al: A phase II study of high-dose cyclophosphamide, thiotepa, and carboplatin with autologous marrow support in women with measurable advanced breast cancer responding to standard-dose therapy. J Clin Oncol 1992;10:102–110.

510. Peters WP, Ross M, Vredenburgh JJ, et al: High-dose chemotherapy and autologous bone marrow support as consolidation after standard-dose adjuvant therapy for high-risk primary breast cancer. J Clin Oncol 1993;11:1132–1143.

511. Stemmer SM, Cagnoni PJ, Shpall EJ, et al: High-dose paclitaxel, cyclophosphamide, and cisplatin with autologous hematopoietic progenitor-cell support: A phase I trial. J Clin Oncol 1996;14:1463–1472.

512. Antman KH, Rowlings PA, Vaughan WP, et al: High-dose chemotherapy with autologous hematopoietic stem-cell support for breast cancer in North America. J Clin Oncol 1997;15:1870–1879.

513. Rahman ZU, Frye DK, Buzdar AU, et al: Impact of selection process on response rate and long-term survival of potential high-dose chemotherapy candidates treated with standard-dose doxorubicin-containing chemotherapy in patients with metastatic breast cancer. J Clin Oncol 1997;15:3171–3177.

514. Rowlings PA, Williams SF, Antman KH, et al: Factors correlated with progression-free survival after high-dose chemotherapy and hematopoietic stem cell transplantation for metastatic breast cancer. JAMA 1999;282:1335–1343.

515. Rizzieri DA, Vredenburgh JJ, Jones R, et al: Prognostic and predictive factors for patients with metastatic breast cancer undergoing aggressive induction therapy followed by high-dose chemotherapy with autologous stem-cell support. J Clin Oncol 1999;17:3064–3074.

516. Bezwoda WR, Seymour L, Dansey RD: High-dose chemotherapy with hematopoietic rescue as primary treatment for metastatic breast cancer: A randomized trial. J Clin Oncol 1995;13:2483–2489.

517. Stadtmauer EA, O'Neill A, Goldstein LJ, et al: Conventional-dose chemotherapy compared with high-dose chemotherapy plus autologous hematopoietic stem-cell transplantation for metastatic breast cancer. N Engl J Med 2000;342:1069–1076.

518. Rodenhuis S, Richel DJ, Van der Wall E, et al: Randomised trial of high-dose chemotherapy and haemopoietic progenitor-cell support in operable breast cancer with extensive axillary lymph-node involvement. Lancet 1998;352:515–521.

519. Hortobagyi GN: High-dose chemotherapy for primary breast cancer: Facts versus anecdotes. J Clin Oncol 1999;17:25–29.

520. Nichols CR, Rosti G: Dose-intensive therapy for germ cell neoplasms. Semin Oncol 1992;19(Suppl 2):145–149.

521. Legros M, Dauplat J, Fleury J, et al: High-dose chemotherapy with hematopoietic rescue in patients with stage III to IV ovarian cancer: Long-term results. J Clin Oncol 1997;15:1302–1308.

522. Stiff PJ, Bayer R, Kerger C, et al: High-dose chemotherapy with autologous transplantation for persistent/relapsed ovarian cancer: A multivariate analysis of survival for 100 consecutively treated patients. J Clin Oncol 1997;15:1309–1317.

523. Elias A: Hematopoietic stem cell transplantation for small cell lung cancer. Chest 1999;116(Suppl):531S–538S.

524. Matthay KK, O'Leary MC, Ramsay NK, et al: Role of myeloablative therapy in improved outcome for high risk neuroblastoma: Review of recent Children's Cancer Group results. Eur J Cancer 1995;31:572–575.

525. Shuster JJ, Cantor AB, McWilliams N, et al: The prognostic significance of autologous bone marrow transplant in advanced neuroblastoma. J Clin Oncol 1991;9:1045–1049.

526. Camitta BM, Thomas ED, Nathan DG, et al: A prospective study of androgens and bone marrow transplantation for treatment of severe aplastic anemia. Blood 1979;53:504–514.

527. Bacigalupo A, Bruno B, Saracco P, et al: Antilymphocyte globulin, cyclosporine, prednisolone, and granulocyte colony-stimulating factor for severe aplastic anemia: An update of the GITMO/EBMT study on 100 patients. Blood 2000;95:1931–1934.

528. Champlin RE, Ho WG, Gale RP: A randomized controlled trial of antithymocyte globulin in patients with aplastic anemia. N Engl J Med 1983;308:113–118.

529. Storb R, Champlin RE: Bone marrow transplantation for severe aplastic anemia. Bone Marrow Transplant 1991;8:69–72.

530. Champlin RE, Feig SA, Sparkes RS, Gale RP: Bone marrow transplantation from identical twins in the treatment of aplastic anemia: Implication for the pathogenesis of the disease. Br J Haematol 1984;56:455–463.

531. Young NS, Maciejewski J: Mechanisms of disease: The pathophysiology of acquired aplastic anemia. N Engl J Med 1997;336:1365–1372.

532. Champlin RE, Horowitz MM, van Bekkum DW, et al: Graft failure following bone marrow transplantation for severe aplastic anemia: Risk factors and treatment results. Blood 1989;73:606–613.

533. Storb R, Etzioni R, Anasetti C, et al: Cyclophosphamide combined with antithymocyte globulin in preparation for allogeneic marrow transplants in patients with aplastic anemia. Blood 1994;84:941–949.

534. McGlave PB, Haake R, Kim T, et al: Therapy of severe aplastic anemia in young adults and children with allogeneic bone marrow transplantation. Blood 1987;70:1325–1330.

535. Anasetti C, Storb R, Longton G, et al: Donor buffy coat cell infusion after marrow transplantation for aplastic anemia. Blood 1988;72:1099–1100.

536. Deeg HJ, Anasetti C, Petersdorf E, et al: Cyclophosphamide plus ATG conditioning is insufficient for sustained hematopoietic reconstitution in patients with severe aplastic anemia transplanted with marrow from HLA-A, B, DRB matched unrelated donors. Blood 1994;83:3417–3418.

537. Davies SM, Wagner JE, DeFor T, et al: Unrelated donor bone marrow transplantation for children and adolescents with aplastic anaemia or myelodysplasia. Br J Haematol 1997;96:749–756.

538. Hows J, Szydlo R, Anasetti C, et al: Unrelated donor marrow transplants for severe acquired aplastic anemia. Bone Marrow Transplant 1992;10(Suppl 1):102–106.

539. Lucarelli G, Galimberti M, Polchi P, et al: Bone marrow transplantation in patients with thalassemia. N Engl J Med 1990;322:417–421.

540. Walters MC, Storb R, Patience M, et al: Impact of bone marrow transplantation for symptomatic sickle cell disease: An interim report. Blood 2000;95:1918–1924.

541. Flowers MED, Zanis J, Pasquini R, et al: Marrow transplantation for Fanconi anaemia: Conditioning with reduced doses of cyclophosphamide without radiation. Br J Haematol 1996;92:699–706.

542. Socié G, Gluckman E, Raynal B, et al: Bone marrow transplantation for Fanconi anemia using low-dose cyclophosphamide/thoracoabdominal irradiation as conditioning regimen: Chimerism study by the polymerase chain reaction. Blood 1993;82:2249–2256.

543. Fischer A, Haddad E, Jabado N, et al: Stem cell transplantation for immunodeficiency. Springer Semin Immunopathol 1998;19:479–492.

544. Gerritsen EJA, Vossen JM, Fasth A, et al: Bone marrow transplantation for autosomal recessive osteopetrosis: A report from the Working Party on Inborn Errors of the European Bone Marrow Transplantation Group. J Pediatr 1994;125:896–902.

545. Krivit W, Lockman LA, Watkins PA, et al: The future for treatment by bone marrow transplantation for adrenoleukodystrophy, metachromatic leukodystrophy, globoid cell leukodystrophy and Hurler syndrome. J Inherit Metab Dis 1995;18:398–412.

546. O'Reilly RJ, Brochstein J, Kernan N, et al: HLA A,B,D disparity, SBA-e-T-cell depleted marrow grafts for severe combined immunodeficiency. Blood 1988;72:399.

547. Filipovich AH, Shapiro RS, Ramsay NKC, et al: Unrelated donor bone marrow transplantation for correction of lethal congenital immunodeficiencies. Blood 1992;80:270–276.

548. Flake AW, Roncarolo MG, Puck JM, et al: Treatment of X-linked severe combined immunodeficiency by in utero transplantation of paternal bone marrow. N Engl J Med 1996;335:1806–1810.

549. Kohn DB, Hershfield MS, Carbonaro D, et al: T lymphocytes with a normal ADA gene accumulate after transplantation of transduced autologous umbilical cord blood CD34+ cells in ADA-deficient SCID neonates. Nat Med 1998;4:775–780.

550. Snowden JA, Biggs JC, Brooks PM: Autologous blood stem cell transplantation for autoimmune diseases. Lancet 1996;348:1112–1113.

551. Sullivan KM, Shulman HM, Storb R, et al: Chronic graft-versus-host disease in 52 patients: Adverse natural course and successful treatment with combination immunosuppression. Blood 1981;57:267–276.

Chapter 47

Umbilical Cord Blood Banking and Transplantation

Joanne Kurtzberg

Hematopoietic stem cells from banked umbilical cord blood (UCB) are an alternative source of donor stem cells for use in allogeneic transplantation. This therapy is currently used to treat patients with aggressive or recurrent malignancies, immunodeficiency diseases, certain genetic conditions such as inborn errors of metabolism and hemoglobinopathies, and congenital and acquired bone marrow failure syndromes. In the future, this unique stem cell source may be used in cellular therapies, including reparative and regenerative therapies for diseases of nonhematopoietic tissues.

Donor availability is a major obstacle to the use of bone marrow as the source of reconstituting cells after a transplant. Only 20% to 25% of patients in need of a stem cell transplant have a fully HLA-matched relative who can serve as the donor. For those lacking a related donor, an HLA-matched unrelated, living bone marrow donor is identified for approximately 25% of Caucasian patients through the National Marrow Donor Program and other living donor registries, but a suitably matched unrelated marrow donor is found for less than 10% of patients of ethnic minority backgrounds. For the remaining patients, a fully matched, unrelated stem cell donor is not identified.

Umbilical cord or placental blood, the portion of the infant's blood that remains in the placenta or afterbirth, contains multipotent stem and progenitor cells that circulate throughout fetal life. The placenta produces multiple factors that mobilize these cells into the infant's circulation as they traffic to and from developing organs. After delivery of the baby, residual fetal blood (umbilical cord blood) remaining in the placenta can be harvested and cryopreserved for future use. Cord blood can be collected during the third stage of labor or from the placenta ex utero within approximately 15 to 20 minutes of the delivery. Collection of this blood carries no risk to the mother or baby. Because cord blood can be collected without discomfort or risk, mothers of ethnic minority backgrounds are more likely to donate to cord blood banks than to adult bone marrow registries.

The most important advantage of cord blood stem cells is that they do not need to be fully HLA-matched for a successful transplant. Despite HLA mismatching, allogeneically transplanted cord blood stem cells are less likely to cause acute and chronic graft-versus-host disease (GVHD), a major obstacle to the success of allogeneic bone marrow transplantation. Cord blood is significantly less likely to transmit the infectious diseases transmissible through the blood. Because graft characterization and HLA typing are performed at the time of initial banking, the units are readily available for patients in need of a donor for allogeneic stem cell transplant.

■ Cord Blood Procurement and Banking

Although there are many practices for cord blood banking, all represent variations on a common theme. The blood should be harvested into a closed sterile collection container containing citrate-phosphate-dextrose (CPD) or an equivalent anticoagulant to prevent clotting. Generally, this step is accomplished by sterile puncture of one of the umbilical veins allowing the cord blood to drain by gravity into a bag containing anticoagulant. In the early days of cord blood banking, blood was harvested in open systems, generally into open-mouthed containers. However, this practice resulted in a high rate (20% to 30%) of contamination of the product with bacterial organisms, generally representative of vaginal flora. Heparin was tested as an anticoagulant early on, but CPD has been identified as the anticoagulant with the lowest toxicity to hematopoietic stem and progenitor cells with an activity over a range of collection volumes.

After harvest from the placenta, the collected cord blood can be maintained at room temperature for up to 48 to

72 hours without appreciable cell losses. Most banks deplete the cord blood unit of red blood cells (RBCs) and reduce its volume with hetastarch or other density-gradient solutions. For long-term storage, cells are cryopreserved in dimethyl sulfoxide (DMSO) and stored under liquid nitrogen. Maximal storage time, or expiration date, is unknown, but under stable conditions, the cells are likely to remain viable for decades.

Precautions must be taken to avoid mixing of maternal and fetal blood, which would lead to contamination of the cord blood unit with HLA-disparate, immunocompetent maternal T cells that could cause GVHD in a transplant recipient.[1] Placentas with fetal-maternal shunts, large tears, or any other anomalies that may result in mixing of fetal and maternal blood should be excluded from donation. Despite implementation of these guidelines, it is estimated that small numbers (<1:50,000 cells) of maternal cells are present in most UCB units. This low level of contamination does not appear to cause maternal cell–induced GVHD in most transplant recipients. At our center (Duke University Medical Center), two patients have been seen who developed elevated hepatic transaminases 6 months after transplant. Liver biopsy confirmed the presence of maternal cells in both patients. GVHD prophylaxis was withdrawn to allow the engrafted UCB T cells to reject the maternal cells. The rejection occurred over the subsequent 6 months, and both patients are alive and well approximately 6 years after the transplant.

The two major types of cord blood donations are public or private (directed) donation.[2, 3] In general, public banks are not-for-profit organizations supported by grants and contracts, whereas private banks are supported by revenues collected from the banking family.

Private Cord Blood Banks

Private cord blood banks are generally for-profit private companies providing a service for a fee. Private donations are financed by the family of the donor or recipient and are usually directed to the baby from whom the cord blood was harvested or a specific recipient in their family. In the minority of private donations, a first-degree relative in need of a transplant donor is identified in advance of the baby's birth. There are no established medical indications for UCB banking; however, it is generally agreed that directed donor banking is indicated when a sibling of the baby has a disease amenable to allogeneic transplantation therapy. Because the donation allows for greater mismatching between the donor and recipient, there is a 75% chance that a given unit will be at least a haploidentical match for a full biologic sibling, and a 50% chance that the unit will be a haploidentical match for a half-sibling. The remainder of private or directed donations are undertaken as investments in the unknown potential for cord blood to be used to treat serious illnesses in the future. To date, very few transplants have been facilitated by these private, speculative banking activities.

Private banking companies provide a collection kit to families interested in directed banking. The units are collected by the physician, midwife, or nurse delivering the baby and are shipped back to the company's banking facility. Compensation for the collector varies, ranging from none to monetary reimbursement based on effort expended. Limited testing is performed on the units, and minimal standards are used to determine whether a unit is eligible for processing and banking. Both collection and banking fees and yearly storage fees are generally charged.

Most pediatricians believe that routine cord blood storage in healthy babies is unnecessary.[3] In this regard, it is important to point out that autologous cord blood would not be used for bone marrow transplantation if that child subsequently experienced childhood leukemia, because of concerns about (1) contamination of the cord blood with malignant cells and (2) lack of graft-versus-leukemia (GVL) effects.[4] Directed donation of UCB for another family member is indicated when there is a first-degree relative with a high-risk or refractory pediatric malignancy amenable to treatment with transplantation therapy, a hemoglobinopathy or other transfusion-dependent anemia, congenital or acquired marrow failure or immunodeficiency, or inborn error of metabolism. Over the past decade, our center has performed transplantation in seven patients with matched, related UCB for refractory leukemia (n = 2), thalassemia (n = 3), Krabbe disease (n = 1) or Fanconi anemia (n = 1) and in five patients with haploidentical, related UCB for Blackfan-Diamond anemia, thalassemia, chronic myelocytic leukemia (CML), amegakaryocytic thrombocytopenia, and T-cell acute lymphoblastic leukemia (ALL).

It is interesting to speculate about whether haploidentical, related UCB will be useful in the nonmyeloablative transplantation setting. In that case, it is possible that babies may donate to grandparents, parents, aunts, cousins, and so on, who have adult malignancies or autoimmune disease. Currently, there is insufficient data to address the question of whether haploidentical related cord blood will play a role in the treatment of adults with refractory malignancies or other diseases amenable to treatment with allogeneic stem cell transplantation.

Public Cord Blood Banks

Public banks collect cord bloods from healthy, term placentas after obtaining maternal informed consent. In granting consent, the infant's mother acknowledges that the donation is voluntary and that she gives up all rights of the baby's family to the cord blood for the public good. The mother also agrees (1) to allow review of medical records related to her obstetrical care, the delivery, and the baby's perinatal and pediatric care, (2) to give a detailed family medical history, (3) to relinquish a sample of her own blood for infectious disease testing and HLA typing, and (4) to allow carrier state testing for genetic diseases (hemoglobinopathy screening, inborn errors of metabolism, immunodeficiency syndromes) to be performed on a sample of her baby's cord blood if the potential transplant recipient has one of these diseases. The results of the foregoing tests are not routinely provided to the baby's parents or physicians. However, if a disease potentially putting the infant donor at risk is identified, the parents and the mother's or baby's physician are both notified. In some states, if the results of tests for hepatitis B or C, human T-cell leukemia virus (HTLV) type I or II, or human immunodeficiency virus (HIV) type 1 or 2 are positive, law requires notification of the state Board of Health or Centers for Disease Control and Prevention (CDC).

Public cord blood banks ensure confidentiality and do not allow any contact between the infant donor or the donor's family and the patient receiving the stem cells. Bar-coding systems have been developed for labeling to ensure that confidentiality is maintained. Most banks maintain a confidential link between information about the mother and the bar-code label attached to the unit to allow for future contact with the family if necessary.

Public cord blood banks operate under Investigational New Drug applications (INDs) from the U.S. Food and Drug Administration (FDA) in the United States and equivalent national regulatory agencies in other countries. The banks adhere to good tissue practices and guidelines for cellular and tissue-based products, as published by the FDA in the *Federal Register* on January 8, 2001. Over the past decade, with support from governmental and private sources, unrelated umbilical cord blood has been banked by various investigators for public use.[5-11] Approximately 100,000 units are estimated to be listed in individual public banks worldwide. Establishment of these banks was stimulated by the need for stem cell donors for patients who have malignant diseases and genetic conditions correctable by transplantation therapy who lacked a suitably matched, related donor. Units stored in public banks are available for any patient in need who is medically eligible for transplantation therapy. These units are tested and HLA-typed at the time of banking, rendering them readily available for transplantation therapy when identified as the donor of choice for a patient in need.

The first public bank in the world was established by Dr. Pablo Rubinstein at the New York Blood Center with grant support from the National Heart Lung and Blood Institute (NHLBI) of the National Institutes of Health (NIH).[5] This bank, now known as the Placental Blood Program, has banked more than 16,000 units in the past 11 years and has provided more than 1200 units for transplantation worldwide. In 1996, the NHLBI established the Cord Blood Transplantation Study (COBLT), which initially funded three academic centers to establish the second public bank in the United States. COBLT set up banking sites—at Duke University Medical Center in collaboration with the American Red Cross (The Carolinas Cord Blood Bank), Georgetown University, and the University of California at Los Angeles.[6] Collection of units for the COBLT banks was supported through a contract from the National Heart Lung and Blood Institute through June of 2001, creating an inventory of approximately 8000 units. An additional public bank listing approximately 6000 units was established at Cardinal Glennon Hospital in St. Louis through private and philanthropic sources. The American Red Cross has committed to large-scale public cord blood banking and supports six banks currently operating with multiple collection sites throughout the United States.

Public banks employ a team of specially trained nurses and medical technologists who are responsible for recruiting and screening donors, obtaining maternal consent, medical histories, and blood samples, harvesting the units, and transporting the units to the laboratory for banking. Units are generally collected from term babies born after uncomplicated pregnancy, labor, and delivery. Units are cryopreserved within 48 to 72 hours of collection and are placed in quarantine until test results are known. Because HLA typing is the most expensive part of the banking process, banked units must pass a screening algorithm before HLA typing is performed. After HLA typing is completed, the units are recorded in the search registry so as to be accessible to patients in need of unrelated donors. The average time from UCB harvest to listing on the registry is 4 to 6 weeks.

Public cord blood donation is voluntary. A mother consents (preferably before the onset of labor) to voluntarily donate her baby's cord blood, to allow for testing of maternal blood, fetal blood, or both for infectious and genetic diseases transmitted through blood and stem cells, for testing of the cord blood for stem and progenitor cell content, and for review of the family's medical history and the medical records of both the infant and mother. Screening for homozygous hemoglobinopathies may be performed through direct testing of the cord blood or, in states with mandatory screening, by obtaining the results of the state screening program tests for the infant donor. Maternal donors are excluded if they are known to be infected with hepatitis B or C, HTLV, or HIV viruses, if they have traveled to or lived in countries where HIV, vCJD (mad cow disease) or malaria is endemic, if they practice high-risk behaviors or are known to have positive results of viral serologic or DNA tests for syphilis, hepatitis B or C, HTLV I or II, or HIV 1 or 2.

Detection of cytomegalovirus (CMV) in cord blood presents a unique dilemma. Forty percent to 90% of mothers are seropositive for CMV immunoglobulin (Ig) G before pregnancy. This maternal IgG crosses the placenta, yielding a positive serologic test result in the cord blood. However, the presence of maternal anti-CMV IgG is not indicative of active CMV viremia, disease, or infection. Rather, it represents passive transfer of antibody implying serologic conversion after routine infection earlier in the mother's life. Thus, if the mother's blood tests positive for CMV IgG, the cord blood will test positive, reflecting passive transfer of the maternal IgG. However, this test result in no way indicates that the fetus was exposed to or infected with CMV virus or that the cord blood is contaminated with CMV.

Alternative methods of CMV viral detection in cord blood have been sought. The New York Blood Center's Placental Blood Program routinely performs cultures of donor infants' saliva for CMV virus and blood assays for CMV IgG and IgM in the mothers of these babies. With this approach, the overall incidence of positive saliva culture results was 0.3%. However, this finding did not reliably correlate with titers of CMV IgM in the blood of mothers of babies with positive culture results. Techniques to detect CMV DNA in cord blood cells or plasma are under development but are not yet ready for clinical use. In our experience, 10% of mothers with indeterminate anti-CMV IgM results show evidence of CMV viremia on DNA testing. The significance of this finding is under investigation.

The FDA has recommended that public UCB banks develop look-forward programs to follow donors for the development of diseases that would not be recognized at birth but that could develop later in life and be transmitted to and clinically expressed in a transplant recipient. Most centers do not have the resources to effectively execute proactive follow-up or look-forward programs. As an alternative, they rely on the parents to inform the banks if a donor experiences any serious illnesses during childhood (e.g. cancer, acquired immunodeficiency syndrome [AIDS], genetic diseases, immunodeficiency syndromes). Using these methods, the incidence of development of clinically significant, unanticipated disease in the UCB donor in the first 5 years of life is < 1:10,000 donors.

Publicly banked units are characterized in laboratories committed to excellence in stem cell processing and cryopreservation. UCB units are characterized through the enumeration of cell counts, differential counts to determine mononuclear cell and nucleated red blood cell dosing, viability, ABO and Rh typing, CD34 positivity, CD3 positivity as a measure of T cell content, and clonal hematopoietic progenitor cell content (granulocyte-macrophage and granulo-cyte-erythroid-megakaryocyte-macrophage colony-forming units, erythroid burst-forming units). Bacterial and fungal cultures are routinely performed, and units that test positive are generally excluded from the inventory. Procedures for volume reduction, RBC depletion, and cryopreservation have been standardized and validated.[5, 6] HLA typing is performed on the pellet of RBCs and granulocytes using molecular techniques. Most banks currently use DNA technology to minimally determine antigenic or serologic typing for HLA-A and HLA-B, and DNA or allelic level for HLA-DRB1. Results are transferred to electronic databases that can be accessed by transplant centers searching for donors for their patients.

The COBLT project studied more than 35,000 potential maternal donors and 18,000 collected cord blood units. The study found that the main reason for donor exclusion prior to collection of the cord blood unit was a risk factor for infectious disease exposure in the mother or a positive infectious disease screening test result in the mother before delivery. The main reason for exclusion of the unit after collection for banking was low cell count, low volume, or both. In the 8000 units banked in the COBLT banks, the average number of total nucleated cells was 1×10^9 and the average number of CD34-positive cells was 2.6×10^6.[6] These values represent a 10- to 20-fold decrease from the average numbers of cells used in a typical bone marrow transplant.

Unfortunately, accessing unrelated cord blood units available for transplantation is not a centralized process. There is no current universal registry where units from all umbilical cord blood banks list their inventories. Thus, patients and transplant centers in search of a donor must search banks individually. Most of the larger banks have independent search programs, and some of the smaller banks have net-worked through the National Marrow Donor Program or the American Red Cross. With support from the NHLBI, the Emmes Corporation developed an Internet-based, user-protected computerized search system that can be accessed by the 27 transplant centers participating in the COBLT transplant study. Netcord, an international, collaborative allegiance of 14 public cord blood banks, is developing a hub-based, Internet search engine to facilitate searching of units listed by their organization.

Cord blood has not yet been licensed by the FDA as a product, although some restricted licensing is expected by the year 2003. Public units used for transplantation can be obtained at no cost from NIH-sponsored banks or with an FDA-set fee for cost reimbursement from other public banks in the United States and abroad.

■ Early Experience in Umbilical Cord Blood Transplantation

The proof that an umbilical cord blood unit harvested from a single donor contained sufficient stem cells to rescue a myeloablated patient required an experiment in human trans-plantation. Before the demonstration of successful engraft-ment of UCB, there was great skepticism about the feasibility of the procedure. Transplant experts doubted that cord blood would contain sufficient numbers of cells to enable timely short-term or durable long-term marrow reconstitution. Those believing that engraftment was possible thought that it would hold true only for small children. Many worried that the

immunologic naiveté of cord blood lymphocytes would lead to post-transplant immunodeficiency and the lack of graft-versus-leukemia activity.

The first cord blood transplant in the world was performed in 1988, in a 6-year old boy with Fanconi anemia who received cord blood from his HLA-matched sister, by Dr. Eliane Gluckman at the Hopital Saint-Louis in Paris.[12] This transplant, which was supported by an international, multidisciplinary collaboration among several academic medical centers, a private insurer (Blue Cross/Blue Shield), Hopital Saint-Louis in Paris, and the first private umbilical cord blood company (Biocyte), proved that cord blood con-tained sufficient stem cells to rescue a child and stimulated the use of related, directed donor UCB transplantation for approx-imately 60 additional transplants over the subsequent 5 years. Outcomes of these transplants demonstrated (1) the feasibil-ity of engraftment in children, (2) delayed time to engraftment of neutrophils and platelets compared with results using matched-related bone marrow, and (3) a lower incidence of acute and chronic GVHD compared with results in allogeneic bone marrow transplantation from matched related donors in young children.[12–18]

■ Experience with Unrelated UCB Transplantation

The first unrelated cord blood transplant was performed in a 3-year-old white boy with refractory T-cell ALL by the Pediatric Bone Marrow Transplant Program at Duke University Medical Center in August 1993. The UCB donor was a unit from the New York Blood Center matching four of six HLA antigens.[19] The patient received a cell dose of 4.6×10^7 nucleated cells per kg and engrafted neutrophils on post-transplant day 31 and platelets on post-transplant day 50. He did not experience acute GVHD. Unfortunately, he died of a pulmonary alveolar hemorrhage 61 days after receiving the transplant and could not be evaluated for the longer-term endpoints.

Between September 1993 and November 1995, 24 addi-tional high-risk pediatric patients, ranging in age from 1 to 23 years and weighing 7.4 to 53 kg, were enrolled in a phase I trial of the feasibility of unrelated cord blood transplanta-tion.[15] All patients received myeloablative chemotherapy or chemotherapy plus radiation therapy, and all but one received transplants of grafts mismatched at one to three HLA loci. Cell doses for transplantation ranged from 0.67 to 16.81×10^7 cells/kg. One patient experienced primary graft failure, and one, autologous reconstitution. The median time to neutrophil engraftment (first of three consecutive days to achieve an absolute neutrophil count of 500 cells/μL) was 22 days. The median time to platelet engraftment (defined as achievement of a platelet count of 50,000 cells/μL without transfusion in the previous 7 days) was 82 days. Independence from RBC transfusion was achieved in a median of 55 days. The inci-dence of severe (grade III or IV) acute GVHD was 10%, and no patient experienced extensive chronic GVHD. Forty-four percent (n = 11) of these 25 patients survived event free as of June 2002. One patient, a 23-year-old woman with Fanconi anemia and leukemia, died 5 years after transplantation of a secondary malignancy (squamous cell carcinoma of the head and neck), an event that occurred after publication of the ini-tial report. There have been no other late events. All surviving patients remain durably engrafted, with 100% donor chimerism. Subsequent reports from registries at the New York Blood Center and Eurocord have reproduced these results.[15, 20–22]

Since 1993, more than 2000 unrelated cord blood transplants and more than 400 related cord blood transplants have been performed worldwide to treat children and adults with cancer or genetic diseases;[15, 19–40] the overall success rate ranges between 45% to 75%.[19–34] The results in patients with malignancies parallel results after related and unrelated bone marrow transplantation; younger children with earlier-stage disease demonstrate better prognoses. Patients with nonmalignant diagnoses have higher survival rates (70% to 90%), because of their younger age, rapid graft availability, higher cell dosing, and lack of relapse as a contributing cause of failure.

Since 1995, approximately 150 adults lacking traditional stem cell donors have received unrelated cord blood transplants for treatment of high-risk, refractory malignancies. The overall success rate in this group is 25% to 30%, comparable to the rate for unrelated bone marrow transplantation in adults.[27, 28] Graft failure rates are significantly higher in adults than in children, being estimated at 20% to 25%. The higher rates of graft failure are likely due to the lower cell dosing achievable in larger individuals who receive a single UCB donor unit.

After cord blood transplantation, neutrophil engraftment occurs at a median of 25 days in 90% of children and 80% of adults.[19–40] Cell dose, rather than HLA match, has been identified as the most important factor correlating with clinical outcomes after cord blood transplantation.[15, 19, 20, 22, 34, 35] Patients receiving larger cell doses per kilogram of recipient body weight experience more rapid neutrophil and platelet engraftment, higher probabilities of overall engraftment, earlier immune reconstitution, and superior event-free survival. However, because of the biologic differences in size and thymic function among babies, children, and adults, it has not been possible to completely distinguish between the influence of cell dose and that of age in analysis of clinical outcomes in UCB transplants to date. The use of preparative regimens containing total body irradiation (TBI), which causes injury to the host thymus, also contributes to delays in engraftment and immune reconstitution. Patients prepared for transplantation with non-TBI regimens experience earlier immune reconstitution. The spleen may also serve as a reservoir for donor cells. Patients who undergo transplantation after splenectomy have been observed to experience more rapid platelet and myeloid engraftment.

A major advantage of cord blood stem cells over bone marrow stem cells is that UCB cells are much less likely to cause acute or chronic GVHD. Rates of extensive chronic GVHD are extraordinarily low.[19, 20, 22, 23] The incidence of moderate to severe (grades II to IV) acute GVHD after transplantation of unrelated, partially HLA-mismatched UCB is approximately 40%, with 10% of patients experiencing severe (grade III or IV) disease.[17, 19, 20, 22, 34] The conventional wisdom dictates that UCB stem and T cells are more tolerant of a new host than phenotypically identical cells from "adult" bone marrow or mobilized peripheral blood,[41–50] although the exact mechanisms underlying these observations have yet to be described.

The major cause of failure after an unrelated cord blood transplant in both children and adults is opportunistic infection.[19, 20, 22, 23, 34, 35, 51] The tendency to infection is believed to be due to several factors, including (1) lower cell dosing, which leads to longer periods of neutropenia in the first several weeks after transplant, and (2) defects in neutrophil function as these cells recapitulate neonatal neutrophil function and ontogeny. Cord blood–derived lymphocytes are naive, having never been exposed to common bacterial and viral pathogens. Cord blood lacks T cells with memory of CMV, Epstein-Barr virus, and other common viruses with the potential to reactivate in the transplant recipient. Fatal infections generally occur before 100 days after transplant in children and before 180 days after transplant in adults.

The pace of immune reconstitution relates to patient age as well as cell dose delivered by the graft. Duration of administration of immunoprophylaxis to protect patients against GVHD also affects immune reconstitution. Patients younger than 2 years recover CD4-negative T cells to an absolute count higher than 400 cells/μL and near-normal phytohemagglutinin (PHA) responses by 3 to 4 months after transplant. Children between the ages of 2 and 17 years reach similar endpoints 9 to 12 months after transplant. Adults may never fully recover thymic-dependent immune function and generally take up to three times longer than children to recover protective immune function.[52, 53] The cause of this delay may be the lower capacity of the adult host thymus to contribute to the immune reconstitution process.

It is generally agreed that to improve the success of cord blood transplantation in adults, the dose available from single units must be larger. Current preclinical and clinical research is focusing on ex vivo expansion of cord blood cells as one strategy to enlarge the dose of cells available for transplantation.[54–67] Results of phase I clinical trials are encouraging, but additional studies are required to establish the utility of these approaches.[65–67] Another approach under investigation involves combining multiple units for a single transplant. Although transient mixed chimerism has been observed in a limited number of patients treated in this fashion, durable engraftment occurs with a single UCB unit, and times to engraftment are not different from those observed after transplantation of a single UCB unit. Investigators in Spain successfully combined unrelated cord blood transplantation with haploidentical, related bone marrow transplantation.[68] After myeloablative preparative therapy, their patients received both products for transplantation. The haploidentical cells engrafted early and provided neutrophil reconstitution in a median of 12 to 16 days. Subsequently, the cord blood myeloid and lymphoid cells engrafted over approximately 100 days, rejecting the haplo-related stem cells and providing cells for durable engraftment and immune reconstitution.

Nonablative or "mini" transplants are undergoing testing in adult patients with malignancies who are unable to tolerate full-dose myeloablative therapy. Limited trials using unrelated cord blood in this setting have demonstrated success in 50% of heavily pretreated, older patients with malignant diagnoses.[69, 70] Similar approaches have been suggested for children with nonmalignant diagnoses; however, immune-mediated graft rejection and autologous marrow recovery are major obstacles to the success of this approach in younger immunologically competent patients.

Cord blood transplantation has been especially successful in the treatment of young infants and toddlers with inborn errors of metabolism.[71, 72] In these patients, the cord blood stem cells provide a durable source of donor cells, which produce the defective or missing enzyme in the patient. When performed early in the course of disease, stem cell transplantation prevents further progression and, in some cases, facilitates reversal of organ damage caused prior to transplantation. In patients with neurologic diseases, donor cells engraft and differentiate in the brain 4 to 12 months after transplantation.

In patients with leukodystrophies, cord blood transplantation performed in the presymptomatic phase prevents demyelination in both the central and peripheral nervous systems.[72] In patients with mucopolysaccharidoses, transplantation therapy used before the age of 2 to 3 years results in correction of corneal clouding, hepatocellular damage, and bony deformities and prevents central nervous system damage.[71] Most interestingly, cardiac disease, which is usually caused by atherosclerotic changes in coronary arteries in early childhood, is also ameliorated in such children. In 25 children with mucopolysaccharidosis I, transplantation with unrelated UCB after myeloablative chemotherapy prior to 3 years of age resulted in 100% engraftment and 87% event-free survival.[71]

These observations suggest that cord blood stem cells are capable of transdifferentiation into nonhematopoietic lineages. UCB-derived stem cells may exhibit a greater degree of cellular plasticity than adult bone marrow stem cells. There is reason to believe that over the next decade, cord blood–derived cellular therapies will be developed to treat hepatic, cardiac, and neurodegenerative diseases of adults. In addition, cord blood transplantation from both related and unrelated donors is likely to emerge as a front-line corrective therapy for pediatric patients with hemoglobinopathies, to be given early in the course of the disease and before the onset of chronic organ damage, transfusion-associated iron overload, and alloimmunization from repeated transfusions.

REFERENCES

1. Muller SM, Ege M, Pottharst A, et al: Transplacentally acquired maternal T lymphocytes in severe combined immunodeficiency: A study of 121 patients. Blood 2001;98:1847–1851.
2. Smith FO, Kurtzberg J, Karson EM, et al: Umbilical cord blood collection, storage and transplantation: Issues and recommendations for expectant parents and patients. Cancer Res Ther Control 1999;10:217–226.
3. American Academy of Pediatrics Working Group on Cord Blood Banking, 1998: Cord blood banking for potential future transplantation: Subject review. Pediatrics 1999;104:116–118.
4. Rowley JD: Backtracking leukemia to birth. Nature 1998;4:150–151.
5. Rubinstein P, Dobrila L, Rosenfield RE, et al: Processing and cryopreservation of placental/umbilical cord blood for unrelated bone marrow reconstitution. Proc Natl Acad Sci U S A 1995;92:10119–10122.
6. Fraser JK, Cairo MS, Wagner EL, et al: Cord blood transplantation study (COBLT): Cord blood bank standard operating procedures. J Hematother 1998;7:521–561.
7. Boppana SB, Rivera LB, Fowler KB, et al: Intrauterine transmission of cytomegalovirus to infants of women with preconceptional immunity. N Engl J Med 2001;344:1366–1371.
8. Rendine S, Durtoni ES, di Celle F, et al: Analysis of the Turin Umbilical Cord Blood Bank Registry. Transfusion 2000;40:813–816.
9. Rogers I, Sutherland DR, Holt D, et al: Human UC-blood banking: Impact of blood volume, cell separation and cryopreservation on leukocyte and CD34⁺ cell recovery. Cytotherapy 2001;3:269–276.
10. Stanworth S, Warwick R, Fehily D, et al: An international survey of unrelated umbilical cord blood banking. Vox Sang 2001;80:236–243.
11. Ballen K, Broxmeyer HE, McCullough J, et al: Current status of cord blood banking and transplantation in the United States and Europe. Biol Blood Marrow Transplant 2001;7:635–645.
12. Gluckman E, Broxmeyer HE, Auerbach AD, et al: Hematopoietic reconstitution in a patient with Fanconi's anemia by means of umbilical cord blood from an HLA-identical sibling. N Engl J Med 1989;321:1174–1178.
13. Wagner JE: Umbilical cord blood stem cell transplantation. J Pediatr Hematol Oncol 1993;15:169–174.
14. Wagner JE, Kernan NA, Steinbuch M, et al: Allogeneic sibling umbilical-cord-blood transplantation in children with malignant and non-malignant disease. Lancet 1995;346:214–219.
15. Gluckman E, Rocha V, Boyer-Chammard A, et al: Outcome of cord-blood transplantation from related and unrelated donors. N Engl J Med 1997;337:373–381.
16. Kato S, Nishihira H, Sako M, et al: Cord blood transplantation from sibling donors in Japan report of the national survey. Int J Hematol 1998;67:389–396.
17. Rocha V, Wagner JE, Sobocinski KA, et al: Graft-versus-host disease in children who have received a cord-blood or bone marrow transplant from an HLA-identical sibling. N Engl J Med 2000;342:1846–1854.
18. Gluckman E: Hematopoietic stem-cell transplants using umbilical-cord blood. N Engl J Med 2001;344:1860–1861.
19. Kurtzberg J, Laughlin M, Graham ML, et al: Placental blood as a source of hematopoietic stem cells for transplantation into unrelated recipients. N Engl J Med 1996;335:157–166.
20. Wagner JE, Rosenthal J, Sweetman R, et al: Successful transplantation of HLA-matched and HLA-mismatched umbilical cord blood from unrelated donors: Analysis of engraftment and acute graft-versus-host disease. Blood 1996;88:795–802.
21. Rubinstein P, Carrier C, Scaradavou A, et al: Outcomes among 562 recipients of placental-blood transplants from unrelated donors. N Engl J Med 1998;339:1565–1629.
22. Gluckman E: Current status of umbilical cord blood hematopoietic stem cell transplantation. Exp Hematol 2000;28:1197–1205.
23. Gluckman E, Locatelli F: Umbilical cord blood transplants. Curr Opin Hematol 2000;7:353–357.
24. Gluckman E: Hematopoietic stem-cell transplants using umbilical-cord blood. N Engl J Med 2001;344:1860–1861.
25. Nagarajan R, Neglia J, Ramsay N, et al: Successful treatment of refractory Langerhans cell histiocytosis with unrelated cord blood transplantation. J Pediatr Hematol Oncol 2001;23:629–632.
26. Suminoe A, Matsuzaki A, Hattori H, et al: Unrelated cord blood transplantation for an infant with chemotherapy-resistant progressive Langerhans cell histiocytosis. J Pediatr Hematol Oncol 2001;23:633–637.
27. Goussetis E, Peristeri J, Kitra V, et al: Combined umbilical cord blood and bone marrow transplantation in the treatment of beta-thalassemia major. Pediatr Hematol Oncol 2000;17:307–314.
28. Veys P: Umbilical cord blood transplantation in beta-thalassemia major. Pediatr Hematol Oncol 2000;17:281–283.
29. Gore L, Lane PA, Quinones RR, Giller RH: Successful cord blood transplantation for sickle cell anemia from a sibling who is human leukocyte antigen-identical: Implications for comprehensive care. J Pediatr Hematol Oncol 2000;22:437–440.
30. Mullen CA, Thompson JN, Richard LA, Chan KW: Unrelated umbilical cord blood transplantation in infancy for mucopolysaccharidosis type IIB (Hunter syndrome) complicated by autoimmune hemolytic anemia. Bone Marrow Transplant 2000;25:1093–1097.
31. Ziegner UH, Ochs HD, Schanen C, et al: Unrelated umbilical cord stem cell transplantation for X-linked immunodeficiencies. J Pediatr 2001;138:570–573.
32. Yoshimasu T, Tanaka R, Suenobu S, et al: Prompt and durable hematopoietic reconstitution by unrelated cord blood transplantation in a child with Fanconi anemia. Bone Marrow Transplant 2001;27:767–769.
33. Rocha V, Cornish J, Sievers EL, et al: Comparison of outcomes of unrelated bone marrow and umbilical cord blood transplants in children with acute leukemia. Blood 2001;97:2962–2970.
34. Barker JN, Davies SM, DeFor T, et al: Survival after transplantation of unrelated donor umbilical cord blood is comparable to that of human leukocyte antigen-matched unrelated donor bone marrow: Results of a matched-pair analysis. Blood 2001;97:2957–2961.
35. Migliaccio AR, Adamson JW, Stevens CE, et al: Cell dose and speed of engraftment in placental/umbilical cord blood transplantation: Graft progenitor cell content is a better predictor than nucleated cell quantity. Blood 2000;96:2717–2722.
36. Laughlin MJ, Rizzieri DA, Smith CA, et al: Hematologic engraftment and reconstitution of immune function post unrelated placental cord blood transplant in an adult with acute lymphocytic leukemia. Leukemia Res 1998;22:215–219.

37. Laughlin MJ, Barker J, Bambach B, et al: Hematopoietic engraftment and survival in adult recipients of umbilical-cord blood from unrelated donors. N Engl J Med 2001;344:1815–1822.
38. Sanz GF, Saavedra S, Planelles D, et al: Standardized, unrelated donor cord blood transplantation in adults with hematologic malignancies. Blood 2001;98:2332–2338.
39. Lau FY, Wong R, Chui CH, et al: Successful engraftment in two adult patients with severe aplastic anemia using nonmyeloablative conditioning followed by unrelated HLA-mismatched cord blood transplantation. J Hematother Stem Cell Res 2001;10:309–311.
40. Laughlin MJ: Umbilical cord blood for allogeneic transplantation in children and adults. Bone Marrow Transplant 2001;27:1–6.
41. Anasetti C: Young is better if enough. Blood 2001;97:2921.
42. Rubinstein P: HLA matching for bone marrow transplantation—how much is enough? N Engl J Med 2001;345:1842–1843.
43. Ohnuma K, Isoyama K, Ikuta K, et al: The influence of HLA genotyping compatibility on clinical outcome after cord blood transplantation from unrelated donors. J Hematother Stem Cell Res 2000;9:541–550.
44. Harris DT, Schumacher MJ, Locascio J, et al: Phenotypic and functional immaturity of human umbilical cord blood T lymphocytes. Proc Natl Acad Sci U S A 1992;89:10006–10010.
45. Clerici M, DePalma L, Roilides E, et al: Analysis of T helper and antigen-presenting cell functions in cord blood and peripheral blood leukocytes from healthy children of different ages. J Clin Invest 1993;91:2829–2836.
46. Harris DT, LoCascio J, Besencon FJ: Analysis of the alloreactive capacity of human umbilical cord blood: Implications for graft-versus-host disease. Bone Marrow Transplant 1994;14:545–553.
47. Roncarolo MG, Vaccarino E, Saracco P, et al: Immunologic properties of cord blood. In Broxmeyer HE (ed): Cellular Characteristics of Cord Blood and Cord Blood Transplantation. Bethesda, MD, American Association of Blood Banks Press, 1998, pp 67–82.
48. Chalmers IMH, Janossy G, Contreras M, et al: Intracellular cytokine profile of cord and adult blood lymphocytes. Blood 1998;92:11–18.
49. Gaddy J, Broxmeyer HE: Cord blood natural killer cells: Implications for cord blood transplantation and insights into natural killer cell differentiation. In Broxmeyer HE (ed): Cellular Characteristics of Cord Blood and Cord Blood Transplantation. Bethesda, MD, American Association of Blood Banks Press, 1998, pp 83–112.
50. Liu E, Tu W, Law HKW, et al: Changes of CD14 and CD1a expression in response to IL-4 and granulocyte-macrophage colony-stimulating factor are different in cord blood and adult blood monocytes. Pediatr Res 2001;50:184–189.
51. Carvajal E, Verdeguer A, Fernandez JM, et al: Herpesvirus-6 encephalitis complicated by Wernicke-Korsakoff syndrome in a pediatric recipient of unrelated cord blood transplantation. J Pediatr Hematol Oncol 2001;23:626–628.
52. Giraud P, Thuret I, Reviron D, et al: Immune reconstitution and outcome after unrelated cord blood transplantation: A single paediatric institution experience. Bone Marrow Transplant 2000;25:53–57.
53. Klein AK, Patel DD, Gooding JE, et al: T-cell recovery in adults and children following umbilical cord blood transplantation. Biol Blood Marrow Transplant 2001;7:454–466.
54. Miller JS, McCullar V, Punzel M, et al: Single adult human CD34$^+$/Lin$^-$/CD38$^-$ progenitors give rise to natural killer cells, B-lineage cells, dendritic cells and myeloid cells. Blood 1999;93:96–106.
55. Qiu L, Meagher R, Welhausen S, et al: Ex vivo expansion of CD34$^+$ umbilical cord blood cells in a defined serum-free medium (QBSF-60) with early effect cytokines. J Hematother Stem Cell Res 1999;8:609–618.
56. Kinoshita T, Koike K, Mwamtemi HH, et al: Retinoic acid is a negative regulator for the differentiation of cord blood-derived human mast cell progenitors. Blood 2000;95:2821–2828.
57. Doerner M, Roecklein B, Torok-Storb B, et al: Expansion and transduction of nonenriched human cord blood cells using HS-5 conditioned medium and FLT3-L. J Hematother Stem Cell Res 2000;9:759–765.
58. Shih CC, DiGiusto D, Forman SJ: Ex vivo expansion of transplantable human hematopoietic stem cells: Where do we stand in the year 2000? J Hematother Stem Cell Res 2000;9:621–628.
59. Lewis ID, Almeida-Porada G, Du J, et al: Umbilical cord blood cells capable of engrafting in primary, secondary, and tertiary xenogeneic hosts are preserved after ex vivo culture in a noncontact system. Blood 2001;97:3441–3449.
60. Gluckman Eliane: Current status of umbilical cord blood hematopoietic stem cell transplantation. Exp Hematol 2000;28:1197–1205.
61. Almeida-Porada G, Brown RL, MacKintosh FR, et al: Evaluation of serum-free culture conditions able to support the ex vivo expansion and engraftment of human hematopoietic stem cells in the human-to-sheep xenograft model. J Hematother Stem Cell Res 2000;9:683–693.
62. Woods EJ, Liu J, Derrow CW, et al: Osmometric and permeability characteristics of human placental/umbilical cord blood CD34$^+$ cells and their application to cryopreservation. J Hematother Stem Cell Res 2000;9:161–173.
63. Robinson S, Mosley RL, Parajuli P, et al: Comparison of the hematopoietic activity of flt-3 ligand and granulocyte-macrophage colony-stimulating factor acting alone or in combination. J Hematother Stem Cell Res 2000;9:711–720.
64. Nielsen SD, Husemoen LLN, Sorensen TU, et al: FLT3 ligand preserves the uncommitted CD34$^+$ CD38$^-$ progenitor cells during cytokine prestimulation for retroviral transduction. J Hematother Stem Cell Res 2000;9:695–701.
65. Sasayama N, Kashiwakura I, Tokushima Y, et al: Expansion of megakaryocyte progenitors from cryopreserved leukocyte concentrates of human placental and umbilical cord blood in short-term liquid culture. Cytotherapy 2001;3:117–126.
66. Shpall EJ, Quinones R, Giller R, et al: Transplantation of ex vivo expanded cord blood: A Phase I/II feasibility study. In Press, Blood Bone Marrow Transplant 2002.
67. Jaroscak J, Goltry K, Smith A, et al: Augmentation of umbilical cord blood transplantation with ex vivo expanded cells: Results of a phase I trial using the Aastrom Replicell system. Submitted, Blood, 2002.
68. Fernandez MN, Regidor C, Cabrera R, et al: Cord blood transplants: Early recovery of neutrophils from co-transplanted sibling haploidentical progenitor cells and lack of engraftment of cultured cord blood cells, as ascertained by analysis of DNA polymorphisms. Bone Marrow Transplant 2001;28:355–363.
69. Rizzieri DA, Long GD, Vredenburgh JJ, et al: Successful allogeneic engraftment of mismatched unrelated cord blood following a nonmyeloablative preparative regimen. Blood 2001;98:3486–3488.
70. Chen BJ, Cui X, Chao NJ: Addition of a second, different allogeneic graft accelerates white cell and platelet engraftment after T-cell-depleted bone marrow transplantation. Blood 2002;15:2235–2240.
71. Staba S, Martin PL, Szabolcs P, et al: Correction of Hurler syndrome with unrelated umbilical cord blood transplantation. Biol Blood Bone Marrow Transplant 2002;8:98.
72. Kurtzberg J, Richards K, Wenger D, et al: Correction of Krabbe disease neonatal hematopoietic stem cell transplantation. Biol Bone Marrow Transplant 2002;8:97.

Chapter 48

Mononuclear Cell Preparations

Iain J. Webb

Mononuclear cell preparations collected from bone marrow have been used as a source of hematopoietic progenitor cells to support myeloablative therapy for various malignant and nonmalignant disorders for more than 40 years.[1, 2] Mobilized mononuclear cells collected from the peripheral blood and mononuclear cells collected from the umbilical cord have also been used as sources of hematopoietic progenitor cells. In addition, with the identification of the graft-versus-leukemia effect, mononuclear cells are increasingly being used in adoptive immunotherapy approaches, primarily as donor lymphocyte infusions. This chapter reviews sources of hematopoietic progenitor cells and other mononuclear cell preparations as well as collection and processing methods.

◾ Hematopoietic Progenitor Cell Components

Hematopoietic progenitor cells (HPCs) may be isolated from bone marrow, mobilized peripheral blood, and umbilical cord blood (UCB). Centers have increasingly been using mobilized autologous as well as allogeneic peripheral blood instead of bone marrow–derived HPCs. In addition, many centers are actively investigating the use of UCB as an alternative source of HPCs.

Progenitor cells collected from the peripheral blood have in most centers replaced bone marrow as the HPC source of choice for autologous transplantation and increasingly for allogeneic transplantation. Prior to collection, the patient or allogeneic donor is given an agent to mobilize the progenitor cells into the peripheral blood. Patients are treated with a cytokine such as granulocyte (G) colony-stimulating factor (CSF) (G-CSF) or granulocyte-macrophage CSF (GM-CSF) to mobilize stem cells into the peripheral blood, in many cases after they receive chemotherapy. The cells are collected in the outpatient setting. After chemotherapy, the patient undergoes

leukapheresis once the cell counts recover from the nadir. Circulating peripheral blood CD34+ cell levels may be used to predict the yield.[3, 4] If cytokines are used without prior chemotherapy, collection is begun on a predetermined day during their administration. If peripheral blood collections are to be used for allogeneic transplantation, collection is begun on the fourth or fifth day of G-CSF administration.

For autologous transplantation, the advantages of peripheral blood over bone marrow have been well documented.[5] They include more rapid engraftment, decreased need for transfusions, lower incidence of infection and rate of antibiotic use, and shorter hospital stay. Engraftment may also be more rapid with allogeneic peripheral blood than with allogeneic bone marrow. Peripheral blood components typically contain at least 1 log more T cells than bone marrow components, however, potentially increasing the risk for graft-versus-host disease (GVHD). Nevertheless, the incidence of acute GVHD has not been found to be significantly elevated.[6] The reasons for this finding are unclear, but it may in part be due to the effects of the G-CSF on T cells. However, reports have suggested that chronic GVHD may be more common in recipients of peripheral blood components.[7]

HPC units collected from placental or umbilical cord blood have received much attention. Although many units have been banked for potential autologous or intra-family use, most UCB transplants have been allogeneic. Gluckman and associates[8] first reported the clinical use of UCB-derived HPCs in 1989. Since that time, hundreds of UCB transplants have been performed in North America and Europe.[9] After the birth of a child, UCB is collected from the umbilical cord, placental veins, or both. Initial reports suggested that UCB transplants may be performed across HLA barriers with less risk of GVHD than would be anticipated if a bone marrow donor with the same HLA type were used.[10] If this diminished risk of GVHD is confirmed in subsequent studies, UCB could become an attractive alternative for patients requiring allogeneic transplantation who do not have an HLA-matched donor. However, the dose of UCB-derived HPCs necessary for an adult recipient remains to be defined, and larger studies are required to determine the appropriate indications for use of these components.

■ Donor Lymphocyte Infusions

When it became clear that hematopoiesis could reliably be established through the use of allogeneic cells, efforts were undertaken to find ways to minimize the toxicities associated with myeloablative therapy as well as to decrease the incidence and severity of GVHD, a major cause of morbidity and mortality in allograft recipients. Depletion of T cells from the donor graft and intensification of prophylactic immunosuppression were evaluated as methods to decrease the incidence of or to prevent GVHD.

It subsequently became apparent that recipients of T cell–depleted grafts were at higher risk of relapse of the disease being treated[11] and that disease response to transplant therapy was often associated with the occurrence of GVHD.[12] Although they precipitated further clinical research into the control of GVHD, these observations provided convincing evidence for the existence of a graft-versus-leukemia (GVL) effect. Efforts have been focused on improving the understanding of this phenomenon, with the intent to harness GVL but avoid GVHD, thus minimizing toxicity while improving outcomes. Attempts have thus been made to minimize the GVHD-related and non–GVHD-related toxicity occurring at the time of HPC transplantation.

Furthermore, treatment options for disease relapse after allogeneic transplantation of HPCs are limited. Salvage chemotherapy is rarely effective in providing long-term remissions and is associated with significant toxicity. Second transplants have a markedly higher incidence of morbidity and mortality owing to the cumulative effects of high-dose chemotherapy and irradiation. Consequently, there has been much interest in the clinical application of GVL to patients whose disease has progressed following HPC transplantation. Approaches utilizing cellular therapy to treat and prevent relapse with donor lymphocyte infusions (DLIs) have subsequently been initiated.

Use in Patients with Relapse

DLIs are frequently used to treat patients who experience relapse after allogeneic HPC transplantation. Complete hematologic and cytogenetic responses can be achieved in more than 75% of patients with stable-phase chronic myelogenous leukemia (CML) who are treated with DLIs at relapse.[13, 14] Response is best in patients in the earliest stages of relapse. For example, the European Group for Blood and Marrow Transplantation (EBMT) documented complete remissions in 73% of 84 patients with relapsed CML (Table 48.1).[13] Eighty-seven percent of patients remained in remission at 3 years, and GVHD of grade II or higher developed in 41% of patients, with myelosuppression in 34% of patients. Clinical features of GVHD were associated with the attainment of remission, suggesting a relationship between GVHD and the GVL effect of lymphocyte infusions.

DLIs have also been used to treat other patients experiencing relapse after allogeneic transplantation. Significant responses and complete remissions have also been noted in a variety of other malignant hematologic diseases, including multiple myeloma, chronic lymphocytic leukemia (CLL), non-Hodgkin lymphoma, myelodysplastic syndrome, and acute leukemia. Collins and associates[14] reviewed the experience of 25 North American bone marrow transplantation (BMT) programs in 1997. Aggregate reports revealed that complete responses were seen in 60% of patients with CML. The response rates were higher in patients with cytogenetic and chronic-phase relapse (75.7%) than in patients with accelerated-phase (33.3%) or blastic-phase (16.7%) relapse. Overall, 89.6% of patients remained in complete remission at 2 years. Complete remission was less common in patients with acute myelogenous leukemia (AML) (15.4% of 39 patients) and acute lymphocytic leukemia (ALL) (18.2% of 11 patients). Complete remissions were also seen in two of four assessable patients with myeloma and in two of five assessable patients with myelodysplasia. Among patients with CML, response was more common if the patients were in chronic phase and had demonstrated chronic GVHD after HPC transplantation. Responses were correlated with the development of acute and chronic GVHD after DLI, which occurred in 60% and 60.7% of DLI recipients, respectively. In addition, 18.6% of DLI recipients experienced pancytopenia, the second most common adverse effect associated with DLI.

Table 48.1 Rate of Complete Remission after Donor Lymphocyte Infusion for Relapse in Patients with Leukemia Who Underwent Bone Marrow Transplantation

Diagnosis	No. of Evaluable Patients	Patients with Complete Remissions	
		No.	Percentage
Chronic myelogenous leukemia			
All stages	75	54	72
Cytogenetic relapse	17	14	82
Hematologic relapse	50	39	78
Accelerated blast	8	1	12.5
Polycythemia vera	1	1	100
Acute myelogenous leukemia	17	5	29
Myelodysplastic syndrome	4	1	5
Acute lymphocytic leukemia	12	0	0
Total	109	61	56

Modified from Kolb HJ, Schattenberg A, Goldman JM, et al: Graft-versus-leukemia effect of donor lymphocyte transfusion in marrow grafted patients. European Group for Blood and Marrow Transplantation Working Party Chronic Leukemia. Blood 1995;86:2041–2050.

DLI and Novel Treatment Strategies

Attempts to minimize GVHD and transplant-related toxicity while maintaining GVL have included nonmyeloablative conditioning regimens as well as T-cell depletion in combination with DLI. As previously noted, T-cell depletion has been associated with increased risk of relapse after allogeneic transplantation. One approach to overcome this higher risk of relapse associated with T-cell depletion is to use DLI as a T-cell "add-back" at some point weeks to months after HPC infusion.

In a retrospective analysis of patients with chronic-phase CML treated with allogeneic marrow BMT, outcomes in 46 patients receiving T cell–depleted (TCD) grafts and 40 patients receiving standard immunosuppressive therapy were compared.[15] The two groups of patients received similar myeloablative regimens and had similar pretreatment characteristics. Incidences of grade 2 to 4 acute GVHD (15% vs. 37%, $P = .026$) and chronic GVHD (18% vs. 42%, $P = .024$) were lower in the TCD group, but the estimated 3-year probability of relapse was higher in this group. Twenty-three patients (20 in the TCD group and 3 in the non-TCD group) were assessable for response to DLI. After DLI, 17 of 20 patients in the TCD group and 2 of 3 patients in the non-TCD group achieved complete remission. Overall survivals at 3 years were similar—72% for the TCD group and 68% for the non-TCD group ($P = .38$)—suggesting that DLI can restore the GVL effect that is decreased by T-cell depletion.

Efforts are currently under way to develop strategies that will minimize GVHD at the time of transplantation through the use of T-cell depletion of the HPC component while maximizing GVL through the administration of DLI at some point after transplantation.

Methods are also in development to induce the GVL effect without the use of high doses of chemotherapy or radiotherapy used in a conventional myeloablative BMT. Donor cell engraftment can be achieved through the use of nonmyeloablative conditioning regimens, with significantly less morbidity and mortality than are seen after conventional allogeneic BMT.[16] This approach is now being used for patients with hematologic malignancies as well as some solid tumors. However, mixed chimerism frequently results and may predispose to relapse. Mixed chimerism can be converted to full donor chimerism by infusion of donor lymphocytes. The use of DLI in this setting may induce or amplify a GVL effect. Consequently, nonmyeloablative transplantation with DLI infusion at a later date is currently undergoing clinical evaluation.

Evidence of a graft-versus-tumor response exists not only for hematologic malignancies but also for solid tumors.[17, 18] Childs and colleagues[19] reported a series of 19 patients with metastatic renal cell carcinoma who received nonmyeloablative peripheral blood stem cell transplants from sibling donors. Seventeen of the donors were fully HLA matched, and two were mismatched at one HLA locus. In addition to cyclosporine, the recipients of the mismatched grafts received anti-thymocyte globulin (ATG). After the tapering of the cyclosporine dosage, 8 patients were eligible for DLI if they had stable or progressive disease and no evidence of grade 2 to 4 GVHD. Responses were seen in 10 of the 19 patients (53%) at a median of 4 months after transplantation. Of interest, the likelihood of a response was significantly higher if GVHD was present.

In addition, Ueno and associates[20] reported a series of ten patients with breast cancer who had received allogeneic peripheral blood stem cell transplants. These ten patients received HLA-matched sibling donor allografts, were stable or responding to standard therapy, and had tumor infiltration of the liver, at least 20% tumor involvement of the bone marrow, or both. Conditioning included cyclophosphamide, carmustine, and thiotepa. One patient, who showed a complete response prior to therapy, remained in this condition after receiving the transplant. In addition, there were three partial responses, and five patients had stable disease. Of interest, there was evidence of a graft-versus-tumor response in two patients who had progressive disease after transplant. Of four patients whose immunosuppression was reduced, two showed response in the liver, with the development or exacerbation of GVHD.

Although these novel transplantation strategies have to date been utilized in a limited number of patients and diseases, there is enough evidence of success to warrant their further investigation and optimization.

Toxicity

DLI may produce remissions in patients with CML whose disease relapsed after BMT. However, the use of DLI may produce significant complications, most commonly pancytopenia and GVHD. In early reports, pancytopenia occurred in more than 50% of cases.[21] The mechanism is not understood, but the phenomenon may represent a form of transfusion-associated GVHD.[22] In this clinical situation, the likelihood of pancytopenia is associated with the extent of donor chimerism in the recipient's bone marrow prior to DLI. This association suggests that the donor lymphocytes are ablating the recipient's hematopoietic cells and that pancytopenia develops if adequate donor HPC function has not been established to maintain normal peripheral blood cell counts. The development of cytopenias is correlated with response and occurs at a similar point after infusion. Pancytopenia may be prolonged and has been reported to cause death. If cytopenias are recognized at an early stage, they can be treated by the collection and administration of additional HPCs from the donor.

Initial studies of DLI reported a high incidence of acute GVHD (80%); however, subsequent studies have reported a lower incidence of significant GVHD (40%).[13, 21] Chronic GVHD is noted in a significant number of patients who do not demonstrate manifestations of acute GVHD. In part because of the high incidence of GVHD, the mortality rate after DLI in early studies was as high as 22%.[21]

Attempts have also been made to decrease the risk of GVHD by changing the dosing regimen for administration of the DLI as well as by manipulating the DLI components themselves. Some groups have chosen to infuse serial doses of DLI until response is achieved.

My colleagues and I have successfully utilized T-cell depletion of donor bone marrow as a means to abrogate GVHD and have similarly depleted DLI of CD8+ T-cells in an attempt to reduce the incidence of GVHD while preserving GVL.[23] Our approach has been to use (1) serial incubations with anti-CD6+ cell monoclonal antibody (MoAb) and baby rabbit complement (BRC) to deplete T cells from bone marrow[24–27] and (2) serial incubations with anti-CD8+ cell MoAb and BRC to deplete T cells from lymphapheresis collections. At our institution utilizing DLIs depleted of CD8+ cells, increasing numbers of CD4+ cells were infused.[23]

Serial cohorts of patients received 0.3, 1.0, or 1.5×10^8 CD4+ cells/kg. Disease responses after CD4+ DLI were documented in 15 of 19 patients (79%) with early-phase CML relapse, in 5 of 6 patients (83%) with relapsed multiple myeloma, and in 1 patient with myelodysplasia. Overall, 12 of 38 patients (32%) who could be evaluated for toxicity experienced acute or chronic GVHD. However, 6 of 27 patients (22%) receiving 0.2×10^8 CD4 cells/kg experienced GVHD, compared with 6 of 11 patients (55%) who received 1.0×10^8 or more CD4 cells/kg ($P = .07$). Neutropenia and thrombocytopenia developed in 7 patients who showed response to DLI but was transient in all but 1. This patient had prolonged cytopenia, which resolved after the infusion of additional bone marrow collected from the donor. Cytopenias and cytogenetic response in the patients with CML occurred at medians of 12 and 13 weeks after treatment with DLI, respectively. Treatment-related mortality was low (3%), with one death related to infection in the setting of immunosuppression for GVHD.

All patients in this trial who experienced GVHD demonstrated tumor regression, but the presence of GVHD was not required for patients to achieve a response, because 48% of patients with responses never showed evidence of GVHD. Because of the relatively low risk of toxicity associated with the infusion of defined numbers of CD4+ donor cells, further studies can be undertaken in the setting of persistent minimal residual disease to prevent relapse after allogeneic BMT.

The pathogenesis of GVL is poorly understood. Indeed, the lymphocyte populations responsible or GVL, transfusion-associated GVHD, and post–HPC transplantation GVHD have not been determined. Depletion of either CD6+ or CD8+ lymphocytes from donor bone marrow has been shown to lessen GVHD at the time of allogeneic transplantation,[24, 28] and CD4+ cells have been implicated in GVL.[29] Further experiments to identify the role of donor lymphocyte populations in GVHD are necessary.

Component Assessment

Assays must be performed on HPC components to determine the component quality and to quantitate the HPC content. In addition, the T-cell content of DLIs should be determined and, in many centers, is controlled. Further, if procedures are performed to alter the number, function, or both of specific cell populations, these changes must be quantified.

The number and type of T cells in DLI components is frequently determined. Assessments of the mononuclear cell, nucleated cell, CD34+ cell, granulocyte-macrophage (GM) colony-forming unit (CFU) (GM-CFU), granulocyte-erythroid-macrophage-megakaryocyte CFU (GEMM-CFU), and long-term culture-initiating cell (LTC-IC) contents have been used to evaluate HPC quality and content. Enumeration of CD34+ cells using flow cytometry analysis is commonly performed as a measure of HPC quality. As with the other assays, CD34+ cell enumeration methods vary among centers, making it difficult to characterize an HPC component adequately to achieve hematologic engraftment.[30, 31] Standardized protocols for CD34+ cell enumeration have been proposed in an attempt to limit variability and permit comparison of HPC content of components collected and infused at different centers.[32] Methodologies to determine absolute cell concentrations, instead of percentages, may further improve the accuracy of the CD34+ cell enumeration procedure.[33]

In addition to assays performed to quantitate HPC content, components must be tested for contaminants, such as bacteria. Contamination rates increase with component manipulation such as negative selection and may be associated with clinical sequelae. For this reason, bacterial cultures should be part of the quality control for HPC collection, processing, cryopreservation, thawing, and reinfusion procedures.[34]

Lastly, patient outcome is the most critical indicator of component quality. Accordingly, engraftment must be monitored prospectively in HPC recipients, and any adverse patient outcomes must be evaluated to determine whether characteristics of the HPC component or its processing may have been associated with these sequelae. In recipients of DLI, the incidence of cytopenias and GVHD should be similarly followed.

Processing and Storage of Mononuclear Cell Components

Autologous and, occasionally, allogeneic HPC components are collected before the patient receives myeloablative therapy and are cryopreserved. Cells are suspended in a mixture of an electrolyte solution, a protein source, and a cryoprotectant such as dimethyl sulfoxide or hydroxyethyl starch.[35] Cryopreserved cells are infused rapidly when thawed, the freezing solution being infused along with the cells. Premedication is required to minimize toxicities.[36–38]

For allogeneic transfusion, acute hemolysis associated with infusion of an ABO-incompatible component is a defined risk.[39] If there is a major ABO incompatibility, defined as the presence of antibodies against donor red blood cells (RBCs) in the recipient's plasma, procedures are often performed to remove the RBCs from the donor HPCs before infusion. If there is a minor ABO incompatibility, in which the donor plasma contains isohemagglutinins against recipient RBCs, the component is washed or volume-reduced to remove plasma. Alternatives to these procedures include plasma or RBC exchange in the recipient and infusion of sources of donor blood group antigens to absorb recipient antibodies.[40, 41]

Increasingly, laboratories are performing more extensive procedures in an attempt to deplete unwanted cell populations from the HPC component. Tumor cells are removed from autologous components to decrease the risk for relapse, and T lymphocytes are removed from allogeneic components to abrogate acute GVHD. The majority of these procedures are performed with either negative or positive selection methods.

Positive selection of HPC components enriches the cell population to be retained while nonspecifically depleting all other cell populations. The systems currently available for positive selection utilize MoAbs directed against the CD34 antigen, which is expressed on HPCs. Cells are incubated with the anti-CD34 MoAb; separation is then achieved through the use of biotin-avidin, magnetic beads, or high-speed cell sorting.[42–45] Fifty percent or more of the CD34+ cells are usually retained, and CD34+ cell purities in excess of 70% can be achieved. Positive selection has been reported to result in a greater than 3-log depletion of tumor cells in patients with multiple myeloma.[46]

In contrast, negative selection targets the cells to be removed from the component while preserving other cell populations.[47] The methods for negative selection include attempts to separate cells on the basis of physical characteristics, in vitro sensitivity to chemotherapeutic agents, or MoAb-mediated targeting of cell-surface antigen. For example, density-gradient centrifugation and centrifugal elutriation have been used to separate cells on the basis of size. Trials have used 4-hydroxycyclophosphamide or mafosfamide to kill tumor cells. Cells can bind to MoAbs conjugated to magnetic beads, dense particles, or surfaces and then physically separated from the other cell populations within a component. In addition, MoAbs may be used to destroy tumor cells or T cells via conjugation with toxins or complement-mediated lysis.[48]

In general, DLIs are given soon after collection and are often not cryopreserved. As already indicated, DLI cell content may be adjusted to enable infusion of a specific dose of cells. Alternatively, negative selection procedures may be performed to deplete certain cell subsets, such as CD8+ cells.[23]

Whether any of these extensive procedures results in clinical benefit remains controversial. There is indirect evidence that tumor depletion is associated with improved outcome,[48–51] but there have been no randomized trials confirming this. Similarly, T-cell depletion can decrease the risk of GVHD, but whether it improves long-term outcomes is unclear.[15] Consequently, all of these procedures should be performed in the context of clinical trials.

Standards and Regulations

The regulations associated with HPC processing and administration are in evolution. Principles of current good manufacturing practice (cGMP) and total quality management (TQM) can be applied to HPC and DLI components. In 1991, the 14th edition of American Association of Blood Banks (AABB) *Standards for Blood Banks and Transfusion Services* was extended to include HSCs. In 1996, the AABB published a separate document, *Standards for Hematopoietic Progenitor Cells*, to expand and replace Section Q of the *Standards for Blood Banks and Transfusion Services*.[52, 53] These standards include sections dealing with donor selection, component collection, processing, testing, labeling, storage, transportation, issue, infusion, and record-keeping for HPCs, including autologous as well as allogeneic bone marrow, peripheral blood progenitor cells, and UCB.

Also, the Foundation for the Accreditation of Cell Therapy (FACT), formed in 1993, conducts programs for inspection and accreditation of HPC collection and processing facilities as well as transplantation programs. The FACT *Standards* represent a consensus document for organizations working together in the field of clinical conduct of hematopoietic progenitor cell transplantation, including the International Society for Hematotherapy and Graft Engineering (ISHAGE), and the American Society for Blood and Marrow transplantation (ABMT).[54] The U.S. Food and Drug Administration (FDA) is currently reviewing the regulation of HPC components and issued a comprehensive draft document on its approach to regulation in February 1997.[55] The FDA has not yet finalized its approach to the regulation of this rapidly developing field but, as a first step, has required that all cell- and tissue-processing facilities register and report their activities.[56] Standardized procedures for quality control of HSC products, similar to those in use for cellular blood components, are required to ensure adequate safety of myeloablative therapy. The FDA has outlined good tissue practice (GTP) to meet these goals.[57]

Future Directions

There are several areas requiring active investigation into the use of HPC components. First, definitive trials are necessary to clarify whether there is any clinical benefit associated with CD34+ cell selection and tumor cell or T-cell depletion. Second, building on platforms by which cells have been expanded but differentiated,[58] and using new cytokines and developing systems, we may be able to expand primitive HPC populations. Expanded populations would be useful for infusion in patients whose autologous grafts contain insufficient numbers for transplantation. In addition, the ability to expand HPCs could make UCB components available to more recipients with less perceived risk. In addition, expanded cells may be useful for gene therapy approaches.

Much effort has been expended to use HPC as a strategy for clinical gene therapy. Stable expression of a transgene in a primitive HPC would, in theory, be an ideal way to replace missing gene products in a patient. Despite numerous attempts, however, no durable results had been achieved. With the 2000 report by Cavazzana-Calvo and associates[59] of the successful treatment of severe combined immune deficiency with gene therapy, interest was renewed, and this therapeutic approach will be the focus of much activity in the years to come.

Advances have also been made in our understanding of the biology as well as potential clinical applications of pluripotent and non-hematopoietic stem cells, which in the foreseeable future will translate into novel therapies. With the proliferation of reports identifying the ability of stem cells to differentiate into musculoskeletal, neural, and hepatic tissue, the use of stem cell–based cellular products to treat benign diseases is assured.[60–62] These advances may lead to strategies to heal a severed spinal cord, cure Parkinson's disease and muscular dystrophy, and restore function to the liver and other organs.

Last but not least, mononuclear cells may be used as starting material to produce adoptive immunotherapy components other than donor lymphocyte infusion. They can be used to produce antigen-presenting cells (APCs) such as dendritic cells (DCs) as well as antigen-specific or cytotoxic lymphocytes (CTLs). Dendritic cells, APCs commonly derived from peripheral blood collections, are increasingly being used in cancer vaccines.[63, 64] In addition, attempts have been made to develop ex vivo systems to produce CTL clones that can recognize specific antigens and destroy cells infected by viruses, bacteria, or parasites as well as target cells expressing a malignant cell surface phenotype. These engineered CTL clones have been shown to be highly effective in animal models and have subsequently been developed for use in human diseases. Clinical trials to treat Epstein-Barr virus, cytomegalovirus, malaria, and solid tumors have already been initiated.

REFERENCES

1. Thomas ED, Lochte HLJ, Lu WC, et al: Intravenous infusion of bone marrow in patients receiving radiation and chemotherapy. N Engl J Med 1957;257:491--496.
2. Thomas ED, Storb R: Technique for human marrow grafting. Blood 1970;36:507–515.
3. Remes K, Matinlauri I, Grenman S, et al: Daily measurements of blood CD34+ cells after stem cell mobilization predict stem cell yield and posttransplant hematopoietic recovery. J Hematother 1997;6:13–19.

4. Fontao-Wendel R, Lazar A, Melges S, et al: The absolute number of circulating CD34(+) cells as the best predictor of peripheral hematopoietic stem cell yield. J Hematother 1999;8:255–262.

5. Gillespie TW, Hillyer CD: Peripheral blood progenitor cells for marrow reconstitution: Mobilization and collection strategies [see comments]. Transfusion 1996;36:611–624.

6. Bensinger WI, Martin PJ, Storer B, et al: Transplantation of bone marrow as compared with peripheral-blood cells from HLA-identical relatives in patients with hematologic cancers. N Engl J Med 2001;344:175–181.

7. Storek J, Gooley T, Siadak M, et al: Allogeneic peripheral blood stem cell transplantation may be associated with a high risk of chronic graft-versus-host disease. Blood 1997;90:4705–4709.

8. Gluckman E, Broxmeyer HA, Auerbach AD, et al: Hematopoietic reconstruction in a patient with Fanconi's anemia by means of umbilical-cord blood form an HLA-identical sibling. N Engl J Med 1989;321:1174–1178.

9. Rubinstein P, Carrier C, Scaradavou A, et al: Outcomes among 562 recipients of placental-blood transplants from unrelated donors [see comments]. N Engl J Med 1998;339:1565–1577.

10. Rocha V, Wagner JE Jr, Sobocinski KA, et al: Graft-versus-host disease in children who have received a cord-blood or bone marrow transplant from an HLA identical sibling. Eurocord and International Bone Marrow Transplant Registry Working Committee on Alternative Donor and Stem Cell Sources. N Engl J Med 2000;342:1846–1854.

11. Marmont AM, Horowitz MM, Gale RP, et al: T-cell depletion of HLA-identical transplants in leukemia. Blood 1991;78:2120–2130.

12. Horowitz MM, Gale RP, Sondel PM, et al: Graft-versus-leukemia reactions after bone marrow transplantation. Blood 1990;75:555–562.

13. Kolb HJ, Schattenberg A, Goldman JM, et al: Graft-versus-leukemia effect of donor lymphocyte transfusions in marrow grafted patients. European Group for Blood and Marrow Transplantation Working Party Chronic Leukemia. Blood 1995;86:2041–2050.

14. Collins RH Jr, Shpilberg O, Drobyski WR, et al: Donor leukocyte infusions in 140 patients with relapsed malignancy after allogeneic bone marrow transplantation. J Clin Oncol 1997;15:433–444.

15. Sehn LH, Alyea EP, Weller E, et al: Comparative outcomes of T-cell-depleted and non-T-cell-depleted allogeneic bone marrow transplantation for chronic myelogenous leukemia: Impact of donor lymphocyte infusion. J Clin Oncol 1999;17:561–568.

16. Khouri IF, Keating M, Korbling M, et al: Transplant-lite: Induction of graft-versus-malignancy using fludarabine-based nonablative chemotherapy and allogeneic blood progenitor-cell transplantation as treatment for lymphoid malignancies. J Clin Oncol 1998; 16:2817–2824.

17. Ueno NT, Hortobagyi GN, Champlin RE: Allogeneic peripheral blood progenitor cell transplantation in solid tumors. Cancer Treat Res 1999;101:133–156.

18. Bay JO, Choufi B, Pomel C, et al: Potential allogeneic graft-versus-tumor effect in a patient with ovarian cancer. Bone Marrow Transplant 2000;25:681–682.

19. Childs R, Chernoff A, Contentin N, et al: Regression of metastatic renal-cell carcinoma after nonmyeloablative allogeneic peripheral-blood stem-cell transplantation [see comments]. N Engl J Med 2000;343:750–758.

20. Ueno NT, Rondon G, Mirza NQ, et al: Allogeneic peripheral-blood progenitor-cell transplantation for poor-risk patients with metastatic breast cancer. J Clin Oncol 1998;16:986–993.

21. Antin JH: Graft-versus-leukemia: No longer an epiphenomenon. Blood 1993;82:2273–2277.

22. Webb IJ, Anderson KC: Transfusion-associated graft-versus-host disease. In Popovsky MA (ed): Transfusion Reactions. Bethesda, MD, American Association of Blood Banks, 1996, pp 185–204.

23. Alyea EP, Schlossman RL, Canning C, et al: CD8-depleted donor lymphocyte infusions mediate graft-versus multiple myeloma effect [abstract 1021]. Blood 1996;88:258a.

24. Soiffer RJ, Murray C, Mauch P, et al: Prevention of graft-versus-host disease by selective depletion of CD6-positive T lymphocytes from donor bone marrow. J Clin Oncol 1992;10:1191–1200.

25. Soiffer RJ, Ritz J: Selective T cell depletion of donor allogeneic marrow with anti-CD6 monoclonal antibody: Rationale and results. Bone Marrow Transplant 1993;12:S7–S10.

26. Soiffer RJ, Fairclough D, Robertson M, et al: CD6-depleted allogeneic bone marrow transplantation for acute leukemia in first complete remission. Blood 1997;89:3039–3047.

27. Soiffer RJ, Mauch P, Fairclough D, et al: CD6+ T cell depleted allogeneic bone marrow transplantation from genotypically HLA nonidentical related donors. Biol Blood Marrow Transplant 1997;3:11–17.

28. Champlin R, Ho W, Gajewski J, et al: Selective depletion of CD8+ T lymphocytes for prevention of graft-versus-host disease after allogeneic bone marrow transplantation. Blood 1990;76:418–423.

29. Faber LM, van Luxemburg-Heijs SAP, Veenhof WFJ, et al: Generation of CD4+ cytotoxic T-lymphocyte clones from a patient with severe graft-versus-host disease after allogeneic bone marrow transplantation: Implications for graft-versus-leukemia reactivity. Blood 1995;86:2821–2828.

30. Brecher ME, Sims L, Schmitz J, et al: North American multicenter study on flow cytometric enumeration of CD34+ hematopoietic stem cells. J Hematotherapy 1996;5:227–236.

31. Johnsen HE, Knudsen LM: Nordic flow cytometry standards for CD34+ cell enumeration in blood and leukapheresis products: Report from the Second Nordic Workshop. Nordic Stem Cell Laboratory Group (NSCL-G). J Hematotherapy 1996; 5:237–245.

32. Sutherland DR, Anderson L, Keeney M, et al: The ISHAGE guidelines for CD34+ cell determination by flow cytometry. J Hematother 1996;5:213–226.

33. Kenney M, Chin-Yee I, Weir K, et al: Single platform flow cytometric absolute CD34+ cell counts based on the ISHAGE guidelines. Cytometry 1998;34:61–70.

34. Webb IJ, Coral FS, Andersen JW, et al: Sources and sequelae of bacterial contamination of hematopoietic stem cell products: Implications for safety of hematotherapy and graft engineering. Transfusion 1996;36:782–788.

35. Rowley SD: Hematopoietic stem cell processing and cryopreservation. J Clin Apheresis 1992;7:132–134.

36. Davis J, Rowley SD, Santos GW: Toxicity of autologous bone marrow graft infusion. Prog Clin Biol Res 1990;333:531–540.

37. Stroncek DF, Fautsch SK, Lasky LC, et al: Adverse reactions in patients transfused with cryopreserved marrow. Transfusion 1991;31:521–526.

38. Dhodapkar M, Goldberg SL, Tefferi A, Gertz MA: Reversible encephalopathy after cryopreserved peripheral blood stem cell infusion. Am J Hematol 1994;45:187–188.

39. Greeno EW, Perry EH, Ilstrup SJ, Weisdorf DJ: Exchange transfusion the hard way: Massive hemolysis following transplantation of bone marrow with minor ABO incompatibility. Transfusion 1996;36:71–74.

40. Nussbaumer W, Schwaighofer H, Gratwohl A, et al: Transfusion of donor-type red cells as a single preparative treatment for bone marrow transplants with major ABO incompatibility. Transfusion 1995;35:592–595.

41. Webb IJ, Soiffer RJ, Andersen JW, et al: In vivo adsorption of isohemagglutinins with fresh frozen plasma in major ABO-incompatible bone marrow transplant. Biol Blood Marrow Transplant 1997;3:267–272.

42. Shpall EJ, Jones RB, Bearman SI, et al: Transplantation of enriched CD34-positive autologous marrow into breast cancer patients following high-dose chemotherapy: Influence of CD34-positive peripheral-blood progenitors and growth factors on engraftment. J Clin Oncol 1994;12:28–36.

43. McNiece I, Briddell R, Stoney G, et al: Large-scale isolation of CD34+ cells using the Amgen cell selection device results in high levels of purity and recovery. J Hematother 1997;6:5–11.

44. Tricot G, Gazitt Y, Leemhuis T, et al: Collection, tumor contamination, and engraftment kinetics of highly purified hematopoietic progenitor cells to support high dose therapy in multiple myeloma. Blood 1998;91:4489–4495.

45. Webb IJ, Schlossman RL, Jiroutek M, et al: Predictors of high yield and purity of CD34+ cell selected peripheral blood progenitor cells, collected from patients with multiple myeloma. Cytotherapy 1999;1:175–182.

46. Schiller G, Vescio R, Freytes C, et al: Transplantation of CD34+ peripheral blood progenitor cells after high-dose chemotherapy for patients with advanced multiple myeloma. Blood 1995;86:390–397.

47. Champlin R: Purging: The separation of normal from malignant cells for autologous transplantation. Transfusion 1996;36:910–918.

48. Freedman AS, Neuberg D, Mauch P, et al: Long-term follow-up of autologous bone marrow transplantation in patients with relapsed follicular lymphoma. Blood 1999;94:3325–3333.

49. Rill DR, Buschle M, Foreman NK, et al: Retrovirus-mediated gene transfer as an approach to analyze neuroblastoma relapse after autologous bone marrow transplantation. Hum Gene Ther 1992;3:129–136.

50. Brenner MK, Rill DR, Moen RC, et al: Gene-marking to trace origin of relapse after autologous bone-marrow transplantation. Lancet 1993;341:85–86.

51. Sharp JG, Kessinger A, Mann S, et al: Outcome of high-dose therapy and autologous transplantation in non-Hodgkin's lymphoma based on the presence of tumor in the marrow or infused hematopoietic harvest. J Clin Oncol 1996;14:214–219.

52. Menitove JE (ed): Standards for Hematopoietic Progenitor Cells. Bethesda, MD, American Association of Blood Banks, 1996.

53. Klein H (ed): Standards for Blood Banks and Transfusion Services, 17th ed. Bethesda, MD, American Association of Blood Banks, 1996.

54. Standards for Hematopoietic Progenitor Cell Collection, Processing, and Transplantation, North American edition. Omaha Neb Foundation for the Accreditation of Hematopoietic Cell Therapy, 1996.

55. Proposed approach to regulation of cellular and tissue-based products: Availability and public meeting. Fed Regist 1997;62:9721–9722.

56. Human cells, tissues, and cellular and tissue-based products: Establishment registration and listing. Fed Regist 2001;66:5447–5469.

57. Current good tissue practice for manufacturers of human cellular tissue-based products: Inspection and enforcement. Fed Regist 2001;66:1508–1559.

58. Stiff P, Chen B, Franklin W, et al: Autologous transplantation of ex vivo expanded bone marrow cells grown from small aliquots after high-dose chemotherapy for breast cancer. Blood 2000;95:2169–2174.

59. Cavazzana-Calvo M, Hacein-Bey S, de Saint Basile G, et al: Gene therapy of human severe combined immunodeficiency (SCID)-XI disease. Science 2000;288:669–672.

60. Eglitis MA, Mezey E: Hematopoietic cells differentiate into both microglia and macroglia in the brains of adult mice. Proc Natl Acad Sci U S A 1997;94:4080–4085.

61. Ferrari G, Cusella-De Angelis G, Coletta M, et al: Muscle regeneration by bone marrow-derived myogenic progenitors. Science 1998;279:1528–1530.

62. Petersen BE, Bowen WC, Patrene KD, et al: Bone marrow as a potential source of hepatic oval cells. Science 1999;284:1168–1170.

63. Kugler A, Stuhler G, Walden P, et al: Regression of human metastatic renal cell carcinoma after vaccination with tumor cell-dendritic cell hybrids [see comments]. Nature 2000;6:332–336.

64. Gong J, Nikrui N, Chen D, et al: Fusions of human ovarian carcinoma cells with autologous or allogeneic dendritic cells induce antitumor immunity. J Immunol 2000;165:1705–1711.

Index

Note: Page numbers followed by b indicate boxed material. Page numbers followed by f indicate figures. Page numbers followed by t indicate tables.